The Quantitative Analysis of Drugs

The Quantitative Analysis of Drugs

by

D. C. GARRATT
D.Sc. (Lond.), Ph.D., Hon. M.P.S., F.R.I.C.
Chief Analyst, Boots Pure Drug Co. Ltd.

Assisted by

L. BREALEY, B.Sc., Ph.D., F.R.I.C.
(*Physical Assays*)
C. A. JOHNSON, B.Sc., B.Pharm., F.P.S., F.R.I.C.
(*Chemical Assays*)
K. L. SMITH, M.P.S.
(*Bio-Assays*)
G. SYKES, M.Sc., F.R.I.C.
(*Microbiology*)

THIRD EDITION

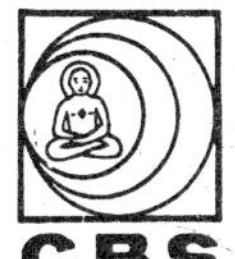

CBS
CBS Publishers & Distributors Pvt. Ltd.
New Delhi • Bengaluru • Chennai • Kochi • Kolkata • Mumbai
Hyderabad • Nagpur • Patna • Pune • Vijayawada

ISBN : 81-239-0754-0

First Indian Edition: 2001
Reprint: 2003, 2004, 2005, 2008

This edition has been published in India by arrangement with John Wiley & Sons Ltd., USA.

Published by **Satish Kumar Jain** and produced by **Varun Jain** for
CBS Publishers & Distributors Pvt. Ltd.,
4819/XI Prahlad Street, 24 Ansari Road, Daryaganj, New Delhi - 110002
delhi@cbspd.com, cbspubs@airtelmail.in • www.cbspd.com
Ph.: 23289259, 23266861, 23266867 • Fax: 011-23243014

Corporate Office: 204 FIE, Industrial Area, Patparganj, Delhi - 110 092
Ph: 49344934 • Fax: 011-49344935
E-mail: publishing@cbspd.com • publicity@cbspd.com

Branches:
- ***Bengaluru:*** 2975, 17th Cross, K.R. Road, Bansankari 2nd Stage, Bengaluru - 70 • Ph: +91-80-26771678/79 • Fax: +91-80-26771680 E-mail: cbsbng@gmail.com, bangalore@cbspd.com
- ***Chennai:*** No. 7, Subbaraya Street, Shenoy Nagar, Chennai - 600030 Ph: +91-44-26681266, 26680620 • Fax: +91-44-42032115 E-mail: chennai@cbspd.com
- ***Kochi:*** Ashana House, 39/1904, A.M. Thomas Road, Valanjambalam, Ernakulum, Kochi • Ph: +91-484-4059061-65 Fax: +91-484-4059065 • E-mail: cochin@cbspd.com
- ***Kolkata:*** 6-B, Ground Floor, Rameshwar Shaw Road, Kolkata - 700014 Ph: +91-33-22891126/7/8 • E-mail: kolkata@cbspd.com
- ***Mumbai:*** 83-C, Dr. E. Moses Road, Worli, Mumbai - 400018 Ph: +91-9833017933, 022-24902340/41 • E-mail: mumbai@cbspd.com

Representatives:

- Hyderabad: 0-9885175004
- Patna: 0-9334159340
- Jharkhand: 0-9811541605
- Nagpur: 0-9021734563
- Pune: 0-9623451994
- Uttarakhand: 0-9716462459

Printed at:
J.S. Offset Printers, Delhi (India)

PREFACE TO THIRD EDITION

In the present volume—as in previous editions—the intention of the author is to survey comprehensively all medicinal drugs commonly in use together with their pharmaceutical preparations.

The last five years has seen a very rapid advance in the field of pharmaceutical analysis and the need for revision of the previous edition has become evident. Further, the claims for incorporation of all methods used in the examination of drugs—chemical, physical, microbiological and biological—cannot be denied any longer since each type of determination is sometimes necessary for the adequate control of medicinal preparations.

The author's practice in this book has always been to select from experience those methods likely to prove most serviceable rather than produce a compendium of all published methods. Because of the rapid increase in the techniques available for pharmaceutical analysis, the need for specialisation has grown and the author has realised the impracticability of keeping in touch with all the practical details which are so valuable to the analyst. To overcome this difficulty and to enhance the value of the book, he has obtained the collaboration of specialist colleagues in the various fields of activity now included in the book. Each contributor is, in the author's opinion, an authority in his sphere of work and the author's thanks are due to Dr. L. Brealey (physical assays), Mr. C. A. Johnson (chemical assays), Mr. K. L. Smith (bio-assays) and Mr. G. Sykes (microbiology) for their painstaking work; inevitably the greatest burden fell on Mr. Johnson who devoted much time and energy to the task.

About one half of the previous edition has been completely re-written, a few monographs have been deleted and the remainder of the book has been revised; a considerable amount of new material has been added and many new appendices avoid repetition in the main text. A considerable amount of experimental work has been necessary to adopt colorimetric methods to the use of spectrophotometric measurements at specific wavelengths.

The various pharmacopœias and codices have a major influence on the control of the purity of drugs and any textbook on drug analysis must take cognisance of the methods in current official publications. The necessarily frequent publication of new pharmacopœias is occasioned by the new drugs available rather than by advances in analytical chemistry; this edition is correlated with the *British Pharmacopœia* 1958 and the *United States Pharmacopeia* XVI, but since it includes the latest trends in analytical techniques its contents should cover official methods for quantitative determinations in future editions of official books. However, since standards may become out-of-date it has been decided not to include them in this edition.

The author again desires to thank the General Medical Council for permission to include material from the *British Pharmacopœia* and the Pharmaceutical Society of Great Britain for permission to include material from the *British Pharmaceutical Codex*. The Association of Official Agricultural Chemists has also granted permission to utilise information from their *Official Methods of Analysis*.

The author wishes to thank numerous journals, particularly *The Analyst* and *The Journal of Pharmacy and Pharmacology* for permission to publish information. The Society for Analytical Chemistry has also been generous in permitting access to its Analytical Methods Committee reports when in the press.

During revision the author has had the benefit of assistance of colleagues other than those already mentioned. He wishes to thank Mr. W. L. Sheppard, B.Sc., F.R.I.C., for the revised monographs on Vitamin A and Vitamin D, Mr. P. G. Marshall, M.A., for the appendix on Infra-red Spectroscopy, Mr. G. Brewer, A.I.L., for checking the references, Mr. K. Hazzledine for line drawings and numerous associates for personal contributions; these include Messrs. P. Atherton, A.R.I.C., D. A. Elvidge, B.Sc., F.R.I.C., W. H. Harper, and Miss N. F. Mullholland, B.Sc. Others are acknowledged in the text.

Finally, the author's grateful thanks are given to Miss C. King, B.Sc., for preparation of the index, for very patient proof-reading and assistance in preserving uniformity of style and also to Miss I. Ladden, B.Pharm., for compilation of manuscripts and proofs for the printers; their enthusiastic help was invaluable.

D. C. GARRATT

CONTENTS

ABBREVIATIONS

Publications

A.B.C.M.	The Association of British Chemical Manufacturers
A.O.A.C.	Methods of Analysis of the Association of Official Agricultural Chemists 9th edn., (1960)
Acta Chem. Scand.	Acta Chemica Scandinavica
Acta Pharm. Sinica	Acta Pharmaceutica Sinica: also known as Yao Hsueh Hsueh Pao
Acta Pharmacol. Toxicol.	Acta Pharmacologica et Toxicologica. København
Amer. J. Pharm.	American Journal of Pharmacy
Amer. J. Sci.	American Journal of Science
Amer. Soc. Testing Materials, Spec. Tech. Publ.	American Society for Testing Materials, Special Technical Publication
Anal. Chem.	Analytical Chemistry
Anal. Chim. Acta	Analytica Chimica Acta
Analyst	Analyst
Ann. Appl. Biol.	Annals of Applied Biology
Ann. Chim. Anal. et Chim. Appl.	Annales de Chimie Analytique et de Chimie Appliquée
Ann. Chim. Appl. (Roma)	Annali di Chimica Applicata (Roma)
Annalen	Annalen der Chemie, Justus Liebigs
Antibiotics & Chemotherapy	Antibiotics & Chemotherapy
Arch. Biochem. Biophys.	Archives of Biochemistry and Biophysics
Arch. Pharm.	Archiv der Pharmazie
Atti Congr. Naz. Chim. Pura ed Appl.	Atti del Congresso Nazionale di Chimica Pura ed Applicata
B.M.J.	British Medical Journal
B.N.F.	British National Formulary (1960)
B.P.	British Pharmacopœia (1958)
B.P.C.	British Pharmaceutical Codex (1959)
B.S.	British Standard
B. Vet. C.	British Veterinary Codex (1953)
Ber.	Berichte der Deutschen Chemischen Gesellschaft
Biochem. J.	Biochemical Journal
Biometrika	Biometrika
Boll. Chim.-Farm.	Bollettino Chimico-Farmaceutico. Milano
Brit. J. Anæsthesia	British Journal of Anæsthesia
Brit. J. Ind. Med.	British Journal of Industrial Medicine
Brit. J. Nutrition	British Journal of Nutrition
Bul. Soc. Sţi. Bucureşti	Buletinul Societătii de Stiinţe din Bucureşti
Bull. Narcotics	Bulletin on Narcotics, United Nations, Department of Social Affairs

ABBREVIATIONS

Bull. Sci. Pharmacol.	Bulletin des Sciences Pharmacologiques. Paris
Bull. Soc. Chim. France	Bulletin de la Société Chimique de France
C & D	Chemist and Druggist
Českosl. Farm.	Československá Farmacie
Chem. Anal. (*Warsaw*)	Chemia Analityczna (Warszawa)
Chem. & Ind.	Chemistry and Industry
Chem. Eng. Mining Rev.	Chemical Engineering and Mining Review. Melbourne
Chem. Listy	Chemicke Listy
Chem. Weekblad	Chemische Weekblad
Chem. Zvesti	Chemicke Zvesti
Chemiker-Ztg.	Chemiker-Zeitung
Chim. et Ind. (*Paris*)	Chimie et Industrie (Paris)
Chimia (*Switz.*)	Chimia (Switzerland)
Compt. Rend.	Comptes Rendus Hebdomadaires des Scéances de l'Académie dès Sciences
D.A.B.	Deutsches Arzneibuch, 6 Ausgabe German Pharmacopœia, 6th Edition
Dansk. Tidsskr. Farm.	Dansk Tidsskrift for Farmaci
Determination of Trace Elements, *S.A.C.*	The Society for Analytical Chemistry. Analytical Methods Committee. Trace Elements in Fertilisers and Feeding-Stuffs Sub-Committee. Determination of Trace Elements, with Special Reference to Fertilisers and Feeding-Stuffs (Cambridge), W. Heffer and Sons Ltd., 1963
Drug Standards	Drug Standards
Drugg. Circ.	Druggists' Circular, New York
Dtsch. Apoth.-Ztg.	Deutsche Apotheker-Zeitung
Endocrinology	Endocrinology
FAO Plant Protection Bulletin	Food and Agriculture Organisation of the United Nations, FAO Plant Protection Bulletin
F.D.A.	United States Food and Drug Administration
Federation Proc.	Federation Proceedings
Giorn. Farm. Chim.	Giornale di Farmacia, di Chimica e di Scienze affini
Helv. Chim. Acta	Helvetica Chimica Acta
Ind. Eng. Chem.	Industrial and Engineering Chemistry
Ind. Eng. Chem., Anal. Edn.	Industrial and Engineering Chemistry, Analytical Edition
Int. Sugar J.	International Sugar Journal
J.A.O.A.C.	Journal of the Association of Official Agricultural Chemists
J. Agric. Food Chem.	Journal of Agricultural and Food Chemistry
J. Amer. Chem. Soc.	Journal of the American Chemical Society
J. Amer. Oil Chemists' Soc.	Journal of the American Oil Chemists' Society
J. Amer. Pharm. Ass.	Journal of the American Pharmaceutical Association

ABBREVIATIONS

J. Amer. Pharm. Ass., Sci. Edn.	Journal of the American Pharmaceutical Association, Scientific Edition
J. Appl. Chem.	Journal of Applied Chemistry
J. Biol. Chem.	Journal of Biological Chemistry
J. Chem. Educn.	Journal of Chemical Education
J. Chem. Soc.	Journal of the Chemical Society
J. Chromatog.	Journal of Chromatography
J. Endocrinology	Journal of Endocrinology
J. Fed. Insts. Brewing	Journal of the Federated Institutes of Brewing, London
J. Ind. Eng. Chem.	Journal of Industrial and Engineering Chemistry
J. Inst. Petrol.	Journal of the Institute of Petroleum
J. Org. Chem.	Journal of Organic Chemistry
J. Pharm. Chim.	Journal de Pharmacie et de Chimie
J. Pharm. Pharmacol.	Journal of Pharmacy and Pharmacology
J. Pharm. Sci.	Journal of Pharmaceutical Sciences
J. Pharmacol.	Journal of Pharmacology and Experimental Therapeutics
J. Roy. Soc., N.S.W.	Journal of the Royal Society of New South Wales
J. Roy. Statist. Soc., Suppl.	Journal of the Royal Statistical Society, Supplement
J. Sci. Food Agric.	Journal of the Science of Food and Agriculture
J. Soc. Chem. Ind.	Journal of the Society of Chemical Industry
J. Soc. Chem. Ind., Japan	Journal of the Society of Chemical Industry, Japan
Lez. Chim. Org.	Lezioni di Chimica Organica
Microchem. J.	Microchemical Journal
Mikrochemie	Mikrochemie vereinigt mit Mikrochimica Acta
Mikrochemie. Pregl-Festschr.	Mikrochemie. Pregl-Festschrift
Mikrochim. Acta	Mikrochimica Acta
Mitt. Dtsch. Pharm. Ges. (publ. in *Arch. Pharm.*)	Mitteilungen der Deutschen Pharmazeutischen Gesellschaft und der Pharmazeutischen Gesellschaft der DDR. Included in Archiv der Pharmazie
N.F.	National Formulary XI (1960)
Nature	Nature
Naturwissenschaften	Naturwissenschaften
P.E.O.R.	Perfumery and Essential Oil Record
Ph. I.	Pharmacopœa Internationalis (International Pharmacopœia) First Edition
Pharm. Acta Helv.	Pharmaceutica Acta Helvetiæ
Pharm. J.	Pharmaceutical Journal
Pharm. Soc.	The Pharmaceutical Society of Great Britain
Pharm. Weekblad	Pharmaceutische Weekblad
Pharm. Zentralhalle	Pharmazeutische Zentralhalle
Pharm. Ztg.	Pharmazeutische Zeitung

ABBREVIATIONS

Proc. Feigl Anniversary Symp.	Analytical Chemistry 1962. Philip W. West *et al.*, eds. The Proceedings of the International Symposium held at Birmingham University (U.K.), April 1962 in honour of FRITZ FEIGL to commemorate his 70th birthday. (Amsterdam), Elsevier Publishing Company, 1963
Proc. Roy. Soc. (London)	Proceedings of the Royal Society (London)
Pyrethrum Post	Pyrethrum Post
Quart. J. Pharm.	Quarterly Journal of Pharmacy and Pharmacology
Rec. Trav. Chim.	Recueil des Travaux Chimiques des Pays-Bas
S.A.C.	Society for Analytical Chemistry
S.I.	Statutory Instrument
Sci. Pharm.	Scientia Pharmaceutica
Science	Science
Soap Sanit. Chemicals	Soap and Sanitary Chemicals
Spectrochim. Acta	Spectrochimica Acta
Spice Mill	Spice Mill
Talanta	Talanta
Trans. Faraday Soc.	Transactions of the Faraday Society
U.S.P.	Pharmacopeia of the United States XVI (1960)
Y.B. Pharm.	Year-Book of Pharmacy
Z. Anal. Chem.	Zeitschrift für Analytische Chemie
Z. Angew. Chem.	Zeitschrift für Angewandte Chemie
Z. Anorg. Chem.	Zeitschrift für Anorganische Chemie
Z. Elektrochem.	Zeitschrift für Elektrochemie
Z. Öffentl. Chem.	Zeitschrift für Öffentliche Chemie
Z. Untersuch. Lebensm.	Zeitschrift für Untersuchung der Nahrungs- und Genussmittel sowie der Gebrauchsgegenstände
Zavod. Lab.	Zavodskaya Laboratoriya

General

A	angstrom units
$[\alpha]_D$	specific rotation
amp.	ampère
At.Wt.	atomic weight
b.p.	boiling-point
B.S.S.	British Standard sieve
cm	centimetre
cm^{-1}	wave number (frequency of radiation)
°(optical)	angular degree
°(temperature)	degree Centigrade
°F	degree Fahrenheit
°K	degree Kelvin
dm	decimetre
E	extinction
EDTA	ethylenediamine tetra-acetic acid, used as the di-sodium salt

ABBREVIATIONS

e.m.f.	electro-motive force
f.p.	freezing-point
g	gramme
I.U.	International Unit
in.	inch
l	litre
lb	pound
LD50	a dose lethal to 50 per cent of the organisms
m	meta
M	molar (concentration)
m.p.	melting-point
mA	milliampère
MeV	mega-electronvolt
mg	milligramme
ml	millilitre
mm	millimetre
mμ	millimicron = 10^{-6} millimetre
mV	millivolt
Mol.Wt.	molecular weight
μA	microampère
μg	microgramme
μl	microlitre
N	normal (concentration)
N.P.L.	National Physical Laboratory
N.T.P.	normal temperature and pressure
o	ortho
p.	page
p	para
p.p.m.	parts per million
p.s.i.	per square inch
pH	hydrogen ion exponent
pK	dissociation constant
r.p.m.	revolutions per minute
R_F	relative band speed
S.C.E.	standard calomel electrode
s.w.g.	standard wire gauge
sp.gr.	specific gravity
sq.cm.	square centimetre
u	unit
V	volt
v/v	volume in volume
w/v	weight in volume
w/w	weight in weight

THE QUANTITATIVE ANALYSIS OF DRUGS

ACETIC ACID

CH_3COOH Mol. Wt. 60·05

Although the percentage of total acid present may be determined by direct titration with N alkali to phenolphthalein, 1 ml N = 0·06005 g, the purity of glacial acetic acid is best determined by specific gravity and freezing-point. All likely impurities cause a lowering of both freezing-point and specific gravity, with the exception of small percentages of water which have the effect of raising the specific gravity of concentrated acetic acid. Richmond and England[1] constructed tables correlating these constants with percentages of acid, and the following values taken from their figures may be used for interpolation.

TABLE 1

ACID PER CENT	FREEZING-POINT	SPECIFIC GRAVITY
100	16·6°	1·056
99·5	15·65°	1·0569
99·0	14·74°	1·0582
98·5	13·90°	1·0594
98·0	13·12°	1·0606
97·5	12·38°	1·0617
97·0	11·68°	1·0627
96·5	11·00°	1·0637
96·0	10·34°	1·0646

Between 95 and 100 per cent purity the following relationship was found between freezing-point and specific gravity: (16·63 − f.p.) × 0·00144 = sp. gr. − 1·0555.

Propionic acid, which they consider the most common impurity in glacial acetic acid, depresses both specific gravity and freezing-point, and the percentage of propionic acid can be calculated by dividing the difference between the specific gravity calculated equivalent to the freezing-point and that found by 0·00135. It is stated that the precautions necessary in the determination of freezing-point are (*a*) to cool only to about one degree below the freezing-point, and (*b*) not to expose too much to moisture.

Dilute acetic acid may be estimated by direct titration with 0·5N sodium hydroxide, using phenolphthalein as indicator, 1 ml 0·5N = 0·030025 g.

The titration of aniline in acetic acid with perchlorate, using either a potentiometric or visual end-point, was applied by Ellerington and Nicholls[2] to the determination of acetic anhydride in mixtures of acetic anhydride and acetic acid. The acetic anhydride is allowed to react with excess of standard aniline solution in glacial acetic acid, the excess of aniline being titrated with perchloric acid in acetic acid. The end-point is determined potentiometrically or by using a suitable indicator such as crystal violet.

Into a clean and thoroughly dry 100-ml graduated flask weigh sufficient sample to contain approximately 1 g of acetic anhydride and dilute to volume with glacial acetic acid. By pipette, put into a 150-ml stoppered flask 50·0 ml of standardised aniline in acetic acid solution. Add by pipette 20·0 ml of the prepared solution of the sample in acetic acid, allow to stand for a minimum of forty minutes, and titrate the excess of aniline with standard perchloric acid in glacial acetic acid.

$$\text{Acetic anhydride per cent} = \frac{(B - T) \times 0{\cdot}01021 \times F \times 100}{0{\cdot}2 \times W}$$

B = volume in ml of standard perchloric acid solution equivalen to 50·0 ml of aniline in acetic acid
T = titre in ml of perchloric acid solution after reaction
F = factor of 0·1N perchloric acid solution
W = weight of sample taken.

ACETATES

Although **ammonium acetate,** $C_2H_3O_2(NH_4)$, Mol. Wt. 77·09, can be estimated by either of the usual methods: (*a*) by distillation of the ammonia in sodium hydroxide solution into excess of standard acid, or (*b*) by adding excess standard alkali, boiling until free from ammonia and back titrating; it is most conveniently determined by utilising the reaction of ammonia with formalin; neutral hexamethylenetetramine is produced and the acetic acid is titrated.

To 1 to 2 g of ammonium acetate in water add 10 ml of 40 per cent formaldehyde solution (which is usually acid and must be previously neutralised to phenolphthalein); titrate with N alkali to phenolphthalein. 1 ml N = 0·07709 g $C_2H_3O_2(NH_4)$.

This method is of general applicability for ammonium salts, as for example **ammonium citrate,** $C_6H_5O_7(NH_4)_3$, Mol. Wt. 243·2. 1 ml N = 0·08107 g.

Potassium acetate, $C_2H_3O_2K$, Mol. Wt. 98·15, and **sodium acetate,** $C_2H_3O_2Na,3H_2O$, Mol. Wt. 136·1, are estimated by titration of the alkaline solution obtained by charring a known weight of the material in a platinum dish and dissolving the residue in water; methyl orange is used as indicator. 1 ml 0·5N acid = 0·04907 g potassium acetate and 0·06804 g sodium acetate.

For lead acetate, see p. 377.

Strong Solution of Ammonium Acetate, *B.P.C.* Prepared by neutralising acetic acid with ammonium bicarbonate and ammonia; it contains about 57 per cent of ammonium acetate. This is assayed by the formalin method described above, using 5 ml of solution in 50 ml of water.

ACETIC ANHYDRIDE, $(CH_3CO)_2O$, Mol. Wt. 102·09.

The following method of determination is accurate but close attention to detail is necessary.

> Dissolve about 2 g, accurately weighed, in 50 ml of N sodium hydroxide in a stoppered flask, and allow to stand for one hour; titrate the excess of alkali with N hydrochloric acid, using phenolphthalein solution as indicator. Calculate the number of ml of N sodium hydroxide required for 1 g; call this quantity '*a*.'
>
> Dissolve about 2 g, accurately weighed, in 20 ml of dry benzene in a stoppered flask, cool in ice, and add a cold solution of 10 ml of dry aniline in 20 ml of dry benzene; allow the mixture to stand for one hour, add 50 ml of N sodium hydroxide and shake vigorously; titrate the excess of alkali with N hydrochloric acid, using phenolphthalein solution as indicator. Calculate the number of ml of N sodium hydroxide required for 1 g; call this quantity '*b*.'
>
> $$(a - b) \times 10{\cdot}2 = \text{percentage of } C_4H_6O_3.$$

A rapid but less accurate method of evaluation is that of Radcliffe and Medofski[3] using direct titration. Then if p be the weight of the sample used and q the weight of acetic acid found from the number of millilitres of N alkali used, the weight of anhydride present is 5·6641 $(q - p)$. This method assumes that only acetic acid and acetic anhydride are present.

DETERMINATION OF ACETYL GROUPS

Two principles have been used in the determination of acetyl groups:

(i) treatment with an excess of alkali, allowing to stand for some hours or refluxing and titrating excess alkali with acid.

Methods depending on this principle are not suitable for general application because they cannot be used for analysis of substances that are decomposed by strong alkali and they cannot be applied to compounds that possess acidic properties either in themselves or as a result of hydrolysis.

At room temperature and below only *O*-acetyl groups are attacked; at higher temperatures *N*-acetyl groups are also determined.

(ii) hydrolysis with alkali, distillation of the acetic acid from a sulphuric or phosphoric acid solution and collection of the acid in an excess of alkali.

Kuhn and Roth[4] developed a procedure in which hydrolysis and subsequent distillation of acetic acid were carried out in a single flask. The main objection appears to be that the design of the apparatus permits the carry-over of sulphuric acid, either in mist or droplet form if rapid distillation or bumping occurs.

Wiesenberger[5] drew attention to the slowness of Kuhn and Roth's method and to errors associated with it in a review of methods available for determination of acetyl groups. Later[6] he evolved a method with a claimed high degree of accuracy and precision. This method is now widely used and accepted for determination of acetyl groups and saponification methods are not viewed with favour. The apparatus used by Wiesenberger is described in British Standard 1428 : Part C 2 : 1954. Wiesenberger's method splits off *N*-acetyl groups with sulphuric or phosphoric acid and *O*-acetyl groups with aqueous or methanolic sodium hydroxide solution. The resulting acetic acid is then isolated by a number of successive distillations and titrated with 0·01N sodium hydroxide using phenolphthalein indicator. Reference to the British Standard quoted above will show that elaborate precautions have been taken to prevent carry-over of other acids and it is clear that unless this type of apparatus is used and the technique of distillation followed in detail unsatisfactory results will be obtained. For the initial treatment of most *O*-acetyl compounds any one of the four hydrolysing solutions mentioned above is satisfactory. Wiesenberger's original method was intended for micro (3–10 mg of sample) application, but it is also reported to be 'highly satisfactory' for semi-micro work (20–30 mg of sample). In this case double the quantities of reagents used in the original method[5] are used and the titration of the acid is carried out with 0·05N sodium hydroxide. Precise details of a suitable method are not possible since the hydrolysing reagent will vary from substance to substance, but for a fairly simple *O*-acetyl compound the following procedure might be employed:

> Introduce 20 to 30 mg of sample into the Wiesenberger flask and add an anti-bumping device (a small piece of platinum is commonly employed) followed by 4 ml of 4N sodium hydroxide (aqueous). Heat for thirty minutes at 150° to 155°, allow to cool somewhat and then immerse the flask in an ice-bath. Run 2 ml of specially-prepared sulphuric acid solution (see below) down the condenser tube, followed by 6 ml of water. Then detach the flask from the condenser using a total of 3 ml of water to rinse down the condenser and the joint surface of the flask. Connect the distillation head to the flask and clamp the condenser at an angle of 45° for distillation of the acetic acid. Place 2 ml of water in the funnel above the flask and trap. With the flame of a micro-burner under the flask continue heating until vapour has condensed in the vapour trap

and reaches the distillation temperature as shown by the appearance of condensate in the spray trap. Remove the flame, whereupon the condensate in the spray trap is sucked back into the flask. Apply the flame again to the flask and continue distillation until 6 ml of distillate has been collected in a measuring cylinder. Remove the burner, run the 2 ml of water in the funnel into the flask and top up the funnel again with 2 ml of water. Collect another 2 ml of distillate and continue alternate additions and collection of 2-ml portions until 25 ml of distillate has been collected. Transfer the condensate to a 100-ml conical flask to await titration. Meanwhile add 5 ml of water to the flask and distil into the now empty cylinder. Follow this by a further 5 ml which is distilled off in 1-ml portions to ensure a complete rinsing out of the whole apparatus. The total volume of condensate is now 35 ml. Boil the solution for seven to eight seconds to expel carbon dioxide, cool rapidly and titrate immediately with 0·05N sodium hydroxide to the first faint pink colour of phenolphthalein. 1 ml of 0·05N sodium hydroxide = 2·152 mg of CH_3CO.

Sulphuric Acid Solution. A dilute solution is prepared as follows and volatile acids are distilled off. Add 100 ml of concentrated microanalytical reagent quality acid carefully, with cooling, to 210 ml of water in a 750-ml round-bottomed flask. Allow the mixture to stand for one hour, then when the diluted acid has cooled, insert the distillation head of the acetyl apparatus in the neck of the flask and attach to the condenser. Bring the contents of the flask to the boil and collect 10 ml of distillate and discard it. Introduce another 5 ml of water through the funnel into the flask and collect a further 5 ml of distillate in a clean 25-ml measuring cylinder. Continue this process until 25 ml of distillate has been collected, then transfer the liquid to a clean, quartz, 100-ml conical flask and titrate with 0·01N sodium hydroxide. Collect a further 25 ml of distillate, adding 5 ml of water to the acid before distilling off each successive 5 ml, so that the volume of liquid in the flask remains substantially constant. Each 25 ml of distillate should require not more than 0·02 ml of the alkali to neutralise it; if the titre is higher continue distillation to complete the removal of the volatile acids. Stop the distillation when this is so and when the acid solution has cooled to room temperature store it in a glass-stoppered bottle with the neck covered with a dust cap.

1. Richmond, H. D., and England, E. H., *Analyst*, 1926, **51,** 283.
2. Ellerington, T., and Nicholls, J.J., *Analyst*, 1957, **82,** 233.
3. Radcliffe, L. G., and Medofski, S., *J. Soc. Chem. Ind.*, 1917, **36,** 628.
4. Kuhn, R., and Roth, H., *Ber.*, 1933, **66,** 1274.
5. Wiesenberger, E., *Mikrochemie*, 1942, **30,** 176.
6. Wiesenberger, E., *Mikrochemie*, 1947, **33,** 51.

ACETONE

$(CH_3)_2CO$ Mol. Wt. 58·08

Messinger's method of determination in which iodoform is produced with potassium hydroxide and iodine is known to give high results in the presence of ethanol. Haughton[1] also found the method to give high results with specially purified acetone and is inclined to the opinion that a small portion of the acetone reacts with the alkaline iodine to form formic acid instead of iodoform.

The modification by Rakshit,[2] replacing potassium hydroxide by lime water, is more accurate:

> Place a portion of the sample to be examined, containing about 0·05 g of acetone, in a 750-ml flask and add 300 ml of freshly prepared lime water; loosely close the flask with a rubber bung and heat to about 35°. Add 5 ml of 0·2N iodine, drop by drop, and shake the liquid for five minutes; then similarly add a further 5 ml of iodine solution and shake, and so on until 40 ml of iodine solution has been used. The gradual introduction of the iodine is necessary, because if all of it is added at once the reaction is not complete. If, during the addition of iodine, the colour persists after thorough shaking, more lime solution should be used. Ten minutes after the final addition of iodine add a few drops of starch solution, cool and add 15 ml of N sulphuric acid, and titrate the excess of iodine with 0·1N sodium thiosulphate, 1 ml 0·1N iodine = 0·00193 g.

The error due to ethanol was found to be slight, and a mean of fifty analyses showed that 0·8 ml of 0·2N iodine was absorbed by 1 ml of ethanol. In practice it has been found to be unnecessary to add the iodine as slowly as is directed.

Acetone may also be estimated by the method that is used for the determination of aldehydes and ketones by means of hydroxylamine hydrochloride; this forms oximes, liberating the acid, which can be titrated direct. It is a very rapid process, Pemberton, Card and Craven[3] finding that the titration can be completed in aqueous solution within a minute or two. In their opinion not more than three-quarters of the hydroxylamine salt should be decomposed, and under these conditions a constant factor must also be used for a given indicator depending on the hydrolysis of acetoxime at the end-point acidity. The factor for methyl orange-xylene cyanol (pH 3·7) was found to be 0·983 and for 4·5 indicator, 0·988. Haughton prefers the factor 0·974 for methyl orange-xylene cyanol.

Maltby and Primavesi[4] consider ethanolic solution with bromophenol blue as indicator preferable, since they found the reaction to go to completion under the conditions used. The reagent is 2 per cent hydroxylamine hydrochloride in approximately 85 per cent ethanol neutralised to bromophenol blue. Sufficient sample is taken to require about 20 ml of 0·2N alkali and a standard volume of 70 ml of reagent. At the same time an equal volume of reagent is taken in another flask to act as a blank and any water or ethanol added with the sample must be added to the blank in equal amount, since the colour of the indicator depends on the concentration of both water and ethanol. Titration is performed after five minutes' reaction. Care must be taken during the assay against the volatility of acetone.

For estimation of small quantities of ethanol in acetone, Craven[5] adapts Agulhon's reaction to quantitative use. It was observed that 1 ml of pure acetone with 3 ml of a reagent containing 0·5 g of potassium dichromate in 100 ml of pure colourless nitric acid (sp. gr. 1·310) develops a green colour only after three hours, whereas with 0·5 per cent of ethanol or formaldehyde present, a blue colour appears within a minute or two. The dilution is found which will just fail to reach the full blue colour in five minutes when taking 1·0 ml of the sample with increasing amounts of reagent, 1 ml of Agulhon's reagent = 0·00117 g C_2H_5OH.

Adams and Nicholls[6] in a paper on the analysis of mixtures containing acetone, ethanol and *iso*propyl alcohol found that for low strengths, where the total proportion does not exceed 10 per cent by volume, the apparent proof strength and refraction of the mixture are practically additive factors. When only two known substances are present the quantities of each can be calculated by proportion from the two determinations of specific gravity and immersion refractometer reading. With three known substances present, when one can be determined by any independent process, allowance can be made for it in the strength and refraction of the solution, and the proportions of the other two can then be calculated. These workers also modified Penzoldt's specific qualitative test for the detection of acetone (depending on the formation of indigotin by condensation) to provide a quantitative colorimetric method for small amounts. Their method is rapid and is limited to dilutions of 0·01 per cent of acetone. For low concentrations of acetone the precipitation of indigotin is not apparent for some time, but a yellow to greenish-blue colour develops, depending on the proportion of acetone present, and this is suitable for quantitative determination. The detailed method is as follows:

> To an aliquot portion of the distillate to be tested (containing not more than 0·02 g acetone and diluted with water to 10 ml) add 1 ml of a 1 per cent solution of *o*-nitrobenzaldehyde in 50 per cent pure ethanol. After mixing, add 0·5 ml of 30 per cent sodium hydroxide solution and allow the test solution to stand for about fifteen minutes, avoiding strong daylight. At the end of this time compare the colour with that developed in a set of standard acetone solutions, containing from 0 to 20 mg of acetone in 10 ml, which have been similarly treated at the same time.

The range of the colours produced is very marked, and it is possible to have as many as twenty readily differentiated standards within the range suggested.

Nicholls[7] also gives a useful table for specific gravity and immersion refractometer readings of dilute mixtures of acetone and water, which is reproduced below. If from the specific gravity of a dilute pure aqueous

TABLE 2

ACETONE g/100 ml	EQUIVALENT PROOF STRENGTH	REFRACTOMETER READING AT 60° F
0	0	15·5
1	1·63	17·45
2	3·24	19·4
3	4·83	21·35
4	6·45	23·4
5	8·12	25·5
6	9·80	27·65
7	11·44	29·6
8	13·15	31·55
9	14·93	33·7
10	16·73	35·75

solution of acetone the apparent proof strength be determined from the Official Tables,* the factor 0·760 will give a percentage by volume of acetone not differing by more than 0·1 per cent from the correct value.

For **traces** of acetone Pemberton, Card and Craven[3] recommend the iodoform reaction of Messinger, which they state will detect nephelometrically 5 p.p.m. of acetone in an aqueous solution saturated with sodium chloride.

(*Cf.* Ethyl Alcohol and Isopropyl Alcohol.)

1. HAUGHTON, C. O., *Ind. Eng. Chem. Anal. Edn.*, 1937, **9**, 167.
2. RAKSHIT, J., *Analyst*, 1916, **41**, 245.
3. PEMBERTON, E. S., CARD, S. T., and CRAVEN, E. C., *J. Soc. Chem. Ind.*, 1935, **54**, 163T.
4. MALTBY, J. G., and PRIMAVESI, G. R., *Analyst*, 1949, **74**, 498.
5. CRAVEN, E. C., *J. Soc. Chem. Ind.*, 1933, **52**, 239T.
6. ADAMS, C. A., and NICHOLLS, J. R., *Analyst*, 1929, **54**, 2.
7. NICHOLLS, J. R., *Analyst*, 1929, **54**, 9.

* Tables Showing the Relation Between the Specific Gravity of Spirits at 60°/60° F and the Percentage of Alcohol by Weight and by Volume. (H.M. Stationery Office.)

ACETYLSALICYLIC ACID

$C_6H_4.OCOCH_3.COOH$ Mol. Wt. 180·2

Acetylsalicylic acid (aspirin) is usually estimated by hydrolysis to salicylic and acetic acids by means of excess of 0·5N alkali and back titration with acid, using phenolphthalein or phenol red as indicator. 1 ml 0·5N = 0·04504 g. Other methods are: (*a*) direct titration by dissolving a weighed quantity in cold neutral ethanol, diluting with water and titrating with 0·5N alkali to phenolphthalein; hydrolysis is very slow until after addition of an excess of alkali and introduces no error in the normal time of titration, 1 ml 0·5N = 0·09008 g, (*b*) titration of the salicylic acid formed in the hydrolysed mixture, by taking an aliquot part containing approximately 0·05 g and titrating with 0·1N bromine by the method described under Salicylic Acid (p. 558). 1 ml 0·1 N = 0·003003 g aspirin. Particular note should be made of the errors to be avoided when determining salicylic acid by this method after extraction from mixtures with chloroform and ether.

The difference between the amount of alkali used in direct titration and one half of that used for the back-titration method above, has been suggested as an indication of the amount of free salicylic acid present; however, with the quantities of the latter found in commercial samples the difference of titration using 1 g of sample would only fall within normal experimental error.

The *B.P.* test for free salicylic acid is a modification of the method of Jones,[1] and the limit of impurity allowed is equivalent to 0·05 per cent of salicylic acid in the aspirin.

> Dissolve 1 g of salicylic acid in 60 ml of ethanol, adjust the volume to 100 ml with water; dilute 10 ml of this solution to 1 litre as a standard, making 1 ml = 0·1 mg of acid. Dissolve 0·6 g of aspirin in a measuring cylinder in 9 ml of ethanol and dilute with water to 90 ml. Take two similar Nessler cylinders; into one pour 60 ml of the solution, into the other the remaining 30 ml with 3 ml of ethanol and adjust to the volume of the first. There is thus a difference of 200 mg in the amount of aspirin in the two solutions. Add 1 ml of 1 per cent acid ferric ammonium sulphate solution to each, mix and match the colour by adding the standard salicylic acid solution from a burette. Each ml of standard is equivalent to 0·05 per cent of salicylic acid in the sample.

This determination should be carried out without delay to avoid hydrolysis of the aspirin. Appreciable amounts of free salicylic acid above the *B.P.* limit do not give accurate figures of the amount present. Nutter-Smith[2] pointed out that certain substances, notably tartaric and citric acids, mask the ferric salicylate colour reaction by forming non-ionised salts with the iron, and 1 per cent citric acid will mask the presence of about 0·2 per cent of free salicylic acid.

ACETYLSALICYLIC ACID

Determination of free salicylic acid in the aspirin in preparations such as tablets should include a separation procedure if phosphate ions are present, since this interferes in the colorimetric method:

> Transfer a suitable quantity of the powdered tablets to a separator, add 50 ml of chloroform and 10 ml of water, shake well and allow to settle. Filter about 20 ml of the chloroform layer through a dry filter paper rejecting the first 5 ml of filtrate, and allow 10 ml of the filtrate to evaporate to dryness by exposing a large surface to a current of dry air at room temperature before proceeding with the colorimetric assay.

In discussing a limit test for free salicylic acid in aspirin, Edwards and colleagues[3] studied the kinetics of the hydrolysis of the aspirin and conditions for formation and stability of the ferric salicylate complex. In studying the ferric salicylate test it was concluded that time is a very important factor and that quantitative tests should be made at a constant pH. The concentration of substances in the test solution should be controlled. In studying interference it was noted that, as well as citrate, phosphate and sulphate exerted an inhibiting effect on colour formation. The kinetics of the hydrolysis showed the necessity to correct for the degree of hydrolysis occurring in the course of direct determination for free salicylic acid thus making it essential to fix temperature and weight. However, in the method where interfering substances are present, no hydrolysis correction need be made, provided the time for extraction and colour measurement is relatively small (about ten minutes). This is because the partition of aspirin between benzene and ferric ammonium sulphate solution is such that the final aspirin concentration in the ferric ammonium sulphate solution can be neglected. The extraction procedure proposed for estimating salicylic acid in aspirin preparations is as follows:

> Place 0·2 g of dry powdered sample in a clean dry 100-ml separator plugged just above the tap with a small piece of cotton wool, and extract with four portions, each of 10 ml, of benzene, collecting the benzene extracts in a second dry separator. Extract the combined extracts with 5 ml of a solution containing 5 ml of a 0·2 per cent ferric ammonium sulphate solution and 5 ml of a buffer solution (0·08M acetic acid and 0·32M ammonium monochloroacetate) made up to 45 ml with water. Run off the aqueous layer into a 50-ml graduated flask containing 2 ml of dehydrated ethanol. Repeat the extractions until there is no further pink coloration in the aqueous layer. When the salicylic acid has been completely extracted from the benzene, pour the rest of the buffered ferric ammonium sulphate solution, if any, into the graduated flask and make the solution up to the mark, shaking so that adequate mixing is ensured. If necessary, remove traces of benzene in this solution by filtration through a wetted filter paper, discarding the first portion of the filtrate. Collect a further portion and measure the maximum extinction (E) of this solution in a 4-cm cell at about 530 mμ. The salicylic acid concentration is then read from a calibration curve, the data for which is given in Table 3.

TABLE 3

RELATIONSHIP BETWEEN SALICYLIC ACID CONCENTRATION AND EXTINCTION COEFFICIENT AT 530 mμ*

SALICYLIC ACID μg/50 ml	E at 530 mμ (4-cm cell)
200	0·188
400	0·358
600	0·545
800	0·720
1000	0·895
1200	1·078

* *Comparison cell solution:* 2 ml dehydrated ethanol, 5 ml 0·2 per cent ferric ammonium sulphate solution, 5 ml buffer solution all made up to 50 ml.

Test cell solution: Comparison solution plus salicylic acid.

Aspirin can be separated from many other organic substances in chloroform solution by extraction with sodium bicarbonate solution.

A simple determination of aspirin in mixtures is by its hydrolysis with sodium citrate and titration of the liberated acid to phenolphthalein. This method can be applied direct to **Mixture of Aspirin,** *B.P.C.* (containing 3·43 per cent of aspirin with suspending agents).

> Reflux 20 ml of mixture with 2 g of sodium citrate for thirty minutes, wash the condenser with warm water, collecting the washings in the flask and titrate with 0·5N sodium hydroxide using phenolphthalein as indicator. 1 ml 0·5N = 0·04505 g $C_9H_8O_4$.

Mixture of Aspirin for Infants, *B.P.C.* Contains 3·66 per cent of aspirin with suspending agents, flavouring and colour. It can be assayed by first extracting the aspirin from 20 ml with four quantities each of 30 ml of ether and evaporating the extracts to dryness before adding 20 ml of water to the residue and completing by the sodium citrate hydrolysis given above.

Tablets of Aspirin, *B.P.* Usually contain 5 grains of the acid.

The best method for the determination of acetylsalicylic acid is by following the *B.P.* method given under Acetylsalicylic Acid without extraction but using a quantity of the material obtained by powdering the 20 tablets used in determining the average weight. A rapid determination for routine purposes is to disintegrate three tablets with 2 or 3 ml of water in a flask, then adding 20 ml of ethanol neutralised to phenolphthalein and titrating direct with 0·5N sodium hydroxide. Under these circumstances 1 ml 0·5N NaOH = 0·09008 g $C_9H_8O_4$. For the estimation of free salicylic acid a quantity of tablet equivalent to 0·6 g of aspirin is dissolved in ethanol and any starch or talc which may be present is filtered off.

Compound Tablets of Aspirin, *B.P.C.* Contain 3½ grains of aspirin, 2½ grains of phenacetin and ½ grain of caffeine.

The following method will estimate all the ingredients on one weighed portion after taking a sample of 20 tablets, determining the average weight and powdering.

> Completely extract 0·5 g of powdered tablets with chloroform. To the residue after evaporation of the chloroform, or to 0·5 g of original powder if free from diluent, add 10 ml of dilute sulphuric acid and reflux under an efficient condenser for one hour. Cool the solution obtained and transfer it to a separator with a small quantity of water and chloroform. Wash down the inside of the condenser with water, adding the washings to the bulk in the separator. Extract with chloroform four or five times, transferring the extracts to a second separator.
>
> To the aqueous residue of *p*-phenetidin in the first separator carefully add an excess of sodium bicarbonate and then 10 to 20 drops of acetic anhydride and shake well. Extract the precipitated phenacetin with chloroform and remove the solvent in a weighed open-necked flask. Volatilise any acetic acid by addition of ethanol in small portions, evaporating in a current of warm air, dry the residue at 105° and weigh the phenacetin.
>
> Extract the chloroform in the second separator three times with dilute sodium hydroxide solution and then with water. Evaporate the chloroform and weigh the anhydrous caffeine after drying at 105°.
>
> The sodium hydroxide solution will contain the salicylic acid. Acidify with dilute hydrochloric acid and extract with four portions of ether. After drying the ether extracts with anhydrous sodium sulphate, evaporate the solvent nearly to dryness on a water-bath and finally to dryness either by a current of air or by tilting the flask and 'pouring out' ether vapour as the flask is rotated. Dry the residue in a desiccator and weigh the salicylic acid. Convert to aspirin by the factor 1·305.

Useful check methods are (*a*) titration of the aspirin direct in dilute ethanol, or by the sodium citrate hydrolysis method given above; (*b*) a total nitrogen determination by the Kjeldahl method will check the figures found for phenacetin and caffeine.

Compound aspirin tablets are sometimes made with caffeine citrate. The citric acid can be determined by the difference of acidity found by direct titration and that calculated from the weight of salicylic acid obtained in the method described above. 1 ml 0·5N NaOH = 0·03502 g $C_6H_8O_7,H_2O$.

Soluble Tablets of Aspirin, *B.P.* Contain 5 grains of aspirin with citric acid and calcium carbonate.

The total acetylsalicylic acid can be determined by boiling a portion of the powdered sample with dilute sulphuric acid under a reflux condenser, extracting the liberated salicylic acid with ether, evaporating the ether below 30°, dissolving the residue in 20 ml of 0·5N sodium hydroxide and making up to a definite volume. An aliquot part is brominated as given under Salicylic Acid (p. 558).

Tablets of Aspirin and Phenacetin, *B.P.C.* Contain $3\frac{1}{2}$ grains of aspirin and $2\frac{1}{2}$ grains of phenacetin. These tablets are assayed by dissolving in dilute sodium hydroxide solution, extracting the phenacetin with chloroform, then heating the aqueous residue to hydrolyse the aspirin and determining the salicylic acid, either by extraction with ether after acidification as given under Compound Tablets of Aspirin, or by bromination as given under Salicylic Acid. The sodium citrate hydrolysis method given above for the determination of aspirin can also be applied directly to this preparation.

Tablets of Aspirin, Phenacetin and Codeine, *B.P.* (Compound Tablets of Codeine). Contain 4 grains of aspirin, 4 grains of phenacetin and $\frac{1}{8}$ grain of codeine phosphate.

Although selection from the modifications of assays given above for the various compound aspirin tablets can be used the usual assay is the following:

> Shake a portion of powdered tablets with excess alkali and extract with chloroform. Determine the aspirin in the aqueous residue as given under Tablets of Aspirin and Phenacetin. Wash the chloroform extracts with dilute acid, evaporate and weigh the phenacetin. Make the acid washings alkaline with ammonia, extract with chloroform, evaporate and weigh or titrate the codeine.

Since the amount of codeine present is comparatively small, use of a single weighed portion of material suitable for the ingredients in larger proportions will tend to give errors from weighing or titrating small amounts of codeine. It is preferable, although longer, to weigh out a separate 5-g portion of sample for the latter, eliminating the other ingredients as above. The *B.P.* direction to extract the codeine with standard acid and back-titrate is not recommended; it has not been repeated for **Soluble Tablets of Aspirin, Phenacetin and Codeine,** *B.P.* (the same ingredients with citric acid and calcium carbonate).

Many methods have appeared in the literature during recent years which depend upon chromatographic or ion-exchange separation of the ingredients. The following method[4] has been found to be very satisfactory for routine determination of both Compound Codeine Tablets and Soluble Compound Codeine Tablets.

> Take a sample of 20 tablets, determine the average weight and powder. Take about 4 g of the powder, accurately weighed, and boil under reflux with 60 ml of 70 per cent ethanol for five minutes. Wash down the condenser with 10 ml of 70 per cent ethanol. Shake well and strain the warm solution through a loose, cotton-wool plug into a 100-ml graduated flask. Wash the first vessel with two 10-ml portions of 70 per cent ethanol and run the washings through the plug into the flask. Cool the solution, dilute to volume, shake and filter, rejecting the first 20 ml of filtrate. Place

a 20-ml aliquot on a previously prepared ion-exchange column of re-precipitated alginic acid (see page 461, mesh fraction 72–85 B.S., saturated with 70 per cent ethanol: On washing with ethanol, the column material contracts slightly and it must then be compacted by firm pressure on the top glass-wool plug) and allow it to run into the column taking about ten minutes and washing in with small volumes of 70 per cent ethanol. Open the tap wide and wash with successive small volumes of 95 per cent ethanol, taking care to wash down the walls, until a total volume of about 100 ml has passed through.

Codeine phosphate. Wash the column with 100 ml of water and elute the codeine to volume into a 100-ml graduated flask with N hydrochloric acid at a flow rate of 3–5 ml per minute. Measure the extinction (E) of a 1-cm layer at the maximum at about 285 mμ using N hydrochloric acid as reference.

$$\text{codeine phosphate per tablet} = \frac{100 \times w \times E}{20 \times W \times E_1}\ \text{g}$$

E = observed extinction
E_1 = E(1 per cent, 1 cm) at 284·5 mμ of codeine phosphate (if unknown assume a value of 39. For accurate results the figure for the batch used should be determined).
w = average weight of a tablet
W = weight of powdered tablets taken.

Phenacetin and aspirin. Evaporate the bulked ethanolic effluents from the column almost to dryness. Add 15 ml of dilute sulphuric acid and reflux for seventy minutes. Wash down the condenser with water, transfer, with washing to a 1-litre graduated flask, cool and dilute to 1 litre. Dilute 10-ml and 5-ml aliquots to volume in 200-ml graduated flasks. Measure the extinction (E) of a 1-cm layer of these dilutions at 301 mμ and 221 mμ respectively using water in the comparison cell.

$$\text{aspirin per tablet} = \frac{w(266E_1 - 6{\cdot}90E_2)}{100W}\ \text{g}$$

$$\text{phenacetin per tablet} = \frac{w(437E_2 - 155E_1)}{100W}\ \text{g}$$

E_1 = observed extinction at 301 mμ
E_2 = observed extinction at 221 mμ
w = average weight of a tablet
W = weight of powdered tablets taken.

Extraction with 70 per cent ethanol was selected because of the satisfactory solubility of all three components in this medium. Determination of the aspirin and phenacetin by a two-point procedure on the suitably diluted eluate from the column is not satisfactory because the positions of their respective absorption maxima preclude an accurate estimation in this way, furthermore the aspirin, having been subjected to boiling aqueous ethanol is partially hydrolysed. However, experience has shown that little loss of salicylic acid occurs on evaporation of the ethanol so long as it is not allowed to go to complete dryness. Hydrolysis of the ethanolic solution leads to some formation of ethyl salicylate. The hydrolysis method given makes an accurate two-point method possible, since *p*-phenetidin has an almost negligible absorption at the salicylic acid peak.

The equations for the calculation of aspirin and phenacetin contents are based on E(1 per cent, 1 cm) values for their acid hydrolysates of 270 and 462 at 221 mμ and 190 and 3 at 301 mμ respectively; all samples examined have conformed to these values and they can be regarded as standard. No standard value can be adopted for codeine phosphate (it has been found to vary from 37 to 41) and for accurate results the E(1 per cent, 1 cm) value has to be available for the batch of material used.

Tablets of Aspirin and Dover's Powder, *B.P.C.* Contain 2½ grains each of aspirin and Dover's powder.

The aspirin in this preparation can be determined most readily by the sodium citrate hydrolysis method given above.

For morphine, see p. 489.

Compound Tablets of Aspirin and Dover's Powder, *B.P.C.* Contain 3 grains of aspirin, 1¼ grains of phenacetin and 1 grain of Dover's powder.

The aspirin in these tablets can be determined readily by the sodium citrate hydrolysis method given above.

For phenacetin the method given under Compound Tablets of Aspirin should be used.

For morphine, see p. 489.

ACETYLSALICYLATES

Calcium acetylsalicylate, $C_{18}H_{14}O_8Ca,2H_2O$, Mol. Wt. 434·4, and **lithium acetylsalicylate,** $C_9H_7O_4Li$, Mol. Wt. 186·1, are estimated by weighing their sulphated ash. Caution is necessary when sulphuric acid is added to the ash for sulphating. 1 g $CaSO_4$ = 3·191 g calcium aspirin and 1 g Li_2SO_4 = 3·385 g lithium aspirin.

Calcium acetylsalicylate may contain small puantities of calcium chloride as a stabiliser, since the salts are more easily hydrolysed than the free acid (Coplans and Green[5]).

Aluminium acetylsalicylate, $C_{18}H_{15}O_9Al$, Mol. Wt. 402·3, has become of pharmaceutical interest. It contains a considerable amount of salicylate. The method of determination of both acetylsalicylic acid and salicylic acid is based on that of the *N.F.* except that more chloroform extractions have been found desirable.

Transfer to a 250-ml separator about 100 mg of aluminium aspirin, accurately weighed, add 40 ml of freshly prepared sodium fluoride-hydrochloric acid solution (dissolve 500 mg of sodium fluoride in 100 ml of 0·1N hydrochloric acid) and shake for five minutes. Allow the solution to stand for ten minutes with frequent shaking. Extract with eight portions, each of 20 ml, of chloroform, filtering each extract into a 200-ml graduated flask, dilute to volume with chloroform and mix. Dilute 20 ml of this solution to 100 ml with chloroform and measure the extinction of the diluted solution at 278 mμ and 308 mμ using 1-cm cells and chloroform as the blank.

Calculate the percentage of acetylsalicylic acid and salicylic acid in the sample using the following formulæ.

$$\%\ \text{Acetylsalicylic acid} = 10{,}000\left(\frac{e_1}{E_1} - \frac{E_2}{E_1} \times \frac{e_2}{E_3}\right) \times \frac{100}{W}$$

$$\%\ \text{Salicylic acid} = \frac{10{,}000 e_2}{E_3} \times \frac{100}{W}$$

W = weight of sample taken in mg
e_1 = extinction of sample solution at 278 mμ
e_2 = extinction of sample solution at 308 mμ
E_1 = E(1 per cent, 1 cm) at 278 mμ for acetylsalicylic acid in chloroform solution
E_2 = E(1 per cent, 1 cm) at 278 mμ for salicylic acid in chloroform solution
E_3 = E(1 per cent, 1 cm) at 308 mμ for salicylic acid in chloroform solution.

1. Jones, A. J., *C. & D.*, 1919, 402.
2. Nutter-Smith, A., *Analyst*, 1920, **45**, 412.
3. Edwards, L. J., Gore, D. N., Rapson, H. D. C., and Taylor, Mary P., *J. Pharm. Pharmacol.*, 1955, **7**, 892.
4. Foster, J. S., and Murfin, J. W., private communication.
5. Coplans, M., and Green, A. G., *J. Soc. Chem. Ind.*, 1935, **54**, 805.

ACONITE

Most of the aconite species contain one or more characteristic alkaloids all of which are derivatives of isomeric aconines. The *B.P.C.* aconite is confined to the root (the leaf also contains similar alkaloids) of *A. napellus*, Linn., which contains the crystalline alkaloid **aconitine** (acetylbenzoylaconine), $C_{34}H_{47}O_{11}N$, Mol. Wt. 645·8, with smaller proportions of non-crystalline alkaloids.

Aconitine is easily decomposed, being readily hydrolysed, especially in hydroxylic solvents, and its degradation products are much less potent than the parent alkaloid. Various considerations have emphasised that the physiologically active constituents of the numerous species of aconite require separate and special investigation. The assumption that all the ether-soluble bases are aconitine is obviously incorrect. Methods for the determination of aconite itself have been described; those based on the products of hydrolysis are too uncertain to be considered. Other procedures are based on paper chromatography, such as that described by Mital and Mühlemann[1] who used a system consisting of amyl alcohol, formic acid and benzene for separation and then, after location of the individual alkaloids with Dragendorff's reagent determined the relative amounts spectrophotometrically.

Physiological methods of standardisation are probably of more value although these have not been investigated very fully, the drug having only limited use; but in the course of an investigation for the *S.A.C.* on the assay of aconite it was shown that there is some correlation and the results of chemical assay for total alkaloids will give more than an approximate measure of the therapeutic efficacy of a sample.

The Analytical Methods Committee of the *S.A.C.*[2] found that more consistent results were obtainable when assay was based on the total alkaloidal content rather than upon the ether-soluble portion and recommended the following method. This has been adopted by the *B.P.C.*, the official root now being required to contain a minimum of 0·5 per cent total alkaloids.

> Introduce 10 g of the root, in No. 60 powder, into a stoppered percolator of suitable capacity and add 100 ml of a mixture of three volumes of ether and one volume of chloroform, shake well and set aside for fifteen minutes; add 5 ml of dilute ammonia solution and shake for one minute at ten-minute intervals during one hour. Allow the liquid to percolate into a separator. When the liquid ceases to flow, pack the drug firmly and continue the percolation with further quantities of the solvent until complete extraction of the alkaloids is effected. Test the percolate for complete extraction by collecting separately about 2 ml in a dish, evaporating the solvent, dissolving the residue in a few drops of 0·1N sulphuric acid and adding 1 drop of 0·1N iodine. In the absence of alkaloids of aconite no precipitate or turbidity is formed.
>
> To the percolate add 30 ml of N sulphuric acid, or sufficient to render the mixture faintly acid, shake well, allow to separate and run off the lower layer. Continue the extraction with 10-ml portions of 0·1N sulphuric acid until extraction of the alkaloids is complete, as shown by the iodine test. Wash the mixed acid solutions with about 10 ml of chloroform and run off the latter into a second separator containing 20 ml of 0·1N sulphuric acid, shake, allow to separate and reject the chloroform. Repeat the washing of the liquid in the first separator with two further 5-ml quantities of chloroform, transfer each in turn to the second separator, wash with the same aqueous acid liquid, allow to separate and reject the chloroform layer as before. Transfer the acid liquid from the second separator to the first separator, make just alkaline with dilute ammonia solution and add 2 ml in excess; shake with successive portions of chloroform until complete extraction of the alkaloids is effected, washing each chloroform extract with the same 20 ml of water contained in another separator. Remove the chloroform by distillation, add to the residue 2 ml of dehydrated ethanol, evaporate at a temperature not exceeding 60°, and dry at a temperature below 60° for thirty minutes. Dissolve the residue in 2 ml of neutral 95 per cent ethanol, warm until dissolved, add 20 ml of 0·02N sulphuric acid and 10 ml of water; cool and titrate with 0·02N sodium hydroxide, using methyl red as indicator. 1 ml of 0·02N acid = 0·01291 g of the alkaloids of aconite calculated as aconitine.

Cornwell and Jones[3] showed that the results of the assay were dependent on many factors, and especially that as the ether-soluble alkaloids were not entirely aconitine a variable quantity of these is extracted dependent on the method and proportions of solvents used; further, ethanol must be absent, for if it is present, other basic material is extracted; finally, it was ascertained that the alkaloidal residue is easily decomposed. It is certain that the details of any method used must be strictly adhered to for results to be comparable.

Liniment of Aconite, *B.P.C.* A 1 : 2 percolate of the root in 90 per cent alcohol, containing 3 per cent of camphor.

The following procedure has been found satisfactory for the determination of total alkaloids.

> To 50 ml add 150 ml of water and 5 ml of dilute sulphuric acid. Extract with four portions, each of 50 ml, of ether, wash the combined extracts with 5 ml of 0·1N sulphuric acid and discard the ether. Make the combined aqueous solutions and washing alkaline with ammonia and extract with successive portions of chloroform until extraction is complete, washing each extract with the same 20 ml of water. Evaporate the chloroform at a low temperature, add 2 ml of ethanol to the residue, re-evaporate and dry the residue at 60° for one hour. Dissolve the residue in 20 ml of 0·02N sulphuric acid and titrate with 0·02N sodium hydroxide using methyl red as indicator. 1 ml 0·02N sulphuric acid = 0·01291 g of alkaloids calculated as aconitine.

The camphor present may be estimated by the method of Hampshire and Page, described on p. 156.

> Distil 25 ml of the liniment in steam until 150 ml of distillate has been collected. Wash down the condenser with 75 ml of aldehyde-free ethanol, which dissolves the camphor in the distillate. Dilute to 250 ml, and take 60 ml, containing about 0·2 g of camphor, for the determination.

Liniment of Aconite may be made with industrial methylated spirit, and hence aldehydes present in the alcohol will be precipitated in the assay. An approximate allowance can be made for this; Hampshire and Page in a control experiment on industrial spirit with these proportions obtained a precipitate equivalent to 0·12 per cent of camphor.

Liniment of Aconite, Belladonna and Chloroform, *B.P.C.* (A.B.C. Liniment). Equal parts of the liniments of aconite, belladonna and chloroform, the latter consisting of equal parts of chloroform and camphorated oil.

A good analysis of the liniment is somewhat fortuitous, as the preparation separates easily and average samples are withdrawn with difficulty, therefore care must be taken in mixing before sampling from bulk.

Chloroform is determined on 5 ml of a 10 per cent dilution in ethanol by the volumetric method described on p. 168; also the colorimetric method of Moffit (see Chloroform) has been tried successfully. Camphor is determined by following the method given under Liniment of Aconite.

Calculated from the formula, the preparation should contain 16·6 per cent by volume of chloroform, 6 per cent w/v of camphor and about 51 per cent v/v of alcohol; total alkaloids about 0·16 per cent w/v calculated as hyoscyamine. The fixed oil content is 13·3 per cent v/v, but extractive matter from the aconite and belladonna brings the apparent figure to 14 per cent.

1. MITAL, V. K., and MÜHLEMANN, H., *Pharm. Acta Helv.*, 1956, **31**, 420.
2. *Analyst*, 1942, **67**, 289.
3. CORNWELL, C. W., and JONES, A. J., *Y.B.Pharm.*, 1926, 388.

ADRENALINE

$C_6H_3(OH)_2CHOH.CH_2NHCH_3$ Mol. Wt. 183·2

Adrenaline is the active principle of the suprarenal gland. It may also be prepared synthetically. Adrenaline acts as a base and can be titrated if present in sufficient quantity. The purity of the base can be determined by non-aqueous titration with perchloric acid (see p. 792), 1 ml 0·1N perchloric acid = 0·01832 g.

In N sulphuric acid, adrenaline has an absorption maximum at 278 mμ, E(1 per cent, 1 cm) = 153, and a minimum at 250 mμ, E(1 per cent, 1 cm) = 20.

Barker, Eastland, and Evers[1] in a critical survey of the colour tests which have been proposed for the determination of adrenaline preferred the potassium persulphate reaction as being most specific and comparable with biological estimation when the necessary conditions, including control of temperature and pH, are observed. Rees[2] confirmed the value of the persulphate method since it is applicable in the presence of ascorbic acid, which is present in fresh suprarenal gland. The following is the method recommended but modified for a spectrophotometric finish.

Prepare the necessary reagent, containing in aqueous solution 0·2 per cent potassium persulphate, 1·0 per cent sodium chloride, 0·239 per cent disodium hydrogen phosphate, and 0·937 per cent sodium dihydrogen phosphate; this solution should have pH 5·5, and is stable if kept away from the light and in a cool place. Mix 1 ml of the reagent with 1 ml of the solution to be tested, containing between 0·01 and 0·10 mg of adrenaline, and immediately measure the maximum extinction at 490 mμ, using a 1-cm all-glass cell. Then place the cell in a thermostat at 22° and read the colour again after thirty minutes. The increase in extinction is then compared with that given by a standard solution of adrenaline treated in a similar manner; alternatively, a colour concentration curve can be prepared from a standard adrenaline solution.

For gland extracts adjust the pH of the extract to 5·4 using methyl red as an external indicator.

For gland extracts the persulphate method was found to be the only one to give results comparable with those obtained by biological methods. For the quantitative determination of the glands themselves satisfactory results were obtained by using protein-free trichloracetic acid extracts; in this case the filtrate must not be neutralised before adding the reagent, but the requisite amount of alkali added afterwards and allowance made for the increase in volume.

A simple oxidation of adrenaline with iodine at pH 5·4 to 5·5 is also satisfactory for colorimetric assay, the excess iodine being removed with thiosulphate for quantitative measurement.

A colorimetric method of determination of adrenaline in pharmaceutical products containing bisulphite was developed by Doty.[3] The colour developed reaches maximum intensity quickly and is constant for some hours.

Iron Reagents. (*a*) Ferrous sulphate solution is prepared by dissolving 1·5 g of ferrous sulphate in 200 ml of water containing 0·3 ml of dilute hydrochloric acid and 1·0 g of sodium bisulphite. (*b*) To 10 ml of this solution add 0·5 g of sodium citrate and 0·5 g of sodium bisulphite.

Buffer Reagent. Dissolve 50·4 g of sodium bicarbonate in about 480 ml of water to which has been added 10 ml of strong ammonia solution and 22·5 g of amino-acetic acid. Adjust the final volume to 500 ml and the pH to 8·0.

Pipette 10 ml of the solution into a comparison tube (or flask), add 0·1 ml of the iron-citrate reagent (*b*) followed by 1·0 ml of the buffer reagent. After mixing the solution, allow to stand for twenty minutes and examine it in a suitable spectrophotometer to determine the extinction at about 540 mμ. The concentration of adrenaline is read directly from a calibration curve, prepared in a similar manner with a standard adrenaline solution.

Cobefrin (3,4-dihydroxyphenylpropanolamine) reacts identically as adrenaline in this procedure.

Methods have been described whereby adrenaline and noradrenaline may be determined simultaneously in the same solution. The methods are based on observations of Weil-Malherbe and Bone[4] who found that, when adrenaline and noradrenaline are condensed with ethylenediamine, the fluorescence due to the adrenaline derivative is about five times that of the noradrenaline derivative at 550 mμ. At 500 mμ however the fluorescence of the two compounds is similar. Many modifications of the procedure have been suggested and it has been criticised because of its non-specificity (catechol and many other related substances will also give rise to fluorescent compounds when condensed with ethylenediamine).

Another technique depends upon the fact that, on oxidation with manganese dioxide or potassium ferricyanide at pH 5 to 6, adrenaline and noradrenaline are converted to adrenochrome and noradrenochrome respectively. At pH 3 to 4 however only adrenaline is oxidised. Such a differential method would obviously be unsatisfactory for determination of a small amount of noradrenaline in the presence of a large excess of adrenaline.

Although good agreement is found between colorimetric and biological methods when assaying freshly-prepared adrenaline solutions, on aged solutions or solutions that have been subjected to a certain amount of heat during sterilisation results obtained by colorimetric methods are frequently higher than those obtained by biological methods. Since this is most probably because the *l*-adrenaline has been partly converted to the much less potent *d*-isomer and the enantiomorphic forms of a substance give precisely the same colour reactions a method based on the determination of optical rotation would seem applicable. Such methods have been described by Rosenblum, Goldman and Feldman[5] and by Hellberg[6] who from optical rotation measurements calculated the amount of *l*-isomer present over and above that nullified by the *d*-isomer and then calculated the total *l*-isomer as the geometric mean of this figure and the amount of both isomers determined by Doty's method.[3]

However, inherent in these methods are the assumptions that no chromogenic substances, other than adrenaline, are present and that the rotatory power of the solutions is due solely to *l*-adrenaline which precludes their use for routine testing of samples in which the nature of the other materials present is unknown. For such samples Welsh[7] has produced a method in which the adrenaline is converted quantitatively to the triacetyl derivative which may be determined qualitatively as well as quantitatively by polarimetry, and this method has been adopted by the *U.S.P.* for Epinephrine Solution, Inhalation, Injection, and Sterile Suspension and Epinephrine Bitartrate Ophthalmic Ointment. It is described in detail under Solution of Adrenaline.

Similar considerations apply to noradrenaline where again the *l*-isomer is more potent than the *d*-isomer and Norepinephrine Acid Tartrate Injection *U.S.P.* is assayed by the above method using values of 1·1423 and 80 for the gravimetric and rotatory factors, respectively.

l-Noradrenaline is usually present in adrenaline obtained from natural sources and Welsh[7] has given a method whereby the mixed triacetyl derivatives of adrenaline and noradrenaline may be separated by partition chromatography using water supported on Celite as the stationary phase and benzene as the mobile phase. Subsequent hydrolysis of the separated noradrenaline derivative enables the total $(d + l)$ noradrenaline content of the original sample to be determined colorimetrically after oxidisation to noradrenochrome by the method of von Euler and Hamberg.[8]

For analysis of solutions containing adrenaline the net error due to using the rotatory and gravimetric factors applicable to adrenaline is less than 1 per cent and may be ignored.

Higuchi, Sokoloski, and Schroeter,[9] while acknowledging the fact that Welsh's method represents a major step forward in solving the problem of determining adrenaline in the presence of its degradation products, criticise the method in certain respects and suggest improvements. The authors state that the acetylated product obtained by Welsh's method is usually not pure triacetyl adrenaline but contains other acetylation products, and this leads to variable errors; an improvement is effected by reducing the acetylation time to two minutes, which is adequate for conversion of adrenaline to its triacetyl derivative. A further modification proposed is that, instead of extracting the triacetyl derivative with chloroform, the reaction mixture is buffered and stabilised by the addition of citric acid and then mixed to a slurry with Celite and transferred to a chromatographic column prepared by mixing Celite with pH 4, 0·1M citrate buffer and *iso*-octane and draining off the *iso*-octane. The triacetyl adrenaline is then eluted with chloroform and, since most of it is contained between the twentieth and thirtieth ml of eluate, the first 10 ml of eluate is discarded and exactly 50 ml collected for gravimetric and polarimetric analysis. The authors recommended that the above modifications be adopted in the *U.S.P.* but this has not been implemented in either the *U.S.P.* XVI or in its first supplement.

Adrenaline acid tartrate, $C_9H_{13}O_3N,C_4H_6O_6$, Mol. Wt. 333·3. As with adrenaline base, the acid tartrate may be titrated in non-aqueous media with perchloric acid (see p. 792). 1 ml 0·1N perchloric acid = 0·03333 g. In N sulphuric acid, adrenaline acid tartrate has an absorption maximum at 278 mμ, E(1 per cent, 1 cm) = 82, and a minimum at 250 mμ, E(1 per cent, 1 cm) = 11.

Eye-drops of Zinc Sulphate and Adrenaline, *B.P.C.* Contain 50 per cent of Adrenaline Solution and 0·25 per cent of zinc sulphate.

The adrenaline may be determined by the iodine method given under Injection of Adrenaline using 4 ml of sample.

For zinc, see p. 697.

Injection of Adrenaline, *B.P.* Contains adrenaline acid tartrate equivalent to 0·10 per cent adrenaline, with sodium metabisulphite and sodium chloride. Oxidation with iodine is applicable for colorimetric determination.

To 2 ml of sample add 2 ml of phthalate buffer solution at pH 5·4 and dilute to 100 ml. To 10 ml of this diluted solution add 9·0 ml of 0·01N iodine, allow to stand for ten minutes and then add 1 ml of 0·01N sodium thiosulphate. Compare the intensity of colour developed with that of a standard solution of adrenaline similarly treated.

The ferrous sulphate-citrate method given above is also applicable to this preparation after diluting 5 ml of the sample to 100 ml with water.

A direct spectrophotometric assay is satisfactory when the absorption characteristics of the adrenaline acid tartrate used are known.

Dilute 3 ml of the injection to 100 ml with water. Measure the maximum extinction (E) of a 1-cm layer of the dilution at about 278 mμ using water as the blank. Per cent adrenaline acid tartrate = $E/3 \times 100/A$

where A = E(1 per cent, 1 cm) at 278 mμ of adrenaline acid tartrate in water.

Unofficial injections of adrenaline formulated with 0·5 per cent phenol are prepared commercially. The following method will determine both constituents.

Place 5 ml of the sample on to an oxycellulose or alginic acid column and wash with three portions, each of 25 ml, of water, collecting the eluate in a 100-ml graduated flask. Make up to volume with water and dilute 10 ml to 100 ml with water (solution A).

Elute the adrenaline with four quantities, each of 25 ml, of N sulphuric acid, collecting the eluate in a 100-ml graduated flask until the flask is filled to the mark (solution B).

Determine the phenol in solution A by measuring the maximum extinction (E) of a 1-cm layer at about 269 mμ using water as the blank.

$$\text{phenol} = \frac{E}{5} \times \frac{100}{10} \times \frac{100}{A} \text{ per cent}$$

where A = E(1 per cent, 1 cm) at 269 mμ for phenol in water.

Determine the adrenaline acid tartrate in solution B by measuring the maximum extinction (E_1) of a 1-cm layer at about 278 mμ using N sulphuric acid as the blank.

$$\text{adrenaline acid tartrate} = \frac{E_1}{5} \times \frac{100}{A_1} \text{ per cent}$$

where A_1 = E(1 per cent, 1 cm) at 278 mμ for adrenaline acid tartrate in N sulphuric acid.

Injection of Lignocaine and Adrenaline, *B.P.* Contains the equivalent of 0·00125 per cent w/v of adrenaline.

The adrenaline is determined by a modification of the ferrous sulphate-citrate assay given on p. 20.

To 10 ml of the injection add 20 mg of sodium metabisulphite, 0·1 ml of freshly-prepared ferrous sulphate-citrate solution and 1 ml of the buffer reagent. Mix, allow to stand for ten minutes and extract with 10 ml of ether. Reject the ether after separation and measure the extinction at 540 mμ. Calculate the adrenaline content by reference to a curve prepared by treating suitable quantities of a standard solution of adrenaline acid tartrate by the same process.

Injection of Procaine and Adrenaline, *B.P.* Contains the equivalent of 0·002 per cent w/v of adrenaline.

The adrenaline is determined as Lignocaine and Adrenaline Injection omitting the ether extraction.

Solution of Adrenaline, *B.P.* Contains the equivalent of 0·1 per cent of adrenaline, 0·4 per cent of chlorbutol, 0·1 per cent of chlorocresol, 0·8 per cent of sodium chloride, and 0·1 per cent of sodium metabisulphite.

The adrenaline in this solution is most suitably determined by the ferrous sulphate-citrate method detailed above, after diluting 5 ml to 100 ml with water.

ADRENALINE

The tri-acetyl derivative method of Welsh[7] for the determination of *l*-adrenaline in the presence of decomposition products (p. 21), as applied to Epinephrine Solution *U.S.P.* is as follows:

Pipette 30 ml into a 125-ml separator and remove the chlorbutol by extracting with three 25-ml quantities of carbon tetrachloride, shaking for one minute each time and separating the carbon tetrachloride layer. Discard the carbon tetrachloride extracts and rinse the stopper and the mouth of the separator with a few drops of water. Add 0·2 ml of starch mucilage and then destroy the bisulphite by adding dropwise, with swirling, a solution prepared by dissolving 0·5 g of iodine and 1·5 g of potassium iodide in 25 ml of water until the blue colour formed persists. Immediately afterwards add just sufficient 0·1N sodium thiosulphate to discharge the blue colour. (*N.B.*—Proceed with the assay from this point without delay.)

Add to the liquid in the separator 2·10 g of sodium bicarbonate, preventing it from coming into contact with the mouth of the separator, and swirl until most of the sodium bicarbonate has dissolved. By means of a 1-ml syringe, rapidly inject 1·0 ml of acetic anhydride directly into the contents of the separator and immediately stopper the separator and shake vigorously until evolution of carbon dioxide has ceased (seven to ten minutes), releasing the pressure as necessary through the stop-cock. Allow to stand for five minutes and extract with six 25-ml quantities of chloroform, filtering each extract through a small plug of cotton wool previously rinsed with chloroform, into a beaker.

Evaporate the combined extracts on a water-bath under a jet of air to about 3 ml, completely transfer the residue with small portions of chloroform to a tared 50-ml beaker, and heat again to evaporate the solvent completely. Heat further at 105° for thirty minutes, cool in a desiccator and weigh the residue of triacetyl adrenaline. Add 5·0 ml of chloroform, cover the beaker, gently swirl until the residue is completely dissolved, and determine the specific rotation, R, using a 2-dm, semi-micro polarimeter tube.

$$\text{mg adrenaline in 30 ml of sample} = (0{\cdot}5 + 0{\cdot}5R/93) \times W \times 0{\cdot}5923$$

where W is the weight of triacetyl adrenaline in mg, R is its specific rotation (in degrees without regard to sign), 0·5923 is a gravimetric conversion factor and 93 is the rotatory factor found using residues obtained in the assay of purified synthetic *l*-adrenaline bitartrate.

Compound Spray of Adrenaline and Atropine, *B.P.C.* A complex preparation containing 0·83 per cent of adrenaline acid tartrate.

It has been found that metabisulphite in excess interferes with the persulphate colour reaction. This can be avoided by acidifying with a known amount of N acid, passing nitrogen through to remove the sulphur dioxide and then adding an equivalent of N sodium hydroxide to neutralise.

As mentioned above, for many preparations of adrenaline oxidation with a trace of iodine in solution buffered at pH 5·4 to 5·5 gives a satisfactory colorimetric assay. This can be applied to Compound Spray of Adrenaline and Atropine after removal of sulphur dioxide.

Dilute 5 ml to 250 ml with water, pipette 15 ml into a small flask, add

3 ml of 0·5N hydrochloric acid and pass nitrogen through for four hours. Add 1 ml of solution of standard pH 5·4 followed by 12 ml of 0·1N sodium hydroxide. Transfer to a 50-ml graduated flask and make up to volume with water. To 10 ml of this dilution add 8 ml of 0·02N iodine, allow to stand for ten minutes, add 2 ml of 0·1N sodium thiosulphate and mix well. Compare the colour intensity with that produced when 15 ml of a standard solution of adrenaline acid tartrate containing 0·167 g of $C_9H_{13}O_3N,C_4H_6O_6$ in 1 litre is similarly treated.

The papaverine in this preparation can be extracted from hydrochloric acid solution with chloroform (p. 497) and the atropine methonitrate precipitated in the aqueous residues as reineckate (p. 120).

Noradrenaline acid tartrate, $C_8H_{11}O_3N,C_4H_6O_6,H_2O$, Mol. Wt. 337·3, is assayed similarly to adrenaline by non-aqueous titration using 0·15 g, 1 ml 0·1N perchloric acid = 0·03193 g anhydrous. **Isoproterenol hydrochloride,** $C_{11}H_{17}O_3N,HCl$, Mol. Wt. 247·7 (1 ml 0·1N = 0·02477 g) and **hydroxyamphetamine hydrobromide,** $C_9H_{13}ON,HBr$, Mol. Wt. 232·1 (1 ml 0·1N = 0·02321 g) are also assayed in the *U.S.P.* by non-aqueous titration.

ISOPRENALINE SULPHATE, $(C_{11}H_{17}O_3N)_2,H_2SO_4,2H_2O$, Mol. Wt. 556·6.

Isoprenaline sulphate is a synthetic drug similar in action to adrenaline; it is administered both by inhalation as sprays and orally as tablets. Its quantitative determination by colorimetric methods follows that for adrenaline, although some preparations do not react normally with the iron-citrate reagent.

In water isoprenaline sulphate has an absorption maximum at 280 mμ, E(1 per cent, 1 cm) = 100, and a minimum at 249 mμ, E(1 per cent, 1 cm) = 9.

Spray of Isoprenaline Sulphate, *B.P.C.* Contains 1·0 per cent of isoprenaline sulphate with propylene glycol and sodium metabisulphite in water.

Dilute 5 ml of spray to 50 ml. To 3 ml of the dilution in a 100-ml flask add 2 ml of solution of standard pH 5·4 and make up to volume with water. To 10 ml of this solution add 8 ml of 0·02N iodine and allow to stand for ten minutes. Add 2 ml of 0·1N sodium thiosulphate and mix. Compare the intensity of colour developed with that produced when 5 ml of a standard solution of isoprenaline sulphate containing 1·00 g per 100 ml is similarly treated.

For a spectrophotometric assay:

Dilute 5 ml of sample to 100 ml with water and further dilute 10 ml of this solution to 100 ml with water. Measure the maximum extinction of a 1-cm layer at about 280 mμ using water as the blank.

Compound Spray of Isoprenaline Sulphate, *B.P.C.* A complex preparation containing 1·0 per cent of isoprenaline sulphate. The isoprenaline can be determined by the iodine method given above under Spray of Isoprenaline Sulphate.

The papaverine in this preparation can be extracted from hydrochloric acid solution with chloroform (p. 497) and the atropine methonitrate precipitated in the aqueous residues as reineckate (p. 120).

Tablets of Isoprenaline Sulphate, *B.P.* Usually contain 10 mg of isoprenaline sulphate in a lactose base. The determination follows that given above for sprays.

> Dissolve an amount of powdered tablets to contain about 50 mg of isoprenaline sulphate in 100 ml of water containing 3·5 ml of 0·5N hydrochloric acid, filter and dilute to 200 ml. To 10 ml add 2 ml of pH 5·4 buffer and dilute to 100 ml. Continue the determination by the method given under Spray of Isoprenaline Sulphate and calculate the weight in each tablet of average weight.

The ferrous sulphate-citrate assay given above under adrenaline is applicable to this preparation after shaking an appropriate amount of powdered tablets with water for fifteen minutes, diluting to a suitable volume and filtering.

A simple spectrophotometric assay follows that for Spray of Isoprenaline Sulphate after dissolving an amount of powdered tablets, equivalent to 100 mg of isoprenaline sulphate, in 200 ml of water and diluting 10 ml of this solution to 100 ml with water.

1. Barker, J. H., Eastland, C. J., and Evers, N., *Biochem. J.*, 1932, **26,** 2129.
2. Rees, H. G., *Quart. J. Pharm.*, 1936, **9**, 659.
3. Doty, J. R., *Anal. Chem.*, 1948, **20**, 1166.
4. Weil-Malherbe, H., and Bone, A. D., *Biochem. J.*, 1952, **51**, 311.
5. Rosenblum, H., Goldman, R., and Feldman, H., *J. Amer. Pharm. Ass., Sci. Edn.*, 1949, **39**, 255.
6. Hellberg, H., *J. Pharm. Pharmacol.*, 1955, **7**, 191.
7. Welsh, Ll. H., *J. Amer. Pharm. Ass., Sci. Edn.*, 1955, **44,** 507.
8. Von Euler, U. S., and Hamberg, U., *Science*, 1949, **110**, 561.
9. Higuchi, T., Sokoloski, T. D., and Schroeter, L. C., *J. Amer. Pharm. Ass., Sci. Edn.*, 1959, **48,** 553.

ALKALI METALS

(Potassium, Sodium and Lithium)

CHEMICAL METHODS

Potassium

Of the usual processes employed for the determination of potassium that by means of perchloric acid is the most suitable. Procedures have been described using tetraphenylboron as precipitant (see p. 31) but it should be remembered that this method is subject to considerable interference, especially when ammonium salts are present.

The method used in the Fertilisers and Feeding Stuffs Regulations (1960), for the determination of potash as perchlorate in guanos and mixed fertilisers, will give generally concordant results. It is summarised below:

> Gently incinerate 10 g of the sample at a temperature not exceeding 500° in order to char organic matter, if present, and then heat for ten minutes with 10 ml of concentrated hydrochloric acid and finally boil with 300 ml of water. Add 10 g of calcium oxide made into a paste with water and gently boil for half an hour. Cool, make up to 500 ml and filter. Make 250 ml of filtrate just acid with hydrochloric acid and heat to boiling-point. To the boiling solution add barium chloride solution drop by drop until there is no further precipitation. Make alkaline with ammonia, add excess of ammonium carbonate and then, while boiling, a little ammonium oxalate; cool, make up to 500 ml and filter. Evaporate to dryness 100 ml of the filtrate in a porcelain or platinum dish. Heat the residue gently over a low flame until all ammonium salts have been expelled, the temperature being carefully kept below that of low redness. (This preliminary treatment is necessary to eliminate metals other than alkalies.) Moisten the residue with concentrated hydrochloric acid, evaporate to dryness, take up the residue in water and filter again.
>
> To the filtrate in a platinum dish or porcelain basin add about 7 ml of 20 per cent perchloric acid solution (sp. gr. 1·125, free from chloric acid). Evaporate the mixture on a hot-plate or sand-bath until white fumes are copiously evolved.
>
> Redissolve the precipitate in hot water, add a few drops of perchloric acid solution and concentrate the whole again to the fuming stage. After cooling, stir the residue in the basin thoroughly with 20 ml of 95 per cent ethanol. Then allow the precipitate to settle and pour the clear liquid through a dry filter paper, draining the precipitate as completely as possible. Redissolve the precipitate on the paper and in the basin with hot water, add 2 ml of perchloric acid solution and again evaporate to the fuming stage. Cool and stir thoroughly with 20 ml of ethanol, allow to settle and pour the clear liquid through a weighed sintered-glass or Gooch crucible, draining the precipitate as completely as possible from the liquid before adding the washing solution. Wash the precipitate by decantation with ethanol saturated with potassium perchlorate at the temperature at which it is used, pouring the washings through the

crucible on which the whole of the precipitate is finally collected; dry at 100° and weigh. $KClO_4 \times 0{\cdot}34 = K_2O$.

Sodium

When the percentage constituents of a mixture of sodium and potassium are required, the potassium is usually determined by the method mentioned above and the sodium calculated by difference.

The available methods for the direct determination of sodium are not so well established as those for potassium and much criticism has been made of the various methods. Tabern and Shelberg[1] have applied Kahane's method of using an acid ethanolic solution of magnesium uranyl acetate to sodium salts of organic acids, and its successful use for the determination of sodium in calcium sodium lactate and of sodium bromide in the presence of up to six times its weight of potassium bromide has been confirmed by Liversedge.[2] A slightly modified method was used by Liversedge, the triple magnesium salt being precipitated in a large granular form readily retained by a sintered-glass crucible. Phosphates, if present, must first be removed.

Precipitating reagent: 100 g of magnesium acetate, 32 g of uranyl acetate, 20 ml of glacial acetic acid and 500 ml of 90 per cent ethanol made up to 1 litre with water, heated on a steam-bath to effect solution and filtered after cooling.

To the substance, containing between 5 and 10 mg of sodium dissolved in 5 to 10 ml of water or ethanol, add 3 ml of precipitating reagent for each mg of sodium expected. Place the beaker in ice-cold water and stir occasionally with a glass rod during half an hour and allow to stand a further half an hour. Filter the precipitate through a sintered-glass crucible (1G3) and wash with 5 to 10 ml of the reagent, followed by 10 ml of 95 per cent ethanol. Dry between 105° and 110°; 1 g of triple salt = 0·0153 g Na.

Lithium

Lithium in pharmaceutical salts is treated as the other alkali metals, *i.e.* it is assayed for its acidic radical, and lithium salts are described under the appropriate acid.

Methods of separation of lithium depend, almost without exception, on the solubility of lithium salts and the insolubility of the salts of the other alkali metals in organic solvents. The method of determination adopted by Brown and Reedy[3] has been selected as being relatively simple; it gives reasonable accuracy and is essentially:

Evaporate a solution of the chlorides (sodium, potassium, barium and strontium do not interfere with the determination, but calcium must be absent) to dryness in a small beaker and volatilise ammonium salts by heat. Grind up the residue with a small glass rod and add 25 ml of dry acetone containing 1 drop of concentrated hydrochloric acid (to dissolve lithium hydroxide); stir the mixture well and allow to settle. Pour the clear supernatant liquid through a small filter paper into a platinum dish and wash the residue and paper with small portions of dry acetone. After dissolving the residue of mixed chlorides in a small quantity of water, evaporating and regrinding the residue, repeat the extraction. This treatment liberates any lithium chloride which may be occluded in the crystals; two extractions completely remove the lithium chloride if the total weight of chlorides is below 0·5 g.

Evaporate the combined filtrates to dryness, slowly heat the residue to remove organic matter and add a few drops of concentrated sulphuric acid before heating to dull redness, cooling and weighing as sulphate, $Li_2SO_4 \times 0{\cdot}1263 = Li$.

FLAME PHOTOMETRIC METHODS

The alkali metals are easily determined by flame photometric methods which are always less time-consuming than chemical methods and offer the same order of accuracy. The precise procedure used will depend on the type of equipment which is available but certain generalisations can be made which are applicable to all instruments. These elements are easily excited and have relatively low ionisation potentials so a low temperature flame is always indicated and air-coal gas, air-propane and air-hydrogen are most convenient. As the resonance lines appear in the visible region of the spectrum filter instruments can be used so long as spectral interferences are negligible or can be corrected for. If a monochromator instrument is used such corrections are more easily and accurately made.

Potassium

The strongest lines of potassium are the doublet 7660/7690 A which is almost always used for analytical purposes, although the blue line at 4044 A can be useful also. Self-absorption is of little importance but ionisation is quite a serious problem if a hot flame is used.

The most important spectral interferences arise from barium, sodium, cæsium and rubidium. Of these the most serious is likely to be that of sodium but this can be reduced considerably by using a dense didymium filter which absorbs strongly at 5890 A and therefore reduces the light from the main sodium lines.

Moderate concentrations (up to 0·1N) of mineral acids in the solutions used do not have much effect on the emission but this depends to some extent on the instrument used and standards should always contain the same anions as the samples as far as this is possible.

Sodium

The doublet at about 5890 A is always used for the determination of sodium. At concentrations above 2 to 3 p.p.m. it suffers from strong self-absorption and it is wise to work at concentrations of not more than 10 p.p.m.

ALKALI METALS

Very few spectral interferences are encountered mainly because of the very high sensitivity of sodium. Calcium is the most important interfering element and when filter instruments are used its effect may be serious. It can however be eliminated by adding aluminium to sample and standard solutions. The amount required will depend on many factors and must be determined by experiment.

The effect of acids is similar to that under potassium and similar precautions should be applied.

Lithium

Lithium exhibits a strong resonance line at 6708 A and this is almost always used for its determination. It is less easily ionised than the other alkalis but as flame temperatures are made higher LiOH is increasingly produced in the flame so that the relative radiation at 6708 A is reduced. Cool flames as stated above should therefore be used. Calibration curves are reasonably linear up to concentrations of about 20 p.p.m. and so if the instrument has sufficient sensitivity it is wise to work at maximum concentrations of 10 p.p.m. or thereabouts.

Spectral interferences can be expected from relatively large concentrations of barium, strontium, calcium, and sodium, although the use of the cool flame will reduce the effect of the first three to a minimum. These interferences will of course be most severe with filter instruments and corrections must be applied in the usual ways. When background correction is being applied with a monochromator instrument by measuring the intensity to one side of the line, care must be exercised to avoid the weak lithium line at 6100 A, the ends of the band systems of CaO and the oxide or hydroxide systems of strontium and barium.

Moderate excesses of most acids do not affect the intensity of lithium lines very much but it is usually easy to arrange that samples and standards contain the same acids in the same concentrations and it is wise to keep these concentrations as low as is reasonable.

ALKALI SALTS

The determination of the salts of the alkalies is almost invariably made by estimating the acidic radical, either directly or by the alkalinity of the ash after destroying the organic part by heat; hence they are described under the appropriate acids.

ALKALI CARBONATES AND BICARBONATES

Except lithium carbonate, which is relatively insoluble and is first dissolved in an excess of acid and back titrated, these compounds, as pharmaceutical chemicals, are all determined by direct titration with standard acid, using methyl orange or screened methyl orange as indicator. **Lithium carbonate,** Li_2CO_3, Mol. Wt. 73·89, 1 ml N = 0·03695 g; **potassium bicarbonate,** $KHCO_3$, Mol. Wt. 100·1, 1 ml 0·5N = 0·05005 g; **potassium carbonate,** $K_2CO_3,1\frac{1}{2}H_2O$, Mol. Wt. 165·2, 1 ml 0·5N = 0·03455 g anhyd.; **sodium bicarbonate,** $NaHCO_3$, Mol. Wt. 84·01, 1 ml 0·5N = 0·04200 g; **sodium carbonate,** $Na_2CO_3,10H_2O$, Mol. Wt. 286·2, 1 ml 0·5N = 0·07155 g; **anhydrous sodium carbonate,** Na_2CO_3, Mol. Wt. 106·0, 1 ml 0·5N = 0·0265 g.

For formulations such as mixtures and mouth-washes the direct titration method referred to above is usually applicable; where much organic matter is present (mixtures containing rhubarb or ipecacuanha, for example) a preliminary evaporation to dryness and ignition is necessary.

Effervescent Tablets of Potassium, *B.P.C.* Each tablet contains 500 mg of potassium bicarbonate, 300 mg of potassium acid tartrate with anhydrous citric acid, sucrose and saccharin.

These tablets can be assayed for potassium by flame photometry. Since there are no interfering ions, tetraphenylboron precipitation is also applicable:

Dissolve an amount of powdered tablets equivalent to about one-quarter of a tablet in a mixture of equal volumes of acetate buffer solution, pH 3·7 (see p. 116) and water and dilute to 200 ml with the mixture in a graduated flask. Transfer a 10-ml aliquot of this solution to a dry beaker, add, with swirling, 15 ml of 0·01M sodium tetraphenylboron, allow to stand for five minutes and filter through a dry, sintered-glass crucible. Pipette 20 ml of the filtrate into a flask, add 0·50 ml of bromophenol blue indicator and titrate the excess sodium tetraphenylboron with 0·005M cetylpyridinium chloride to the blue end-point. Repeat the operation omitting the sample. 1 ml 0·01M sodium tetraphenylboron = 0·0003910 g potassium.

ALKALI HYDROXIDES

Although sodium carbonate is relatively insoluble in ethanol, potassium carbonate has been found to be appreciably soluble; hence the method for determination of the purity of potassium hydroxide by the requirement of a minimum total alkali with a maximum carbonate is incorrect when the latter is obtained as ethanol-insoluble.

The *B.P.* avoids this error by precipitating the carbonates with barium chloride and then titrating the hydroxides with N hydrochloric acid, without filtration, to phenolphthalein (*a*); the titration can be continued to bromophenol blue (*b*) for carbonate, 1 ml N HCl = 0·06911 g K_2CO_3 and 0·05300 g Na_2CO_3; total alkali $(a + b)$, 1 ml N = 0·05611 g KOH and 0·0400 g NaOH. **Potassium hydroxide,** KOH, Mol. Wt. 56·11; **sodium hydroxide,** NaOH, Mol. Wt. 40·00.

The well-known method for titrating hydroxide and carbonate in one solution by the use of two indicators can be employed. It is used by the *U.S.P.* and saves a considerable amount of time. The method is only applicable when the carbonate present is small in quantity, as loss of carbon dioxide must be prevented; the solution should be dilute and the titration conducted in the cold:

> Dissolve about 1·5 g of the hydroxide in about 40 ml of recently-boiled and cooled distilled water. Cool to 15° and titrate with N sulphuric acid, using phenolphthalein as indicator and avoiding violent agitation. When the colour of the indicator is discharged, *i.e.* when the hydroxide is neutralised and half the carbonate (by conversion into bicarbonate), note the volume of acid required (a ml). Add methyl orange and continue the titration to a permanent pink colour (when the remaining half of the carbonate is neutralised), b ml. Then $(a - b)$ ml = hydroxide, $2b$ ml = carbonate and $(a + b)$ ml = total alkali.

1. Tabern, D. L., and Shelberg, E. F., *Ind. Eng. Chem., Anal. Edn.*, 1931, **3,** 278.
2. Liversedge, S. G., *Quart. J. Pharm.*, 1937, **10,** 364.
3. Brown, M. H., and Reedy, J. H., *Ind. Eng. Chem., Anal. Edn.*, 1930, **2,** 304.

ALUMINIUM

Al At. Wt. 26·98

The determination of aluminium by precipitation with oxine has now been largely superseded by the more rapid method of titration with EDTA, a number of different procedures having been suggested. The method is not quite so straightforward as with many other metals because aluminium complexes with EDTA somewhat slowly and this makes a direct titration very difficult. Taylor[1] has described a method of direct titration which depends upon complexing the aluminium solution at a pH of 6 and a temperature above 70° using hæmatoxylin as indicator. Results by this method may vary within about 1 per cent of the theoretical figure and for routine purposes the method suffers from the disadvantages that the sample solution must be placed in the burette and that titration must be carried out in hot solution.

An adaptation of the method described by Ter Haar and Bazen[2] has been applied to pharmaceutical preparations.[3] This depends upon complexing the aluminium with an excess of EDTA and titrating the excess EDTA using thorium nitrate as the titrant and alizarin S as indicator. Now, however, metal indicators operating in the acid pH range are available and this has resulted in the development of a more satisfactory procedure, based upon titration of the excess EDTA with lead nitrate solution using xylenol orange as indicator. A study of the effect of conditions on this determination has been made[4] and it has been found that the following factors all control the rate at which aluminium is complexed by EDTA: (1) the time of reaction, (2) the temperature at which the reaction proceeds, (3) the excess of complexing reagent which is present during reaction, and (4) the salt concentration at the time of reaction. These factors are interdependent so that in a solution where the minimum of acid has been used to dissolve the sample and where a large excess of EDTA is present a quantitative result may be obtained by allowing to stand for only ten minutes in the cold at the complexing stage. If, however, the acid concentration is increased it becomes necessary to leave the reaction mixture to stand for a longer time in the cold or to heat the solution. The method described below for dried aluminium hydroxide gel is based upon these considerations.

Traces of aluminium are of little significance in pharmaceutical analytical work but may be determined by the use of aluminon (ammonium aurine tricarboxylate) which forms a lake with aluminium at a pH of about 4 to 5. Procedures have been suggested by Lampitt and Sylvester,[5] Strafford and Wyatt,[6] Chenery,[7] and Rolfe, Russell and Wilkinson.[8] It is essential that experimental conditions are very carefully controlled in order to obtain a quantitative result.

Potash alum, $KAl(SO_4)_2,12H_2O$, Mol. Wt. 474·4, **ammonium alum** $NH_4Al(SO_4)_2$, $12H_2O$, Mol. Wt. 453.3, and **aluminium sulphate,** $Al_2(SO_4)_3,18H_2O$, Mol. Wt. 666·4, may be determined by the following method.

To a solution containing about 0·35 g, accurately weighed, of potash alum (or an equivalent amount of the other salts) in 100 ml of water, add 30 ml of 0·05M EDTA. Warm on a water-bath for ten minutes, cool, and add about 1 g of hexamine and 5 drops of xylenol orange solution. Titrate with 0·05M lead nitrate until the yellow colour changes to pink. Each ml of 0·05M EDTA is equivalent to 0·02372 g of $KAl(SO_4)_2,12H_2O$; 0·02266 g of $NH_4Al(SO_4)_2$, $12H_2O$; 0·01666 g of $Al_2(SO_4)_3$, $18H_2O$.

Sulphate ions interfere with the EDTA titration using thorium as a back titrant because of complex formation.

Aluminium hydroxide gel and **dried aluminium hydroxide gel** may be assayed by the following method:

Dissolve about 4 g of the gel or 0·4 g of the dried gel, accurately weighed, in 2 ml of concentrated hydrochloric acid by rotating the flask to ensure that the whole of the sample is moistened by the acid and then warming on a water-bath until the sample is dissolved. Cool and dilute to 100 ml with water. To 25 ml of this solution add 50 ml of 0·05M EDTA and neutralise to congo red paper by the dropwise addition of sodium hydroxide solution. Warm on a water-bath for thirty minutes, cool, add 3 g of hexamine and titrate with 0·05M lead nitrate, using xylenol orange solution as indicator. Each ml of 0·05M EDTA is equivalent to 0·002549 g of Al_2O_3.

If excess of acid is used to dissolve the gel the salt concentration during the complexing stage becomes too high and low results may be obtained. In practice solution is brought about much more rapidly and efficiently if only 2 to 3 ml of acid is used to dissolve 0·4 g of dried gel than if 10 to 15 ml is used. Results obtained by the EDTA method may be significantly lower than those obtained by precipitation of hydroxide followed by ignition. The classical gravimetric procedure may give erroneously high results unless meticulous attention is paid to the conditions of ignition. In addition, commercial samples of aluminium hydroxide gel contain quite high proportions of impurities such as calcium, magnesium, silicon, and iron. All these impurities would contribute to a higher result being obtained by the precipitation procedure but only iron would affect the EDTA method. Very large quantities of magnesium may be tolerated with no effect on the EDTA assay. If calcium is present in a quantity equivalent to the amount of aluminium, or in greater amount, the xylenol orange end-point using hexamine (3 g) as buffer becomes unsatisfactory. If the buffering conditions are made more rigid, however, the end-point is very sharp and quantitative recoveries of aluminium are obtained even in the presence of a three-fold excess of calcium. This can be achieved by adding 7 g of hexamine and 5 ml of dilute hydrochloric acid after the complexing and cooling stage of the assay. The small amounts of calcium (up to about 1 per cent) likely to be present in commercial samples of gel do not appear to have any effect on the sharpness of the end-point.[4]

An important control for aluminium hydroxide gel is the determination of neutralising capacity. It is important that the gel lowers the acidity of the stomach rapidly and maintains this condition over a long period of time. A number of tests have been suggested for the evaluation of this characteristic[9,10,11]. One which has been investigated endeavours to simulate *in vivo* reaction. The aluminium hydroxide gel is added to an artificial gastric juice heated at 37°, the mixture being kept well stirred. The pH is recorded after thirty seconds, two minutes, four minutes, six minutes, eight minutes, and ten minutes. At this point 20 ml of the liquid is withdrawn and is replaced by 20 ml of gastric juice. The pH determinations are repeated until changes indicate that the antacid is no longer effective.

The test of the *B.P.* is a compromise in which the gel is added to 100 ml of water heated to 37° and, after thorough dispersion, 100 ml of 0·1N hydrochloric acid, also heated to 37°, is added. The pH of the solution is measured after ten minutes, fifteen minutes, and twenty minutes and limiting values are prescribed. More standard hydrochloric acid is then added and, after maintaining at 37° for one hour, the resulting solution is back titrated with 0·1N sodium hydroxide.

Aluminium hydroxide gel is subject to bacterial contamination, particularly of water-borne types including the genus *Pseudomonas*, and the growth of such organisms can give rise to off-odours and off-flavours. In order to avoid this, a preservative such as chloroform should be added.

Aluminium Powder, *B.P.C.* Consists principally of metallic aluminium with some oxide. It is lubricated with stearic acid during manufacture which serves to protect it from oxidation.

Weigh 0·2 g into a 500-ml flask fitted with a rubber stopper carrying a 150-ml separator, an inlet tube connected to a cylinder of carbon dioxide and an outlet tube dipping into a water-trap, the two tubes extending only a short way into the flask. Add 60 ml of water that has been recently boiled and cooled and swirl to disperse the sample. Stopper the flask, displace the air with carbon dioxide and add, through the separator, a solution prepared, immediately before use, by dissolving 56 g of ferric alum in air-free water, adding 7·5 ml of concentrated sulphuric acid and diluting to 100 ml with air-free water. Maintaining an atmosphere of carbon dioxide, shake the flask gently, heat to boiling and boil for five minutes after the sample has dissolved. Increase the carbon-dioxide rate to a fairly rapid flow and cool rapidly to 20°. Transfer rapidly to a 250-ml graduated flask, dilute to volume with air-free water and mix. Immediately add 15 ml of concentrated phosphoric acid to exactly 50 ml of the solution and titrate with 0·1N potassium permanganate. 1 ml 0·1N = 0·000899 g of metallic aluminium.

Calculate the percentage with reference to the substance freed from lubricant and volatile matter. The lubricant can be determined by dissolving the metal in hydrochloric acid, filtering, washing, drying the paper and beaker and extracting the stearic acid with acetone.

Dusting-powder of Alum and Zinc for Infants, *B.P.C.* Contains 1 part of potash alum with 2 parts each of talc and zinc oxide.

Alum is determined officially by precipitation of sulphate with barium chloride. A better method is as follows:

Weigh 2 g into a flask, add 100 ml of water, stopper the flask and shake for about five minutes. Filter into a 500-ml flask, washing the first flask and the filter with a further 100 ml of water and, to the combined filtrate and washings, add 40 ml of 0·05M EDTA and neutralise to congo red with sodium hydroxide solution. Heat on a water-bath for fifteen minutes, cool, add 1 to 2 g of hexamine and titrate the excess EDTA with 0·1M zinc solution using xylenol orange as indicator. 1 ml 0·05M EDTA = 0·001349 g Al.

Solution of Aluminium Acetate, *B.P.C.* Prepared from aluminium sulphate, acetic acid and calcium carbonate and contains 1·8 per cent Al.

Dilute 10 ml to 100 ml with water in a graduated flask. To 10 ml add 40 ml of 0·05M EDTA, 90 ml of water and 0·15 ml of methyl red indicator. Neutralise with N sodium hydroxide, added dropwise, warm on a water-bath for thirty minutes and cool. Add 1 ml of dilute nitric acid (this is necessary, as otherwise there is insufficient acid to produce the required buffering action). Then add 5 g of hexamine and titrate with 0·05M lead nitrate using xylenol orange as indicator. 1 ml 0·05M = 0·001349 g Al.

Tablets of Aluminium Hydroxide, ***B.P.*** Contain dried aluminium hydroxide gel and peppermint oil.

Weigh and powder 20 tablets, avoiding frictional heat, and dissolve, as completely as possible, an amount of the powder equivalent to about 0·4 g of the dried gel by warming on a water-bath with a mixture of 3 ml of concentrated hydrochloric acid and 3 ml of water. Complete as for the gel from ' Cool and dilute . . .'.

1. Taylor, M. P., *Analyst*, 1955, **80,** 153.
2. Ter Haar, K., and Bazen, J., *Anal. Chim. Acta*, 1954, **10,** 23.
3. Brookes, H. E., and Johnson, C. A., *J. Pharm. Pharmacol.*, 1955, **7,** 836.
4. Gartside, B., and Johnson, C. A., unpublished work.
5. Lampitt, L. H., and Sylvester, N. D., *Analyst*, 1932, **57,** 418.
6. Strafford, N., and Wyatt, P. F., *Analyst*, 1943, **68,** 319.
7. Chenery, E. M., *Analyst*, 1948, **73,** 501.
8. Rolfe, A. C., Russell, F. R., and Wilkinson, N. T., *J. Appl. Chem.*, 1951, **1,** 170.
9. Armstrong, J., and Martin, M., *J. Pharm. Pharmacol.*, 1953, **5,** 672.
10. Gore, D. N., Martin, B. K., and Taylor, M. P., *J. Pharm. Pharmacol.*, 1953, **5,** 686.
11. Brindle, H., *J. Pharm. Pharmacol.*, 1953, **5,** 692.

AMPHETAMINE

$C_6H_5.CH_2.CH(NH_2).CH_3$ Mol. Wt. 135·2

The base is official in the *B.P.* and is assayed by determination of its basicity after solution in an excess of 0·1N hydrochloric acid and back titration with alkali to methyl red. 1 ml 0·1N = 0·01352 g.

Another method of assay which can be used is that given under methylamphetamine below. 1 g residue × 0·8076 = $C_9H_{13}N$.

Amphetamine sulphate and **dexamphetamine sulphate,** $(C_9H_{13}N)_2$, H_2SO_4, Mol. Wt. 368·5. These are best determined by the following distillation method which is official in the *B.P.*

Transfer about 0·4 g, accurately weighed, to a round-bottomed flask fitted for distillation, add 120 ml of water and 2 ml of 20 per cent sodium hydroxide solution. Distil into 50 ml of 0·1N hydrochloric acid until the volume in the flask is reduced to about 5 ml. Titrate the excess acid with 0·1N sodium hydroxide, using methyl red. 1 ml 0·1N = 0·01843 g $(C_9H_{13}N)_2,H_2SO_4$.

It is most important in this determination that the volume in the distillation flask should be reduced to a small amount. Saturation of the liquid with sodium chloride seems to offer no advantage, the volume must still be reduced to a low level.

An alternative but less satisfactory method is to extract the base from alkaline solution with successive quantities of ether to which, after washing with a little water, is added a known excess of 0·1N hydrochloric acid; after evaporation of the ether the excess of acid is back-titrated.

In 0·1N sulphuric acid amphetamine sulphate has an absorption maximum at about 257 mμ, E(1 per cent, 1 cm) = 10.

Tablets of Amphetamine Sulphate, *B.P.* Usually contain 5 mg of amphetamine sulphate.

The official assay requires an extraction into ether from an alkaline sodium chloride-saturated solution followed by re-extraction of the base with hydrochloric acid and subsequent steam distillation as described for the parent substance. The distillation is necessary because it is difficult to remove alkali completely by washing the ethereal extracts. For routine purposes a direct distillation from the tablet is possible but in the presence of certain diluents or of ammonium salts the official method is necessary.

Non-aqueous titration may also be used for the determination, the following method being satisfactory for many formulations.

To an accurately weighed sample of powdered tablets equivalent to about 0·15 g of amphetamine sulphate add 20 ml of glacial acetic acid and warm to dissolve as completely as possible. Filter through a plug of glass wool into a flask, repeatedly washing the tablet base residue with warm glacial acetic acid and filtering as before, using about 50 to 60 ml in all. Titrate with 0·05N perchloric acid using crystal violet as indicator. 1 ml 0·05N = 0·01843 g $(C_9H_{13}N)_2,H_2SO_4$.

Another method for rapid routine determination employs a spectrophotometric finish when the absorption characteristics of the amphetamine sulphate used are known.

Transfer an amount of the powdered tablets equivalent to 25 mg of amphetamine sulphate to a separator containing 30 ml of water and 5 ml of 0·1N sodium hydroxide and shake to dissolve. Extract with four 30-ml portions of anæsthetic ether and wash the combined ether extracts with 2 ml of water. Run the ether solution into a wide-mouthed flask containing 20 ml of 0·1N sulphuric acid and evaporate the ether on a water-bath. Cool, transfer to a 50-ml graduated flask and make up to volume with 0·1N sulphuric acid. Centrifuge a portion of the solution and measure the maximum extinction of a 1-cm layer of the clear supernatant liquid at about 257 mμ using 0·1N sulphuric acid as reference and calculate the percentage of amphetamine sulphate in the original sample.

METHYLAMPHETAMINE, $C_6H_5.CH_2.CH(NH.CH_3).CH_3$, Mol. Wt. 149·2.

This is official in the *B.P.C.* with a method of assay based on solution of a known weight in ethanol, evaporation in the presence of excess hydrochloric acid, and drying of the hydrochloride formed to constant weight, 1 g residue × 0·8036 = $C_{10}H_{15}N$.

Methylamphetamine hydrochloride, $C_6H_5.CH_2.CH(NH.CH_3).CH_3$, HCl, Mol.Wt. 185·7. Methylamphetamine hydrochloride is determined by the method for amphetamine sulphate. 1 ml 0·1N hydrochloric acid = 0·01857 g.

Determination may also be based on titration of the chloride ion or by non-aqueous titration.

Injection of Methylamphetamine Hydrochloride, *B.P.* A sterile solution in water. The assay is by the method of steam distillation given above using a volume equivalent to about 0·1 g of methylamphetamine hydrochloride.

Tablets of Methylamphetamine Hydrochloride, *B.P.* Usually contain 5 mg of methylamphetamine hydrochloride. The official assay is the distillation method given for amphetamine sulphate.

ANEURINE HYDROCHLORIDE

$C_{12}H_{17}ON_4SCl,HCl$ Mol. Wt. 337·3

The methods of assay for aneurine in complex galenicals have been developed from the original colorimetric or fluorimetric methods necessary for the small concentrations present in natural sources; microbiological methods can also be used for small amounts. For tablets and injection solutions where the amounts are greater Adamson and Handisyde[1] have shown that a gravimetric technique is more accurate. Titration in non-aqueous solvents is also applicable (see p. 792).

Colorimetric methods such as that of Auerbach[2] based on the reaction with diazotised *p*-aminoacetophenone are unreliable because of the reactivity of extraneous material, but Ballard and Ballard[3] have made it suitable for tablets and solutions where traces of inorganic salts and a relatively large proportion of dextrose made no difference.

Diazotate reagent: Cool 10 ml of a 0·06 per cent solution of *p*-aminoacetophenone solution in 0·2N hydrochloric acid to 5°, add 3 ml of a 0·2 per cent sodium nitrite solution and mix. After three minutes add 3 ml of 2N sodium hydroxide and mix by shaking. Use between two and five minutes after preparation.

For solutions: Prepare a dilution of the sample to contain about 0·1 mg of aneurine hydrochloride per ml and having an acid concentration equivalent to 0·01N. Transfer 5 ml to a 50-ml graduated flask, add 10 ml of 50 per cent ethanol, mix, add 5 ml of diazotate reagent and again mix. Place in a water-bath at 20° for twelve minutes and then dilute to 50 ml with *iso*propyl alcohol. Determine the extinction at 520 mμ in a 1-cm cell, subtract the value of a reagent blank and read off the amount of aneurine from a calibration curve.

For tablets: Finely powder twenty tablets and weigh accurately an amount of powder expected to contain about 10 mg of aneurine into a 100-ml conical flask. Add exactly 5 ml of dilute hydrochloric acid and 10 ml of water, heat to boiling and boil gently for four minutes. Cool, add $(x - 1)$ ml of N sodium hydroxide, transfer to a 100-ml graduated flask and dilute to 100 ml with water. (The value of x is the number of ml of N sodium hydroxide required to neutralise the hydrochloric acid in a control determination, after cooling.) Use 5 ml of this solution for a determination as described for simple solutions.

The method of choice because of its specificity is the oxidation of aneurine by alkaline ferricyanide to thiochrome, a strongly fluorescent substance. For natural products, such as foodstuffs, the procedure adopted is digestion with pepsin in order to release the aneurine from the tissues, followed by digestion with taka-diastase to hydrolyse that fraction of the vitamin present as pyrophosphate. The conditions of oxidation generally accepted are those of Harris and Wang,[4] although modifications of the preliminary treatment have been developed based on the adsorption of the aneurine on a base-exchange zeolite. Where the aneurine is present uncombined and not difficult to extract, digestion with dilute hydrochloric acid and centrifuging is all that is necessary for extraction. The greatest difficulties with the thiochrome method result from the quenching effect of interfering substances on the fluorescence; these are almost entirely eliminated with the adsorption technique.

The Analytical Methods Committee of the *S.A.C.* have issued a report[5] on the chemical assay of aneurine based mainly on the work of Daglish,[6] Hazel Williams and Wokes,[7] and Elvidge.[8]

Adsorption Column. Base-exchange tubes: These are to be made of glass, the upper part being not less than 15 cm long and 0·8 to 1·0 cm in internal diameter and the lower part being narrow-bore tubing of suitable length. The lower end may be fitted with a tap or other method of controlling the rate of flow. A reservoir to contain at least 30 ml may be attached to the upper part.

Base-exchange silicate: This consists of an artificial zeolite such as Decalso F (Permutit Co. Ltd., London) in the form of a granular powder of 60- to 90-mesh size, tested for its suitability for adsorbing and eluting aneurine under the given conditions (at least 90 per cent 'recovery' of aneurine should be obtained under the given conditions). Activate the base-exchange silicate as follows: Place a convenient quantity (100 to 500 g) of the base-exchange silicate in a suitable beaker, add sufficient hot 3 per cent acetic acid solution to cover the material and maintain the temperature at about 100° for ten to fifteen minutes, stirring frequently. Allow the mixture to settle and decant the supernatant liquid. Repeat the washing three times with hot 25 per cent potassium chloride solution, and finally wash with boiling water until the last washing gives no reaction for chloride. Dry the material at approximately 100° and store in a well-closed container.

Enzyme Solution. Prepare a fresh solution from a suitable source of phosphatase. (Taka-diastase, diluted with lactose, Parke Davis & Co., London; or Clarase, Takamine Laboratories, Clifton, N.J., U.S.A., have been found suitable.) Suspend, with thorough shaking, 6 g of the enzyme preparation in 2·5M sodium acetate (205 g anhydrous sodium acetate per litre) and dilute to 100 ml with additional sodium acetate solution. Each batch of material used as a source of phosphatase should be tested for aneurine by this fluorimetric method and the necessary correction applied.

Fluorimeter. This may be of the direct reading type, measuring in deflections, or the null-point type, measuring in densities.* The exciting radiation must be within the 300 to 400 mμ range; it is most conveniently obtained at suitable intensity by the use of a high-pressure mercury-vapour lamp, type MB, in conjunction with a primary filter. A secondary filter† transmitting mainly light between 400 and 450 mμ is placed between the fluorescent solution and the photo-cell.

Stock Aneurine Solution, 100 *μg per ml*. Prepare this from the British Standard preparation, or a sub-standard of equal purity. Dissolve a weighed amount of aneurine hydrochloride equivalent to 50 mg of the International Standard in sufficient 0·2N hydrochloric acid to make 500 ml. This solution is stable for several months if stored in a refrigerator (*i.e.* below 5°).

Standard Aneurine Solution. Dilute 5 ml of stock aneurine solution, warmed to room temperature, to 100 ml with water. Transfer 10 ml of this dilution to a flask containing 200 ml of approximately 0·1N sulphuric acid and 12·5 ml of sodium acetate solution and dilute to 250 ml with water. The final concentration of aneurine is 0·2 μg per ml. This solution is stable for at least a week if stored in a refrigerator.

Stock Quinine Sulphate Solution, 100 *μg per ml*. Dissolve 0·025 g of quinine sulphate, *B.P.* in sufficient 0·1N sulphuric acid to make 250 ml. This solution is stable if stored in a dark brown bottle at a temperature below 5°.

Quinine Standard, 1 *μg per ml*. Dilute 10 ml of stock quinine sulphate solution to 1 litre with 0·1N sulphuric acid. Any solution which has been exposed to ultra-violet light in the fluorimeter should be discarded.

Extraction. The material to be assayed, if solid, should pass a No. 30 B.S. sieve or a finer sieve, and should be well mixed just before withdrawal of the sample to ensure homogeneity. Accurately weigh or pipette into a large boiling-tube a sample (not more than 5 g) estimated to contain not more than 50 μg of aneurine. Add 65 ml of approximately 0·1N hydrochloric acid or sulphuric acid. Digest the sample for thirty minutes in a water-bath with frequent mixing. The liquid must remain at a pH below 4·5 during the digestion. If at the end of the digestion it is not distinctly acid to bromocresol green indicator, the extract should be discarded and a further quantity of the sample extracted with stronger acid. Cool the extract to below 50° and adjust the pH to between 4 and 4·5 by addition of 2·5M sodium acetate using bromocresol green as the external indicator. Add 5 ml of freshly prepared enzyme suspension, mix, and incubate at 45° to 50° for three hours, or at 37° overnight with addition of a drop of sulphur-free toluene. Cool to room temperature,

* Some null-point type instruments read also in 'transmission.' Here transmission $= \frac{1}{\text{antilog. density}}$.

† Chance OX1, 1·5 to 2·0 mm thick, has been found suitable for the primary filter, and Chance OB2 (blue), 1·5 to 2·0 mm thick for the secondary filter.

centrifuge the mixture until the supernatant liquid is clear and transfer the supernatant liquid to a 100-ml graduated flask. Wash the residue by centrifuging successively with 10 ml, 10 ml and 5 ml of 0·1N hydrochloric acid or sulphuric acid. Add the washings to the supernatant liquid and dilute the whole to volume with water. This is the 'original extract.'

Purification. Plug the bottom of an adsorption column with glass wool, which should be lightly packed, and fill the column with 5 g of activated base-exchange silicate suspended in water. Allow the water to drain almost entirely but leave enough to cover the base-exchange silicate, and pour in 5 ml of 3 per cent acetic acid. Allow to drain as before.

Transfer 25 ml of the 'original extract' to the column by means of a pipette. Discard the filtrate that has percolated through the column. Wash the column with three successive portions, about 10 ml each, of boiling water and discard the washings.

After washing the column, pour through 10 ml of almost boiling acid potassium chloride (25 per cent potassium chloride containing 8·5 ml of concentrated hydrochloric acid per litre) from a supply kept in a boiling water-bath. Collect the eluate in a stoppered 25-ml graduated cylinder. Add a second 10-ml portion when all of the first portion has entered the base-exchange silicate and collect the eluate in the same cylinder. When this second portion has drained through, cool the eluate to room temperature, dilute to 25 ml with acid potassium chloride solution and mix well. This is the 'sample eluate.'

Oxidation to Thiochrome. In this and all subsequent stages undue exposure of the solutions to direct daylight or other source of ultra-violet light must be avoided.

(*a*) Pipette 5 ml of sample eluate into each of two separators.

(*b*) Start a stream of nitrogen or air bubbling through the solution in vessel number 1, add 5 ml of alkaline potassium ferricyanide solution (3 ml of 1 per cent potassium ferricyanide solution diluted to 100 ml with 15 per cent sodium hydroxide just before use) and then add 25 ml of water-saturated *iso*butyl alcohol the current of nitrogen or air still being continued. Shake (or continue vigorous bubbling) for ninety seconds.

(*c*) Start a stream of nitrogen or air bubbling through the solution in vessel number 2, then add 5 ml of 15 per cent sodium hydroxide solution, followed by 25 ml of water-saturated *iso*butyl alcohol, then continue as in step (*b*). This is the 'unknown blank.'

(*d*) Repeat steps (*a*), (*b*) and (*c*) with 5 ml of standard aneurine solution in place of the sample eluate. The solution from step (*c*) is the 'standard blank.'

Caution: The oxidation of all solutions used in a given assay should be carried out in immediate succession to avoid changes in experimental conditions. Similar precautions must be taken in the reading of their fluorescence.

Separation of Thiochrome Solution and Measurement of its Fluorescence. After the solutions have stood for a few minutes to allow complete separation, add 1 ml of ethanol to the upper layer in each vessel and stir the upper layer gently until it is clear, taking care to avoid disturbing the aqueous layer.

Take off each upper layer into a cell and measure its fluorescence against that of the quinine standard, if a null-point fluorimeter is being used, or as direct deflections if a deflection instrument is being used. The blank should exhibit only faint fluorescence.

'Recovery' Experiment. Repeat the above procedure, including the steps of extraction, purification, conversion to thiochrome, separation of thiochrome solution and measurement of fluorescence, with a recovery experiment made by adding to another portion of the sample that is the same weight as that previously taken, a volume of stock aneurine solution containing an amount of aneurine similar to the amount expected in that weight of sample.

Calculation. If the fluorescence has been measured on an instrument employing a density scale, convert all densities into antilogs and take reciprocals of these. (If the instrument reads 'transmissions' use those readings instead of reciprocals of antilog density. Here U, U_B, S and S_B are the readings themselves.)

Let U = reciprocal for unknown
U_B = reciprocal for unknown blank
S = reciprocal for standard
S_B = reciprocal for standard blank
V = volume of original solution put through base-exchange silicate.

If the fluorescence intensities have been measured as deflections, these are employed instead of the reciprocals of antilogs. Then the aneurine content of the sample in μg per g =

$$\frac{U - U_B}{S - S_B} \times \frac{1}{5} \times \frac{25}{V} \times \frac{100}{\text{g of sample taken}}.$$

The factor 1/5 converts the reading to μg per ml instead of μg per 5-ml aliquot. Since the final volume of eluate is 25 ml the factor $25/V$ corrects for volume changes during adsorption and elution. If the suggested 25 ml is adsorbed, this factor becomes unity.

Note. This calculation assumes that the fluorescence of the thiochrome solution in the unknown is less than that of the quinine standard. If it is not, the assay should be repeated using a smaller amount of the material.

Use of Recovery Experiment Data. Calculate the percentage recovery of the added aneurine from the following formula:

$$\frac{A_R - A_U}{A_A} \times 100$$

where

A_U = aneurine content of sample in μg per g calculated as above
A_R = aneurine content of sample with added aneurine calculated as above
A_A = μg of aneurine added to each gram of sample.

This percentage recovery provides an indication of the effect of disturbing factors, including the quenching effect of impurities, but should not be relied upon to make a satisfactory correction for interfering factors. In general, if the percentage recovery falls below 80, the result of the assay should be considered unsatisfactory.

Fluorescent grease must not be used to lubricate taps; glycerol or silicone may be used. The water-saturated *iso*butyl alcohol is obtained by steam-distilling the commercial material in an all-glass apparatus; the fluorescence of the distillate should not be more than that of a solution of quinine sulphate in 0·1N sulphuric acid containing 0·01 μg per ml.

Visual measurement of the thiochrome fluorescence is possible using narrow non-fluorescent tubes, the contents of which are matched in a dark room with an ultra-violet lamp. The test solution and a strong aneurine standard are oxidised and extracted under exactly similar conditions together with a blank from which the ferricyanide has been omitted; a measured volume of the test solution is matched against addition of the standard to the blank. The tubes are inclined at an angle of 60°, but they must not be exposed longer than necessary, since the fluorescence is unstable in ultra-violet light. The final comparison is made when the volumes have been equalised.

The direct measurement of the ultra-violet absorption of aneurine has been used for determination of aneurine by various workers and, although rapid, has been criticised both for the poor reproducibility of the absorption under specified conditions and in the fact that the absorption of a solution of aneurine which has partly decomposed by fission of the molecule closely follows that of the original substance.

Aneurine can also be assayed microbiologically (see p. 813) and this is the method of choice when the content is below the level of about 5 μg per g.

To extract the aneurine, weigh accurately about 5 g of the sample, suspend it in 50 ml of 0·1N sulphuric acid in a covered conical flask, heat in a water-bath for thirty minutes, cool and add 2·5M sodium acetate until the pH value lies between 4·5 and 5·0 (using an external indicator). Then add about 0·1 g of Mylase P (a mixed enzyme preparation) followed by a few drops of toluene and incubate at 37° for twenty-four hours. Steam for fifteen minutes, adjust the pH value to 6·5 with 2N sodium hydroxide, transfer to a 100-ml graduated flask and make up to volume with water. For test purposes, filter an aliquot of this solution and dilute with water so that the solution contains an estimated aneurine concentration of about 0·02 μg per ml.

Because of the possibility of interfering substances, it is necessary to include an aneurine-free 'blank' in the dilutions of the standard. For this purpose, add 4 ml of a freshly prepared 10 per cent solution of sodium sulphite to 25 ml of the filtered solution from the graduated flask, adjust the pH value with N sulphuric acid to about 5·4 and autoclave in steam at 121° (15 lb. steam pressure) for fifteen minutes. After cooling add sufficient 10 vol. hydrogen peroxide (0·5 to 1 ml is the usual amount) to neutralise exactly the excess of sodium sulphite. An external indicator, made by mixing equal volumes of 1 per cent starch suspension, 50 per cent sulphuric acid and 5 per cent potassium iodide solution, is needed for this. After neutralising, adjust the pH value back to 6·5 with 2N sodium hydroxide and make up to 50 ml in a graduated flask. To a portion of this blank solution add sufficient of a 0·1 per cent solution of aneurine standard so that when diluted to a concentration equivalent to that of the test solution prepared above, the aneurine content is 0·02 μg per ml. Proceed with the assay as outlined on pp. 815 to 826.

Aneurine can also be assayed by the plate-diffusion method (see p. 814) but this is much less sensitive and requires concentrations in the range 5 to 0·5 μg per ml to give a satisfactory dose-response curve.

The amounts of aneurine present in tablets and ampoule solutions are sufficient for gravimetric determination. Adamson and Handisyde[1] have investigated the use of silicotungstic acid as a precipitating reagent; under the assay conditions prescribed no precipitate is given by manufacturing intermediates and decomposition products of aneurine nor by various cations and other vitamins; errors introduced by tablet excipients are within the limits of precision of the method. The time of boiling after adding the precipitant is significant and it is important to note that some substances give a precipitate on cooling so that it is essential to filter hot. There is a tendency for large amounts of other water-soluble vitamins to co-precipitate and results up to 3 per cent too high are liable in a poly-vitamin preparation, but addition of the precipitant drop by drop minimises the effect.

Injection solutions: Dilute the solution to contain 0·5 mg of aneurine per ml and pipette 50 ml of this into a 250-ml conical flask. Add 2 ml of concentrated hydrochloric acid, bring to the boil rapidly, add 2 ml of a 10 per cent solution of silicotungstic acid (previously filtered through a No. 4 sintered-glass crucible), and boil gently for two minutes. Filter immediately in a tared No. 4 sintered-glass crucible and wash the precipitate with almost boiling dilute hydrochloric acid (1 vol. of concentrated acid diluted to 20 vol. with water), then once with 5 to 10 ml of water, and finally with two 5-ml quantities of acetone. Suck dry at the pump, and heat to constant weight at 100° to 105°. Weight of precipitate × 0·1936 = weight of anhydrous aneurine.

Tablets: To 250 ml of water add 10 ml of concentrated hydrochloric acid, and into about 60 ml of this mixture drop a number of tablets estimated to contain about 50 mg of aneurine. Allow the tablets to disintegrate, and to stand for one hour with occasional shaking. After allowing to settle, filter the extract into a 100-ml graduated flask, and re-extract the insoluble matter with successive portions of the dilute acid, filtering each extract into the graduated flask until the volume is made up to 100 ml. After mixing the combined extracts, pipette out 50 ml into a 250-ml conical flask, bring to the boil, and precipitate with 2 ml of 10 per cent silicotungstic acid, collecting, washing and weighing the precipitate as above.

When the tablets have a high aneurine content, they may be disintegrated and made up to volume in the graduated flask, since the volume error introduced by the insoluble matter is relatively small. The actual volume of the insoluble matter may be calculated, and hence its significance assessed, by the usual two-dilution method.

Vannatta and Harris[9] suggested certain minor modifications of the Adamson and Handisyde method. These were: a slight difference in the excess of reagent added, an increase in boiling time from two to three minutes, addition of silicotungstic acid to the initial wash liquid, and drying for three hours at 80° rather than to constant weight. The method of Vannatta and Harris gives a slightly higher result. The precision of the methods is similar but which is the more accurate would be difficult to say.

A further modification is to equilibrate the silicotungstate to its fully hydrated form in which it is said to be stable under normal atmospheric conditions, by leaving it for twenty-four hours in a desiccator at 60 per cent relative humidity. Under such conditions of drying the factor of 0·1929 × weight of precipitate should be used.

Injection of Aneurine Hydrochloride, *B.P.* A sterile solution containing 25 mg of aneurine hydrochloride in 1 ml of water for injection. For assay either the fluorimetric technique on a suitable dilution or the silicotungstic acid precipitation method given above can be used. For the latter, 1 ml of injection is diluted to 50 ml for assay.

Tablets of Aneurine Hydrochloride, *B.P.* The usual strength of this tablet is 3 mg and no difficulty is experienced in following either the fluorimetric or silicotungstic acid methods given above. It must be realised that the results of assay by the latter method may give rather different figures from the fluorimetric method.

Compound Tablets of Aneurine, *B.P.C.* Contain 1 mg each of aneurine hydrochloride and riboflavine and 15 mg of nicotinamide.

Although the fluorimetric method given above is applicable to this preparation the method of Foster and Murfin described in more detail under Strong Compound Tablets of Aneurine can be applied, but for this simpler preparation the following technique may be used:

Powder the sample and shake an accurately weighed quantity of powder equivalent to about 7 tablets with 50 ml of acetic acid (0·5 per cent v/v) for thirty minutes. Filter (pH should be between 3 and 4) and reject the first 10 ml of filtrate.

Transfer 10 ml of this solution to the alginic acid column with the flow rate adjusted to 1 ml per minute. When nearly all the solution has passed through wash the column with small portions of water at the same flow rate. Wash the column with 200 ml of water.

Elute the nicotinamide with 500 ml of 0·005N hydrochloric acid, dilute to 1 litre and measure the extinction of a 1-cm layer at about 261 mμ. Calculate the weight of nicotinamide in a tablet of average weight using an E(1 per cent, 1 cm) of 411 at 261 mμ.

Elute the aneurine hydrochloride with 150 ml of 2N hydrochloric acid and measure the extinction of a 1-cm layer at about 246 mμ. Calculate the weight of aneurine hydrochloride in a tablet of average weight using an E(1 per cent, 1 cm) of 416 at 246 mμ.

For riboflavine see p. 552.

Strong Compound Tablets of Aneurine, *B.P.C.* Contain 5 mg of aneurine hydrochloride, 2 mg of riboflavine, 20 mg of nicotinamide and 2 mg of pyridoxine hydrochloride.

ANEURINE HYDROCHLORIDE

Although the fluorimetric method given above is applicable to this preparation, Foster and Murfin[10] successfully applied alginic acid to the quantitative separation of aneurine, nicotinamide and pyridoxine when present in admixture, with subsequent assay of these separated components spectrophotometrically. Preparation of the alginic acid is described under Nux Vomica (p. 461).

Prepare an absorption column by the following method. Soak 4 g of prepared alginic acid in water until the swelling is complete. Insert a small plug of glass wool just above the top of an absorption tube, 15 cm long and 2 cm in internal diameter. Stir the alginic acid mixture and transfer to the absorption tube. Allow to settle and plug the top of the column with glass wool. Wash the column with successive portions of 2N hydrochloric acid until the extinction of a 1-cm layer of the washings at 245, 261, and 291 mμ is less than 0·005. Finally wash with successive portions of water until the washings are neutral to litmus.

Powder the sample and shake an accurately weighed quantity of the powder equivalent to about 7 tablets with 100 ml of acetic acid 0·5 per cent v/v for thirty minutes. Filter (pH should be between 3 and 4) and reject the first 10 ml of filtrate.

Transfer 10 ml of this solution to the column with the flow rate adjusted to 1 ml per minute. When nearly all the solution has passed through wash the column with small portions of water at the same flow rate. Wash the column with 200 ml of water.

For nicotinamide and pyridoxine hydrochloride: Elute the pyridoxine hydrochloride and nicotinamide with 500 ml of 0·005N hydrochloric acid. Measure the extinction of a 4-cm layer at 291 mμ. Dilute 25 ml of this solution to 50 ml with the solvent and measure the extinction of a 1-cm layer at 261 mμ.

Calculate the weight of pyridoxine hydrochloride in each tablet of average weight. The mg per tablet of pyridoxine hydrochloride is given by the formula:

$$\frac{(29{\cdot}25C - 1{\cdot}28B)}{(\text{No. of tab. equiv. taken})}$$

Calculate the weight of nicotinamide in each tablet of average weight. The mg per tablet of nicotinamide is given by the formula:

$$\frac{(243B - 3{\cdot}44C)}{(\text{No. of tab. equiv. taken})}$$

B = extinction of a 1-cm layer at 261 mμ
C = extinction of a 4-cm layer at 291 mμ

Assay for aneurine hydrochloride: Elute the aneurine hydrochloride with 250 ml of 2N hydrochloric acid and measure the extinction of a 1-cm layer at 246 mμ. Calculate the weight of aneurine hydrochloride in a tablet of average weight using an E(1 per cent, 1 cm) of 416 at 246 mμ.

For riboflavine see p. 552.

Capsules of Vitamins, *B.P.C.* A multi-vitamin capsule.

The determination of the vitamins follows the general method given under each.

There is evidence of the absorption of aneurine in the capsule envelope, hence for this constituent the whole capsules should be dissolved and an aliquot used for determination.

Thiamine mononitrate, $C_{12}H_{17}N_5O_4S$, Mol. Wt. 327·4, is assayed in the *U.S.P.* by a method similar to the fluorimetric method given above; using aneurine hydrochloride as a standard it is necessary to multiply by 0·9706 to convert to mononitrate.

Dried Yeast, *B.P.C.* Dried yeast consists of unicellular fungi belonging to the family Saccharomycetaceæ which have been dried so as to avoid decomposition of the vitamins present and which should be free from viable cells. It is a source of the vitamin B complex. For aneurine the determination follows the *S.A.C.* method outlined above using 1 g of sample.

For determination of riboflavine see p. 553, and for nicotinic acid see p. 443.

1. ADAMSON, D. C. M., and HANDISYDE, F. P., *Quart. J. Pharm.*, 1948, **21**, 370.
2. AUERBACH, M. E., *J. Amer. Pharm. Ass., Sci. Edn.*, 1940, **29**, 313.
3. BALLARD, C. W., and BALLARD, E. J., *J. Pharm. Pharmacol.*, 1949, **1**, 330.
4. HARRIS, L. J., and WANG, Y. L., *Biochem. J.*, 1941, **35**, 1050; *Chem. & Ind.*, 1942, **61**, 27.
5. *Analyst*, 1951, **76**, 127.
6. DAGLISH, C., *Quart. J. Pharm.*, 1947, **20**, 257.
7. WILLIAMS, Hazel, and WOKES, F., *Quart. J. Pharm.*, 1947, **20**, 240.
8. ELVIDGE, W. F., *Quart. J. Pharm.*, 1947, **20**, 263.
9. VANNATTA, E. E., and HARRIS, L. E., *J. Amer. Pharm. Ass., Sci. Edn.*, 1959, **48**, 30.
10. FOSTER, J. S., and MURFIN, J. W., *J. Pharm. Pharmacol.*, 1961, **13**, 126T.

ANTHRAQUINONE-CONTAINING DRUGS

The purgative activity of drugs containing anthraquinones can be assessed by comparing the purgation produced in mice after oral dosing with that produced by a sample of the drug serving as a standard.

After dosing the mice are observed and the responses scored either as the number showing a purgative effect (quantal effect) or as the number of 'wet fæces' excreted per mouse (graded effect) and potency estimates with their limits of error calculated by the methods given on page 841.

Miller and Alexander[1] have described the conduct of the test for **senna** based on the quantal effect produced in mice. Healthy mice weighing 20 to 30 g are selected for test from a colony having free access to food and water during the preceding twenty-four hours and are transferred to individual cages constructed so that the fæcal excretions may fall freely on to white absorbent paper placed 1 to 2 cm beneath the cages. They are observed after thirty minutes and any which are excreting fæces wet enough to stain the paper are removed. Those remaining are divided into groups of 16 and are dosed respectively with the standard and test preparations at two levels. The drug is administered in a constant volume of 0·5 ml by means of a stomach tube attached to a tuberculin syringe. The mice are observed after five hours and the number showing any purgative effect are recorded.

An assay method using the graded effect has been described by Lou.[2] Male mice weighing not less than 18 g are observed for three hours and any passing wet fæces removed. Those remaining are divided into groups of 10 to receive respectively the standard and test preparations at 2 levels. The number of wet fæces excreted by the mice, either singly or in pairs, is recorded after not less than twelve hours.

Miller and Alexander made their standard solutions by adding 50 ml of boiling water to 2 g of senna powder, allowing this to cool to room temperature and decanting the supernatant fluid after centrifuging. They found that doses corresponding to 8 and 16 mg of senna provided suitable dose levels for the standard preparation. Lou triturated the powdered senna with boiling water, made up to volume with cold water, and administered the drug as a suspension giving doses corresponding to 10 and 20 mg.

We have found that when the whole drug is administered in suspension mice which require doses of 5 and 10 mg for quantal response assays would require doses of 15 and 30 mg when the graded response is to be used.

The method of Lou has also been applied by Lou and Fairbairn to the assay of **rhubarb**[3] and **cascara.**[4] The dose levels needed were of the order 40 and 180 mg respectively.

Much work has been undertaken during the last few years in attempts to produce a satisfactory chemical or physical method for the determination of the purgative activity of anthraquinone-containing drugs. Of the various purgative drugs in this category, senna has received most attention since it would appear to offer the best chance of success. The original method for senna on which much subsequent work has been based was published by Kussmaul and Becker.[5] This depends upon extraction and separation procedures followed by a colorimetric determination by the Bornträger reaction in which a solution containing the aglycones resulting from hydrolysis of the anthraquinone-glycosides is heated with sodium hydroxide and hydrogen peroxide. A version of this method is given below and is based on one published by Fairbairn and Michaels[6] in which an extraction with sodium bicarbonate solution was introduced so that only those aglycones with carboxylic acid groupings on the anthracene nucleus are determined. This type of method has been found to be capable of a reasonable degree of reproducibility between laboratories but the value of the results as an assessment of purgative activity is doubtful. The isolation by Vickers[7] of a glycoside that gives the colour reaction and yet has a negligible biological activity and the subsequent publication by Crellin and co-workers[8] detailing several new glycosides of senna strengthen the suspicion with which any purely chemical or physical assessment of purgative activity must be viewed. In addition to this, observations in the authors' laboratories have shown that the intensity of colour produced when the final alkaline solution is heated depends to a considerable degree on the amount of hydrogen peroxide present, the colour being most intense when the final alkaline solution is heated without any oxidising agent present.

The method of Fairbairn and Michaels is as follows:

First prepare an infusion of the sample as follows. For whole pod, or pod in coarse powder, weigh 10 g into a 500-ml graduated flask (the whole pod should first be cut into strips, 2 to 3 mm wide), add about 450 ml of boiling water and allow to stand in a water-bath for ten minutes, shaking frequently. Remove from the bath, adjust the pH to between 6 and 7 with N sodium hydroxide, cool immediately, dilute to volume with water and filter. For pod in fine powder, weigh 1 g into a 100-ml graduated flask, add about 90 ml of boiling water and complete as above.

Pipette 10 ml of the filtered infusion into a separator, adjust the pH to about 3 with N hydrochloric acid and remove the free anthraquinones by extracting, first with 60 ml and then with 40-ml quantities of ether, until the last extract is colourless. Combine the extracts and wash with small quantities of acidified water (at about pH 3), adding the washings to the original aqueous layer. Add to the aqueous solution half its volume of 5N hydrochloric acid, heat in a water-bath for fifteen minutes and cool, when the aglycones will separate as a brown flocculent precipitate. Add 80 ml of ether, shake and allow to settle. Separate the aqueous layer and pour off the ether layer into another separator, leaving behind the brown residue that forms as a layer between the ether and water layers. Dissolve the residue in a small quantity of 30 per cent sodium hydroxide solution and add the separated aqueous layer (which contains excess of acid) to the resulting solution. Continue the extraction, with 40-ml quantities of ether, in a similar manner (the repeated solution in alkali is necessary to avoid occlusion of aglycone in the intermediate layer) until the last ether extract is colourless, indicating complete extraction of the aglycones.

Extract the combined ether extracts with small quantities of N sodium bicarbonate until the last extract is colourless. Combine the bicarbonate solutions, add ether and acidify with 5N hydrochloric acid. When effervescence has ceased, shake to extract, run off the aqueous layer and filter the yellow ether layer into a graduated flask. Dissolve any brown residue in sodium hydroxide solution as before, re-acidify and repeat the extraction with 20 ml of ether. Continue to extract in this way, with 20-ml quantities of ether, until extraction is complete and then dilute the combined extracts to volume with ether.

Pipette a suitable volume of the ether solution into a separator and extract with small quantities of N sodium hydroxide. Combine the extracts, add 0·2 ml of 3 per cent hydrogen peroxide solution for every 10 ml of alkaline liquid and heat in a water-bath for four to five minutes. Cool, make up to a suitable volume with N sodium hydroxide and measure the extinction of the resulting solution at the absorption maximum at about 520 mμ. Derive the aglycone content from a standard curve constructed from the mean of standard curves for sennoside A and sennoside B, prepared after hydrolysing with hydrochloric acid, extracting and oxidising as above.

Many other chemical approaches have been suggested to the solution of this difficult problem, but in our opinion none is satisfactory.

The problems associated with the assay of senna are, if anything, more complex in the cases of cascara, rhubarb and **aloes.** At the present time no reliable chemical assessment of these drugs is available.

Aloin is a mixture of crystalline substances obtained from aloes and receives little attention from the standardisation viewpoint in the *B.P.C.* An amorphous variety of aloin which does not conform to the *B.P.C.* description has appeared in commerce and Lister and Pride[9] have suggested means by which the varieties may be differentiated, including a paper chromatographic procedure. For crystalline aloin they report that a 1-cm layer of a 0·0025 per cent solution (freshly prepared) in water, calculated for the anhydrous material, has an extinction of about 0·55 at 298 mμ and about 0·61 at 354 mμ. To exclude amorphous material they stipulate that the ratio of the extinction at 354 mμ to that at 298 mμ should be greater than 1·0.

1. Miller, L. C., and Alexander, E. B., *J. Amer. Pharm. Ass., Sci. Edn.*, 1949, **38,** 417.
2. Lou, T. C., *J. Pharm. Pharmacol.*, 1949, **1,** 673.
3. Lou, T. C., and Fairbairn, J. W., *J. Pharm. Pharmacol.*, 1951, **3,** 225.
4. Lou, T. C., and Fairbairn, J. W., *J. Pharm. Pharmacol.*, 1951, **3,** 295.
5. Kussmaul, W., and Becker, B., *Helv. Chim. Acta*, 1947, **30,** 59.
6. Fairbairn, J. W., and Michaels, I., *J. Pharm. Pharmacol.*, 1950, **2,** 807.
7. Vickers, C., *J. Pharm. Pharmacol.*, 1961, **13,** 509.
8. Crellin, J. K., Fairbairn, J. W., Friedmann, C. A., and Ryan, H. A., *J. Pharm. Pharmacol.*, 1961, **13,** 639.
9. Lister, R. E., and Pride, R. R. A., *J. Pharm. Pharmacol.*, 1959, **11,** 278T.

ANTIBIOTICS

PENICILLINS

The first penicillin to be used was an amorphous material consisting largely of the calcium, potassium or sodium salt of benzylpenicillin but containing also varying small amounts of the salts of similar antimicrobial acids. This material is no longer encountered, having been entirely replaced by the crystalline salts and other derivatives of benzylpenicillin as well as the more recent penicillins based on β-aminopenicillamic acid.

The principal penicillins of present importance are benzylpenicillin, sodium or potassium salt (penicillin G); procaine benzylpenicillin; benzathine penicillin; benethamine penicillin; phenoxymethylpenicillin, potassium or calcium salt (penicillin V); methicillin sodium; phenethicillin sodium; penicillamine hydrochloride.

Only microbiological methods of assay were available originally, but they have been largely replaced by chemical or physical ones. Microbiological methods are still useful, however, for confirmatory work (indeed, they are still the only means by which *potency* can be determined) and they are particularly valuable with preparations, such as ointments and lozenges in which the penicillin content is relatively low, and also in materials such as feed supplements.

BENZYLPENICILLIN AND ITS SALTS

Most chemical methods of assay for the benzylpenicillin salts depend upon hydrolytic cleavage of the β-lactam ring to give penicilloic acid. This cleavage can be brought about either by alkali or by the enzyme penicillinase. If the cleavage is brought about by penicillinase in a previously neutral and unbuffered solution the resulting acid may be titrated with alkali to give a measure of the penicillin present (see under penicillinase method, below). Alternatively, and more commonly, the liberated penicilloic acid is determined through its ability to take up iodine, a property not possessed by the parent molecule. The method was originally suggested by Alicino[1] but it has undergone various modifications and revisions from time to time. The following procedure is one which is in common use in this country at the present time.

Dissolve about 60 mg, accurately weighed, in water and dilute to 50 ml. Transfer 10 ml to a 250-ml stoppered flask, add 5 ml of N sodium hydroxide and allow to stand for thirty minutes in a water-bath at 30°. Acidify with 5·5 ml of N hydrochloric acid, add 30 ml of 0·02N iodine, close the flask with a stopper moistened with water and allow to stand in a water-bath at 30° for fifteen minutes, protected from light. Titrate the excess of iodine with 0·02N sodium thiosulphate, using starch mucilage, added towards the end of the titration, as indicator. Carry out a blank determination by transferring 10 ml of the penicillin solution to a stoppered flask, adding 30 ml of 0·02N iodine and titrating immediately with 0·02N sodium thiosulphate. The difference between the two titrations represents the amount of iodine that has reacted with the total penicillins present. Each ml of 0·02N iodine is approximately equivalent to 0·764 mg of total penicillin as the sodium salt, or to 0·798 mg as the potassium salt.

Carry out the assay simultaneously using the Standard Preparation of penicillin to determine the exact equivalent of each ml of 0·02N iodine and from this calculate the result of the assay.

It might be expected that one molecule of penicillin, after hydrolysis, would absorb eight atoms of iodine,[2] but by experiment it is found that a variable amount is absorbed, depending on the exact conditions and this makes it necessary for a Standard Preparation and for standard conditions to be used. The method has two principal advantages, first, it has a high degree of specificity since non-penicillin impurities are to a large extent allowed for in the blank determination and secondly, the relatively large iodine absorption makes the method highly sensitive. It will be noted, however, that in the procedure given above the blank determination is not a true control for the unhydrolysed penicillin solution must be titrated immediately after addition of the standard iodine; thus any slowly-absorbing impurities which may be present are not given time to react as they are in the determination itself where they are in contact with an excess of iodine for fifteen minutes at 30°. This treatment of the blank must be adopted because, in the original work of Alicino, it was shown that iodine is slowly absorbed during the waiting period, probably because of breakdown of the penicillin. It is reported that this breakdown can be avoided by buffering the solution, and in fact the *U.S.P.* uses a phosphate buffer of pH 6·0. Other workers use an acetate buffer, pH 4·5, and under these conditions the blank solution may be treated in exactly the same way as the test solution, except that the hydrolysis period with sodium hydroxide is omitted.

Total penicillins may also be determined by the penicillinase method. For this method buffering substances should not be present as these reduce the sensitivity of the assay and the amount of penicillin being determined should be at least 10 mg. The method is particularly suitable for the assay of salts of penicillin and can be used for the procaine derivative.[3]

Adjust the penicillinase to pH 7·5 using phenol red as indicator. Prepare a colour control by mixing 1 ml of this with 10 ml of distilled water containing 0·2 ml of phenol red indicator. Weigh accurately 50 mg of the penicillin sample, dissolve in 10 ml of water also containing 0·2 ml of phenol red indicator, and adjust the pH value to match that of the control. Add 1 ml of penicillinase and allow to stand at room temperature for thirty minutes. Titrate with 0·01N sodium hydroxide until the colour of the solution again matches that of the control. Allow to stand for some minutes longer to ensure that the reaction is completed, and titrate further if necessary. Calculate the potency of the preparation on the basis that 1 ml of 0·01N sodium hydroxide is equivalent to 6023 I.U. of penicillin.

If the indicator is present in the standard alkali a better colour comparison is obtainable at the end-point.

A spectrophotometric method has been described[4] which depends upon the controlled degradation of penicillin to penicillenic acid. This is carried out by heating with sodium acetate-acetic acid buffer solution of pH 4·6 to which a trace of copper sulphate has been added. In the absence of copper sulphate reproducible results are not obtainable. The extinction at 322 mμ (the maximum absorption peak for penicillenic acid) gives a measure of the penicillin present. The method is as follows:

Extract a quantity of the preparation (with water for benzylpenicillin) so as to give a solution containing between 160 and 190 units per ml. To a 20-ml aliquot of this solution add 50 ml of acetate buffer and then place 5-ml aliquots into each of five boiling-tubes. Place four of these tubes into a water-bath so that the level of liquid in the tubes is below that of the boiling water and allow to remain for exactly twenty-five minutes. Remove the tubes from the bath, cool and make up to 10 ml with acetate buffer in stoppered cylinders. In the meantime dilute the contents of the fifth (unheated) tube in the same way. Measure the extinction of the solutions in a 1-cm cell at 322 mμ using water in the comparison cell. Subtract the blank (unheated) solution from the mean value for the other four solutions and calculate the potency of the preparation by comparing the E(1 per cent, 1 cm) value so obtained with that obtained for a pure sample of the appropriate penicillin.

Acetate buffer. This is 0·4M sodium acetate containing 0·45 p.p.m. of copper.

The method has been applied to tablets, ointments, lozenges, injections and suspensions, but for rapid determination the penicillinase method is to be preferred.

Other methods which have been suggested for total penicillins include one in which potassium ferricyanide is used as an oxidising agent, the excess ferricyanide being back-titrated with ceric sulphate[5] and a method in which the β-lactam structure of penicillin is reacted with an amine dye [*N*-(1-naphthyl-4-azobenzene)ethylenediamine] to give a coloured condensation product.[6]

Investigation into methods for the estimation of individual penicillins has been considerable. Generally, at present, one or other of the microchromatographic techniques is most satisfactory with the possible exception of the assay of **benzylpenicillin** ($C_{16}H_{17}O_4N_2SNa$, Mol. Wt. 356·4 and $C_{16}H_{17}O_4N_2SK$, Mol. Wt. 372·5) in relatively pure samples by precipitation of the *N*-ethylpiperidinium salt; the following procedure is recommended:

Dissolve about 120 mg in 5 ml of water in a 15-ml centrifuge tube and cool in ice-cold water. Add 5 ml, accurately measured, of amyl acetate, previously saturated with the *N*-ethylpiperidinium salt of benzylpenicillin cooled in ice-water and filtered. Add 0·5 ml of phosphoric acid solution (20 per cent of the *B.P.* acid) stopper with a wet cork, shake immediately for fifteen seconds and centrifuge for thirty seconds. Pipette off the aqueous layer completely and add to the centrifuge tube 0·5 g of freshly ignited, powdered anhydrous sodium sulphate. Stir, allow to stand in ice-water for five minutes, centrifuge for thirty seconds and replace in ice-cold water for five minutes. Pipette off a 3-ml aliquot, representing three-fifths of the weight of penicillin, into a suitable tared centrifuge tube containing a thin glass rod slightly curved at the end. Add 3 ml of acetone (containing not more than 0·3 per cent of water) previously saturated with the *N*-ethylpiperidinium salt of benzylpenicillin, cooled in ice-water and filtered. Add 1·5 ml of *N*-ethylpiperidine solution (to make mix 2 ml of *N*-ethylpiperidine and 8 ml of amyl acetate) previously saturated with the *N*-ethylpiperidinium salt of benzylpenicillin, cooled in ice-water and filtered. Stir, close the mouth of the tube with a rubber thimble, place the tube inside a test-tube, close this with a cork and stand in ice-cold water for two hours. Remove the centrifuge tube and centrifuge for one minute. Break the surface to dislodge any particles at or above the surface of the liquid and again centrifuge for one minute. Decant off the supernatant liquor and wash the precipitate by stirring with 2 ml of a solution containing equal volumes of acetone and amyl acetate, saturated with the *N*-ethylpiperidinium salt of benzylpenicillin, cooled in ice-water and filtered. Centrifuge for one and a half minutes and decant. Wash twice by stirring with 2 ml of ether, centrifuging for one and a half minutes and decanting. Smear the deposit over the inside of the tube by means of the curved glass rod and dry at room temperature *in vacuo* to constant weight, the tube being placed in a nearly horizontal position. 1 g of residue = 0·7962 g of $C_{16}H_{17}O_4N_2SNa$ or 0·8322 g of $C_{16}H_{17}O_4N_2SK$.

It must be emphasised that this method is only suitable for the assay of benzylpenicillin in samples consisting substantially of benzylpenicillin. The assay should be repeated using the Standard Preparation of benzylpenicillin (dried crystalline sodium salt obtainable from the National Institute for Medical Research, assayed in terms of International Standard penicillin). The result should indicate that 95·8 per cent of the Standard is sodium benzylpenicillin; if a lower value (but not less than 93·0 per cent) is obtained the assay may be considered valid and a proportionate correction should be applied to the result obtained on the sample under test. The purity of reagents is essential, particularly for the *N*-ethylpiperidine. The temperature is important and should be ice cold whenever possible. If penicillin X (*p*-hydroxybenzylpenicillin) is present the method may give an erroneous result, since a non-quantitative precipitation of the salt of penicillin X takes place.[7]

For the microbiological assay of benzylpenicillin and its preparations to determine their potency, see p. 813.

A colorimetric method for the estimation of one or more species of penicillin in a mixture was described by Baker, Dobson and Martin.[8] It is based on the fact that the relatively stable hydroxamic acid derivatives of the various penicillins show different partition coefficients between *iso*propyl ether-*iso*propyl alcohol and phthalate buffer, at a given pH, and can therefore be separated by paper chromatography.

Quantitative figures are obtained by developing the chromatograms with ferric chloride, extracting the iron complexes with butyl alcohol, measuring the extinction in a colorimeter and reading the penicillin concentration from a standard curve. This colorimetric method is suitable for crude or pure salts of penicillin; a convenient amount for quantitative estimation is 1 mg.

Dip a Whatman No. 4 paper in 0·10M potassium hydrogen phthalate and air-dry. It should be dry enough to gain rather than lose water when it is placed in the chromatogram box. To retain heptyl penicillin hydroxamic acid on a reasonable length of paper while the other penicillins are adequately developed, the lower third of the paper should be dipped in phthalate buffer of pH 6·2. Whatman No. 1 paper will give satisfactory chromatograms but a much longer time of development is then required.

Dissolve 10 to 40 mg of penicillin salt in 1 ml of a mixture of equal volumes of 4N hydroxylamine hydrochloride and 3N sodium hydroxide. 10 μl of this solution is applied as a spot to the chromatogram and air-dried. Ten such spots are required for a quantitative analysis and can be accommodated on a sheet 15 cm wide.

Mobile Phase. The mobile phase is *iso*propyl ether containing 15 per cent v/v of *iso*propyl alcohol. To each 100 ml of the mixture add 2·4 ml of 0·10M potassium hydrogen phthalate to give approximate saturation with respect to the stationary phase. The mixture should be free from aldehydes or peroxides; distillation of the solvents from saturated bisulphite or 5N sodium hydroxide ensures this.

Apparatus. The apparatus consists of a perspex box 15 $\times$ 25 $\times$ 60 cm with a gabled lid, so that liquid condensing on the top does not drip on to the chromatograms. The walls of the box are lined with cotton cloth, over which both phases are pumped continuously by a diaphragm pump delivering 1,500 ml per minute. The liquids are drawn from the bottom of the box, and, in setting up the apparatus, special attention is paid to ensuring that both phases are circulated.

Place the papers, already spotted with hydroxamic acids and hanging from an empty trough, in the chromatogram box and start the pump. After thirty minutes fill the trough with 50 ml of the mobile phase. Remove the paper six hours later, air-dry and spray with 2 per cent ferric chloride solution in 0·01N hydrochloric acid.

Cut the chromatograms across into strips, each containing the ten spots from one species of penicillin, which will have an average area of 75 sq. cm. Macerate each strip with 1 ml of 20 per cent ferric chloride in 0·1N hydrochloric acid, 10 ml of *n*-butanol, 2 g of anhydrous sodium sulphate and 0·6 g of sodium chloride. Hold the tubes in a water-bath at 20° until measured. The paper and salt can be packed at the bottom of the tube with a glass rod so that 7 to 8 ml of butanol can be poured off for colorimetric measurement, which is made in any suitable colorimeter.

The extinction of the butanol solution prepared in this way increases with temperature, and the extraction and measurement should be made at a constant temperature; the colour appears to be stable for many hours.

Procaine Benzylpenicillin, $C_{16}H_{18}O_4N_2S,C_{13}H_{20}O_2N_2,H_2O$, Mol. Wt. 588·7. This salt is composed of one molecule of procaine base and one molecule of benzylpenicillin with one molecule of water of crystallisation. The assay of procaine presents no serious difficulties. Although nitrite titration has been recommended the simplest method is titration with standard acid after alkaline chloroform extraction.

Transfer about 0·1 g, accurately weighed, to a separator, add 20 ml of water and 5 ml of 10 per cent sodium carbonate decahydrate solution. Extract by shaking with successive quantities, each of 25 ml, of chloroform until complete extraction of the procaine is effected, washing each chloroform extract with the same 5 ml of water. Transfer the mixed chloroform extracts to a second separator, add 20 ml of 0·01N sulphuric acid, shake thoroughly, allow to separate, run off the chloroform layer into a third separator and wash with 5 ml of water. Titrate the excess of sulphuric acid in the aqueous solution and washings with 0·01N sodium hydroxide using methyl red as indicator. 1 ml 0·01N sulphuric acid = 0·002363 g of procaine base, $C_{13}H_{20}O_2N_2$.

The procaine may also be determined colorimetrically using *N*-(1-naphthyl)ethylenediamine (see Procaine, p. 190).

Benzylpenicillin may be determined by the standard *N*-ethylpiperidine method (above) using 120 mg of the sample, but to ensure reasonably accurate results the sample should be finely powdered so that initial solution is not delayed. 1 g of residue = 1·315 g of $C_{16}H_{18}O_4N_2S$, $C_{13}H_{20}O_2N_2,H_2O$.

The determination of total penicillins is not easy. The *U.S.P.* uses the direct iodimetric assay as applied to benzylpenicillin after dissolving the sample in methanol, but this may lead to results which are 3 to 5 per cent low, due to interaction of procaine with iodine. Wild[9] suggested the use of silicotungstate as a procaine precipitant before application of the iodimetric method but details given in his method required clarification. Based on the original, the following modification has been found by us to be satisfactory.

Standardisation of silicotungstic acid: Dissolve 3 g of the acid in water and titrate with 0·1N sodium hydroxide, using thymol blue as indicator, until a definite, permanent, yellow colour appears. Let the ml of 0·1N alkali required be '*A*.'

Dissolve 0·463 g of procaine hydrochloride and 0·606 g of sodium benzylpenicillin in water and dilute to 500 ml in a graduated flask. Pipette 50 ml of this solution into a 150-ml beaker and add 1 g of sodium chloride. Prepare a solution of sodium silicotungstate by dissolving 2·5 g of the silicotungstic acid in ($A \times 1{\cdot}15$) ml of 0·1N sodium hydroxide and diluting to 50 ml in a graduated flask. Using this solution as titrant and a 10-ml burette, titrate the procaine penicillin solution, stirring well. When the precipitate coagulates, indicating that the end-point is near, add the titrant 2 drops at a time, stirring and allowing to settle after each addition, until a 0·5-ml portion of the clear supernatant liquid gives no turbidity when mixed with 0·5 ml of 0·1N iodine in a test-tube. This gives an approximate titration figure since some of the mixture has been removed. Repeat the titration, adding the volume of titrant required for the first titration before testing with iodine. Let the ml of titrant required be '*B*.'

Prepare a reagent by dissolving ($B \times 0{\cdot}60$) g of the silicotungstic acid together with 10 g of sodium chloride in ($A \times B \times 0{\cdot}24$) ml of 0·1N sodium hydroxide, boiling gently for ten minutes to complete solution.

Cool, transfer to a 100-ml graduated flask and dilute to volume with water.

Determination of procaine penicillin: Weigh 0·1 g of the sample into a 100-ml graduated flask, dissolve in 60 to 70 ml of water and add, by pipette, 10 ml of the silicotungstic acid reagent. Dilute to volume with water, mix thoroughly and filter through dry filter paper into a dry flask.

Pipette 10 ml of the filtrate into a stoppered flask and complete the iodimetric determination of total penicillins described above, beginning with 'add 5 ml of N sodium hydroxide . . .'.

Repeat the iodimetric procedure using 10 ml of a standard solution of sodium benzylpenicillin in place of the 10 ml of filtrate, multiply the titration figure by 1·6520 to give the exact equivalent of each ml of 0·02N iodine in terms of procaine penicillin monohydrate and from this calculate the result of the assay.

The potency of procaine penicillin and of its preparations is determined microbiologically by the method given on p. 814, using Standard Preparation of Penicillin as the standard. In using this method it is important to ensure, on account of the relatively low solubility of procaine penicillin (1 in 200 in water), that an adequate amount of buffer solution is added to the weighed sample to dissolve it completely. Some prepared procaine penicillins may be difficult or slow to dissolve; this can be overcome by first wetting the sample with a few drops of acetone before adding the buffer solution.

Benzathine pencillin, $C_{16}H_{20}N_2(C_{16}H_{18}O_4N_2S)_2$, Mol. Wt. 909·2. This salt, *NN'*-dibenzylethylenediamine dibenzylpenicillin, is characterised by an extremely low solubility in water. Parker and Donegan[10] obtained satisfactory assay with iodine after first decomposing the salt with alkali. A correct blank titration is obtained by treating an aqueous suspension with iodine solution without alkali treatment.

Treat a weighed quantity (W) of about 500 mg with 1 to 2 ml of N sodium hydroxide and wash into a 500-ml flask with water. Shake until solution is complete, in 2 to 3 minutes, and then dilute to volume with water. Pipette 5-ml aliquots into three stoppered flasks and treat with 5 ml of N sodium hydroxide. After allowing to stand for at least ten minutes treat each successively with 5·5 ml of N hydrochloric acid and 20 ml of 0·01N iodine and allow to stand for exactly fifteen minutes. Titrate the excess of iodine with 0·01N sodium thiosulphate and average the titrations (S). Determine a blank by weighing 4 to 6 mg of the sample, washing into a stoppered flask with 10 to 15 ml of water and adding 20 ml of 0·01N iodine. Titrate immediately with 0·01N sodium thiosulphate (B).

$$\text{The potency of the sample} = \frac{(B - S) \times 66{\cdot}15}{W} \text{ I.U./mg}$$

$$\text{and the purity} = \frac{\text{potency (I.U./mg)}}{13{\cdot}07} \text{ per cent.}$$

The dibenzylethylenediamine content can be determined readily by treating a suspension of the salt with excess of alkali in the presence of sodium chloride and extracting the free base with ether.

Decompose a weighed quantity of about 100 mg with 1 ml of N sodium hydroxide and wash into a separator with 15 to 25 ml of water. Add 1 to 2 g of sodium chloride and shake with 30 ml of ether. Separate and repeat the extraction with 20 ml of ether. Wash the mixed ethers three times with 10-ml portions of 10 per cent sodium chloride solution. Then shake the ether with 25 ml of 0·01N hydrochloric acid, run off the acid and wash the ether with 20 ml of water. Titrate the mixed acid extracts with 0·01N sodium hydroxide using bromophenol blue as indicator.

$$\text{Purity} = \frac{\text{ml acid absorbed} \times 12}{100 \times \text{wt. of sample}}$$

A more satisfactory method for determination of the benzathine moiety is by non-aqueous titration as follows:

Shake 1 g thoroughly with 30 ml of brine and 10 ml of 20 per cent sodium hydroxide and then extract with four 50-ml quantities of ether. Combine the extracts, wash with three 10-ml quantities of water, extract the washings with 25 ml of ether and add the extract to the main ether solution. Evaporate the ether solution to low volume, add 2 ml of dehydrated ethanol and evaporate to dryness. Add 50 ml of glacial acetic acid to the residue and titrate with 0·1N perchloric acid using as indicator 1 ml of a 0·2 per cent solution of α-naphtholbenzein in glacial acetic acid. Carry out a blank determination omitting the sample. The difference between the two titrations represents the amount of perchloric acid required to neutralise the liberated base. 1 ml 0·1N = 0·01202 g $C_{16}H_{20}N_2$.

The *U.S.P.* makes use of a spectrophotometric determination of benzathine in this material, based on the extinction of a 0·05 per cent solution in methanol at 263 mμ.

To determine the potency of benzathine penicillin and of its preparations, the microbiological assay is employed using the Standard Preparation of Penicillin as standard. Because of the very low solubility of benzathine penicillin in water (about 1 in 6,000) a solution-aid is necessary and formamide or dimethylformamide is used.

Weigh about 20 mg of the sample, or an amount calculated to contain about 20,000 units of penicillin and dissolve in about 5 ml of formamide or dimethylformamide. Make up to 200 ml with buffer solution pH 7 and proceed with the assay as given on p. 814.

Benethamine Penicillin, $C_{15}H_{17}N,C_{16}H_{18}O_4N_2S$, Mol. Wt. 545·7. Benethamine penicillin is the *N*-benzylphenethylamine salt of benzylpenicillin and its potency is determined by microbiological assay (p. 814) using the Standard Preparation of Penicillin as standard.

The *N*-benzylphenethylamine content can be determined by extraction with ether in alkaline solution.

Shake 0·1 g thoroughly with 20 ml of water, 2·5 ml of 10 per cent sodium carbonate decahydrate solution and 20 ml of ether, allow to separate and extract the aqueous layer with two further 20-ml quantities of ether. Combine the ether extracts, wash with three 5-ml quantities of water and then extract the ether layer with 25 ml of 0·01N sulphuric acid. Wash the ether layer with three 5-ml quantities of water, adding the washings to the acid extract and titrate the excess acid with 0·01N borax using methyl red and methylene blue solution as indicator. 1 ml 0·01N H_2SO_4 = 0·002113 g $C_{15}H_{17}N$.

PHARMACEUTICAL PREPARATIONS OF BENZYLPENICILLINS

Microbiological methods have been extensively used in the past for many preparations of penicillin but there is now an increasing application of chemical procedures. The penicillinase titration method of Royce, Bowler and Sykes[3] is very useful, particularly for solution-tablets and oral tablets provided that these have not been formulated with buffer substances. Assays on penicillin mixtures with insoluble substances, such as sulphonamide powders, can be done directly on the suspension in water, or, preferably, after separating the insoluble matter. The various preparations of penicillin in oily bases, ointments, etc. can be assayed directly by suspending a weighed quantity in water with indicator and adding an equal volume of chloroform; the mixture is shaken gently, adjusted to pH 7·5 and penicillinase added. It must be titrated continuously during the inactivation period to keep the penicillin in the aqueous phase. The method is not suitable for lozenges.

The iodimetric method of assay is favoured for many official purposes and it can be applied, with very little sample preparation, to injections, tablets and solution-tablets. For ointments and similar preparations it is not directly applicable since high results may be obtained due to iodine absorption by the base. For preparations of this type Boymond[11] has recommended iodimetric determination after mixture with benzene and extraction with water.

Procaine penicillin preparations may be determined by the spectrophotometric method described by Stock[4] (see above) but because of its low solubility in water, methanol is used as the extracting solvent. Procaine absorbs strongly in the ultra-violet and exhibits a maximum at 292 mμ. The absorption at 322 mμ (the maximum for penicillenic acid) is still significant and for pure procaine penicillin the irrelevant absorption amounts to 23 per cent of the total. However, if the absorption is measured at 322 mμ both before and after the heating period, then the increase is entirely due to the penicillin present.

Where microbiological assays are preferred to determine the potency of a preparation, the following notes are of interest:

(*a*) Procaine penicillin. Some samples may be slow and difficult to dissolve; this can be overcome by first wetting the sample with a few drops of acetone before adding the buffer solution.

(*b*) Ointments, oily suspensions, etc. The penicillin is separated from the oily phase by first dissolving a weighed or measured amount of the sample in a suitable volume of ether and removing the penicillin by extracting with three approximately equal amounts of buffer solution, pH 7. The extracts are then combined and the assay continued as on p. 814.

(*c*) Preparations such as lozenges containing sugars as diluents yield erroneous assays by the standard method. To overcome this, add either an equivalent amount of glucose to the standard penicillin solution or 0·5 per cent of glucose to the assay plate medium.

PHENOXYMETHYLPENICILLIN, $C_{16}H_{18}O_5N_2S$, Mol. Wt. 350·4 (Penicillin V)

Total penicillins in this substance and in its calcium or potassium salts may be determined by a slight modification of the iodimetric method already described, while phenoxymethylpenicillin is determined spectrophotometrically. This may be done by dissolving in dilute sodium bicarbonate solution (water in the case of the salts) and measuring the extinction value at 268 mμ (as in the *B.P.*) or by dissolving in methanol and measuring at 276 mμ (as in the *U.S.P.*). Recommended methods are as follows:

> For total penicillins: Weigh 60 mg into a 50-ml graduated flask, add 1 ml of saturated sodium bicarbonate solution and 2 ml of water and allow to stand, with occasional shaking, for five to ten minutes until solution is complete. Add 40 ml of water and, with constant shaking, 0·5 ml of N hydrochloric acid and dilute to volume with water. Complete the assay described above (benzylpenicillin) beginning with 'Transfer 10 ml to a stoppered flask . . .'.
>
> From the result of the second assay (using standard) determine the amount of total penicillins, calculated as $C_{16}H_{17}O_4N_2SNa$, equivalent to each ml of 0·02N iodine, multiply it by 0·9832 to obtain the amount of total penicillins, calculated as $C_{16}H_{18}O_5N_2S$, equivalent to each ml of 0·02N iodine and from this calculate the result of the first assay.

Although opinions vary concerning the absolute potency of pure benzylpenicillin, on the evidence available it seems reasonable that for the purpose of this assay, the Standard Preparation of Penicillin containing 1,670 units per mg, may be assumed to be 100·0 per cent pure.

> For phenoxymethylpenicillin: Dissolve 0·1 g in 4 ml of 5 per cent sodium bicarbonate solution, dilute to 500 ml with water and determine the extinction at 268 mμ, using 1-cm cells. E(1 per cent, 1 cm) at 268 mμ of phenoxymethylpenicillin is 34·8.

Phenoxymethylpenicillin calcium, $(C_{16}H_{17}O_5N_2S)_2$ Ca, $2H_2O$, Mol. Wt. 774·9 and **phenoxymethylpenicillin potassium,** $C_{16}H_{17}O_5N_2SK$, Mol. Wt.

388·5, are both official substances and they are controlled for total penicillin content and for phenoxymethylpenicillin content by the methods described above.

Tablets of Phenoxymethylpenicillin, *B.P.*, may contain phenoxymethylpenicillin or its calcium or potassium salt; the content of active material may be determined by the iodimetric assay. Similar considerations apply to capsules.

MODIFIED PENICILLINS

Continuous research is being carried out to produce modified penicillins with more potent or more specific activity than the antibiotics at present available, or to overcome the penicillin-resistance which certain strains of organisms have built up. A number of these modified penicillins, such as methicillin and phenethicillin is already available and it seems likely that more will appear within the next few years. Little has been published on the analytical chemistry of these substances but it is probable that hydrolysis with sodium hydroxide followed by titration of the excess alkali could be used for determination of the sodium or potassium salts of the substances mentioned above; penicillamine hydrochloride may be determined by the iodimetric assay.

Microbiological methods are not used with the newer penicillins, except for their clinical estimation in blood, etc., because being mainly synthetic and of a different basic structure each possesses different antibacterial properties, hence each would require its own separate standard. The potencies of the new type penicillins cannot be properly related to those of benzylpenicillin for assay purposes.

TETRACYCLINES

The most important tetracycline antibiotics in use are tetracycline itself, chlortetracycline (aureomycin) and oxytetracycline (terramycin).

TETRACYCLINE HYDROCHLORIDE, $C_{22}H_{24}O_8N_2,HCl$, Mol Wt. 480·9.

A microbiological assay is the method of choice (see p. 813) but spectrophotometric methods are also applicable. One spectrophotometric method is based on the formation of a yellow colour with an absorption maximum at 380 mμ when tetracycline is dissolved in 0·25N sodium hydroxide,[12] another on the orange-brown colour (maximum absorption 490 mμ) formed on mixing a dilute hydrochloric acid solution of the sample with ferric chloride solution. The former method which is described below is also applicable to oxytetracycline but not to chlortetracycline while the ferric chloride reaction, which is given in detail under oxytetracycline, applies to all three.

Weigh about 25 mg of the hydrochloride of the antibiotic into a 250-ml graduated flask, dissolve in 50 ml of water and dilute to volume with water. Transfer a 15-ml aliquot to a 100-ml graduated flask, add 70 ml of water and 5·0 ml of 5N sodium hydroxide and dilute to volume with water. Exactly six minutes after the addition of the alkali determine the extinction at 380 mμ, with water as blank and read the content of tetracycline, or oxytetracycline, from a standard curve prepared by treating a series of standards exactly as above and plotting extinction against content of tetracycline, or oxytetracycline.

The colour produced with chlortetracycline, under the conditions described above, fades rapidly and for the determination of tetracycline in mixtures with chlortetracycline containing up to 20 per cent of the latter antibiotic the above method may be applied directly. However, for mixtures of the two antibiotics in which chlortetracycline is the major constituent, the extinction due to the chlortetracycline, with an absorption maximum at 345 mμ, must be taken into account. In this case the tetracycline will give a shelf at 380 mμ superimposed on the chlortetracycline band and since the height of this shelf depends on the concentration of tetracycline, small amounts of tetracycline may be determined using a standard curve prepared with mixtures of the two antibiotics of known concentration.

CHLORTETRACYCLINE HYDROCHLORIDE, $C_{22}H_{23}O_8N_2Cl,HCl$, Mol. Wt. 515·4 (Aureomycin).

This material is also determined officially by a microbiological method (p. 813) but a number of different types of physico-chemical assay are possible.

(i) A blue fluorescence, due to the formation of *iso*chlortetracycline, is obtained by the action of alkali. This principle has been utilised in methods by Levine, Garlock and Fischbach[13] and by Chiccarelli, Van Gieson and Woolford;[14] Levine's recommended procedure is given below. The rate at which the fluorescence is developed and its intensity depend upon the pH of the solution, hence the solution must be highly buffered and at a pH at which the rate of conversion is sufficiently slow at room temperature to permit measurement of the initial, or blank, fluorescence. The rate of reaction increases with temperature and the developed fluorescence is reasonably stable, especially at lower concentrations of chlortetracycline.

Prepare a buffer reagent of pH 7·6 by dissolving 16 g of dibasic potassium phosphate and 2 g of monobasic potassium phosphate in water and adjusting to 90 ml.

To 10 ml of solution containing 2·5 to 35 μg of aureomycin, add 2·0 ml of buffer reagent. Mix and measure the fluorescence immediately. Heat in a water-bath for five minutes, cool and read the fluorescence in from fifteen minutes to one hour. Deduct the blank and calculate the aureomycin by reference to a standard curve prepared by treating suitable aliquots of a standard solution of aureomycin hydrochloride as described above.

(ii) On heating with dilute sulphuric acid chlortetracycline is degraded to give a product having a characteristic ultra-violet absorption spectrum. This method was developed by Hiscox[15] who heated the chlortetracycline in N sulphuric acid at 100° for eight minutes. The difference in extinction at specified wavelengths is proportional to the amount of antibiotic present in solution.

To a 5-ml aqueous aliquot containing 100 to 500 μg of aureomycin in a boiling-tube add 5 ml of 2N sulphuric acid. Heat in boiling water for eight minutes, cool and make up to 25 ml. Measure the extinction of the solution at 274 mμ and 350 mμ; the difference is proportional to the aureomycin present in solution.

By experiment a regression line was established using this method: $Y = 15{\cdot}43X + 0{\cdot}124$ where Y = μg of aureomycin per ml of the final solution and X = difference in extinction.

(iii) A commonly used method and one which has proved reliable in routine practice, is based on the conversion of chlortetracycline by heating in acid solution to anhydrochlortetracycline which has an absorption maximum at 445 mμ. A second portion of the sample is heated in a solution which is buffered at pH 7·5 and this results in the formation of *iso*chlortetracycline which is stable in acid solution and has no absorption at 445 mμ and can, therefore, be used as a blank. This method has been developed by Chiccarelli and co-workers to the determination of chlortetracycline in animal feed supplements[16] and in pharmaceuticals.[17] The procedure, as applied to the antibiotic itself, is as follows:

Weigh out about 0·05 g, transfer to a 500-ml graduated flask, add about 300 ml of water and shake until the sample is completely dissolved. Make up to volume with water. Prepare a similar solution from a Reference Standard of chlortetracycline hydrochloride. Into each of two 50-ml graduated flasks pipette 10 ml of the sample solution and into two further flasks pipette 10 ml of standard solution.

To one of the sample solutions and one of the standard solutions add, in order, 12 ml of 5N hydrochloric acid, 15 ml of a buffer solution pH 7·5 (prepared by dissolving 178 g of dipotassium phosphate and 22 g of potassium dihydrogen phosphate in 1 litre of water), 2 ml of freshly prepared 10 per cent sodium bisulphite and 3 ml of 0·4N sodium hydroxide. Place the flasks in boiling water for exactly seven minutes and cool immediately.

To the remaining sample and standard solutions add, in order, 15 ml of buffer solution pH 7·5, 2 ml of 10 per cent sodium bisulphite and 3 ml of 0·4N sodium hydroxide. Place the flasks in boiling water for exactly five minutes, add 12 ml of 5N hydrochloric acid, mix and continue heating for a further two minutes. Cool the flasks immediately. Dilute all solutions to volume with water and measure the extinctions of the acid-treated sample and standard solutions at 445 mμ in a 1-cm

> cell using as blanks the sample and standard solutions heated with pH 7·5 buffer only.
>
> Calculate the percentage of chlortetracycline hydrochloride in the sample by direct comparison with the standard.

The aureomycin content of animal feed supplements may be determined by extracting a quantity containing about 10 mg with about 70 ml 0·25N hydrochloric acid for thirty minutes, diluting with water to 100 ml, then treating a filtered portion of this solution exactly as described above.

For feeds and feed supplements, extraction for microbiological assay is with acid-acetone (40 ml concentrated hydrochloric acid and 1,300 ml of acetone diluted to 2 litres with water). A control standard is necessary containing unfortified or inactivated feed material. The assay organism recommended is *Bacillus cereus* (NCIB 9231).

For preparation of inactivated feeds for standards:

> Suspend a 20 g sample of the fortified feed in 100 ml of acid-acetone mixture, shake for one hour and separate in a centrifuge. Neutralise a 25-ml portion of the supernatant solution with N sodium hydroxide using methyl orange as indicator and make up to 100 ml in a graduated flask with phosphate buffer solution, pH 4·5 Measure 25 ml of this solution into a 50-ml beaker, add 2·5 ml of N sodium hydroxide and boil gently for fifteen minutes. Cool and add 2·5 ml of N hydrochloric acid. Transfer quantitatively to a 50-ml graduated flask and add a known amount of a solution of the chlortetracycline standard equal to the amount estimated to be present in the test sample. Make up to volume with phosphate buffer solution and from this prepare further final dilutions as required in the assay.

Demethylchlortetracycline hydrochloride, $C_{21}H_{21}O_8N_2Cl,HCl$, Mol. Wt. 501·3. This is standardised microbiologically (see Appendix VII).

OXYTETRACYCLINE DIHYDRATE, $C_{22}H_{24}O_9N_2,2H_2O$, Mol Wt. 496·5 and **OXYTETRACYCLINE HYDROCHLORIDE,** $C_{22}H_{24}O_9N_2,HCl$, Mol. Wt. 496·9 (Terramycin).

A microbiological method (see p. 813) is prescribed by the *B.P.* although the *U.S.P.* XV (for oxytetracycline itself) relied on a version of the colorimetric method with ferric chloride (see below). The microbiological determination of potency in the *B.P.* is augmented by a spectrophotometric assay:

> Dissolve 20 mg in sufficient *B.P.* solution of standard pH 2·0 to produce 100 ml. Dilute 10 ml to 100 ml with the buffer solution and measure the extinction of the resulting solution at the maximum at about 353 mμ, using 1-cm cells. E(1 per cent, 1 cm) of oxytetracycline dihydrate or oxytetracycline hydrochloride at 353 mμ is 284.

When ferric chloride is added to a solution of oxytetracycline hydrochloride an orange-brown colour is produced.[18] A reliable version of this method is that applied to animal-feed supplements by the Analytical Methods Committee of the *S.A.C.*[19]

Weigh an amount of sample containing the equivalent of about 0·03 to 0·05 g of oxytetracycline free base into a 250-ml beaker and add 50 ml of 10 per cent v/v acetic acid. Allow to stand for twenty minutes, stirring gently with a magnetic stirrer and then filter quantitatively through paper in a Buchner funnel until a clear filtrate is obtained. (It may be necessary to re-filter through the funnel once or twice.) Wash the filter paper with 10 ml of water and then adjust the filtrate to a pH of 2·0 ± 0·05 with a few drops of concentrated hydrochloric acid, using a pH meter. Transfer the solution quantitatively to a 100-ml graduated flask with 0·01N hydrochloric acid and dilute to volume with 0·01N hydrochloric acid.

Transfer a 5-ml aliquot of the solution to each of two tubes and then to the first tube (the blank) add 15 ml of 0·01N hydrochloric acid and to the second tube add 5 ml of 0·01N hydrochloric acid and 10 ml of a 0·05 per cent solution of ferric chloride hexahydrate in 0·01N hydrochloric acid. Mix and allow to stand at 20° to 25° for twenty minutes. Measure the extinction of the solution in the second tube at 490 mμ, using matched 1-cm cells, with the blank solution in the comparison cell.

Calculate the content of oxytetracycline free base by reference to a standard curve prepared by using suitable volumes of a standard solution of oxytetracycline hydrochloride in 0·01N hydrochloric acid covering the range 0 to 2,000 μg.

Phosphates, fluorides, thiocyanates and other substances that combine with ferric iron interfere and therefore, if present, must be removed before carrying out the determination.

For feeds and supplements, extraction for microbiological assay is with acid methanol (20 ml of concentrated hydrochloric acid diluted to 1 litre with methanol). A control standard is necessary containing unfortified or inactivated feed material. The assay organism recommended is *Bacillus cereus* (NCIB 9231).

For preparation of inactivated feeds for standards:

Suspend a 20 g sample of the fortified feed in 100 ml of acid methanol, shake for one hour and separate in a centrifuge.

Prepare a column with an equal mixture of sodium carbonate and Silflow. Pack the column dry and tamp down before use.

Pour about 50 ml of the solution above on the dry column and allow it to percolate. Adjust the inactivated extract to pH 4·5 with N hydrochloric acid and transfer 20 ml to a 50-ml graduated flask. Add a known amount of a solution of the oxytetracycline standard equal to the amount estimated to be present in 4 g of the test sample and make up to volume with phosphate buffer solution. From this prepare further final dilutions as required in the assay.

A number of other methods have been described for determination of the tetracyclines, mainly colorimetric ones based on colour formation with various metal ions or with complex molecules such as phospho- and arseno-molybdates but these have not found widespread acceptance in routine practice. It has also been shown that tetracyclines may be titrated non-aqueously with perchloric acid in dioxan.[20]

Pharmaceutical preparations of the tetracyclines are mainly confined to capsules, tablets and injections and the methods given above are usually applicable with little or no modification. For official purposes extensive use is made of microbiological assays.

STREPTOMYCINS

Streptomycin and dihydrostreptomycin have very similar chemical structures and so many of the chemical methods which are available are equally applicable to both antibiotics. Certain procedures have a measure of specificity however and may be used for the determination of one of the substances in the presence of the other. The *B.P.* relies upon microbiological assay (see p. 813) for determination of the potency of both these antibiotics, which are official in the form of their sulphates.

STREPTOMYCIN SULPHATE, $(C_{21}H_{39}O_{12}N_7)_2,3H_2SO_4$, Mol. Wt. 1457·4

When subjected to alkaline hydrolysis streptomycin yields maltol, 2-methyl-3-hydroxy-γ-pyrone, quantitatively and this fact may be used in the assay of streptomycin, the maltol being determined either spectrophotometrically (maximum absorption at 322 mμ) or colorimetrically (after reaction with ferric iron to give a purple-red colour). Dihydrostreptomycin will not yield maltol under the conditions given below so that streptomycin can be determined in its presence as, for example, in Streptoduocin for Injection, *U.S.P.* which contains equal amounts of the two antibiotics.

Pipette a volume of sample containing 2·5 g (2,500,000 units) of streptomycin sulphate into a 100-ml graduated flask and dilute to volume with water. Dilute a 5-ml aliquot of this solution to 500 ml with water in a graduated flask, then transfer a 5-ml aliquot of this final dilution to a test-tube and add exactly 1 ml of 2N sodium hydroxide. Mix and place the tube in a water-bath. Exactly three minutes after the addition of the alkali, remove the tube from the bath and cool under a cold-water tap for exactly three minutes. At the end of this time add, by pipette, 4 ml of a 1 per cent solution of ferric ammonium sulphate in 0·75N sulphuric acid, shake and allow to stand. After exactly ten minutes, measure the extinction at 550 mμ, using 2-cm cells with water in the comparison cell. Read the concentration of streptomycin in the final 5-ml aliquot prepared from the sample from a standard curve.

The standard curve is prepared as follows: Transfer suitable volumes, covering the range 0 to 2·0 mg of a standard solution of streptomycin sulphate containing 0·5 mg per ml, to a series of test-tubes and dilute each to 5 ml with water. Treat the contents of each tube exactly as described above from 'add exactly 1 ml of 2N sodium hydroxide . . .' and ending with '. . . water in the comparison cell.' Prepare a curve by plotting streptomycin sulphate content against extinction.

Ashton, Foster and Fatherley[21] have developed a colorimetric reaction based on the streptidine moiety of the molecule which is therefore applicable to both streptomycin and dihydrostreptomycin. Other antibiotics, notably penicillin and its compounds, do not interfere, so that the method is useful for the determination of one or other of the streptomycins in the samples of mixed antibiotics. The colour is not permanent, the rate of fading depending on the relative concentration of the three reagents.

Either dissolve the sample in water or dilute liquid samples to give a solution containing between 100 and 400 units of dihydrostreptomycin per ml (0·1 to 0·4 mg per ml of dihydrostreptomycin base). Transfer 2 ml of the sample solution to a test tube (6 × 1 inch), add 15 ml of water and then 1 ml of 0·4 per cent diacetyl solution, 1 ml of 20 per cent potassium hydroxide solution and 1 ml of 10 per cent solution of α-naphthol in dehydrated ethanol, in that order. Mix the contents of the tube by inversion after each addition. Start timing when the diacetyl solution is added. Precisely forty minutes later determine the extinction at 525 mμ in a 1-cm cell against water. Prepare a standard graph from suitable dilutions of a standard dihydrostreptomycin solution, using the same procedure for colour development as described for the sample. Determine the potency of the diluted sample solution from the standard graph. A standard graph should be prepared for each determination to allow for differences in room temperature, reagents, and so on.

No effect on the colour intensity was obvious when the solutions contained high concentrations of sodium sulphate, sodium citrate, calcium chloride, 0·2 per cent sodium benzylpenicillin, 0·03 per cent procaine benzyl penicillin or 0·03 per cent penethamate hydriodide.

DIHYDROSTREPTOMYCIN SULPHATE, $(C_{21}H_{41}O_{12}N_7)_2,3H_2SO_4$, Mol. Wt. 1461·5

Hiscox[22] has shown that when dihydrostreptomycin is heated in dilute sulphuric acid solution a maximum appears in the absorption spectrum at 265 mμ. Under identical conditions, streptomycin develops maxima at 245 and 315 mμ and a minimum at 285 mμ. Provided the conditions described below are strictly followed dihydrostreptomycin may be determined in the presence of small amounts of streptomycin, but larger amounts of the latter material, as well as other antibiotics, will interfere.

Transfer to a test-tube a volume of an aqueous solution containing between 1 and 3 mg of dihydrostreptomycin and, if necessary, dilute to 3 ml with water. Then add 3 ml of 0·5N sulphuric acid, connect the flask to an air condenser and reflux gently on a water-bath for two hours. Cool, transfer to a 25-ml graduated flask with water and dilute to volume with water. Measure the extinctions at 265 mμ and 280 mμ and read the dihydrostreptomycin content corresponding to the difference between the two extinctions from a standard curve. The standard curve is prepared by treating suitable amounts of pure dihydrostreptomycin, covering the range 0 to 3 mg, exactly as above and plotting the difference between the two extinctions against concentration.

The method based on colour formation with diacetyl and α-naphthol in alkaline solution, described above for streptomycin, is equally applicable to the dihydro-compound.

OTHER ANTIBIOTICS

CHLORAMPHENICOL, $C_{11}H_{12}O_5N_2Cl_2$, Mol. Wt. 323·1

A number of chemical and physical methods is available for the determination of this substance, although the *B.P.* relies entirely on physical constants as a means of control of the purity of the drug. The *U.S.P.*, on the other hand, prescribes a microbiological method of assay. The E(1 per cent, 1 cm) of a solution in water is 298 at 278 mμ and use may be made of this for the determination of chloramphenicol in formulated products such as eye-drops, ear-drops and capsules. Chloramphenicol can also be determined by a colorimetric method based upon reduction of the nitro-group with zinc, stannous chloride or, better, sodium dithionite followed by diazotisation and coupling with *N*-(1-naphthyl)ethylenediamine. The following method includes a pre-extraction stage to free chloramphenicol from interfering substances.[23]

Pipette a suitable volume (2 to 5 ml) of a solution containing between 10 and 50 μg of chloramphenicol into a separator and add 5 ml of 0·2M phosphate buffer (pH 6·0). Extract with two 25-ml portions of a mixture of 2 volumes of chloroform and 1 volume of ethyl acetate and filter the organic layers through dry filter paper into a flask. Evaporate the solvents on a water-bath under a jet of air and dissolve the residue in 3 ml of 0·1N sodium hydroxide. Add 25 mg of sodium dithionite, mix and allow to stand at room temperature for fifteen minutes. Then add 0·5 ml of 5 per cent sodium nitrite solution followed by 5 to 10 drops of concentrated hydrochloric acid and, after one to three minutes, 1 ml of 5 per cent sulphamic acid solution. Remove any fumes above the surface of the liquid by aspiration, add 0·5 ml of a 0·5 per cent aqueous solution of *N*-(1-naphthyl)ethylenediamine dihydrochloride and dilute with water to a known volume to give a convenient extinction. Allow to stand for two hours and measure the extinction of the solution at 558 mμ against a reagent blank. (If the final solution is turbid, shake with a small volume of chloroform and centrifuge before measuring the extinction.) Read the chloramphenicol content from a standard curve prepared by treating a series of standard solutions of chloramphenicol, covering the range 10 to 50 μg, exactly as above and plotting the chloramphenicol content against extinction.

Chloramphenicol is also reducible at the dropping mercury electrode and an example of the use of this approach is its determination in **Paint of Chloramphenicol and Crystal Violet,** *B. Vet. C.*, which contains 10 per cent of chloramphenicol and 0·5 per cent of dye in alcoholic solution.

Prepare a 0·25 per cent v/v solution of the sample in water and mix a suitable volume of this solution with an equal volume of buffer solution, pH 4·0, prepared by mixing 80 ml of 0·2N acetic acid with 20 ml of 0·2N sodium acetate. Add 0·1 g of powdered thymol and transfer a suitable amount of the mixture so obtained to a polarograph cell that has a mercury pool anode. Maintain the solution at a temperature of 25° and bubble through it oxygen-free nitrogen that has previously been passed through water, until the solution is deoxygenated. Record a polarogram to about −1·1 volt, correcting the diffusion current for the residual current.

Dissolve 0·10 g of chloramphenicol in 1 ml of 95 per cent ethanol and dilute with equal volumes of the buffer solution, pH 4·0 and water to give a solution containing 125 μg of chloramphenicol per ml. Record the polarogram of this solution under the conditions described above and calculate the chloramphenicol content of the sample by comparing the diffusion currents of the two solutions.

Ear-drops of Chloramphenicol, *B.P.C.* Usually contain 5 per cent in propylene glycol.

The antibiotic may be determined both in this preparation and in **Eye-drops of Chloramphenicol** by diluting a suitable volume with water to give a final concentration of about 0·001 per cent w/v and measuring the extinction at the maximum at about 278 mμ using 1-cm cells, E(1 per cent, 1 cm) of chloramphenicol = 298.

Eye Ointment of Chloramphenicol, *B.P.C.* Usually contains 1 per cent in a fatty base.

In this preparation a microbiological method of assay is preferable (see p. 813) because of interference from the base with the ultra-violet absorption method.

Chloramphenicol cinnamate, $C_{20}H_{18}O_6N_2Cl_2$, Mol. Wt. 453·3 may be assayed microbiologically (see p. 813) or by measuring the extinction of a 0·00075 per cent solution in dehydrated ethanol at the maximum at about 276 mμ using 1-cm cells. E(1 per cent, 1 cm) = 709.

Chloramphenicol palmitate, $C_{27}H_{42}O_6N_2Cl_2$, Mol. Wt. 561·6 may be assayed microbiologically (see p. 813) or by the extinction of a 0·003 per cent solution in dehydrated ethanol, measured at the maximum at about 271 mμ using 1-cm cells, E(1 per cent, 1 cm) = 178.

NEOMYCIN

Unlike other antibiotics, neomycin, always prepared as the sulphate, consists of a mixture of several components, the three main ones being neomycin B, neomycin C and neamine (neomycin A). Of these, neomycins B and C are the most important, but so far they have not been separated with any certain degree of purity, hence it is not possible to give even an empirical formula for neomycin. Similarly, the ratios of the amounts of the components can vary, and so a microbiological assay (see p. 813) is at present preferred to a chemical one, although chemical assays have been described for neomycins B and C (see below). In the absence of a suitable reference standard of accepted and known purity all assay procedures are perforce based on standard material of arbitrarily chosen potency, and so they lack the precision of other antibiotic assays.

Neomycin sulphate normally contains 80 to 85 per cent of neomycin B, 15 to 20 per cent of neomycin C and usually less than 2 per cent of neamine, along with traces of other unknown, but biologically active, fractions. The relative activities of the three main components differ according to the assay organism and conditions employed, but in general neomycin C has a rather lower activity than has neomycin B, and neamine a very low activity, probably only one-tenth to one-fiftieth that of neomycin B. Because of this various assays employing different organisms have been proposed, each with the intention of selecting the most active fractions to the exclusion of the less potent ones. Thus, the *B.P.* recommends *Bacillus pumilus* as the assay organism and the *U.S.P.* requires the use of either *Staphylococcus aureus* or *Klebsiella pneumoniæ*; certain strains of *Sarcina lutea* are alleged to be selective for neomycin B. In practice, the differences found are comparatively small, amounting usually to only 1 or 2 per cent.

A chemical assay procedure for total neomycins B and C, proposed by Dutcher *et al.*,[24] is based on the observation that both when heated with strong mineral acid yield furfural as one of the decomposition products. The quantitative estimation of the furfural is best made by measurement of the intensity of the absorption maximum at 280 mμ, provided there are no interfering substances present. The optimum conditions are the following:

> Prepare a standard solution containing 1 mg of neomycin base per ml by dissolving an equivalent amount of the hydrochloride (73·0 per cent base on anhydrous salt) or sulphate (66·5 per cent base on anhydrous salt) in water. Measure duplicate samples of 0·5 and 0·25 ml of standard solution into boiling-tubes and prepare duplicate tubes containing 0·5 and 0·25 ml of the unknown solution, which should be adjusted to within 500 to 1,500 μg of neomycin base per ml.
>
> To the solutions of standard and unknown add either 4·5 or 4·75 ml of 40 per cent by volume sulphuric acid to bring the final volume to 5·0 ml. Mix and place vertically in a water-bath for one and a half hours and then cool. If the standard curve has been prepared by a similar procedure, it is unnecessary to adjust the final volume before measuring the absorption. Read the extinction of the solutions at 280 mμ.

The control standards are run as checks to be certain that they fall within 5 per cent of the values found for the standard curve. From the observed extinction of the unknown solutions, the amount of neomycin base in the sample can be read from the standard curve.

The above method cannot be applied directly to pharmaceutical preparations because coloured constituents and some other substances interfere but Morgan, Honig, Warren and Levine[25] have devised a method in which the interfering substances and degradation products are removed by column chromatography, after which the neomycin is hydrolysed with acid and the furfural thus obtained is determined colorimetrically after complexing with *p*-bromoaniline.[26] The method has been described in detail since on examination it has proved to be of value for routine control of neomycin preparations. However, on checking the relation between chemical and biological activity of the recovered base it has been found that the recoveries only relate to the chemical method and that the potency (by microbiological test) has been partly destroyed in the manipulative procedure; this loss has been shown due to the action of ammonia. It has also been found necessary to use about 200 ml of ammonia solution to elute the base from the column instead of the recommended 100 ml. The method, as applied to different preparations, is as follows:

Apparatus: This consists of a glass chromatographic tube, with a tap at its lower end, connected, by means of rubber tubing, to a separator for use as a reservoir for washing the column. The tube should be 18 in. long and should be of diameter ⅜ in. for the lower 6 in. and 1⅜ in. for the upper 6 in. and should have a bulb 2 in. in diameter with its top 6 in. from the top of the tube.

Preparation of chromatographic column: Add about 20 glass beads and 12 g of dry IRC 50 resin to the tube and pass about 120 ml of N sulphuric acid through the resin bed, collecting the effluent, dropwise, in a 250-ml beaker containing 3 drops of phenolphthalein indicator, until the effluent in the beaker is colourless. Back-wash the resin with 150 ml of water and allow the washings to drain from the column. Rinse the beaker thoroughly, transfer 3 drops of phenolphthalein indicator to it and pass 100 ml of N sodium hydroxide through the column until the effluent collected in the beaker is pink. Again back-wash the column with 150 ml of water and allow the washings to drain from the column. The column is now ready for use.

Chromatographic procedure: Introduce the sample solution (for preparation see below) to the top of the chromatographic column and allow to flow through the column with the flow rate adjusted to 8 to 10 ml per minute. Wash the column with 100 ml of water and then elute the neomycin with about 100 ml of a dilute ammonia solution prepared by diluting 2 volumes of strong ammonia solution with 15 volumes of water, adjusting the flow rate to 5 to 7 ml per minute. Collect the eluate in a 100-ml graduated flask and dilute to volume with water.

Development and measurement of colour: Pipette a 5-ml aliquot of the eluate into a 50-ml round-bottomed flask containing 3 glass beads and, at the same time, into a second similar flask, also containing 3 glass beads, pipette 5 ml of an aqueous solution of *U.S.P.* Neomycin Reference Standard, prepared to contain 0·100 mg of neomycin base per ml. To each flask add, by pipette, 25 ml of xylene and 3·0 ml of 80 per cent v/v sulphuric acid solution. Connect each flask to a reflux condenser and heat by means of electric heating mantles adjusted so that both flasks reflux at exactly the same rate. Reflux for exactly sixty minutes and then disconnect the heating mantles and allow the flasks (still attached to the condensers) to cool to room temperature. Then disconnect without disturbing the phases and treat the contents of each flask, respectively, as follows. Decant the xylene layer into a 125-ml separator containing about

2 g of anhydrous sodium acetate and a small, glass-wool plug in its stem. Stopper the separator and shake for thirty seconds. Separate off the xylene layer and pipette 3 ml into a large test-tube. Pipette 3 ml of the xylene into a third test-tube for the blank.

To each tube add 15·0 ml of *p*-bromoaniline reagent (prepared by adding 8·0 g of *p*-bromoaniline to a mixture of 380 ml of thiourea-saturated glacial acetic acid, 10 ml of 20 per cent sodium chloride solution, 5 ml of 5 per cent oxalic acid solution and 5 ml of 10 per cent disodium phosphate solution in an amber-coloured bottle, shaking, stoppering the bottle and allowing to stand overnight before use; the solution should be used within one week). Shake the test-tube laterally and allow to stand in the dark for forty-five minutes.

Measure the extinctions of the sample and standard solutions at 526 $\pm$ 2 mμ, using 5-cm cells with the blank solution in the comparison cell in each case. Calculate the neomycin content by comparison.

Preparation of solution for analysis.

Reagent: Citric-hydrochloric acid solution: Dissolve 10·0 g of citric acid in water, add 35·0 ml of concentrated hydrochloric acid and dilute to 200 ml with water.

Solutions: Pipette a volume of sample containing about 10 mg of neomycin base into a 500-ml flask containing about 250 ml of water and mix. Adjust the pH to 4·0 with 0·1N hydrochloric acid or 4 per cent sodium bicarbonate solution.

Lotions, Ointments: Weigh an amount of sample equivalent to about 10 mg of neomycin base into a 500-ml flask containing 100 to 150 ml of hot citric-hydrochloric acid solution. Allow to cool, and shake for five minutes. Then add 4 g of Celite, swirl and filter with gentle suction through a Whatman No. 40 filter paper covered with 2 to 3 g of Celite in a Buchner funnel. Wash the filter with about 200 ml of water and adjust the pH of the combined filtrate and washings to 4·0 by the addition of sodium bicarbonate powder.

Tablets: Transfer an amount of powdered tablets equivalent to 0·5 g of neomycin base to a 500-ml flask containing 200 ml of hot citric-hydrochloric acid solution. Shake for five minutes and then add 4 g of Celite and swirl. Filter bright with gentle suction through a Whatman No. 40 filter paper covered with 2 to 3 g of Celite in a Buchner funnel. Wash with about 150 ml of water, transfer the combined filtrate and washings to a 500-ml graduated flask and dilute to volume with water. Transfer a 10-ml aliquot of this solution to a flask containing about 250 ml of water and adjust the pH to 4·0 with 0·1N hydrochloric acid or 4 per cent sodium bicarbonate solution.

Creams: Weigh an amount of sample equivalent to about 10 mg of neomycin base into a separator, with the aid of 100 ml of hot citric-hydrochloric acid solution, and allow to cool to about 40°. Add 50 ml of chloroform, stopper the separator and invert, releasing any excess pressure in the separator immediately. Repeat the inversion, followed by release of pressure until it is possible to shake the mixture continuously and then shake for three minutes, releasing the stopper occasionally. Remove the stopper, allow the layers to separate at room temperature and then run the organic layer into a second separator containing 50 ml of 0·1N hydrochloric acid and shake for thirty seconds. Allow the layers to separate, run the organic layer into a third separator containing 50 ml of 0·1N hydrochloric acid and again shake for thirty seconds.

Allow the layers to separate and discard the organic layer. Repeat the extraction and washing with two further 50-ml quantities of chloroform, and discard the chloroform. Transfer the aqueous solution from the first separator to a 500-ml flask and rinse the separator with the acid solutions from the other two separators, adding the rinsings to the flask. Add 4 g of Celite and swirl. Filter bright through a Whatman No. 40 filter paper covered with 2 to 3 g of Celite in a Buchner funnel, wash the filter with about 200 ml of water and adjust the pH of the combined filtrate and washings to 4·0 (±1) by the addition of sodium bicarbonate powder.

Pan and Dutcher[27] have described a method for the separation of acetylated neomycin B and C by paper chromatography.

An increasing number of other antibiotics are now being used and the table given below lists some of the more important ones; in the majority of cases a microbiological method is preferable (see Appendix VII for details) but some chemical or physical procedures are available and these are referred to in the table.

TABLE 4

ANTIBIOTIC	FORMULA	MOL. WT.	ASSAY
Bacitracin, *B.P.*			Microbiological.
Zinc Bacitracin			For potency: Microbiological. For zinc: see p. 687.
Cycloserine	$C_3H_6O_2N_2$	102·1	Light absorption of 0·001 per cent solution in 0·1N HCl at maximum at 219 mμ. See also * below.
Erythromycin, *B.P.*	$C_{37}H_{67}O_{13}N$	733·95	Light absorption after dilute alkaline hydrolysis. E(1 per cent, 1 cm) 236 mμ = 85.
Erythromycin Ethyl Carbonate, *U.S.P.*	$C_{40}H_{71}O_{15}N$	806·0	Microbiological.
Erythromycin Glucoheptonate, *U.S.P.*	$C_{37}H_{67}O_{13}N,C_7H_{14}O_8$	960·1	Microbiological.
Erythromycin Lactobionate, *U.S.P.*	$C_{37}H_{67}O_{13}N,C_{12}H_{22}O_{12}$	1092·3	Microbiological.
Erythromycin Stearate, *U.S.P.*	$C_{37}H_{67}O_{13}N,C_{18}H_{36}O_2$	1018·4	Microbiological. Contains an excess of stearic acid.

TABLE 4 (*contd.*)

ANTIBIOTIC	FORMULA	MOL. WT.	ASSAY
Erythromycin Estolate	$C_{52}H_{97}O_{18}NS$	1056·4	For potency: Microbiological. For lauryl sulphate: See † below.
Erythromycin Ethyl Succinate			Microbiological.
Erythromycin Propionyl Ester			Microbiological.
Griseofulvin	$C_{17}H_{17}O_6Cl$	352·8	Light absorption of 0·001 per cent solution in ethanol at 291 mμ. E(1 per cent, 1 cm) 291 mμ = 686. See also ‡ below.
Novobiocin Calcium, *B.P.*	$(C_{31}H_{35}O_{11}N_2)_2Ca,2H_2O$	1299·4	Microbiological.
Novobiocin Sodium, *B.P.*	$C_{31}H_{35}O_{11}N_2Na$	634·6	Microbiological.
Nystatin, *U.S.P.*	$C_{46}H_{77}O_{19}N$	948·1	Microbiological.
Oleandomycin	$C_{35}H_{61}O_{12}N$	687·9	Microbiological.§
Oleandomycin Phosphate, *N.F.*	$C_{35}H_{61}O_{12}N,H_3PO_4$	785·9	Microbiological.§
Triacetyl-oleandomycin, *N.F.*			Potency: Microbiological.§ For acetyl groups: see p. 3.
Polymyxin B Sulphate, *B.P.*			Microbiological.
Tyrothricin, *N.F.*			Microbiological.
Viomycin Sulphate			Microbiological.

* Colorimetric determination of cycloserine.[28]

Colour reagent: Mix equal volumes of a 4 ± 0·5 per cent aqueous solution of sodium nitroprusside (prepared not more than two weeks before use and stored in the dark) and 4N sodium hydroxide; the reagent must be used within fifteen minutes.

Determination: Prepare a solution of the sample in 0·1N sodium hydroxide to contain 25 to 150 μg of cycloserine per ml. Transfer a 1-ml aliquot to a test-tube, add 3 ml of N acetic acid followed by 1·0 ml of the colour reagent, mix and allow to stand at room temperature for ten minutes. Measure the extinction at 625 mμ against a reagent blank and read the cycloserine content from a standard curve prepared by carrying out the procedure on varying amounts of pure cycloserine. (If the extinction is too high to read, repeat the determination using a smaller weight of sample; the colour complex must not be diluted.)

Since this assay is specific for the ring structure of cycloserine, derivatives of cycloserine with the same ring structure can also be determined by this method. Among the compounds that do not interfere are benzylpenicillin, streptomycin, dihydrostreptomycin, bacitracin, chlortetracycline, neomycin, glucose, lactose and sucrose.

† Erythromycin Estolate: Determination of lauryl sulphate.

Dissolve about 0·5 g in 25 ml of dimethylformamide, add 2 drops of a 0·3 per cent solution of thymol blue in methanol and titrate with freshly standardised 0·1N sodium methoxide. 1 ml 0·1N = 0·0002663 g lauryl sulphate.

‡ Griseofulvin—determination in blood by the spectrofluorimetric method of Bedford, Child and Tomich.[29] The only known metabolite, 6-desmethyl-griseofulvin, does not fluoresce and the extraction procedure recommended does not remove fluorescent substances from the blood. More recently, however, it has been shown by the same workers[30] that certain drugs, such as acetylsalicylic acid and quinine, may cause high results. The method is based on extraction of the antibiotic into ether, evaporation of the extract to dryness and solution of the residue in 1 per cent aqueous ethanol. The fluorescence of this solution is compared with that of a standard griseofulvin solution, both solutions being activated at 295 mμ and analysed at 450 mμ.

§ Using *Klebsiella pneumoniæ*, ATCC 10031.

The following antibiotics are also available commercially: amphotericin B, framycetin sulphate, gramicidin, *N.F.*, and kanamycin sulphate. Each of these can be assayed microbiologically for potency by the plate-diffusion method using a suitable medium, organism and pH value in the agar.

1. ALICINO, J. F., *Ind. Eng. Chem., Anal. Edn.*, 1946, **18**, 619.
2. SMITH, E. L., *Analyst*, 1948, **73**, 197.
3. ROYCE, A., BOWLER, C., and SYKES, G., *J. Pharm. Pharmacol.*, 1952, **4**, 904.
4. STOCK, F. G., *Analyst*, 1954, **79**, 662.
5. HISCOX, D. J., *Anal. Chem.*, 1949, **21**, 658.
6. SCUDI, J. V., *J. Biol. Chem.*, 1946, **164**, 183.
7. MADER, W. J., and BUCK, R. R., *Anal. Chem.*, 1949, **21**, 664.
8. BAKER, P. B., DOBSON, F., and MARTIN, A. J. P., *Analyst*, 1950, **75**, 651.
9. WILD, A. M., *J. Appl. Chem.*, 1951, **1**, 329.
10. PARKER, G., and DONEGAN, L., *J. Pharm. Pharmacol.*, 1954, **6**, 167.
11. BOYMOND, P., *Pharm. Acta. Helv.*, 1947, **22**, 353.
12. WOOLFORD, M. H., Jnr., and CHICCARELLI, F. S., *J. Amer. Pharm. Ass., Sci. Edn.*, 1956, **45**, 400.
13. LEVINE, J., GARLOCK, E. A., Jnr., and FISCHBACH, H., *J. Amer. Pharm. Ass., Sci. Edn.*, 1949, **38**, 473.
14. CHICCARELLI, F. S., VAN GIESON, P., and WOOLFORD, M. H., Jnr., *J. Amer. Pharm. Ass., Sci. Edn.*, 1956, **45**, 418.
15. HISCOX, D. J., *J. Amer. Pharm. Ass., Sci. Edn.*, 1951, **40**, 237.
16. CHICCARELLI, F. S., WOOLFORD, M. H., Jnr., and TROMBITAS, R. W., *J.A.O.A.C.*, 1957, **40**, 922.
17. CHICCARELLI, F. S., *J. Amer. Pharm. Ass., Sci. Edn.*, 1959, **48**, 263.
18. MONASTERO, F., MEANS, J. A., GRENFELL, T. C., and HEDGER, F. H., *J. Amer. Pharm. Ass., Sci. Edn.*, 1951, **40**, 241.
19. *Analyst*, 1963, **88**, in the press.
20. YOKOYAMA, F., and CHATTEN, L. G., *J. Amer. Pharm. Ass., Sci. Edn.*, 1958, **47**, 548.
21. ASHTON, G. C., FOSTER, M. C., and FATHERLEY, M., *Analyst*, 1953, **78**, 581.

22. HISCOX, D. J., *Anal. Chem.*, 1951, **23,** 923.
23. LEVINE, J., and FISCHBACH, H., *Antibiotics & Chemotherapy*, 1951, **1,** 59.
24. DUTCHER, J. D., HOSANSKY, N., and SHERMAN, J. H., *Antibiotics & Chemotherapy*, 1953, **3,** 534.
25. MORGAN, J. W., HONIG, A. B., WARREN, A. T., and LEVINE, S., *J. Pharm. Sci.*, 1961, **50,** 668.
26. RICE, E. W., *Anal. Chem.*, 1951, **23,** 1501.
27. PAN, S. C., and DUTCHER, J. D., *Anal. Chem.*, 1956, **28,** 836.
28. JONES, L. R., *Anal. Chem.*, 1956, **28,** 39.
29. BEDFORD, C., CHILD, K. J., and TOMICH, E. G., *Nature*, 1959, **184,** 364.
30. CHILD, K. J., BEDFORD, C., and TOMICH, E. G., *J. Pharm. Pharmacol.*, 1962, **14,** 374.

ANTIHISTAMINES

Most of the antihistamines are salts of organic bases and their determination is generally either by base extraction or non-aqueous titration.

(A) Extraction

(*a*) extract with ether from sodium hydroxide solution, evaporate, dissolve the residue in 2 ml of ethanol and excess of 0·1N hydrochloric acid; titrate with methyl red or screened methyl red as indicator.

(*b*) extract with ether from ammonia solution, evaporate and complete as in (*a*).

TABLE 5

ANTIHISTAMINE	FORMULA	MOL. WT.	ASSAY METHOD	1 ML 0·1N EQUIVALENT
Antazoline Hydrochloride, *B.P.*	$C_{17}H_{19}N_3,HCl$	301·8	A(*c*), B(*a*) or B(*c*)†	0·03018 g
Tablets, *B.P.*			A(*f*)	
Antazoline Methanesulphonate, *B.P.C.*	$C_{17}H_{19}N_3,CH_3SO_3H$	361·5	A(*c*)	0·03615 g
Antazoline Phosphate, *N.F.*	$C_{17}H_{19}N_3,H_3PO_4$	363·4	B(*a*) or B(*d*)	0·03634 g
Carbinoxamine Maleate, *N.F.*	$C_{16}H_{19}ON_2Cl,C_4H_4O_4$	406·9	B(*a*)	0·02034 g
Chlorcyclizine Hydrochloride, *B.P.*	$C_{18}H_{21}N_2Cl,HCl$	337·3	B(*d*) in dioxan	0·01687 g
Tablets, *B.P.*			Total nitrogen	0·01687 g
Chlorothen Citrate, *N.F.*	$C_{14}H_{18}N_3SCl,C_6H_8O_7$	488·0	B(*d*)	0·02440 g
Chlorpheniramine Maleate, *B.P.C.*	$C_{16}H_{19}N_2Cl,C_4H_4O_4$	390·9	B(*d*)	0·01954 g
U.S.P.			B(*a*)	
Cyclizine Hydrochloride, *B.P.C.*	$C_{18}H_{22}N_2,HCl$	302·9	B(*d*)	0·01514 g

TABLE 5 (*contd.*)

ANTIHISTAMINE	FORMULA	MOL. WT.	ASSAY METHOD	1 ML 0·1N EQUIVALENT
Dimenhydrinate, *B.P.C.*	$C_{17}H_{21}ON,C_7H_7O_2N_4Cl$	470·0	A(*d*) for base = for salt.‖	0·02554 g 0·04700 g
Diphenhydramine Hydrochloride, *B.P.*	$C_{17}H_{21}ON,HCl$	291·8	A(*d*) B(*a*)†	0·02918 g
Capsules, *B.P.*			A(*d*)	
Doxylamine Succinate, *U.S.P.*	$C_{17}H_{22}ON_2,C_4H_6O_4$	388·5	U.V.‡	
Meclozine Hydrochloride, *B.P.C.*	$C_{25}H_{27}N_2Cl,2HCl$	463·9	Total nitrogen	0·02319 g
U.S.P.	$C_{25}H_{27}N_2Cl,2HCl,H_2O$	481·9	B(*c*)	
Mepyramine Maleate, *B.P.*	$C_{17}H_{23}ON_3,C_4H_4O_4$	401·5	A(*e*) B(*a*)†	Wt. × 1·407 0·02007 g
Tablets, *B.P.*			A(*a*)*	0·04015 g
Methapyrilene Hydrochloride, *N.F.*	$C_{14}H_{19}N_3S,HCl$	297·9	B(*d*)	0·01489 g
Phenindamine Tartrate, *B.P.*	$C_{19}H_{19}N,C_4H_6O_6$	411·5	B(*b*)§	0·04115 g
U.S.P.			B(*a*)	
Tablets, *B.P.*			B(*b*)*§	
Pheniramine Maleate, *N.F.*	$C_{16}H_{20}N_2,C_4H_4O_4$	356·4	B(*a*)	0·01782 g
Promethazine Hydrochloride *B.P.*	$C_{17}H_{20}N_2S,HCl$	320·9	A(*a*)	0·03209 g
U.S.P.			B(*a*)	
Tablets, *B.P.*			A(*a*)*	
Promethazine Theoclate, *B.P.C.*	$C_{17}H_{20}N_2S,C_7H_7O_2N_4Cl$	499·1	A(*b*) for base = for salt.¶	0·02844 g 0·04991 g
Thenyldiamine Hydrochloride, *N.F.*	$C_{14}H_{19}N_3S,HCl$	297·9	B(*d*)	0·01489 g
Thonzylamine Hydrochloride, *N.F.*	$C_{16}H_{22}ON_4,HCl$	322·8	B(*d*)	0·01614 g
Tripelennamine Hydrochloride, *B.P.*	$C_{16}H_{21}N_3,HCl$	291·8	B(*a*)	0·01459 g
Tripelennamine Citrate, *U.S.P.*	$C_{16}H_{21}N_3,C_6H_8O_7$	447·5	B(*a*)	0·02238 g
Triprolidine Hydrochloride, *B.P.C.*	$C_{19}H_{22}N_2,HCl,H_2O$	332·9	B(*a*)	0·01574 g anhyd.

* After solution in dilute hydrochloric acid.
† Not official, but recommended.
‡ Measure extinction in comparison with standard.
§ After extraction with chloroform from sodium carbonate solution.
‖ The theoclic acid may be determined separately as follows:

To a mixture of 50 ml of water, 3 ml of dilute ammonia solution and 6 ml of 10 per cent ammonium nitrate solution add 0·8 g of sample, warm on a water-bath for five minutes and add 25 ml of 0·1N silver nitrate. Warm for fifteen minutes, shaking frequently, cool, dilute to 200 ml with water and allow to stand for sixteen hours. Filter, wash the residue with water, neutralise the combined filtrate and washings to litmus paper with concentrated nitric acid and add 3 ml of the acid in excess. Titrate the excess silver nitrate with 0·1N ammonium thiocyanate using ferric alum as indicator. 1 ml 0·1N silver nitrate = 0·02146 g $C_7H_7O_2N_4Cl$.

¶ The theoclic acid may be determined separately by diluting the combined aqueous solution and washings from A(*b*) to 50 ml with water, adding 6 ml of 10 per cent ammonium nitrate and completing as in ‖ from the words 'warm on a water-bath for five minutes . . .'.

(*c*) extract with chloroform from sodium hydroxide solution, evaporate and complete as in (*a*).
(*d*) dissolve in sodium chloride solution and assay as in (*a*).
(*e*) extract with ether from sodium hydroxide solution, evaporate and weigh the base.
(*f*) extract with ether from sodium hydroxide solution, wash the ether extracts free from alkali, then extract with excess of 0·1N hydrochloric acid and titrate back with 0·1N sodium hydroxide using methyl red as indicator.

Any of these methods may be used for the other antihistamines, the choice being personal preference.

(B) Non-aqueous titration with 0·1N perchloric acid using (*a*) crystal violet (*b*) oracet blue B (*c*) quinaldine red (*d*) potentiometric end-point (see pp. 792 and 864).

The official methods of analysis of antihistamines and *B.P.* or *B.P.C.* preparations of them can be summarised conveniently in tabulated form. The letters in the table denoting method of determination refer to those outlined above.

ANTIMONY

Sb At. Wt. 121·75

In those salts of the metal that are used pharmaceutically, antimony is present in the trivalent state and may be determined either by oxidation with iodine or polarographically.

Dissolve from 0·5 to 2 g of the substance in water or dilute hydrochloric acid, add about 5 g of sodium potassium tartrate to keep antimony in solution and then a slight excess of sodium bicarbonate or 2 g of borax. Titrate at once with 0·1N iodine. 1 ml 0·1N = 0·007288 g Sb_2O_3.

Trivalent antimony is liberated from organic and inorganic complexes when these are treated with M hydrochloric acid and the resulting solution is then suitable for the direct polarographic determination of the element. The base electrolyte recommended by Page and Robinson[1] consists of M hydrochloric acid containing 0·1 per cent gelatin as a maximum suppressor. In pharmaceutical samples containing antimony potassium tartrate, antimony has been determined by diluting suitably into a base electrolyte of 1·25N hydrochloric acid with methyl red as a maximum suppressor. Under these conditions the reduction wave of the antimony is at −0·15V versus the S.C.E.

A general method for the estimation of antimony, either in organic combination or as an inorganic salt, is the bromate titration method. It is preferable to the method of titration with iodine in the presence of bicarbonate unless the material being estimated is a fairly pure salt, since the solution being titrated may be coloured somewhat and there is often difficulty in the use of starch as indicator. The bromate method is applicable in the presence of arsenic.

Destruction of organic matter may be obtained by wet combustion (p. 851), care being taken always to have nitric acid present so long as organic matter remains undestroyed and not to heat the sulphuric acid above the 'just-fuming' stage, otherwise antimony compounds may be volatilised. To the sulphuric acid solution obtained, add 30 ml of 1 : 1 hydrochloric acid and boil for half a minute, cool somewhat, dilute to 200 ml and saturate with hydrogen sulphide while still warm. To effect solution of inorganic material, dissolve in concentrated hydrochloric acid and if completely dissolved reduce and titrate as below; if any insoluble matter remains, fuse with sodium peroxide and sodium carbonate, extract with hydrochloric acid and precipitate the antimony in the bulked hydrochloric acid solutions with hydrogen sulphide. Dissolve the sulphide precipitate obtained, from either the organic or inorganic material, in 1 : 1 hydrochloric acid containing potassium chlorate (this is preferable to bromine, which is completely expelled only with difficulty), add 100 ml of concentrated hydrochloric acid and boil until free from chlorine. Cool, reduce the antimony by the addition of 5 to 10 g of sodium sulphite, reduce to 60 ml by boiling (arsenic is volatilised by this procedure), rinse down with warm water, add 20 ml of concentrated hydrochloric acid, boil and titrate with 0·1N bromine, using at first 2 drops of methyl orange as indicator. Titrate to a disappearance of colour, add a further drop of indicator, continue the titration cautiously with vigorous stirring and finally add a further drop to check completion of the reaction. 1 ml 0·1N = 0·006088 g Sb.

Traces of antimony are detected and estimated by the colorimetric method of Clarke.[2] If necessary organic matter may be destroyed by the method of Bamford,[3] which prevents appreciable loss by volatilisation and leaves the antimony in hydrochloric acid solution for the Reinsch method of isolation.

Cut up finely a weighed sample of the material for examination and mix it in a silica basin with sufficient magnesium oxide to give a definitely alkaline reaction. Then cover with a saturated solution of magnesium nitrate. Heat the mixture on a sand-bath, with frequent stirring, until the material has dried and charred. Crush up the charred mass and heat strongly, if necessary, until the ash is quite white, moisten the ash, when cold, with water and add sufficient hydrochloric acid to dissolve the magnesium oxide and give a definitely acid reaction.

Clarke's method[2] was worked out for small amounts of antimony in tin but the method is equally applicable to its determination in other substances.

ANTIMONY

To a solution containing the antimony in 1 : 1 hydrochloric acid, add about 2 g of oxalic acid and heat to boiling, add 1 g of sodium hypophosphite and boil the solution for ten minutes (Burns[4]). Cool, add a strip of copper foil which has been cleaned by warming in dilute nitric acid (sp. gr. 1·2) and well washed. Continue the boiling for one and a half to two hours; wash the copper strip with warm 5 per cent hydrochloric acid and then with water. Dissolve the deposit from the strip by covering it with water, adding about 1 g of sodium peroxide and warming. Pour off the solution from the strip and wash the latter with water. Pass hydrogen sulphide into the solution for a short time and set aside on a water-bath until the small precipitate of copper sulphide has coagulated. Filter, washing the paper with a dilute solution of ammonium nitrate or sodium sulphate. To the filtrate add 5 ml of concentrated sulphuric acid and after the addition of a few drops of nitric acid near the end stage, evaporate the solution just to fuming point; after cooling add 15 ml of water, when a clear solution should be obtained. Determine the antimony colorimetrically in this approximately 20 ml of solution as follows: Put the reagents into a 100-ml Nessler cylinder in the order given: 10 ml of 1 per cent gum acacia, 5 ml of 20 per cent potassium iodide, 1 ml of 10 per cent aqueous pyridine, 1 ml of a dilute solution of sulphur dioxide (one-tenth saturated) and 60 ml of cold 1 : 3 sulphuric acid. Then add the solution obtained as described above, rinsing the beaker with not more than 5 ml of water. Run standard antimony solution (0·0001 g/ml) into another Nessler cylinder containing similar quantities of reagents (except that 80 ml of 1 : 3 sulphuric acid are used instead of 60 ml) until the colours match after the solution has been well stirred and a final adjustment has been made to make the volumes in the Nessler cylinders equal.

Comparison is made by viewing the cylinders vertically over a white tile inclined at an angle to act as a light reflector. Not more than 10 ml of standard should be required; if the solution contains too much antimony for accurate comparison or a turbidity is produced, the procedure is repeated with an aliquot portion of this turbid solution; the turbidity disappears and the colour can be matched against a fresh standard. The standard antimony solution contains 0·2668 g of antimony potassium tartrate in 1 litre of 10 per cent sulphuric acid.

Rhodamine B has been successfully used for the colorimetric determination of traces of antimony. The following method for biological materials is by Maren[5] with small modifications by Freedman;[6] the amount of sulphuric acid used in the digestion should be constant.

To not more than 15 g of blood or tissue, or 50 ml of urine or plasma in a Kjeldahl flask, add 5 ml of concentrated nitric acid, 20 ml of 18N sulphuric acid, a few glass beads and one drop of secondary octyl alcohol, and allow the digestion to start spontaneously. Heat the flask cautiously until the vigorous reaction is over, and then increase the heat. If charring occurs, add 1 or 2 ml of nitric acid to the cooled digest and continue to heat, repeating this operation as often as may be necessary. When no further charring is evident, increase the heat. If iron is present the solution will be yellow when hot but colourless, with frequently a granular precipitate, when cold. When the cooled solution is colourless or only slightly yellow and no further charring occurs, add 2 drops of perchloric acid and heat strongly until fumes of sulphur trioxide are evolved. If the liquid chars or becomes yellow, add more nitric acid and repeat the treatment with perchloric acid. Finally add 3 ml of water and heat again to fuming point.

Immerse the flask in a cold water-bath and add 5 ml of 6N hydrochloric acid. Add 8 ml of 3N phosphoric acid and sufficient solid sodium pyrophosphate to remove any yellow colour due to iron. Add 5 ml of 0·02 per cent rhodamine B solution, shake the flask and cool. Do not interrupt the procedure at any point after addition of the phosphoric acid. Rinse the liquid into a separating funnel with 10 ml of benzene and shake for three minutes.

Separate the aqueous layer and collect the benzene layer, which is coloured red if any antimony is present, in a test-tube, and set it aside for several minutes for water to separate. Ensure complete removal of the antimony by extraction with a further 10 ml of benzene. Place 6 to 8 ml in a 1-cm cell and read the colour intensity using a green filter, Spectrum green 604.

To construct a standard reference curve add incremental values from 0 to 40 μg of antimony to 5 ml of sulphuric acid, treat this with nitric and perchloric acid, and continue in the manner already described. To prepare the standard antimony solution, dissolve 0·2668 g of antimony potassium tartrate in 10 per cent sulphuric acid and make up to 1 litre with the acid. This solution contains 100 μg of antimony per ml. Dilute as required to prepare working standards of 10 and 1 μg per ml.

Methylfluorone (methyltrihydroxyfluorone) is a useful reagent for the determination of traces of antimony. For estimation in the presence of interfering substances the antimony is separated as gaseous stibine[7] and collected in an absorbing solution consisting of methylfluorone in aqueous silver sulphate solution. It is important that each standard be distilled into silver sulphate solution in a similar manner to the test, since the intensity of colour obtained from a given quantity of antimony under these conditions is less than that derived by the addition of antimony directly to the absorption solution.

This procedure has been found useful for the determination of antimony in titanium dioxide and for its estimation in various organic substances; a preliminary wet combustion of organic materials is necessary.

Transfer 100 ml of cold solution containing 15 per cent v/v of sulphuric acid to an eight-ounce wide-mouthed reagent bottle fitted with a rubber stopper carrying a delivery tube. (The delivery tube is fitted with a rolled lead acetate paper inserted between the bottle and the first bend to prevent spray being carried over; the delivery end is fitted with a fine detachable drawn out jet which reaches to within 1 cm of the bottom of an absorption vessel such as a 50-ml Nessler cylinder.) Add 10 g of granulated zinc, stopper, and pass the generated gas through an absorption solution for at least ninety minutes (preferably overnight) at room temperature and preferably in the dark. The absorption solution is prepared by adding to 25 ml of a 0·2 per cent aqueous solution of silver sulphate, in the order shown, 2 ml of starch mucilage, 0·5 ml of a 0·01 per cent solution of tartaric acid, 0·25 ml of N sulphuric acid, and 1 ml of a 0·01 per cent solution of methylfluorone in 95 per cent ethanol containing 0·2 per cent v/v of sulphuric acid. Compare any colour produced in the absorption solution with standards prepared by treating suitable aliquots of a standard antimony solution in a similar manner (0·02668 g antimony potassium tartrate in 100 ml of water; 1 ml diluted to 100 ml = 0·001 mg Sb per ml). The procedure is most suitable for the range 25 to 200 p.p.m. of antimony.

ANTIMONY SALTS

The tartrated antimony salts are estimated by the iodine titration method given on p. 78, after dissolving about 0·5 g in water. **Antimony potassium tartrate,** $C_4H_4O_7SbK$, Mol. Wt. 324·9, 1 ml 0·1N = 0·01625 g; **antimony sodium tartrate,** $C_4H_4O_7SbNa$, Mol. Wt. 308·8, 1 ml 0·1N = 0·01544 g.

Sodium antimonylgluconate is a trivalent antimony derivative. The total antimony is determined after wet combustion by reduction with potassium iodide in the presence of tartaric acid, boiling off the iodine completely, making alkaline with sodium hydroxide, then just acid with dilute sulphuric acid, and titrating in bicarbonate solution with 0·05N iodine. 1 ml = 0·003044 g Sb. Trivalent antimony can be determined polarographically as described above directly on the material.

Sodium stibogluconate is a pentavalent antimony compound and the antimony is determined as for the total antimony in sodium antimonylgluconate.

Stibophen, $C_{12}H_4O_{16}S_4SbNa_5,7H_2O$, Mol. Wt. 895·3, is pentasodium antimony biscatechol-3,5-disulphonate.

The trivalent antimony in this preparation can be determined without destruction of organic matter by dissolving about 0·5 g in dilute acetic acid, adding an excess of 0·05N iodine and titrating back with thiosulphate after standing for five minutes. 1 ml 0·05N = 0·003044 g trivalent Sb.

Determination of sulphur has been tried by the flask combustion method, with low results and corrosion of the platinum gauze.

Injection of Stibophen, *B.P.* Contains 6·4 per cent w/v of stibophen with sodium acid phosphate in water for injection.

The presence of sodium metabisulphite in certain formulations interferes with the determination of trivalent antimony by iodine titration but this difficulty may be overcome by the addition of 3 ml of formaldehyde to the solution acidified with hydrochloric acid and allowing to stand for five minutes before titration.

1 Page, J. E., and Robinson, F. A., *J. Soc. Chem. Ind.*, 1942, **61**, 93.
2. Clarke, S. G., *Analyst*, 1928, **53**, 373.
3. Bamford, F., *Analyst*, 1934, **59**, 101.
4. Burns, R. H., *Analyst*, 1935, **60**, 220.

5. MAREN, T. H., *Anal. Chem.*, 1947, **19,** 487.
6. FREEDMAN, L. D., *Anal. Chem.*, 1947, **19,** 502.
7. HANDS, J. J. H., and YARDLEY, J. T., Organic Reagents for Metals, Vol. 1, Hopkin & Williams Ltd., 5th Edn. 1955, p. 109.

ARSENIC

As At. Wt. 74·92

If the arsenic is present in the trivalent form and sufficient is present, say 0·05 to 0·10 g as As_2O_3, the iodine oxidation method of determination may be employed.

> To a slightly acid solution (excess of acid or alkali being neutralised to phenolphthalein) add 2 g of sodium bicarbonate, to neutralise the hydriodic acid liberated during the titration, and titrate with 0·1N iodine. 1 ml 0·1N = 0·004945 g As_2O_3.

Unless the arsenic solution is pure and free from other iodine absorbing substances, the method is unreliable. **Arsenic trioxide,** As_2O_3, Mol. Wt. 197·8, 1 ml 0·1N = 0·004945 g, is assayed after solution in dilute sodium hydroxide and neutralisation with N hydrochloric acid. In this case, Ferrey[1] found the use of sodium phosphate gave more consistent results than sodium bicarbonate.

Another suitable method for the determination of arsenious compounds is by iodate titration; this is particularly useful for the determination of arsenic isolated by hydrochloric acid distillation, the amount of mineral acid being adjusted to be equivalent to about 50 per cent of strong acid before titration. The method is described in detail under Halogen Acids, p. 292. 1 ml 0·05M iodate = 0·009895 g As_2O_3.

If arsenic has to be freed from interfering substances before estimation, use is made of the volatility of its chloride at low temperatures as compared with other metallic chlorides. The Analytical Methods Committee of the *S.A.C.*[2] recommends the distillation process described below; it stresses the importance of using the relative quantities that are specified, in order to obtain success. In the presence of organic matter it is generally necessary to resort to destructive wet oxidation to bring the material into a suitable condition in which the arsenic can be satisfactorily determined. General Methods for Destruction of Organic Matter are given in Appendix XI, p. 851, and of these Methods of Wet Decomposition (1)A, (1)B, (1)C and (1)D with continuation (1)(b)1 are suitable for use in the determination of arsenic, the particular method being chosen to suit the type of sample to be analysed. In no circumstances should more than 10 ml of concentrated sulphuric acid be used.

The essential details for distillation are as follows. If less than 8 to 10 ml of sulphuric acid has been used in the wet decomposition it should be supplemented before continuing.

If necessary, transfer the colourless liquid obtained by wet oxidation to the flask of a distillation apparatus, consisting of a 100-ml or 200-ml Kjeldahl flask of resistance glass or silica, with a ground-in condenser, into which has been blown a tap funnel as shown in Fig. 1 (it is an advantage to have the condenser interchangeable with the condensing extension to the decomposition flask so that the arsenic can be distilled from the same flask in which the wet decomposition was carried out).

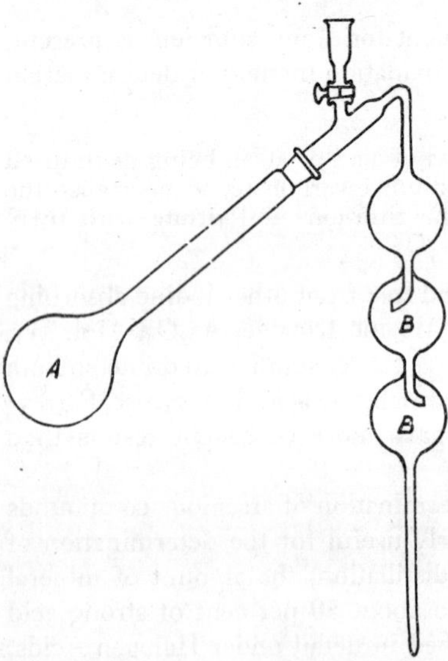

FIG. 1

Kjeldahl flask. Flask A has a capacity of 100 or 200 ml and a neck length of 7 to 8 inches; bulbs B of condenser are of 25-ml capacity, total length of condenser being 18 to 20 inches. The unlettered bulb should be of 25-ml capacity for the three-bulb type of condenser or should be omitted in the two-bulb version.

Without inserting the condensing arm evaporate the solution to fuming and then allow to cool. Add 7 ml of water, cool, add 5 g of a mixture made up in the following proportions, 5 g of sodium chloride, 0·5 g of hydrazine sulphate, and 0·02 g of potassium bromide (this can be made up in bulk and will keep indefinitely in a stoppered bottle), avoiding contamination of the ground portion of the neck of the flask, and fit the condenser, moistening the joint with water to prevent leakage. Clamp the apparatus so that the condenser is vertical, with its tip reaching just short of the bottom of a 25-ml measuring cylinder containing 15 ml of water, which is cooled in ice and water. Add 10 ml of concentrated hydrochloric acid to the contents of the flask through the tap funnel, and carefully close the tap.

Heat the flask with a micro-burner at a rate such that the contents are brought to boiling in not less than thirty minutes. After the condenser has become full of steam, continue to heat the flask so that the distillation proceeds smoothly for three to five minutes for small amounts or longer, until the volume is reduced by about half, for appreciable amounts of arsenic. During the whole of this procedure, and particularly at the moment when the steam reaches the cold water in the receiver, care should be taken to prevent a suck back. The distillation must not be taken too far, *i.e.* fumes of sulphur trioxide must not appear. When the distillation is complete open the tap, remove the burner, and disconnect the condenser. Wash down the condenser once with a few millilitres of water, collecting the washings in the cylinder. Evaporate the distillate to dryness on a water-bath, dissolve the residue by warming in 3 ml of concentrated sulphuric acid and dilute to 25 ml with water. Determine the arsenic in this solution by a suitable method dependent on the quantity likely to be present. If present in sufficient amount this may be done by titration with 0·1N iodine in sodium bicarbonate solution or by 0·05M iodate, as already described.

For smaller quantities of arsenic, a method suitable for filling in the gap between ordinary titration or precipitation and stain methods for traces is that due to Ramberg (Cox[3]), by titration with dilute potassium bromate solution. The method is suitable for quantities down to 0·01 mg of arsenious oxide.

Destroy any organic matter by the recommended method, not allowing the atmosphere in the flask to be free from red fumes whilst organic matter remains; cool, and remove nitrous fumes by adding 25 ml of saturated ammonium oxalate solution and reboiling until white fumes appear. After cooling, add 20 ml of water, 50 ml of concentrated hydrochloric acid, 2 g of ferrous sulphate and 10 to 15 mg of potassium bromide. If any yellow or brown colour appears at this stage, nitrogen acids are present and the experiment must be rejected. Distil the mixture in the special all-glass apparatus described above, the distillate being collected in 150 ml of water. Distil a volume of 20 to 25 ml in ten minutes. To the distillate add 1 drop of 1 : 5,000 methyl orange solution and then titrate slowly at a temperature of 35° to 40° with potassium bromate solution (0·1485 g per litre; 1 ml = 0·20 mg As). The end-point is quite sharp and is reached when the red colour of the methyl orange is discharged. Add the bromate solution a drop at a time towards the end of the titration. Apply a correction for the blank on the reagents; this should not exceed 0·2 to 0·3 ml.

The blank determination must be made since even the number of drops of methyl orange used in the titration will affect the results considerably —presumably the ethanol of the reagent being oxidised by the bromine. Quinoline yellow (4 drops of a 0·5 per cent aqueous solution) has been found satisfactory by Belcher[4] as a reversible indicator in bromometric titrations.

Evans' method[5] for the determination of small quantities (2 to 5 mg) of arsenic by reduction to metal is particularly useful for preparations where relatively large amounts of iron are present. It is preferable not to destroy the organic matter as it does not interfere when in moderate quantities. The following procedure is a slight modification of the original method:

Dissolve an amount of material equivalent to about 4 mg of arsenic in equal parts of concentrated hydrochloric acid and water, filter, if necessary, through asbestos in a Gooch crucible, washing with 1 : 1 hydrochloric acid to make the total volume 140 ml. Add 12 g of sodium hypophosphite and 0·5 g of copper sulphate and boil gently under an air reflux condenser for fifteen minutes. Cool somewhat and filter through a small Gooch crucible, using a minimum of asbestos. Wash successively with 50 ml of 1 in 4 hydrochloric acid containing 2·5 per cent of sodium hypophosphite and 25 ml of 5 per cent ammonium chloride solution. Then hold the crucible over a large beaker and allow 0·02N iodine to drip slowly into it from a burette, stirring the asbestos with a glass rod to break up the mat, until 20 ml have been added. Place the crucible in the beaker and allow to stand for three minutes. Remove the Gooch crucible and wash down with 200 ml of water (previously blued with a crystal of potassium iodide, starch solution and 0·02N iodine). Add 2 g of sodium bicarbonate and 10 ml of 0·02N arsenic in slightly acid solution (or sufficient to discharge the colour). Continue the titration with 0·02N iodine. A blank determination is necessary and the process must be carried through without interruption. 1 ml 0·02N iodine = 0·0003957 g As_2O_3.

An unsatisfactory feature in the method is the relatively slow rate of solution of arsenic in dilute iodine solution; Haslam and Wilkinson[6] showed that the titration technique was unnecessarily complicated. The precipitated arsenic can be filtered onto a medium containing a large proportion of oxycellulose and that, after addition of an excess of standard iodine to the arsenic-oxycellulose mixture, the excess can be titrated directly with standard arsenite solution. The filtering medium is prepared by digesting about twenty 11-cm Whatman No. 40 filter papers on a water-bath for about four hours with 400 ml of water containing 4 ml of concentrated hydrochloric acid and 20 ml of saturated bromine water; the pulped material thus prepared is stored in a bottle and small amounts of it are washed thoroughly with water before use in the filtration of precipitated arsenic. To keep the precipitated arsenic in a finely-divided condition so that it will readily dissolve in the iodine solution, it is better to mix a little of the well-washed filter paper pulp with the precipitate. The washed arsenic precipitate and filter paper pulp are transferred to a glass-stoppered bottle with 50 ml of water and thoroughly disintegrated before adding successively 2 g of potassium iodide, 2 g of sodium bicarbonate and excess of 0·01N iodine. After thoroughly shaking to ensure complete solution of the precipitate the excess is titrated with 0·01N sodium arsenite. The end-point, which is that at which the yellow of the iodine changes to the white of the pulp, is quite sharp.

Traces of arsenic may be determined either by the molybdenum blue or Gutzeit methods. For determination of arsenic contents from 1·5 to 15 μg in the sample taken the molybdenum blue method is recommended by the Analytical Methods Committee of the *S.A.C.*,[2] the details are as follows:

Destroy any organic matter by the recommended method. If the total heavy metal content of the test solution exceeds 1,000 μg or if an excessive amount of insoluble material is present in the test solution distil the arsenic as described above.

(*a*) If the distillation procedure has not been carried out, dilute the solution from the destruction of organic matter with 15 ml of water, boil gently for a few minutes, cool to about 70°, add 10 ml of concentrated hydrochloric acid, and allow to cool. Transfer the solution to a

100-ml conical flask, filtering if the solution is not clear and rinsing in with the minimum amount of water.

(*b*) If the distillation procedure has been carried out, transfer the distillate, without further addition of hydrochloric acid, to a 100-ml conical flask, rinsing in with the minimum amount of water.

Warm the solution from (*a*) or (*b*) to about 40°, add 2 ml of thioglycollic acid solution (12 g of 90 per cent v/v thioglycollic acid diluted to 100 ml with water), mix well and set aside to cool for fifteen minutes. Then cool the solution more rapidly (*e.g.* in a bath of ice and water) to room temperature, add 1 ml of potassium iodide-ascorbic acid solution (15 g of potassium iodide and 2·5 g of ascorbic acid dissolved in sufficient water to produce 100 ml), wash down the sides of the flask with a few millilitres of water, and mix carefully. Transfer the solution to a 100-ml calibrated separating funnel containing a few millilitres of chloroform, washing out the flask with several small portions of water. The volume of the solution at this stage should be 45 to 50 ml.

Add 5 ml of dithiocarbamate reagent (1 g of pure crystalline diethylammonium diethyldithiocarbamate dissolved in 100 ml of redistilled or analytical reagent grade chloroform) shake vigorously for forty seconds, remove the stopper, and wash it with a few drops of chloroform. Allow the layers to separate, and then run the lower layer into a clean 25-ml separating funnel, taking care not to allow any of the aqueous layer to enter the tap of the first funnel. Wash the aqueous layer twice with about 0·5 ml of chloroform, without mixing, and add the washings to the main extract. Extract the aqueous layer with a further 2-ml portion of dithiocarbamate reagent, shaking for thirty seconds, and allow the layers to separate. Run the chloroform layer into the second funnel, washing twice with 0·5 ml of chloroform, as before, and adding the washings to the main extract. Reject the aqueous layer.

Add 10 ml of N sulphuric acid to the combined extracts, shake for five seconds, and allow the layers to separate. Run the chloroform layer into a 50-ml conical flask, wash the sulphuric acid layer with two small portions of chloroform, without mixing, and add the washings to the chloroform solution in the flask. During this operation care must be taken not to allow any of the aqueous layer to enter the tap of the funnel.

Add 2·0 (±0·02) ml of acid molybdate solution (for preparation see below), measured accurately from a tube pipette, to the chloroform solution, close the mouth of the flask with a glass bulb, and evaporate the chloroform on a boiling water-bath, conducting the evaporation slowly and carefully so that as little as possible of the acid residue is sprayed up the sides of the flask. When the chloroform has been removed, transfer the flask to a hot-plate, and evaporate until fumes of perchloric acid appear, accompanied by a sudden reaction. Continue to heat for about one minute (not longer), allow to cool, and remove the glass bulb, washing it with a few drops of water. Evaporate the contents of the flask just to fuming again, without the glass bulb in position. All traces of organic matter should have disappeared by this stage.

Insert into the flask a 'cold finger' condenser consisting of a small test-tube with a flanged mouth, fitting loosely in position, the bottom being about 10 to 15 mm from the bottom of the flask, filled almost to the brim with cold water; the outside of the condenser must be clean and dry. Place the flask on the hot-plate (a hot-plate with a surface temperature of approximately 250° is suitable for this operation), heat for ten minutes at a temperature such that a 'blanket' of fumes about half fills the flask and the temperature of the water in the condenser rises to about 90° (±5°) at the end of the ten-minute heating period. Then allow the solution to cool.

For determination of arsenic wash down the condenser and the sides of the flask with 7·0 ml of N sulphuric acid and then with 2·0 ml of water (use a tube pipette for both additions). Close the flask with a glass bulb, and boil until the total volume is reduced to 6 or 7 ml and free chlorine has been removed. Cool the solution, which should be clear and colourless at this stage, add 1·0 ml of a 0·030 per cent w/v solution of hydrazine sulphate in water, mix, and drain the flask into a stoppered 10-ml calibrated cylinder or flask, rinsing the conical flask with 1 or 2 millilitres of water and using the washings to dilute the solution to the 10-ml mark. Mix thoroughly by shaking, and return the solution to the 50-ml conical flask. Close the mouth of the flask with a glass bulb, and heat the flask on a boiling water-bath for fifteen minutes. Remove the flask from the bath, and allow to cool for thirty minutes. If any fading due to the presence of excess of chlorine is observed, the solution should be re-boiled and the reduction with hydrazine sulphate repeated.

Measure the extinction of the test solution at 840 mμ using a spectrophotometer and 2-cm cells with, in the comparison cell, a blank solution prepared in exactly the same way as the test solution but omitting the sample. As a check on the procedure, the extinction of the blank solution measured against a solution consisting of 2 ml of the acid molybdate solution and 8 ml of N sulphuric acid should be 0·0 to 0·05 measured on the spectrophotometer, a 2-cm cell being used at a wavelength of 840 mμ. The use of specially purified reagents reduces the blank considerably.

Read the number of micrograms of arsenic equivalent to the observed extinction from the calibration graph established as described below.

For preparation of calibration graph introduce 0, 0·2, 0·5, 1·0, 1·5, and 2·0 ml of standard arsenic solution (1 ml = 10 μg As freshly prepared by diluting 10 ml of strong arsenic solution to 1 litre; strong arsenic solution contains 0·417 g $Na_2HAsO_4,7H_2O$ per 100 ml) into respective 50-ml conical flasks and add to each 2·0 ml of acid molybdate solution and 7 ml of N sulphuric acid. Mix well, and heat the flasks on a hot-plate until the volume has been reduced to 5 to 6 ml. Cool the solutions, to each add 1·0 ml of a 0·030 per cent w/v solution of hydrazine sulphate in water, mix, and drain the flasks into 10-ml stoppered cylinders, rinsing the flasks with a small amount of water, and use the washings to dilute the main solutions to the 10-ml mark. Mix thoroughly, and return each solution to its original 50-ml conical flask. Close the mouth of each flask with a glass bulb, and heat the flasks on a boiling water-bath for fifteen minutes; then allow them to cool for thirty minutes. Measure the extinction of each solution in turn against the first solution (containing no added arsenic) in a spectrophotometer at 840 mμ, a 2-cm cell being used. Construct a graph relating the extinction value to the number of micrograms of arsenic.

Acid molybdate solution. Mix exactly 250 ml of 10N sulphuric acid (accurately standardised) with exactly 250 ml of a 7 per cent w/v solution of ammonium molybdate, $(NH_4)_6Mo_7O_{24},4H_2O$, in water. Filter into a 1-litre graduated flask, washing the filter with water, add exactly 250 ml of 4N perchloric acid (accurately standardised) and dilute to 1 litre at 20° with water. Store in a polythene bottle.

The molybdenum-blue method may be extended for determination of amounts of arsenic down to 0·5 μg (as As) if the reagents are specially purified by extraction with diethylammonium diethyldithiocarbamate solution before use.

In the opinion of the Analytical Methods Committee of the *S.A.C.*[2] the molybdenum-blue method is considered to have inherent advantages over the Gutzeit method, which may be regarded as an estimation rather than a determination, since it depends on the evaluation of the intensity of a stain on a test-paper and the judgments of individual analysts may differ slightly. Nevertheless, within this limitation and provided that the details of the method are strictly observed, the Gutzeit method is adequate in many circumstances, particularly when it is necessary to ascertain whether or not an arsenic content exceeds a certain limit. It is also less intricate and time-consuming than the molybdenum-blue method.

The modification of the Gutzeit method recommended is the following:

The Gutzeit apparatus consists of a wide-mouthed bottle of 120-ml capacity, closed by a rubber bung through which passes a glass tube. This tube has a total length of 200 mm and an internal diameter of exactly 4·0 mm (external diameter about 5·5 mm) and is drawn out at the lower end to a diameter of about 2 mm. A hole about 3 mm in diameter is blown in the side near the constricted part. The tube passes through the bung so that, when it is inserted in the bottle containing 70 ml of liquid, the constricted end is above the surface of the liquid and the hole is below the bottom of the bung. The tube has a shallow projection, 0·4 to 0·5 mm thick, at its upper end, which fits into a slight depression in a cap consisting of a short tube of the same internal diameter as the lower tube. The contacting edges of the two tubes are flanged and ground smooth at right angles to the tube so as to fit closely. The short upper tube has a grooved top, and the lower tube two projections, in order that the upper tube may be secured to the lower by means of a rubber band. The device for holding the test-paper disc is shown in detail in Fig. 2.

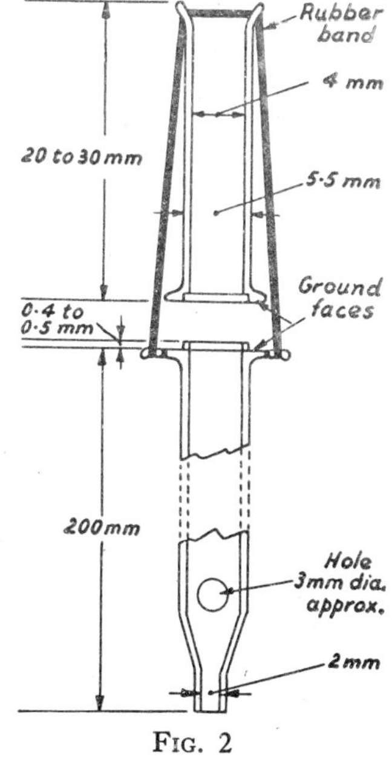

FIG. 2

Destroy the organic matter by the recommended method and carry out the distillation procedure described previously. Dilute the distillate to 50 ml in a graduated flask and mix. Pack the glass tube of the apparatus lightly with cotton wool (previously moistened with a 10 per cent w/v solution of lead acetate in water and dried) so that the upper surface of the cotton wool is 25 to 30 mm below the top of the tube. Place a piece of mercuric chloride paper (filter paper, similar in substance and texture to a Whatman No. 1 filter paper, that has been soaked in a saturated aqueous solution of mercuric chloride, dried in a warm atmosphere without exposure to daylight and stored in the dark until required) against the ground end of this tube with the smooth face of the filter paper downwards to form a diaphragm between it and the upper tube, and fasten the tubes together by means of the rubber band.

Alternatively any other method of attaching the mercuric chloride paper may be used provided that the whole of the evolved gas passes through the paper, that the portion of the paper in contact with the gas is a circle 4·0 mm in diameter, and the paper is protected from sunlight during the test.

If the expected arsenic content of the test solution is more than 5 μg, mix an aliquot (not more than 25 ml) of the test solution such as would contain from 2 to 5 μg of arsenic with concentrated hydrochloric acid in the proportions—

$$x \text{ ml of sample solution} : \left(8 - \frac{16x}{50}\right) \text{ ml of hydrochloric acid}$$

Dilute the solution to 60 ml with water, and add 1 ml of hydrochloric acid-stannous chloride reagent (see below) and 1 g of potassium iodide.

If the expected arsenic content of the test solution is 5 μg or less, mix the whole of the test solution with 1 ml of hydrochloric acid-stannous chloride reagent and 1 g of potassium iodide, and dilute to 60 ml with water.

At the same time add 1 ml of hydrochloric acid-stannous chloride reagent and 1 g of potassium iodide to a blank solution prepared in exactly the same way as the test solution but omitting the sample. (This blank test must be made to ensure that the apparatus and all the reagents give no visible stain.)

Transfer the diluted test and blank solutions to separate wide-mouthed bottles and add 10 g of zinc (zinc pellets containing 0·06 per cent of copper, or granulated zinc containing 0·01 to 0·02 per cent of copper) to each. Immediately place the prepared glass tubes in position, protecting them from sunlight throughout the remainder of the test. Allow the reaction to proceed without the application of external heat for fifteen minutes, and then transfer the bottles to a water-bath maintained at 35° to 40° for thirty minutes.

Compare in normal daylight the stain produced on the mercuric chloride paper with a series of freshly made standard stains prepared by adding known amounts of standard arsenic solution (1 ml = 5 μg As, freshly prepared by diluting 1 ml of strong solution to 100 ml with water; strong arsenic solution contains 0·066 g of As_2O_3 dissolved in 50 ml of arsenic-free concentrated hydrochloric acid and diluted to 100 ml) to tests carried out under the same conditions as are applied to the sample. A suitable range for the series of standard stains is 0·5 to 5·0 μg of arsenic.

Stannous chloride solution. Dissolve 65 g of stannous chloride, $SnCl_2$, $2H_2O$, in 180 ml of water and 200 ml of concentrated hydrochloric acid, sp. gr. 1·18. Boil the solution until its volume has been reduced to 200 ml, cool, filter through a fine-grained filter paper, and keep in a well stoppered bottle.

This solution must comply with the following test:

To 10 ml add 8 ml of water and 8 ml of arsenic-free concentrated hydrochloric acid, and distil 16 ml. To the distillate add 50 ml of water and 2 drops of the stannous chloride solution, and apply the general test; the stain produced must not be deeper than a 1-ml standard stain, showing that the proportion of arsenic present does not exceed 0·5 p.p.m.

*Hydrochloric acid-stannous chloride reagent.** Mix 10 ml of the above stannous chloride solution with 90 ml of arsenic-free concentrated hydrochloric acid.

The separation of arsenic by distillation has not been considered necessary by the *B.P.* or *B.P.C.* for most of the official substances and a simplified procedure is used. It is adequately explained with details and modifications for all those substances required to pass the limit test in the *B.P.* Appendix VI. It is doubtful whether the official test does determine the actual amount in many cases. With the tendency to limit the test to only a few chemicals likely to retain traces in commercial practice, a full procedure would seem desirable.

In an examination of foodstuffs contaminated by certain organic arsenicals, Williams[7] found that in the absence of more than 0·05 g sodium chloride, simple digestion with sulphuric acid, potassium sulphate and a catalyst of copper sulphate gave results as close to theoretical for traces of arsenic as by the conventional wet oxidation method with sulphuric and nitric acids. This method is useful for routine testing. Points of interest in the method are that special reduction of the arsenic before the Gutzeit test is unnecessary, whereas after nitric acid oxidation prior reduction must be carried out and sometimes hydrogen evolution causes spray acid to pass the lead acetate paper and gives irregular staining; this is prevented by insertion of a ½-inch pad of asbestos below the lead acetate paper. Details of the technique are the following:

Digest a suitable quantity of material with 10 g of potassium sulphate, 2 ml of 10 per cent copper sulphate solution and 20 ml of concentrated sulphuric acid, or sufficient to allow 8 ml for every gram of dry organic matter in the portion taken. When clear, dilute the liquid with about 70 ml of water and boil until free from any odour of sulphur dioxide, cool and dilute to 100 ml. Take a suitable aliquot portion from this for the Gutzeit test, diluting to 50 ml with a solution containing 10 per cent of potassium sulphate, 0·2 per cent of copper sulphate and 10 per cent by volume of sulphuric acid. After addition of 0·5 ml of stannous chloride AsT carry out the test as given in the *B.P.* using the asbestos pad as described above and prepare standard stains under similar conditions for comparison.

The *B.P.* arsenic test is only used as a limiting test and for quantitative

* *Note.* This reagent contains a concentration of stannous chloride ten times greater than that of stannated hydrochloric acid AsT of the *B.P.*

measurement is not so good as the 'strip' modification, in which the stains are produced on strips of mercuric chloride paper, the lengths and intensities of the stain being proportional to the amount of arsenic present. The apparatus (the actual dimensions of which are not important as long as comparative tests are carried out in apparatus of the same dimensions) consists of a wide-mouthed bottle holding about 120 ml, fitted with a rubber bung through which passes a glass tube, about 15 cm long and about 7 mm internal diameter. On to the top end of the tube, which is tapered, is fused a glass tube about 6 cm long and 3 mm internal diameter. The wider tube is packed to within 5 cm of the bottom end with lead acetate wool. A strip of mercuric chloride paper, about 8 cm long and sufficiently wide just to pass down the narrow tube, is inserted and either allowed to rest on the top of the lead acetate wool or, better, is bent at the upper end to retain its position about 5 mm above the lower end of the tube. The rate of evolution of hydrogen must be regulated by use of the same amount of free acid, zinc and water for each test in order to obtain comparative stains. Standard stains may be preserved for comparison by sealing them between dry microscope slides and keeping them protected from light or by dipping in hot melted paraffin. If the paper is treated with a solution of potassium iodide, the stain is blackened and more easily measured, and after drying may be preserved as above. If any doubt exists as to whether the stain produced in the test is due to arsenic, it should be treated with hot concentrated hydrochloric acid. If due to arsenic it will be intensified to a brick red, whilst if due to antimony or phosphine it will be destroyed. The strip method is official in the *U.S.P.*, where mercuric bromide papers are preferred.

If the standard stains are mounted on cardboard in such a way that the lower edges are in alignment, the upper edges of the stain should then form a continuous curve. Subsequently test stains can be determined by placing the strips in alignment with the standard strips and moving the former until the upper edge of the stain coincides with the curve.

Arsenical Solution, *B.P.C.* Contains 1·0 per cent w/v of arsenic trioxide which is determined by titration with 0·1N iodine in the presence of excess of sodium bicarbonate.

ARSENATES

Arsenates are not officially recognised in pharmacy, those in use are iron arsenate (see Iron Salts) and anhydrous **sodium arsenate,** Na_2HAsO_4, Mol. Wt. 185·9. The latter is assayed by reduction to arsenite with hydriodic acid in the presence of a high concentration of hydrochloric or sulphuric acid to prevent reversal of the reaction.

To 0·25 g of sodium arsenate add 50 ml of 1 : 1 hydrochloric acid and

3 g of potassium iodide; titrate the liberated iodine with 0·1N thiosulphate. 1 ml 0·1N = 0·009297 g Na_2HAsO_4.

If, after titration, the mixture is nearly neutralised with sodium hydroxide and finally with a slight excess of sodium bicarbonate, it may then be titrated with 0·1N iodine. In the opinion of Corfield and Woodward[8] this latter titration gives more accurate results.

FitzGibbon[9] prefers reduction to arsenite and then titration with iodine in the presence of bicarbonate.

To about 0·35 g of sodium arsenate add 20 ml of water and 5 ml of concentrated sulphuric acid, followed by 2 ml of 0·1N iodine and 0·2 g of finely-powdered amorphous phosphorus. Heat the mixture to boiling-point and maintain at this temperature until reduction is complete (approximately three minutes) and the solution is colourless. Filter the mixture whilst still warm through a Gooch crucible and wash the residue with three portions of 10 ml of water. Nearly neutralise the solution with strong alkali and titrate with 0·1N iodine after the addition of excess sodium bicarbonate.

ORGANIC ARSENICALS

A number of organic compounds of arsenic are official in the *B.P.* and *B.P.C.*, some of which are controlled by regulations made under the Therapeutic Substances Act and are assayed biologically for maximum toxicity and therapeutic potency. The following table summarises the compounds which are official in the *B.P.* or *B.P.C.*

TABLE 6

SUBSTANCE	FORMULA	MOL. WT.	METHOD OF ANALYSIS (see below)	1 ML 0·1N IODINE =
Acetarsol, *B.P.*	$C_8H_{10}O_5NAs$	275·1	(*a*)(*b*)	0·01375 g
Carbarsone, *B.P.*	$C_7H_9O_4N_2As$	260·1	(*a*)	0·01300 g
Neoarsphenamine, *B.P.C.* (Novarsenobenzene)	$C_{13}H_{13}O_4N_2SAs_2Na$	466·1	(*a*)	0·003746 g As
Oxophenarsine hydrochloride, *B.P.C.*	$C_6H_6O_2NAs,HCl$	235·5	(*a*)	0·003746 g As 0·01178 g*
Tryparsamide *B.P.*	$C_8H_{10}O_4N_2AsNa,\frac{1}{2}H_2O$	305·1	(*a*)	0·01480 g†

* Also by direct titration in acid solution with 0·1N iodine.
† Anhydrous.

The methods of assay employed for organic arsenic compounds consist of 'wet oxidation' of the organic matter and either direct titration of the arsenate formed or reduction to arsenite and subsequent titration.

(*a*) The general method given by the *B.P.* is based on the iodometric method of Little, Cahen and Morgan.[10]

The *B.P.* method differs mainly in using larger quantities of acids.

ARSENIC

Heat just at boiling-point a quantity of material containing approximately 0·05 g of arsenic with 7·5 ml of sulphuric acid and 1·5 ml of fuming nitric acid in a 600-ml Kjeldahl flask for one hour. Cool slightly, add 15 drops of fuming nitric acid and heat for a further five minutes; add cautiously 5 g of ammonium sulphate and when nitrogen ceases to be evolved, cool and dilute with water to about 100 ml. Add 1 g of potassium iodide, allow to stand and then concentrate the solution to about 50 ml by boiling, taking care to avoid loss of solution by spraying. Add just sufficient 0·01N sodium thiosulphate to decolorise the solution, then add 60 ml of water. Make the solution faintly alkaline to litmus paper with sodium hydroxide solution then faintly acid with dilute sulphuric acid and finally alkaline with sodium bicarbonate. Titrate with 0·1N iodine using mucilage of starch as indicator. 1 ml 0·1N = 0·003746 g As.

It may be necessary to add a further quantity of nitric acid in the oxidation stage for some compounds and with the larger amount of sulphuric acid a nearly colourless solution can be obtained by concentration, after the addition of potassium iodide, to about 50 ml. Concentration to 40 ml often causes precipitation of a yellow deposit not decomposed by thiosulphate.

(*b*) Acetarsol may be decomposed more readily by Newbery's method.[11] This method is somewhat quicker and is recommended with minor modifications for all official arsenicals by Ballard.[12] The modified method is as follows:

Weigh accurately into a 250-ml conical flask an amount of sample expected to contain from 0·08 to 0·09 g As. If (*a*) soluble in water, dissolve in 30 ml of water; (*b*) insoluble in water, dissolve in 5 ml of N sodium hydroxide and 20 ml of water and add 5 ml of N sulphuric acid; (*c*) containing chloride, dissolve in 50 ml of water. Place several glass beads in the flask and a small funnel in the neck, add 8 g of ammonium persulphate and boil briskly until colourless and for two minutes longer. (In the case of sodium cacodylate heat for about five minutes after ebullition commences.) Add cautiously 50 ml of approximately N oxalic acid and boil vigorously for five minutes. Add cautiously 40 ml of dilute sulphuric acid and 10 ml of potassium iodide solution. Boil vigorously until the volume is reduced to about 40 ml. Cool, just remove the pale yellow colour by the addition of approximately 0·1N sodium sulphite drop by drop (1 to 3 drops usually) and immediately add about 60 ml of water. Add 1 drop of phenolphthalein solution and sufficient sodium hydroxide test solution to render just alkaline. Add 10 ml of dilute sulphuric acid, mix, cool, neutralise with sodium bicarbonate, add up to 5 g in excess and titrate with 0·1N iodine. If starch solution is used add it just before the end-point is reached.

To 40 ml of sodium hydroxide test solution add 80 ml of dilute sulphuric acid, 1 drop of phenolphthalein solution and dilute sulphuric acid until colourless; then add 10 ml of acid in excess, 10 ml of potassium iodide solution and cool. Neutralise with sodium bicarbonate and add up to 5 g in excess. Titrate with 0·1N iodine and deduct the reading from that obtained above. 1 ml of 0·1N iodine = 0·003746 g As.

(*c*) Kahane[13] offers a general method which he states gives good results with a wide range of organic arsenic compounds.

Destroy the organic matter in 0·2 to 0·4 g by heating with small quantities of an oxidising mixture of strong sulphuric, nitric and perchloric acids. When a colourless liquid results and fumes of sulphuric acid appear, cool, add 0·25 g of hydrazine sulphate and heat the liquid for ten minutes to reduce the arsenic to the trivalent form and to decompose any excess of reducing agent. Add 20 ml of water and cool; add 0·1 to 0·2 g of potassium bromide and titrate with potassium bromate solution until a faint yellow colour of free bromine is obtained. 1 ml 0·1N bromate = 0·003746 g. As.

(*d*) Sodium cacodylate may be titrated with 0·5N acid, using methyl orange as indicator, after neutralising to phenolphthalein if necessary. 1 ml 0·5N = 0·0800 g $Na(CH_3)_2AsO_2$.

The determination of the sodium content of organic arsenicals containing this metal may be required in pharmaceutical analysis and the following method is applicable:

To about 0·5 g of substance add 1 ml of sulphuric acid and wet combust in the usual way with nitric acid. To the residue add 5 ml of water and evaporate to white fumes. Add 1 g of hydrazine hydrochloride and 30 ml of a mixture of 20 ml of hydrochloric acid and 10 ml of water. Boil down to 5 ml repeat the evaporation twice with 20-ml quantities of hydrochloric acid and finally evaporate to as low a volume as possible. Wash into a platinum dish, add a slight excess of ammonia, evaporate to dryness, ignite and weigh the sodium sulphate. $Na_2SO_4 \times 0{\cdot}3238$ = Na.

1. FERREY, G. J. W., *Pharm. J.*, 1931, **127,** 10.
2. *Analyst*, 1960, **85,** 629.
3. COX, H. E., *Analyst*, 1925, **50,** 3.
4. BELCHER, R., *Anal. Chim. Acta*, 1951, **5,** 30.
5. EVANS, B. S., *Analyst*, 1929, **54,** 523.
6. HASLAM, J., and WILKINSON, N. T., *Analyst*, 1953, **78,** 390.
7. WILLIAMS, H. A., *Analyst*, 1941, **66,** 228.
8. CORFIELD, C. E. and WOODWARD, Elsie, *Y. B. Pharm.*, 1921, 342.
9. FITZGIBBON, M., *Analyst*, 1933, **58,** 469.
10. LITTLE, H. F. V., CAHEN, E., and MORGAN, G. T., *J. Chem. Soc.*, 1909, **95,** 1477.
11. NEWBERY, G., *J. Chem. Soc.*, 1925, **127,** 1751.
12. BALLARD, C. W., *Quart. J. Pharm.*, 1946, **19,** 226.
13. KAHANE, E., *J. Pharm. Chim.*, 1934, **19,** 116.

ASCORBIC ACID

(Vitamin C)

$C_6H_8O_6$ Mol. Wt. 176·1

The chemical assay of ascorbic acid depends on the marked reducing properties of the vitamin and simple titration with standard iodine solution can be employed for the pure isolated compound. 1 ml 0·01N

= 0·0008805 g. This method can also be used for routine control of products known not to contain other reducing substances (Bacharach, Cook and Smith[1]). Other titrants using its reducing properties are ceric ammonium sulphate, as described under Ascorbic Acid Tablets, or potassium iodate.

Dissolve 0·17 g in 10 ml of water, add 50 ml of concentrated hydrochloric acid and cool. Run in 47 ml of 0·01M potassium iodate from a burette, swirling continuously, cool, add 5 ml of chloroform, stopper the flask and shake vigorously. Continue the titration, shaking vigorously after each addition of iodate, until the violet colour of the chloroform layer is just discharged. 1 ml 0·01M = 0·003522 g $C_6H_8O_6$.

Generally ascorbic acid is determined in animal or vegetable extracts by its reducing action on the dyestuff 2,6-dichlorophenolindophenol, the results by this method being closely in agreement with those obtained biologically. It is not, however, truly specific, the same reaction being given by glutathione and cysteine.

If possible, rapid extraction and titration is desirable, as errors may be introduced in plant products by oxidases partially destroying the ascorbic acid during sampling and grinding; oxidation is also prevented by the use of metaphosphoric acid during extraction.

In the opinion of Harris and Olliver[2] the following precautions are to be observed to obtain satisfactory results in determination of ascorbic acid by titration against 2,6-dichlorophenolindophenol. Take the average of the determinations on several samples from one batch. If possible avoid mincing or chopping which may invalidate the result because of destruction of ascorbic acid by the liberated oxidases, but otherwise grind in the presence of sand and under cover of 5 per cent metaphosphoric acid and centrifuge. Because extraction is more complete when a small sample is taken, titration on a micro-scale is more accurate than the use of a macromethod. Copper-free water must be used. The titration should be completed within one minute. A strongly acid solution gives most accurate results and titration of the unknown solution against a fixed amount of the dye gives a more easily detectable end-point than the titration carried out in the reverse manner. If dehydroascorbic acid is present it can be determined by a second titration after passing sulphuretted hydrogen through another portion of the solution, stoppering, allowing it to stand overnight at 0° and then bubbling oxygen-free nitrogen through the solution while it is connected to a vacuum pump and again titrating; the difference in titration gives the amount of dehydroascorbic acid. The authors could detect significant amounts of dehydroascorbic acid only in a few natural materials; they are of the opinion that the large amounts claimed by various workers is due to slow and incomplete extraction, permitting oxidation to occur. The presence of combined ascorbic acid was also discounted.

The presence of sulphur dioxide interferes with the determination of ascorbic acid and it should be removed by adding 5 ml of acetone to 20 ml of an acid extract, forming an acetone bisulphite compound,[3] then titrating in the usual way after three or four minutes, taking a little longer over it than normally as ascorbic acid reduces the dye more slowly in 20 per cent acetone than in water. For citrus juices the following procedure may be used:

Prepare the indicator solution by making a 0·08 per cent solution of 2,6-dichlorophenolindophenol in copper-free water, filter and keep in the dark. The strength diminishes more rapidly in daylight; after some time it gives a solution which during titration deposits a bluish precipitate and interferes with the end-point, it must then be discarded. The dye solution should be standardised at least daily and preferably just before use against freshly prepared ascorbic acid solution (50 mg/100 ml in 20 per cent metaphosphoric acid) which in turn has been standardised against 0·01N iodine.

Take a portion of material containing 2 to 3 mg of ascorbic acid (for concentrated juices a 10 per cent w/v solution in dilute metaphosphoric or acetic acid is made and aliquots used for titration), add a few drops of glacial acetic acid and 2 ml of acetone in a deep porcelain dish. Titrate with the dye solution from a 10-ml semi-microburette until the red colour is not further discharged after a few seconds. Alternatively, determine by potentiometric titration using a dead-stop end-point (see p. 867).

A modification of the titration method for ascorbic acid must be used in fruit juices, such as blackcurrant, where the colour would normally interfere. McHenry and Graham[4] propose the following titration technique:

Place 2 ml of chloroform in a Gerber tube, add a suitable volume of the liquid being tested and introduce the dye carefully into the upper layer. Pass purified carbon dioxide through the top layer to mix the juice and dye. Invert the Gerber tube and shake, so that the chloroform can take up any excess of the dye. Centrifuge the Gerber tube simultaneously with one containing juice and chloroform only, comparing the colours of the chloroform layers. Take the appearance of the faintest trace of pink in the chloroform layer as the completion of the titration.

Tablets of Ascorbic Acid, *B.P.* Usually contain 25 mg. The excipient in this preparation will not interfere with a direct use of the reducing properties of ascorbic acid.

Dissolve a weight of powdered tablets equivalent to 0·15 g of ascorbic acid as completely as possible in a mixture of 30 ml of water and 20 ml of dilute sulphuric acid and titrate with 0·1N ceric ammonium sulphate using *o*-phenanthroline ferrous complex solution as indicator. 1 ml 0·1N = 0·008806 g $C_6H_8O_6$.

For preparation of 0·1N ceric ammonium sulphate and *o*-phenanthroline ferrous complex, see under Iron, p. 349.

Capsules of Vitamins, *B.P.C.* Contain 15 mg of ascorbic acid in a complex mixture of vitamins and oily excipient.

> Shake a weighed quantity of the liquid expressed from the sample, equivalent to about 75 mg of ascorbic acid with 25 ml of freshly prepared 20 per cent metaphosphoric acid solution until completely dispersed, centrifuge and filter. Wash the residue with successive portions of a 5 per cent solution of trichloroacetic acid until the volume of the combined filtrate and washings is exactly 100 ml. Titrate a 2·5-ml aliquot of this solution with 2,6-dichlorophenolindophenol solution (as used for Syrup of Black Currant), avoiding oxidation by air.

Syrup of Black Currant, ***B.P.C.***

The principle of the technique described above for highly coloured juices has been adopted for the official assay. Briefly the method is as follows:

> To about 5 g add 20 ml of 25 per cent metaphosphoric acid solution, 20 ml of acetone and dilute to 100 ml. To 3-ml portions of the dilution in pointed centrifuge tubes add measured amounts (0·4 to 0·7 ml) of dye solution (20 mg per 100 ml in pH 7·2 buffer made by diluting 35 ml of 0·2N sodium hydroxide and 50 ml of 0·2M potassium dihydrogen phosphate to 200 ml). Mix with a fine stream of carbon dioxide, then add 3 ml of chloroform and re-mix. Repeat the titration with measured quantities about the approximate end-point shown in the preliminary titration. The end-point is taken as the amount of dye solution used in the first tube which shows a faint pink coloration.

The *B.P.C.* uses a solution of the sodium salt of 2,6-dichlorophenolindophenol such that 1 ml is equivalent to 0·2 mg of ascorbic acid but the dye solution is best standardised without further dilution immediately before use against pure ascorbic acid.

N-Bromosuccinimide was proposed[5] as a titrant of ascorbic acid and the suggested method has been adapted by Evered[6] to the determination of ascorbic acid in highly coloured solutions such as blackcurrant juices. The method has been tried by the writers but anomalous results have been obtained on certain samples where figures were considerably higher than those obtained by the official dichlorophenolindophenol method; these anomalous results were confirmed in other laboratories on the same samples and are probably due to the presence of added colouring matter.

Ascorbic acid is sometimes formulated together with ferrous salts or trace amounts of copper and in such cases the dichlorophenolindophenol method cannot be used.[7] A method based on the formation of the 2,4-dinitrophenylhydrazones of oxidation products of ascorbic acid is, however, applicable.[8] Ascorbic acid is oxidised to dehydroascorbic acid by mild oxidising agents and the reaction product in turn undergoes a rapid spontaneous transformation to diketogulonic acid in solutions at a pH below 1·0 or in neutral or alkaline media; both these oxidation products form a bis-2,4-dinitrophenylhydrazone derivative which, on treatment with 85 per cent sulphuric acid, undergoes a molecular rearrangement to form a stable reddish-brown product having a light absorption maximum at about 500 mμ. Bromine is a suitable oxidising agent for ascorbic acid and, by carrying out determinations before and after oxidation, the method may be used to give a measure of both the ascorbic acid that has undergone natural oxidation and the total ascorbic acid originally present. Little interference is encountered from the presence of large excesses of sucrose or other sugars since the osazones formed are decomposed by the high acid concentration used.

LEMON JUICE

The value of lemon juice lies in its ascorbic acid content, but a genuine juice has chemical characteristics to which it should conform. Free citric acid may be determined by direct titration of 20 ml with 0·5N potassium hydroxide using phenolphthalein as indicator. 1 ml 0·5N = 0·035 g $C_6H_8O_7,H_2O$. Genuine lemon juice also contains small quantities of sugar, phosphate and potash salts and may be preserved with alcohol.

There is no known method for accurately determining fruit juice content. For the determination of citrus juices in beverages it is shown by Stern[9] that the percentage and alkalinity of the ash is of no value because of the influence of the alkalinity from sodium benzoate or sulphites added as preservatives and saccharin added in the presence of sodium bicarbonate. The phosphoric anhydride content is independent of these factors and the following table summarises the data for the range to be expected in natural juices.

TABLE 7

VARIETY	P_2O_5 PER CENT W/V		
	MAXIMUM	MINIMUM	AVERAGE
Lemon	0·042	0·019	0·027
Orange	0·062	0·028	0·043
Grapefruit	0·052	0·024	0·035
Lime	0·030	0·016	0·022

Results for concentrated juices, calculated to natural juice strength are in accordance with these figures.

Determinations are carried out on the ash by precipitation with ammonium molybdate in the presence of ammonium nitrate, boiling the washed precipitate with excess of 0·5N sodium hydroxide to expel all ammonia, cooling and back titrating with 0·5N sulphuric acid, using phenolphthalein as indicator. The colorimetric determination of phosphate is also useful for fruit juices (see p. 532).

Fruit juices, and particularly orange juice, are liable to contamination with yeasts of the osmophilic type, which under certain circumstances may cause gaseous fermentation. Not all osmophilic yeasts give rise to gas production, but obviously those doing so are the least desirable. With freshly made material, the numbers of yeast cells present may be quite small, hence the amount of sample needed to detect viable yeasts in such material will be greater than with older material.

Dissolve 10 g of bacteriological peptone, 500 g of glucose, 1 g of sodium acid phosphate and 1 g of citric acid in water and make up to 1 litre. Distribute in about 20-ml amounts in tubes or bottles, each containing a Durham tube (for detecting the evolution of gas) and sterilise at 115° (10 lb steam pressure) for twenty minutes.

To each of a sufficient number of such tubes or bottles (depending on the size of sample to be examined) add about 10 ml of the test sample and incubate at about 25°. A minimum sample of 20 ml should be examined. Incubation is normally for fourteen days, but gas production frequently becomes evident after about seven days. At the end of the incubation period subculture from each container on a glucose agar slope (1 per cent glucose in nutrient agar at pH 6–6·5) and incubate for a further three days to detect the presence of non-gas-producing yeasts or to confirm the presence of gas-producing ones.

1. BACHARACH, A. L., COOK, P. M., and SMITH, E. L., *Biochem. J.*, 1934, **28**, 1038.
2. HARRIS, L. J., and OLLIVER, M., *Biochem. J.*, 1942, **36**, 155.
3. MAPSON, L. W., *Biochem. J.*, 1942, **36**, 196.
4. MCHENRY, E. W., and GRAHAM, M., *Biochem. J.*, 1935, **29**, 2013.
5. BARAKAT, M. Z., *et al.*, *Anal. Chem.*, 1955, **27**, 536.
6. EVERED, D. F., *Analyst*, 1960, **85**, 515.
7. CHAPMAN, D. G., ROCHON, O., and CAMPBELL, J. A., *Anal. Chem.*, 1951, **23**, 1113.
8. ROE, J. H., MILLS, M. B., OESTERLING, M. J., and DAMRON, C. H., *J. Biol. Chem.*, 1948, **174**, 201.
9. STERN, I., *Analyst*, 1943, **68**, 44.

BARBITONES

There are some thirty or forty barbitone derivatives employed therapeutically. Nearly all of them are 5,5-disubstituted derivatives of the parent substance barbituric acid, $CO:(NH.CO)_2:CH_2$. Many are combined with analgesics, but the combination is so weak that the barbiturates may be separated by an appropriate technique, generally by simple extraction.

Barbiturates act in solution as acidic substances and, although themselves relatively insoluble in water, they form very soluble sodium derivatives. Their quantitative determination depends upon extraction from acidified aqueous solution with solvents and identification by physical tests, such as melting-point, micro-crystalline form, etc. Methods of assay based on titration of the acidic nature of the imido hydrogen in the nucleus of these derivatives or precipitation of the only slightly dissociated silver salt with liberation of the nitric acid have not given concordant results, small differences in the conditions of test upsetting the determination.

Titration in non-aqueous solvents has been applied to barbiturates using various solvents and titrants (see Appendix III).

Ryan, Yanowski and Pifer[1] titrated the sample in dimethylformamide with 0·1N lithium methoxide using thymol blue as indicator. Small volumes of dimethylformamide were used (favouring a high ratio of benzene to solvent at the end-point) as it had been found that this sharpened the end-point slightly.

Chatten[2] found that with dimethylformamide as solvent the end-point faded rapidly even when the titration flask was protected from the atmosphere. He recommends chloroform as solvent to which 1 ml of methanol has been added per 50 ml of chloroform (to prevent the precipitation of barbiturate salts that occurs with chloroform alone) and employed as titrant 0·1N potassium hydroxide in anhydrous methanol. This reagent in our hands gave poor end-points when the titration volume exceeded about 5 ml.

Leavitt and Autian[3] investigated the use of tetra-*n*-butylammonium hydroxide as titrant and employed both a potentiometric and a visual method of determining the end-point. They found that the potentiometric method gave a sharp inflection at the end-point when benzene-*iso*propyl alcohol or benzene-chloroform solvent was used and a modified calomel electrode enhanced the inflection in a majority of the determinations carried out. They state that the visual method, employing thymol blue as the indicator, gave the desired accuracy and precision necessary for routine control purposes.

The official methods are not consistent. In the *B.P.* about 0·2 g is dissolved in 40 ml of dimethylformamide and titrated with 0·1N lithium methoxide using quinaldine red as indicator; precautions are taken against the effect of carbon dioxide and a blank is determined with the lithium methoxide. The *B.P.C.* uses considerably less solvent, 15 ml, for about 0·4 g of substance, thus providing a more suitable titration volume, but requires no protection against carbon dioxide. The latter conditions are in keeping with the findings of Ryan *et al.*[1] Prior neutralisation of the titration system as given under the Appendix on non-aqueous titration should always be carried out. However, in our opinion, the conditions for titration of barbitones by non-aqueous methods are so critical that as an assay for determination of purity they are not justified.

Determination of the alkali in the sodium salts of diethyl and phenylethyl barbituric acid is possible in 50 to 60 per cent ethanol using bromophenol blue as indicator.

BARBITONES

The following method is also generally applicable to the sodium salts of the barbiturates:

> Transfer about 0·5 g to a 150-ml separator and dissolve in 25 ml of water; add 20 ml of chloroform and 2 drops of methyl orange solution. Titrate with 0·1N hydrochloric acid, shaking during the titration.

It is preferable to assay these derivatives by extraction of the acid since this is more specific.

The quantitative extraction of the lower alkyl derivatives, such as diethyl barbituric acid, from aqueous solution is difficult as the partition coefficients are not high. By determination of the K values for barbitone it can be shown that ethyl acetate is undoubtedly the best of the common solvents for extracting these derivatives, with ether and ether-chloroform as good substitutes. More complex mixed solvents such as chloroform, ethanol and ether are favoured by some workers; they offer little advantage over ether for rapidity of extraction and the residues are less pure. Ether extracts are usually very pure and barbiturates can be extracted direct from urine with this solvent.

Barbiturates must not be kept in contact with strong alkalies for any length of time as hydrolysis quickly takes place, giving a complex mixture of products.

The barbitones given in Table 8 are official.

Barbiturates precipitate with xanthydrol (Fabre[4]) and alkaline cobalt solutions, but the quantitative application is not sufficiently accurate to be considered more than a very approximate determination. Also, these reagents are not specific (Mohrschulz[5]). The work of Dille and Koppanyi[6] illustrates the colorimetric determination of small amounts of barbitones with cobalt.

> Extract the barbiturate or dissolve it in chloroform. To 2 ml of this solution add 0·1 ml of 1 per cent cobalt acetate in dehydrated methanol and 0·6 ml of 5 per cent v/v *iso*propylamine in dehydrated methanol. Compare, in a colorimeter, the reddish-violet colour produced with standard solutions containing the barbiturate under consideration. The concentration of the standard must be near that of the unknown, concentrations containing 0·04 to 0·12 per cent being appropriate. The standards must only be kept for a few hours in stoppered tubes.

Theobromine and theophylline shows a positive reaction, but none of the common chloroform-soluble drugs combined with barbiturates were found to interfere. Results were accurate to within 6 per cent.

Allobarbitone may be determined by bromination as in the Koppeschaar method (see Phenol, p. 513), the bromine giving an additive compound with the unsaturated allyl groups; hence 1 ml 0·1N bromine = 0·005205 g. Ten minutes' contact with the reagent is sufficient.

TABLE 8

BARBITONE	FORMULA	MOL. WT.	M.P. ACID °C	FACTOR†	ABSORPTION	
					SOLUTION IN 0·1N NaOH λ(max.) mμ	E(1%, 1 cm)
Allobarbitone, *B.P.C.* [5,5-diallylbarbituric acid]	$C_{10}H_{12}O_3N_2$	208·2	172–174	0·02082	—	—
Amylobarbitone, *B.P.* [5-*iso*amyl-5-ethylbarbituric acid]	$C_{11}H_{18}O_3N_2$	226·3	155–158	0·02263	245	293
Amylobarbitone Sodium, *B.P.*	$C_{11}H_{17}O_3N_2Na$	248·3	—	1·097		
Barbitone, *B.P.C.* [5,5-diethylbarbituric acid]	$C_8H_{12}O_3N_2$	184·2	189–192	0·01842	244	324
Barbitone Sodium, *B.P.*	$C_8H_{11}O_3N_2Na$	206·2	—	1·119		
Butobarbitone, *B.P.* [5-*n*-butyl-5-ethylbarbituric acid]	$C_{10}H_{16}O_3N_2$	212·3	122–125	0·02123	246	330
Cyclobarbitone, *B.P.* [5-ethyl-5-*cyclo*hex-1-enylbarbituric acid]	$C_{12}H_{16}O_3N_2$	236·3	171–175	0·02363	251	296
Hexobarbitone, *B.P.C.* [5-*cyclo*hex-1′-enyl-1,5-dimethylbarbituric acid]	$C_{12}H_{16}O_3N_2$	236·3	145–147	0·02363	—	—
Hexobarbitone Sodium *B.P.C.*	$C_{12}H_{15}O_3N_2Na$	258·3	—	1·093		
Methylphenobarbitone, *B.P.C.* [5-ethyl-1-methyl-5-phenylbarbituric acid]	$C_{13}H_{14}O_3N_2$	246·3	178–181	0·02463	—	—
Pentobarbitone Sodium, *B.P.* [Na salt of 5-ethyl-5-(1-methylbutyl)barbituric acid]	$C_{11}H_{17}O_3N_2Na$	248·3	about 128	1·097	242	321
Phenobarbitone, *B.P.* [5-phenyl-5-ethylbarbituric acid]	$C_{12}H_{12}O_3N_2$	232·2	174–177	0·02322	253	320
Phenobarbitone Sodium, *B.P.*	$C_{12}H_{11}O_3N_2Na$	254·2	—	1·095		
Quinalbarbitone (Secobarbital), *U.S.P.* [5-allyl-5-(1-methylbutyl)barbituric acid]	$C_{12}H_{18}O_3N_2$	238·3	—	0·01191*	—	—
Quinalbarbitone Sodium, *B.P.*	$C_{12}H_{17}O_3N_2Na$	260·3	—	1·092		
Thialbarbitone Sodium, *B.P.C.* [Na salt of 5-allyl-5-*cyclo*hex-2′-enyl-2-thiobarbituric acid]	$C_{13}H_{15}O_2N_2SNa$	286·3	about 138	1·083	—	—
Thiopentone Sodium, *B.P.* [Na salt of 5-ethyl-5-(1-methylbutyl)-2-thiobarbituric acid, 100 + Na_2CO_3, 6]	—	—	about 157	—	—	—

Elixir of Phenobarbitone, *B.P.C.* Contains phenobarbitone 0·46 per cent w/v with orange, glycerin and colouring matter.

The phenobarbitone can be determined accurately by the following method, which avoids the emulsions given by a more direct procedure.

Add 50 ml to 50 ml of solvent ether in a separator, shake, separate and run off the ethereal layer. Shake with two further 50-ml portions of ether, mix the ethereal extracts, wash with a little water and shake with a mixture of 5 ml of 2N sodium hydroxide and 25 ml of water. Separate, reserve the aqueous portion and shake the ethereal layer with two successive 5-ml portions of water. Add the aqueous extracts to the reserved liquid, acidify with dilute hydrochloric acid and extract with four successive 25-ml portions of ether. Bulk the extracts, remove the ether, dry at 105° and weigh the residue of $C_{12}H_{12}O_3N_2$.

Considering the nature of the assay and the amount of extractable excipient, the *U.S.P.* assay of tablets containing free barbitones is unnecessarily complicated and an accurate determination is made by direct extraction of the active ingredient from the powdered tablets with a solvent, usually ether. The possibility of significant amounts of excipient in the recovered barbitone can be checked by a melting-point determination; this should be within one or two degrees of the minimum *B.P.* or *B.P.C.* figure. The following official tablets containing barbitones are assayed in this way: **Tablets of Amylobarbitone,** *B.P.*, **Tablets of Barbitone,** *B.P.C.*, **Tablets of Butobarbitone,** *B.P.*, **Tablets of Cyclobarbitone,** *B.P.*, **Tablets of Methylphenobarbitone,** *B.P.C.*, and **Tablets of Phenobarbitone,** *B.P.* Chloroform is a much better extracting solvent than ether for methylphenobarbitone.

Cyclobarbitone decomposes on storage, particularly in tablets, so that the extraction method of assay is unsatisfactory under these conditions. A bromometric assay as given under Salicylic Acid (p. 558) will indicate the residual content more correctly although the precautions enumerated must be observed to avoid erratic results. **Cyclobarbitone Calcium,** $C_{24}H_{30}O_6N_4Ca$, Mol. Wt. 510·6, is considered more stable and is official in the *N.F.* with a bromometric assay.

For the substance dissolve 0·5 g in a mixture of 5 ml of water and 5 ml of glacial acetic acid in a flask, warming if necessary, cool, add 50 ml of 0·1N bromine and 10 ml of concentrated hydrochloric acid and stopper immediately. Allow to stand in ice for fifteen minutes with occasional shaking, add 10 ml of 10 per cent potassium iodide and allow to stand in ice for a further ten minutes. Titrate the liberated iodine with 0·1N sodium thiosulphate using starch, added towards the end of the titration, as indicator. 1 ml 0·1N bromine = 0·01277 g.

For the tablets weigh an amount of powdered tablets equivalent to about 0·5 g of cyclobarbitone calcium into a 100-ml glass-stoppered cylinder, add 10 ml of 4 per cent sodium hydroxide solution and 40 ml of water and shake mechanically for thirty minutes. Transfer quantitatively to a 100 ml graduated flask with water, dilute to volume with water, mix and filter. Pipette 25 ml of the filtrate into a glass-stoppered flask and continue as described above from the addition of bromine solution, adding 30 ml of 0·1N bromine.

Phenobarbitone is often compounded with other drugs such as stilbœstrol, theobromine and aminophylline in tablet formulations. A simple infra-red method of assay has been found useful on such materials.[7] The samples are made up in chloroform solution and the carbonyl stretching absorption band at 1,740 cm^{-1} is utilised.

Capsules of Amylobarbitone Sodium, *B.P.*, **Tablets of Amylobarbitone Sodium,** *B.P.* **Tablets of Barbitone Sodium,** *B.P.*, **Tablets of Pentobarbitone Sodium,** *B.P.*, and **Tablets of Phenobarbitone Sodium,** *B.P.* The tablets are liable to absorb carbon dioxide rapidly on exposure and liberate a considerable proportion of free barbiturate, extractable with ether from the powdered material.

The excipients in these preparations do not interfere with a direct extraction with solvent from acidified solutions; preliminary washing with ether in alkaline solution may cause losses in the assay due to formation of emulsions.

Bodin[8] has applied direct argentimetric potentiometric titration to phenobarbitone and its sodium salt in preparations containing a variety of standard diluents. He eliminates uncertainty in the end-point potential by determining the potential of a standard blank solution (saturated with silver carbonate) for each sample just prior to titration and using this as the end-point potential for titration of the sample. Stearates, halides and ammonium salts interfere and special consideration must be given to samples containing polyethylene glycols, alcohol, or hexamine. He includes a procedure for removal of stearates from tablets.

Prepare a standard blank solution by mixing 10·0 ml of 95 per cent ethanol, 50 ml of a 3 per cent solution of anhydrous sodium carbonate (analytical-reagent grade) and 1·00 ml of 0·01N silver nitrate solution with sufficient water to make 100 ml. Determine the potential of this solution, using silver and saturated calomel electrodes connected by a saturated potassium nitrate, agar salt bridge.

Weigh (or measure) an amount of sample equivalent to about 200 mg of phenobarbitone and mix with exactly 10 ml of 95 per cent ethanol. Add 50 ml of a 3 per cent solution of anhydrous sodium carbonate and sufficient water to make 100 ml and titrate with 0·1N silver nitrate solution to the standard blank potential. To correct for the blank, subtract 0·1 ml from the volume of 0·1N silver nitrate solution used.

For tablets and capsules (stearates present). Weigh an amount of sample equivalent to about 500 mg of phenobarbitone and transfer to a 250-ml graduated flask with exactly 25 ml of 95 per cent ethanol. Add 25 ml of water and swirl the flask until the undissolved solid is evenly dispersed. Add 125 ml of a 3 per cent solution of anhydrous sodium carbonate, shake and dilute to volume with water. Filter, preferably with suction, through a fine, retentive filter paper, rejecting the first 25 ml of the filtrate and collecting the remainder in a dry receiver. Titrate 100-ml portions of the filtrate with 0·1N silver nitrate to the standard blank potential. Correct for the blank as before.

For **Elixir of Phenobarbital,** *U.S.P.* Mix 50 ml of the sample with 50 ml of a 3 per cent solution of anhydrous sodium carbonate. Prepare a blank solution consisting of 7·0 ml of dehydrated ethanol, 50 ml of the 3 per cent sodium carbonate solution, 1·00 ml of 0·01N silver nitrate and sufficient water to make 100 ml. Determine the potential of the blank solution and titrate the sample solution to this potential. Correct for the blank as before.

Tablets of Belladonna and Phenobarbitone, *B.P.C.* Each tablet contains approximately 49 mg of phenobarbitone and 26 mg of dry extract of belladonna. The *B.P.C.* assay for phenobarbitone is as follows:

Weigh an amount of powdered tablets equivalent to about 0·13 g of phenobarbitone, dissolve in 10 ml of 0·1N sodium hydroxide and saturate the solution with sodium chloride. Make acid to litmus paper with concentrated hydrochloric acid and extract with 15-ml quantities of ether until extraction is complete. Extract the combined extracts with four 20-ml quantities of a mixture of 6 ml of 20 per cent sodium hydroxide solution and 76 ml of brine, combine the aqueous extracts and make acid to litmus paper with concentrated hydrochloric acid. Extract with 15-ml quantities of ether until extraction is complete, combine the ether extracts and wash with two 2-ml quantities of water, rejecting the washings. Filter the ether solution, wash the filter with ether, evaporate the ether from the combined extracts and washings and dry the residue of phenobarbitone to constant weight at 105°.

Tablets of Quinalbarbitone Sodium, *B.P.* These tablets are nearly always supplied sugar-coated; they should be completely disintegrated in the presence of a little sodium hydroxide and then filtered before extraction with ether from acidified solution.

PHENYTOIN SODIUM, $C_{15}H_{11}O_2N_2Na$, Mol. Wt. 274·3

Assayed by extraction of the diphenylhydantoin with a mixture of 4 volumes of chloroform and 1 volume of *iso*propyl alcohol. 1 g residue = 1·087 g sodium derivative.

Tablets of Phenytoin Sodium, *B.P.* Usually contain 100 mg.

For assay disintegrate 20 tablets by digesting with 50 ml of water, add 5 ml of N sodium hydroxide and filter. To an aliquot of the filtrate equivalent to about 0·2 g of phenytoin sodium add 25 ml of water and 10 ml of dilute hydrochloric acid and extract the diphenylhydantoin directly as above.

1. Ryan, J. C., Yanowski, L. K., and Pifer, C. W., *J. Amer. Pharm. Ass., Sci. Edn.*, 1954, **43,** 656.
2. Chatten, L. G., *J. Pharm. Pharmacol.*, 1956, **8,** 504.
3. Leavitt, D. E., and Autian, J., *Drug Standards*, 1958, **26,** 33.
4. Fabre, R., *J. Pharm. Chim.*, 1922, **26,** 241; 1923, **27,** 204.
5. Mohrschulz, W., *Quart. J. Pharm.*, 1934, **7,** 725.
6. Dille, J. M., and Koppanyi, T., *J. Amer. Pharm. Ass.*, 1934, **23,** 1079.

7. Garratt, D. C., and Marshall, P. G., *J. Pharm. Pharmacol.*, 1954, **6,** 950.
8. Bodin, J. I., *J. Amer. Pharm. Ass., Sci. Edn.*, 1956, **45,** 185.

BELLADONNA

A considerable amount of literature is available on the determination of the alkaloidal content of belladonna, most of the methods suggested being variations of the general process of extraction from the leaf by a solvent in the presence of alkali, followed by acid extraction and finally solvent extraction from alkaline solution. The variations usually differ from the general method in the first part of the process (*i.e.* extraction of the alkaloids from the plant) which is the most difficult operation.

BELLADONNA HERB (Belladonna Leaf)

Good quality herb contains 0·4 to 1·0 per cent of alkaloids, mainly hyoscyamine.

The method of the *B.P.* is as follows:

> Reduce a sufficient quantity to a fine powder (No. 85), weigh 10 g of the powder into a flask and add 50 ml of a mixture of 4 volumes of ether and 1 volume of 95 per cent ethanol. Shake thoroughly, allow to stand for ten minutes and then add a mixture of 1·5 ml of dilute ammonia solution and 2 ml of water and shake frequently during one hour. Transfer the mixture to a small percolator plugged with cotton wool and, when the liquid ceases to flow, pack firmly and continue the percolation, first with 25 ml of the ether/ethanol mixture, and then with ether until the alkaloids are completely extracted. (The total time of percolation should not exceed three hours.) Evaporate the percolate on a water-bath until the volume is reduced to about 20 ml and then transfer to a separator, washing the flask with three 10-ml quantities of chloroform and adding the washings to the separator. Extract, first with 20 ml of 0·5N sulphuric acid, and then with successive 10-ml portions of a mixture of 3 volumes of 0·1N sulphuric acid and 1 volume of 95 per cent ethanol until the alkaloids are completely extracted. Combine the acid solutions and wash, first with 10 ml and then with two 5-ml quantities of chloroform, extracting each chloroform washing in turn with the same 20 ml of 0·1N sulphuric acid in another separator. Reject the chloroform. Combine the acid solutions, make distinctly alkaline with dilute ammonia solution and extract with successive quantities of chloroform until the alkaloids are completely extracted, washing each extract separately, with the same 10 ml of water. Combine the extracts, evaporate most of the chloroform and then transfer to a shallow open dish and evaporate the remainder of the chloroform. Add 2 ml of dehydrated ethanol to the residue, evaporate to dryness and dry at 100°, weighing at intervals of one hour until two successive weighings do not differ by more than 1 mg. Dissolve the residue in 2 ml of chloroform, add 10 ml of 0·05N sulphuric acid, warm to remove the chloroform,

cool and titrate the excess acid with 0·05N sodium hydroxide using methyl red as indicator. 1 ml 0·05N sulphuric acid = 0·01447 g of alkaloids, calculated as hyoscyamine.

Although this type of method has been used with confidence by analysts for many years, a recent collaborative trial, involving fourteen laboratories, has shown that widely discordant results may be obtained. Investigation into the cause of these discrepancies has shown that the percolation stage gives rise to a considerable amount of variation between laboratories: although the *B.P.* specifies the use of a fine powder higher results are obtained (at least when assaying the root) if moderately fine powder (in which the majority of the sample is between 44- and 85-mesh) is used. Another serious cause of error may be in the heating stage, intended to remove volatile bases; if atropine sulphate is treated by the final extraction stage of the *B.P.* process the yield may be more or less low according to the amount of air that has access to the residue during heating. Thus, if the residue is heated in a small oven a higher result (although not quite theoretical) will be obtained than if it be heated on a water-bath with free interchange of air over the surface. A modification of the later stages of the assay that has given higher and more consistent yields is the following:

Make distinctly alkaline to litmus paper with dilute ammonia solution and then add 2 ml of the ammonia in excess and extract with successive 25-ml quantities of chloroform until the alkaloids are completely extracted, as indicated by testing with Dragendorff's reagent (Mayer's reagent, as used in the *B.P.* method, is not sufficiently sensitive). Wash each chloroform extract, separately, with the same 10 ml of water and filter into a 250-ml, beaker-flask through a cotton-wool plug, previously well washed with chloroform. Evaporate the chloroform from the combined extracts on a water-bath (do not use a current of air) until the volume is reduced to 1 to 2 ml and then evaporate to dryness at room temperature using, if necessary, a very gentle current of air. Transfer the flask to a vacuum desiccator containing phosphorus pentoxide and evacuate at room temperature for fifteen minutes. Dissolve the residue in 4 to 5 ml of chloroform, add 10 ml of 0·05N sulphuric acid, cover the flask with a small watch-glass and carefully remove the chloroform by heating over a small flame. Rinse the watch-glass with a little water, collecting the rinsings in the flask, cool, and titrate the excess acid with 0·05N sodium hydroxide using screened methyl red as indicator.

It has been shown[1] that many volatile bases that might be expected to be present in belladonna (particularly in samples of root with a high proportion of 'crown') are removed by this process. Tropine is not removed, but it is extremely unlikely that the official heating process brings about a quantitative separation of hyoscyamine and tropine. The *U.S.P.* treatment at this stage of the assay is to heat for fifteen minutes on a water-bath but with free access of air the same possibility of loss exists as with the *B.P.* method. It might be thought that the duration and temperature of contact with and the strength of alkali used in the initial extraction procedure would affect the results obtained, but comparative assays, identical in all respects except that the *B.P.* cold percolation (where 1·5 ml of 10 per cent ammonia solution is used with 50 ml of organic solvent for a one-hour maceration period) was used in one case and the *U.S.P.* hot extraction (using 8 ml of 30 per cent ammonia solution with 30 ml of organic solvent for an overnight maceration period) in the other, gave very similar results. At the present time no reliable recommendations for a full procedure can be given.

To overcome the possibility of errors arising from partial decomposition of the alkaloids, Reimers[2,3] has proposed a hydrolytic method for the determination of solanaceous alkaloids and it is claimed that this method avoids errors which may arise from incomplete removal of volatile bases, the presence of non-volatile, non-alkaloidal bases (for example, tropine and oscine) and the retention of ammonia by the alkaloidal extract.

A comparison of the direct titration and hydrolytic methods has been made by Drey.[4] For the official drugs he concluded that the hydrolytic and non-hydrolytic methods are in good agreement but that with certain *Duboisia* and *Datura* species the hydrolytic method gave lower and more realistic results. Even if the heating period to remove volatile bases is extended to eight or ten hours, the direct titrimetric method of the *B.P.* give high results for *Duboisia myoporoides*. Although the authors did not apply their method to Indian belladonna they considered it probable that application of the hydrolytic method would be advantageous in this case also.

The procedure recommended by Drey is as follows:

> Reduce a sufficient quantity to a No. 60 powder and extract 25 g of the powder, in two separate portions, each of 12·5 g, by the *B.P.* method given above, increasing all quantities of solvent by 25 per cent. Combine the final chloroform extracts, evaporate to low volume and then dilute to exactly 50 ml with chloroform and mix. Pipette 20 ml of this solution into a shallow, open dish, evaporate to dryness and titrate the alkaloids with 0·05N sulphuric acid as in the *B.P.* assay. Dilute the titrated liquid to about 35 ml with water, add 10 ml of 2N sodium hydroxide and evaporate for fifteen minutes on a water-bath. Cool, neutralise with dilute hydrochloric acid and add 0·05 ml of the acid in excess. Transfer to a separator and extract, first with four 25-ml portions and then with two 20-ml portions of a mixture of 1 volume of *iso*propyl alcohol and 3 volumes of chloroform, washing each extract with the same 15 ml of water. Combine the extracts, evaporate the solvent and dissolve the residue in 15 ml of warm water. Cool the solution and titrate with 0·02N sodium hydroxide using phenolphthalein as indicator.

Dry Extract of Belladonna, *B.P.* Contains 1 per cent of the alkaloids of belladonna, calculated as hyoscyamine.

As the preparation contains powdered herb, emulsification due to particles of solid suspended matter is liable to occur unless precautions are taken to avoid it. In the *B.P.* assay it is difficult to wash the 3 g of extract into a separator completely with 12 ml of liquid; if the extract is weighed on to a small piece of glazed paper, the whole can be dropped into a dry separator and the necessary amount of ethanol and water added. By taking care to compress tightly with a glass rod the cotton-wool plug through which the chloroform solution is filtered, most of the suspended matter is removed.

> Weigh 3 g into a separator, washing in with 12 ml of a mixture of equal volumes of 95 per cent ethanol and water and shake well and frequently during about thirty minutes. Add 2 ml of dilute ammonia solution and extract with successive 25-ml quantities of chloroform until the alkaloids are completely extracted, running each chloroform extract in turn into a second separator through a tightly-packed cotton-wool plug previously rinsed with chloroform. (Usually four extractions will be sufficient.) Extract the chloroform solution with successive portions of a mixture of 3 volumes of 0·2N sulphuric acid and 1 volume of 95 per cent ethanol until complete extraction of the alkaloids is effected. Combine the acid extracts and complete as described under Belladonna Herb, above, beginning with the words 'wash, first with 10 ml and then with two 5-ml quantities of chloroform . . .'.

Green Extract of Belladonna, *B.P.C.* Contains 1 per cent by weight of alkaloids.

A soft extract of belladonna herb, assayed in the *B.P.C.* by the *B.P.* method for Dry Extract of Belladonna.

Below is given a more rapid method for determination:

> Weigh about 2 g into a dish, mix with 5 to 10 ml of water and transfer to a separator without filtering. Wash in with water to make a total of about 15 ml. Wash the dish with 30 ml of chloroform and add it to the liquid in the separator. Finally, add a few drops of ammonia to any residue in the dish to effect solution. Continue as for Belladonna Herb. The chloroform separates at once and is free from emulsions.

Glycerin of Belladonna, *B.P.C.* A mixture of Green Extract of Belladonna with glycerin and containing 0·5 per cent by weight of alkaloids.

> Weigh, by difference, about 10 g into a separator, add 15 ml of water, 5 ml of ethanol and make slightly alkaline with ammonia. Extract the alkaloids with 30-ml portions of chloroform. Treat the combined chloroform solutions with three portions of dilute acid, make the acid extracts alkaline, and extract the alkaloids as usual with chloroform. Wash, evaporate, dry and titrate as given under Belladonna Herb.

The *B.P.C.* assay is as for Dry Extract of Belladonna using approximately 6 g of sample, accurately weighed.

Tincture of Belladonna, *B.P.* Contains 0·30 per cent of the alkaloids of belladonna.

The *B.P.* assay is as follows:

> Evaporate 100 ml on a water-bath until the volume is reduced to about

10 ml and, if necessary, add sufficient 95 per cent ethanol to dissolve any separated substance. Transfer to a separator with a little water, add 10 ml of water and 2 ml of dilute ammonia solution and extract with successive quantities of chloroform until the alkaloids are completely extracted. Combine the chloroform extracts and extract with successive quantities of 0·2N sulphuric acid until complete extraction of the alkaloids is effected. Combine the acid extracts and complete as described under Belladonna Herb, above, beginning with the words 'wash, first with 10 ml and then with two 5-ml quantities of chloroform . . .'.

Because the percolation stage is unnecessary this galenical would be expected to give inter-laboratory results that are in closer agreement than those obtained with belladonna itself. Evaporation of the tincture should not be taken so far as 10 ml, however; it should only proceed at a temperature below 70° until it cannot be continued without deposition of chlorophyll and resinous matter.

BELLADONNA ROOT

The total alkaloids vary from 0·3 to 0·8 per cent.

The *B.P.C.* assay for total alkaloids is exactly as for Belladonna Herb and the remarks made above apply equally to the root.

Janniah[5] obtained a highly-coloured alkaloidal residue from some Indian belladonna roots by the *B.P.* assay, but eliminated most of the colour by adding 1 g of powdered tragacanth and 2 to 3 ml of water to the concentrated and cooled ether-ethanol percolate and shaking for about five minutes. After filtration and washing through a tight cotton-wool plug he continued the assay of the *B.P.* (except for the substitution of hydrochloric acid for sulphuric acid).

Liquid Extract of Belladonna, *B.P.C.* Contains 0·75 per cent of the alkaloids of belladonna.

Some care is required during the preliminary extraction stage of the assay to avoid serious emulsification.

Liniment of Belladonna, *B.P.C.* Contains 0·375 per cent of belladonna alkaloids and 5 per cent of camphor.

The *B.P.C.* assay calls for no comment, the preliminary extraction with chloroform in acid solution satisfactorily eliminating camphor and resinous matter.

Another method of assay which gives separations free from emulsions is:

> Introduce 20 ml of liniment into a separator, add 30 ml of water and make slightly alkaline with ammonia. Extract three times with a mixture of 7 volumes of ether and one volume of chloroform. Extract the combined solvents with three portions of dilute acid, make the acid extracts alkaline and extract the alkaloids as usual with chloroform. Wash, evaporate and titrate as directed under Belladonna Herb.

Liniment of Belladonna contains 5 per cent of camphor. This may be determined by the method of Hampshire and Page (p. 156), with the preliminary process of distilling 40 ml of liniment in steam until 150 ml of distillate has been collected, washing down the condenser with 85 ml of aldehyde-free ethanol and diluting to 250 ml; 50 ml of the diluted distillate is taken for the determination.

An alternative procedure is the gas chromatographic method as used for Liniment of Camphor (p. 159).

Plaster-mass of Belladonna. Consists of a soft extract of belladonna mixed with Plaster Mass of Lead with Colophony.

The following method of assay was recommended by Wing[6] for application to plasters with resin bases.

Weigh into a tared flask 15 g of plaster, dissolve in 40 ml of chloroform. Remove the chloroform on a water-bath until the residue is of a thick consistency. Add 2 ml of dilute sulphuric acid and 50 ml of water. Heat with constant stirring to remove the remaining chloroform and boil for two minutes. Cool immediately to room temperature. Adjust the weight with water to 76 g plus the weight of plaster taken. Filter and transfer 50 ml, representing two-thirds of the weight of the plaster being assayed, to a separator. Shake with 10 ml of chloroform, washing the chloroform after separation with 5 ml of 0·1N sulphuric acid. Repeat with a further 10 ml of chloroform, wash with the same portion of 0·1N acid and reject the chloroform solutions. Make the bulked acid solutions alkaline with ammonia and extract the alkaloids with four successive 35-ml portions of chloroform. Wash the combined chloroform solutions with 5 ml of water, evaporate the chloroform and dry the residue for half an hour at 100°. Complete the assay as for Belladonna Herb. 1 ml 0·02N acid = 0·005788 g of hyoscyamine. To the amount indicated by the titration add 0·003 g to correct for loss of hyoscyamine.

The author stated that no detectable loss resulted when the alkaloids were heated in acid solution and ascribed at least part of the loss of alkaloid, and hence the somewhat large correction factor, to incomplete extraction due to solubility of hyoscyamine in the aqueous phase. Since an aliquot is taken an assumption is implied as to the amount of the mass that dissolves.

Plaster of Belladonna. Consists of elastic or non-elastic cotton cloth spread with Belladonna Plaster Mass. Wing[6] applied the method for plaster mass (above) to the spread plaster with resin basis. In his opinion the *N.F.* method for spread plaster (below) made with rubber basis is inapplicable, the lead salts formed interfering with separation of the alkaloids.

Weigh into a beaker 30 g of a spread plaster cut into small pieces. Add 50 ml of chloroform, warm and stir until the plaster dissolves and transfer the solution to a tared flask. Repeat with successive portions of 20, 20 and 10 ml of chloroform. Dry the fabric and weigh. Remove the chloroform from the mixed solutions on a water-bath until of a thick consistency and continue as for Belladonna Plaster Mass.

The *N.F.* method is nevertheless found by some workers to be satisfactory for the plaster with the rubber base and briefly is as follows:

Cut about 10 g of the weighed plaster into small strips and place in a 150-ml flask. Add 50 ml of chloroform and shake until the mass is disintegrated. Pour off the chloroform into a beaker and wash the cloth with two further portions each of 25 ml of chloroform, then with 50 ml of ethanol containing 1 ml of dilute ammonia solution and finally with 40 ml of ethanol. Stir the bulked solvents gently but thoroughly and allow to stand until any coagulum has separated into a compact mass. Dry the cloth, allow natural moisture regain and weigh to obtain the weight of plaster mass by difference. Filter the solution into a separator through a small pledget of cotton wool. Knead the coagulum with a glass rod to force out retained solution and rinse with 10 ml of ethanol. Extract the alkaloids from the chloroform-ethanol solution by repeated extraction with approximately 0·5N acid. Complete the assay by making distinctly alkaline with ammonia and extracting the alkaloids with chloroform; evaporate, dry and titrate in the usual manner.

The alkaloids may need a further purification by re-extracting with acid, washing the acid solution with chloroform and then completing the assay in the usual way.

In our opinion, however, no satisfactory method exists for the determination of belladonna in plaster mass and plasters. The proportion of alkaloid is so small and the associated materials are so difficult to remove without loss of alkaloid, that the result of a lengthy assay can, at best, only be regarded as an approximation to the true alkaloidal content.

Allport and Wilson[7] have proposed the use of Vitali's reaction for the rapid determination of the alkaloids in belladonna and stramonium for control purposes. The method is not applicable to *Hyoscyamus niger* or its galenical preparations. In order to obtain constant results experimental details must be followed. It must be noted that the colour produced is affected by the presence of other organic bases and hence the prescribed method is not accurate if Indian belladonna has been used in the galenical. An alkaloidal assay can be completed within an hour and the results are said to compare favourably with those obtained by the official methods. The most likely cause of delay is tardy percolation which is liable to arise when working with finely powdered drugs, but the difficulty can be circumvented by mixing with prepared sawdust and exercising special care to avoid tight packing in the percolator. The details of the final colorimetric assay are given under Atropine.

ATROPINE, $C_{17}H_{23}O_3N$, Mol. Wt. 289·4

Morin[8] suggested the use of Vitali's reaction for the determination of small amounts of atropine and it was studied by Allport and Wilson[7] for its application to routine examination of belladonna preparations. The details of the colorimetric assay of hyoscyamine are given below.

For simple alkaloidal solutions or tablets take an aliquot part in water, containing between 1·6 and 2·4 mg of atropine, make ammoniacal and extract with small portions of chloroform to give a final volume of 10 ml. To this extract in a stoppered cylinder add 20 ml of 6 per cent acetic acid in approximately 5 per cent ethanol, shake, separate, pipette off about 5 ml of the upper layer and filter through a dry filter paper. Transfer exactly 1 ml of the filtrate to an evaporating dish (5 cm diameter) evaporate just to dryness on a water-bath and immediately add from a dropping pipette 0·2 ml of fuming nitric acid (sp. gr. 1·5 AnalaR grade); the use of the fuming acid, containing at least 95 per cent of nitric acid, is essential. Ensure that the acid makes contact with the whole of the alkaloidal residue, and evaporate to dryness leaving the dish on the water-bath for three minutes altogether. Add about 3 ml of acetone (AnalaR grade) stir to dissolve the residue and transfer to a standard stoppered measuring cylinder of 10 ml capacity; wash the dish with further small quantities of acetone and transfer them to the measure until the latter contains exactly 10 ml of solvent. Allow the contents of the measure to cool, if necessary adjust the volume to 10 ml with acetone, add 0·1 ml of a 3 per cent solution of AnalaR potassium hydroxide in AnalaR methanol (prepared not more than a fortnight beforehand), insert the stopper, invert the cylinder once and allow to stand exactly five minutes, the slight haze produced by the addition of the alkali disappears before the colour is measured. Transfer a portion of the purple liquid to a 1-cm cell and record the colour intensity in a photoelectric absorptiometer. Prepare a calibration curve with quantities of 0·025 mg to 0·15 mg of pure hyoscyamine subjected to the whole procedure.

Attempts to omit the step involving acetic acid were unsuccessful.

Allport and Jones[9] confirmed that atropine reacts quantitatively the same as hyoscyamine and that the method is also applicable to hyoscine, the intensity of the colours produced by equal weights of hyoscyamine and hyoscine being inversely proportional to their molecular weights.

Ashley[10] has confirmed the findings of other workers that this method gives accurate and reproducible results only when the reagents, reaction times and water content of the acetone are rigidly controlled; not more than 0·2 per cent of water should be present in the acetone. In its application to the determination of hyoscine, pyridine of analytical reagent quality is preferred; provided the water content of the solvent does not exceed 0·17 per cent w/v, the intensity of the colour is approximately 20 per cent greater than that produced using acetone. It was also observed that the colour is affected by light so that solutions should be kept in the dark prior to colour measurement and 0·5 per cent potassium hydroxide in methanol is preferred to the stronger solution used by Allport and Wilson. The modified method gave accurate results with official preparations containing hyoscine hydrobromide.

A new approach to the Vitali type of reaction has been made by Freeman.[11] After nitration the residue is dissolved in dimethylformamide and tetramethylammonium hydroxide is used for making alkaline. The recommended method, which can be applied to pure solutions containing hyoscyamine and related alkaloids or to their galenicals, after partial purification by the method of Allport and Wilson, is:

Evaporate a measured quantity of solution, containing about 0·05 to 0·15 mg of alkaloid, to dryness on a water-bath and nitrate the residue by the addition of 0·2 to 0·3 ml of fuming nitric acid. Remove the nitric acid by evaporation and transfer the residue to a 10-ml graduated flask with the aid of small quantities of dimethylformamide. Add 0·3 ml of a 25 per cent w/w aqueous solution of tetramethylammonium hydroxide and dilute to volume with dimethylformamide. Allow to stand for five minutes and measure the extinction at 540 mμ using 1-cm cells with dimethylformamide in the comparison cell. The calibration curve is linear.

In our hands the method was found to be capable of giving an accurate estimate of the atropine content of tablets, but with a spread of about 15 per cent. The exact conditions of nitration do not appear to be critical, but it is important that the nitrated sample is not heated any longer than necessary, otherwise charring may occur.

Although the presence of atropine does not interfere with the colorimetric determination of morphine, the minutest trace of the latter disturbs the colour reaction for atropine. To eliminate interference from morphine it is oxidised with ferric chloride and the atropine then extracted:

Transfer a measured quantity of the aqueous solution expected to contain approximately 1 mg of atropine into a small separator, dilute with water until the volume of the liquid approximates to 5 ml, add 0·5 ml of a solution of ferric chloride (5 per cent w/v of $FeCl_3$ in water) and allow to stand for two minutes. Add 2 g of sodium citrate, shake until dissolved, render the mixture alkaline by adding 0·5 ml of dilute ammonia solution and proceed with the extraction and colorimetric determination of atropine as already described.

A completely new approach to the determination of small amounts of nitrogenous bases (including tropine alkaloids) in aqueous solutions such as eye-drops and injections has been published by Johnson and King.[12] Precipitation with tetraphenylboron at pH 3·7 is used; the excess of the latter is then determined by back-titration with a standard solution of quaternary ammonium salt to a visual end-point. Melting-points of the organic tetraphenylboron salts may be used in the identification of many of these compounds. An assay, including standardisation of reagents, can be completed in half an hour and the accuracy of the method was shown to compare very favourably with that of many of the official methods for the compounds examined.

No interference was obtained from *p*-hydroxybenzoic acid esters, phenol, chlorbutol, chlorocresol and chloroxylenol in concentrations at which these materials are used as fungistats, bactericides and bacteriostats in aqueous eye-drop and injection solutions. Phenylmercuric nitrate (0·002 per cent w/v) which is sometimes used in these preparations as a bactericide produced a small positive error. The extent of this error will depend on the sample size and the compound being determined, but when contained in the preparations examined was in the range +0·2 to +1·0 per cent.

Uncoated tablet materials, lactose, liquid glucose, mannitol, stearic acid, starch, calcium stearate, talc and sucrose could be tolerated in the precipitation solution without interference. As gelatin and polyvinylpyrrolidone precipitate with sodium tetraphenylboron it is not possible to apply the method to tablets containing these materials.

Preliminary extraction of the organic bases from oily eye-drops, ointments and suppositories is necessary before applying the general method. Extraction is made from an organic solvent with 2N acetic acid followed by pH 3·7 buffer solution. Acid extracts obtained in this way from Theobroma Oil *B.P.C.*, Basis for Eye Ointments *B.P.* and Castor Oil *B.P.* contained no interfering materials.

The general method is the following:

Reagents:

Bromophenol blue solution: Dissolve 0·1 g of bromophenol blue in a mixture of 3·0 ml of 0·05N sodium hydroxide and 5 ml of 90 per cent ethanol, warming to assist solution, and dilute to 250 ml with 20 per cent ethanol.

Buffer solution, pH 3·7: Dissolve 10 g of anhydrous sodium acetate in about 300 ml of water, add 1 ml of bromophenol blue solution and then add glacial acetic acid until the colour of the indicator changes from blue to green (usually 35 to 40 ml required). Dilute to 500 ml with water.

0·005M Cetylpyridinium chloride: Dissolve 1·80 g of cetylpyridinium chloride in 10 ml of 95 per cent ethanol and dilute to 1 litre with water. Store in an amber-coloured bottle.

0·01M Sodium tetraphenylboron: Dissolve 3·42 g of sodium tetraphenylboron in 50 ml of water, add 0·5 g of aluminium hydroxide gel, *B.P.* and shake for twenty minutes. Dilute to 300 ml with water, add and dissolve 16·6 g of analytical reagent grade sodium chloride and allow to stand for thirty minutes. Filter clear (re-filter the first 20 to 30 ml of filtrate if cloudy), using suction, through two thicknesses of Whatman No. 42 filter paper, wash the filter with water and dilute the filtrate to 1 litre with water. Adjust the pH to between 8·0 and 9·0 with 0·1N sodium hydroxide, using narrow range Universal pH papers. Store in an amber-coloured flask.

0·01M Potassium chloride: Dissolve 0·1491 g of analytical-reagent grade potassium chloride, previously dried at 150° for one hour, in 100 ml of buffer solution, pH 3·7, and dilute to exactly 200 ml with water.

Determination:

First determine the molarity of the cetylpyridinium chloride solution as follows. Pipette 10 ml of 0·01M potassium chloride into a clean, dry beaker, add 15 ml of 0·01M sodium tetraphenylboron, swirling during the addition, and allow to stand for five minutes. Filter into a dry flask through a dry No. 4 sintered-glass crucible. Pipette 20 ml of the filtrate into a 150-ml flask, add 0·50 ml of bromophenol blue solution, dilute to 50 ml with water and titrate with 0·005M cetylpyridinium chloride to a blue end-point. Let the ml required be '*Ts*'. To a further 15 ml of 0·01M sodium tetraphenylboron add 4 ml of buffer solution, pH 3·7 and 0·50 ml of bromophenol blue solution and titrate with 0·005M cetylpyridinium chloride to the same end-point. Let the ml required be '*B*.'

The molarity, M, of the cetylpyridinium chloride solution is given by the relationship $M = 10{\cdot}00\, M_1\, (B - 5/4\, T_S)$, where M_1 is the molarity of the potassium chloride solution.

Pipette 10 ml of a sample solution (prepared as described under the individual preparation) into a clean, dry beaker and continue as described above beginning with the words 'add 15 ml of 0·01M sodium tetraphenylboron, . . .' and ending with the words '. . . to a blue end-point.' Let the ml required be 'T_E.' Each ml of the difference $(B - 5/4\, T_E)$ is equivalent to 'y' g of the substance being determined, where 'y' is the equivalent weight for 1 ml of 0·01M cetylpyridinium chloride.

Atropine sulphate, $(C_{17}H_{23}O_3N)_2,H_2SO_4,H_2O$, Mol. Wt. 694·9. In N sulphuric acid atropine sulphate has the following light absorption characteristics:

Maxima	E(1 per cent, 1 cm) 251·5 mμ	= 5·00
	E(1 per cent, 1 cm) 257 mμ	= 5·95
	E(1 per cent, 1 cm) 263 mμ	= 4·60
Minima	E(1 per cent, 1 cm) 254 mμ	= 4·40
	E(1 per cent, 1 cm) 261 mμ	= 3·90

These figures are given in some detail because atropine has a very low absorption.

Eye-drops of Atropine Sulphate, *B.P.C.* A 1 per cent solution of atropine sulphate with 0·75 per cent sodium chloride in water.

Dilute 5 ml to 50 ml with N sulphuric acid. Measure the maximum extinction of a 1-cm layer of this solution at about 257 mμ using N sulphuric acid as reference and calculate the percentage of atropine sulphate in the original sample. In order to establish the position and E value of the peak, readings should be made at intervals of 0·5 mμ.

The tetraphenylboron method given above can be used after preparing the sample solution by adding 10 ml of buffer solution, pH 3·7, to 4 ml of the eye-drops in a 20-ml graduated flask and diluting to volume with water. 1 ml cetylpyridinium chloride = 0·001737 g.

Eye Ointment of Atropine, *B.P.* Atropine sulphate, 1·0 per cent, in simple eye ointment.

Allport[13] examined the deterioration of atropine eye ointments on storage and concluded that those made with atropine sulphate maintain their strength fairly well, but when atropine alkaloid itself is used deterioration is more rapid, particularly when the ointment is stored in glycero-gelatin capsules.

For assay, dissolve about 4 g of ointment by the aid of gentle heat in chloroform and dilute sulphuric acid. Transfer to a separator and extract with portions of dilute sulphuric acid, wash the combined acid extracts with chloroform and then make them just alkaline with ammonia. Re-extract the alkaloids with chloroform, wash, evaporate to dryness and titrate as usual. 1 ml 0·05N acid = 0·01737 g atropine sulphate.

Light petroleum (b.p. 40° to 60°) is also recommended for dissolving the ointment before acid extraction.

The tetraphenylboron method given above can be used after preparing the sample solution as follows:

Dissolve about 8 g, with warming, in 20 ml of solvent ether and extract first with 15 ml of 2N acetic acid, followed by two quantities, each of 10 ml, of buffer solution, pH 3·7, and then 5 ml of the buffer. Filter each extract in turn through a small plug of cotton wool, gently warm the combined extracts, to remove traces of organic solvent, cool and dilute to 50 ml with buffer solution in a graduated flask. 1 ml cetylpyridinium chloride = 0·001737 g.

Eye Ointment of Atropine and Cocaine, *B.P.C.*1954. Atropine sulphate 0·25 per cent and cocaine hydrochloride 0·25 per cent in simple eye ointment.

Nicholls[14] has found that cocaine can be separated from most other alkaloids by extracting the former with light petroleum from solutions made alkaline with sodium bicarbonate. Hence the two alkaloids present in this ointment can be assayed by first extracting the total alkaloids into acid solution as under Eye Ointment of Atropine, and then adding an excess of sodium bicarbonate and light petroleum and extracting the cocaine. Finally, on making the aqueous solution alkaline to ammonia, the atropine may be isolated as usual. See also Cocaine, p. 186.

Injection of Atropine Sulphate, *B.P.* A 0·06 per cent solution of atropine sulphate in water which may or may not contain a bactericide.

If no bactericide is present or if one which does not absorb in the ultraviolet is included then the atropine sulphate may be determined by measuring the maximum extinction at about 257 mμ without dilution and comparing the value obtained with that of a solution of atropine sulphate in water. If, however, phenol, cresol, or chlorocresol have been used then the following method is applicable.

Pipette 30 ml of the injection solution on to a previously prepared oxycellulose or alginic acid column (see p. 461) and allow to pass through the column at a flow rate of 1 to 3 ml per minute. Wash with at least three portions of 25 ml of water, collecting the eluate and washings. Dilute this fraction suitably with water and determine the bactericide spectrophotometrically (see p. 519).

Elute the atropine from the column with successive portions of N sulphuric acid, collecting the eluate in a 25-ml flask, until the flask is filled to the mark. Measure the maximum extinction of a 1-cm layer at about 257 mμ using N sulphuric acid as reference and calculate the percentage of atropine sulphate in the original sample.

Tablets of Atropine Sulphate, *B.P.* Usually contain 1/100 grain of atropine sulphate.

Weigh an amount of powdered tablets equivalent to about 20 mg atropine sulphate, add 40 ml of water and 5 ml of dilute sulphuric acid and shake occasionally during two hours. Filter, wash the filter with water and, using the combined filtrate and washings, make alkaline with dilute ammonia and extract without delay and as rapidly as possible with successive quantities of chloroform. Wash the combined extracts with water, evaporate to dryness and titrate as usual using 0·02N acid and alkali. 1 ml 0·02N acid = 0·006949 g $(C_{17}H_{23}O_3N_2)_2,H_2SO_4,H_2O$.

The tetraphenylboron method given above can be used after preparing the sample solution by dissolving 40 powdered tablets, with gentle warming, in 12·5 ml of buffer solution, pH 3·7, and centrifuging if necessary before making up to volume with water in a 25-ml graduated flask. 1 ml of cetylpyridinium chloride = 0·001737 g.

The separate determination of hyoscine, hyoscyamine and atropine in a mixture is of considerable interest. Rowson[15] has investigated this problem and has proposed the following method based on the observation that at pH 8·5 hyoscine is quickly and completely extracted by chloroform whereas atropine is extracted with difficulty; the hyoscyamine extracted is calculated from the optical rotation of the mixed alkaloids after correction for the hyoscine content. The specific rotation of *l*-hyoscyamine was taken as −22° and *l*-hyoscine as −18°.

The method has been tried on *Hyoscyamus muticus* leaf with concordant repeat determinations, but it has not been investigated sufficiently to determine whether accurate results are attainable.

Extract the total alkaloids with chloroform in the presence of an excess of ammonia. Remove the solvent and dry the residue in a current of air on a water-bath for fifteen minutes. Dissolve the residue in a measured quantity of ethanol and determine the optical rotation of the solution. Calculate the *l*-hyoscyamine content after correcting for the *l*-hyoscine present as shown by the separation described below.

Titrate an aliquot portion of the ethanolic solution with 0·02N hydrochloric acid using methyl red as indicator and from this titre calculate the total alkaloidal content. To the titration liquid add the exact equivalent of sodium bicarbonate and shake out with 15 ml quantities of chloroform, three portions being found sufficient for a titre of 10 ml. Remove the solvent, titrate the residue and continue the process until two consecutive titrations differ by not more than 0·2 ml of 0·02N acid; from this figure calculate the hyoscine. 1 ml 0·02N = 0·006064 g. The difference between total alkaloidal content and the sum of the hyoscyamine and hyoscine gives the amount of atropine present.

Atropine methonitrate, $C_{17}H_{23}O_3N,CH_3NO_3$, Mol. Wt. 366·4. The alkaloidal base is not precipitated from solutions of this compound but Vitali's colorimetric reaction can be applied to the determination of small quantities in tablets and solutions after either extraction with ethanol and evaporation or direct solution in 6 per cent acetic acid for application of Allport and Wilson's method described above.

The substance can be assayed by non-aqueous titration (p. 792) and forms an insoluble compound with ammonium reineckate.

Dissolve about 0·1 g in 40 ml of water and add 20 ml of dilute sulphuric acid followed by 30 ml of 1 per cent ammonium reineckate solution. Mix and allow to stand for thirty minutes. Filter through a tared Gooch crucible and wash with water saturated with atropine methoreineckate until free from sulphate. Wash with 3 ml of water followed by 2 ml of 95 per cent ethanol and dry over P_2O_5 *in vacuo* to constant weight. 1 g of residue = 0·5884 g $C_{18}H_{26}O_6N_2$.

Eye-drops of Atropine Methonitrate. Contain 1 per cent of atropine methonitrate and 0·75 per cent of sodium chloride.

The tetraphenylboron method given above can be used for assay after preparing the sample solution by adding 10 ml of buffer solution, pH 3·7, to 4 ml of the eye-drops in a 20-ml graduated flask and diluting to volume with buffer. 1 ml of cetylpyridinium chloride = 0·001832 g.

HOMATROPINE HYDROBROMIDE, $C_{16}H_{21}O_3N,HBr$, Mol. Wt. 356·3

The assay of the alkaloidal base in this salt follows the conventional lines of extraction with chloroform from ammoniacal solution and titration of the dried alkaloid using methyl red as indicator. 1 ml 0·05N acid = 0·01781 g $C_{16}H_{21}O_3N,HBr$. It can be assayed by non-aqueous titration (p. 792) using 0·5 g. 1 ml 0·1N perchloric acid = 0·03563 g. **Homatropine methylbromide,** $C_{17}H_{24}O_3NBr$, Mol. Wt. 370·3 can also be assayed by this method. 1 ml 0·1N perchloric acid = 0·03703 g.

Eye-drops of Homatropine, *B.P.C.* Contain 2 per cent of homatropine hydrobromide.

The tetraphenylboron method given above can be used for assay after preparing the sample solution by adding 10 ml of buffer solution, pH 3·7, to 3 ml of the eye-drops in a 20-ml graduated flask and diluting to volume with buffer. 1 ml of cetylpyridinium chloride = 0·001782 g.

Eye-drops of Cocaine and Homatropine, *B.P.C.* Contain 1 per cent of cocaine hydrochloride and 2 per cent of homatropine hydrobromide.

The alkaloids cannot be separated but a total alkaloidal figure can be obtained by the tetraphenylboron method after preparing the sample solution by the method given under Eye-drops of Homatropine.

HYOSCINE HYDROBROMIDE, $C_{17}H_{21}O_4N,HBr,3H_2O$, Mol. Wt. 438·3

The salt of an alkaloid obtained from various solanaceous plants. The base can be extracted with chloroform from ammoniacal solution and is titrated to methyl red. 1 ml 0·05N acid = 0·02192 g $C_{17}H_{21}O_4N,HBr,3H_2O$.

Eye-drops of Hyoscine Hydrobromide, *B.P.C.* Contain 0·25 per cent.

This preparation can be assayed by the tetraphenylboron method given above, using 10 ml of a solution prepared by mixing 5 ml of the sample with 5 ml of buffer solution, pH 3·7. 1 ml of cetylpyridinium chloride = 0·002192 g.

Eye Ointment of Hyoscine, *B.P.* Usually contains 0·25 per cent of hyoscine hydrobromide.

This preparation can be assayed by the method given under Atropine Eye Ointment using a weight of sample equivalent to about 25 mg of hyoscine hydrobromide. 1 ml 0·05N sulphuric acid = 0·02192 g $C_{17}H_{21}O_4N,HBr,3H_2O$.

Injection of Hyoscine Hydrobromide, *B.P.* Usually contains 0·04 per cent.

The preparation can be assayed by direct extraction of the base from a volume equivalent to about 20 mg of hyoscine hydrobromide with chloroform from ammoniacal solution. The extraction should be carried out without delay. 1 ml 0·02N hydrochloric acid = 0·008767 g $C_{17}H_{21}O_4N,HBr,3H_2O$.

Tablets of Hyoscine Hydrobromide, *B.P.* Usually contain 1/200 grain.

The assay follows the methods given under Tablets of Atropine Sulphate.

Hyoscyamine hydrobromide, $C_{17}H_{23}O_3N,HBr$, Mol. Wt. 370·3 and **hyoscyamine sulphate,** $(C_{17}H_{23}O_3N)_2,H_2SO_4$, Mol. Wt. 676·8, again follow the conventional alkaloid base determination as indicated under Homatropine hydrobromide. 1 ml 0·02N = 0·007402 g $C_{17}H_{23}O_3N,HBr$ and 0·006768 g $(C_{17}H_{23}O_3N)_2,H_2SO_4$.

1. Allen, J., private communication.
2. Reimers, F., *Dansk Tidsskr. Farm.*, 1944, **18,** 217.
3. Reimers, F., *Quart. J. Pharm.*, 1948, **21,** 470.
4. Drey, R. E. A., *J. Pharm. Pharmacol.*, 1958, **10,** 241T.
5. Janniah, S. L., *Analyst*, 1939, **64,** 590.
6. Wing, W. T., *Quart. J. Pharm.*, 1938, **11,** 489.
7. Allport, N. L. and Wilson, E. S., *Quart. J. Pharm.*, 1939, **12,** 399.
8. Morin, C., *J. Pharm. Chim.*, 1936, **23,** [viii], 545.
9. Allport, N. L. and Jones, N. R., *Quart. J. Pharm.*, 1942, **15,** 238.
10. Ashley, M. G., *J. Pharm. Pharmacol.*, 1953, **4,** 181.
11. Freeman, F. M., *Analyst*, 1955, **80,** 520.
12. Johnson, C. A., and King, R. E., *J. Pharm. Pharmacol.*, 1962, **14,** 77T.
13. Allport, N. L., *Quart. J. Pharm.*, 1935, **8,** 429.
14. Nicholls, J. R., *Analyst*, 1936, **61,** 155.
15. Rowson, J. M., *Quart. J. Pharm.*, 1944, **17,** 226.

BENZOIC ACID

C_6H_5COOH Mol. Wt. 122·1

The quantitative examination of benzoic acid in pharmaceutical preparations is comparatively simple, and the acid is usually present in sufficient quantity to estimate by direct titration or by weight after isolation.

The *B.P.* method of estimation is by direct titration in ethanol; phenolphthalein or phenol red may be used as indicator, the colour change being quite sharp in the presence of ethanol, phenolphthalein being less sensitive. 1 ml 0·5N NaOH = 0·06106 g. Benzoic acid may also be titrated in a non-aqueous medium such as dimethylformamide, an alkaline methoxide or tetrabutylammonium hydroxide being used as titrant (see p. 793).

When benzoic acid is extracted by ether from an acidified solution and the solvent evaporated, care must be taken to avoid loss by volatilisation. Lerrigo[1] found that after spontaneous evaporation from moist ether and air-drying at room temperature no volatilisation occurred; at 40° to 50° only a very slight loss of benzoic acid resulted, but at 70° the loss from 0·5 g was more than 0·020 g per hour.

The extraction and estimation of small quantities of benzoic acid present as preservative may be required in the analysis of galenicals such as cough syrups. Several methods are available, the determination having received considerable attention because of the need for accurate assay for purposes of the Preservative Regulations.[2] Direct extraction of the benzoic acid from acidified solution is not usually practicable and it is generally isolated by steam distillation. The technique followed is that of Monier-Williams.[3]

Introduce a convenient weight of the sample, 30 to 100 g, into a 500-ml flask and if a liquid, saturate with salt at the rate of about 40 g to every 100 ml of water present. If the sample is not liquid mix it with water to the required consistency and saturate the mixture with salt. Make the mixture distinctly acid with phosphoric acid and rapidly steam distil into 10 ml of N sodium hydroxide contained in a porcelain basin, the latter avoiding difficulties in extraction due to solution of silica during the subsequent evaporation. Collect a total distillate of 500 ml in about one and a half hours. Then evaporate the distillate to a volume of about 20 ml, cool to about 40° and treat with a 5 per cent solution of potassium permanganate until a pink colour persists. Cool the solution, decolorise with sulphur dioxide and acidify. Then transfer the solution to a separator, washing in with water to give a volume of about 60 ml. Saturate the liquid with salt and then extract with four portions each of 15 ml of a mixture of equal volumes of ether and light petroleum (b.p. 40° to 60°). Transfer each extraction to a test-tube 15 to 16 cm in length and 1·5 to 1·8 cm internal diameter and successively evaporate at about 30°, a current of air being blown over the surface.

Wash the benzoic acid adhering to the sides down to the lower portion of the tube with a few drops of ether and again evaporate at low temperature.

This isolated benzoic acid may not be pure and purification by sublimation is recommended by Monier-Williams. The product is then weighed, the following technique being that given in the original paper:

> About 2 g of pure dry sand is introduced into the tube so that the greater part of the benzoic acid is covered by sand. This sand must previously have been well washed with *aqua regia* and then with distilled water, and finally ignited. The object of the sand is to regulate heat transference during sublimation and to provide a large surface from which the benzoic acid can volatilise. A disc of filter paper, cut rather larger than the diameter of the test-tube, is pushed down into the tube, preferably by means of a cork borer, until it is about $\frac{3}{4}$ inch above the level of the sand. The tube is lightly corked, not air-tight, and placed upright in an air-oven so that the lower 4 cm of the tube is inside the oven. An ordinary air-oven can be fitted up for this purpose by making holes in the top just large enough to take the test-tube and fitting a copper plate inside the oven at the right height to serve as a rest for the tubes. The tubes can be held upright in the holes by a little asbestos paper packing. Unless the tubes fit tightly, convection currents will interfere with the even deposition of the sublimate. Sublimation is carried out for one to one and a half hours at a temperature of about 160°. A copper air-oven measuring 8 inches in each direction, maintains a temperature of approximately 160° without automatic regulation, when heated with the full flame of a Bunsen burner. After one to one and a half hours' sublimation the tube is removed, allowed to cool, and the lower part cut off between the sand layer and the filter paper disc; this is carefully removed from the tube and any crystals on it returned to the tube. The part of the tube containing the sublimate is now dried, either in a desiccator or in a current of dry air. The tube is then weighed, the sublimate dissolved out with ether, and the tube reweighed.

This determination of benzoic acid is not specific; it must be remembered that any cinnamic acid present would be oxidised to benzoic acid by permanganate.

Fairly pure residues from extraction may be titrated directly with 0·05N sodium hydroxide using phenol red as indicator (1 ml 0·05N = 0·0061 g of $C_7H_6O_2$), or determined colorimetrically by a method based on Mohler's nitration test; Illing[4] examined this reaction and recommended the technique:

> Introduce the benzoic acid residue as the sodium salt into a boiling-tube and heat in a beaker of boiling brine until the liquid is driven off and all drops of condensation water have disappeared. Cool, add 0·1 g of potassium nitrate and 1 ml of concentrated sulphuric acid. Place the tube in boiling water for twenty minutes. Cool and add 2 ml of water. Hold the tube under running water and add carefully 10 ml of 15 per cent ammonia solution followed by 2 ml of a 2 per cent hydroxylamine hydrochloride solution. Mix well and place in a beaker of water at 65° for five to six minutes. Cool and match the colour with that developed by mixing the amounts of iron ammonium alum and potassium thiocyanate solution given below for varying quantities of benzoic acid.

Should the prepared meta-diaminobenzoic acid solution require to be diluted the dilution is made with a solution prepared in the following manner:

Add 20 ml of concentrated sulphuric acid to 40 ml of water containing 2 g of potassium nitrate; cool the liquid while 200 ml of water containing 100 ml of strong ammonia is carefully added. Finally add to the solution 40 ml of water in which 0·8 g of hydroxylamine hydrochloride is dissolved.

TABLE 9

BENZOIC ACID mg	IRON AMMONIUM ALUM SOLUTION (1 G PER LITRE) ml	POTASSIUM THIOCYANATE SOLUTION (2 PER CENT) ml	VOLUME MADE UP TO ml
0·1	0·2	0·2	15
0·25	0·3	0·3	15
0·5	0·5	0·5	15
0·75	0·7	0·6	15
1·0	1·0	0·8	15
2·0	1·5	1·5	15
3·0	2·0	1·5	15
4·0	2·0	2·3	15
5·0	3·0	2·5	15
6·0	4·0	3·5	50
7·0	4·0	4·5	50
8·0	4·5	3·5	50
9·0	5·0	4·0	50
10·0	5·5	5·5	50

Compound Ointment of Benzoic Acid, *B.P.C.* Contains 6 per cent of benzoic acid and 3 per cent of salicyclic acid in a mixture of emulsifying wax and paraffins.

To determine the benzoic and salicylic acids:

Dissolve exactly 2·5 g of ointment in a mixture of ether and ethanol, previously neutralised to phenolphthalein, and determine the total acidity with 0·1N sodium hydroxide.

For salicylic acid, dissolve exactly 2·5 g in ether and extract completely with saturated sodium bicarbonate solution, washing each extract with ether. After cautious acidification with dilute hydrochloric acid, extract with ether, evaporate carefully, dissolve the residue in N sodium hydroxide and determine by bromination (see p. 558). 1 ml 0·1N bromine = 0·002302 g. Calculate the ml of 0·1N sodium hydroxide equivalent to the salicylic acid found (1 ml 0·1N = 0·01381 g) and deduct from the titration figure for total acidity. 1 ml 0·1N = 0·01221 g benzoic acid.

Blake[5] has described a non-aqueous titration method whereby the benzoic and salicyclic acids may be determined separately by differential titration with sodium methoxide in a medium of dimethylformamide. In our experience, sensitive apparatus is necessary to indicate the separate voltage steps.

BENZOATES

The *B.P.* method for estimating sodium benzoate is a modification of Henville's method,[6] using bromophenol blue as indicator instead of methyl orange as recommended by him. The former indicator has a range similar to methyl orange and may be used advantageously for titration of strong bases combined with weak acids.

To a solution of about 3 g of sample dissolved in 50 ml of water in a separator and neutralised, if necessary, to phenolphthalein, add 50 ml of ether, shake and titrate to bromophenol blue with 0·5N acid until the indicator changes to green. Then separate the aqueous layer, wash the ether with water, add 20 ml of fresh ether to the aqueous layer and washings, and continue the titration with constant shaking until the end-point is reached, only a few drops being required in the second stage.

1 ml 0·5N = 0·06958 g **ammonium benzoate,** $C_7H_5O_2NH_4$, Mol. Wt. 139·2, and 0·07205 g **sodium benzoate,** $C_7H_5O_2Na$, Mol. Wt. 144·1.

The alkali in sodium benzoate can be determined by titration after ignition by the general method for alkali salts of organic acids.

Char completely about 1·5 g of the salt in a platinum dish, add an excess of 0·5N acid, boil, filter and wash. Ignite the filter paper and residue to a white ash and add it to the filtrate obtained from the first ignition. Titrate the excess of acid with 0·5N alkali to methyl orange. 1 ml 0·5N = 0·07205 g of sodium benzoate.

A modification of this technique is to char completely, then moisten with acetic acid, tilt the dish to drain the carbonaceous residue, evaporate to dryness in this position and continue the ignition.

If required the benzoic acid content may be determined by weighing or titrating the residue obtained after extraction with ether in acid solution, taking the precautions given under Benzoic Acid.

1. Lerrigo, A. F., *Analyst*, 1926, **51,** 405.
2. The Preservatives in Food Regulations, S.I., 1962, No. 1532.
3. Public Health and Medical Subjects, No. 39.
4. Illing, E. T., *Analyst*, 1932, **57,** 224; 1939, **64,** 586.
5. Blake, M. I., *J. Amer. Pharm. Ass., Sci. Edn.*, 1957, **46,** 287.
6. Henville, D., *Analyst*, 1927, **52,** 149.

BENZOIN

The estimation of free and total balsamic acids, due to Cocking, is described under Tolu Balsam (p. 643). In the case of benzoin, the alcoholic extract from about 2·5 g of the resin should be used for the estimation of free balsamic acids instead of the original gum as used in the assay for the total acids. *B.P.* benzoin contains a minimum of 25 per cent of total balsamic acids calculated on the dry alcohol-soluble matter. There is no official limit for free balsamic acids but a good Sumatra benzoin contains 19 to 29 per cent, calculated on the dry alcohol-soluble matter; alcohol-insoluble matter should not exceed 20 per cent.

Siam benzoin contains no cinnamic acid and is almost entirely soluble in 90 per cent ethanol. It is included in the *U.S.P.* and the limits for benzoin under that authority include a minimum of 75 per cent alcohol-soluble extractive for Sumatra benzoin and 90 per cent for Siam benzoin. The *U.S.P.* assay for alcohol-soluble extract is taken from the method of Bennett and Bickford.[1]

> Extract 2 g of sample for five hours in a Soxhlet thimble with 95 per cent ethanol containing about 0·1 g of sodium hydroxide. Dry the insoluble matter and weigh. To this weight add the water content of the drug determined by toluene distillation. The alcohol-soluble extract is calculated by difference.

Acid value 105 to 163 (see Tolu Balsam), ester value 47 to 83, saponification value 169 to 223 (all calculated on dry alcohol-soluble matter) were standards in the *B.P.* 1948 but are not now official requirements. In the opinion of Parry[2] these acid and ester values, which are to be determined on the sample, but calculated to the alcohol-soluble matter, will certainly exclude many pure samples of Sumatra benzoin.

Inhalation of Benzoin, *B.P.C.* Contains a mixture of benzoin and storax in strong alcohol.

The minimum total balsamic acids calculated from those present in the individual drugs should be 3·75 per cent.

Tincture of Benzoin, *B.P.C.* A simple 10 per cent tincture of benzoin in 90 per cent alcohol.

The total balsamic acids should be determined, using 25 ml of tincture; it contains theoretically at least 1·98 per cent w/v.

Compound Tincture of Benzoin, *B.P.* (Friars' Balsam). A tincture prepared from benzoin, storax, tolu and aloes.

The full examination of this galenical should be undertaken, as some commercial preparations are made from inferior and partially-exhausted drugs.

The total solids should be at least 18 per cent w/v, and are best determined by diluting 10 ml of the tincture to 50 ml with ethanol, evaporating 5 ml of the dilution and drying the residue in an oven at 100° until a constant loss of 1 mg per hour is obtained. Cocking[3] preferred a determination of total solids by drying *in vacuo* over sulphuric acid and found an average difference of 1·94 per cent for this method, compared with drying for one hour in an oven; he calculated the minimum total solids as 18·16 per cent w/v, allowing for maximum moisture and insoluble matter. Other figures found included acid value 61·3 to 77·8, ester value 88·8 to 123·8, and saponification value 156·1 to 198·1, all calculated on the total solids.

Free and total balsamic acids should be determined, using 10 ml of tincture for each assay. Figures obtained experimentally for a series of tinctures from a reliable source showed 7·4 to 9·6 per cent total acids and 3·9 to 5·0 per cent free acids, whilst obviously inferior samples from other sources gave 4·18 to 5·98 per cent and 1·96 to 3·29 per cent for total and free acids respectively; the total solids in these latter examples were not low. The minimum total balsamic acids calculated from those present in the individual drugs used in the preparation is 4·6 per cent.

1. Bennett, T. N., and Bickford, C. F., *J.A.O.A.C.*, 1928, **11**, 386.
2. Parry, E. J., *C. & D.*, 1932, **117**, 251.
3. Cocking, T. T., *Quart. J. Pharm.* 1928, **1**, 337.

BISMUTH

Bi At. Wt. 208·98

The many methods and their modifications available for the estimation of bismuth have mainly been devised for its determination in ores and complex inorganic mixtures; little difficulty should be experienced in the assay of pharmaceutical bismuth compounds.

In forensic work wet combustion should be employed to destroy organic matter as bismuth is appreciably volatilised when organic matter containing it is charred.

General methods for the estimation of bismuth present in quantity include direct weighing as sulphide; precipitation as sulphide, conversion to carbonate and ignition to oxide; and precipitation as phosphate. Recently the use of EDTA as a titrant for bismuth has considerably simplified the determination of this metal in pharmaceutical mixtures. Bismuth forms a complex at pH 1 to 2 and at this degree of acidity few other metals likely to be encountered (with the exception of iron) interfere; bismuth may therefore be selectively titrated in the presence of, say, aluminium, magnesium, or calcium. Various methods available have been discussed by Brookes and Johnson[1] and the following general procedure is recommended:

Dilute a suitable aliquot of a solution in nitric acid, containing about 120 mg of bismuth, to 50 ml with water ensuring that only sufficient acid is present to prevent precipitation of the metal. Add 0·1 g of sulphamic acid and allow to stand for two minutes. Add 2 drops of catechol violet indicator and, if the solution is violet in colour, add dilute ammonia solution drop by drop until the characteristic deep blue colour is obtained. Titrate with 0·05M EDTA until the solution turns violet-red, dilute with 200 ml of water, add a further 6 to 8 drops of the indicator solution (the solution reverts to its original blue colour on dilution) and continue the titration. The colour of the solution changes through violet, red and orange, followed by a sharp change to bright yellow at the end-point. 1 ml 0·05M EDTA = 0·01045 g Bi.

The two-stage dilution in the assay given above is used to prevent precipitation of basic bismuth salts. It is said that such precipitation can also be avoided by addition of glycerol to the titration liquid. This practice is adopted in a number of official methods, but in our opinion the end-point, although adequate, is not so good as with the dilution technique described above.

When this method is applied to a substance such as bismuth carbonate a result which is as much as 1 per cent lower than that obtained by ignition may be expected; this is due to the fact that the EDTA method gives bismuth alone, whereas the residue after ignition will also contain the alkali and alkaline earth metals which are usually present.

Where phosphate precipitation is required the method of Schœller and Waterhouse[2] is recommended. The advantages claimed for the phosphate precipitation include the definite composition of the precipitate, which is unchanged by ignition and not readily reduced, and its heavy, crystalline nature which enables it to be filtered rapidly. It was found that the conditions for quantitative precipitation of the phosphate required careful adjustment, but, if the details are followed precisely, it is a rapid and satisfactory method of estimation.

To a cold bismuth solution containing approximately 0·1 g of metal and an indefinite amount of nitric acid, but free from chlorides, in a total bulk of less than 100 ml, add strong ammonia solution until a slight permanent precipitate is obtained. Add 2 ml of concentrated nitric acid (which should dissolve the precipitate at once). Heat the clear liquid to boiling and, whilst boiling, precipitate with a 10 per cent diammonium phosphate solution, added from a burette (at a rate of about 30 drops per minute, which may be increased once the bismuth phosphate is thrown down), slow addition favouring the formation of a coarsely crystalline precipitate. A considerable excess of phosphate solution should be used (30 ml of 10 per cent solution for 0·1 g), and stirring must be continued throughout the addition to prevent bumping. Dilute the solution with boiling water to about 300 ml and allow to settle for fifteen minutes on a water-bath. Decant the clear liquid through a 9-cm No. 40 Whatman filter paper or a Gooch crucible; stir the precipitate twice with a hot 3 per cent ammonium nitrate solution containing a few drops of nitric acid per litre, transfer to the filter, complete the washing, dry the precipitate and gently ignite. If a filter paper is used, detach the precipitate as completely as possible before charring the paper at a low temperature in a porcelain crucible. $BiPO_4 \times 0{\cdot}6875 = Bi$.

Precipitated bismuth, *B.P.C.*, is determined by EDTA titration after solution of about 0·35 g, accurately weighed, in a mixture of 2 ml of concentrated nitric acid and 4 ml of water and diluting to 50 ml.

Traces of bismuth may be estimated colorimetrically as bismuth potassium iodide in acid solution and in the presence of sulphurous acid, small amounts of other metals not interfering. An excess of sulphurous acid must be avoided as it produces a yellow colour with potassium iodide.

Haddock[3] has shown that the yellow bismuth compound formed with potassium iodide can be quantitatively extracted by organic solvents, and in the presence of considerable quantities of highly coloured ions and other interfering metals it is possible to determine very small amounts of bismuth by this method. Lead and thallium in quantities greater than 0·5 mg are the only two elements which interfere seriously; other interfering metals (antimony, copper, silver, mercury, tin), especially those which react with soluble iodides, are removed by extracting the bismuth with diphenylthiocarbazone in chloroform before proceeding to the colorimetric determination.

To the neutral or acid solution free from organic matter, add 2 g of citric acid, make alkaline with ammonia, cool and add 2 g of potassium cyanide. Shake the mixture with four portions, each of 15 ml of a 0·1 per cent solution of diphenylthiocarbazone in chloroform. Wash each extract with the same 10 ml of water contained in another separator and evaporate the chloroform. Heat the residue with 1 ml of concentrated sulphuric acid and destroy organic matter by adding 30 per cent hydrogen peroxide solution drop by drop; after cooling dilute to 20 ml with water and eliminate any sulphur dioxide formed from the acid by the cautious addition of a very weak iodine solution. To the resulting liquid (or to the original acid solution of mixtures not containing interfering metals) add 4 drops of an approximately 5 per cent sulphurous acid solution, 2 ml of 30 per cent hypophosphorous acid and 5 ml of fresh 10 per cent potassium iodide solution. Shake the liquid thoroughly with successive 3-ml portions of a mixture of three parts of amyl alcohol and one part of ethyl acetate until the final extract is almost colourless, collecting the extracts in a small graduated cylinder. Prepare a standard colour by adding a known amount of a 0·001 per cent solution of bismuth to the aqueous solution and again extracting with the organic solvent as before; several other standards may be prepared similarly. Adjust each of the series of extracts to the same volume (about 6 ml for 10 to 40μg of bismuth and 10 to 12 ml for 40 to 100μg). Filter through small plugs of cotton-wool before comparison either in 10-ml Nessler cylinders or a suitable colorimeter.

It was found that the bismuth could be determined directly in the presence of considerable quantities of manganese, cobalt, chromium, cadmium and nickel so long as the standard colour was prepared as directed above.

BISMUTH SALTS

Bismuth salts are now determined officially either by phosphate precipitation or by EDTA titration. The table below summarises the methods of assay used for the *B.P.* and *B.P.C.* bismuth salts and methods applicable to some other salts:

TABLE 10

BISMUTH SALT	AMOUNT TAKEN FOR DETERMINATION	METHOD
Carbonate, *B.P.C.*	0·5 g	EDTA
Glycollylarsanilate, *B.P.C.*	0·5 g	Phosphate after heating on a water-bath with 10 ml HNO_3 until light colour
Oxychloride, *B.P.*	0·2 g	Phosphate
Oxyiodide	0·35 g	EDTA after heating to dryness with HNO_3 until iodine expelled and dissolving in HNO_3
Salicylate	0·3 g	EDTA
Sodium Tartrate, *B.P.*	0·5 g	Phosphate
Subgallate, *B.P.C.*	0·8 g	EDTA after ignition at 500°
Subnitrate, *B.P.C.*	0·5 g	EDTA

Injection of Bismuth Oxychloride, *B.P.* A sterile suspension containing 10 per cent of bismuth oxychloride with sodium chloride and chlorocresol.

For assay determine the weight of injection in a sufficient number of containers and dissolve in a sufficient quantity of concentrated nitric acid. Evaporate to dryness, moisten the residue with concentrated sulphuric acid and ignite at a temperature not exceeding 500°. Dissolve the residue in just sufficient concentrated nitric acid to prevent precipitation of the metal when the solution is diluted to a suitable volume with water. Using a volume of the resulting solution equivalent to about 2 g of the sample, complete as in the general method for determination of bismuth given above, p. 127.

Injection of Bismuth Sodium Tartrate, *B.P.* A sterile solution of bismuth sodium tartrate and usually contains 60 mg per ml.

For assay evaporate to dryness a volume expected to contain about 0·5 g of bismuth sodium tartrate, moisten the residue with concentrated sulphuric acid and ignite at a temperature not exceeding 500°. Dissolve the residue in a mixture of 2 ml of concentrated nitric acid and 4 ml of water and complete by the general method for determination of bismuth given above, p. 127, from 'add 0·1 g of sulphamic acid. . . .'.

Compound Lozenge of Bismuth, *B.P.C.* Contains bismuth carbonate, calcium carbonate and heavy magnesium carbonate in sucrose and acacia. All three active ingredients may be determined[1] with EDTA as follows:

Take a sample of 20 lozenges, determine the average weight and powder the lozenges.

For bismuth, determine by the general method for the determination of bismuth, p. 127, using 2 g of powdered lozenges.

For calcium and magnesium, ignite about 2 g of the powdered lozenges at a temperature not exceeding 500° until all the carbon is removed and then dissolve the residue in a mixture of 6 ml of water and 3 ml of concentrated nitric acid. Add 2 ml of dilute hydrochloric acid and 150 ml of water and then add dilute ammonia solution until the solution remains just acid to litmus paper. Boil for two minutes, cool to 15°, filter into a 250-ml graduated flask and dilute to volume with water. Proceed as described for the determination of calcium and magnesium in Compound Mixture of Calcium Carbonate for Infants (p. 154) using two 50-ml aliquots of the solution instead of the two 20-ml aliquots of solution A directed in that assay.

Compound Powder of Bismuth, *B.P.C.* A mixture of 1 part each of bismuth carbonate and sodium bicarbonate with 3 parts each of calcium carbonate and magnesium carbonate.

The method given under Compound Lozenge of Bismuth is clearly applicable to this preparation, except that there is no necessity to ignite in the determination of calcium and magnesium. The present *B.P.C.* method is based upon precipitation of the bismuth with potassium iodide and determination of total and soluble alkali.

For bismuth: dissolve about 1·5 g in dilute nitric acid, add dilute ammonia solution until a slight permanent precipitate and just redissolve with dilute nitric acid. To the cold solution add potassium iodide solution with constant stirring until in excess as shown by a slight yellow colour, dilute to about 250 ml with boiling water and boil until almost colourless. Adjust the pH to 4·2 with sodium acetate, filter on a sintered glass filter, wash and dry at 105°. 1 g residue = 0·5939 g Bi.

The solubility of the other salts in the bicarbonate solution gives high results for a titration of the filtrate for sodium bicarbonate unless the carbon dioxide is eliminated by boiling; an appreciable error may also be caused owing to the solubility of magnesium carbonate if the volume of water used for extraction and washing is not limited, hence:

For total alkali: Dissolve 2 g in 50 ml of N hydrochloric acid, boil, cool and titrate with N sodium hydroxide using phenolphthalein as indicator.

For bicarbonate: Boil 10 g of an aqueous suspension of the powder with 150 ml of water for ten minutes, cool, filter, washing the residue with 100 ml of warm water, and titrate the filtrate to bromophenol blue.

The magnesium in the filtrate by experiment was found to be equivalent to less than 0·1 per cent of sodium bicarbonate.

1. Brookes, H. E., and Johnson, C. A., *J. Pharm. Pharmacol.* 1955, **7,** 846.

2. Schœller, W. R., and Waterhouse, E. F., *Analyst*, 1920, **45**, 435.
3. Haddock, L. A. *Analyst*, 1934, **59**, 163.

BORIC ACID

H_3BO_3 Mol. Wt. 61·84

The methods of determining boric acid in drugs have been conveniently summarised by Scott Dodd[1] and they have been critically studied by him. Substances containing over 8 per cent of glycerides or glycerol should not be strongly ignited even with excess of alkali, as some loss of boric acid may occur. Fats must be removed by light petroleum or benzene, re-extracting these solvents with alkali. If carbonates are present carbon dioxide must be expelled in acid solution before titration; phosphates must also be eliminated. Appreciable loss results from lengthy evaporation of acidified solutions of boric acid, but if solutions are dilute no loss occurs when they are boiled for five minutes.

Free boric acid has a very low dissociation constant, the direct-titration curve being between about pH 6 and 11, and strong acids, such as mineral acids, can be titrated in the presence of boric acid with an indicator having a colour change below 6 (such as methyl orange, pH 2·9 to 4·0 and methyl red, pH 4·2 to 6·3). Other acids must be neutralised before titration of boric acid, but errors are likely in attempting to neutralise concentrated solutions owing to buffering. When glycerol or mannitol is added to a solution of boric acid an acid complex is formed and the dissociation constant is increased considerably, the complexes being about as strong as acetic acid. Mannitol is more suitable than glycerol in forming the acid complex with boric acid as it is more likely to be neutral, less is required, and it gives a sharper end-point. According to Scott Dodd there is some indication that more definite combination occurs with mannitol. Many polyatomic alcohols and some sugars can be used and Gilmour[2] recommends technical invert sugar instead of glycerol as a reagent for titration because it reacts equally well and is much cheaper. Sciarra and Zapotocky[3] have carried out a comparative study on various substances that may be used in the titration and show that, in both visual and potentiometric methods of titration, mannitol, fructose, invert sugar and propylene glycol can all be used successfully to replace glycerol. They recommend that potentiometric titrations should be used for samples containing boric acid where the end-point of the titration is not definitely shown by an indicator or when a coloured substance interferes in the detection of the end-point. In our hands this has worked quite satisfactorily and the recommended method is as follows:

Mix 50 ml of a solution containing about 0·2 g of boric acid with a solution of 5 g of mannitol in 50 ml of water, stir the solution mechanically and titrate potentiometrically with 0·1N sodium hydroxide using glass and calomel electrodes.

The titration curve of the acid complex lies between pH 3 and 7·2 approximately, so that an indicator with pH change slightly higher than 7·2 can then be used to titrate the boric acid. Phenolphthalein (pH 8·2 to 9·2) and phenol violet (pH 8 to 10) are satisfactory and the *B.P.* has adopted phenolphthalein in the case of boric acid. If glycerol is used it should be first neutralised to phenolphthalein and at least 30 per cent by volume must be present when neutralisation point is reached, and the *B.P.* method of estimation of boric acid using 2 g of sample in 50 ml of water with 100 ml of glycerol, titrating with N sodium hydroxide, allows for this. 1 ml N = 0·06184 g H_3BO_3.

Accurate estimation of boric acid is also obtainable by distillation in acid solution with methanol vapour (Alcock[4]).

In the presence of organic matter moisten the sample with 10 ml of 2N sodium hydroxide. If much fat is present, it should be removed with ether. Evaporate the water on a water-bath and ash; there is no need to burn away all the carbon. Transfer the ash from the dish to a distilling flask with as little water as possible, dissolve the ash with a few ml of dilute sulphuric acid by warming. Add methyl red and 30 per cent sodium hydroxide solution until alkaline. Concentrate the liquid to 1 or 2 ml over a Bunsen flame, with continuous agitation. After cooling, add 60 ml of methanol and methyl red indicator. Drop in concentrated sulphuric acid until the solution is strongly acid. Distil with methanol vapour, taking care not to allow the residue in the flask to become too concentrated. Collect the distillate in sufficient N sodium hydroxide to maintain an alkaline reaction. Distil off the methanol from the receiving flask and titrate the boric acid in the usual way after neutralisation to methyl orange and boiling to remove carbon dioxide.

Estimation of boric acid by ignition to boric oxide is not practicable, a slow volatilisation taking place (Bagshaw[5]).

For **small amounts** of boron, up to 30 μg in the final solution, the carmine method of Hatcher and Wilcox[6] can be recommended.

Weigh accurately a suitable quantity of the sample into a 25-ml silica dish. Add 0·1 g of calcium oxide for each g of material, mix well and thoroughly moisten with water, evaporate the mixture to dryness and ash the residue as completely as possible in a muffle furnace at 450° to 500° for three hours. Cool and treat the residue with 10 ml of 2N hydrochloric acid. Remove any undissolved material by filtration or centrifuging for five to ten minutes, and dilute the solution to exactly 25 ml with distilled water.

Transfer 2 ml of the sample solution to a beaker and cautiously add 10 ml of concentrated sulphuric acid, mix, and cool. Add 10 ml of carmine solution (prepared by dissolving 0·05 g in 100 ml of concentrated sulphuric acid, leaving the mixture overnight or until dissolved) mix and set it aside for six to seven hours or overnight for colour development. Carry out a blank procedure with all the reagents used.

Measure the extinctions of the test and blank solutions in a spectrophotometer at a wavelength of 585 mμ using a 1-cm cell. Read the number of micrograms of boron equivalent to the observed extinction values of the test and blank solutions from a previously prepared calibration graph and so obtain a net measure of boron in the sample.

Establish the calibration graph as follows: Measure appropriate amounts of standard boron solution (0·5716 g boric acid per litre, 1 ml = 100 μg boron) into a series of 25-ml silica dishes and carry out the whole procedure as described above. The amounts should be chosen so that the 2 ml aliquots taken from the 25-ml volumes cover the range 0 to 30 μg boron. Measure the extinction values at a wavelength of 585 mμ using 1-cm cells, and construct a graph relating the extinctions to the number of micrograms of boron.

Eye Lotion of Boric Acid, *B.P.C.* A simple solution of 3·43 per cent w/v of boric acid in purified water. This can be titrated directly with N sodium hydroxide using 50 ml with an equal volume of glycerol.

Compound Eye Lotion of Zinc Sulphate, *B.P.C.* A solution of boric acid, 2·29 per cent and zinc sulphate, 0·34 per cent in purified water.

For analysis take 50 ml of the liquid, add 0·4 g of sodium carbonate dissolved in water, boil, filter and wash. To the filtrate add methyl orange and a slight excess of 0·5N hydrochloric acid. Boil for five minutes, neutralise, add an equal volume of glycerol and titrate the boric acid with 0·5N alkali to phenolphthalein or phenol violet. Dry the precipitated zinc carbonate and ignite gently to oxide in a porcelain crucible. $ZnO \times 3{\cdot}534 = ZnSO_4,7H_2O$.

Boric Acid Gauze, Lint, *B.P.C.*, and **Cotton Wool.** The *B.P.C.* preparation is standardised to contain 3 to 7 per cent of boric acid.

Place the specified quantity in a stoppered bottle, add 50 ml of boiling water and 40 ml of glycerol. Titrate with 0·2N alkali to phenol violet. 1 ml 0·2N = 0·01237 g H_3BO_3.

It is important to use an unexposed portion of the material and care must be taken to cut out the quantity for estimation so as not to shake off boric acid in handling.

Ointment of Boric Acid, *B.P.C.* Contains 1 per cent of boric acid in a mixture of paraffins containing a little beeswax and cetostearyl alcohol.

The boric acid may be determined by direct titration, but in this case the end-point is somewhat obscure.

Weigh about 5 g of ointment into a wide-mouthed flask, add 50 ml of a previously neutralised 50 per cent solution of glycerol, warm the flask on a water-bath until the fat has melted and the hot mixture has been thoroughly agitated. Titrate with 0·1N alkali to phenolphthalein or phenol violet. 1 ml 0·1N = 0·006184 g.

In the *N.F.* method of titration the ointment is melted with water, shaken frequently for fifteen minutes, filtered and the fats washed with hot water before titrating an aliquot part of the filtrate.

For another method of estimation:

> Dissolve a weighed quantity of ointment in light petroleum, wash the solution a number of times with water and titrate the combined aqueous washings.

It should be noted that boric acid ointment is often not completely homogeneous.

COMPOUND BORIC ACID POWDERS

Three dusting powders containing boric acid are included in the *B.P.C.*, *i.e.* **Boric Talc,** 5 per cent of boric acid and 10 per cent of starch in talc; **Compound Salicylic Acid Dusting Powder,** 3 per cent of salicylic acid and 5 per cent of boric acid in talc; and **Compound Zinc Dusting Powder,** containing 5 per cent boric acid, 25 per cent zinc oxide, 35 per cent starch and 35 per cent purified talc. **Boric Acid and Starch Dusting Powder,** containing 25 per cent of boric acid is official in the *B.Vet.C.*

In the presence of salicylic acid the powder must first be treated with dilute alkali, filtered, acidified and extracted with ether before determining the boric acid in the aqueous residues. In the absence of zinc oxide, boric acid can be titrated directly; in the presence of zinc oxide the boric acid is extracted with cold water for titration and the zinc oxide determined in the water-insoluble portion by solution in an excess of N acid and back titration with alkali to methyl orange in the presence of 2 g of ammonium chloride.

A full analysis of Compound Zinc Dusting Powder is given below:

> Determine the boric acid in the cold water-soluble portion by titration in the presence of 50 per cent of glycerol with 0·5N alkali to phenolphthalein or phenol violet. To the residue add dilute hydrochloric acid, heat to boiling and filter. Wash, dry the talc at 105° and weigh. Determine the zinc in the acid filtrate by titration (p. 696). The starch figure is usually obtained by difference, but may be assayed using the cold hydrochloric acid method described under Starch (p. 577) which gives a close approximation.

In stored preparations some combination may occur between zinc oxide and boric acid in the presence of moisture and low results would then be obtained for boric acid by direct aqueous extraction before titration; it is then necessary to dissolve the whole in an excess of acid and precipitate the zinc with sodium carbonate and filter before determining the boric acid. Unless a freshly prepared material is under examination it is advisable always to treat the sample in this way.

Poultice of Kaolin, *B.P.* A mixture of kaolin, 52·7, boric acid, 4·5, volatile matter, 0·3 and glycerin, 42·5 parts.

BORIC ACID

Good results for a complete analysis can be obtained by the following procedure:

Mix about 1 to 1·5 g with hot water, filter through a weighed Gooch crucible, wash and dry the residue of kaolin at 105°. (Ignition gives low results from loss of water of hydration.)

Warm about 20 g of poultice with water until thoroughly disintegrated, aiding dispersion by rubbing with a glass rod. Add an equal bulk of glycerol and titrate direct with 0·5N alkali to phenolphthalein or phenol violet for boric acid. 1 ml 0·5N = 0·03092 g.

Heat about 30 g of poultice with water until thoroughly disintegrated, filter through a Büchner funnel, washing the residue repeatedly with hot water. Evaporate the total filtrates to under 50 ml, cool, make up accurately to 50 ml and take the specific gravity of the glycerol solution. From the specific gravity found subtract that due to the percentage of boric acid actually present in the solution (subtraction for each 1 per cent boric acid = 0·0035) and calculate the percentage of glycerol from the table in the Appendix. (*Note.* The percentages of glycerol in the tables are w/w; multiply by the corrected specific gravity of the solution to obtain per cent w/v and divide by 2 for the actual weight of glycerol in the weight of poultice taken for assay. Allow a minimum of 98 per cent for *B.P.* glycerin.)

As the glycerol can be extracted practically pure, it should be possible to use the chemical method of estimation given under Glycerin.

The percentage unaccounted for in the above assay represents volatile matter and extraneous moisture.

BORATES

Borax, $Na_2B_4O_7,10H_2O$, Mol. Wt. 381·4. Borax hydrolyses in aqueous solution to boric acid and sodium hydroxide and hence has an alkaline reaction. When borax is titrated with a strong acid to methyl orange or methyl red, the end-point is quite sharp and occurs when the acid is entirely in the free state, as boric acid is quite unaffected by these indicators. The *B.P.* method is by this titration. 1 ml 0·5N = 0·09536 g. It can then be titrated as described above under Boric Acid. The second titration should be double that of the first; any disagreement would indicate excess of boric acid or alkali, and this fact is used for mixtures of borax and sodium bicarbonate such as **Alkaline Nasal Solution-tablets,** *B.P.C.* and **Compound Thymol Solution-tablets,** *B.P.C.* Ashing to eliminate interference from dye is necessary in the latter product.

Glycerin of Borax, *B.P.C.* A solution of borax, 12 per cent w/w in glycerin.

This preparation has an acid reaction due to interaction of the borax with the glycerol to form sodium metaborate and glyceryl borate, which latter hydrolyses to boric acid.

For estimation dissolve about 15 g in water, neutralise to methyl orange, add glycerol or mannitol and titrate with 0·5N alkali to phenolphthalein or phenol violet. 1 ml 0·5N = 0·04768 g borax.

Honey of Borax, *B.P.C.* A solution of borax, 10 per cent, in glycerin and honey.

If a mixed indicator of methyl orange and xylene cyanol is used in the preliminary neutralisation, the end-point can be seen in most cases and direct determination of the boric acid is then possible without ashing. Otherwise, for determination of the borax, ash about 2 g in the presence of an equal weight of anhydrous sodium carbonate, dissolve in hot water and titrate by the method given above for boric acid after neutralising to methyl orange.

As the optical activity of sugars differs in borax solution from that of aqueous solution, the activity being restored after acidification by a strong acid (Levy and Doisy[7]), the optical activity of the honey must be determined after acidification. Strong acids rapidly invert sucrose; hence, although only a little sucrose should be present, the rotation of a 20 per cent w/v solution must be observed as soon as possible after dilution. Any error by inversion would be quite small for genuine honey (limits $[\alpha]_D + 2{\cdot}6°$ to $- 12{\cdot}8°$).

Compound Powder of Borax for Nasal Wash, *B.P.C.* Equal parts of borax, sodium bicarbonate, sucrose and sodium chloride. The ingredients can be estimated in the following way:

Dissolve about 2·5 g in water and titrate to methyl orange with 0·5N acid. Boil for a few minutes, cool, add an equal volume of glycerol and titrate to phenolphthalein with 0·5N alkali. The number of ml of 0·5N alkali in the second titration × 0·04768 = g borax. From the first titration take half the volume of the second titration, the remaining volume in ml × 0·04201 = g sodium bicarbonate. Estimate sodium chloride in about 0·3 g by Volhard's method, described under Halogen Acids, p. 290. 1 ml 0·1N $AgNO_3$ = 0·005845 g.

Sodium perborate, $NaBO_2.H_2O_2,3H_2O$, Mol. Wt. 153·9.

For determination dissolve 0·3 g in 50 ml of water and either (*a*) acidify strongly with sulphuric acid and titrate with 0·1N potassium permanganate or (*b*) add 2 g of potassium iodide and 10 ml of dilute sulphuric acid and titrate the liberated iodine with 0·1N thiosulphate. 1 ml 0·1N = 0·007694 g. The latter method is preferable.

1. Scott Dodd, A., *Analyst*, 1929, **54,** 645, 715; 1930, **55,** 23.
2. Gilmour, G. van B., *Analyst*, 1921, **46,** 3.
3. Sciarra, J. J., and Zapotocky, J. A., *J. Amer. Pharm. Ass., Sci. Edn.*, 1955, **44,** 370.
4. Alcock, R. S., *Analyst*, 1937, **62,** 522.
5. Bagshaw, C. R., *Analyst*, 1918, **43,** 138.
6. Hatcher, J. T., and Wilcox, L. V., *Anal. Chem.*, 1950, **22,** 567.
7. Levy, M., and Doisy, E. A., *J. Biol. Chem.*, 1929, **84,** 749.

CAFFEINE

$C_8H_{10}O_2N_4,H_2O$ Mol. Wt. 212·2

Caffeine is a very weak base and its salts are decomposed by water; hence it can be extracted from both acid and alkaline solution (more easily from the latter) by chloroform and this is generally employed as the method of estimation, the extracted anhydrous caffeine being weighed. Caffeine is only slightly soluble in ether and this solvent is unsuitable for its extraction. As caffeine is moderately soluble in water, the small partition between solvents demands a large number of extractions before the material is quantitatively removed. Caffeine is very susceptible to decomposition by strong alkali and should be extracted immediately from alkaline solution.

Caffeine is very resistant to acids and to clean it from other organic matter it may be warmed with strong acids without decomposition. By completely digesting with sulphuric acid as in the Kjeldahl method for nitrogen, caffeine is quantitatively oxidised and a nitrogen figure ($N \times 3{\cdot}466 =$ anhydrous caffeine) is a good check method for its determination. Such a method may be employed direct on Compound Syrup of Glycerophosphates.

In our experience the non-aqueous titration of purine derivatives as bases has not been very satisfactory and with perchloric-acetic acid we obtained very unsatisfactory end-points for caffeine. Satisfactory potentiometric titration has been claimed[1] however, using a mixed solvent of acetic acid and acetic anhydride.

Estimation of *B.P.* caffeine in galenicals can only be approximate as the commercial article effloresces and contains varying quantities of moisture, an average moisture figure being 7 per cent; this figure may be used for calculation of the original *B.P.* caffeine from a weighed quantity of the anhydrous base; the *B.P.* maximum is 8·5 per cent. Anhydrous caffeine is also available commercially.

The estimation of caffeine in mixtures and compound tablets is given under the various galenicals in which it occurs, *e.g.* Compound Tablets of Aspirin, etc.

According to Daoust[2] small amounts of caffeine can be determined by precipitation as phosphomolybdate and solution in acetone for colorimetric measurement. Aspirin or phenacetin do not interfere but the reaction is not specific for caffeine. Although precipitation of larger amounts may be convenient, a 3 mg aliquot of caffeine precipitated in a volume of 25 ml is most suitable for colorimetric measurement; a large excess of precipitating reagent should be avoided.

To an amount of powdered tablet containing approximately 30 mg of caffeine add 100 ml of water and heat just to boiling. Transfer to a boiling water-bath, add, with stirring, 10 ml of dilute hydrochloric acid (1 : 1) and then, drop by drop, 2 ml of 20 per cent phosphomolybdic acid. Continue heating for fifteen to twenty minutes until the heavy yellow precipitate coagulates. Filter hot through a sintered-glass filter of medium porosity and wash with 30 ml of cold dilute hydrochloric acid (1 : 9). Dissolve the precipitate in acetone and dilute to 100 ml with acetone. Dilute 10 ml of this solution to 25 ml with acetone for measurement of the absorption at 440 mμ. Determine the amount of caffeine present by reference to a standard graph prepared by similar treatment of 1 to 5 ml aliquots of a standard solution containing 1·0 mg of anhydrous caffeine per ml.

CAFFEINE SALTS

As caffeine is a very weak base its salts are readily hydrolysed by water and caffeine may be extracted directly by a solvent (but preferably immediately after making alkaline); the combining acid may be titrated as free acid even in the presence of the caffeine. **Caffeine citrate,** $C_8H_{10}O_2N_4,C_6H_8O_7$, Mol. Wt. 386·3. Citric acid may be titrated direct with 0·5N sodium hydroxide to phenolphthalein. 1 ml 0·5N = 0·06439 g caffeine citrate.

Caffeine is very soluble in alkali benzoates and salicylates, and mixtures with these salts are prepared. Examples of these mixtures are: **caffeine and sodium benzoate** and **caffeine and sodium salicylate.** The caffeine is determined by extraction with chloroform in alkaline solution and, after acidification, the aromatic acids are extracted from the residual aqueous liquid with ether and titrated with 0·1N alkali after evaporation. 1 ml 0·1N = 0·0144 g $C_7H_5O_2Na$ and 0·0160 g $C_7H_5O_3Na$.

Caffeine and sodium iodide is an intimate mixture of equal parts of caffeine with sodium iodide. Caffeine is extracted by chloroform in alkaline solution in the usual way. Sodium iodide is determined in the aqueous residues from the caffeine extraction by iodate titration.

Elixir of Caffeine Iodide, *B.P.C.* Contains 9·14 per cent w/v of caffeine and sodium iodide with sodium iodide, liquorice and chloroform in decoction of coffee.

The preparation is standardised on its anhydrous caffeine content, allowance being made for the caffeine in the decoction of coffee. Alkaline extraction, although normally more rapid than from acid solution, is not satisfactory since intractable emulsions are formed with chloroform.

To 10 ml of elixir in a separator add 5 ml of dilute hydrochloric acid; extract with six 30 ml portions of chloroform, washing each extract successively with the same 10 ml of water contained in a second separator. Evaporate the solvent, dry at 105° and weigh the residue of anhydrous caffeine.

The sodium iodide is preferably determined by the Volhard method.

THEOBROMINE, $C_7H_8O_2N_4$, Mol. Wt. 180·2, (3,7-dimethylxanthine).

Theobromine can be converted quantitatively into caffeine by the method of Self and Rankin[3] with a slight excess of dimethyl sulphate in the presence of sodium hydroxide. The process has been found of general value for the determination of theobromine and is described in detail later under theobromine and sodium salicylate to which it was first applied.

The formation of silver-theobromine is the principle involved in the method of Boie,[4] the accuracy of which has been verified and it is applied in the *B.P.C.* to theobromine.

Weigh 0·3 g into a flask, add 120 ml of water and boil gently until dissolved. Cool, add 20 ml of 0·1N silver nitrate and 1·5 ml of phenol red indicator and titrate the liberated nitric acid with 0·1N sodium hydroxide to a deep red-violet colour. 1 ml 0·1N = 0·01802 g $C_7H_8O_2N_4$.

Theobromine and sodium salicylate consists of a mixture of sodium salicylate and sodium theobromine in approximately equimolecular proportions.

Boie's method given above has been adapted to this preparation by the *N.F.*, the alkalinity being first neutralised. The following modification will allow a determination of the alkalinity.

Dissolve 0·5 g of theobromine and sodium salicylate in 100 ml of hot water, add 15 ml of 0·1N sulphuric acid and boil to remove carbon dioxide. Cool to 40°, add 1·5 ml of phenol red solution and a measured quantity of 0·1N sodium hydroxide until the mixture is alkaline (2 to 3 ml required). Titrate with 0·1N sulphuric acid until the colour of the indicator changes to lemon yellow. The amount of 0·1N sodium hydroxide deducted from the total 0·1N acid is a measure of the alkalinity. To this solution add 20 ml of 0·1N silver nitrate and titrate the liberated nitric acid with 0·1N sodium hydroxide to a deep red-violet colour. 1 ml 0·1N = 0·01802 g theobromine. The approach of the end-point is indicated by incipient precipitation of silver oxide.

The salicylic acid may be determined by extraction with ether or chloroform (see p. 557) after precipitation of most of the theobromine.

The *B.Vet.C.* method, adopted from the *B.P.* 1953, is that of Self and Rankin mentioned above.

Dissolve 1 g of theobromine and sodium salicylate in 10 ml of water in a small stoppered flask, add 2 ml of N sodium hydroxide and 0·6 ml of dimethyl sulphate and shake continuously for five minutes. Allow to stand for half an hour, shaking frequently, then add 3 ml of N sodium hydroxide and 10 ml of water; shake well for two minutes. Transfer to a separator with chloroform and a little water, and extract the caffeine immediately by shaking with successive portions of chloroform, washing each extract with about 10 ml of water contained in a second separator. Evaporate the chloroform, dry at 105° and weigh. 1 g anhydrous caffeine = 0·9278 g of theobromine ($C_7H_8O_2N_4$).

Tne original method has been criticised in using insufficient alkali for complete reaction, an increase to 4 ml of N sodium hydroxide on the first addition being recommended. It is essential that the caffeine produced in the reaction should be extracted as soon as possible after formation, since it is quickly decomposed by strong alkali.

Although the method has generally given excellent results, occasionally inexplicably high figures have been obtained. These have been found due to the slow volatility of methyl salicylate formed during the reaction. If an open dish is used for the evaporation of the chloroform such errors are avoided.

Parkes and Parkes[5] employed a 5 per cent solution of phenol in chloroform for the extraction of theobromine; the solubility in this is about eight times that in chloroform. After evaporation of the chloroform from the mixed solvent solution the phenol is removed by holding the flask in the fingers and rotating it over a small flame while sucking a gentle current of air through it with a filter pump.

Theobromine can be separated from caffeine by the formation of insoluble silver-theobromine, $C_7H_7O_2N_4Ag$, on addition of silver nitrate; or, in a mixture of the two, caffeine can be extracted in alkaline solution with chloroform, theobromine being left as the sodium salt in aqueous solution.

Tablets of Phenobarbitone and Theobromine, *B.P.C.* Contain 5 grains of theobromine and $\frac{1}{2}$ grain of phenobarbitone.

The theobromine can be determined by the silver method of Boie given above, after washing out the phenobarbitone with ether. Since theobromine is slightly soluble in ether, a definite volume of solvent must be used and a correction applied. The official assay is essentially as follows:

For theobromine: Determine the average weight of 20 tablets, powder and transfer about 0·7 g to a stoppered flask. Add 50 ml of ether, shake for a few minutes and filter into a small separator, washing the flask and filter with four 12-ml portions of ether and reserving the ethereal solution. Place the filter and contents in the original flask and dissolve the residue of theobromine in 150 ml water and 25 ml (or a sufficient quantity) of 0·1N sulphuric acid. Boil vigorously for two minutes, cool to 40° and add 1·5 ml of phenol red solution. Make distinctly alkaline by addition of a slight excess of 0·2N sodium hydroxide and adjust the reaction of the solution by carefully adding 0·1N sulphuric acid dropwise until the bluish-red colour just becomes distinctly yellow. Add 50 ml of 0·1N silver nitrate and titrate the liberated acid slowly with 0·2N sodium hydroxide to a deep red-violet colour. 1 ml 0·2N = 0·03603 g of $C_7H_8O_2N_4$. To the weight of theobromine found add 0·006 g to correct for its solubility in ether.

For phenobarbitone: To the ethereal solution reserved from the above assay add 20 ml of a solution containing 1 per cent w/v of sodium hydroxide in brine and shake. Allow to separate, transfer the aqueous layer to a second separator and extract the ethereal layer with further portions of the sodium hydroxide-brine solution, transferring each extract to the second separator. Shake the solution with two 15-ml quantities of ether, shaking each separated ethereal liquid with the same 3 ml of water in a second separator and reject the ethereal liquids. Add the washing to the alkaline liquid, acidify with hydrochloric acid and completely extract the phenobarbitone with successive 15-ml portions of ether. Mix the ethereal solutions and wash with two 2-ml quantities of water. Mix the aqueous washings and shake with 10 ml of ether. Mix the ethereal solutions, filter and wash the filter with ether; evaporate the solvent and dry the residue to constant weight at 105°.

A rapid method for routine examination is the following:

To a weight of powder equivalent to three tablets add 20 ml of ethanol, shake to dissolve the phenobarbitone, filter through a Gooch crucible, wash the precipitate twice with 20 ml portions of ethanol followed by 10 ml of water. Dry at 105° and weigh the theobromine. Evaporate the filtration washings, dissolve the residue in dilute sodium hydroxide and transfer to a separator, acidify and extract the phenobarbitone with ether. Evaporate, dry and weigh.

This method is not applicable if starch has been used in the tablet.

THEOPHYLLINE, $C_7H_8O_2N_4$, Mol. Wt. 180·2 or $C_7H_8O_2N_4$, H_2O, Mol. Wt. 198·2, (1,3-dimethylxanthine).

Theophylline behaves analytically like theobromine. It can be quantitatively methylated to caffeine by the method of Self and Rankin given above and it forms an insoluble silver compound. However, sodium acetate is sometimes present and will interfere with the silver determination unless the acetic acid is volatilised with excess of standard sulphuric acid.

Theophylline can be extracted quantitatively from acid solution with a mixture of chloroform and *iso*propyl alcohol.

Aminophylline (Theophylline with Ethylenediamine). This substance is prepared by evaporating a solution of theophylline in ethylenediamine to dryness.

Reimers[6] showed that theophylline can be extracted in acid solution from this preparation with a mixture of chloroform and *iso*propyl alcohol. Although *iso*propyl alcohol is a little better solvent, ethanol can be used but further extraction is then necessary.

Dissolve about 0·5 g in 20 ml of water in a separator and slightly acidify to bromocresol green with dilute hydrochloric acid. Add 5 g of sodium chloride and extract with four successive 25 ml portions of a mixture of 3 volumes chloroform and 1 volume *iso*propyl alcohol. Wash each extract with the same 10 ml of water, evaporate the solvent, dry the residue of anhydrous theophylline at 105° and weigh.

The ethylenediamine can be titrated directly using about 0·5 g and titrating with 0·1N hydrochloric acid. Bromocresol green is a satisfactory indicator, titrating to about pH 4·6 (blue-green), but the best end-point is obtained with '4·5' indicator, the end-point being very distinct at the grey tint. 1 ml 0·1N = 0·003005 g $C_2H_4(NH_2)_2$.

Precipitation of theophylline as the silver compound, which is filtered off, is a useful method particularly for tablet formulations:

> After titration of ethylenediamine, add 25 ml of 0·1N silver nitrate to the titrated liquid, warm on a water-bath for fifteen minutes and then cool in ice-water for thirty minutes. Filter, by suction, through a hardened filter paper in a Buchner funnel, wash the residue with three 10 ml quantities of water and titrate the combined filtrate and washings with 0·1N sodium hydroxide using methyl red as indicator. 1 ml 0·1N = 0·01802 g $C_7H_8O_2N_4$.

Another rapid method is the volumetric method of the *U.S.P.*; a slight modification of the original technique by using a sintered-glass filter is preferable. This method is applicable to Meralluride and Injection of Mersalyl.

> Dissolve 0·25 g on a water-bath in 50 ml of water with 8 ml of dilute ammonia solution. Add excess 0·1N silver nitrate and continue the warming for fifteen minutes. Cool to between 5° and 10° for twenty minutes, filter, preferably through a filtering crucible under reduced pressure and wash the precipitate with three 10 ml quantities of water. Acidify the combined filtrate and washings with concentrated nitric acid, adding 3 ml of the acid in excess and titrate the excess silver nitrate with 0·1N ammonium thiocyanate using ferric ammonium sulphate indicator. 1 ml 0·1N = 0·01802 g $C_7H_8O_2N_4$.

The results by this method are slightly more erratic than the longer gravimetric method since 0·1 ml of 0·1N silver nitrate is equivalent to 0·72 per cent of theophylline when 0·25 g is taken for assay.

Reimers[6] suggested that on drying at 125° the residue will be theophylline, the moisture and ethylenediamine being driven off. Experiments have shown that this test gave only slightly high results and is a useful check; some eight hours' drying is necessary.

Injection of Aminophylline, *B.P.* Usually a 2·5 per cent solution in water for injection.

The assay is the silver precipitation method exactly as the parent substance using a volume equivalent to 0·5 g of aminophylline, if necessary diluted to 20 ml with water.

Tablets of Aminophylline, *B.P.* The usual strength of these tablets is 0·1 g of theophylline with ethylenediamine. The assay is exactly as for the parent substance given above using about 0·5 g of the powdered sample.

1. Anastasi, A., Gallo, U., and Novacic, L., *J. Pharm. Pharmacol.*, 1955, **7**, 263.
2. Daoust, R. A., *J. Amer. Pharm. Ass., Sci. Edn.*, 1953, **42**, 744.
3. Self, P. A. W., and Rankin, W. R., *Quart. J. Pharm.*, 1931, **4**, 346.
4. Boie, H., *Pharm. Ztg.*, 1930, **75**, 968.
5. Parkes, A. E., and Parkes, H. A., *Analyst*, 1937, **62**, 791.
6. Reimers, F., *J.A.O.A.C.*, 1937, **20**, 631.

CALCIUM

Ca At. Wt. 40·08

The classical method for calcium is by gravimetric determination as oxalate. A hot solution of calcium salt in hydrochloric acid is treated with ammonium oxalate or oxalic acid and neutralised with ammonia; the precipitate is washed with dilute ammonium oxalate solution and is then ignited to calcium carbonate or oxide, or is converted to calcium sulphate by treatment with sulphuric acid. An alternative volumetric finish is to dissolve the precipitated oxalate in sulphuric acid and titrate with potassium permanganate.

If calcium is precipitated from cold ammoniacal or neutral solution by the addition of oxalate, an extremely finely divided precipitate is obtained. Precipitation from hot ammoniacal solution yields a coarse-grained precipitate which can be filtered fairly readily, but the best results are obtained by adding alkali after the addition of oxalate. A precipitate obtained in this way may be contaminated with oxalic acid or ammonium oxalate but this does not matter if it is to be ignited; slightly high results are to be expected if the precipitate is titrated with permanganate. The method of homogeneous precipitation has much to commend it and this yields an extremely coarse-grained precipitate. Excess of oxalate is added to an acid solution of the calcium salt followed by urea, the solution is then heated to just below its boiling-point when the urea slowly hydrolyses producing ammonia and hence a slow precipitation of calcium oxalate. Almost all metals except magnesium and the alkali metals must be absent. Co-precipitation is a very important factor in gravimetric calcium determinations since the solubility of magnesium oxalate is relatively small and a sharp separation is not easily obtained. Two difficulties exist (i) actual precipitation of the magnesium oxalate and (ii) occlusion of magnesium oxalate in the precipitate of calcium oxalate. The problem is further aggravated because calcium oxalate has an appreciable solubility in magnesium solutions. The danger of actual precipitation of magnesium oxalate may be lessened by avoiding boiling the solution and by using a considerable excess of ammonium oxalate which increases solubility due to formation of complex magnesium oxalate ions (calcium does not form such complex ions). Co-precipitation of alkali metals is also a tiresome problem. These metals are carried down as oxalates, sodium being much more strongly co-precipitated than potassium. The presence of a high concentration of sodium ions calls for double precipitation although long digestion of the precipitated ions tends to decrease the weight of co-precipitated ions. Taking all these factors into consideration the following method of precipitation is recommended:

Dilute an aqueous solution containing up to about 200 mg of calcium ions to 200 ml with water. Add methyl red indicator and 5 ml of concentrated hydrochloric acid, followed by 50 ml of a warm 6 per cent solution of ammonium oxalate (if magnesium is not to be determined afterwards this amount of oxalate can be doubled). Heat to 70° or 80° and add a 10 per cent solution of ammonium hydroxide dropwise until the indicator just changes to yellow. Allow to stand without further heating for one hour (not longer if magnesium is present) then filter; wash the precipitate with a 0·1 per cent solution of ammonium oxalate and then dissolve it in 50 ml of hot 10 per cent hydrochloric acid. Wash the paper with hot 1 per cent hydrochloric acid and dilute to 200 ml. Add 1 g of ammonium oxalate, heat nearly to boiling and re-precipitate, as above, allowing to stand for one or two hours. Filter off the precipitate, wash with cold 0·1 per cent solution of ammonium oxalate and weigh as carbonate by igniting at 500° or as oxide by igniting at 1000° to 1100°.

If a volumetric finish is preferred the precipitate should be dissolved by passing about 100 ml of hot dilute sulphuric acid through the filter in small quantities at a time, heating the solution so obtained to about 70°, and titrating with 0·1N potassium permanganate, maintaining the solution at about 70° throughout the titration.

For most work in pharmaceutical analysis classical methods have now been superseded by complexometric titration. Determination of calcium by itself presents little difficulty and two basic procedures are applicable, (i) titration at pH 10 in ammonia buffer using solochrome black as indicator and (ii) titration at pH 12 to 13, either in diethylamine using alizarin black (diadem chrome black) or in potassium hydroxide solution using Patton and Reeder's indicator. Provided a small quantity of complexed magnesium is included for titration (i) sharp and satisfactory end-points are obtained by these methods and there is no significant difference in the results obtained at the two pH values if a pure calcium compound is titrated. Difference in the two results would be expected if the calcium salts were contaminated with magnesium, when the titration at pH 10 would include both ions and that at the higher value the calcium only.

The recommended method for the determination of calcium salts in the absence of other ions, is, therefore, as follows:

Dissolve a suitable quantity of calcium salt, to contain about 0·05 g Ca, in about 150 ml of water. Add 4 ml of 8N potassium hydroxide and about 0·2 g of Patton and Reeder's indicator (containing ascorbic acid—see Appendix II). Titrate with 0·05M EDTA to a pure blue end-point.

A suitable alternative is to use 20 ml of diethylamine instead of the potassium hydroxide and a few drops of Acid Alizarin Black SN as indicator. Many other indicators have been recommended for the titration of calcium when it occurs by itself and the choice is a matter of personal preference.

When magnesium is also present the calcium can be determined specifically by adjusting the solution to pH 12 or 13 when magnesium hydroxide precipitates and calcium remains in solution to be titrated by the complexing agent. Although this was one of the first methods to be established in complexometric analysis it is still far from satisfactory. A number of possible sources of error exist:

(i) Some calcium may be co-precipitated with magnesium hydroxide, (ii) magnesium hydroxide may dissolve to some extent in the EDTA thus giving a tendency to high results and sluggish end-points, (iii) the indicator used may be adsorbed onto the magnesium hydroxide precipitate making the end-point difficult to detect. Removal of the magnesium hydroxide by filtration may seem to be an obvious way to avoid some of these difficulties but in practice such a procedure is unsatisfactory. Many indicators have been suggested for the complexometric titration of calcium in the presence of magnesium. Some of these have been critically examined by Belcher, Close and West,[1] but their investigation was limited to the use of 0·01M titrant and to solutions in which the ratio of the magnesium to calcium was not greater than 1 : 1. In pharmaceutical work, however, magnesium is often present in excess of calcium and a stronger titrant is frequently employed. In a comparison of a number of indicators including murexide, alizarin black, methylthymol blue, calcon, calcein and Patton and Reeder's indicator, it has been shown that calcon is satisfactory where the amount of magnesium does not exceed that of calcium, but some difference of opinion exists where magnesium is present in excess. Patton and Reeder's reagent is favoured by many workers and is said to give a somewhat sluggish, but detectable end-point when magnesium is present in five-fold excess and when the titration is carried out at the 0·05M level. Calcein and methylthymol blue give unsatisfactory end-points whilst alizarin black is not suitable in the presence of large quantities of magnesium. Opinion regarding murexide is rather mixed; this was the original indicator used by Schwarzenbach and it has given good service for a number of years. When the concentration of magnesium present is low the end-point is detectable but not very good and recovery of calcium is of about the right order. When the magnesium is present in considerable excess, however, calcium recovery is low and detection of the end-point is a matter of considerable experience. Some improvement is obtained by using murexide screened with naphthol green. It will be realised that the choice of a method for determining calcium in the presence of magnesium may be a matter of individual preference since none of those described at the present time is free from criticisms.

Calcium may be determined by flame photometry but in common with the other alkaline earth metals it is considered one of the more difficult elements to determine by flame photometric methods because so many extraneous anions and cations cause variations in the intensity of its flame emission. However, with modern instrumentation the difficulties can usually be overcome and most samples can be examined satisfactorily.

The useful emission of calcium comprises the resonance line at 4227 A and molecular bands usually ascribed to CaO at about 5540 A and 6200 A.

The choice of wavelength depends on the equipment used; with filter instruments one of the molecular bands is employed but with a monochromator the atomic line is sometimes preferred. The total emission increases with flame temperature and the relative intensities of the line and bands also vary, the hotter the flame the greater is the dissociation of molecules and therefore the higher the intensity of the atomic line.

The elements which give rise to the most serious spectral interferences are sodium and barium. Of these sodium is the more important because it is present in so many of the samples in which calcium is determined. When relatively large amounts are present it causes an elevation of general background and this interferes with determinations when either filter or monochromator instruments are used. Filters also permit a significant amount of light through from the adjacent part of the spectrum to that wavelength of maximum transmission. Interference filters are usually better in this respect than optical filters but even so those which are used to isolate the bands at 5540 A or 6200 A will leak a considerable amount of light from the sodium doublet at 5890 A. Monochromators are therefore better in this respect but it must be remembered that in addition to the general background elevation, scattered light must be taken into account and this may be considerable. Whatever type of instrument is used sodium interference can be reduced considerably by using a didymium filter but one is always still faced with the problem of compensating for continuous background elevation. This is best accomplished by utilising a recording monochromator instrument and a base-line technique for measuring the line or band intensity. If a recorder is not available, then the background can be measured to one side of the line. With a filter instrument, however, the only satisfactory method is to standardise with solutions containing precisely the same amount of sodium as the sample.

By far the most serious interference effects in the determination of calcium are due to anions such as phosphate, sulphate, arsenate and oxalate, and to elements such as aluminium, beryllium, boron, chromium, iron and molybdenum which can exist as anions in the flame. These all give rise to reductions in line intensities, probably due to the formation of compounds which are either of low volatility or are not dissociated.

Several methods have been described for dealing with this problem. The first is useful when varying amounts of phosphate are present in the samples. When increasing amounts of phosphate are added to solutions containing a fixed amount of calcium, the intensity is reduced in the manner shown in Fig. 3. Leyton[2] showed that the point where the curve flattens corresponds approximately to a molar ratio of calcium to phosphate of 1 : 1 and suggested that this might be due to the formation of $Ca_3(PO_4)_2$ and the height of the horizontal portion of the curve depends on the dissociation of the molecule. This view is supported by the fact that the limiting intensity in the presence of excess phosphate varies with flame temperature. Advantage can be taken of this phenomenon when unknown quantities of phosphate are present in analytical samples, it is necessary only to add an excess of phosphoric acid or ammonium phosphate to samples and standards. The intensity of the calcium emission and therefore sensitivity is of course reduced in this technique and it can be seen in Fig. 4 that with an air-acetylene flame this reduction may amount to about 40 per cent. For many types of sample the method can be recommended and is considered superior to those which depend upon eliminating phosphate by precipitation or ion exchange.

Some methods depending on the addition of dextrose[3] or EDTA[4] to solutions containing sulphate or phosphate have been described and it is known that in biological solutions containing protein the phosphate does

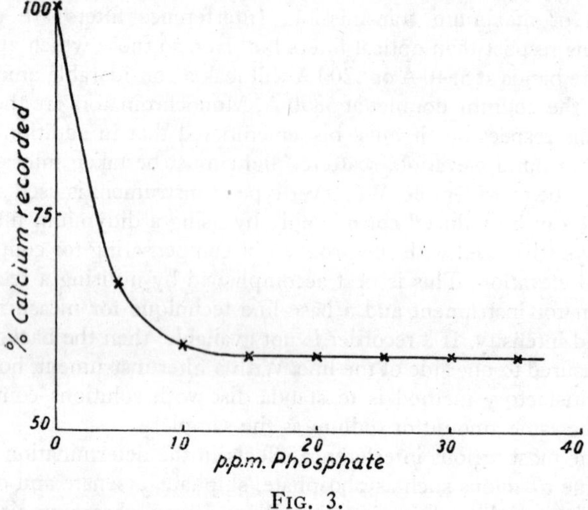

FIG. 3.

not inhibit the calcium emission as much as would be expected. The efficiency of EDTA addition has been ascribed to the complexing effect but it would be interesting to compare the effect of a number of organic materials which give rise to excess carbon, for it is by no means certain that an organic complex can exist in the flame.

The interference due to metals which can exist as anions in the flame is often of a much more serious nature than that due to phosphate and sulphate. For example the addition of 100 p.p.m. of aluminium to a solution containing 5 p.p.m. of calcium causes complete suppression of the calcium emission. However, if an excess of strontium, magnesium or lanthanum is added the calcium emission is completely restored. Fig. 4 shows this in a series of recordings; it can be seen that the strontium causes an elevation of the background but the intensity of the CaO band, using a base line method of measurement is exactly the same in chart recordings A, C and E, G. This phenomenon can easily be explained on the basis of the law of mass action, and can be used as the basis of two analytical procedures. If no recording instrument is available, a series of standards is produced, each containing an excess of strontium and varying quantities of calcium

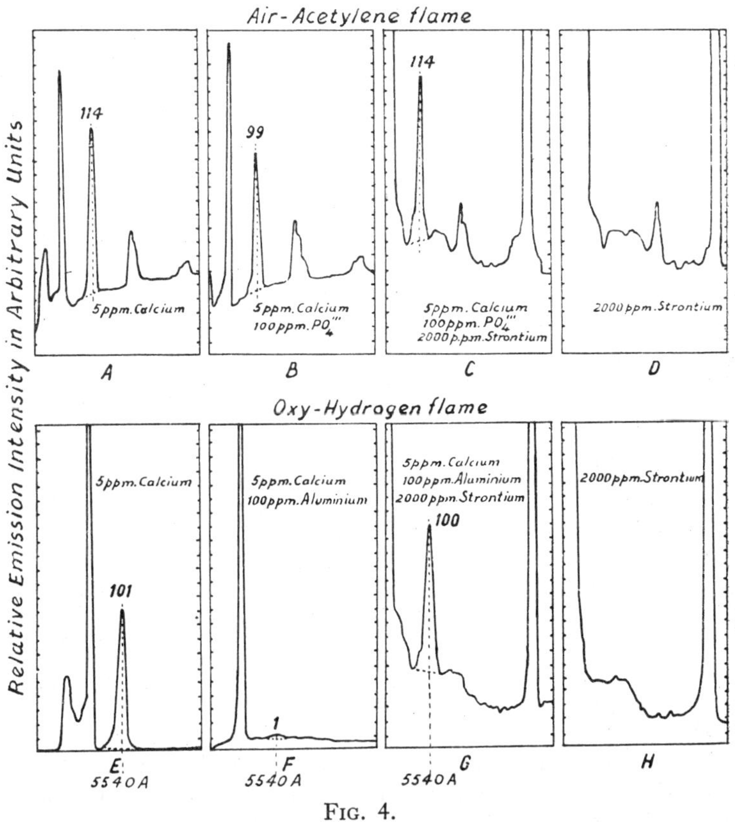

FIG. 4.

from zero upwards. The instrument is set to zero with the standard containing no calcium, and a 100 per cent reading with the strongest standard with respect to calcium. A standard curve is prepared in the normal way and used to determine the calcium in a solution containing the same amount of strontium as the standard. If, however, a recording instrument is available then a standard curve can be produced from solutions which do not contain strontium and used to estimate the calcium in solutions containing aluminium and strontium. This is a great saving in strong strontium solutions which are quite valuable when prepared free of calcium. This type of buffering with strontium, lanthanum, or magnesium is also effective in eliminating the interfering effects of phosphate, sulphate and other elements and has been widely used in the authors' laboratory. Standard addition techniques (see p. 872) are often very useful particularly when the samples contain a number of different interfering ions; they are indicated particularly when only a small number of samples are to be examined and a full scale investigation is not warranted.

It can be seen now that although calcium presents many problems in flame photometry, methods can usually be found provided suitable equipment is available. A fairly hot or hot flame is always indicated and ideally a recording monochromator instrument is required if samples of any complexity are to be examined.

Calcium may be determined by atomic absorption spectrophotometry. This technique has been used for the estimation of calcium in biological fluids[5,6,7] and agricultural materials.[8,9] It is a speedy method, superior to the more tedious chemical determination by oxalate precipitation and more specific than the EDTA titration method. The accuracy is of the order of ± 2 per cent and sensitivity limits have been reported[10] at 0·08 to 1 p.p.m. of calcium in solution. The interference problems are very similar to those experienced with the emission method although not quite so formidable.

Suitable apparatus has been described by various authors.[11,12] It consists of a calcium hollow cathode tube, atomiser and burner assembly, monochromator or spectrograph and electronic detection and readout equipment. The calcium hollow cathode tubes are available commercially* and are usually modulated to emit light at 50 or 100 cycles per second. Suitable atomisers and chambers provide a mist of the solution which is passed into a stainless-steel burner and vaporised with an air/acetylene flame. The monochromator or spectrograph isolates the resonance line at 4227 A and a photomultiplier is used with an A.C. amplifier to give a reading proportional to the calcium line intensity on a meter. The instrument is set to read 100 per cent transmission at 4227 A with water in the flame and is then calibrated with standard calcium solutions. Readings obtained from sample solutions are converted to concentration from the standard curve of calcium absorption versus concentration. Modulated instruments are used to eliminate interferences arising from background emission. Long-path burners[13] from 7 to 12 cm in length are used to give maximum sensitivity; reduction of sensitivity has been achieved by rotation of the burner thus varying the length of the absorption path.

The types of interference are similar to those associated with the flame emission method, being caused in the main by ionisation and formation of non-volatile compounds. Both ionisation of the calcium atoms in the flame

* Tubes available from either Adam Hilger Limited, London, England, or Ransley Glass Instruments, Melbourne, Australia.

and the formation of compounds with phosphate, sulphate, silicate, aluminium, etc. will reduce the concentration of ground state atoms, thus reducing the absorption.

Calcium ionisation in the flame may be reduced or eliminated by adding an excess of sodium or potassium to the solutions. For the calcium suppression by phosphate, sulphate, silicate and alumina excess concentrations of a competing cation or anion may be added *e.g.* Sr, La, Mg, SO_4, etc. Finally the protein interference of calcium in blood sera solutions has been overcome by the use of EDTA as a complexing reagent.

The magnitude of the interference effects is dependent upon the type of flame, the flame height and temperature. Most authors prefer the air/acetylene to the cooler flames such as air/coal gas and air/propane. The best sensitivity and least phosphate interference was found to be 4 to 5 mm above the burner top. The variety of instrumentation used for the method necessitates individual investigation to determine the optimum conditions with a particular equipment.

The atomic absorption method is in some ways superior to the flame photometry method since spectral radiation interferences do not occur.

Small quantities of calcium may be determined by flame photometry or atomic absorption. In the absence of suitable apparatus, milligram quantities may be determined by making use of picrolonic acid which forms an insoluble calcium salt. A neutral solution is treated with lithium picrolonate, the insoluble calcium salt is filtered off and the excess picrolonate titrated with cetylpyridinium bromide using bromophenol blue as indicator.[14]

Evers[15] devised a roughly quantitative test for the determination of calcium in the presence of large proportions of magnesium such as in magnesium salts.

> Dissolve 2 g of the salt in 25 ml of 25 per cent w/w sulphuric acid; add 50 ml of industrial spirit or 95 per cent ethanol. Allow to stand overnight, filter and wash the precipitate with a mixture of 2 volumes of ethanol and 1 volume of 25 per cent sulphuric acid, ignite and weigh as calcium sulphate.

The results were slightly low as calcium sulphate appears to possess a small solubility in the solution, but a correction allowance gives a more accurate determination. In addition to the use of the method as a limit test for calcium in magnesium salts, since the results are unaffected by the presence of iron or phosphate, it has been applied to the determination of calcium in such preparations as Compound Syrup of Iron Phosphate.

Recently a sensitive specific colour reagent for microgram quantities of calcium in solution has been described. This is di-(*o*-hydroxyphenylimino) ethane, also known as glyoxal-bis-(2-hydroxyanil) and this has been adapted to the quantitative determination of small quantities of calcium in magnesium carbonate by Leonard.[16]

CALCIUM

Reagents:

Calcium-free magnesium carbonate. Dissolve 24·6 g of analytical reagent grade magnesium sulphate (heptahydrate) in 200 ml of water and add 20 per cent sodium hydroxide solution until a precipitate just forms. Heat the mixture to 80° and add, while stirring, a hot solution of 10·6 g of anhydrous sodium carbonate in 200 ml of water. Allow to cool, filter off the precipitate, wash thoroughly with water and dry at 110°.

Calcium-free magnesium carbonate solution. Slurry 0·5 g of calcium-free magnesium carbonate with 25 ml of water, dissolve by the addition of 22·5 ml of 0·5N hydrochloric acid, boil gently for five minutes to expel carbon dioxide, cool and dilute to 250 ml with water in a graduated flask.

Glyoxal-bis-(2-hydroxyanil) reagent. This is a 0·5 per cent solution, prepared by dissolving 0·25 g of glyoxal-bis-(2-hydroxyanil) in about 20 ml of methanol, warming gently to assist solution and cooling, and diluting to 50 ml with methanol.

Standards:

Concentrated standard calcium solution. Dissolve 1·001 g of dry, analytical reagent grade calcium carbonate in 25 ml of N hydrochloric acid, boil to expel carbon dioxide, cool and dilute to exactly 1 litre with water.

Dilute standard calcium solution. Dilute a 10 ml aliquot of the concentrated solution to exactly 1 litre with water. This solution contains 4·0 μg of Ca per ml.

Method:

Dissolve 0·5 g of the sample in 22·5 ml of 0·5N hydrochloric acid, boil the solution for five minutes to remove carbon dioxide, cool and dilute to 250 ml with water in a graduated flask. Transfer a 5 ml aliquot of this solution to the first of three 25-ml graduated flasks and at the same time transfer a 5 ml aliquot of the calcium-free magnesium carbonate solution to each of the second and third flasks. To the third flask (the internal standard) add a volume of dilute standard calcium solution (0 to 7 ml) to contain approximately the same amount of calcium as is expected to be present in the 5 ml aliquot of the sample solution and dilute to 12 ml by adding a measured volume of water. To each of the first and second flasks add 7 ml of water and treat the contents of each flask, respectively, as follows. Add 0·70 ml of N sodium hydroxide, 0·25 ml of glyoxal-bis-(2-hydroxyanil) reagent and 10·0 ml of a mixture of equal volumes of 95 per cent ethanol and *n*-butanol and dilute to volume with water. Mix thoroughly, allow to stand for fifteen minutes and then centrifuge at 2000 r.p.m. for three minutes.

Measure the extinctions at 520 mμ of the supernatant liquids from the first and third flasks, using 2-cm cells with the supernatant liquid from the second flask in the comparison cell in each case. From a standard curve, read the μg of calcium equivalent to the extinction of the sample solution, corrected if necessary for the extinction of the internal standard. If the sample contains an excessive amount of calcium repeat using a smaller aliquot of the sample solution diluted to 5·0 ml with the calcium-free magnesium carbonate solution.

Prepare the standard curve as follows. Into each of a series of eight 25-ml graduated flasks pipette 5 ml of the calcium-free magnesium carbonate solution and then add, respectively, 0 ml, 1 ml, 2 ml, 3 ml, 4 ml,

5 ml, 6 ml and 7 ml of dilute standard calcium solution. Dilute the contents of each flask to 12 ml by the addition of a measured volume of water and complete as described above from 'treat the contents of each flask . . .' measuring the extinctions at 520 mμ of the solutions from the second to the eighth flasks, using 2-cm cells with the solution from the first flask in the comparison cell in each case and prepare a curve by plotting extinctions against μg of Ca.

Calcium hydroxide, $Ca(OH)_2$, Mol. Wt. 74·0. The *B.P.* method of assay has been devised to determine the hydroxide only, apart from the carbonate present. As calcium hydroxide is only sparingly soluble in water but much more soluble in solutions of sugars, after disintegrating about 3 g of the sample with 10 ml of neutral ethanol, the hydroxide is dissolved by adding 490 ml of 10 per cent sucrose solution and shaking vigorously for five minutes and then frequently during four hours. After filtration of an aliquot part from undissolved carbonate, the alkali is titrated with N hydrochloric acid, using phenolphthalein as indicator. 1 ml N = 0·03705 g $Ca(OH)_2$.

Calcium carbonate, $CaCO_3$, Mol. Wt. 100·1, may be determined by dissolving in excess of standard hydrochloric acid, boiling and back titrating with sodium hydroxide after cooling, using methyl orange as indicator. 1 ml N = 0·05005 g.

Calcium chloride, $CaCl_2,6H_2O$, Mol. Wt. 219·1, 1 ml 0·1N $KMnO_4$ or 0·05M EDTA = 0·01095 g; **calcium gluconate,** $C_{12}H_{22}O_{14}Ca,H_2O$, Mol. Wt. 448·4, 1 ml 0·1N $KMnO_4$ or 0·05 M EDTA = 0·02242 g and **calcium mandelate,** $C_{16}H_{14}O_6Ca$, Mol. Wt. 342·4, 1 ml 0·1N $KMnO_4$ or 0·05M EDTA = 0·01712 g can be assayed for their calcium content either by precipitation as oxalate and titration with permanganate or by EDTA titration, both described above.

Calcium phosphate of commercial standard consists essentially of a mixture of tribasic and dibasic salts. The *B.P.C.* estimation depends on the precipitation of calcium oxalate under suitable conditions of pH which prevent phosphate precipitating with too high a pH, or the incomplete separation of the oxalate in solutions in which the pH is too low.

Dissolve 0·2 g in 50 ml water and 2 ml hydrochloric acid, add 25 ml of dilute solution of ammonium acetate (7·2 per cent) and a slight excess of ammonium oxalate. After coagulating the precipitate by heat as usual, filter, wash, suspend in water acidified with dilute sulphuric acid, heat to 60° and titrate with 0·1N permanganate. 1 ml = 0·00517 g $Ca_3(PO_4)_2$.

For EDTA titration:

Dissolve 1 g in 10 ml of concentrated hydrochloric acid by warming on a water-bath. Dilute with 50 ml of water, cool, transfer to a 250 ml graduated flask and dilute to volume with water. Take 25 ml in a 500 ml flask, add 30 ml of 0·05M EDTA, 10 ml of ammonia buffer solution and 100 ml of water and titrate with 0·1N zinc to solochrome black as indicator. 1 ml 0·05M EDTA = 0·005170 g $Ca_3(PO_4)_2$.

CALCIUM

Calcium hydrogen phosphate, $CaHPO_4,2H_2O$, Mol. Wt. 172·1, is the pure dibasic salt and is determined by the same methods. 1 ml 0·1N = 0·008605 g $CaHPO_4,2H_2O$.

Injection of Calcium Gluconate, *B.P.* Contains about 10 per cent of calcium gluconate but up to 5 per cent of it may be replaced by a suitable calcium salt as stabiliser. The calcium content can be determined by the direct EDTA titration method given above.

Compound Mixture of Calcium Carbonate for Infants, *B.P.C.* This preparation contains 1·83 per cent each of calcium carbonate, magnesium carbonate and sodium bicarbonate with flavouring.

The sodium bicarbonate can be determined by the method given under Compound Powder of Magnesium Carbonate (p. 395) using 30 g.

The following method may be used for determination of the calcium. The total calcium and magnesium is determined in an aliquot by EDTA titration, the calcium precipitated as oxalate from a further aliquot and the residual magnesium titrated to give the calcium by difference.

Weigh 15 g into a 100-ml graduated flask, add the minimum volume of dilute hydrochloric acid necessary to effect solution without the aid of heat and then dilute to volume with water (solution A).

Transfer a 20 ml aliquot of solution A to a flask, dilute to about 50 ml with water and neutralise with 20 per cent sodium hydroxide solution. Add 5 ml of ammonia buffer solution and titrate with 0·05M EDTA using solochrome black as indicator. Let the ml 0·05M EDTA required be '*a*' ml.

Transfer a further 20 ml aliquot of solution A to a beaker, dilute to about 50 ml with water and add 1 g of ammonium chloride and 1 g of ammonium oxalate. Neutralise with dilute ammonia solution, add 5 ml of the ammonia in excess, boil for five minutes and allow to stand for two hours. Filter, wash the beaker and residue with hot water and combine the filtrate and washings. Add 5 ml of ammonia buffer solution and titrate with 0·05M EDTA using solochrome black as indicator. Let the ml 0·05M EDTA required be '*b*' ml. 1 ml 0·05M EDTA, (*a*–*b*), = 0·005005 g $CaCO_3$; (*b*) = 0·001216 g Mg.

Solution of Calcium Hydroxide, *B.P.* (Lime Water)

Titrate 25 ml with 0·1N acid using phenolphthalein as indicator. 1 ml 0·1N = 0·003705 g $Ca(OH)_2$.

For other salts of calcium see the appropriate monographs on the acids.

Compound Syrup of Ferrous Phosphate, *B.P.C.*

In this and similar syrups containing both iron and calcium the following oxalate-precipitation method is applicable:

Weigh 20 g into a beaker, add 150 ml of water and 3 g of citric acid and heat to the boiling-point. Make alkaline to litmus paper with dilute ammonia solution, add 20 ml of 33 per cent w/w acetic acid and then, to the boiling solution add 50 ml of 2·5 per cent ammonium oxalate solution and boil gently for two hours. Filter, wash the residue with water, dry, moisten with concentrated sulphuric acid and ignite gently to constant weight. 1 g of residue = 0·2944 g Ca.

1. Belcher, R., Close, R. A., and West, T. S., *Talanta*, 1958, **1,** 238.
2. Leyton, L., *Analyst*, 1954, **79,** 497.
3. Pro, M. J., and Mathers, A. P., *J.A.O.A.C.*, 1954, **37,** 945.
4. Wirtschafter, J. D., *Science*, 1957, **125,** 603.
5. Willis, J. B., *Spectrochim. Acta*, 1960, **16,** 259.
6. Willis, J. B., *Anal. Chem.*, 1961, **33,** 556.
7. Allan, J. E., *Spectrochim. Acta*, 1962, **18,** 605.
8. David, D. J., *Analyst*, 1959, **84,** 536.
9. David, D. J., *Analyst*, 1960, **85,** 495.
10. Gatehouse, B. M., and Willis, J. B., *Spectrochim. Acta*, 1961, **17,** 710.
11. Box, G. F., and Walsh, P., *Spectrochim. Acta*, 1960, **16,** 255.
12. David, D. J., *Analyst*, 1958, **83,** 655.
13. Clinton, O. E., *Spectrochim. Acta*, 1960, **16,** 985.
14. Washbrook, C. C., *Analyst*, 1950, **75,** 621.
15. Evers, N., *Analyst*, 1931, **56,** 293.
16. Leonard, M. A., *J. Pharm. Pharmacol.*, 1962, **14,** 63T.

CAMPHOR

$C_{10}H_{16}O$ Mol. Wt. 152·2

The estimation of camphor in the crude or refined product is best done by difference, after subtracting the percentage of impurities, *i.e.* dirt, non-volatile matter, water and oil, which are determined by the following methods:

Dirt and Non-volatile Matter. Weigh the residue after volatilisation in an open dish on a hot-plate.

Moisture. Determine by the Dean and Stark method, given in Appendix V (p. 803).

Oil. Lane[1] suggested the determination of the iodine value by Wijs' method to calculate the oil content, using a figure of 1·4 as iodine value for natural camphor and 130 for the oil. Salamon[2] obtained a figure of 0·1 on a carefully purified camphor, and for oils which had been freed from camphor as much as possible by expression and fractionation an iodine value of 86 to 91 was found; in his opinion not more than 5 per cent of camphor was present in these oils and he suggested an iodine value of 100 for the oil free from camphor. Salamon used the Wijs' method, taking 1·5 g of camphor or 0·2 g of oil for the determination and allowing one hour contact with the reagent. The Rosenmund-Kuhnhenn method (see Iodine Value, p. 754) has been suggested by Yamada and Koshitaka[3] for determining the iodine value in order to calculate the oil content.

The determination of camphor in galenicals has been the subject of much investigation, methods depending either on the optical rotation of natural camphor or on its ketonic nature being likely to be replaced by gas-liquid chromatography (see below).

Methods involving the optical rotation of camphor are of little value as synthetic camphor, which is practically devoid of rotatory power, is now used and the rotations of solutions of natural camphor differ according to the solvent. In ethanolic solution the highest specific rotatory power is obtained by measurement of a weak solution of camphor in strong ethanol; formulæ have been derived to calculate the percentage from rotation in given solvents (Partheil and Van Haaren; Schoorl[4]).

Densities and refractive indices of solutions of camphor have also been recommended as means for determination, but the errors inherent in such methods are obvious.

Methods of assay involving the ketonic nature of camphor and the formation of oxime, phenylhydrazone or semicarbazone and weighing the product give low results owing to incomplete precipitation and the volatility of the compound; volumetric hydroxylamine methods suffer from the former defects, although Mital and Gaind[5] claim good recoveries in pharmaceutical preparations with a volumetric method in which hydroxylamine hydrochloride is used. For spirit, liniment and solution of camphor in turpentine, the following procedure is applicable.

> Reflux the sample (containing 0·2 g of camphor) for four hours with 20 ml of aldehyde-free 95 per cent ethanol, 10 ml of a 4 per cent solution of hydroxylamine hydrochloride in aldehyde-free 90 per cent ethanol and 0·3 g of sodium bicarbonate. Cool, rinse the condenser with 20 ml of light petroleum (b.p. 50° to 60°), collecting the rinsings in the flask and titrate the mixture first with 0·2N hydrochloric acid to dimethyl yellow and then with 0·2N potassium hydroxide to phenolphthalein. Carry out a control omitting the camphor and adding 5 ml of steam-distilled turpentine oil before refluxing for the spirit and solution and 1 g of arachis oil before refluxing for the liniment. Calculate the amount of camphor present from the difference in the volume of 0·2N potassium hydroxide used in the two titrations. 1 ml of 0·2N = 0·0304 g camphor.

Hampshire and Page[6] evolved a useful practical method for the determination of camphor in galenicals using 2,4-dinitrophenylhydrazine as a precipitant. Precipitation is quicker and the hydrazone produced found to be much less volatile. The method was found by the authors to give fairly accurate results with pure camphor, both natural and synthetic. However, its precision is not sufficiently good for its application to the assay of camphor itself as in the *B.P.* and the minimum standard of 96 per cent for a material which might be expected to be very pure underlines the shortcomings of the assay procedure. The general method is:

> Dissolve about 0·2 g of camphor, accurately weighed by difference, in 25 ml of aldehyde-free ethanol in a 300-ml conical flask and slowly add, with constant shaking, 75 ml of the reagent (prepared by dissolving

1·5 g of 2,4-dinitrophenylhydrazine in a mixture of 10 ml of concentrated sulphuric acid and 10 ml of water, diluting with water to 100 ml and filtering; the reagent decomposes on standing and must be made up just before use). Then heat the mixture on a water-bath under a reflux condenser for four hours, allow it to cool, dilute with 2 per cent v/v sulphuric acid to 200 ml (weaker acid allows crystallisation of the excess of base from the solution) and allow to stand for twenty-four hours. Collect the precipitate on a weighed Gooch crucible with paper mat, or on a sintered-glass filter, wash it with successive quantities of 10 ml of cold distilled water until the washings are no longer acid, and dry at 80°; 1 g of camphor 2,4-dinitrophenylhydrazone corresponds to 0·458 g of camphor.

The original method in which the ethanol was distilled from the reaction mixture before diluting is an unnecessary complication. Andersen[7] determined the correction for solubility of camphor dinitrophenylhydrazone with both natural and synthetic camphor, and found no significant differences if ethanol is not removed. The solubility correction is about 0·2 per cent. Drying of the nitrophenylhydrazone at 105° is satisfactory.

The process can be applied to the determination of camphor in galenicals, but, except for Spirit of Camphor, direct determination is not feasible, and separation is necessary. Separation by steam distillation was found very satisfactory, only traces of other reacting substances being carried over.

Steam-distil a quantity of the galenical containing about 1 g of camphor, using a double-surface condenser and cooling the receiver in ice. The camphor (which distils after any ethanol present) partly deposits in the condenser. When about 150 ml of distillate has been collected, stop the process and wash down the condenser with a sufficient quantity of aldehyde-free ethanol to dissolve the camphor in the distillate. The volume of ethanol used must be known in order that the concentration of ethanol in the reaction mixture may be adjusted to 25 per cent v/v. Take an aliquot part of the distillate, containing about 0·2 g of camphor, for the determination.

Instead of using aldehyde-free ethanol for dilution and in view of the fact that many galenicals containing camphor are made with industrial methylated spirit, this form of ethanol may be used for dilution so long as a control experiment is carried out with the same amount of ethanol. A determination on a liniment of aconite made with industrial methylated spirit and no camphor gave a precipitate equivalent to 0·12 per cent w/v of camphor; but many industrial spirits contain less aldehyde, especially those purified for analytical use, one sample only showing aldehyde equivalent to 0·022 per cent of camphor.

Camphor has been determined by Baines and Proctor[8] in a number of essential oils and pharmaceutical preparations using a gas chromatographic technique. It was necessary, for some of the samples, to use a special injection system (see p. 877) in order to prevent non-volatile materials in the samples from entering the column. The apparatus employed a thermal conductivity detector with 4 in. platinum wires 0·001 in. diameter of nominal resistance 25 ohms, the wires in the channels being matched to within 0·1 ohm. The bridge current was 200 mA and the output recorded on a 2·5 mV recorder. 2 per cent of ethylbenzene was added to standards and samples as an internal standard and the operating conditions were as follows: Column length, 7 ft; column diameter, 4 to 5 mm; column temperature, 130°; stationary phase, 20 per cent of squalane on 100 to 120 mesh Celite; sample size, nominally 30 μl; carrier gas, 4 : 1 (by volume) hydrogen : nitrogen mixture at 100 ml/min. Under these conditions the retention volumes were, camphor 1200 ml, ethyl benzene 270 ml.

Liniment of Camphor, *B.P.* (Camphorated Oil). A 20 per cent w/w solution of camphor in arachis oil.

If properly prepared there should be no loss of camphor during manufacture.

The *B.P.* includes an assay in which the camphor is determined by the loss on heating about 2 g in an open dish on a water-bath until no odour of camphor is discernible, the residue being cooled in a desiccator before weighing. Prolonged heating of the residue tends towards low results due to a gain in weight by the oil.

If natural camphor has been used a rapid estimation with a fair degree of accuracy is by direct polarisation of the liniment in a 1-dm tube. The observed rotation in degrees × 1·962 = per cent w/w of camphor.

The *N.F.* Liniment of Camphor (made with cottonseed oil) is assayed as follows:

> Place approximately 5 ml of camphor liniment in a dried and weighed 120-ml Erlenmeyer flask and weigh accurately. Connect the flask with a U-shaped drying tube, place the flask and tube in an air-oven, maintained at 110°, and pass a steady stream of carbon dioxide through the U-tube into the flask for two hours. The orifice of the gas delivery tube should be about 15 mm above the surface of the liniment. Remove the flask, blow out the remaining carbon dioxide with dry air, cool the flask in a desiccator and weigh. The loss in weight is not less than 19 per cent and not more than 21 per cent of the camphor liniment taken for the assay.

Overbye and Schœtzow[9] proved the necessity for carbon dioxide protection during heating, the camphor figure obtained without this precaution being 1·5 to 2·0 per cent low.

Determination of camphor by loss would allow partial substitution by other volatile matter such as light mineral oil, and a direct determination of camphor is preferable. It can be carried out by the method of Hampshire and Page (above), although experience of this method has shown that it tends to give somewhat low results of the order of 96 per cent recovery.

> Distil about 5 g in a current of steam until 120 ml of distillate has

been collected. It will be necessary to use a splash bulb to prevent particles of oil being carried over into the distillate. Wash down the condenser with 100 ml of aldehyde-free ethanol and dilute the product to 250 ml. Take 50 ml of dilution for the determination.

The fixed oil remaining after the removal of volatile matter should be examined for purity, especially for the absence of heavy mineral oil.

The gas chromatographic procedure is applicable to this product:

To 4 ml of sample add 0·400 ml of ethylbenzene and make up to 20 ml with acetone. Place 30 μl of this solution on to a column as described above and from the chromatogram calculate the camphor content of the sample using the peak area ratio method (see p. 878).

Ammoniated Liniment of Camphor, *B.P.C.* A mixture of camphor and ammonia in alcohol containing oil of lavender. Ammonia may be determined by adding 5 ml to an excess of 0·5N acid and back-titrating with 0·5N sodium hydroxide to methyl red. 1 ml 0·5N = 0·008515 g.

For chemical estimation of camphor dilute 10 ml of liniment with 20 ml of ethanol, acidify with dilute sulphuric acid, the liquid being cooled in ice to prevent loss of camphor. Distil in steam until 150 ml of distillate has been collected. Wash down the condenser with a total of 75 ml of ethanol to dissolve the camphor in the distillate. Then dilute to 250 ml and take 50 ml, containing about 0·2 g of camphor, for the determination as above.

For gas chromatographic assay, add 0·400 ml of ethylbenzene to 10 ml of sample, make up to 20 ml with acetone and continue as under Liniment of Camphor.

To apply their method to ammoniated liniment of camphor, liniment of soap, and liniment of turpentine, Mital and Gaind[5] found a previous steam distillation was necessary and the following method may be used.

Dilute the sample (containing 2·5 g of camphor) to 50 ml with steam-distilled turpentine oil, add 50 ml of water, acidify with dilute sulphuric acid to methyl orange and steam-distil. Separate the oily layer of the distillate, wash the condenser and separator with 50 ml of ethanol and extract the aqueous layer with 30 ml of ether. Bulk the oil, ethanolic solution and ether, dilute to 250 ml with ethanol and use a 20 ml aliquot for the estimation given above.

The authors claim recoveries of from 96 to 102 per cent when using this method.

Spirit of Camphor, *B.P.C.* A simple solution of camphor, 10 per cent w/v, in 90 per cent alcohol.

The chemical method for determination of camphor given above under Camphor, may be applied directly, without modification, using 2 ml of spirit and diluting to 25 ml with ethanol. The gas chromatographic procedure can be used exactly as given under Ammoniated Liniment of Camphor.

A rapid colorimetric method for camphor in the spirit has been described by Blake and Hopkins.[10]

Dissolve 0·125 g of *p*-dimethylaminobenzaldehyde in 65 ml of concentrated sulphuric acid and 35 ml of water. Add 7 ml of this reagent by burette to an aliquot of a dilution of the sample in chloroform to contain between 0·6 and 7·5 mg of camphor. Stopper, shake and allow to stand two hours for colour development and measure the extinction at 460 mμ.

Prepare a standard curve in a similar manner from aliquots of a prepared solution of camphor in chloroform in the range 0·6 to 7·5 mg of camphor.

1. LANE, K. W., *J. Soc. Chem. Ind.*, 1922, **41,** 32T.
2. SALAMON, M. S., *Analyst*, 1923, **48,** 536.
3. YAMADA, S., and KOSHITAKA, T., *J. Soc. Chem. Ind. Japan*, 1928, **31,** 142B.
4. PARTHEIL, A., and VAN HAAREN, A., *Arch. Pharm.*, 1900, **238,** 164; SCHOORL, N., *Pharm. Weekblad*, 1927, **64,** 338.
5. MITAL, H. C., and GAIND, K. N., *J. Pharm. Pharmacol.*, 1956, **8,** 37.
6. HAMPSHIRE, C. H., and PAGE, G. R., *Quart. J. Pharm.*, 1934, **7,** 558.
7. ANDERSEN, K. K., *Quart. J. Pharm.*, 1938, **11,** 264.
8. BAINES, C. B., and PROCTOR, K. A., *J. Pharm. Pharmacol.*, 1959, **11,** 230T.
9. OVERBYE, D. A., and SCHŒTZOW, R. E., *J. Amer. Pharm. Ass.*, 1935, **24,** 961.
10. BLAKE, M. L., and HOPKINS, L. V., *Drug Standards*, 1959, **27,** 39.

CANTHARIDES

The numerous modifications of the assay of cantharides are all the same in principle. Since cantharides contains cantharidin partly free and partly as a salt of cantharidic acid which is insoluble in chloroform or benzene, extraction must be made in acid solution, the acid liberated being converted into a lactone. As the extracting medium dissolves fatty matter, the cantharidin is washed with solvent in which it is insoluble, light petroleum being usually employed. Free cantharidin is volatile in steam or ethanol vapour and must be dried at low temperatures, at least below 65°.

Guthrie and Brindle,[1] in an examination of the methods of different pharmacopœias, found the final residues of cantharidin to be impure and the greatest error to be caused in the removal of the fat. They claimed that the best method of separating the cantharidin from the bulk of the fat was by boiling with water, and they evolved a method based on their findings:

Triturate 10 g of cantharides in moderately coarse powder with 1 ml of concentrated hydrochloric acid. Transfer completely to a continuous extraction apparatus using cotton wool to remove the last traces of powder. Add the cotton wool to the powder. Completely exhaust with 100 ml of chloroform (two hours). Transfer the chloroform solution to a 300-ml wide-necked flask, rinsing the extraction flask with a few millilitres of chloroform. Remove the greater part of the chloroform by evaporation on a boiling water-bath and expel the last few millilitres by a current of air. Add 70 ml of water and boil for five minutes under a reflux condenser. Immediately filter the mixture of water and fat through a moistened filter paper, 5 cm in diameter, into a previously warmed separator. Return the fat with the filter paper to the flask and repeat the boiling and filtering as before using 50, 50 and 40 ml of water successively. Allow the mixed aqueous extracts to cool and add 2 ml of concentrated hydrochloric acid. Extract with three separate quantities of 30, 25 and 20 ml of chloroform. Wash the combined chloroform extracts with 10 ml of water and remove the chloroform by evaporation as above, finally drying in a current of air at 60°. Add to the residue 5 ml of a mixture of light petroleum (3 volumes) and dehydrated ethanol (1 volume) previously saturated with cantharidin and allow to stand for half an hour in the closed flask. Carefully decant the liquid and treat with two further quantities each of 5 ml of the mixture. Dry the residue in an oven at 60° for half an hour, cool and weigh.

Cantharidin, $C_{10}H_{12}O_4$, Mol. Wt. 196·2, may be extracted from galenicals in acid solution with chloroform.

The determination of **small amounts** was investigated by Guthrie and Brindle.[2] For quantities of 10 mg or more a precipitation as barium cantharidate at about pH 8·0 is recommended as a gravimetric method; the process was applied to a variety of solutions containing other substances from which the cantharidin could be extracted with chloroform after acidification with hydrochloric acid.

To the solution containing the cantharidin add phenolphthalein and 0·1N sodium hydroxide until a pink colour persists. Then add 0·1N hydrochloric acid until only a very faint pink colour remains. Add barium chloride solution drop by drop with constant stirring until an excess is present. After allowing to stand overnight filter off the precipitate, using a sintered-glass filter, wash with water, dry at 105° and weigh. Barium cantharidate × 0·561 = cantharidin.

Since cantharidin is often employed in very dilute solution the barium precipitation was adapted to volumetric determination which is applicable to amounts too small to be weighed. Amounts of barium down to 0·1 mg can be determined reasonably accurately by determining the excess of barium used in precipitation.

Adjust the solution to about pH 8·0 by the addition of sodium hydroxide solution, if necessary, until a pink colour forms with phenolphthalein and then carefully add very weak hydrochloric acid until a very faint pink colour just persists. Add an accurately measured volume of standard barium chloride solution (0·02 to 0·05 per cent of $BaCl_2,2H_2O$) ensuring an excess of barium chloride and adjust the total volume. After allowing to stand for six hours decant the liquid through a small plug of cotton wool and use an aliquot part of the filtrate for the determination of the excess of barium chloride. Determine the barium chloride by adding an excess f 0·004N or 0·01N potassium chromate solution, allow to stand for three hours and centrifuge, or allow to stand for longer and carefully decant the clear liquid. Determine the excess of potassium chromate in an aliquot portion by adding a few crystals of potassium iodide and 2 ml of 10 per cent hydrochloric acid and titrating with 0·002N sodium thiosulphate solution. Carry out a blank determination of the potassium chromate solution using the same volume. 1 mg of barium chloride = 0·941 mg of cantharidin.

For cantharidin hair lotions containing only a very small proportion of cantharidin it is necessary to apply a purification by sublimation before using the volumetric determination given above; this process would appear to be applicable to a wide variety of preparations.

Acidify a volume of the preparation corresponding to about 0·5 to 1·0 mg of cantharidin with 1 ml of concentrated hydrochloric acid and extract with three portions (15, 10 and 5 ml) of chloroform. Remove the chloroform under reduced pressure or in a current of air at 40°. Transfer the residue of impure cantharidin by means of acetone solution to a metal lid such as is often used for closing wide-necked bottles. After evaporating the acetone at 40°, cover the contents with a thin watch glass containing water to act as a condenser. Float this on a mercury bath at 105° to 110°. Remove the watch glass and substitute by another at intervals until examination under the microscope shows that no more cantharidin crystals are forming. The time required for complete sublimation varies from forty-five minutes to two hours. Dissolve the sublimed cantharidin from the watch glasses by means of acetone, add water containing a little sodium hydroxide, remove the acetone by boiling and adjust the pH to about 8·0. Complete the volumetric determination as usual.

If oil or fat is present a preliminary separation of the cantharidin by extraction with boiling water is necessary, the aqueous solution being acidified and extracted with chloroform and the process completed as described above.

1. Guthrie, G. A., and Brindle, H., *Quart. J. Pharm.*, 1942, **15**, 61.
2. Guthrie, G. A., and Brindle, H., *Quart. J. Pharm.*, 1943, **16**, 249.

CAPSICUM

The traditional assessment of capsicum is by means of a pungency test. Obviously such a test leaves much to be desired and a method is now available for the determination of capsaicin which is known to be the only substance responsible for the pungency of capsicum. The method given below, which is based on one recommended by the joint Pharmaceutical Society/Society for Analytical Chemistry Committee on methods of assay of crude drugs[1] depends upon extraction of the capsaicin and its determination by a spectrophotometric difference method. The recommended method is as follows.

Reduce a sufficient quantity to a moderately fine powder (No. 30) and extract 5 g in a soxhlet apparatus for at least six hours (or until exhausted) with analytical-reagent grade dehydrated methanol. Transfer the extract to a 100-ml graduated flask with more of the dehydrated methanol and dilute to volume with the same solvent.

Transfer a 10-ml aliquot of this solution to a 150-ml separator and add 15 ml of the dehydrated methanol, 15 ml of water, 2 g of sodium chloride and 5 ml of 0·1N sodium hydroxide. Shake well to mix and then extract with three quantities each of 10 ml of light petroleum (b.p. 80° to 100°). Combine the extracts, wash with 10 ml of 60 per cent v/v methanol (prepared from dehydrated methanol) and add the washings to the aqueous layer; discard the light petroleum layer. Filter the bulked aqueous layer through a cotton-wool plug into a beaker-flask, wash the filter with 10 ml of the 60 per cent methanol, combine the filtrate and washing and evaporate the solvent on a water-bath. Dilute the solution to about 50 ml with water and adjust the pH to between 7·0 and 7·5 by the addition of 0·1N hydrochloric acid, using either a pH meter or phenol red external indicator. Transfer the solution to a separator and extract with six quantities each of 20 ml of ether (peroxide-free, as tested by the *B.P.* method for Anæsthetic Ether). Combine the ether extracts, wash with 10 ml of water and discard the washings. Add 20 ml of the dehydrated methanol to the combined ether extracts and evaporate to low volume (about 1 ml) on a water-bath. Transfer to a 100-ml graduated flask with dehydrated methanol and dilute to volume with the same solvent. Add 0·05 g of purified carbon (prepared by shaking 10 g of activated carbon with 100 ml of dehydrated methanol, filtering through a sintered-glass crucible and drying at 105°), shake thoroughly, filter through a Whatman No. 542 filter paper and reject the first 20 ml of the filtrate.

Pipette 10 ml of the filtrate into a 25-ml graduated flask, add 5·0 ml of freshly prepared 0·1N sodium hydroxide, shake well, cool and dilute to volume with dehydrated methanol (Solution A).

Pipette a further 10 ml of the filtrate into a second 25-ml graduated flask, add 5·0 ml of 0·05N hydrochloric acid, shake well, cool and dilute to volume with the dehydrated methanol (Solution B). At the same time prepare two blank solutions by diluting, with the dehydrated methanol, 5·0 ml of the 0·1N sodium hydroxide to 25 ml (Solution C) and 5·0 ml of the 0·05N hydrochloric acid to 25 ml (Solution D).

Measure the extinction of Solution C at 248 mμ and at 296 mμ, using 1-cm cells with Solution D in the comparison cell. Similarly measure the extinction of Solution A at 248 mμ and at 296 mμ, using 1-cm cells with Solution B in the comparison cell. Deduct the corresponding blank readings.

Calculate the capsaicin content of the sample from the corrected values of E(1 per cent, 1 cm) at each wavelength, assuming a value of 313 for the E(1 per cent, 1 cm) difference at 248 mμ and a value of 127 for the E(1 per cent, 1 cm) difference at 296 mμ. If the results differ by less than 5 per cent the capsaicin content of the sample is a mean of the two figures.

The above method can be applied to oleoresin of capsicum, which usually contains between 8 and 12 per cent of capsaicin, by the following method.

Dissolve 0·25 g in 2 ml of anæsthetic ether and dilute to exactly 100 ml with analytical-reagent grade dehydrated methanol. Transfer a 10-ml aliquot of this solution to a 150-ml separator and continue by the method for capsicum beginning with the words 'add 15 ml of the dehydrated methanol, 15 ml of water . . .'.

For Capsicum Ointment the following procedure can be applied.

Heat 3 g on a water-bath with 30 ml of water, add 10 ml of 3 per cent barium hydroxide solution and heat to boiling-point with continuous stirring. Cool and filter through a moistened filter-paper. Transfer the residue and filter to the original vessel and repeat the extraction twice, finally washing the filter with 50 ml of water. Combine the filtrates and washings and continue by the method given for capsicum beginning with the words 'adjust the pH to between 7·0 and 7·5 by the addition of 0·1N hydrochloric acid . . .'.

The method is also applicable to Tincture of Capsicum as follows.

To 10 ml in a 150-ml separator add 15 ml of analytical reagent grade dehydrated methanol, 15 ml of water, 2 g of sodium chloride and 5 ml of 0·1N sodium hydroxide, shake well to mix and continue by the method for capsicum beginning with the words 'extract with three quantities, each of 10 ml, of light petroleum (b.p. 80° to 100°) . . .'.

Capsaicin is the vanillylamide of *iso*-decenoic acid (8-methyl-*N*-vanillylnon-6-enamide); synthetic compounds that have a close chemical similarity to capsaicin also have pungent properties and are used in place of, or in addition to, naturally occurring material. The method given above will not differentiate between capsaicin and a synthetic compound such as *N*-vanillylnonanamide. A method has been suggested by Datta and Susi[2] for the quantitative differentiation between natural capsaicin and the synthetic material, based on infra-red measurements at 970 cm^{-1}; the peak at this wavelength is due to a *trans* double bond present in the fatty acid moiety of the natural compound, and appears to be unique for capsaicin. Datta and Susi only applied their method to mixtures of pure materials but it is possible that a quantitative determination of capsaicin in capsicum could be worked out which would detect adulteration with synthetic capsaicin-like material.

1. Joint Committee of the Pharmaceutical Society and the Society for Analytical Chemistry on Methods of Assay of Crude Drugs: Report of the Capsicum Panel, *Analyst*, 1959, **84,** 603.
2. Datta, P. R., and Susi, H., *Anal. Chem.*, 1961, **33,** 148.

CARBROMAL

$C_7H_{13}O_2N_2Br$ Mol. Wt. 237·1

Carbromal (2-bromo-2-ethylbutyrylurea) is easily hydrolysed by alkali and the bromide then determined; aqueous alkali is preferable. Although the flask combustion method could be used for this determination there is no obvious advantage over the simple hydrolysis procedure.

To about 0·5 g add 20 ml of 0·5N aqueous sodium hydroxide and boil under reflux for one hour. Cool, acidify with dilute nitric acid and determine the bromide by Volhard's method described under Halogen Acids, p. 290. 1 ml 0·1N = 0·02371 g.

Tablets of Carbromal, *B.P.* Usually contain 5 grains of carbromal. The tablets may be assayed either by the hydrolysis method given above or by direct extraction of the powdered tablets with ether or preferably acetone; the latter is the official method. The residue should be dried at 80° as it is slightly volatile at 100°.

BROMVALETONE, $C_6H_{11}O_2N_2Br$, Mol. Wt. 223·1, (2-brom*iso*valerylurea)

Bromvaletone reacts similarly to carbromal and the assay is the same. 1 ml 0·1N = 0·02231 g.

Tablets of Bromvaletone. Contain 5 grains of bromvaletone. The assay follows that given above under Tablets of Carbromal, ether being the most suitable solvent.

A mixture of carbromal and bromvaletone has been encountered. The proportions of bromine or nitrogen are insufficiently different to be used to calculate the amounts of each present. A determination of the melting-points of mixtures of known proportions in 10 per cent differences after evaporation from ether solution will give a graph for comparison with the unknown mixture. A mixed melting-point of this and the calculated mixture will check the accuracy of the assessed figure.

CHLORAL HYDRATE

$CCl_3.CH(OH)_2$ Mol. Wt. 165·4

Alkali easily decomposes chloral into chloroform and alkali formate and the method of estimation of the purity of the compound is by the use of this reaction.

Dissolve about 4 g in 10 ml of water, add 30 ml of N sodium hydroxide; allow the mixture to stand for two minutes and titrate back with N acid, using phenolphthalein as indicator. 1 ml N = 0·1654 g.

The conditions must be strictly adhered to and low laboratory temperatures must be avoided; also the reaction mixture must not be heated, otherwise the excess of alkali decomposes the chloroform formed and high results are obtained. This was confirmed by Harrington, Boyd and Cherry[1] who showed that some hydrolysis of the chloroform occurred at room temperature in the excess of alkali present. If, after neutralisation of the excess alkali, the chloride formed is titrated with 0·1N silver nitrate using potassium chromate as indicator, a correction for this hydrolysis is possible. Since 3 mols. of sodium chloride produced are equivalent to 4 mols. of sodium hydroxide required for the chloroform hydrolysis, 2/15 of the silver nitrate titration must be deducted from the N sodium hydroxide absorbed in the original hydrolysis.

The formate resulting from alkaline hydrolysis may be determined by reduction with mercuric chloride or permanganate, but the methods are more tedious and subject to errors; no advantage is gained by their use.

Another method of estimation is to convert the chloroform thus produced into potassium chloride by long contact with ethanolic potash (see Chloroform, p. 168); mixtures are best left overnight before refluxing. 1 ml 0·1N silver nitrate = 0·005514 g. However, low results have been reported for this method.

Self[2] preferred the following method as being more convenient than heating with ethanolic potash.

> Boil 0·1 g with either 1 g of aluminium powder in 15 ml of 33 per cent acetic acid and 40 ml of water, or with 2·5 g of zinc filings (No. 20 powder) in 15 ml of glacial acetic acid and 40 ml of water for thirty minutes under reflux. Wash down the condenser, filter through cotton wool and determine the chlorine by Volhard's method. 1 ml 0·1N $AgNO_3$ = 0·005514 g.

Rupp[3] suggested a further method of estimation dependent on the reaction between iodine and the formate obtained with alkali.

> To 10 ml of a 1 per cent solution of chloral hydrate add 25 ml of 0·1N iodine and then 2 ml of N sodium hydroxide. After ten minutes acidify and titrate the excess of iodine with 0·1N sodium thiosulphate.

Kolthoff[4] prefers to use sodium carbonate as the alkali, which would appear to be less likely to act on the chloroform produced.

Mixture of Chloral, *B.P.C.* Contains 9·14 per cent w/v of chloral hydrate. It is best assayed by Self's method given above, using about 1 g of the mixture.

Mixture of Chloral and Potassium Bromide for Infants, *B.P.C.*, a compound mixture containing 3·33 per cent of chloral hydrate and 4·57 per cent potassium bromide and **Mixture of Potassium Bromide and Chloral,** *B.P.C.*, containing 4·57 per cent of potassium bromide and 2·29 per cent of chloral hydrate, may both be assayed by Self's method given above. From the total halogen the potassium bromide (determined by a direct Volhard) must be subtracted before calculating the chloral hydrate content.

Syrup of Chloral, *B.P.C.* A 20 per cent w/v solution of chloral hydrate in syrup and water.

Provided the sample is fresh and made closely to formula the chloral may be determined by decomposition with alkali and back titration as described above, using 20 ml of syrup; however, a large excess of chloral hydrate may retard the reaction and give a low result. After keeping, the syrup is unstable, the free chloral hydrate content decreases on storage due to the formation of a chloral and glucose complex and the end-point of the titration is indefinite. The original chloral hydrate can be determined by Self's method (above) using about 0·6 g and calculating the proportion of chloral hydrate by weight in volume from the weight per ml.

BUTYLCHLORAL HYDRATE, $C_4H_7O_2Cl_3$, Mol. Wt. 193·5

Butylchloral hydrate does not yield chloroform on reacting with alkali, the products of decomposition being dichloropropylene, hydrochloric acid and formic acid. In mixtures, estimation follows the lines of that for chloral hydrate. Back titration with acid after heating with N aqueous potassium hydroxide for half an hour gives unreliable figures, but a Volhard determination of the chloride formed by this treatment is satisfactory; only one chlorine atom is replaced. 1 ml 0·1N silver nitrate = 0·01935 g.

1. Harrington, T., Boyd, T. H., and Cherry, G. W., *Analyst*, 1946, **71,** 97.
2. Self, P. A. W., *Pharm. J.*, 1907, **25,** 4.
3. Rupp, E., *Pharm. Zentralhalle*, 1923, **64,** 151.
4. Kolthoff, I. M., *Pharm. Weekblad*, 1923, **60,** 2.

CHLOROFORM

$CHCl_3$ Mol. Wt. 119·4

For the chemical estimation of chloroform in solutions containing appreciable quantities, its reaction with ethanolic potash to form potassium chloride and potassium formate is employed. Simple spiritous solutions may be determined direct, but for mixtures of low chloroform content or those containing interfering ingredients the chloroform must first be distilled.[1]

Add a quantity of the mixture, to contain approximately 0·1 g of chloroform, to 75 ml of ethanol and 1 g of calcium carbonate contained in a distilling flask, avoiding loss of chloroform by taking care not to agitate the mixture and to keep the tip of the pipette just below the surface of the liquid. Distil approximately 70 ml through an efficient condenser, the end of which dips below the surface of a solution of ethanolic potash (the strength of potash solution required is discussed below). Wash down the condenser with 10 to 15 ml of water into the receiver. Estimate the chloroform in the distillate by the method described below.

Where the ingredients do not interfere (or for the distillates obtained as above):

Quickly weigh an amount of the mixture, or introduce an aliquot part of an ethanolic dilution, to contain 0·1 g of chloroform, into a weighed stoppered flask containing alcoholic potash (the *A.O.A.C.* requires a very strong solution to be used, containing 35 g of potash in 100 ml of methanol, but this is unnecessary and good results are obtainable using 0·5N ethanolic potash). Allow the mixture to stand for some hours, overnight being preferable, and then reflux on a water-bath for an hour or two; or boil the mixture, without preliminary standing, under a very efficient reflux condenser for four hours on a water-bath. Cool, dilute with water, acidify with nitric acid and complete by the Volhard method (see p. 290). 1 ml 0·1N $AgNO_3$ = 0·003980 g; or determine the silver chloride gravimetrically, AgCl × 0·27765 = $CHCl_3$. A control experiment must be carried out on the ingredients.

Chloroform can be saponified completely in fifteen minutes in a Lintner pressure bottle immersed in a water-bath, using 30 per cent potassium hydroxide in ethanol (30 g and 30 ml of water up to 100 ml with ethanol). Robinson[2] has examined the conditions under which chloroform in aqueous solution can be completely hydrolysed by potassium hydroxide at room temperature. His preferred conditions involve mixing the chloroform solution with aqueous potassium hydroxide (to give 3·5M) in a vessel which is filled almost to the stopper and allowed to stand for six hours at 20°. The chloride is then determined by the Volhard method. Robinson states that removal of a sample solution containing chloroform by sucking into a bulb-pipette can result in losses of up to 8 per cent of the chloroform withdrawn.

Soap liniments containing chloroform should be acidified with aqueous sulphuric acid before distilling.

Small quantities of chloroform may be determined within the limited degree of accuracy attainable by colorimetric methods by that of Moffit,[3] which is useful in the presence of other readily decomposed chloro-compounds such as carbon tetrachloride:

First distil a small volume (usually 3 to 5 ml) of the sample under examination with 75 ml of industrial methylated spirit and collect 50 ml of distillate. Measure 10 ml of a 2 per cent w/v solution of β-naphthol in 40 per cent cold potassium hydroxide solution into each of several Nessler cylinders (the success of the test depends upon the strength of the potash solution). To each cylinder add measured volumes of a standard chloroform solution (0·5 per cent by volume of chloroform dissolved in industrial methylated spirit) to contain 0·001 to 0·003 ml of chloroform and add sufficient industrial spirit to make the total volume 11·0 ml (preferably add the methylated spirit before the chloroform and deliver both with the tip of the pipette dipping slightly below the surface of the liquid). Similarly treat aliquot parts of the sample distillate, shake the cylinders and allow them to stand for from five to ten minutes, when the blue colour developed is compared. It is essential that comparison be made within a few minutes.

Cole[4] similarly employs the pink colour produced between chloroform and pyridine in the presence of strong sodium hydroxide as a quantitative colorimetric method for the determination of small amounts of chloroform.

Chloroform may be determined in all kinds of aqueous solutions, pastes and suspensions by the gas chromatographic procedure of Brealey, Elvidge and Proctor.[5] A special injection system was used by the authors and an improved version has been made by Brealey and Baines[6] (see p. 877), in order to prevent the non-volatile material, present in many samples, from reaching the column. Using this equipment chloroform is determined either directly or after dilution with water.

The apparatus employed a thermal conductivity detector similar to that described under Camphor (p. 157) and the method is as follows:

Prepare standards containing 0·1, 0·2 and 0·4 per cent chloroform and add *n*-propanol in the ratio 1 : 100 by volume. Dilute the samples with water if necessary to bring the chloroform content within the range 0·1 to 0·4 per cent and add *n*-propanol in the ratio 1 : 100 by volume. Chromatograph the samples and standards under the following conditions: column length, 3 feet 6 inches; column diameter, 4 to 5 mm; column temperature, 88°; stationary phase, 20 per cent of Carbowax 1500 (polyethylene glycol) on 36 to 85 mesh 'Chromosorb'; carrier gas, nitrogen at 40 ml per minute; temperature of injection system (flash heater) 145°; sample size, about 30 μl.

Under these conditions, the retention volume for chloroform is 169 ml and for *n*-propanol 238 ml. The water is eluted after the *n*-propanol, giving a negative peak and elution is complete after twenty minutes from the start. The chloroform content of the sample is calculated using the peak height method (see p. 879) by reference to the standards.

It has been found in routine practice that the calibration curve relating the ratio of the peak heights of chloroform and *n*-propanol to chloroform concentration is linear and reasonably reproducible from day to day. It has become standard practice therefore to use only one standard containing 0·2 per cent chloroform and this is run each day as a check.

Emulsion of Chloroform, *B.P.C.* This preparation separates so rapidly as to make sampling or analysis impossible with any degree of accuracy.

Spirit of Chloroform, *B.P.* Chloroform 5 per cent by volume in 90 per cent alcohol.

About 1 to 1·5 g should be taken for the direct volumetric determination of chloroform as given above. It may also be determined by the gas chromatographic procedure.

Tincture of Chloroform with Morphine, *B.P.C.* See under Opium.

CARBON TETRACHLORIDE, CCl_4, Mol. Wt. 153·8

The determination of carbon tetrachloride follows the lines of that for chloroform except that decomposition with alcoholic potash is much more difficult. The use of strong potash (35 g potassium hydroxide in methanol to make 100 ml) and heating under pressure is necessary.

Use about 0·1 g of carbon tetrachloride, allow to stand with the potash solution in a Lintner pressure flask for one hour, then heat in a boiling water-bath for a further hour, allow to cool and proceed as under Chloroform. 1 ml 0·1N $AgNO_3$ = 0·003846 g.

CHLORBUTOL, $C_4H_7OCl_3,\frac{1}{2}H_2O$, Mol. Wt. 186·5

Chlorbutol is trichlor-*tert*-butyl alcohol with variable amounts of water of crystallisation (usually $\frac{1}{2}H_2O$). Determination is similar to that for other chloro-compounds decomposed by alcoholic potash (see Chloroform). It is more easily decomposed by alkalies and so requires a shorter contact period.

Dissolve about 0·2 g in 5 ml of ethanol, add 5 ml of 20 per cent sodium hydroxide solution and heat under reflux on a water-bath for fifteen minutes, cool, dilute with 20 ml of water acidified with nitric acid and determine the chloride in the usual way. 1 ml 0·1N $AgNO_3$ = 0·005916 g $C_4H_7OCl_3$, or 0·006216 g $C_4H_7OCl_3,\frac{1}{2}H_2O$.

BROMOFORM, $CHBr_3$, Mol. Wt. 252·8

Bromoform is decomposed by alcoholic potash under the same conditions as chloroform and its assay is based on this reaction (see above). For mixtures of low bromoform content or those containing interfering ingredients the bromoform must first be distilled.

IODOFORM, CHI_3, Mol. Wt. 393·8

The determination of iodoform, both in the solid form and in mixtures, is accomplished by direct decomposition with acidified silver nitrate.

Although the reaction mixture is usually directed to be heated under reflux for one hour, the writers have obtained excellent results by the method of Kunke,[7] which requires only a comparatively short digestion in the cold and is applicable to galenicals:

Weigh in a conical flask a sufficient quantity of material to contain about 0·2 to 0·25 g of iodoform. Add 40 ml of 95 per cent ethanol, swirl and, if necessary, warm gently to dissolve the iodoform. Filter if necessary, re-extracting the residue and washing the filter paper with small quantities of ethanol so as to obtain the iodoform quantitatively in the filtrate. Immediately add 40 ml of 0·1N silver nitrate and finally 10 ml of concentrated nitric acid. Swirl gently for five minutes and allow to stand at room temperature for two to three hours with occasional swirling. Titrate the excess of 0·1N silver nitrate with 0·05N potassium thiocyanate, using ferric ammonium sulphate as indicator. 1 ml 0·1N = 0·01312 g of CHI_3.

As Glass[8] has observed, care must be taken that the end-point of the titration is decided upon with all the accuracy possible, since 0·1 ml of 0·1N solution affects the result by 0·66 per cent when using 0·2 g of iodoform. A gravimetric determination may be made by collecting the silver iodide precipitate and drying it in the usual manner, $AgI \times 0{\cdot}5590 = CHI_3$.

Iodoform may be determined by the flask combustion technique (see p. 796). The method for iodine-containing substances should be followed using a sample weight of about 10 mg. 1 ml 0·02N sodium thiosulphate = 0·0004374 g CHI_3.

Iodoform Gauze

To determine the iodoform, weigh about 5 g of gauze in a beaker, macerate with portions of ethanol until all the iodoform is extracted and assay the mixed ethanolic extracts as above.

Compound Paint of Iodoform (Whitehead's Varnish). This contains 10 per cent w/v of iodoform in an ethereal solution of benzoin, storax and balsam of tolu.

Iodoform is determined by the general chemical method, using 2 ml in 40 ml of ethanol, or, better, 40 ml of a 1 in 20 dilution in ethanol, but after allowing the reaction mixture to stand for two or three hours it is filtered and the precipitate washed with 50 per cent ethanol. This modification is necessary to enable the end-point of the titration to be seen.

Suppository of Iodoform. Each contains 0·2 g of iodoform in cocoa butter.

Since iodoform is very soluble in cocoa butter, extraction before assay is not quantitative. A direct assay in the presence of the melted fat is quite satisfactory:

To about 5 g of suppository, in a stoppered flask, add 40 ml of warm ethanol, melt the fat and shake well. Add 40 ml of 0·1N silver nitrate, followed by 10 ml of nitric acid and allow to stand for two hours, shaking occasionally and maintaining the temperature just to keep the fat melted. Titrate the excess of silver nitrate with 0·1N potassium thiocyanate using solution of ferric ammonium sulphate as indicator. 1 ml 0·1N = 0·01312 g of CHI_3.

TRICHLOROETHYLENE, $CHCl{:}CCl_2$, Mol. Wt. 131·4

Kelly, O'Connor and Reilly[9] obtained quantitative hydrolysis of trichloroethylene by heating with 25 per cent aqueous potassium hydroxide solution in a sealed Carius tube for one hour at 150°. From 8 to 12 ml of the alkali solution should be used for each gram of trichloroethylene present. The potassium chloride formed is determined by the Volhard method. 1 ml 0·1N $AgNO_3$ = 0·00438 g.

1. Matchett, J. R., *J.A.O.A.C.*, 1931, **14,** 360.
2. Robinson, E. A., *Anal. Chim. Acta*, 1960, **23,** 305.
3. Moffit, W. G., *Analyst*, 1933, **58,** 2.
4. Cole, W. H., *J. Biol. Chem.*, 1926, **71,** 173.
5. Brealey, L., Elvidge, D. A., and Proctor, K. A., *Analyst*, 1959, **84,** 221.
6. Brealey, L., and Baines, C. B., private communication.
7. Kunke, W. F., *J.A.O.A.C.*, 1931, **14,** 370.
8. Glass, N., *Quart. J. Pharm.*, 1935, **60,** 351.
9. Kelly, D. F., O'Connor, M., and Reilly, J., *Analyst*, 1941, **66,** 489.

CHROMIUM

Cr At. Wt. 52·00

The determination of chromates or dichromates may be conveniently carried out by their reaction with an excess of a standard solution of a ferrous salt, the excess being titrated with 0·1N permanganate; it is the converse of the usual titration of ferrous salts with dichromate (see Iron). The oxidation of acidified iodide solutions and titration of the liberated iodine with 0·1N sodium thiosulphate is often employed, but this method is said to be subject to disturbing influences owing to the slowness of the reaction and partial oxidation of hydriodic acid by air. The acidified dichromate solution may be freed from air by the addition of two portions, each of 0·2 g, of sodium bicarbonate and allowing the mixture to stand for five minutes after the addition of 1 g of potassium iodide, with a current of carbon dioxide passing through the flask, before diluting and completing the titration of the liberated iodine with 0·1N thiosulphate.

Sully[1] proposes the use of a copper catalyst to improve the speed and accuracy of the reaction; in the presence of copper, acetic acid can replace mineral acid. The proportion of catalyst recommended is 5 ml of 0·001N copper sulphate for 20 ml of 0·1N dichromate, the titration to be conducted in the presence of 5 ml of glacial acetic acid at a temperature not above 25°; subtraction of 0·05 ml for the catalyst is necessary.

Chromium trioxide, CrO_3, Mol. Wt. 100·0. Assayed by the iodine method. 1 ml 0·1N = 0·00333 g.

Traces of chromium may be determined by the diphenylcarbazide reaction.[2] Organic matter may be destroyed by ashing at 600° with twice its weight of lime, the residue being dissolved in dilute hydrochloric acid and filtered.

Evaporate a portion of the solution, containing 20 to 50 μg of chromium, with a few drops of concentrated phosphoric acid to fumes. Cool and oxidise with 1 ml of 1 per cent potassium permanganate solution by heating on a water-bath for twenty minutes. Make slightly alkaline with dilute sodium hydroxide solution, add 5 per cent sodium azide solution drop by drop to decolorise the excess of permanganate and allow to simmer on a hot-plate for ten minutes. Cool, filter, acidify with 5 ml of dilute sulphuric acid, add 2·5 ml of diphenylcarbazide solution (0·25 per cent in 25 per cent ethanol) and make up to 25 ml. Allow the solution to stand for five minutes and measure the extinction at 540 mμ in a spectrophotometer. Carry out a blank determination. Read the number of milligrams of chromium equivalent to the observed extinction of test and blank from a calibration graph.

Establish the calibration graph from appropriate amounts of standard chromium solution covering the range 0 to 20 μg to which 5 ml of dilute sulphuric acid and 2·5 ml of diphenylcarbazide solution have been added before making up to 25 ml. (Standard chromium solution contains 0·3740 g K_2CrO_4 per litre and is diluted 1 to 50 when required, 1 ml = 2 μg chromium.)

Potassium dichromate, $K_2Cr_2O_7$, Mol. Wt. 294·2. Assayed by the iodine method given above. 1 ml 0·1N = 0·004904 g.

1. Sully, B. D., *J. Chem. Soc.*, 1942, 366.
2. Saltzman, B. B., *Anal. Chem.*, 1952, **24,** 1016.

CINCHONA

The species of cinchona officially recognised in the *B.P.C.* were *C. calisaya* Weddell, *C. ledgeriana* Moens, *C. officinalis* Linn., *C. succirubra* Pavon, and hybrids of either of the last two species with either of the first two. They contain from 5 to 10 per cent of total alkaloids, mainly quinine, cinchonidine, cinchonine and quinidine.

Commercial cinchona barks are usually special hybrid strains which yield up to 10 per cent, or sometimes more, of quinine with a low proportion (say 2 per cent) of other alkaloids.

The extraction of the alkaloids from cinchona is difficult and, as the bark contains colouring matter and substances which cause emulsification, the quantitative determination is not easy. A continuous extraction assay is needed, such as that of Self and Corfield;[1] this is probably the most satisfactory process.

Mix thoroughly about 10 g in No. 60 powder, accurately weighed, with a mixture of 7·5 ml of strong lead subacetate solution and 12·5 ml of water and allow to stand for one hour; add 50 ml of ammoniacal ethanol (containing 2·5 per cent of strong ammonia solution), mix well, and allow to stand for a further hour; transfer to an apparatus for the continuous extraction of drugs with a little more of the ammoniacal ethanol and exhaust, the extraction being continued for about four hours. Evaporate off the greater portion of the ethanol, add 10 ml of N sulphuric acid and 40 ml of water, heat to boiling, and cool. Filter through a tightly-packed plug of cotton wool, previously moistened with water, into a separator. Shake the contents of the separator vigorously with three 20-ml portions of chloroform and separate, washing each portion with the same portion of a mixture of 5 ml of N sulphuric acid and 15 ml of water. Make the mixed acid solutions alkaline with dilute ammonia solution and shake with successive portions of chloroform until the alkaloids are completely extracted. Wash the chloroform with a little water, evaporate to dryness, add 5 ml of ethanol, re-evaporate and dry to constant weight at 105°.

There is no need to dry the bark as it grinds easily to No. 60 powder. The lead subacetate is needed to decompose the cinchotannic acids and precipitate cinchona red and other non-alkaloidal material which would otherwise give an impure alkaloidal residue. Excess lead is coagulated and removed by boiling with dilute sulphuric acid after extraction. During the continuous extraction ammonia is generally lost and it is advisable to pour a little more ammonia through the condenser on to the marc and continue the extraction for a further hour. Quinine is very soluble in ammonia and it is advisable to continue chloroform extractions more times than is usual for most other alkaloidal assays. It is essential to add ethanol to quinine residues before drying and weighing if consistent figures are to be obtained.

The assay for quinine and cinchonidine is dependent on the precipitation of these alkaloids as tartrates; careful adjustment of the pH to the neutral sulphates is required, hæmatoxylin or litmus being the most suitable indicators. The method is described under Totaquine (p. 176); if applied to the alkaloids obtained in the above assay of the bark the quantities of reagents must be adjusted for the weight of residue.

Howard[2] has pointed out the inadvisability of titration of cinchona alkaloids, for (i) the average molecular weight is arbitrary and any assumed figure may be far from correct; (ii) the alkaloids are of high molecular weight, and hence a small error in titration causes a large error in the result; (iii) the dissociation of the alkaloids in varying degrees gives an incorrect end-point.

Extract of Cinchona, *B.P.C.* 1954. A soft extract made with strong alcohol and containing 10 per cent of total cinchona alkaloids.

The following method of assay is, in detail, that devised by Self and Corfield.[3] They found that by this process emulsions can be avoided, however vigorously the mixtures be shaken, provided that the volumes of all the reagents prescribed are used as directed. It is possible, however, that the proportions given may be unsuitable for any preparations which are not made strictly according to the *B.P.C.* 1954 formula (which uses strong alcohol in the extraction of the bark). Sodium hydroxide has been found preferable to ammonia as it dissolves cinchona red much more readily and produces a liquid which is practically free from solid particles, but the alkali should be well mixed with the aqueous solution before adding chloroform.

Mix about 2 g, accurately weighed, with 5 ml of water and 5 ml of 95 per cent ethanol, add 1 ml of N hydrochloric acid, and extract with successive 20-ml portions of chloroform by shaking vigorously for two minutes, washing each extract with the same 5 ml of N sulphuric acid; retain the two aqueous solutions separately, reject the chloroform extracts, and add to each aqueous solution 2·5 ml of sodium hydroxide solution. Extract the solutions successively with the same 20-ml portions of chloroform by shaking for two minutes, until extraction is complete; combine the extracts, wash with a little water, reject the washings, evaporate off the chloroform, add 5 ml of 95 per cent ethanol, re-evaporate, and dry the residue of total alkaloids to constant weight at 105°.

If emulsions are formed the following modification may be tried:

Weigh out about 1 g of extract and, if emulsification occurs with the chloroform, add a little glycerol (0·5 ml at a time) up to 2 ml and then if necessary a little ethanol, avoiding an excess and using plenty of chloroform. Usually four extractions with chloroform are sufficient, but two acid washings are preferable to single washing. Bulk the acid washings but keep them separate from the main liquors and continue as in the above method. Complete extraction of the alkaloids is usually obtained with four portions of chloroform, but sometimes many more are required.

Liquid Extract of Cinchona, *B.P.C.* 1954. Prepared by diluting the soft extract to contain 5 per cent of cinchona alkaloids.

The method of assay is exactly the same as that for Extract of Cinchona, from which it is prepared. Use about 5 g of the liquid extract. Calculate the proportion of alkaloids w/v from the specific gravity; the preparation is too viscous to measure accurately.

TOTAQUINE

The League of Nations Malaria Commission[4] defined totaquine as a preparation standardised to contain 70 per cent of crystallisable alkaliods, of which quinine should constitute not less than 15 per cent, with not more than 20 per cent amorphous alkaloids, 5 per cent of mineral matter and 5 per cent of moisture. It was introduced as a cheap substitute for quinine and no particular cinchona species is prescribed as a source provided it has the required composition, but the composition permits it to be made by extraction of the total alkaloids of *C. succirubra* or *C. robusta.*

The method of assay is a modification of Chick's method[5] by Goodson and Henry,[6] and requires some considerable skill to obtain accurate results.

For quinine and total crystallisable alkaloids. Dissolve 2 g in a mixture of 20 ml of N sulphuric acid, 40 ml of water and 40 ml of ethanol (95 per cent). Heat to boiling, and add 0·1N sodium hydroxide, keeping the liquid hot during the addition, until the solution is just faintly alkaline to litmus paper. Cool, add 0·1N sulphuric acid drop by drop until the solution is slightly acid to litmus paper, boil for one or two minutes, cool and, if necessary, again make slightly acid to litmus paper; boil and filter into a tared flask. Wash out the original vessel and the filter with boiling water until the alkaloids have been completely extracted, adding the washings to the original filtrate. Evaporate the filtrate until it weighs about 120 g, add 30 g of powdered sodium potassium tartrate, shake until dissolved, and set aside for twenty-four hours. Filter off the precipitate through a hardened filter, and wash the flask and filter with 80 ml of a 25 per cent w/v solution of sodium potassium tartrate in water, added in portions. Reserve the filtrate and washings for the determination of cinchonine. Return the filter with the precipitate to the flask, add 40 ml of 20 per cent solution of sodium hydroxide and 80 ml of chloroform, and set aside, shaking from time to time, until complete solution is effected. Separate the chloroform solution, and wash the flask and the aqueous liquid with further quantities of chloroform until the alkaloids have been completely extracted. Wash the mixed chloroform solutions with a little water. Remove the chloroform, add 5 ml of 95 per cent ethanol, and evaporate. Dry the residue of quinine and cinchonidine to constant weight at 100°.

Determine the quinine in the mixture of the two alkaloids by a determination of methoxyl (see p. 434), 1·0 per cent of methoxyl is equivalent to 10·45 per cent of anhydrous quinine.

Transfer the filtrate and washings reserved from the precipitated tartrates to a separator containing 80 ml of ether and 20 ml of 20 per cent solution of sodium hydroxide, and shake. Run off the aqueous layer into a second separator, and shake it with two further quantities, each of 80 ml, of ether. Bulk the mixed ethereal solutions, wash with a little water, and extract the alkaloids by shaking with successive quantities of 10, 10 and 5 ml of N sulphuric acid, and finally with 10 ml of water. To the mixed acid and aqueous liquids, add 25 ml of ether and 30 ml of N sodium hydroxide, shake and set aside for one hour. Collect the precipitated cinchonine on a tared filter, using a little water to completely transfer the precipitate to the filter; separate the ether from the filtrate and again run the ether through the precipitate on the filter. Shake the aqueous liquid again with two separate quantities of 25 ml of ether and use these ethereal washings to wash the precipitate. Dry the residue of cinchonine to constant weight at 100°. To the weight obtained, add 80 mg to correct for loss of cinchonine due to its solubility in ether.

Run the ethereal filtrate from the cinchonine into a separator; wash out the filter flask with a little water and ether, and add the washings to the liquid in the separator. Separate the aqueous layer, and extract the alkaloid from the ethereal solution by shaking with successive quantities of 10, 10, 5 and 5 ml of a 10 per cent solution of glacial acetic acid, which have been previously used to wash out any alkaloid remaining in the filter flask or the stem of the funnel. Heat the mixed acetic acid solutions to the boiling-point, neutralise with dilute solution of ammonia, and add 5 g of potassium iodide. Allow to stand overnight, and decant the clear supernatant liquid through a filter, warm the precipitate with 5 ml of 50 per cent ethanol, filter off the liquid, and wash the crystalline residue onto the filter with 5 ml of 50 per cent ethanol. Dry the residue of quinidine hydriodide to constant weight at 100°. To the weight obtained, add 8 mg to correct for loss of quinidine hydriodide due to its solubility. Each g of quinidine hydriodide is equivalent to 0·7171 g of quinidine.

The sum of the percentages of quinine, cinchonidine cinchonine and quinidine gives the percentage of crystallisable alkaloids.

Chick's original method included a separation of the quinine as sulphate:

Treat the total alkaloids with warm water slightly acidified with dilute sulphuric acid until perceptibly acid. Add water to make 70 ml for each 1 g of alkaloids taken, heat and add very dilute sodium hydroxide, with stirring, until the mixture is neutral with a faint tendency to acidity. Digest at 85° for five minutes, cool and leave at 15° for one hour. Filter through a small counterpoised double filter, wash carefully with water at 15° until the washings measure 90 ml for each 1 g of mixed alkaloids. Dry at 100° and weigh. To the weight add 0·000817 g for each 1 ml of filtrate and washings. The weight divided by 0·855 is the equivalent of crystallised sulphate.

The quinine sulphate so obtained contains cinchonidine sulphate, which, although more soluble, crystallises out with it. A recrystallisation as quinine chromate is said to free the quinine substantially from cinchonidine.

Another method in common use, that of calculating the proportions of quinine and cinchonidine from the optical rotation of a mixture of the two, requires considerable skill in making the polarimetric determinations so as to avoid large errors, and there is some doubt as to the exact figures which should be assumed for the rotations of the quinine and cinchonidine bases.

The precipitate is usually contaminated with small quantities of dextrorotatory alkaloids and the mixed tartrate precipitate should be recrystallised before taking a polarimetric reading; recrystallise by dissolving the tartrates in a minimum of boiling 10 per cent tartaric acid solution, filtering hot through activated charcoal, neutralising hot with sodium hydroxide solution to litmus or hæmatoxylin and allowing to crystallise overnight. Furthermore, considerable difficulty may be experienced in reading the rotation of the precipitates. The *N.F.*X. gave a method which is briefly:

Dissolve 0·250 g of the dried precipitate in 2·0 ml of N hydrochloric acid and sufficient water to 25 ml. Add 10 mg of activated charcoal, slowly invert three times and filter at once through a small dry filter into a dry flask rejecting the first few ml of filtrate; then polarise in a 1-dm tube at 25° in sodium light. Calculate the percentage anhydrous quinine by the following formula:

$$\frac{(M - 80{\cdot}5) \times 0{\cdot}79 \times T}{0{\cdot}505 \times S}$$

M = observed angular rotation in minutes.
T = wt of dried tartrate precipitate.
S = wt of totaquine taken for assay.

Goodson and Henry[6] concluded that the discrepancy occurring between the specific rotation and that calculated from the composition of the mixture as determined by methoxyl determination was due to cinchonine precipitated with the quinine and cinchonidine. This can be avoided by precipitation of the tartrates from slightly acid solutions, or their reprecipitation prior to taking polarimetric readings as described above.

The amount of ether used for extraction of the cinchonine may be insufficient for samples of totaquine containing high proportions (40 to 50 per cent) of this alkaloid.

For determination of amorphous alkaloids (quinoidine, quinicine, cinchonicine, etc.):

After filtration of the quinidine hydriodide, add dilute sulphuric acid to the filtrate and evaporate nearly to dryness; make alkaline and extract completely with ether. Dry and weigh the alkaloidal residue, and subtract the weights correcting for solubilities in the determination of crystallisable alkaloids.

QUININE SALTS

As an antimalarial, quinine has now been largely replaced by synthetic drugs and many of the salts have gone out of use; all the salts of quinine may be assayed for their quinine content as follows:

Dissolve about 0·2 to 0·3 g in a little dilute sulphuric acid, transfer to a separator and make distinctly alkaline with sodium hydroxide. Extract with successive portions of chloroform, washing each portion with 5 ml of water contained in a second separator. Evaporate the chloroform solutions, add 5 ml of ethanol and again evaporate; dry at 105° and weigh.

Toal and Jones[7] have shown that ethanol treatment is necessary after chloroform evaporation from quinine alkaloids, and drying at 105° is complete in one to two hours, further heating causing decomposition.

Quinine salts may be determined by non-aqueous titration (see p. 792).

The pure alkaloid **Quinine,** $C_{20}H_{24}O_2N_2,3H_2O$, Mol. Wt. 378·5, can be titrated quite satisfactorily to methyl red or bromocresol purple. 1 ml 0·05N = 0·01622 g anhydrous quinine.

The quinine salts and preparations in Table 11 are official in the *B.P.*

The various salts of quinine are incorporated into a number of official preparations such as syrups and tablets. The simpler formulations can be assayed by a spectrophotometric method based upon the absorption characteristics in the ultra-violet. For example, in N sulphuric acid, quinine hydrochloride has two absorption maxima at 250 mμ and 347 mμ, the E(1 per cent, 1 cm) values being about 730 and 140 respectively. However, this technique is not applicable to the more complex samples such as Easton's Syrup or Tablets without first extracting the quinine and a

TABLE 11

QUININE SALT	FORMULA	MOL. WT.	QUININE FACTOR
Bisulphate	$C_{20}H_{24}O_2N_2,H_2SO_4,7H_2O$	548·6	1·302 anhyd. 1·691 cryst.
Tablets, *B.P.**			
Dihydrochloride	$C_{20}H_{24}O_2N_2,2HCl$	397·4	1·225
Injection, *B.P.*	0·3 g per ml		
Hydrochloride	$C_{20}H_{24}O_2N_2,HCl,2H_2O$	396·9	1·112 anhyd. 1·223 cryst.
Tablets, *B.P.*†			
Sulphate	$(C_{20}H_{24}O_2N_2)_2,H_2SO_4,2H_2O$	783·0	1·151 anhyd. 1·207 cryst.
Tablets, *B.P.*†			

* For assay, see below.
† Method of assay the same as for Quinine Bisulphate Tablets.

fluorimetric procedure is of greater value. It is convenient therefore to use such a method for all determinations.

Dilute or extract the sample with 0·1N sulphuric acid to give a final concentration of quinine suitable for the fluorimeter being used; usually about 0·5 μg per ml is satisfactory. The excitation radiation must be within the range 300 to 400 mμ and is most conveniently obtained by the use of a high-pressure mercury vapour lamp and a filter to isolate the line at 355 mμ. A secondary filter transmitting light between 420 and 450 mμ is used between the fluorescent solution and the detector. Calibrate the instrument with a standard solution or solutions of quinine in 0·1N sulphuric acid and measure the fluorescence intensity of the sample.

Ammoniated Solution of Quinine, *B.P.C.* A mixture of quinine sulphate, dilute solution of ammonia and 60 per cent alcohol.

For quinine. Dilute 20 ml with water, extract direct with portions of chloroform, wash the chloroform with a little water, evaporate, add 5 ml of ethanol, re-evaporate, dry at 105° for two hours and weigh.

For ammonia. Titrate 20 ml with 0·5N hydrochloric acid, using methyl red as indicator. 1 ml 0·5N = 0·0085 g NH_3.

Tablets of Quinine Bisulphate, *B.P.* Usually contain 5 grains of quinine bisulphate and are sugar-coated.

For chemical assay, complete disintegration of the tablets with dilute hydrochloric acid is necessary. After filtration from acid-insoluble matter an aliquot part is first washed in acid solution with chloroform before making alkaline and extracting the quinine in the usual way.

For fluorimetric assay:

Shake an accurately weighed quantity of the powdered tablet material containing about 150 mg of quinine bisulphate with about 100 ml of 0·1N sulphuric acid for thirty minutes and dilute to 250 ml with the same solvent. Dilute 10 ml of this solution to 250 ml and further dilute 5 ml to 250 ml both with 0·1N sulphuric acid. Proceed with the general method given above.

Quinidine sulphate, $(C_{20}H_{24}O_2N_2)_2,H_2SO_4,2H_2O$, Mol. Wt. 783·0, is assayed for its quinidine content by the method used for quinine salts.

Tablets of Quinidine Sulphate, *B.P.* Usually contain 3 grains of quinidine sulphate.

No difficulty is experienced in the chemical assay. A quantity of powdered tablets, equivalent to about 0·3 g of quinidine sulphate, is dissolved in acid and preferably filtered before extracting the base in the usual way.

Quinidine formulations can be assayed by a fluorimetric method analogous to that for quinine.

SYNTHETIC ANTIMALARIALS

For treatment of malaria, quinine has now been largely replaced by synthetic antimalarials and the most important are listed in Table 12. Most are salts of organic bases and, in general, the free bases can be extracted with ether or chloroform from ammoniacal or sodium hydroxide solution and either weighed after drying or dissolved in excess of standard acid and titrated. Nitrite titration is applicable in some cases and non-aqueous titration with perchloric acid (p. 792) with others; the latter is recommended for mepacrine hydrochloride after adding 10 ml of 5 per cent mercuric acetate in glacial acetic acid (to prevent interference from chloride) and 25 ml of chloroform, swirling until the precipitate dissolves.

Mepacrine hydrochloride is assayed in the *U.S.P.* by precipitation as insoluble dichromate with titration of excess reagent.

Dissolve about 0·25 g, accurately weighed, in water. Add 10 ml of a solution of 25 g of sodium acetate and 10 ml of glacial acetic acid in sufficient water to give 100 ml, followed by exactly 50 ml of 0·1N potassium dichromate. Dilute to 100 ml with water in a graduated flask and filter. To 50 ml of filtrate add 15 ml of concentrated hydrochloric acid, 20 ml of 5 per cent potassium iodide solution and allow to stand for five minutes. Dilute and titrate with 0·1N sodium thiosulphate using starch solution as indicator. Repeat the assay without the mepacrine hydrochloride as a blank. 1 ml 0·1N $K_2Cr_2O_7$ = 0·008482 g of $C_{23}H_{30}ON_3Cl,2HCl,2H_2O$.

The assay of **proguanil hydrochloride** depends on the precipitation of a copper complex of the base[8] and the official method is as follows:

Dissolve about 0·6 g, accurately weighed, in 50 ml of water by warming gently, cool to 10° and add ammoniacal cupric chloride solution with stirring until the solution retains a deep blue colour. Allow the precipitate to stand for not less than one hour, then filter through a tared

TABLE 12

SYNTHETIC ANTIMALARIAL	FORMULA	MOL. WT.	ASSAY METHOD
Amodiaquine Hydrochloride, *B.P.*	$C_{20}H_{22}ON_3Cl,2HCl,2H_2O$	464·8	Extraction with chloroform in NH_3, drying at 105°. Wt. × 1·205 (anhyd.)
Tablets, *B.P.*	Usually 0·2 g		
Chloroquine Phosphate, *B.P.*	$C_{18}H_{26}N_3Cl,2H_3PO_4$	515·9	Extraction with ether in NaOH and titration 1 ml 0·1N HCl = 0·02579 g
Injection, *B.P.*	40 mg of base per ml		
Tablets, *B.P.*	Usually 0·25 g		
Chloroquine Sulphate, *B.P.*	$C_{18}H_{26}N_3Cl,H_2SO_4,H_2O$	436·0	Extraction with ether in NaOH and titration 1 ml 0·1N HCl = 0·02090 g (anhyd.)
Injection, *B.P.*	40 mg (as base) per ml		
Tablets, *B.P.*	Usually 0·2 g		
Hydroxychloroquine Sulphate, *B.P.*	$C_{18}H_{26}ON_3Cl,H_2SO_4$	434·0	Extraction with chloroform in NH_3, drying at 105°. Wt. × 1·292
Tablets, *B.P.*	Usually 0·2 g		
Mepacrine Hydrochloride, *B.P.*	$C_{23}H_{30}ON_3Cl,2HCl,2H_2O$	508·9	Extraction with chloroform in NH_3, drying at 105°. Wt. × 1·282 (anhyd.) *or* Non-aqueous titration to crystal violet 1 ml 0·1N $HClO_4$ = 0·02365 g (anhyd.) See also *U.S.P.* method
Tablets, *B.P.*	Usually 0·1 g		
Mepacrine Methane-sulphonate, *B.P.C.*	$C_{23}H_{30}ON_3Cl,2CH_3.SO_3H,H_2O$	610·2	Extraction with chloroform in NaOH, drying at 105°. Wt. × 1·481 (anhyd.)
Primaquine Phosphate, *B.P.*	$C_{15}H_{21}ON_3,2H_3PO_4$	455·4	Nitrite titration 1 ml 0·1M $NaNO_2$ = 0·04554 g
Tablets, *B.P.*	Usually 7·5 mg (as base)		
Proguanil Hydrochloride, *B.P.*	$C_{11}H_{16}N_5Cl,HCl$	290·2	Precipitation of copper complex dried at 130°
Tablets, *B.P.*	Usually 0·1 g		
Pyrimethamine, *B.P.*	$C_{12}H_{13}N_4Cl$	248·7	Non-aqueous titration to quinaldine red 1 ml 0·1N $HClO_4$ = 0·02487 g
Tablets, *B.P.*	Usually 25 mg		

In all preparations the method of assay is the same as that for the drug.

sintered-glass crucible of porosity 3, fitted with an asbestos pad. Wash the precipitate with 100 ml of a mixture of 1 part of dilute ammonia solution and 5 parts of water, followed by cold water, until the washings are colourless. Dry to constant weight at 130°; 1 g residue = 1·020 g $C_{11}H_{16}N_5Cl,HCl$.

For assay of the tablets, shake a quantity of the powdered tablets equivalent to 1 g of proguanil hydrochloride with 100 ml of water continuously for one hour, filter and determine by the method given above using 50 ml of the filtrate.

Chlorproguanil hydrochloride, $C_{11}H_{15}N_5Cl_2,HCl$, Mol. Wt. 324·7 can be assayed similarly using 100 ml of water to dissolve the sample and drying the copper complex at 105°. 1 g residue = 1·0175 g chlorproguanil hydrochloride.

1. SELF, P. A. W., and CORFIELD, C. E., *Quart. J. Pharm.*, 1930, **3**, 410.
2. HOWARD, B. F., *Y.B. Pharm.*, 1923, 691.
3. SELF, P. A. W., and CORFIELD, C. E., *Quart. J. Pharm.*, 1931, **4**, 335.
4. League of Nations, Malaria Commission, CM/*Malaria*/167(1).
5. CHICK, O., 'Allen's Commercial Organic Analysis', 5th edition, 1929, **7**, 426.
6. GOODSON, J. A., and HENRY, T. A., *Quart. J. Pharm.*, 1932, **5**, 161.
7. TOAL, J. S., and JONES, A. J., *Quart. J. Pharm.*, 1935, **8**, 401.
8. STAGG, H. E., *J. Pharm. Pharmacol.*, 1949, **1**, 391.

CITRIC ACID

$C_3H_4(OH)(COOH)_3,H_2O$ Mol. Wt. 210·1

Citric acid can be titrated directly with N alkali to phenolphthalein or, preferably, to thymol blue which gives a more distinct end-point. 1 ml N = 0·06404 g anhydrous acid or 0·07005 g monohydrate.

Lampitt and Rooke[1] examined the various methods available for the determination of citric acid and concluded that the pentabromoacetone method (depending on the oxidation of the acid by permanganate to acetonedicarboxylic acid, which then reacts with bromine to form pentabromoacetone) was the most convenient and reliable. A careful research into the procedure evolved the following technique which is claimed to be capable of yielding results of a high degree of accuracy. This has been confirmed by the writers, who have been able to recover almost theoretical yields of citric acid from standard mixtures containing also tartaric acid and sucrose:

To 50 ml of a solution containing a maximum of 0·1 g of citric acid add 10 ml of 1 : 1 by volume sulphuric acid and 5 ml of 37·5 per cent w/v potassium bromide solution. (Except for pure citric acid and milk serum, 10 ml of freshly-prepared bromine water should also be added and any precipitate formed from acetonedicarboxylic acid filtered off after half an hour's standing.) Add 5 per cent w/v potassium permanganate solution dropwise from a burette with constant shaking until a brown precipitate persists, 10 ml being usually required for 0·1 g of citric acid. Allow the mixture to stand at room temperature for one hour, further addition of permanganate being made if the brown precipitate disappears. Add slowly, sufficient 20 per cent w/v ferrous sulphate solution in 1 per cent sulphuric acid until a pale yellow solution containing a white precipitate is obtained, and then cool the mixture in an ice-chest overnight (sixteen hours).

Remove the precipitate by filtration through a sintered-glass crucible (size 10G4), wash out the reaction flask with the filtrate to remove the last traces of precipitate and pass the washings through the crucible. Then wash the precipitate in the crucible with portions of 10, 10 and 5 ml of cold water. Note the volume of the filtrate. Dry the crucible to constant weight in a vacuum desiccator (about sixteen hours); dissolve the precipitate out of the crucible with ethanol followed by 20, 10 and 10 ml portions of ether; again dry the crucible in the vacuum desiccator and weigh, the loss in weight being taken as pentabromoacetone.

$$\text{Citric acid (anhydrous)} = 0{\cdot}424\left(W + \frac{0{\cdot}005V}{100}\right),$$

where W represents the difference in weight of the crucible before and after treatment with ethanol and ether, and V is the original volume of filtrate from the reaction mixture, less the total volume of washings.

Anhydrous citric acid × 1·0937 = citric acid monohydrate.

CITRATES

The alkali citrates are estimated by the general method for salts of organic acids, *i.e.*:

> Ignite a known weight in a platinum dish, add water and standard acid to the charred mass, boil, filter and titrate the excess of acid in the filtrate with standard alkali to methyl orange or methyl red.

An alternative method is to boil with water after ignition, then filter and wash; ignite the filter paper and residual carbonaceous matter to a white ash and add the ash to the previous filtrate before titrating to methyl orange with standard acid. The method can be used for **potassium citrate,** $C_6H_5O_7K_3,H_2O$, Mol. Wt. 324·4, 1 ml 0·5N = 0·05407 g; **sodium citrate,** $C_6H_5O_7Na_3,2H_2O$, Mol. Wt. 294·1, 1 ml 0·5N = 0·04902 g; **lithium citrate,** $C_6H_5O_7Li_3,4H_2O$, Mol. Wt. 282·0, 1 ml 0·5N = 0·04700 g; and **sodium acid citrate,** $C_6H_6O_7Na_2,1\frac{1}{2}H_2O$, Mol. Wt. 263·1, 1 ml 0·5N = 0·06578 g. A sodium citrate containing $5\frac{1}{2}$ molecules of water of crystallisation is also obtainable commercially.

Citrates of alkali metals may be determined by non-aqueous titration with standard perchloric acid in acetic acid using crystal violet or α-naphtholbenzein as indicator (see p. 792).

1. LAMPITT, L. H., and ROOKE, H. S., *Analyst*, 1936, **61**, 654.

COCA

Coca consists of the dried leaves of *Erythroxylum coca*, Lam. (Bolivian or Huanuco leaf), or *E. truxillense*, Rusby (Peruvian or Truxillo leaf), and contains esters of ecgonine, e.g. methyl benzoylecgonine (cocaine), methyl cinnamylecgonine (cinnamyl cocaine), methyl-α-truxillylecgonine and methyl-β-truxillylecgonine (α- and β-truxillines). Generally Peruvian leaf contains more alkaloid but a smaller proportion of cocaine than Bolivian leaf, the total alkaloids being 0·5 to 1·5 per cent.

The assay of coca leaves and of crude cocaine is the subject of the Bulletin of the Health Organisation of the League of Nations Extract No. 6.[1] For the leaves the following method is recommended:

Determine the moisture content on leaves ground to pass through a 2-mm sieve, drying about 2 g at 103° to 105°. Triturate 20 g in a mortar with 20 ml of 2N sodium carbonate and allow to stand for half an hour with occasional stirring. Then extract the mixture continuously with ether for a few hours, allow it to stand overnight in contact with ether and again extract until a total of eight hours' extraction has been given. Then extract the ethereal solution with 20, 15 and 10 ml of 0·1N hydrochloric acid; filter each extract through cotton wool. To the combined acid extracts add 30 ml of 2 : 1 ether and light petroleum, followed by 1 g of sodium bicarbonate in small amounts at a time. After shaking and separating, re-extract the aqueous solution with three further 30-ml quantities of mixed solvent. Dry the combined extracts, filter and evaporate. Dissolve the residue in 5 ml of neutral 95 per cent ethanol and titrate with 0·1N acid, with methyl orange as indicator, then add 50 ml of water and complete the titration. 1 ml 0·1N acid = 0·0185 g ecgonine = 0·0303 g cocaine.

As a check, the combined acids (benzoic, cinnamic, truxillic) may be determined. To the solution from the titration of the alkaloids, add 5 ml of 2N sodium hydroxide and boil the mixture until the volume is reduced to about 10 ml. Continue the boiling under reflux for a further five minutes, then acidify with hydrochloric acid and extract with three 30-ml portions of 2 : 1 ether and light petroleum mixture. Dry the combined extracts with sodium sulphate, remove the solvent under slightly reduced pressure, the temperature being kept below 30°. Dissolve the residue in 5 ml of neutral 95 per cent ethanol and titrate with 0·1N sodium hydroxide to phenolphthalein. 1 ml 0·1N alkali = 0·0185 g ecgonine.

In a report of the United Nations Commission of enquiry on the Coca leaf[2] it was observed that no true crystals of cocaine were obtained with platinic chloride on the residue from the ether-light petroleum when dissolved in dilute acid. The crystals which were obtained were hybrids, not characteristic of cocaine. The difficulty was overcome by shaking the mixed solvent extract with 10 ml of a 2 per cent aqueous solution of potassium permanganate. After separation of the layers the permanganate was discarded and the organic layer treated as in the original method.

This treatment had no effect on the subsequent acidimetric titration of the cocaine. It was also noted that the addition of about 10 per cent of 95 per cent ethanol to the ether used in the extraction of coca leaves tends to reduce emulsions and thus shortens the time required for analysis without affecting the results.

A method for the determination of ecgonine in coca leaves is also described in the United Nations report:

> Extract a 10 g sample of leaves by the method described in the official determination of coca leaves, but using ethyl ether containing approximately 10 per cent of 95 per cent ethanol and an extraction time of four hours. Follow the method for coca leaves until the residue is obtained after evaporation of the ether-light petroleum extract. Then, to the residue contained in a 150-ml beaker, add 5 ml of concentrated nitric acid and 5 ml of phosphotungstic acid solution (10 g phosphotungstic acid in 90 ml of water and 10 ml of concentrated nitric acid). Warm the solution on a water-bath with occasional stirring to effect granulation of the precipitate, allow to cool by standing for one hour or overnight and then filter through a sintered-glass crucible. Wash the ecgonine phosphotungstate with 1 per cent nitric acid solution and finally with 10 ml of cold water. Dry for one hour at 100°, cool, and weigh. The weight of phosphotungstate divided by 3·64 and multiplied by 10 gives the percentage of ecgonine in the leaves.

Coca as such now finds little use in pharmacy, the isolated cocaine being more suitable for use. In the locality where it is grown for export it is the practice to isolate a crude mixture of alkaloids by treating the leaves with lime and percolating with naphtha or benzene. This mixture at destination is evaluated for its total ecgonine content, since pure ecgonine is isolated, methylated and benzoylated to give cocaine. The following method may be used to assay the crude cocaine for ecgonine content:

> Weigh 1 g of the well-mixed sample into a conical flask fitted with a ground-glass joint and a long air-condenser. Add 15 ml of concentrated hydrochloric acid and boil the solution gently for forty-five minutes so that the fumes condense as much as possible. Cool, rinse the condenser into the flask with water and rinse the contents of the flask into a separator, using water and ether. Shake out the acids with ether, using five portions. Wash the ether extracts with a little water and wash the water with a little ether and add the washings to the rest of the aqueous liquid. Evaporate the dissolved ether from the latter by heating for a short time on a water-bath in a flask having a funnel inserted in the neck; transfer to a tared glass dish. Evaporate and dry in a water-oven until the weight is constant (the residue is hygroscopic and special precautions must be taken in weighing). Dissolve the residue in a little ethanol and titrate with 0·1N sodium hydroxide using phenolphthalein as indicator.
>
> Reduce 1 g to ash and weigh; treat with dilute hydrochloric acid, evaporate to dryness and heat in a water-oven until of constant weight. Subtract this weight from that found in the first experiment. Also titrate the ash with 0·1N sodium hydroxide and deduct from the figure previously found. If required, calculate the difference to cocaine. 1 ml 0·1N ≡ 0·0303 g of cocaine; ecgonine hydrochloride × 1·368 = cocaine.

The method of assaying raw cocaine for ecgonine alkaloids recommended by the Health Organisation of the League of Nations[1] is polarimetric:

Determine the moisture content of crude cocaine by drying about 1 g in a vacuum desiccator. To determine the ecgonine content, dissolve about 0·5 g in 15 ml of 2N hydrochloric acid and boil the solution under reflux for five hours. After cooling slowly over a period of at least two hours, filter through a plug of cotton wool and wash the wool with small quantities of 2N acid until the filtrate measures 25 ml at 20°. Mix well and measure the optical rotation in a 2-dm tube. Calculate the percentage of ecgonine in the raw cocaine by the formula

$$\frac{a \times 25}{2 \times 57} \times \frac{100}{w} \text{ or practically } \frac{22a}{w}$$

where a = optical rotation and w = weight of cocaine; specific rotatory power of ecgonine = +57°. Cocaine = ecgonine × 1·64.

As a check on the ecgonine content the combined acids may be determined. Dissolve about 0·5 g of the raw cocaine in 5 ml of acetone and 5 ml of 2N sodium hydroxide and boil under reflux for fifteen minutes. Evaporate the acetone, transfer the aqueous solution to a separator with about 15 ml of water, acidify with 10 ml of 2N hydrochloric acid and proceed as given under coca leaves (above).

COCAINE, $C_{17}H_{21}O_4N$, Mol. Wt. 303·4

Nicholls[3] has pointed out that as cocaine is a relatively weak base, the free alkaloid can be extracted with an immiscible solvent, after addition of sodium bicarbonate, whilst other alkaloids and local anæsthetics, which are stronger bases, are not extracted. Also cocaine in slightly acid solution is not appreciably affected by permanganate, whilst almost all other alkaloids and local anæsthetics are attacked. For carrying out the oxidation:

Dissolve the extracted residue in 0·1N sulphuric acid and add a solution of 3 per cent potassium permanganate in 0·5N sulphuric acid until an excess is indicated by the colour. After the solution has been decolorised with oxalic acid add sodium bicarbonate in excess and extract any cocaine with light petroleum immediately after the addition of the bicarbonate. Oxidation can be hastened by keeping the solution in a water-bath at about 60°.

Hence in cases where traces of other alkaloids are extracted, the extract may be treated as above to decompose interfering substances.

If permanganate oxidation has not been used, any other alkaloid remaining in the solution from which the cocaine has been extracted, may be liberated with excess of ammonia and extracted as usual.

In N sulphuric acid cocaine has an absorption maximum at 234 mμ, E(1 per cent, 1 cm) = 397.

Small quantities of cocaine may be determined by use of the fact that on mild alkaline hydrolysis it yields methanol; the sensitivity is approximately 2 mg of alkaloid. Only substances yielding methanol on hydrolysis will interfere, hence procaine will not affect the determination. The following details are described by Young:[4]

> Weigh 25 to 50 mg of alcohol-free sample into a small distilling flask and add 2 ml of 2 per cent aqueous sodium hydroxide solution and 5 ml of water. Connect the flask to a condenser with a ground glass joint and distil the contents into a previously calibrated Nessler cylinder until 2 ml of distillate is collected. Introduce 0·4, 0·6 and 1·0 ml portions of a standard cocaine solution (50 mg of pure cocaine hydrochloride in 10 ml water) into separate distillation flasks and collect 2 ml distillates in Nessler cylinders. Add to the test and standard distillates 0·25 ml of 24 per cent ethanol and 2·75 ml water followed by 2 ml of potassium permanganate solution and allow to stand with occasional shaking for ten minutes. Add 2 ml of oxalic acid reagent and 5 ml of Schiff's reagent and allow to stand for two hours. Compare the colour developed by the sample with those of the primary standards. To obtain an accurate determination make a final comparison with a series of standards in 0·1 ml increments in the region of the nearest primary standard.

The reagents used are those described under Ethyl Alcohol, p. 250.

Eye-drops of Cocaine and Mercuric Chloride, *B.P.C.* (Factory Eye Drops). Contain cocaine, approximately 0·5 per cent, and mercuric chloride in castor oil.

Normal assay is possible; no interference is caused by the presence of mercuric chloride. The extracted cocaine is white and crystalline.

> Transfer about 10 g, accurately weighed, with the aid of 40 ml of ether to a separator containing 15 ml of 0·1N hydrochloric acid. Shake, run off the aqueous layer into a second separator and shake the ether layer with further quantities of 15 ml of 0·1N hydrochloric acid until complete extraction of the alkaloid is effected. Wash the mixed aqueous solutions with two portions, each of 10 ml, of ether. Reserve the aqueous solution, wash the mixed ethereal solutions with 10 ml, of water and reject the ether. To the aqueous solution add a slight excess of dilute solution of ammonia and shake with successive quantities of ether until complete extraction of the alkaloid is effected. Wash the mixed ethereal solutions with two portions, each of 10 ml, of water. Remove the ether, add 10 ml of ethanol, evaporate and dry at 80°. Dissolve the residue in 5 ml of 0·05N sulphuric acid and titrate with 0·05N sodium hydroxide, using methyl red as indicator. 1 ml 0·05N = 0·01517 g of $C_{17}H_{21}O_4N$.

Cocaine hydrochloride, $C_{17}H_{21}O_4N,HCl$, Mol. Wt. 339·8

Eye-drops of Cocaine, *B.P.C.* Contain 2 per cent of cocaine hydrochloride with sodium chloride and parahydroxybenzoates.

The tetraphenylboron method given under Atropine, p. 116, can be used for this preparation, preparing the solution by adding 10 ml of buffer solution, pH 3·7, to 3 ml of the sample in a 20-ml graduated flask and diluting to volume with water. 1 ml cetylpyridinium chloride = 0·001699 g.

Lamellæ of Cocaine, *B.P.* 1953. Contain 1·3 mg of cocaine hydrochloride.

Dissolve 10 discs in N sulphuric acid and make up to 250 ml. Dilute 10 ml of this solution to 100 ml with the same solvent. Measure the maximum extinction of a 1-cm layer at about 234 mμ using the N sulphuric acid as blank. Calculate the amount of cocaine in each disc.

LOCAL ANÆSTHETICS

A large number of synthetic local anæsthetics are available and the more important of these are listed in the table below, which also indicates the methods of assay which are used.

In general the free bases of those local anæsthetics which occur as salts may be extracted in ammoniacal sodium carbonate or sodium hydroxide solution with ether or chloroform but care must be taken during evaporation of the solvent. Prolonged heating of the isolated bases should be avoided as some of them appear to be slightly volatile at 100°. They are preferably dried in a vacuum desiccator at room temperature; the residues obtained are generally oily but slowly crystallise on standing. The bases may also be titrated with 0·1N acid using methyl red or bromocresol green as indicator.

Two methods which are quite widely applicable to many local anæsthetics are non-aqueous titration (perchloric acid to crystal violet, p. 792) and titration with sodium nitrite (0·5 g in 75 ml water and 10 ml hydrochloric acid, titrating with 0·1M nitrite and determining the end-point using the dead-stop technique, p. 867). A few materials such as benzocaine may be determined by both methods but in most cases either one or the other is applicable. Lignocaine hydrochloride, for example, gives a satisfactory end-point by the non-aqueous method but cannot be determined by titration with nitrite; procaine hydrochloride on the other hand is satisfactorily titrated with nitrite but gives rise to a precipitate during titration in non-aqueous medium which obscures the end-point. Certain compounds such as amethocaine hydrochloride cannot be determined by either method.

Local anæsthetics, such as procaine, which are stronger bases may be completely separated from cocaine by the extraction of the latter with light petroleum in sodium bicarbonate solution by the method of Nicholls (above). Permanganate oxidation, as described on p. 186, completely destroys these local anæsthetics, no extractable matter being obtained. Orthocaine is also phenolic and not removed from solution in sodium hydroxide but easily from sodium bicarbonate solution. The base is very weak and salts are hydrolysed in solution, so that much of it can be extracted in acid solution.

A colorimetric method for the determination of materials containing a primary aromatic amine (such as benzocaine) is based upon diazotisation and coupling with *N*-(1-naphthyl)ethylenediamine hydrochloride. It has been adapted for assay of benzocaine, procaine hydrochloride, butacaine

TABLE 13

LOCAL ANÆSTHETIC	FORMULA	MOL. WT.	ASSAY METHOD
Amethocaine Hydrochloride, *B.P.*	$C_{15}H_{24}O_2N_2$,HCl	300·8	Extraction with ether in Na_2CO_3 and titration. 1 ml 0·1N HCl = 0·03008 g.
Injection, *B.P.*			As for drug.
Benzocaine, *B.P.*	$C_9H_{11}O_2N$	165·2	Nitrite titration. 1 ml 0·1M $NaNO_2$ = 0·01652 g.
Ointment, Compound, *B.P.C.*			As for drug after solution in light petroleum and extraction with four portions of dilute HCl.
Butacaine Sulphate, *B.P.C.*	$(C_{18}H_{30}O_2N_2)_2,H_2SO_4$	711·0	Nitrite titration. 1 ml 0·05M $NaNO_2$ = 0·03555 g.
Butethamine Hydrochloride, *N.F.*	$C_{13}H_{20}O_2N_2$,HCl	272·8	Extraction with chloroform in NH_3 and titration. 1 ml 0·1N HCl = 0·02728 g.
Cinchocaine, *B.P.C.*	$C_{20}H_{29}O_2N_3$	343·5	
Cinchocaine Hydrochloride, *B.P.*	$C_{20}H_{29}O_2N_3$,HCl	379·9	Non-aqueous titration 1 ml 0·1N $HClO_4$ = 0·01900 g.
Lozenges, *B.P.C.*			Extraction with ether in Na_2CO_3 and titration. 1 ml 0·1N HCl = 0·03799 g.
Lignocaine (Lidocaine, *U.S.P.*)	$C_{14}H_{22}ON_2$	234·3	Solution in excess 0·1N acid and titration to methyl red. 1 ml 0·1N H_2SO_4 = 0·02343 g.
Lignocaine Hydrochloride, *B.P.*	$C_{14}H_{22}ON_2$,HCl,H_2O	288·8	Non-aqueous titration. 1 ml 0·1N $HClO_4$ = 0·02708 g. (anhyd.)
Injection, *B.P.*			Extraction with ether in Na_2CO_3 and titration. 1 ml 0·05N HCl = 0·01444 g. (monohyd.)
Injection with Adrenaline, *B.P.**			As injection.
Naepaine Hydrochloride, *N.F.*	$C_{14}H_{22}O_2N_2$,HCl	286·8	Extraction with chloroform in NH_3 and titration. 1 ml 0·1N HCl = 0·02868 g.
Orthocaine, *B.Vet.C.*	$C_8H_9O_3N$	167·2	
Phenacaine Hydrochloride, *N.F.*	$C_{18}H_{22}O_2N_2$,HCl,H_2O	352·9	Extraction with chloroform in NH_3 and weighing. Wt. × 1·122 (anhyd.)
Piperocaine Hydrochloride, *U.S.P.*	$C_{16}H_{23}O_2N$,HCl	297·8	Extraction from brine with ether in NaOH and titration. 1 ml 0·1N HCl = 0·02978 g.
Procainamide Hydrochloride, *B.P.*	$C_{13}H_{21}ON_3$,HCl	271·8	Nitrite titration. 1 ml 0·1M $NaNO_2$ = 0·02718 g.
Injection, *B.P.*			As for drug.
Procainamide Sulphate, *B.P.C.*	$(C_{13}H_{21}ON_3)_2,H_2SO_4$	568·8	Nitrite titration. 1 ml 0·1M $NaNO_2$ = 0·02844 g.
Procaine Hydrochloride, *B.P.*	$C_{13}H_{20}O_2N_2$,HCl	272·8	Nitrite titration. 1 ml 0·1M $NaNO_2$ = 0·02728 g.
Injection with Adrenaline, *B.P.*†			Extraction with *iso*propyl alcohol. 1 : chloroform 3 in Na_2CO_3 and titration. 1 ml 0·1N HCl = 0·02728 g.

* Adrenaline determined by the ferrous sulphate-citrate method (p. 20) with a washing with 10 ml of ether after development of colour.

† Adrenaline determined by the ferrous sulphate-citrate method (p. 20), Chlorocresol by the 4-aminophenazone method (p. 514).

sulphate, and butyl aminobenzoate by Bandelin and Kemp.[5] It is not specific but cocaine and ephedrine do not interfere.

To a prepared solution containing approximately 100 μg of benzocaine in 0·1N hydrochloric acid add 1 ml of freshly prepared 0·5 per cent sodium nitrite solution, mix and allow to stand for three minutes. Add 1·5 ml of a 1 per cent solution of sulphamic acid in water, stopper the flask and shake well. Add 2·5 ml of a 0·2 per cent solution of *N*-(1-naphthyl)ethylenediamine hydrochloride in 0·1N hydrochloric acid and make up to 50 ml with 0·1N hydrochloric acid.

Measure the extinction of the solution at the absorption maximum at about 545 mμ, using matched 5-mm cells with water in the comparison cell.

Read the number of milligrams of benzocaine equivalent to the observed extinction of the test solution from a calibration graph prepared by treating amounts of standard benzocaine solution covering the range 80 to 120 μg in the same way. (Standard benzocaine solution contains 10 mg per litre in 0·1N hydrochloric acid.)

The tetraphenylboron method for small quantities of bases, given under Atropine, p. 116, has also been applied successfully to some preparations of local anæsthetics. Procaine in Injection of Procaine and Adrenaline can be determined by diluting 2 ml of sample to 20 ml with dilute buffer solution, pH 3·7, and taking 10 ml for the assay; each ml of cetylpyridinium chloride is equivalent to 0·001364 g. Amethocaine, however, tends to give high results if the reagent is added in large excess, probably due to the tendency to partial formation of a di-tetraphenylborate.

To study decomposition of procaine hydrochloride solutions, Bullock[6] found the method of Schou and Abildgaard[7] most satisfactory. Since the investigation of the quality of a procaine solution may sometimes be necessary, the method used is given below:

To 10 ml of the partially decomposed solution in a separator add 0·5 g of sodium carbonate and remove undecomposed procaine base and diethylaminoethanol by shaking three times with 20-ml portions of a mixture of 1 volume of *iso*propyl alcohol and 3 volumes of chloroform. Wash the mixed solvent with 5 ml of water in a second separator. Add the water to the first separator, after washing with a fresh quantity of 5 ml of mixed solvent.

Estimate the bases in the volatile solvent by shaking with 10 ml of 0·1N hydrochloric acid, separating and back titrating with 0·1N sodium hydroxide using methyl red and methylene blue as indicator. The quantity of acid (A) is proportional to the total procaine present before any decomposition occurred. Add 2N hydrochloric acid to the residual alkaline liquid in the first separator until a red colour is given with methyl orange and then extract the *p*-aminobenzoic acid with three portions of the above mixed volatile solvent. Wash, filter and evaporate. Dissolve the residual acid in water and titrate with 0·1N sodium hydroxide to phenolphthalein. Since 1 molecule of procaine, on decomposition, gives 1 molecule of *p*-aminobenzoic acid, the quantity of sodium hydroxide used (B) is proportional to the procaine which has been decomposed. Therefore percentage decomposition is $B/A \times 100$.

The following technique was evolved by Allport and Jones[8] for the colorimetric determination of small quantities of procaine in injections and tablets. Adrenaline, ephedrine, boric acid, chlorbutol, sodium sulphite, ammonium chloride, sodium chloride and sodium phosphate, as the substances normally dispensed with procaine, were shown not to interfere, but it should be noted that the method is not applicable to solutions preserved with cresols or other phenols.

Transfer a measured quantity of the injection, or an aqueous solution of the tablets, expected to contain between 0·02 and 0·10 mg of procaine base, into a 10-ml stoppered measuring cylinder and, if necessary, dilute with water to 5 ml. Add 1 ml of N hydrochloric acid and 0·5 ml of a freshly-prepared 1 per cent aqueous solution of sodium nitrite, mix, and allow to stand for thirty seconds. Add 1 ml of a 15 per cent aqueous solution of ammonium sulphamate, shake vigorously, allow to stand for thirty seconds, add 1 ml of a freshly-prepared 1 per cent solution of the refined acid sodium salt of 1-amino-8-naphthol-3,6-disulphonic acid in 20 per cent w/v aqueous sodium hydroxide, mix and dilute to 10 ml with water.

Measure the extinction of the solution at 520 mμ by means of a suitable absorptiometer and read the number of milligrams of procaine equivalent to the observed extinction from a calibration graph prepared by treating amounts of standard procaine solution in 0·1N hydrochloric acid, covering the range 0·02 to 0·10 mg, in the same way. Procaine base $\times$ 1·155 = procaine hydrochloride.

An alternative method for the determination of procaine in injection solutions is as follows:

Weigh an amount of sample equivalent to about 25 mg of procaine hydrochloride into a 100-ml graduated flask, dissolve in 50 ml of water, dilute to volume with water and mix.

Pipette 4 ml of this solution into a 100-ml graduated flask and into another 100-ml graduated flask pipette 2 ml of an accurately prepared 0·05 per cent solution of procaine hydrochloride in water. To each flask add 50 ml of a buffer solution (prepared by mixing 11·90 ml of 0·2M hydrochloric acid and 88·10 ml of 0·2M potassium chloride) and then add 5 ml of a 1 per cent solution of *p*-dimethylaminobenzaldehyde in 95 per cent ethanol (prepared not more than three days before use and stored in an amber-coloured bottle), dilute to volume with water and mix.

Measure the extinction of each solution at the absorption maximum at about 454 mμ, using 1-cm cells with a reagent blank solution in the comparison cell in each case.

Eye-drops of Amethocaine, *B.P.C.* Contain 1 per cent of amethocaine hydrochloride with sodium chloride.

As indicated above the tetraphenylboron method is applicable to this preparation, provided the excess of reagent is controlled. If to 3 ml of sample exactly 7 ml of buffer solution, pH 3·7, is added, followed by 15 ml of 0·01M sodium tetraphenylboron and the method given under Atropine, p. 116, is continued, good results will be obtained. Each ml of cetylpyridinium chloride is equivalent to 0·001504 g.

Compound Lozenges of Benzocaine, *B.P.C.* Contain 0·097 per cent of benzocaine with menthol and borax in a sugar base.

Somewhat high results for benzocaine were obtained by direct extraction of the lozenge mixture with ether owing to slight solubility of other substances; these can be washed out with water. Benzocaine is appreciably volatile in the oven at 100°.

> Take a sample of twenty lozenges and determine the average weight. Powder the sample and extract about 0·5 g, accurately weighed, with ether in a continuous extraction apparatus until complete extraction is effected. Transfer the ethereal extract to a separator and wash with three portions, each of 20 ml, of water. Evaporate the ether in a tared flask at a low temperature, dry in a vacuum desiccator and weigh the residue of benzocaine.

Removal of the menthol from the residue may be slow, high results are also possible if stearic acid has been used as a lubricant. Direct titration with nitrite (see under benzocaine) is satisfactory and the colorimetric method with *N*-(1-naphthyl)ethylenediamine may be used. Non-aqueous titration is not applicable because of the presence of borax.

1. Bulletin of the Health Organisation of the League of Nations, Extract No. 6. Abs. *Analyst*, 1938, **63,** 828.
2. Report of the Commission of Enquiry on the Coca Leaf, May 1950 (United Nations Economic and Social Council, 12th Session) Special Supplement No. 1 (E/1666, E/CN.7/AC.2/1).
3. Nicholls, J. R., *Analyst*, 1936, **61,** 155.
4. Young, J. L., *J.A.O.A.C.*, 1948, **31,** 781.
5. Bandelin, F. J., and Kemp, C. R., *Ind. Eng. Chem., Anal. Edn.*, 1946, **18,** 470.
6. Bullock, K., *Quart. J. Pharm.*, 1938, **11,** 407.
7. Schou, S. A., and Abildgaard, J., *Pharm. Acta Helv.*, 1935, **10,** 38.
8. Allport, N. L., and Jones, N. R., *Quart. J. Pharm.*, 1942, **15,** 238.

COLCHICUM

Both the **corm** and the **seed** of colchicum (*C. autumnale* Linn.) contain the alkaloid colchicine (0·4 per cent and 0·3 to 0·6 per cent respectively) and are assayed similarly, so they can be considered together. Only the corm is official in the *B.P.*

The *B.P.* method, as with many other official alkaloidal processes, is that evolved by Self and Corfield.[1] It was found that colchicine could easily be purified by extraction of inert material with ether, in which colchicine is almost insoluble. Slight emulsification may occur in the first two washings with ether, but this may be disregarded, any emulsion being transferred to the next stage together with the clear aqueous layer. A bright solution for final extraction is obtained by coagulation with 20 per cent sodium sulphate solution and a little talc before filtering. The final extraction with chloroform needs a considerable number of shakings owing to the high solubility of colchicine in water, but little or no tendency to emulsification will be found. It will be noted that, in the assay of the corm, the alkaloidal residue still contains a little water-insoluble impurity which is separated and its weight subtracted. The detailed method is as follows:

Weigh 20·0 g, in coarse powder, into a flask, add 30 ml of 95 per cent ethanol and heat on a water-bath for about fifteen minutes. Transfer to an apparatus for the continuous extraction of drugs and extract with 90 per cent ethanol for three hours. Cool the extract, allow to stand for half an hour and then filter, washing the filter with 90 per cent ethanol until the alkaloids are completely extracted. Combine the filtrate and washings, evaporate to dryness on a water-bath and wash the residue into a separator with 20 ml of a 20 per cent solution of sodium sulphate decahydrate and 50 ml of ether. Shake thoroughly, allow the layers to separate, run the lower layer into a second separator and again shake and allow the layers to separate. Wash the dish and extract the contents of the two separators in the same way, first with two 5-ml quantities of the sodium sulphate solution and then with three 5-ml quantities of water. Combine all the aqueous liquids, heat on a water-bath until the ether is completely expelled, cool, add 0·2 g of powdered talc and dilute to exactly 50 ml with the sodium sulphate solution. Allow to stand for about one hour, shaking frequently, and filter, rejecting the first 5 ml of filtrate. Transfer exactly 40 ml of the filtrate, representing 16 g of the sample, to a separator, add 50 ml of ether, shake and allow the layers to separate. Wash the ether layer with three 5-ml quantities of water, combine the aqueous liquids, add 50 ml of chloroform and shake. Then add 2 ml of N sodium hydroxide, shake thoroughly, allow the layers to separate and run the lower layer into another separator containing 2 ml of 0·1N sodium hydroxide and 15 ml of water. Shake, allow the layers to separate and filter the chloroform solution through a double filter. Continue the extraction with further quantities of chloroform, washing each extract with the alkaline liquid and filtering, as before. Combine the chloroform extracts in a shallow dish, evaporate the chloroform and add two 2-ml quantities of 95 per cent ethanol, evaporating after each addition. Dry the residue over phosphorus pentoxide at a pressure not exceeding 5 mm of mercury for three hours and weigh. Add 10 ml of water to the weighed residue, allow to stand for a few minutes and filter through a small filter, washing the dish and filter with small quantities of water until the alkaloids are completely extracted. Dissolve any insoluble matter on the filter in a little 95 per cent ethanol, transfer to the dish containing the remainder of the insoluble matter, evaporate, dry over phosphorus pentoxide at a pressure not exceeding 5 mm of mercury for three hours and weigh. The difference between the two weights is the weight of alkaloids of colchicum corm present in the sample.

The following notes on the *B.P.* method may be of value:

(*a*) After evaporation of the ethanolic extract, lumps are formed which sometimes occlude a little alkaloid; thorough washing of the dish is only possible with the aid of a drop of ethanol.

(*b*) The sodium sulphate solution used is a little too strong and ether abstracts water giving a precipitate of solid sodium sulphate.

(*c*) Vigorous shaking with chloroform is necessary before adding the sodium hydroxide to remove the last traces of resin acids.

(*d*) A low temperature is desirable for drying the residue of crude colchicine before water extraction. At high temperatures some of the water-soluble alkaloid resinifies and is then difficult to extract completely; drying at 60° is recommended.

(*e*) The weighed alkaloidal residue from the seed does not need further purification.

(*f*) The *B.P.* method for extracting the colchicine from the impure alkaloidal residue from the corm may not remove it entirely, and it is better to add a drop of chloroform to the residue before adding 10 ml of warm water. After evaporating off the chloroform, the solution is cooled and filtered, repeating three times.

Self and Corfield[1] considered the *N.F.*X method to be slow and tedious in application, although extraction is complete and the alkaloid obtained pure. The chief defects are that the filtration of the lead subacetate solution is slow, chloroform extraction must be repeated a number of times to ensure complete removal of the colchicine, and emulsions are frequently encountered.

Nevertheless, many analysts prefer the *N.F.* method, in spite of its disadvantages and conversely find the *B.P.* method tedious, especially in the water washings. A modification of the *N.F.* method with which the originator was able to avoid some of its faults, especially those of emulsification and slow filtration, was suggested by Ragg:[2]

> Mix 15 g of powdered seed or corm with 30 ml of ethanol and heat on a water-bath for fifteen minutes. Transfer to a continuous extraction apparatus and extract for three hours. Cool, allow to stand for half an hour and filter, washing the filter with ethanol until free from alkaloid. Evaporate the filtrate to a soft extract. Transfer to a 300-ml cylinder, washing in completely with about 200 ml of hot water at about 70°. Add 16 ml of strong lead subacetate solution *B.P.* and make up to 300 ml; shake occasionally for half an hour, then cool and make up accurately to 300 ml. Add 3 to 4 g of kieselguhr, shake and filter through a Buchner funnel on which a $\frac{1}{4}$ to $\frac{1}{2}$ inch layer of kieselguhr has been spread to prevent the lead precipitate clogging the filter. To the total filtrate add 5 g of powdered sodium phosphate, shake to dissolve and leave for half an hour. Siphon off the clear liquid, add 1 g of kieselguhr and filter again. Take 150 ml of filtrate (= 7·5 g of seed or corm) and either transfer directly to a separator and extract the alkaloid completely with chloroform, running the extracts through a double filter paper; or evaporate to 20 ml, wash into a separator and extract with chloroform. Either method gives the same result. Evaporate to dryness, re-evaporate with two portions, each of 1 ml, of ethanol and dry to constant weight at 60°.

Liquid Extract of Colchicum (Corm), *B.P.* Contains 0·3 per cent of alkaloids.

For assay: (*a*) By the *B.P.* method:

Evaporate 20 ml to dryness and continue as in Colchicum Corm, washing the residue into a separator with 20 per cent sodium sulphate solution.

Or (*b*) By the method proposed by Ragg (above):

Transfer 15 ml directly into a 300-ml graduated cylinder, add 200 ml of hot water and continue as in the method given, adding 16 ml of strong solution of lead subacetate.

Tincture of Colchicum, *B.P.* Contains 0·03 per cent of alkaloids.

This is made by diluting the liquid extract; hence for assay evaporate 200 ml to low bulk and continue as under Liquid Extract.

COLCHICINE, $C_{22}H_{25}O_6N$, Mol. Wt. 399·4

In ethanol colchicine has an absorption maximum at about 243 mμ, E(1 per cent, 1 cm) = 760 and at about 349 mμ, E(1 per cent, 1 cm) = 433. Because of its sensitivity to light all solutions are made up in amber-coloured glassware.

Tablets of Colchicine, *B.P.* Generally contain 0·25 mg. of colchicine in a lactose base.

The tablets are best assayed by ultra-violet absorption.

Weigh accurately a quantity of powdered tablet material equivalent to about 1 mg of colchicine and transfer to a 100-ml amber-coloured flask. Add about 50 ml of ethanol and shake for 30 minutes. Make up to volume with ethanol, mix, centrifuge a portion of the solution and measure the maximum extinction of a 1-cm layer at about 349 mμ using ethanol as the blank. Calculate the colchicine content of each tablet.

1. Self, P. A. W., and Corfield, C. E., *Quart. J. Pharm.*, 1932, **5**, 347.
2. Ragg, L. W., private communication.

COLOPHONY

(Resin)

In the opinion of Parry[1] the iodine value of colophony is so definitely established that it should be included as a standard figure. The Wijs iodine value ranges from 118 to 128 and the acid value from 150 to 180. It is advantageous to use an ethanolic alkali in titration of the acid value or a considerable amount of ethanol as solvent. The ester value is low (10 to 20).

Resin in Soaps

The determination of resin acids in soaps depends on the fact that fatty acids are esterified under the conditions of the experiment whilst resin acids are unaffected. Determination by the original Twitchell process[2] has been shown to be liable to considerable error, and improvements on this method, which are also simpler in procedure, have been devised. Among them is that of McNicoll:[3]

> Dissolve about 2 g of mixed fatty and resin acids in 20 ml of a 4 per cent solution of naphthalene-β-sulphonic acid in dry methanol and heat under a reflux condenser for thirty minutes, adding a few pieces of porous plate to ensure regular ebullition, and using an electric plate or a Bunsen burner under an asbestos wire gauze as the source of heat. Conduct a blank experiment at the same time with 20 ml of the sulphonic acid solution. Cool the contents of both flasks and titrate with 0·5N ethanolic potash, using phenolphthalein as indicator. 1 ml 0·5N = 0·163 g of resin acids.

The Analytical Methods Committee of the *S.A.C.*[4] has recommended this method for adoption, with the slight modification of titration with 0·2N ethanolic potash. Some small errors are inherent in the process and by experiment the approximate excess of resin acids to be expected was ascertained, from which it was recommended that the resin acids should be calculated as a percentage of the total fatty matter and 1 per cent subtracted, independent of the percentage of resin acid obtained.

For the purpose of calculating the approximate proportion of resin in the soap it may be assumed that resin contains 92 per cent of resin acids. When the percentage of resin is small (less than 5 per cent), results will be less accurate than with larger resin contents. The presence of resin should be established qualitatively by the Liebermann-Storch test. The quantitative method is liable to give erroneous results with certain types of carbolic soaps containing high-boiling tar acids.

Another method is by Wolff and Scholze:[5]

> Dissolve from 2 to 5 g of the mixture of fatty and resin acids in 10 to 20 ml of dry methanol and add 5 to 10 ml of a solution of 1 part of concentrated sulphuric acid in 4 parts of methanol. Boil the mixture for two minutes under a reflux condenser. To the liquid add 5 to 10 times its volume of 7 to 10 per cent sodium chloride solution and extract the fatty esters and resin acids with ether. Wash the combined extracts with dilute sodium chloride solution, add ethanol and titrate the mixture with 0·5N ethanolic potash. With a mean acid value of 160 taken for the resin acids, and a correction of 1·5 per cent allowed for fatty acids that have escaped esterification, the percentage of resin acids is obtained by the formula

$$\frac{\text{ml of } 0{\cdot}5\text{N potash} \times 17{\cdot}76}{\text{wt. of mixture taken}} - 1{\cdot}5.$$

Davidsohn[6] stresses the need for using methanol in the above method, although quite satisfactory results have been obtained with ethanol.

Ointment of Resin, *B.P.C.* Consists of 26 per cent colophony in a base composed of yellow beeswax, olive oil and lard.

Assuming the figures for the constants of resin given above as being normal, the theoretical limits for the ointment would be: saponification value 160 to 170·4, acid value 43·4 to 54·6, unsaponifiable 13·5 to 14·9 per cent, iodine value 64·7 to 76·2. The percentage of resin can be determined approximately by subtracting a value of 6·0 (an average for beeswax and olive oil) from the acid value found and dividing the remainder by 165.

1. PARRY, E. J., *C. & D.*, 1932, **117,** 251.
2. TWITCHELL, E., *Analyst,* 1891, **16,** 169.
3. MCNICOLL, D., *J. Soc. Chem. Ind.*, 1921, **40,** 124T.
4. *Analyst,* 1937, **62,** 868.
5. WOLFF, H., and SCHOLZE, E., *Chemiker-Ztg.*, 1914, **38,** 369.
6. DAVIDSOHN, J., *ibid.*, 1925, **49,** 206.

COPPER

Cu At. Wt. 63·54

The estimation of copper by means of sodium thiosulphate depends upon the precipitation of cuprous iodide by potassium iodide from a faintly acid solution with liberation of iodine:

> To a solution containing the equivalent of about 0·15 g of copper in 50 ml of water or dilute acid, add a slight excess of sodium carbonate and acidify with 5 ml of acetic acid. Add at least 3 g of potassium iodide and titrate immediately with 0·1N sodium thiosulphate until nearly all the iodine has been removed; add mucilage of starch and 1 drop of 0·1N silver nitrate (to make the disappearance of the blue starch-iodide colour sharper) and complete the titration. 1 ml. 0·1N = 0·006354 g Cu.

According to Foote and Vance[1] a modification in which 1 to 2 g of ammonium thiocyanate is added after almost all the liberated iodine has been removed by the thiosulphate gives more exact results although no significant difference has been noted by the present writers.

Also the titration can be made accurate in the presence of arsenic, antimony and iron; but these elements must be oxidised and then the first two prevented from reacting with the potassium iodide by use of an approximately pH 3·7 buffer solution (25 ml of 6N acetic acid and 12 ml of 6N ammonia added to 20 to 40 ml of solution of the substance). The iron is converted into a complex fluoride by the addition of 1 g of sodium fluoride for every 0·1 g of iron immediately before titration.

Copper may be titrated with EDTA (see p. 786) but for general purposes this is not necessary since the cuprous iodide method given above is satisfactory, moreover there is a limit to the amount of copper which may be titrated using a visual indicator because the colour of the copper-EDTA complex is so intense that it masks the indicator change.

Copper can be determined by flame photometry using one or other of the resonance lines at 3247 and 3274 A. A reasonably hot flame is required and air-acetylene, oxygen-acetylene or oxygen-hydrogen mixtures are suitable. The lines lie within an OH band system so that the background is discontinuous whatever gas mixture is used for the flame and this limits the detection sensitivity. Self-absorption occurs so that calibration curves of emission intensity against copper concentration curve towards the concentration axis and the slope reduces as the copper concentration increases. The two lines show this effect to different degrees and although the 3247 A line is more sensitive for low concentrations of copper, the 3274 A line gives a calibration curve with the greater slope at higher concentrations.

Spectral interferences can be expected from relatively large concentrations of nickel and cobalt in the sample solution and it is wise to use narrow slit widths to increase the resolution of the monochromator. Continuous background enhancement occurs when calcium, iron, lithium and sodium are present in the sample but with a recording instrument this effect is easily detected and automatically corrected by the use of a baseline technique (see p. 872).

Phosphoric acid and sulphuric acid depress the copper emission when present in concentrations in excess of 1·0M so if these acids must be present in the sample solution, the same concentration must be added to the standards.

The lower limit of detection is governed by the flame temperature and the level of the background due to the OH molecular band but it is possible easily to detect 1 p.p.m. and to determine 3 p.p.m. of copper using an air-acetylene flame and a recording instrument.

Barbara Russell, Shelton and Walsh[2] have shown that copper can be determined by an atomic absorption technique (see p. 873) and 1 p.p.m. is quoted as the lower limit of detection. Because of the OH molecular band background this method is potentially more sensitive than the flame emission method and the sensitivity can probably be improved.

Small amounts of copper are sometimes of significance and estimation of **traces** can be made with considerable accuracy employing sodium diethyldithiocarbamate, introduced for quantitative measurement by Callan and Henderson.[3] This reagent is not specific for copper and it should be freshly prepared.

Haddock and Evers[4] recommended a method for determining traces of copper in the presence of a large excess of iron without previous removal of the latter. The iron is retained in the aqueous solution by means of ammonium citrate, ferrous iron must be absent and can be oxidised by boiling the solution for a few minutes with a little hydrogen peroxide, whilst the coloured copper thiocarbamate complex is extracted by solvent and the intensity of colour of its solution measured. If EDTA is also present, all interference except that from bismuth is eliminated by chelation. Organic matter may be removed either by incineration or preferably by wet combustion.

To an aliquot of solution containing not more than 50 μg of copper in a volume of not more than 25 ml add 2 g of citric acid and 0·5 g of the disodium salt of EDTA. Add 10 per cent solution of ammonia until the pH is approximately 9 (thymol blue). Add 10 ml of a freshly prepared 0·1 per cent solution of sodium diethyldithiocarbamate and extract immediately with three portions, each of 5 ml, of carbon tetrachloride added from a burette, passing each extract through a small filter of cotton wool. A blank should be run with reagents at the same time. Measure the extinction of the mixed extracts at 435 mμ and obtain the number of micrograms of copper equivalent to the observed extinctions of the test and blank solutions from a calibration graph prepared as follows:

Prepare a standard copper sulphate solution to contain 100 μg of Cu per ml by dissolving 0·3926 g $CuSO_4,5H_2O$ in 2N sulphuric acid, diluted to 1 litre. For use, dilute this solution with 2N sulphuric acid to contain 2 μg per ml. Transfer separate 0, 1, 2·5, 5, 10, 15, 20, and 25 ml portions of this solution made up to 25 ml with 2N sulphuric acid to separators, add 2 g of citric acid and 0·5 g of the disodium salt of EDTA to each and extract with carbon tetrachloride as in the test. Construct a graph relating extinction values to micrograms of copper.

Copper diethyldithiocarbamate is destroyed by cyanide whilst the bismuth complex is not.[5] If, therefore, the carbon tetrachloride layer is shaken with a 5 per cent potassium cyanide solution and does not decolorise, bismuth is present. Jenkins[6] observed that the bismuth complex in carbon tetrachloride is not stable to washing with sodium hydroxide, hence if its presence is indicated by the cyanide test, the original extraction procedure should be repeated but before measurement of the extinction, the carbon tetrachloride solution should be extracted with two portions of 10 ml of N sodium hydroxide.

Another colorimetric method for determination of traces of copper is based upon the use of bis*cyclo*hexanone oxalyldihydrazone. This is a selective and highly sensitive reagent for both cupric and cuprous ions. In alkaline solutions a blue complex is produced in the presence of copper which is stable for several days and is particularly suitable for absorptiometric measurement. The method first described by Nilsson[7] has been modified by Somers and Garraway[8] as follows:

To a suitable volume of copper solution containing 0 to 50 μg of copper (as chloride, nitrate or sulphate), in a 50-ml graduated flask, add 5 ml of 10 per cent ammonium citrate solution, followed by 1 drop of 0·05 per cent neutral red solution. Neutralise to the yellow colour of the indicator by dropwise addition of 3N sodium hydroxide and then add 5 ml of borate buffer (400 ml 0·5M boric acid and 60 ml 0·5M sodium hydroxide or a sufficient volume to give pH 8·1) followed by 0·5 ml of a 0·5 per cent solution of bis*cyclo*hexanone oxalyldihydrazone in 50 per cent w/v ethanol. Adjust the volume to 50 ml with water and measure the blue colour in a 4-cm cell at 595 mμ against a blank prepared from the reagents.

Under the conditions given above the borate buffer maintains the pH within the optimum range of 8·3 to 8·9, the blue complex develops within ten minutes and is stable for three hours. In our experience it is more convenient to increase the volume of bis*cyclo*hexanone oxalyldihydrazone used from 0·5 ml to 2·0 ml and to measure the extinction value in a 1-cm cell. Under these conditions Beer's Law is obeyed over the range 0 to 190 μg. For the modified conditions a calibration graph is prepared by taking suitable aliquots of standard copper solution containing 0·0785 g $CuSO_4,5H_2O$ per litre to give quantities of copper between 20 and 200 μg and carrying out the whole procedure as with the test solution.

COPPER SALTS

The only salts of copper used to any extent in pharmaceutical practice are **copper sulphate,** $CuSO_4,5H_2O$, Mol. Wt. 249·7 and **copper citrate,** $Cu_2C_6H_4O_7,2H_2O$, Mol. Wt. 351·2 (35 to 37 per cent Cu). They may be estimated by the potassium iodide method given above using 0·5 to 1·0 g. 1 ml 0·1N = 0·02497 g $CuSO_4,5H_2O$ and 0·006354 g Cu.

Lotion of Copper and Zinc Sulphates, *B.P.C.* This preparation contains 0·914 per cent of copper sulphate and 1·37 per cent of zinc sulphate dissolved in camphor water.

The classical separation of copper and zinc is lengthy and tedious and involves precipitation of the sulphides. The *B.P.C.* method is based upon electrolytic deposition of first the copper, in an acid medium, and then the zinc, after making alkaline. The copper is first deposited on to a platinum gauze cathode and the increase in weight is noted. The zinc is then deposited on to the coppered platinum and the increase in weight again noted. The main disadvantage of the method lies in the small amounts of metals which are deposited.

The copper can be determined in this preparation by direct application of the cuprous iodide method but until recently no satisfactory method of determining the zinc has been available without prior removal of the copper. A method[9] has now been developed, however, in which the copper is masked with thioglycerol at pH 6·0 and the zinc is titrated with EDTA.

The following procedure is very satisfactory:

For copper, determine by the cuprous iodide method (p. 197) using 10 ml of lotion.

For zinc, to 10 ml of the lotion add 10 ml of a 10 per cent v/v solution of thioglycerol in water and, when precipitation is complete, add 2 ml of dilute hydrochloric acid and 3 g of hexamine, whereupon the precipitate redissolves. Allow to stand for fifteen minutes, add 4 drops of xylenol orange indicator solution and titrate with 0·05M EDTA to the bright yellow colour of the indicator. 1 ml 0·05M EDTA = 0·01438 g $ZnSO_4,7H_2O$.

1. FOOTE, H. W., and VANCE, J. E., *Ind. Eng. Chem., Anal. Edn.*, 1937, **9,** 205.
2. RUSSELL, Barbara J., SHELTON, J. P., and WALSH, A., *Spectrochim. Acta,* 1957, **8,** 317.
3. CALLAN, T., and HENDERSON, J. A. R., *Analyst,* 1929, **54,** 65.
4. HADDOCK, L. A., and EVERS, N., *Analyst,* 1932, **57,** 495.
5. ALLPORT, N. L., and GARRATT, D. C., *J. Soc. Chem. Ind.*, 1948, **67,** 382.
6. JENKINS, E. N., *Analyst,* 1954, **79,** 209.
7. NILSSON, G., *Acta Chem. Scand.*, 1950, **4,** 205.
8. SOMERS, E., and GARRAWAY, J. L., *Chem. & Ind.*, 1957, 395.
9. GARTSIDE, B., private communication.

CRESOL

As pharmaceutical cresol consists of a mixture of isomers in varying proportions with possibly some homologues, the determination of the proportion of the different isomers may be required. It has been ascertained that lysols become less miscible when a high proportion of *meta*-cresol is present in the cresylic acid, although this isomer has a high germicidal value.

The original Raschig method[1] is still employed with slight modification by the *D.A.B.* for the determination of *meta*-cresol in a mixture of the isomers. Under the conditions of the experiment only *meta*-cresol is nitrated, the other isomers being oxidised to oxalic acid. Fox and Barker[2] confirmed the validity of the Raschig process with mixtures made from pure *meta*-cresol and found the best results by the following slightly modified procedure:

Place 10 g of the cresylic acid in a 1,200-ml flask with 15 ml of 98 per cent sulphuric acid and heat on a water-bath until the liquid is viscous when cooled to the room temperature. Spread the liquid in a thin layer over the bottom of the flask by quickly rotating it and then pour 100 ml of nitric acid (sp. gr. 1·40) on to this thin layer. Replace the flask on the water-bath immediately. Allow the violent reaction, which commences in a few seconds, to proceed unchecked. After five minutes pour the reaction mixture into a porcelain dish containing 40 ml of water. Rinse out the flask with 40 ml of water and add to the diluted acids. Allow the mixture to stand for two hours to cool. Break up the cake of crystalline trinitro-*meta*-cresol, filter on a tared filter or Gooch crucible and, after washing the crystals with 100 ml of water, dry at 100° and weigh. Weight of trinitro-*meta*-cresol × 0·5747 = *meta*-cresol.

The product should melt between 102° and 107° and it should be free from tar. The important part of the determination is the initial sulphonation. If less than 25 per cent of *meta*-cresol is present it is better to repeat the determination after adding sufficient pure *meta*-cresol to make the total present up to about 50 per cent. For products containing high percentages of *meta*-cresol of the order of 95 per cent the factor given above should be changed to 0·5799.

If there is more than 10 per cent of phenol in the sample errors are produced owing to contamination of the trinitro-*meta*-cresol with picric acid.

The cresineol method for determination of *ortho*-cresol in commercial cresylic acid has been adopted by the Standardisation of Tar Products Test Committee for refined cresylic acids, based on the work of Potter and Williams.[3] Revised figures (0·4° to 0·7° higher) for the crystallising-points of mixtures were necessary in a modification of the test[4] mainly due to larger quantities of material used in the actual crystallising-point determination, but the effect of use of pure cineole (m.p. 1·2° to 1·4°) is contributory:

Weigh 8·40 g of dry sample and 12·00 g of pure cineole (m.p. 1·2° to 1·4°) into a test-tube 25 mm in diameter, heat the mixture to approximately 5° above the crystallising-point and insert a stirrer and a thermometer (reading from 10° to 70° graduated in 0·1°). Insert the tube in a larger tube to form an air-jacket and immerse the whole in a narrow beaker of water the temperature of which is adjusted to 5° to 10° below the estimated crystallising-point. Take readings every half-minute, the mixture being stirred gently for four or five seconds between each reading until five or more consecutive readings within 0·05° are obtained. If a constant temperature is not obtained plot readings against time intervals and extend the portion of the curve after the rise backwards until it intersects the portion of the curve before the temperature rise; the point of intersection is taken as the true crystallising-point. Excessive cooling should be avoided and a temperature rise of 1° should be regarded as a maximum. Calculate the *o*-cresol from Table 14.

The method is not applicable to an *ortho*-cresol content of less than 40 per cent; in such samples a mixture with an equal weight of pure *ortho*-cresol should be used for the test. Certain cresol mixtures will give slightly abnormal results, but such difficulties do not arise with the ordinary cresylic acids of commerce.

Brooks[5] has shown that *o*, *m*, and *p* cresols can be separated from each other and from phenol and the xylenols by gas chromatography. He used

TABLE 14

o-CRESOL IN SAMPLE	CRYST. POINT OF COMPLEX
40	31·0
45	34·1
50	36·7
55	39·2
60	41·5
65	43·7
70	45·8
75	47·7
80	49·6
85	51·4
90	53·0
95	54·7
100	56·4

a 120-cm × 4·5-mm column of 5 per cent 2,4-xylenyl phosphate on acid washed 100- to 120-mesh Celite at 110°. An argon ionisation detector was employed, the gas inlet pressure was 16 p.s.i. and the sample size did not exceed 0·1 μl.

The determination of cresol in disinfectants follows the methods given under Lysol.

Lysol, *B.P.* (Solution of Cresol with Soap) consists of a solution of cresol in a saponaceous solvent, the latter being prepared from a vegetable oil (usually linseed) and caustic alkali.

The *B.P.* 1948 method of assay for cresol required a larger volume of sample than is often available, and its inclusion was determined by the requirement that the recovered cresol should comply with the standard of the official material; 100 ml of cresol would be needed for the boiling-point test. The complicated manipulation required made a less involved process desirable, especially as the requirement in the *B.P.* monograph that the lysol must be miscible in all proportions up to 10 per cent with water very largely determines the cresol to be used as of *B.P.* quality.

Unfortunately, at present there appears to be no really simple, accurate method available. The following relatively short methods are selected from the many published, but they are all open to criticism if accuracy is required.

(*a*) The *N.F.* method: Mix 50 ml of lysol in a 500-ml distilling flask with 150 ml of purified kerosene. Add 3 g of sodium bicarbonate and distil the mixture into a separator, using an upright condenser, at the rate of not more than 2 drops per second, until the distillate comes over strongly yellow. Run off the lower aqueous layer, shake the kerosene layer with 10 ml of 50 per cent w/w sulphuric acid, allow to stand for two hours and discard the acid layer. Add to the kerosene layer 40 ml of a 15 per cent aqueous sodium hydroxide solution, accurately measured at 25°, shake well for five minutes, then allow to stand until complete separation has taken place and draw off the sodium hydroxide layer into a graduated cylinder. Shake the kerosene layer again with a fresh portion of 20 ml of the sodium hydroxide solution, accurately measured at 25°, and add the separated aqueous layer to the graduated cylinder. Note the volume of the alkaline liquid after adjusting the temperature to 25°, the difference between this volume and the total volume of sodium hydroxide solution used represents the volume of cresol present in 50 ml of lysol.

Edwards and Freak[6] have shown that the nature of the phenol is important for the *N.F.* assumption that 1 ml increase in volume of the alkali is equivalent to 1 ml of cresol.

Experiment has shown that for 50 ml of lysol taken a correction of 0·5 ml should be added to the cresol volume to correct for contraction in the sodium hydroxide solution.

This method has much to recommend it and it has been included in the *B.P.* The following points may be noted:

(i) A little powdered pumice should be added before distillation.

(ii) The distillate may not become yellow but complete distillation is shown by a rapid rise in temperature requiring vigorous boiling.

(iii) A small intermediate layer tends to be formed, containing kerosene, cresol and water; this can be dispersed after running off the lower aqueous layer by adding a little fused calcium chloride and, after dehydration of the intermediate layer, dissolving the residual calcium chloride by the addition of a little water and rejecting the aqueous layer.

(*b*) The *D.A.B.* method: To 40 g of lysol in a 1-litre flask add 120 ml of water and 10 drops of methyl orange. Make acid with sulphuric acid and steam distil until all milkiness in the distillate has disappeared. Stop the cooling of the condenser and distil until steam issues from the end of the condenser. Re-cool and continue distillation for five minutes. For each 100 ml of distillate add 20 g of sodium chloride and shake with 100 ml of light petroleum, separate and repeat the extraction with two portions of 50 ml of light petroleum. Evaporate the solvent, dry the cresol for forty minutes at 100° and weigh.

It has been pointed out by Dodd[7] that all methods involving steam distillation suffer from the defect that higher homologues distil with difficulty, especially in the presence of fatty acids which lower the vapour pressure of tar acids considerably. Also care must be exercised when drying cresols; water is removed with difficulty at 100° and at higher temperatures volatilisation of phenols may take place. Martin[8] suggests that serious errors may occur in distillation methods where volatile fatty acids (such as in coconut oil) are present, but soap made from this oil is not often used as a vehicle for the *B.P.* lysol.

An approximate method by Jordan and Southerden[9] is suitable for routine control purposes:

(*c*) Transfer 50 to 70 g of the sample to a distillation flask, acidify with 30 to 35 ml of dilute sulphuric acid and steam distil until the distillate contains no oily drops and gives no blue colour with ferric chloride. Shake the whole distillate thoroughly to ensure saturation of the aqueous portion and allow to separate. Measure the volume of both layers. Then, assuming that the solubility of cresol is 1 in 50, the cresol is calculated from the following formula:

$$\text{Per cent cresols by wt.} = \frac{100}{\text{wt. taken}}\left(\frac{\text{aqueous volume}}{50} + [\text{cresol layer} \times 1{\cdot}04]\right)$$

The separation is not complete and the accuracy of the method can be improved by 'salting' out the cresol in a separator, transferring the separated cresol layer to a measuring cylinder, washing out the separator with brine to transfer mechanically any residual cresol to the cylinder, adding a few drops of hydrochloric acid and measuring the cresols by volume. With this modification the method approaches in details the *D.A.B.* method given above.

Any of the foregoing chemical assays of lysol can give no measure of its disinfectant and antibacterial properties. These can only be determined by tests using micro-organisms (see below).

Disinfectant Fluids. Coal tar fractions, in the higher boiling ranges comprising cresols, 'cresylic acids' and 'high-boiling tar acids,' are used for making disinfectants other than lysol, namely, the so-called 'black,' 'white' and sanitary fluids. The black fluids are solutions of the cresol fractions in soaps, and the white fluids are emulsions formed with the aid of gelatin, casein, dextrins, etc. Their germicidal efficiencies vary with the particular cresol fraction and the type of soap employed or the nature of the emulgent used; halogenation and the addition of certain types of hydrocarbon 'carriers' also frequently increases germicidal efficacy. Because of these variations, chemical assays again are inadequate for assaying disinfectant fluids, and it is necessary to resort to a microbiological assessment.

Testing Disinfectants (Phenol Coefficient Tests). The tests employed for determining the efficacy of all of the coal tar disinfectants include the **Rideal-Walker test,** the **Chick-Martin test,** the **United States Food and Drug Administration (*F.D.A.*) method** and the **United States Association of Official Agricultural Chemists (*A.O.A.C.*) method,** in which the antibacterial activity of the disinfectant is expressed in terms of its action relative to that of phenol. Each of these tests has much in common, and their main features are set out in the table below. It is necessary to follow precisely the directions as laid down in the approved method in order to get reproducible results. Each test will give a different coefficient

TABLE 15

	RIDEAL-WALKER	CHICK-MARTIN	A.O.A.C. (*Salm. typhi*)	A.O.A.C. (*Staph. aureus*)
Reference	British Standard Specification 541 : 1934 (with later revisions)	British Standard Specification 808 : 1938	*Official Methods of Analysis of the A.O.A.C.*, 8th Ed. p. 88: Washington, D.C.	
Culture	*Salm. typhi* (NCTC 786)	*Salm. typhi* (NCTC 'S' strain)	*Salm. typhi* (Hopkins strain 26) (ATCC 6539)	*Staph. aureus* FDA 209 (ATCC 6538)
Age of culture in broth	5th–14th generation: 23–25 hours at 37°	5th–14th generation: 23–25 hours at 37°	4th generation up to 1 month: 22–26 hours at 37°	4th generation up to 1 month: 22–26 hours at 37°
Culture medium:				
Peptone	Allen & Hanbury Eupeptone No. 1 2%	Allen & Hanbury Eupeptone No. 1 1%	Armour 1%	Armour 1%
Meat extract	Lab-Lemco 2%	Lab-Lemco 1%	Difco 0·5%	Difco 0·5%
Salt	1%	0·5%	0·5%	0·5%
Sterilisation	Bulk: 20 min at 121° 5-ml amounts in tubes: 10 min at 121°	Bulk: 20 min at 121° 10-ml amounts in tubes: 10 min at 121°	10-ml amounts in tubes: 20 min at 121°	10-ml amounts in tubes: 20 min at 121°
Final pH value	7·3–7·5	7·3–7·5	6·8	6·8
Temperature of test	17–18°	20°	20°	(*a*) 20° or (*b*) 37°
Added 'organic' matter	Nil	2·5% yeast suspension	Nil	Nil
End-point of test	Highest dilution killing in 7½ min, not in 5 min	Highest dilution killing in 30 min	Highest dilution killing in 10 min, not in 5 min	Highest dilution killing in 10 min, not in 5 min
Range of normal phenol response level	1–95 to 1–115	1·46 to 2%	1–90 and 1–100	(*a*) 1–60 and 1–70 (*b*) 1–80 and 1–90

Note: The *U.S.F.D.A.* method is essentially the same as the *A.O.A.C.* method, except that the *F.D.A.* method specifies Liebig's beef extract instead of Difco and the *A.O.A.C.* method allows two variations of the culture medium to counteract the bacteriostatic carry-over of substances such as the mercurials and surface-active compounds.

value, and the choice of test will depend on the purpose for which the disinfectant is intended.

The *F.D.A.* and *A.O.A.C.* methods allow the use of two different organisms, *Salmonella typhi* and *Staphylococcus aureus*: recently a modification to the Rideal-Walker test has also been introduced to allow the use of *Staphylococcus aureus* as well as *Salmonella typhi*, this is known as the **Phenol Coefficient** (*Staphylococcus*) **test.** The reason for allowing the use of two different organisms is to ensure that those disinfectant fluids modified by halogenation or by introducing active ingredients other than coal tar acids are not unduly selective in their germicidal action against different types of bacteria.

Procedures. The principle of all of the above tests is that serial dilutions of the test disinfectant and of the standard phenol (dilutions in arithmetic series for the Rideal-Walker, *F.D.A.* and *A.O.A.C.* tests and in logarithmic series for the Chick-Martin test) are inoculated with a given amount of the culture and at intervals one 4-mm loopful of the mixture is transferred to a tube of the culture medium which is incubated at 37° and the growths noted. By equating the 'end-point' dilution of the disinfectant with that of phenol giving the same response, the 'phenol coefficient' of the disinfectant is obtained.

In all cases, the test organisms are stored in the freeze-dried state, but for current use are maintained as stock cultures on agar slopes. These are incubated for the first twenty-four hours at 37° and subsequently kept at room temperature in the dark; subcultures are made at monthly intervals. (It is advisable to start from a fresh freeze-dried tube occasionally.) For use in the test, inoculate from the agar slope into a tube of the prescribed culture medium and incubate at 37°, subculturing at daily intervals for the specified number of generations.

Prepare the phenol test dilutions from a standardised stock 5 per cent solution in distilled water of pure phenol (crystallising-point not less than 40·5°). Prepare the disinfectant test dilutions (usually in a series differing by 10 per cent or thereabouts) from an initial 1 or 2 per cent master dilution in distilled water. In making the master dilution always measure the disinfectant by pipette into the required volume of water and then mix thoroughly; any other procedure might affect the quality of the emulsion formed and hence its disinfecting power.

For the **Rideal-Walker test,** prepare four suitable serial dilutions of the disinfectant and one of the standard phenol in 5-ml amounts in 5 × $\frac{3}{4}$ in. sterile test-tubes, and cool in a water-bath to 17–18°. At half-minute intervals, add 0·2 ml of the twenty-four-hour culture of *Salm. typhi* (also cooled to 17–18°) in turn to each of the tubes, and then at subsequent two and a half, five, seven and a half, and ten minute intervals remove one standard loopful of the mixture to a 5-ml tube of the medium, incubate at 37° for forty-eight to seventy-two hours and record the growths obtained. It may be necessary to repeat the test with another 5 dilutions, but using a different phenol dilution, in order to obtain a satisfactory end-point. Calculate the Rideal-Walker Coefficient by dividing the numerical value of the dilution of the disinfectant which shows growth after two and a half and five minutes but not after seven and a half and ten minutes by that dilution of phenol which shows the same end-point.

For the **Chick-Martin test,** prepare about five suitable dilutions of the disinfectant in a logarithmic series in diminishing stages of 10 per cent and about five of the standard phenol in a similar series starting at a concentration of 2 per cent, all in 2·5-ml amounts in 5 × ⅝ in. sterile test-tubes. Place these tubes in a water-bath at 20° along with a bottle containing 2 ml of the twenty-four-hour culture of *Salm. typhi* and 48 ml of a sterile 5 per cent suspension of yeast ['Yeast for B.S.I. C/10 tests' from the Distillers Co. Ltd., Bristol, England, creamed with water, passed through a 100-mesh sieve, adjusted to pH 7·0, made up with water to contain exactly 5 per cent dry weight of yeast cells, and sterilised to 100-ml amounts in bottles at 121° (15 lb steam pressure) for fifteen minutes]. At half-minute intervals transfer 2·5 ml of the yeast-culture mixture to each 2·5-ml tube of disinfectant or phenol dilution, shake, and after thirty minutes' contact transfer one standard loopful to each of two tubes containing 10 ml of the appropriate culture medium. Incubate at 37° for forty-eight hours and record the results. Calculate the phenol coefficient 'by dividing the mean of the highest concentration of phenol permitting growth in both cultures and the lowest concentration showing absence of growth in both cultures by the corresponding mean concentration of the disinfectant.'

The ***A.O.A.C*** and ***F.D.A.*** methods follow a similar procedure to that of the Rideal-Walker method, except that the test is made at 20° (or 37°), 0·5 ml of the culture is added to each of the 5 ml disinfectant or phenol dilutions, the time intervals for subculturing are five, ten and fifteen minutes, and ten dilution tubes are required for each test, comprising eight of the disinfectant and the two of phenol. For ordinary coal tar disinfectants, the medium as given in the table (p. 206) is satisfactory, but where they contain surface-active compounds of the quaternary ammonium type a 'Letheen' medium is specified, which is the same basic medium with the addition of 0·07 per cent lecithin (Azolectin) and 0·5 per cent Tween 80. The *Staph. aureus* test is made at 20° on disinfectants intended for external use, and at 37° for those intended for personal use or for application to wounds.

In addition to the phenol coefficient tests, a **Use-Dilution Confirmation test** has been introduced in the United States.[10] The purpose of this test is to confirm that the recommended 'use-dilution' of the disinfectant (calculated from the phenol coefficient of the fluid to be equivalent to that of a 5 per cent phenol solution) is in fact satisfactory. If the response in the test is not satisfactory, then an adjustment must be made to the dilutions recommended for use.

Sterilise stainless steel 'penicillin assay' cylinders and immerse in groups of 20 in 20 ml of a forty-eight-hour culture of *Salm. choleræsuis* or a twenty-four-hour culture of *Staph. aureus*, transfer to a filter paper in a petri dish and dry in an incubator for not more than sixty minutes. Drop one cylinder into each of 10 tubes containing 10 ml of the chosen disinfectant dilution and after ten minutes transfer the cylinder to a 10-ml tube of the appropriate nutrient broth. There should be no growth from any of the 10 cylinders after incubation at 37° for forty-eight hours.

Other Cresol-type Disinfectants and Antiseptics. Various non-irritant germicides of low toxicity, and therefore particularly suitable for disinfecting the skin and for application to wounds, contain different amounts of chloroxylenol, dichloroxylenol, benzyl cresols, *o*-phenylphenol, chlorobenzylphenols, special narrow-range boiling fractions of coal tar distillates, etc. They are usually dissolved in a soap, such as castor oil soap, and essential oil solution as they are only sparingly soluble in water. The various phenol coefficient tests, and particularly the Chick-Martin test, are of value in standardising such preparations, but they are of little value in determining their practical efficacy as antiseptics. For such purposes, other more specific tests are required which are beyond the scope of this book.

The official chlorinated compounds are **chlorocresol,** C_7H_7OCl, Mol. Wt. 142·6, **chloroxylenol,** C_8H_9OCl, Mol. Wt. 156·6, and **dichloroxylenol,** $C_8H_8OCl_2$, Mol. Wt. 191·1. These solid phenols are only slowly steam-volatile, but may be extracted from the original product with ether in the presence of sodium carbonate. After re-extraction from the ether with caustic alkali and then with ether from the acidified solution (to free from unsaponified matter), the ether is evaporated and the residue dried in a desiccator. The phenols should be recrystallised from water before identifying by melting-point.

In the determination of halogen in these chlorinated phenols the Stepanow method can be used,

To a portion of sample containing about 0·2 g of chlorocresol contained in a 150-ml flask add 30 to 40 ml of dry ethanol. Connect to an efficient upright Liebig condenser, heat to boiling and add clean, bright sodium metal in small strips dropped down the condenser until 2 g have been added during half an hour. Reflux the mixture until no sodium remains undissolved, dilute with water, filter, acidify with nitric acid and determine the halogen with silver nitrate by Volhard's method (p. 290) or by precipitation and weighing as silver chloride. Conduct a control experiment on the materials used.

Kay and Haywood[11] occasionally found the method to give low results, which were traced to impurities in the ethanol used. An alternative method was proposed, based on fusion with sodium hydroxide and sodium carbonate and determination of the resultant chloride.

Add 0·2 ml of 30 per cent sodium hydroxide solution to each 0·1 g of chlorinated phenol in a platinum crucible. When solution is complete add 5 g of sodium carbonate and mix well. Dry carefully by means of a small flame and then raise to full heat for ten minutes. Extract the chloride in the residue with water and determine by the Volhard method (p. 290).

Chlorocresol can be determined by the 4-aminophenazone method (see p. 514) when present in injection solutions, lotions, etc. It can also be determined in such preparations by use of 2,6-dichloro-*p*-benzoquinone-4-chloroimine.

Dissolve 0·5 g of lotion containing 0·2 per cent of chlorocresol in sufficient 72 per cent ethanol (prepared from industrial methylated spirit that has been refluxed for four hours over potassium hydroxide and distilled) to make exactly 50 ml. Shake well, chill in ice-water and filter. Pipette 10 ml of the filtrate into a 20-ml graduated flask and dilute to 12 ml with the 72 per cent ethanol. Add 2 ml of a 0·012 per cent solution of 2,6-dichloro-*p*-benzoquinone-4-chloroimine in 95 per cent ethanol (refluxed and distilled as above) and 2 ml of a 1·5 per cent aqueous borax solution, mixing after each addition. Allow to stand in the dark for one hour and then dilute to volume with the 72 per cent ethanol. Mix and measure the extinction at 650 mμ in a 2-cm cell; subtract the value of a reagent blank and read off the amount of chlorocresol from a calibration curve.

Chlorocresol and chloroxylenol sometimes occur together in commercial preparations. For the approximate evaluation of these two a method has been devised[12] making use of the fact that the 4-aminophenazone dye resulting from chlorocresol gives a maximum absorption at about 450 mμ whilst that from chloroxylenol gives a maximum at about 520 mμ. The method for determination in an antiseptic cream is as follows:

To 2 g in a 250-ml round-bottomed flask add a large glass bead, 25 ml of dilute hydrochloric acid and 2 ml of ethanol and reflux for one hour. Allow to cool, wash down the inside of the condenser with 10 ml of water, cool thoroughly and transfer to a separator with the aid of 25 ml of ethanol, leaving the paraffin layer in the flask and removing the glass bead. Wash the flask with successive 25-ml portions of chloroform, shaking well to dissolve the paraffin, and add the washings to the separator. Shake well and run the chloroform layer into a second separator. Extract the aqueous layer with two 15-ml quantities of a mixture of two volumes of chloroform and one volume of ethanol. Extract the combined chloroform phases successively with 25 ml, 15 ml and 10 ml of 0·5N sodium hydroxide (these quantities are important and must be adhered to). Combine the alkaline extracts and wash with two 10-ml portions of chloroform, rejecting the chloroform. Swirl, run off any chloroform that collects and decant the alkali into a 1-litre graduated flask, washing in with water. Add 5 ml of 25 per cent ammonium chloride solution and dilute to volume with water. Mix and pipette 50 ml into a separator.

Continue by the 4-aminophenazone method (see p. 514) diluting the extracted colour to 50 ml with chloroform and measure the extinction at 450 mμ and 520 mμ using matched 1-cm cells with a reagent-blank solution in the comparison cell.

Calculate the E(1 per cent, 1 cm) of the mixture at 450 mμ (R_{450}) and the E(1 per cent, 1 cm) of the mixture at 520 mμ (R_{520}) and apply the simultaneous equations:

$$1063A + 177B = 100R_{450}$$
$$394A + 481B = 100R_{520}$$

A = percentage chlorocresol in the sample
B = percentage chloroxylenol in the sample

1063 and 394 are the E(1 per cent, 1 cm) values of chlorocresol at 450 mμ and 520 mμ respectively.
177 and 481 are the E(1 per cent, 1 cm) values of chloroxylenol at 450 mμ and 520 mμ respectively.

Solution of Chloroxylenol, *B.P.* A 5 per cent solution of chloroxylenol in a mixture of terpineol, alcohol and castor oil soap. The chloroxylenol in this preparation can be determined by the above fusion method after evaporation of 5 ml of the sample to dryness with sodium hydroxide or colorimetrically by the 4-aminophenazone method.

1. Raschig, F., *Z. Angew. Chem.*, 1900, 759.
2. Fox, J. J., and Barker, M. F., *J. Soc. Chem. Ind.*, 1920, **39,** 169T.
3. Potter, F. M., and Williams, H. B., *J. Soc. Chem. Ind.*, 1932, **51,** 59T.
4. *J. Soc. Chem. Ind.*, 1938, **57,** 212.
5. Brooks, V. T., *Chem. & Ind.*, 1959, 1317.
6. Edwards, K. B., and Freak, G. A., *J. Soc. Chem. Ind.*, 1920, **39,** 326T.
7. Dodd, A. H., *J. Soc. Chem. Ind.*, 1924, **43,** 93T.
8. Martin, G. F. W., *Analyst*, 1921, **46,** 93T.
9. Jordan, E. J., and Southerden, F., *Pharm. J.*, 1921, **106,** 479.
10. Stuart, L. S., Ortenzio, L. F., and Friedl, J. L., *J.A.O.A.C.*, 1953, **36,** 466.
11. Kay, J., and Haywood, P. J. C., *J. Soc. Chem. Ind.*, 1944, **63,** 382.
12. Savidge, R. A., private communication.

CYANOCOBALAMIN

(Vitamin B_{12})

$C_{63}H_{88}O_{14}N_{14}PCo$ Mol. Wt. 1355·4

Of the direct colorimetric and spectroscopic methods available for the determination of cyanocobalamin, the simplest is that comprising a determination of the extinction at 550 mμ due to the red colour; although this method has obvious limitations it is useful for assaying samples of known origin, particularly if colourless substances having an ultra-violet absorption are present. A more sensitive method involves a determination of the extinction at 361 mμ and this method is official in the *B.P.*

Weigh 2 mg into a 50-ml graduated flask, dissolve in water, dilute to volume with water and mix. Measure the extinction of this solution at the maximum at about 361 mμ, using 1-cm cells with water in the comparison cell. E(1 per cent, 1 cm) of anhydrous cyanocobalamin at 361 mμ = 207.

The above method can be used for aqueous solutions down to a concentration of about 0·001 per cent and, if supplemented by a determination of the ratios of the extinctions at 278 mμ, 361 mμ and 550 mμ or at 341 and 376 mμ,[1] for which definite limits can be fixed, has a measure of specificity.

For samples of biological origin, in which the concentration of the vitamin may be extremely low and which may contain analogues, spectroscopic methods that have greater sensitivity and specificity are necessary and one such method, suitable for concentrations of at least 1 μg of cyanocobalamin per ml, has been proposed by Rudkin and Taylor[2] and is based on the reaction between cyanocobalamin and cyanide in alkaline solution to form a dicyanide complex. This method is as follows:

> To a solution of the sample containing about 200 μg of cyanocobalamin at a concentration of not less than 1 μg per ml, add sufficient solid sodium cyanide to give a final cyanide concentration of 1 per cent and stir until dissolved. If necessary, adjust the pH to between 9·5 and 10·0 by the addition of 10 per cent sodium hydroxide solution. Allow to stand for five hours at room temperature to complete the conversion of cyanocobalamin analogues to the dicyanide complex and then add and dissolve sufficient anhydrous sodium sulphate to give a concentration of 20 per cent, adjust the pH to between 11·0 and 11·5 with 10 per cent sodium hydroxide solution and extract with three quantities of benzyl alcohol, each of volume one-tenth that of the solution. Combine the extracts, add an amount of chloroform equal to one-half their volume and extract with three quantities of water, each of volume one-tenth the volume of the organic layer. Combine the aqueous extracts in a 25-ml graduated flask and dilute to volume with water (Solution A).
>
> To a 10-ml aliquot of Solution A add 2 ml of 10 per cent sodium cyanide solution and at the same time to a second 10-ml aliquot of Solution A add 2 ml of 12·5 per cent potassium dihydrogen phosphate solution to adjust the pH to between 5 and 6. Measure the extinction of each solution at 582 mμ using 2-cm cells and calculate the cyanocobalamin content of the sample from the difference between the two extinctions, using a value of E(1 per cent, 1 cm) = 54 for cyanocobalamin.

In a study by spectrofluorimetry, Duggan, Bowman, Brodie and Udenfriend[3] found that in phosphate buffer pH 7, cyanocobalamin had an activation maximum at 275 mμ and a fluorescence maximum at 305 mμ and that a practical sensitivity of 0·003 μg of cyanocobalamin per ml was obtainable. Since fluorometric methods usually have high sensitivity and specificity, these considerations may enable a valuable method to be developed for the determination of cyanocobalamin, in particular since it may overcome interference by analogues and other cobalamins.

Injection of Cyanocobalamin, *B.P.* Usually contains 50 micrograms of anhydrous material in 1 ml. It may be assayed by the spectrophotometric method, making use of the absorption maximum at 361 mμ. For greater specificity the extinctions should also be measured at 278 mμ and at 550 mμ; the ratio of the extinctions at these two wavelengths to that at 361 mμ should be about 0·57 and 0·3 respectively. Obviously, when carrying out this assay account must be taken of any added bacteriostat; phenol is commonly used and this has no effect on the readings at 361 mμ and at 550 mμ but does affect that at 278 mμ considerably.

In certain mixtures with other vitamins, or in natural products such as liver extracts, feeding stuffs, etc., the only reliable assay may be a microbiological one (see page 813). In the first case the preparation of the sample for assay presents no difficulty and simple dilution to the required level is sufficient, but with the natural products the vitamin may be present in complex-bound forms or as hydroxocobalamin, which is relatively unstable to heat. Both problems can be resolved by treating the sample with cyanide, thus assisting the extraction by breaking the complexes and converting all of the cobalamin to the more stable cyano compound.[4]

To 1 g of the sample in a flask add 30 ml water and 0·05 to 0·5 ml of a 1 per cent solution of sodium cyanide, mix well and adjust the pH value to 4·6–5·0 with N hydrochloric acid. Allow the mixture to stand for thirty minutes, shaking it occasionally, readjust the pH value if necessary, then place the flask in boiling water and leave there until the temperature of the extract has reached 90°. Cool, transfer to a 100-ml graduated flask and make up to volume with water. Clarify if necessary by centrifuging then dilute an aliquot as necessary and proceed with the assay as directed on page 815.

Notes: (1) The amount of cyanide to be added depends on the amount of vitamin B_{12} in the sample and should be such that the residual free cyanide in the final dilutions does not exceed 10 μg per ml.

(2) With material such as gut mucosa and gastric juices even this treatment may not release the vitamin sufficiently to make it available to the test micro-organism. In these cases, a more complicated extraction involving the use of cyanide-activated papain is needed.[5]

HYDROXOCOBALAMIN (Aquocobalamin Chloride)

The absorption spectrum of hydroxocobalamin is similar to that of cyanocobalamin but the peaks occur at different wavelengths and they are displaced somewhat by pH changes; in acid solution the main peaks for hydroxocobalamin occur at 351 mμ and 525 mμ. A suitable spectrophotometric method for the determination of hydroxocobalamin is as follows.

Weigh 2 mg into a 50-ml graduated flask and dissolve in sodium acetate buffer solution, pH 4·5 (prepared by mixing 600 ml of 0·2M acetic acid with 400 ml of 0·2M sodium acetate). Dilute to volume with the buffer solution and mix.

Measure the extinction of this solution at the maximum at about 351 mμ using 1-cm cells with buffer solution in the comparison cell. Calculate the percentage of hydroxocobalamin (with reference to the substance dried *in vacuo* at 105° to constant weight) assuming a value of 190 for the E(1 per cent, 1 cm) of the pure dry substance.

The above determinations should be applied directly to the hydrated sample since Lester Smith and his co-workers[6] have shown that heating at

100° for two hours under reduced pressure (the method used by earlier workers to dehydrate the sample before determining its extinction) causes some decomposition; this accounts for the fact that the E(1 per cent, 1 cm) of 190 which they found is higher than the value quoted in earlier publications.

In trying to find independent criteria for the purity of a reference sample the above workers assessed two highly purified samples of aquocobalamin chloride after quantitative conversion to cyanocobalamin. A known weight of sample was first converted to dicyanocobalamin by adding a trace of cyanide to a solution and allowing to stand for two hours and the solution was then made acid with acetic acid and allowed to stand for a further two hours, in which time the second cyanide group is removed and cyanocobalamin produced. The E(1 per cent, 1 cm) of this solution at 361 mμ was then determined, after suitable dilution. The values obtained (corrected for the small change in molecular weight) were 209 and 210 compared with the accepted value of 207 for cyanocobalamin. This is possibly another approach to the determination of hydroxocobalamin.

1. Bruening, C. F., Hall, W. L., and Kline, O. L., *J. Amer. Pharm. Ass., Sci. Edn.*, 1958, **47,** 15.
2. Rudkin, G. O., and Taylor, R. J., *Anal. Chem.*, 1952, **24,** 1155.
3. Duggan, D. E., Bowman, R. L., Brodie, B. B., and Udenfriend, S., *Arch. Biochem. Biophys.*, 1957, **68,** 1.
4. *S.A.C.* Analytical Methods Committee Report, *Analyst*, 1956, **81,** 132.
5. Gregory, Margaret E., *Brit. J. Nutrition*, 1955, **8,** 340.
6. Smith, E. L., Martin, J. L., Gregory, R. J., and Shaw, W. H. C., *Analyst*, 1962, **87,** 183.

DAPSONE

$C_{12}H_{12}O_2N_2S$ Mol. Wt. 248·3

Dapsone is 4,4′-diaminodiphenyl sulphone and it may be assayed by titration with sodium nitrite using a 'dead-stop' end-point.

> Dissolve about 0·25 g in 30 ml of a mixture of equal volumes of dilute hydrochloric acid and water and titrate electrometrically with 0·1M sodium nitrite using the 'dead-stop' technique (see p. 867). 1 ml 0·1M = 0·01242 g $C_{12}H_{12}O_2N_2S$.

Injection of Dapsone, *B.P.C.* Contains 20 per cent w/v of dapsone in arachis oil.

> Mix an amount to contain about 0·25 g of dapsone with 40 ml of chloroform in a separator and extract first with 60 ml of a mixture of equal volumes of dilute hydrochloric acid and water and then with 10 ml

of water, combining the extracts. Titrate with 0·1M sodium nitrite as above.

Intramammary Injection of Dapsone, *B.Vet.C.* Contains dapsone, 33·3 per cent by weight in a mixture of liquid paraffin and white soft paraffin.

Disperse 1 g in 40 ml of chloroform, add 60 ml of water and 10 ml of concentrated hydrochloric acid and shake until the chloroform layer becomes clear. Titrate electrometrically with 0·1M sodium nitrite, as above.

Intramammary Injection of Dapsone and Penicillin, *B.Vet.C.* Contains dapsone, 33·3 per cent by weight in a mixture of liquid and soft paraffin and benzylpenicillin, usually 50,000 units in each dose.

The assay for dapsone is the same as for Intramammary Injection of Dapsone, above.

For penicillin: Disperse about 1 g, accurately weighed, in 5 ml of carbon tetrachloride and add 100 ml of sterile solution of standard pH 7·0; shake well for fifteen minutes and allow to stand for a further ten minutes. Transfer about 30 ml of the aqueous layer to a sterile 50-ml centrifuge tube and centrifuge for three to five minutes; dilute 10 ml of the clear aqueous solution with sterile solution of standard pH 7·0 to 100 ml and determine microbiologically by the method given in Appendix VII.

Tablets of Dapsone, *B.P.* Usually contain 0·1 g of dapsone.

For assay powder twenty tablets, weigh a quantity to contain about 0·25 g of dapsone, dissolve in 30 ml of a mixture of equal volumes of dilute hydrochloric acid and water and titrate with 0·1M sodium nitrite as above.

SOLAPSONE, $C_{30}H_{28}O_{14}N_2S_5Na_4$, Mol. Wt. 892·9

As obtained commercially solapsone is not of constant composition but is chiefly tetrasodium 4,4′-di-(3-phenyl-1,3-disulphopropylamino)-diphenyl sulphone; it contains water of hydration. The compound is decomposed in acid solution to diaminodiphenyl sulphone (dapsone), the hydrolysis not being quite quantitative even with chemically pure material, it can then be diazotised and determined by titration as above. The acid hydrolysis should not be done under reflux as this would prevent the removal, by volatilisation, of the cinnamic acid produced in the reaction.

Dissolve about 0·5 g of solapsone in 100 ml of water in a wide-necked flask and add 20 ml of dilute hydrochloric acid. Boil the mixture gently for one hour, making up the loss due to evaporation from time to time by addition of water. Cool and titrate electrometrically with 0·1M sodium nitrite using the 'dead-stop' technique (see p. 867). 1 ml 0·1M = 0·04464 g of $C_{30}H_{28}O_{14}N_2S_5Na_4$.

DAPSONE

For colorimetric assay, although the diazo compound can be coupled with *N*-(1-naphthyl)ethylenediamine (see Sulphonamides, p. 609) Dewing and Foster[1] found that for routine assay a more satisfactory determination could be carried out if the acid hydrolysate were treated with sodium nitrite and coupled with dimethyl-α-naphthylamine.

Prepare a series of standard solutions containing 1 to 0·5 mg of 4,4′-diaminodiphenyl sulphone in 100 ml by suitably diluting with water a 1 per cent solution in dilute hydrochloric acid. Treat 10 ml of each standard solution successively with 0·4 ml of concentrated hydrochloric acid, 1 ml of 0·1 per cent sodium nitrite solution, 10 ml of ethanol and 1 ml of a 1 per cent ethanolic solution of dimethyl-α-naphthylamine. Mix thoroughly and after ten minutes measure the extinction at the absorption maximum at about 550 mμ. Prepare a standard curve from the readings obtained.

Prepare a solution of the solapsone under examination, so that it will possess a content of 4,4′-diaminodiphenyl sulphone within the range covered by the standard curve, making due allowance for moisture and for the fact that only 80 per cent recovery is usual. Mix 10 ml of the solution with 0·4 ml of concentrated hydrochloric acid and heat in a water-bath for twenty minutes. Cool, make up the volume to 10 ml with water and treat by the process described above for the standard solutions. After taking the extinction reading use the standard curve to obtain the result of the assay, which may be expressed in terms of anhydrous solapsone or dapsone.

Measurement of the ultra-violet absorption may be used for the assay of dilute aqueous solutions of solapsone in the absence of interfering substances. In aqueous solution E(1 per cent, 1 cm) at 306 mμ is approximately 380, calculated on the anhydrous salt.

Strong Injection of Solapsone, *B.P.C.* Contains 50 per cent of solapsone with a little sodium carbonate in water for injection.

Dilute 10 ml to 100 ml in a graduated flask and, using 10 ml of this solution, carry out the assay described above for solapsone beginning with 'add 20 ml of dilute hydrochloric acid . . .'.

Tablets of Solapsone, *B.P.* Usually contain 0·5 g of solapsone.

Assayed as Solapsone, above, using a weight of powdered tablets to contain about 0·5 g of solapsone.

SODIUM SULFOXONE, $C_{14}H_{14}O_6N_2S_3Na_2$, Mol. Wt. 448·5

Consists of 73 to 81 per cent of disodium di-(*p*-sulphino-methylaminophenyl)sulphone mixed with suitable buffers and inert ingredients.

This material is assayed colorimetrically by diazotising, coupling with *N*-(1-naphthyl)ethylenediamine (see Sulphonamides, p. 609) and measuring the extinction at 560 mμ against a reference standard dapsone.

1. Dewing, T., and Foster, G. E., *Analyst*, 1948, **73**, 558.

DICOPHANE

$C_{14}H_9Cl_5$ Mol. Wt. 354·5

Dicophane, or DDT, is a mixture consisting chiefly of 1,1,1-trichloro-2,2-di-(*p*-chlorophenyl)ethane, this being the most effective insecticidal component present.

To obtain the percentage of *p,p'*-dicophane in the technical product, the following crystallisation method, modified from that of Balaban and Calvert[1] is official and gives results believed to be near to the true figure.

> To about 10 g of sample, accurately weighed, add 50 ml of a solution of pure dicophane in dry ethanol, saturated at 18°, and bring to the boil to effect solution without loss of solvent. Cool slowly and after crystallisation commences allow to crystallise for one hour with occasional swirling and finally allow to stand a further hour at 18° ± 0·5°. Filter through a Gooch crucible or No. 3 sintered-glass filter, washing in with a further 20 ml of saturated DDT solution. Dry to constant weight at 80°.

Cristol, Hayes and Haller[2] considered that use of 75 per cent ethanol saturated with *p,p'*-dicophane as recrystallisation solvent gave more consistent results; a small empirical correction is added.

> Dissolve 2 g of the sample by refluxing with 150 ml of a saturated stock solution of *p,p'*-dicophane in 75 per cent by volume ethanol (maintained when not in use at 25° ± 0·5°) in a 250-ml conical flask. After the sample has completely dissolved, close the flask and allow to cool slowly. Place in a thermostatically controlled bath at 25° and shake intermittently for four hours. Filter on a tared Gooch crucible in the bottom of which is a disc of filter paper. Wash the remainder of the crystals on to the Gooch with 20 ml of the saturated solution. Dry to constant weight at 80°; add a correction of 1·4 per cent to the percentage found to give results in agreement with known mixtures. The melting-point of the separated crystals should be above 106°.

A number of workers have employed dehydrohalogenation with ethanolic alkali as a basis for estimating *p,p'*-dicophane. At ordinary temperatures 0·1N ethanolic alkali will remove HCl quantitatively from the pure substance without further decomposition of the molecule but in commercial samples isomers and other impurities interfere. The most important impurity quantitatively is *o,p'*-dicophane, which may be present to the extent of 8 to 21 per cent; this isomer reacts much more slowly to ethanolic alkali and the amount of chloride liberated under specified conditions can be related to the content of *p,p'*-dicophane by means of a regression equation. Such an equation has been given by Wain and Martin[3] and under the specified conditions should give a close approximation to the *p,p'*-dicophane content:

> Dissolve 0·500 g of the sample in 25 ml of dry ethanol in a 350-ml

conical flask. Stopper the flask and place in a thermostat at 23° and, after temperature equilibrium has been attained, add 25 ml of 0·2N potassium hydroxide in redistilled dry ethanol. Allow the mixture to stand for sixty minutes at 23° then add 25 ml of N nitric acid and determine the liberated chloride by the Volhard method (p. 290). The relationship between the chloride liberated under the specified conditions and the content of *p,p′*-dicophane is expressed as follows:

Per cent *p,p′*-dicophane = (1·56 × mg Cl′ per g of sample) − 58·1.

DDT is included either alone or with other insecticides in many different preparations. Its concentration is usually in the region of 3 to 20 per cent.

Infra-red absorption can be used for its determination, and although the method details are different for each formulation, the following general principles may be applied:

1. DDT alone in powder preparations.

The DDT can usually be extracted with ether and after evaporation of the solvent, the residue is dissolved in carbon disulphide to give a concentration of about 0·5 per cent DDT. A base-line measurement on the band at 1,015 cm^{-1} using cells of 1 mm thickness may then be compared with a similar measurement on a 0·5 per cent standard solution of DDT in carbon disulphide (see p. 885).

2. DDT alone in liquid preparations.

Similar concentrations and measurements to the above may be used, but it is often necessary to remove interfering absorption due to aromatic solvents and emulsifiers. This may sometimes be done by passing the sample through a column of kieselguhr impregnated with oleum as follows:

Triturate 2 ml of concentrated sulphuric acid, 2 ml of oleum and 6 g of kieselguhr and pack tightly into a chromatographic tube of 18 mm internal bore containing light petroleum (b.p. 40° to 60°). Dilute the sample in light petroleum (b.p. 40° to 60°) and transfer an aliquot containing about 50 mg DDT to the column. Elute the DDT with 5 aliquots each of 10 ml of light petroleum (b.p. 40° to 60°) and after evaporation of the solvent dissolve the residue in 10 ml of carbon disulphide for the infra-red measurement.

3. DDT present with other insecticides.

When included with another insecticide such as gamma benzene hexachloride, dieldrin or chlorparacide, DDT is usually present at a concentration several times greater than that of the other material. Therefore, to make simultaneous infra-red measurements of the two insecticides on the same extract, a weaker absorption band than that at 1,015 cm^{-1} must be used. The band at 896 cm^{-1} satisfies this demand and is also in close proximity to the bands at 913 cm^{-1}, 912 cm^{-1} and 883 cm^{-1} which may be used for measurements on dieldrin, gamma benzene hexachloride and chlorparacide respectively. The concentration of DDT in the final solution is usually around 4 per cent and to effect solution carbon tetrachloride must be used as solvent. Cells of 1 mm thickness are required. Dieldrin and chlorparacide are decomposed by the oleum/kieselguhr treatment outlined in 2 above. However, if either of these two materials are present with DDT, interfering absorption may sometimes be removed by filtering the extract of, or the dilution from, the sample in ether through a column of alumina.

Of the numerous colorimetric methods introduced for the determination of **small amounts** of dicophane the modification[4] of that developed by Schechter and Haller[5] used by the *A.O.A.C.* can be recommended. The technique using commercial dicophane as standard material is described herewith.

Prepare sodium methoxide reagent as follows: To 20·0 g of freshly cut sodium in a flask fitted with a reflux condenser, add, in portions down the condenser, sufficient anhydrous methanol to dissolve all the sodium, warming and refluxing if necessary. Transfer to a 500-ml graduated flask, washing in with anhydrous methanol, and dilute to volume with anhydrous methanol. Chill, centrifuge from any carbonate impurity and store in a suitable container to exclude moisture and carbon dioxide. Adjust to 40 g Na per litre (1·74N) by titration with standard acid. Prepare a new standard curve for each fresh batch of the reagent.

Preparation of Standard Curve. Dissolve 40·0 mg of dicophane in benzene and make up to 200 ml (1 ml = 0·20 mg). Measure 0, 1·00, 2·00, 3·00, 4·00 and 5·00 ml of the solution into 50-ml Erlenmeyer flasks and evaporate the solvent on a water-bath. Remove residual vapours with a gentle current of air, and immerse in ice-water (so that the flasks are not resting on the bottom of the ice-water container). When the flasks are thoroughly chilled, slowly add to each 5 ml of chilled nitrating mixture (equal volumes of fuming nitric and concentrated sulphuric acids). Rotate the flasks so that all portions of the residue are wetted, place the ice-water container on a hot plate or water-bath and heat at such a rate that the solutions come to a temperature of about 85° in twenty to thirty minutes. Then place the flasks directly on a water-bath and nitrate for thirty minutes. Remove the flasks and cool under the tap. Treat the contents of each flask, respectively, as follows: slowly pour into a separator containing about 25 ml of ice-cold water and rinse the flask with several portions of ice-cold water, followed by 25 ml of a mixture of one volume of ether and four volumes of light petroleum, adding the rinsings to the separator. Finally rinse with 15 ml of the mixed solvent and pour this rinsing into a second separator. Extract by shaking the first separator vigorously for one minute, allow the layers to separate, run the aqueous layer into the second separator and repeat the extraction. Discard the aqueous layer and combine the solvent layers in the first separator. Add 10 ml of 10 per cent potassium hydroxide solution and shake vigorously for thirty seconds. Run off the aqueous layer and wash the solvent layer with two 15-ml portions of saturated sodium chloride solution. Discard the washings and filter the ether layer through a 0·5-in. layer of glass wool, previously rinsed with ether mixture, into a 125-ml Erlenmeyer flask containing a glass bead. Rinse the separator and filter with a few small quantities of mixed solvent, evaporate the solvent on a water-bath and heat for one hour at 100°. Cool the flask, making sure the interior is thoroughly dry, and dissolve the residue in exactly 25 ml of benzene, stoppering the flask and swirling for one minute to ensure complete solution.

Transfer a 5-ml aliquot to a flask and add exactly 10 ml of the sodium methoxide reagent. Mix well, allow to stand for fifteen minutes and determine the extinction at 600 mμ using matched, stoppered cells with, in the comparison cell, a mixture of one volume of benzene and two volumes of the sodium methoxide reagent. (Readings in the blue at 450 mμ and in the green at 510 mμ should also be made to check the presence of extraneous yellow and red colours when the samples are read.) Prepare a curve by plotting extinction against μg dicophane.

Determination. Pipette an appropriate aliquot of a colourless, fat-free extract of the sample in a suitable solvent into a 50-ml Erlenmeyer flask and evaporate the solvent on a water-bath with the aid of a gentle current of air. When dry, chill thoroughly in ice-water and nitrate, extract and dissolve in benzene as described above under 'Preparation of Standard Curve,' beginning with the words 'When the flasks are thoroughly chilled . . .', but wash the ether mixture with six 10-ml portions of 10 per cent potassium hydroxide solution to ensure removal of interfering oxidation by-products. If the quantity of dicophane is unknown develop and measure the colour as above, in a 5-ml aliquot of the benzene solution using 10 ml of the sodium methoxide reagent. If the extinction is less than 0·20 take a 10- to 15-ml aliquot, evaporate to dryness, dissolve in exactly 5 ml of benzene and develop the colour. If the extinction is greater than 0·80, take a smaller aliquot and dilute to 5 ml with benzene. If the extinction is within the range 0·20 to 0·80 develop the colour in a further 5-ml aliquot. Measure the extinction of the final solution at 600 mμ (and also take readings at 510 mμ and 450 mμ to determine if gross amounts of interfering red or yellow colours are present). Read the total μg dicophane present from the standard curve.

The suitable solvent recommended for the aliquot of the colourless, fat-free extract of the sample required in the determination varies with the product under test and is detailed in the original paper. For general purposes benzene is satisfactory.

The method is empirical, hence the procedure must be followed closely and reagents carefully prepared; the methoxide reagent requires close adjustment of the strength.

Application of Dicophane, *B.P.C.* Contains 2 per cent of dicophane. Dicophane can be determined by its hydrolysable chlorine content:

Boil about 10 g, accurately weighed, under reflux with 20 ml of 5 per cent ethanolic solution of sodium hydroxide for thirty minutes. Add 100 ml of water, acidify with dilute nitric acid and add 10 ml of 0·1N silver nitrate. Shake vigorously, filter, wash and titrate with 0·02N ammonium thiocyanate using iron alum as indicator. 1 ml 0·1N $AgNO_3$ = 0·03545 g $C_{14}H_9Cl_5$.

Dusting Powder of Dicophane, *B.Vet.C.* Contains 5 per cent of dicophane in kaolin.

The dicophane can be determined on about 10 g by the method described above for Application of Dicophane or by the infra-red method given on p. 218. An assay by simple chloroform extraction is also possible.

1. BALABAN, I. E., and CALVERT, A. D., *Ind. Eng. Chem., Anal. Edn.*, 1946, **18**, 339.
2. CRISTOL, S. J., HAYES, R. A., and HALLER, H. L., *Ind. Eng. Chem., Anal. Edn.*, 1945, **17**, 470.
3. WAIN, R. L., and MARTIN, A. E., *Analyst*, 1948, **73**, 479.
4. *A.O.A.C.*, 1960, p. 341.
5. SCHECHTER, M. S., and HALLER, H. L., *J. Amer. Chem. Soc.*, 1944, **66**, 2129.

DIGITALIS

The chemical analysis of digitalis leaf has been the subject of a very considerable volume of literature but as yet the problem remains unresolved. As might be expected, the application of simple, relatively non-specific, colorimetric tests to extracts prepared from the leaves does not give an indication of biological potency since a number of glycosides of differing relative pharmacological activity are present. Attempts to separate the constituent glycosides by chromatographic means, followed by their individual determination, have so far met with only limited success. Moreover, such methods are very lengthy and require skilled technique so that it becomes doubtful whether they could compete with a biological assay on purely economic grounds. Since no reliable method has yet been suggested for the chemical assay of digitalis no attempt is made here to describe a possible procedure. Nor is it within the scope of this book to review the many unsuccessful attempts (for some of which far too ambitious claims have been made) which have been reported. At the time of writing, a biological method of assay provides the only acceptable assessment of potency.

The colorimetric determination of the glycosides has been carried out by three main types of reaction. These consist of (i) *m*-dinitrobenzene which reacts with the lactone group present in all the active glycosides, as well as in some of the inactive ones, (ii) alkaline sodium picrate (the so-called Baljet reagent) which also reacts with the lactone group and (iii) acid-ferric chloride (the so-called Keller-Kiliani reagent) which reacts with digitoxose, the sugar characteristic of all the digitalis glycosides. Detailed methods for the application of these reagents are given below for (i) digoxin (*A.O.A.C.* method), (ii) digitoxin and (iii) digoxin (*U.S.P.* method).

In the absence of a suitable chemical method digitalis must be standardised by means of a biological assay against a standard preparation and for this purpose an International Standard for digitalis is available containing 13·16 units per g.

Among the methods which have been used officially are those based on the determination of the LD 50 in frogs, the determination of the average lethal dose in cats, guinea-pigs and pigeons as well as that based on the emetic effect produced in pigeons. Other methods have been described using the toxic effects against daphnia and the effect on isolated mammalian heart preparations and on the embryonic chick heart. Gold[1] has conducted clinical standardisation and shown that the RT-T segment of the electrocardiogram is sensitive to a 25 per cent change in dosage levels. Gold *et al.*[2] have shown that the cat method provides values which agree well with the human method but that the frog method was unsatisfactory. Braun and Lusky[3] showed that cats could be replaced satisfactorily by pigeons and Braun and Siegfried[4] showed that in five comparisons between cat and guinea-pig methods the agreement was good in four but that in one the difference was greater than 20 per cent.

The method described in the *B.P.* is based on the simultaneous determinations of the average lethal doses in guinea-pigs for standard and the sample being tested. A weighed amount of the standard preparation is transferred to a hard glass-stoppered container of at least 50 ml capacity and 10 ml 80 per cent ethanol added for each g of powder. The upper third of the stopper is lightly greased before insertion and the extraction allowed to proceed with continuous agitation for twenty-four hours at 20° to 30° or for forty-eight hours at 10° to 20°. The contents are centrifuged or filtered through a sintered-glass filter, care being taken to avoid solvent evaporation. If stored in a tightly closed bottle between −5° and +5° the extract may be used for up to one month.

Extracts of the samples being taken are prepared similarly. Dilutions of the extract of the standard and of that of the sample being tested are made with saline solution so that the concentrations of ethanol are equal and do not exceed 10 per cent. These diluted extracts are infused intravenously at a slow uniform rate into guinea-pigs anæsthetised with urethane (0·007 ml/g of a 25 per cent w/v solution injected intraperitoneally) and maintained under artificial respiration.

The concentrations are adjusted so that cardiac arrest occurs between twenty and forty minutes from the commencement of the injection and so that the mean duration of the injection time for standard and unknown do not differ by more than 10 per cent. The amount of digitalis to produce this effect is taken as the lethal dose which may be recorded in terms of units per kg body-weight for the standard and mg per kg for the sample being tested.

The guinea-pigs may be of either sex and should weigh between 200 and 600 g but their weights on any one test should not differ by more than 100 g and the mean body weight of those used on the sample being tested should not differ from that of those used on the standard by more than 10 per cent.

The potency is calculated by equating the average lethal doses for the standard and the sample being tested, and its fiducial limits are calculated by standard statistical methods (see p. 841). The potency of digitalis is considered satisfactory if the estimate lies between 8·5 and 11·5 units per g providing that the fiducial limits ($P = 0{\cdot}95$) of the estimate is not less than 8 nor greater than 12 units per g.

Although the *B.P.* specifies that the extracts should be made at the rate of 1 g of drug to 10 ml of 80 per cent ethanol it has always appeared more convenient to use sufficient ethanol to produce an extract containing 1 u/ml. If the samples being tested are treated similarly it is then much simpler to keep the ethanolic concentrations equal in the subsequent dilutions with saline. The *B.P.* method prescribes that the preparation be injected at a slow uniform rate and this can readily be done by means of a motorised syringe; if such an apparatus is not available and the infusion made from a burette it has been found easier to infuse 0·5 ml within a few seconds at intervals of thirty seconds.

Since the responses in the *B.P.* assay of digitalis are not likely to be obtained at one time a sequential sampling plan based on the cumulative differences in the log lethal doses of the standard and sample being tested may be devised to satisfy the official requirements. The *B.P.* requires that there should be only a 5 per cent probability of accepting material having a potency of less than 80 per cent or more than 125 per cent of that claimed.

It is a reasonable commercial risk to allow a 5 per cent probability of rejecting material having a potency between 95 per cent and 105 per cent of that claimed. Using these limiting conditions and a current estimate (0·004) of the variance of a single difference in the log lethal doses of the standard and the sample being tested the critical values shown in Table 16 may be calculated by applying the appropriate formulæ given on page 848. To reduce the number of entries the critical values are given for every second difference. Appropriate intermediate values apply.

The *B.P.* imposes a further restriction that the potency estimate shall be between 90 and 111 per cent of that claimed; the values to limit this are also given. Up to the twelfth pair of guinea pigs the sequential plan itself controls the material adequately. Beyond that the acceptability of the material is controlled by the estimated potency alone.

The *U.S.P.* method for the standardisation of digitalis is based on the determination of the average lethal dose in pigeons. Ethanolic extracts are made at the rate of 1 g per 10 ml of a mixture of 5 parts ethanol and 1 part water and the extraction is allowed to proceed for 24 ± 2 hours at $25 \pm 5°$ with constant agitation. On the day of the tests these extracts are diluted with normal saline so that the estimated lethal dose per kg of pigeon is 15 ml. Adult pigeons are used for the test and should be as nearly alike as

TABLE 16

CRITICAL VALUES IN A SEQUENTIAL PLAN FOR THE CONTROL OF POWDERED DIGITALIS *B.P.*

GUINEA PIG PAIR No.	ACCEPT IF CUMULATIVE DIFFERENCE IN LOG LETHAL DOSES IS LESS THAN	REJECT IF CUMULATIVE DIFFERENCE IN LOG LETHAL DOSES EXCEEDS
2	—	±0·2771
4	±0·805	±0·3963
6	±0·1997	±0·5155
8	±0·3189	±0·6347
10	±0·4381	±0·7539
12	±0·5573	±0·8731

BEYOND THE TWELFTH PAIR ACCEPT IF ESTIMATED POTENCY LIES BETWEEN 90 AND 111 PER CENT

practicable with respect to breed and weight so that the heaviest weighs less than twice the weight of the lightest. Water is withheld during the period sixteen to twenty-eight hours prior to use. The pigeons are anæsthetised lightly with ether and a level of anæsthesia is maintained for the duration of the test such that the pupillary and corneal reflexes are present and the voluntary musculature is not relaxed to an extent which does not permit the pigeon to make some occasional voluntary movement.

The diluted extracts are injected via the alar vein from a burette calibrated to 0·05 ml, infusing 1 ml per kg body weight within a few seconds at five-minute intervals until the pigeon dies of cardiac arrest. If the number of doses required to produce this is less than 13 or exceeds 19 or if the larger average in one test exceeds the lower by more than 4 doses the data are regarded as preliminary. Not less than 6 pigeons are used for standard and not less than 6 for the assay preparation.

The sample is considered satisfactory if the potency is not less than 0·85 u/100 mg. The required precision is expressed in terms of the confidence interval $L = 2\sqrt{(C-1)(CR^2 + n_T/n_{ST})}$ (see pp. 840 to 842) of the estimated potency and should not exceed 0·3 units.

DIGITOXIN

This, the most potent of the digitalis glycosides, is controlled by the *B.P.C.* on a biological assay, but the *U.S.P.* relies upon column chromatography followed by application of the alkaline picrate reaction. The same type of assay is also applicable to injection solution and tablets of digitoxin. A suitable method, which has been reported to be satisfactory, is as follows:

Reagents:

Formamide. Shake a suitable quantity of formamide with about 10 per cent of its weight of anhydrous potassium carbonate for fifteen minutes and filter. Distil the filtrate in an all-glass apparatus under vacuum at a pressure of about 25 mm of mercury or less. Reject the first portion of distillate containing water and collect the fraction that boils at about 115° at a pressure of 25 mm of mercury or at 101° at a pressure of 12 mm of mercury. Store over concentrated sulphuric acid until the odour of ammonia is no longer perceptible.

Alkaline picrate reagent. Mix 20 ml of 1 per cent aqueous picric acid solution with 10 ml of 5 per cent sodium hydroxide, dilute to 100 ml with water and mix. The reagent is stable for two to three days.

Standard:

Standard digitoxin solution. Dissolve 20·0 mg of *U.S.P.* Digitoxin Reference Standard in 95 per cent ethanol and dilute to exactly 50 ml with 95 per cent ethanol. Dilute a 5-ml aliquot of this solution with 95 per cent ethanol to 50 ml in a graduated flask.

Preparation of chromatographic column:

Insert a small plug of glass wool at the juncture of the tube and the stem of a chromatographic tube that is about 200 mm long and about 25 mm in internal diameter and place a plug of cotton wool above the juncture. Mount in a vertical position and arrange a long-stemmed, glass-stoppered, 500-ml separator to serve as a reservoir.

Stir about 2 g of Celite 545 with 1 ml of water, in a beaker, until fluffy and uniform. Transfer the mixture to the chromatographic tube, pressing down lightly with a flat-ended glass packing rod to a final length of 15–20 mm. Uniformly mix a further 3 g of Celite 545 with a mixture of 2 ml of formamide and 1 ml of water and transfer to the tube. Push a plug of cotton wool lightly and evenly on to the top of the column, sweeping the wall of the tube with it.

Preparation of sample:

Crystalline Digitoxin. Dissolve 20 mg of the sample, accurately weighed, in 20 ml of chloroform. Transfer the solution to a 100-ml graduated flask with the aid of several portions of benzene and dilute to volume with benzene. Transfer a 10-ml aliquot of this solution to the top of the column and when the liquid has passed into the column continue as described below under 'Separation of digitoxin'.

Digitoxin Injection. Pipette a volume of the sample equivalent to about 2 mg of digitoxin into a separator containing 40 ml of water and 1 ml of dilute sulphuric acid. Extract with four 25-ml quantities of chloroform, washing the extracts, successively, with the same 10 ml of water in a second separator. Filter the extracts through a cotton-wool plug, previously rinsed with chloroform, into a beaker and evaporate the chloroform on a water-bath under a jet of air. Add 4 ml of formamide and warm on the water-bath for twenty minutes, stirring frequently. Cool, add 4 ml of water and about 8 g of Celite 545 and mix until the mass appears uniform and does not adhere to the beaker. Transfer the mixture to the tube in several portions, through a funnel with a wide stem, pressing it down with the packing rod. Scrub the beaker with three further quantities, each of 0·5 g, of Celite 545, transferring each portion to the tube and pressing down. Wipe the inside of the beaker with a plug of cotton wool to remove all final traces of Celite and push the plug slowly down on to the top of the sample layer, ensuring that any particles of Celite adhering to the sides of the tube are retained by the cotton wool. (The over-all height of the column should be 120–150 mm.) Continue as described below under 'Separation of digitoxin'.

Digitoxin Tablets. Thoroughly mix an amount of powdered sample containing about 2 mg of digitoxin with 2 ml of water in a beaker. Add 4 ml of formamide, stir thoroughly, cover the beaker with a watch-glass and heat on a water-bath for twenty minutes with frequent stirring. Cool, add 2 ml of water and about 8 g of Celite 545 and stir thoroughly until the mass appears uniform and does not adhere to the beaker. Proceed as described above for Digitoxin Injection, beginning with the words 'Transfer the mixture to the tube. . . .'.

Separation of digitoxin: Elute the digitoxin with a mixture of 3 volumes of benzene and 1 volume of chloroform, washing the wall of the tube with the solvent mixture. Collect the eluate, at a rate not exceeding 4 ml per minute, in a 250-ml graduated flask until nearly 250 ml has been collected. Wash the stem of the tube with a stream of chloroform and dilute to volume with chloroform.

Colorimetric determination: Transfer a 25-ml aliquot of the eluate to a 50-ml Erlenmeyer flask and evaporate the solvents on a water-bath under a jet of air. Moisten the residue with about 0·5 ml of 95 per cent ethanol and again evaporate. Cool the flask, add 5·0 ml of 95 per cent ethanol and allow to stand for fifteen minutes at 25° ± 3° with occasional shaking.

Transfer a 5-ml aliquot of the standard digitoxin solution to a second 50-ml Erlenmeyer flask and 5 ml of 95 per cent ethanol to a third similar flask to serve as a blank. Add 3·0 ml of the alkaline picrate reagent to each flask and mix by swirling, maintaining the temperature at 25° ± 3° and protecting the mixture from intense light. After sixteen minutes determine the extinction of the solutions in the first and second flasks relative to the blank at 495 mμ and calculate the digitoxin content of the sample by comparison.

DIGOXIN, $C_{41}H_{64}O_{14}$, Mol. Wt. 781·0

Digoxin is a crystalline glycoside obtained from *Digitalis lanata*, and no assay is required in the standard of the *B.P.* For the injection and tablets, however, application is made of the Keller-Kiliani reaction. The *U.S.P.* assays Digoxin by an application of the *m*-nitrobenzene reaction and a similar method, based on the work of Honk *et al.*[5] has been adopted by the *A.O.A.C.* For the assay of digoxin injection and tablets the *U.S.P.* also uses the Keller-Kiliani method. Suitable examples of the *m*-dinitrobenzene and Keller-Kiliani methods are given below:

A.O.A.C. m-dinitrobenzene method

Reagent:

Alkaline dinitrobenzene solution. Mix 1 ml of a 10 per cent aqueous solution of tetramethylammonium hydroxide with 140 ml of dry ethanol, titrate a portion of the solution with 0·01N hydrochloric acid to methyl red and adjust the remaining solution to a concentration of 0·008N by dilution with dry ethanol. Immediately before use mix 40 ml of this solution with 60 ml of a 5 per cent solution of *m*-dinitrobenzene in benzene.

Standard:

Standard digoxin solution. Dissolve 25·0 mg of *U.S.P.* Digoxin Reference Standard in hot 95 per cent ethanol, cool and dilute to exactly 100 ml with 95 per cent ethanol. Dilute a 10-ml aliquot of this solution to 100 ml with 95 per cent ethanol in a graduated flask.

Preparation of sample:

Crystalline Digoxin. Prepare a solution in 95 per cent ethanol containing 125 μg of the sample per ml. Pipette 10 ml into a separator, add 50 ml of water and 1 ml of 2N sulphuric acid and extract with three 30-ml portions of chloroform. Wash each extract in a second separator by shaking with 10 ml of water and 1 g of powdered, anion–cation exchange resin (Rohm and Haas Amberlite MB-1, analytical grade, indicator-free, has been found satisfactory) and filter through a plug of cotton wool, previously rinsed with chloroform, into a 100-ml graduated flask. Dilute to volume with chloroform and mix (Assay Solution).

Elixirs and Injections. Pipette a volume of sample containing 1·25 mg of digoxin into a separator and proceed as described above under 'Crystalline Digoxin', beginning with the words 'add 50 ml of water. . . .'.

Tablets. Weigh accurately into a 100-ml beaker an amount of powdered tablets containing 1·25 mg of digoxin. Add 10 ml of 95 per cent ethanol, cover with a watch-glass and heat just to boiling-point on a water-bath. Simmer for twenty minutes with frequent stirring. Cool and transfer quantitatively to a separator with the aid of 30 ml of chloroform and 50 ml of water. Add 1 ml of 2N sulphuric acid and proceed as described above under 'Crystalline Digoxin', beginning with the words 'extract with three 30-ml portions of chloroform. . . .'.

Determination: Pipette 5 ml of standard digoxin solution and 10 ml of Assay Solution into similar flasks and evaporate the solvents on a water-bath under a jet of air. Cool and to each flask add 5 ml of freshly-prepared alkaline dinitrobenzene reagent. Allow to stand for five minutes at a temperature not exceeding 30°, with frequent mixing. Determine the extinction of each solution, relative to a reagent blank, at 620 mμ at one-minute intervals using matched 1-cm cells: mg digoxin in Assay Solution = 1·25 A/A^1, where A is the maximum extinction of the aliquot of the Assay Solution and A^1 is the maximum extinction of the standard.

U.S.P. m-dinitrobenzene method

Reagent: Alkaline dinitrobenzene reagent. Exactly as *A.O.A.C.*

Standard: Standard digoxin solution. Exactly as *A.O.A.C.*

Determination: Transfer 5 ml of a solution in 95 per cent ethanol containing 25 μg of sample per ml (prepared in exactly the same way as the standard solution) to a flask and evaporate to dryness on a water-bath under a jet of air. Cool the residue in a vacuum desiccator for fifteen minutes. Add 5·0 ml of alkaline dinitrobenzene solution and allow to stand, with frequent swirling, for five minutes at a temperature not exceeding 30°. Determine the extinction of the solution at 620 mμ, using matched 1-cm cells with a reagent blank in the comparison cell, repeating the measurement at one-minute intervals until a maximum reading is obtained. Calculate the digoxin content by comparison with the maximum extinction obtained by treating 5 ml of standard digoxin solution in exactly the same way as described for the sample solution.

Keller-Kiliani method

Reagent: Acid-ferric chloride reagent. Mix 60 ml of glacial acetic acid with 5 ml of concentrated sulphuric acid, add 1 ml of a 9 per cent solution of ferric chloride ($FeCl_3,6H_2O$) and cool.

Standard: Standard digoxin solution. Exactly as *A.O.A.C.*

Preparation of sample solution:

Digoxin Injection. Pipette a volume of sample equivalent to about 2·5 mg of digoxin into a separator. Dilute with water to 50 ml, add 1 ml of dilute sulphuric acid and extract with 35 ml of a mixture of 5 volumes of chloroform and 1 volume of *n*-propanol. Run the lower layer into a second separator, wash with 5 ml of water and filter, through a plug of cotton wool previously rinsed with chloroform, into a 100-ml graduated flask. Repeat the extraction and washing procedure with two 30-ml portions of the chloroform/*n*-propanol mixture, dilute the combined extracts to volume with methanol and mix.

Digoxin Tablets. Weigh an amount of powdered sample containing about 2·5 mg of digoxin into a small beaker. Add 5 ml of boiling *n*-propanol, stir vigorously, and allow to cool for twenty minutes, stirring frequently. Transfer quantitatively to a separator, with 30 ml of chloroform and 20 ml of water, add 1 ml of dilute sulphuric acid and shake. Run the lower layer into a second separator, wash with 5 ml of water and filter, through a plug of cotton wool previously rinsed with chloroform, into a 100-ml graduated flask. Repeat the extraction and washing procedure, using two 30-ml quantities of a mixture of 5 volumes of chloroform and 1 volume of *n*-propanol, dilute the combined extracts to volume with methanol and mix.

Determination: Pipette 10 ml of the sample solution and 10 ml of the standard digoxin solution into separate flasks and treat the contents of each flask, respectively, as follows. Just evaporate the solvents on a water-bath under a jet of air and cool the residue in a vacuum desiccator for fifteen minutes. Add 5·0 ml of the acid-ferric chloride reagent, stir with a glass rod, and allow to stand, protected from light, for ten minutes at a temperature not exceeding 30°, stirring frequently. Filter, if necessary, through fine glass wool and determine the extinction, relative to a reagent blank at 590 mμ, using matched 1-cm cells and repeating the measurement at two-minute intervals until a maximum reading is obtained. Calculate the digoxin content of the sample by comparison of the maximum extinction of the sample solution with that of the standard.

Injection of Digoxin, *B.P.* Contains 0·025 per cent w/v of digoxin.

Evaporate 20 ml on a water-bath and dry the residue at 105° for fifteen minutes. Add 5 ml of a mixture of 65 volumes of chloroform and 35 volumes of methanol and dilute to 25 ml with glacial acetic acid (solution A). Dissolve 0·20 g of finely powdered digoxin *B.P.*, 0·58 g of citric acid and 1·43 g of anhydrous sodium phosphate in sufficient glacial acetic acid to produce 100 ml. To 5 ml of this solution, add 10 ml of the chloroform/methanol mixture and dilute to 50 ml with glacial acetic acid (solution B). To 10 ml of solution A add 20 ml of acid-ferric chloride solution (glacial acetic acid containing 2 per cent v/v of concentrated sulphuric acid and 0·005 per cent w/v $FeCl_3$). Allow to stand for one hour in a stoppered flask and compare the extinction of this solution at

590 mμ with that produced by treating 10 ml of solution B in a similar manner.

Tablets of Digoxin, *B.P.* Usually contain 0·25 mg of digoxin.

To a quantity of powdered sample containing about 5 mg of digoxin add 5·0 ml of chloroform/methanol mixture and 20 ml of glacial acetic acid and shake continuously for one hour. Allow to stand and filter the supernatant liquid through a sintered-glass filter (No. 4), rejecting the first few ml of filtrate. Dilute 5 ml of filtrate to 25 ml with the acid-ferric chloride solution and allow to stand for one and a half hours. Compare the extinction of this solution at 590 mμ with that of a solution prepared as follows: To 5 ml of a 0·20 per cent solution of digoxin *B.P.* add 10 ml of chloroform/methanol mixture and sufficient glacial acetic acid to produce 50 ml. Dilute 5 ml of this solution to 25 ml with the acid-ferric chloride solution (described under Injection of Digoxin) and allow to stand for one and a half hours.

1. GOLD, H., *Federation Proc.*, 1944, **3,** 72.
2. GOLD, H., *et al.*, *J. Pharmacol.*, 1941, **73,** 212.
3. BRAUN, H. A., and LUSKY, L. M., *J. Pharmacol.*, 1948, **93,** 81.
4. BRAUN, H. A., and SIEGFRIED, A., *J. Amer. Pharm. Ass., Sci. Edn.*, 1947, **36,** 363.
5. HONK, A. E. H., ALEXANDER, T. G., and BANES, D., *J. Amer. Pharm. Ass., Sci. Edn.*, 1959, **48,** 317.

EFFERVESCENT GRANULES

A number of different types of effervescent granules were once official in the *B.P.C.* but although most of these have been deleted, products of this type are still very popular. The ingredients of principal therapeutic value are mixed with sodium bicarbonate and both tartaric and citric acids; sometimes sucrose is added.

The effervescent granules, as sampled, differ in composition from the formulæ for the original ingredients owing to interaction during preparation with consequent loss of part of the carbon dioxide; the chemical evaluation should be made by the determination of available carbon dioxide and all basic and acidic radicals; by simple calculation to the original formula the analyst will be able to judge if the preparation had been made with the correct proportions of ingredients.

No difficulty is experienced in determining the principal components, *viz.*, caffeine citrate, lithium citrate, magnesium sulphate, sodium phosphate and sodium sulphate. Each can be estimated by the methods described under the monographs on these substances.

Sodium bicarbonate may be calculated from the alkalinity of the ash unless lithium citrate or sodium phosphate is present. A determination of the lithium will enable the sodium to be calculated.

For lithium:

Dissolve about 7 g in water, avoiding loss during effervescence; evaporate to dryness in a platinum dish. Ignite sufficiently to char all organic matter, dissolve as much as possible in hot water and filter. Ignite the filter and the insoluble matter to a white ash and dissolve in dilute hydrochloric acid; add to the main bulk and make the whole slightly acid with hydrochloric acid. Evaporate to dryness and continue by extraction with acetone as under Lithium (p. 28). $Li_2SO_4 \times 1{\cdot}710 = Li_3C_6H_5O_7{,}4H_2O$. If the residue is pulverised while still containing a trace of moisture and then dried completely, the dry residue is obtained in very fine powder.

By this method a yield equivalent to 98·5 per cent of the lithium citrate taken was obtained (after correcting for the purity of the original lithium salt) from a standard preparation of Effervescent Lithium Citrate. The flame photometric method can also be applied.

Citric and tartaric acids may be determined separately with considerable accuracy. The methods given under the monographs on these acids were compared when the acids were present together as in the two common effervescent mixtures, Effervescent Sodium Sulphate, *B.P.C.* 1949, and Effervescent Magnesium Sulphate, *B.P.C.* 1949 (the latter containing sucrose). The results obtained are recorded in Table 17.

TABLE 17

		TARTARIC ACID			CITRIC ACID: LAMPITT AND ROOKE METHOD
		A.O.A.C. METHOD	HARTMANN AND HILLIG METHOD	KING METHOD	
Effervescent Sodium Sulphate (standard preparation).	Added	24·00			21·00
	Found	23·56	24·14	24·30	20·94
Effervescent Magnesium Sulphate (standard preparation).	Added	19·00			12·50
	Found	20·94	*	19·02	12·51

* No result could be obtained, even with the addition of potassium acetate; a large precipitate was formed, but it was not potassium acid tartrate, the titration figure being negligible.

It will be seen from the results that, considering the difficulties of the problem, exceptionally good figures can be obtained by King's method for tartaric acid, and Lampitt and Rooke's method for citric acid, and they are recommended for any similar case.

Sucrose in effervescent preparations cannot readily be determined polarimetrically, since the optical rotation of *d*-tartaric acid is variable, depending on concentration; it is preferable to use the volumetric method given under Sugars.

The determination of **carbon dioxide** in effervescent granules is made by direct absorption. Gravimetric determination is preferable in laboratories where a considerable number of estimations of carbon dioxide are made, since, although the assembling of the apparatus is time consuming, when once set up a considerable saving of time is possible over other methods of determination:

The train consists of a series of stoppered U-tubes and Geissler bulbs as under:

(*a*) U-tube, containing soda-lime to clean indrawn air.
(*b*) A small separating funnel containing dilute sulphuric acid.
(*c*) A wide-mouthed resistance flask closed by a rubber stopper into which is fitted the stem of (*b*) and an outlet tube to
(*d*) A Geissler bulb, containing concentrated sulphuric acid to dry the evolved gas.
(*e*) A U-tube containing glass beads and concentrated sulphuric acid for further drying.
(*f*) A U-tube containing copper-pumice (pumice saturated with a 20 per cent solution of copper sulphate and dried).
(*g*) A U-tube containing concentrated sulphuric acid.
(*h*) A weighed absorption tube containing 'Carbosorb' and about 1 in. of fused calcium chloride granules at the outlet end.
(*i*) A U-tube containing glass beads and concentrated sulphuric acid.
(*j*) An aspirator.

For a determination weigh into the dry flask (*c*) sufficient sample to evolve about 0·1 to 0·15 g of carbon dioxide. Fit the flask on to the rubber stopper, open all taps except (*b*) and commence aspiration. Slowly add the acid from (*b*) and when all has been added close the tap in (*b*) and gradually heat the solution in the flask just to the boiling-point by means of a spirit lamp. Then open (*b*) and aspirate slowly for about twenty minutes. Close the taps in (*h*) and re-weigh. The gain in weight is equivalent to the evolved carbon dioxide.

When not in use, close all taps in the apparatus: frequently renew the acid in (*d*).

Hepburn[1] designed a simple apparatus for the volumetric determination of carbon dioxide, in which the gas, completely evolved from solution under vacuum, is absorbed in baryta water and the residual baryta titrated to phenolphthalein with 0·1N oxalic acid. Standard hydrochloric acid was found to give high results compared with oxalic acid. The time required for absorption was twelve to twenty-four hours. This method has been adopted by the *B.P.C.* for Effervescent Granules.

Edwards, Parkes and Nanji[2] improved the method by a modification of the apparatus, in which the carbon dioxide was made actually to bubble through the baryta solution, thus decreasing the time of absorption to four hours. They found phenol-thymolphthalein (pH 8·3 to 11·0) to be an excellent indicator for the titration of the residual baryta with 0·1N oxalic acid.

The apparatus consists of a tall thick-walled glass vessel, such as a 400-ml absorption tower, fitted with a rubber cork through which passes a tap funnel and a glass tap. The funnel stem runs just through the cork of a stout-walled boiling-tube, of about 50-ml capacity, contained in the tower, and a delivery tube from just inside this cork leads almost to the bottom of the outer vessel.

Weigh a suitable quantity of the sample into the boiling-tube and place 50 ml of 0·1N barium hydroxide and about 50 ml of carbon dioxide-free water (to increase the volume of absorbing liquid) in the outer vessel. Make the apparatus air-tight and then evacuate for about ten minutes by means of suction through the glass tap. Close the tap and run in 20 ml of N hydrochloric acid very gradually from the tap funnel while the apparatus is gently shaken. Allow absorption to continue for four hours with occasional shaking of the apparatus. Then destroy the vacuum by gradually opening the tap of the funnel, and remove the bung and attached tubes, rinsing their surfaces with a little water. Titrate the residual baryta with 0·1N oxalic acid, phenol-thymolphthalein being used as indicator. 1 ml 0·1N = 0·0022 g CO_2.

The use of 0·2N baryta and phenol-thymolphthalein as indicator are improvements on the Hepburn method which can be incorporated in an adaptation, by which the whole apparatus can be placed in an incubator at 37° for three or four hours for more rapid absorption.

The apparatus consists of a thick-walled test-tube 8 × $1\frac{3}{16}$ inches, the side of which is pierced by a hole of about $\frac{1}{4}$-inch diameter, situated 2 inches from the top. The upper end of the tube is encased in a sleeve of rubber doubled back on to the upper edge. The dimensions of the tube are such that they allow it to pass through close to the sides of the neck of an outer vessel containing an interior ledge, against which the rubber can be compressed to form a seal. The test-tube is fitted with a rubber cork through which passes a length of glass tubing having a length of rubber tubing and adjustable pinch-clip attached.

Alternatively the test-tube described above may be supported in the neck of a wide-mouthed bottle of suitable dimensions by means of a wide band of stout rubber tubing drawn over the outside of the bottle, the tube being clamped by a metal band.

Place sufficient material to yield about 0·1 g of carbon dioxide in the test-tube and 50 ml of approximately 0·2N barium hydroxide (in 10 per cent sugar solution) in the outer vessel. Press the rubber firmly against the ledge of the outer vessel and apply suction through the glass tube. When the apparatus is evacuated, close the pinch-clip and gradually introduce 10 ml of dilute hydrochloric acid. Allow the absorption to continue to completion by standing the apparatus in a warm place overnight or at 35° to 40° for four hours. Then restore normal pressure and remove the test-tube, washing the outer surface with a little water. Titrate the residual baryta with 0·2N oxalic acid using phenol-thymolphthalein as indicator. Similarly titrate 50 ml of the barium hydroxide solution and calculate the difference to carbon dioxide. 1 ml 0·2N = 0·0044 g CO_2.

A still more rapid modification is recommended by Cornell,[3] which only requires one- to three-quarters of an hour for the complete evolution of the gas. The apparatus consists of a large and a small Wurtz flask; the larger carries a tap funnel through a rubber stopper, the smaller flask carries a glass tap through a similar stopper. The side arm of the larger flask is inclined to form a straight line with the side arm of the smaller and they are joined by pressure tubing.

Weigh the substance into the larger flask, place 50 ml of 0·25N barium hydroxide in the smaller and exhaust to about 20 mm pressure. Gradually add dilute hydrochloric acid through the tap funnel and, if preferred, place the bulb of the larger flask in a water-bath at 60° to 70° and, similarly, the smaller bulb in a cooling bath. After absorption, titrate the residual baryta as above.

Illing and Whittle[4] modify the use of baryta by absorption of the carbon dioxide in standard sodium hydroxide and addition of excess barium chloride before titration to phenolphthalein. A different apparatus is also described.

1. Hepburn, J. R. I., *Analyst*, 1926, **51**, 622.
2. Edwards, F. W., Parkes, E. B., and Nanji, H. R., *Analyst*, 1935, **60**, 814.
3. Cornell, G. W., *Analyst*, 1936, **51**, 756.
4. Illing, E. T., and Whittle, E. G., *Analyst*, 1939, **64**, 667.

EPHEDRA

The total alkaloids present in ephedra herb amount to about 1·25 to 2 per cent of which about 70 per cent is (—)-ephedrine, the remainder consisting of *pseudo*-ephedrine with small quantities of closely related alkaloids.

Of the methods which have been published, that due to Krishna and Ghose[1] has been recommended by Peyer and Gstirner[2] for its simplicity and uniform results. Methods involving final extraction and evaporation of the base with chloroform should be avoided as ephedrine base reacts on standing with, or evaporation from, this solvent to form the hydrochloride. The *B.P.C.* 1954 adopted the method of Krishna and Ghose with small modifications, which make it more accurate and give results from 15 to 20 per cent higher. Their method has also been recommended as standard by the Analytical Methods Committee of the *S.A.C.*[3]

Shake 20 g frequently during five minutes, in No. 40 powder, with 200 ml of a mixture of 1 volume of chloroform and 3 volumes of ether; add 10 ml of dilute ammonia solution and 1 g of anhydrous sodium carbonate; shake at frequent intervals for four hours, and allow to stand overnight. Transfer to a percolator and continue the percolation, first with 100 ml of the ether-chloroform mixture and then with ether, until the alkaloid is completely extracted; shake the combined percolates with successive portions of 40, 30, 20 and 20 ml of 0·33N hydrochloric acid; to the combined and filtered acid extracts, add N sodium hydroxide until only slightly acid, then add 10 g of anhydrous sodium carbonate and sufficient sodium chloride to saturate the liquid, and shake until dissolved. Extract the alkaline liquid with four successive portions of 60, 50, 50 and 30 ml of ether, and then with 25-ml portions of ether until the extraction of the alkaloid is complete (usually five shakings are sufficient). Allow the combined ether extracts to stand until clear, and decant through a filter into a beaker; warm, and pour off the ether from any crystals which may separate; evaporate the ether to a volume of about 10 ml and then allow the residual solvent to evaporate spontaneously. Dissolve the residue in an excess of 0·1N hydrochloric acid, add 20 ml of water, and titrate the excess of acid with 0·1N sodium hydroxide, using methyl red as indicator. 1 ml of 0·1N hydrochloric acid is equivalent to 0·01652 g of total alkaloids, calculated as $C_{10}H_{15}ON$.

This method can be modified for determination of *l*-ephedrine, provided sufficient of the herb is taken for examination. 100 g is extracted with suitable volumes of reagents, the final acid extractions being evaporated to dryness, redissolved in dilute hydrochloric acid, cleaned with a little activated charcoal, filtered and evaporated. The residue, after treatment with small quantities of dry chloroform, in which *l*-ephedrine hydrochloride is insoluble, is dried at 100° and weighed.

EPHEDRINE, $(C_{10}H_{15}ON)_2,H_2O$, Mol. Wt. 348·5

The alkaloidal base is very volatile and to determine it gravimetrically requires considerable care; the following precautions are necessary:

To an aqueous acid solution containing approximately 0·1 g of alkaloid, the volume of solution being kept low, add excess of solution of ammonia and extract with liberal portions of ether. As the alkaloid is very soluble in water, do not wash the ether extracts but dry them with anhydrous sodium sulphate before evaporating carefully. Dry the alkaloid in a desiccator. As a check after weighing the alkaloid, titrate as usual, using methyl red as indicator. 1 ml 0·1N = 0·01652 g of ephedrine; ephedrine × 1·221 = **ephedrine hydrochloride,** $C_{10}H_{15}ON,HCl$, Mol. Wt. 201·7; ephedrine × 1·297 = **ephedrine sulphate,** $(C_{10}H_{15}ON)_2,H_2SO_4$, Mol. Wt. 428·6. Bromocresol green (Peterson[4]) and bromothymol blue (Moraw[5]) have also been recommended as suitable indicators.

Alternatively, extract the ammoniacal solution of the alkaloid with ether as above, washing each extract with the same 1 ml of water, evaporate to about 10 ml, add excess of 0·1N acid and dilute with water. Evaporate off the residual ether and titrate the excess of acid with 0·1N potassium hydroxide using methyl red as indicator.

In N sulphuric acid, ephedrine hydrochloride has absorption maxima at 251·5, 256·6 and 262·5 mμ, E(1 per cent, 1 cm) = 7·35, 9·40 and 7·25 respectively.

The volatility of ephedrine is a property which is used for assay of galenicals containing the alkaloid or one of its salts and the Analytical Methods Committee of the *S.A.C.*[3] has recommended this procedure for the determination of ephedrine in nasal sprays. The recommended method may find application for determining ephedrine in other preparations provided no other volatile base is present.

Place a suitable weight of the spray, containing about 0·15 to 0·2 g of ephedrine in a steam distillation flask of about 300-ml capacity, fitted with an efficient splash-head. Add 10 g of sodium chloride, 15 ml of 20 per cent sodium hydroxide solution and a little pumice or broken glass. Connect the flask to a condenser and steam distil into a receiver containing 25 ml of 0·05N sulphuric acid. After distillation has begun adjust the volume of the aqueous phase in the flask to between 15 and 30 ml by the application of heat from a small burner and maintain it at this volume. Some sodium chloride should remain undissolved. When about 700 ml of distillate has been collected titrate the excess of acid with 0·05N sodium hydroxide, using methyl red as indicator. Collect a further 50 ml of distillate in a fresh receiver containing a small quantity of water and 1 ml of 0·05N hydrochloric acid and titrate with 0·05N sodium hydroxide. If necessary, continue the distillation until no further alkaloid is removed. Carry out a blank determination using the same quantities of reagents and collecting the same volume of distillate, and make the appropriate correction. Each ml of 0·05N hydrochloric acid neutralised by the volatile base = 0·00826 g of anhydrous ephedrine.

According to Welsh[6] ephedrine can be acetylated quantitatively in aqueous solution to yield a neutral *N*-acetyl derivative which can be extracted with chloroform. The conditions are similar to those employed in the conversion of *p*-phenetidin into phenacetin.

To a solution containing about 0·15 g of ephedrine in 10 ml of water, add sufficient sodium bicarbonate to saturate the solution. Then add a total of 1 ml of acetic anhydride in three approximately equal portions, shaking vigorously after each addition and using due care in releasing pressure developed by carbon dioxide evolution. Allow the reaction mixture to stand fifteen minutes, acidify carefully with dilute sulphuric acid and extract the acetyl-ephedrine immediately with 15-ml portions of chloroform. Wash each extract successively with a dilute solution of sodium bicarbonate, evaporate, dry at 105°, cool and weigh. $C_{12}H_{17}O_2N \times 0{\cdot}9731$ = ephedrine hydrochloride.

Bisulphite interferes with the acetylation and must be eliminated first by addition of a slight excess of iodine in acid solution, followed by decolorisation with thiosulphate. Procaine will also acetylate under the above conditions but forms a basic derivative which can be extracted in alkaline solution with chloroform as a colourless, viscous oil.

Sanchez[7] determined ephedrine by its reaction with alkaline iodine solution at 50° to form iodoform and titration of excess iodine in acid solution. Application of this method to standard solutions of ephedrine hydrochloride has given recoveries within ± 3 per cent of theory. However, when attempting to apply it to the determination of ephedrine hydrochloride in cough mixtures it has proved of no value since gross interference from other alkaloids present (such as codeine and ethylmorphine) would necessitate preliminary separation of ephedrine, probably by steam distillation, and in such a distillate ephedrine can be determined more rapidly and precisely by acidimetric titration.

The identity test of the *B.P.* has been modified for tablets and injections by Allport and Jones[8] to give quantitative results. The colour is stable when extracted by *cyclo*hexane and deeper than in ethereal solution. Lactose interferes because of its reducing action on copper sulphate.

Make an aqueous solution of the tablets so that each ml may be expected to contain between 1 and 1·5 mg of ephedrine base. Transfer 5 ml of this solution to a small separator, add 1 ml of dilute solution of ammonia and 2 ml of methylene chloride (in which lactose is completely insoluble). Shake, allow to separate, draw off the lower layer into another separator and wash with 2 ml of saturated aqueous solution of sodium chloride; after separation, run off the methylene chloride into a dry stoppered weighing bottle. Extract the ammoniacal mixture in the first separator with two further successive 2-ml portions of methylene chloride and, after washing each extract with the same saturated solution of sodium chloride already in the second separator, transfer to the weighing bottle. Add to the mixed methylene chloride extracts 1 ml of a 1 per cent solution of benzoic acid in methylene chloride (to prevent volatilisation of the base) and evaporate the whole to dryness over a boiling water-bath. Add to the residue exactly 1 ml of water, warm gently until solution is effected, allow to cool; add 0·1 ml of a 10 per cent aqueous solution of copper sulphate and 2 ml of a 20 per cent aqueous solution of sodium hydroxide (both of which should have been recently prepared) and mix; add 3 ml of *cyclo*hexane, shake vigorously, transfer to a dry test-tube and allow to separate. Measure the extinction value at 515 mμ of the upper layer, using a 1-cm cell and *cyclo*hexane in the comparison cell. Prepare a calibration graph over the range 4 to 8 mg of ephedrine for calculation of the result.

In order to determine ephedrine in injections, dilute with water so that each ml may be expected to contain between 4 and 8 mg of base and apply the colour test described above to 1 ml of the dilution, commencing with the addition of 0·1 ml of copper sulphate solution.

Elixir of Ephedrine, *B.P.C.* Contains 0·46 per cent w/v of ephedrine hydrochloride in compound syrup.

The standard distillation method given above is applicable for the determination of ephedrine using 50 ml of elixir. In comparison, the *A.O.A.C.*[9] method gave somewhat more erratic recoveries but it is quite a convenient method since it is carried out on a much smaller sample of material.

To 10 ml add 10 ml of water, make slightly alkaline to litmus paper with 20 per cent sodium hydroxide solution, add a further 0·5 ml and extract with six or more successive quantities, each of 20 ml, of ether until extraction is complete. Extract the combined ether extracts with 5 ml of dilute sulphuric acid followed by four successive quantities, each of 5 ml, of water and then wash the combined extracts with 3 ml of chloroform and reject the chloroform. Make the aqueous extracts alkaline to litmus paper with 20 per cent sodium hydroxide solution, add a further 0·5 ml and extract with six successive quantities, each of 15 ml, of chloroform, reserving the extracts. Extract with two further quantities, each of 15 ml, of chloroform, filter these extracts through cotton wool, add 0·1 ml of 32 per cent w/w hydrochloric acid and evaporate to dryness on a water-bath under a jet of air; if a crystalline residue is produced combine it with the reserved extracts with the aid of methanol and repeat the extraction. Filter the reserved extracts through cotton wool, wash the filter with chloroform and to the combined filtrate and washings add 0·2 ml of 32 per cent w/w hydrochloric acid. Evaporate to 2 ml on a water-bath under a jet of air, continue heating continuously without the air jet until the odour of hydrochloric acid is no longer detectable and the residue appears dry; dry the residue of ephedrine hydrochloride for thirty minutes at 110° and weigh.

Mixture of Belladonna and Ephedrine for Infants, *B.P.C.* Contains 0·23 per cent w/v of ephedrine hydrochloride. The ephedrine may be determined by the extraction method given under Elixir of Ephedrine, using 20 ml of mixture.

Nasal Drops of Ephedrine, *B.P.C.* Contain 0·91 per cent w/v of ephedrine hydrochloride. The determination of ephedrine follows the standard distillation method given above using 20 ml of sample.

Tablets of Ephedrine Hydrochloride, *B.P.* Contain ½ grain of ephedrine hydrochloride per tablet.

Although the standard distillation method can be used, it is unnecessarily lengthy. Direct non-aqueous titration with 0·05N perchloric acid to crystal violet (see p. 792) of about 0·15 g of powdered tablets in the presence of mercuric acetate is possible or a physical assay can be used.

Dissolve five tablets in N sulphuric acid and make up to 250 ml. Measure the maximum extinction of a 1-cm layer at about 256·5 mμ using N sulphuric acid as a blank. Calculate the amount of ephedrine hydrochloride in each tablet.

Commercially, preparations are encountered with anhydrous ephedrine, in an oily base, usually containing eucalyptol, camphor and menthol. The ephedrine in such preparations can readily be determined by mixing a suitable volume with glacial acetic acid and toluene and carrying out a direct non-aqueous titration with perchloric acid in glacial acetic acid.

Horák and Gašperík[10] used a method for the determination of ephedrine based on the liberation, by alkaline hydrolysis, of methylamine, which can be determined on the semi-micro scale in the Kjeldahl apparatus and the authors claimed good results when this method was used for the determination of ephedrine hydrochloride in pharmaceutical injections and tablets.

MEPHENTERMINE SULPHATE, $(C_{11}H_{17}N)_2,H_2SO_4,2H_2O$, Mol. Wt. 460·6.

Assayed by base extraction of about 0·4 g with ether from sodium chloride solution after addition of excess of sodium hydroxide, washing the combined ether extracts, adding excess 0·1N hydrochloric acid, removing ether and back-titrating with 0·1N sodium hydroxide to methyl red. 1 ml 0·1N = 0·02123 g anhydrous.

METHOXAMINE HYDROCHLORIDE, $C_{11}H_{17}O_3N,HCl$, Mol. Wt. 247·7

Assayed by non-aqueous titration with 0·1N perchloric acid in the presence of mercuric acetate (see p. 792). 1 ml 0·1N perchloric acid = 0·02477 g.

NAPHAZOLINE HYDROCHLORIDE, $C_{14}H_{14}N_2,HCl$, Mol. Wt. 246·7, and **NAPHAZOLINE NITRATE,** $C_{14}H_{14}N_2,HNO_3$, Mol. Wt. 273·3.

Both assayed by extraction of about 0·3 g of the base from sodium hydroxide solution with chloroform which is washed and evaporated. The residue is dissolved in excess of 0·1N hydrochloric acid and back-titrated with 0·1N sodium hydroxide to methyl red indicator. 1 ml 0·1N = 0·02467 g of the hydrochloride and 0·02733 g of the nitrate.

PHENYLEPHRINE HYDROCHLORIDE, $C_9H_{13}O_2N,HCl$, Mol Wt. 203·7

Phenylephrine hydrochloride can either be determined as in the *B.P.* by addition of excess of 0·1N bromine in the presence of hydrochloric acid and back-titration with 0·1N thiosulphate after fifteen minutes' standing and addition of potassium iodide, 1 ml 0·1N bromine = 0·003395 g or, preferably, by non-aqueous titration with 0·1N perchloric acid in the presence of mercuric acetate (see p. 792) to oracet blue indicator. 1 ml 0·1N perchloric acid = 0·02037 g.

Phenylephrine hydrochloride in preparations, such as nasal sprays, may be determined by a modification[11] of the 4-aminophenazone method (see p. 514). The procedure to be used differs in some important respects from the general method and is, therefore, given below in detail:

Reagent:

4-Aminophenazone solution. Shake 0·5 g of 4-aminophenazone with 100 ml of water and, if necessary, filter. This solution is stable for two to three days if stored protected from light.

Determination:

Pipette a volume of sample containing 0·03 to 1·20 mg of phenylephrine hydrochloride into a 100-ml graduated flask and add 5 ml of freshly prepared 2 per cent potassium ferricyanide solution followed by 5 ml of 4-aminophenazone solution, mixing after each addition. Then add 1 ml of M sodium bicarbonate, make up to volume with water and allow to stand for fifteen minutes.

Prepare a blank solution by carrying out the determination described above omitting the sample.

Measure the extinction of the sample solution, relative to the blank solution, at 500 mμ, using 1-cm cells. Read the concentration of phenylephrine hydrochloride from a calibration curve previously obtained by treating suitable quantities of a standard solution of phenylephrine hydrochloride in water, covering the range 0 to 1·2 mg of phenylephrine hydrochloride, as described above beginning with the words 'add 5 ml of freshly prepared 2 per cent potassium ferricyanide solution . . .' and plotting mg of phenylephrine hydrochloride against extinction.

In our hands, measurement of the extinction after thirty minutes' standing gave more reproducible results.

1. Krishna, S., and Ghose, T. P., *J. Soc. Chem. Ind.*, 1929, **48**, 671.
2. Peyer, W., and Gstirner, F., *Pharm. Ztg.*, 1931, **76**, 1440.
3. *Analyst*, 1948, 73, 312.
4. Peterson, J. B., *Ind. Eng. Chem.*, 1928, **20**, 388.
5. Moraw, H. O., *J. Amer. Pharm. Ass.*, 1928, **17**, 430.
6. Welsh, L. H., *J. Amer. Pharm. Ass., Sci. Edn.*, 1947, **36**, 373; 1952, **41**, 545.
7. Sanchez, J. A., *J. Pharm. Chim.*, 1935, [viii], **22**, 489.
8. Allport, N. L., and Jones, N. R., *Quart. J. Pharm.*, 1942, **15**, 238.
9. *A.O.A.C.*, 1960, p. 473.
10. Horák, F., and Gašperík, J., *Chem. Zvesti*, 1957, **11**, 558.
11. Hiskey, C. F., and Levin, N., *J. Pharm. Sci.*, 1961, **50**, 393.

ERGOT

The assay of ergot has concerned analysts for many years and the continuous steady stream of papers devoted to the subject indicate that a confident solution to the problem has not yet been found. However, little ergot is now used other than for extraction of the alkaloids by manufacturers.

The *B.P.C.* method, based upon the work of Hampshire and Page,[1] does not enjoy the confidence of the majority of workers in this field, particularly in its assay for water-soluble alkaloids. The *B.P.C.* method consists in mixing the dried fat-free drug with ammonia and anæsthetic ether and then extracting the alkaloids by continuous extraction with the latter solvent. Some acetone is added to the ethereal solution (this helps to prevent emulsions in the subsequent extraction) and the alkaloids are extracted with a 1 per cent solution of tartaric acid. Total alkaloids are determined by treating an aliquot portion of the acid solution with dimethylaminobenzaldehyde reagent (see below). Water-insoluble alkaloids are then determined in a second portion of the acid solution by extracting into anæsthetic ether after making alkaline with ammonia, and then back into tartaric acid solution again. Application of the colour reaction to this solution gives water-insoluble alkaloids. By subtraction of this figure from the total alkaloids and application of the appropriate factor, the percentage of water-soluble alkaloids, calculated as ergometrine, can be determined.

The colour reaction with dimethylaminobenzaldehyde, which is almost invariably used for determination of ergot alkaloids, was proposed by Smith.[2] It depends upon the production of a blue coloration when the reagent is mixed with an acidic solution of the alkaloids; the blue colour in the assay is due to the indole group in lysergic acid and the intensity of the colour is the same for equimolecular amounts of all the ergot alkaloids. It is essential that the ergot is entirely defatted and that recently distilled anæsthetic ether is used in the assay, as a trace of peroxide will render the test useless. Formerly ergotoxine ethanesulphonate was used as a standard material, but this has been recognised as a mixture and ergometrine maleate is now preferred.

Ergot, *B.P.C.*, is standardised to contain total alkaloids, minimum 0·19 per cent calculated as ergotamine, of which not less than 15·0 per cent consists of water-soluble alkaloids calculated as ergometrine. **Prepared ergot**, *B.P.C.*, deprived of fat and standardised to contain total alkaloids 0·18 to 0·20 per cent calculated as ergotamine, of which not less than 15·0 per cent consists of water-soluble alkaloids calculated as ergometrine. It must be noted that these standards for water-soluble alkaloids are dependent on the method of assay and lower figures must be expected if the *N.F.* method described below is used.

Ergot has been shown to be liable to rapid deterioration if kept under ordinary conditions of storage.

Foster, MacDonald and Jones[3] applied the principle of paper chromatography to the separation of ergot alkaloids and developed an approximate assay for ergometrine based on the fluorescence of developed chromatograms, compared visually with a series of standard spots prepared at the same time as the sample under test.

Comparison of the results showed that the *B.P.C.* process, in which water-soluble alkaloids are determined by difference, gave much higher figures for ergometrine than the chromatographic method. When some of the final tartaric acid extract obtained by the *B.P.C.* process was submitted to chromatographic analysis ergometrine and ergometrinine were detected and, in addition, lysergic and *iso*lysergic acids. Hence it was concluded that the use of boiling ether for extraction results in partial hydrolysis of the alkaloids with the production of lysergic acid, which is removed with the water-soluble alkaloids and estimated as ergometrine. The *B.P.C.* process therefore is not reliable for determination of the ergometrine content of the drug. The observation that boiling ether causes some destruction of alkaloid was recognised by Hampshire and Page.

Foster, MacDonald and Jones found their results closely comparable with those obtained by the method now included in the *N.F.* which is as follows:

Assay for total alkaloids. (Note: the assay of ergot must be conducted without exposure to daylight, and the alkaline solutions of the alkaloids must receive no more than the minimum necessary exposure to artificial light. The extractions should be timed in such a way that only the acid extracts are allowed to stand overnight, and these should be refrigerated at from 5° to 10° during such storage.) Transfer 10 g of the sample to a 250-ml separator and add 100 ml of a mixture prepared by combining 1 volume of a 10 per cent solution of strong ammonia in methanol with 9 volumes of chloroform (Note 1). Shake vigorously for five minutes, add 50 ml of chloroform and 4 ml of water and mix. When separation is complete filter the extract through glass wool into a flask suitable for rotary vacuum evaporation. Add 25 ml of the methanol-ammonia-chloroform mixture to the separator and shake for five minutes. Add 25 ml of chloroform, mix and, after separation, filter into the flask. Repeat the extraction with a further 25 ml of chloroform. Evaporate the combined extracts to dryness *in vacuo* at a temperature not over 40°. Dissolve the residue in ether and transfer to a 250-ml separator, using a total volume of 80 ml of ether. Wash the flask with 5 ml of 95 per cent ethanol and add the washing to the separator. Extract the alkaloids with four successive portions of 10, 10, 8 and 8 ml of approximately 0·2N sulphuric acid, washing each extract with the same 50 ml of ether in a second separator (Note 2). Filter each portion through a small cotton-wool plug, rinsing the plug with a little water following the last extraction, and collect the aqueous extracts in a 50-ml graduated flask. If at any time during the extraction the aqueous phase does not begin to settle free from emulsion within two to three minutes after shaking, add about 2 ml of 95 per cent ethanol and shake again. Repeat the ethanol additions as required but guard against using more than necessary. Dilute the combined extracts to 50 ml with water, stopper securely and mix. Dilute 5 ml of this solution (Note 3), representing 1 g of ergot, to 25 ml with water and save the remainder of the solution for the assay for ergometrine. To 10 ml of the diluted solution add, dropwise, with vigorous shaking in an ice-bath, 20 ml of *p*-dimethylaminobenzaldehyde solution [prepare as follows: dissolve 125 mg of *p*-dimethylaminobenzaldehyde in a cooled mixture of 65 ml of concentrated sulphuric acid and 35 ml of water and add 0·05 ml of a 9 per cent solution of ferric chloride ($FeCl_3,6H_2O$); the solution should be used within seven days] and allow to stand for thirty minutes. Determine the extinction relative to a blank consisting of 10 ml of water and 20 ml of *p*-dimethylaminobenzaldehyde solution, at 590 mμ using matched 1-cm cells. Express the concentration of total alkaloids as mg of ergotoxine in each g of ergot by comparing the reading with that produced by a solution of ergometrine maleate of such concentration that it will provide an extinction varying from that of the sample by not more than 50 per cent (usually 2 to 4 mg of ergometrine maleate per 100 ml); or from a calibration curve. (1 mg of ergometrine maleate = 1·370 mg of ergotoxine or 1·318 mg of ergotamine.)

Assay for ergometrine. Pipette 20 ml of the concentrated solution of total alkaloids, representing 4 g of ergot, into a 250-ml separator, add 30 ml of water and make slightly alkaline to phenolphthalein with strong ammonia. Extract the ergotoxine-like alkaloids with three successive 30-ml quantities of carbon tetrachloride, washing each extract with the same 20 ml of water in a second 250-ml separator. While making this extraction, completely drain each portion of carbon tetrachloride into the second separator, including any traces of emulsion that cannot be made to separate within fifteen or more minutes. Discard the carbon tetrachloride. Combine the aqueous solutions and extract the ergometrine without delay as follows: Add 40 ml of ether and sufficient sodium chloride to saturate the aqueous phase (about 21 g), and shake for five minutes or until the sodium chloride has completely dissolved. When settled, run off the aqueous phase into the second separator used in the previous extraction. Allow to stand for about five minutes longer, allowing time for the water adhering to the walls of the separator to collect, then run this off also. Pour the ether phase from the mouth of the separator through a cotton-wool plug, previously rinsed with ether, into a third 250-ml separator. Complete the extraction in the same manner, using three successive 30-ml quantities of ether and collecting the ether in the third separator. Extract the ergometrine from the combined ether solutions with a total of four successive 5-ml quantities of approximately 0·2N sulphuric acid, filtering each extract through a small cotton-wool plug into a 100-ml graduated flask. Rinse the plug with a little water, dilute the solution to volume with water, stopper securely and mix. To 10 ml of this solution add 20 ml of *p*-dimethylaminobenzaldehyde solution, mix thoroughly and allow to stand for thirty minutes. Determine the extinction, relative to a blank consisting of 10 ml of water and 20 ml of *p*-dimethylaminobenzaldehyde solution, at 590 mμ, using matched 1-cm cells. Express the concentration of ergometrine as mg of ergometrine maleate in each g of ergot by comparing the reading with that produced by a solution of ergometrine maleate having a concentration which varies from that of the sample by not more than 50 per cent (usually 3 to 5 mg of ergometrine maleate per 100 ml), or from a calibration curve. (1 mg of ergometrine maleate = 0·737 mg of ergometrine.)

Note 1. Chloroform is the best solvent for the alkaloids of ergot. 10 per cent methanol in chloroform is sufficient to render the ammonia solution miscible. The presence of only one liquid phase rather than two is preferable here.

Note 2. Sulphuric acid in dilute solution is a somewhat better solvent for the alkaloids of ergot than is tartaric acid, which was originally proposed.

Note 3. The solution of total alkaloids so obtained must be freshly mixed before taking an aliquot portion, as any traces of precipitate settling out probably contain appreciable amounts of the alkaloids present.

Liquid Extract of Ergot, *B.P.C.* 1954. Prepared by percolation of ergot with tartaric acid and diluted alcohol.

A method of assay based on the *N.F.* procedure above is as follows:

Assay for total alkaloids. Pipette 20 ml of the liquid extract of ergot into a 200-ml graduated flask containing 150 ml of acetone and 2 ml of strong ammonia solution, and mix. Dilute to volume with acetone and shake occasionally during thirty minutes. Filter exactly 100 ml of the liquid through a filter paper, collecting the filtrate in a 150-ml extraction flask. Wash the filter with acetone and add the washings to the flask.

Without delay evaporate the liquid to dryness *in vacuo* at a temperature not above 40°. Dissolve the residue in ether and transfer to a 250-ml separator, using a total volume of 80 ml of ether. Wash the flask with 5 ml of 95 per cent ethanol and add the washing to the separator. Acidify the mixture with 5 ml of approximately 0·2N sulphuric acid and shake. Wash the aqueous phase with 50 ml of ether in a second separator, filter through a small plug of cotton wool and collect in a 50-ml graduated flask. Complete the extraction in the same manner using three successive 8-ml quantities of approximately 0·2N sulphuric acid, collecting each extract in the graduated flask. Finally rinse the cotton-wool plug with a little water, dilute the solution to volume, stopper securely and mix. Proceed as directed in the *N.F.* assay for total alkaloids under Ergot beginning with 'Dilute 5 ml of this solution (Note 3). . . .'. Express the concentration of total alkaloids as mg of ergotamine in each ml of Liquid Extract of Ergot.

Assay for ergometrine. Proceed as directed in the *N.F.* assay for ergometrine under Ergot. Express the concentration of ergometrine as mg of ergometrine maleate in each ml of Liquid Extract of Ergot.

Alexander and Banes[4] have published a new procedure for the assay of ergot. The extraction and preparation of total alkaloids closely follows that of the *N.F.* given above and water-soluble alkaloids are separated by column chromatography. The total and water-soluble alkaloids are then determined colorimetrically with *p*-dimethylaminobenzaldehyde.

Extraction of alkaloids: Weigh 5 g, ground to No. 60 powder, into a 125-ml separator, add 50 ml of extracting solvent (prepared by combining 1 part of a 10 per cent solution of strong ammonia in methanol with 9 parts of chloroform) and shake vigorously for five minutes. Add 50 ml of chloroform and 2 ml of water, shake gently and allow to settle. Draw off the lower layer as completely as possible and filter through glass wool into a 200-ml graduated flask. Add a further 20 ml of extracting solvent to the contents of the separator, mix, add 20 ml of chloroform and shake. Filter the lower layer through the glass wool into the graduated flask and then repeat the extraction procedure once with another 20 ml of extracting solvent and 20 ml of chloroform. Dilute the combined extracts to volume with chloroform and mix.

Preparation of total alkaloid solution: Evaporate a 25-ml aliquot of the chloroform-ammonia extract solution to dryness at a temperature not exceeding 40°. (If desired the dried sample may be stored in a refrigerator overnight before continuation of assay.) Dissolve the residue in 20 ml of ether and transfer to a 125-ml separator with the aid of three 20-ml quantities of ether, followed by two quantities, of 5 ml and 3 ml, respectively, of approximately 0·2N sulphuric acid. (To check for complete transfer add 2 ml of acid to the flask and examine under ultra-violet light. There should be no fluorescence.) Shake the separator and run the acid layer into a 25-ml graduated flask through a plug of glass wool. Extract the ether layer with three successive quantities, of 5 ml, 5 ml and 3 ml, respectively, of 0·2N sulphuric acid, combine the acid extracts in the graduated flask, dilute to volume with water and mix. This solution is the assay preparation of total alkaloids.

Preparation of water-soluble alkaloid solution: Plug the bottom of a chromatographic tube, 20 cm long and 2·5 cm in internal diameter, with glass wool and mount in a vertical position. Stir 5 g of Celite 545 with 5 ml of 0·1N citric acid, in a beaker, until fluffy and uniform. Transfer the mixture to the chromatographic tube, tapping the side of the tube gently to let the mixture settle, and press down firmly and uniformly with a flat-ended glass packing rod. Thoroughly mix 2 g of Celite 545 with 2 ml of water, transfer to the tube and press firmly and uniformly on to the top of the acid trap. Finally place a layer of glass wool on top of the column. Evaporate a 150-ml aliquot of the chloroform-ammonia extract solution to dryness at a temperature not exceeding 40°. There should be no odour of ammonia or solvent. Dissolve the residue in 10 ml of chloroform and transfer quantitatively to the column with the aid of small quantities of chloroform. Wash down the sides of the chromatographic tube with chloroform and then elute the water-insoluble alkaloids with 125 ml of water-saturated chloroform. Inspect for proper retention of water-soluble alkaloids by very briefly holding the column under an ultra-violet lamp. A brightly fluorescent blue ring in the citric acid trap layer indicates that the ergometrine has been properly retained. Discard the eluate and glass-wool cover. Extrude the column containing the sample, by means of a very gentle air pressure, into a 400-ml beaker, stir with 5 ml of 10 per cent sodium bicarbonate and then with sufficient Celite 545 to produce a workable mixture and transfer quantitatively to the chromatographic tube. Rinse the packing rod and stirrer with a small amount of chloroform, collecting the chloroform in a beaker. Add enough Celite 545 to adsorb the chloroform and transfer to the column. Rinse again with chloroform. Pass 75 ml of water-saturated chloroform through the column collecting the eluate in a 125-ml separator containing 5 ml of approximately 0·2N sulphuric acid. Examine the column under an ultra-violet lamp to check for complete removal of water-soluble alkaloids; there should be no fluorescence due to ergot alkaloids.

Shake the mixture of acid and eluate and run the chloroform layer into a second separator (if after standing for fifteen minutes the organic phase does not completely settle out free of emulsion, add about 30 mg of anhydrous sodium sulphate and shake until it dissolves). Pour the acid layer through the mouth of the separator into a 25-ml graduated flask. Rinse the first separator and then the chloroform with three successive quantities, each of 5 ml, of approximately 0·2N sulphuric acid, adding the acid to the graduated flask. Dilute the combined acid extracts to volume with water and mix. This is the assay preparation of water-soluble alkaloids.

Development of colour: Transfer 5-ml aliquots of the assay preparations to separate stoppered Erlenmeyer flasks and at the same time to a third, similar flask transfer a 5-ml aliquot of a standard solution of ergometrine, prepared by dissolving 6·78 mg of ergometrine maleate in 1 per cent tartaric acid and diluting to 250 ml with water. (The standard solution contains the equivalent of 20 μg of ergometrine per ml.) Treat the contents of each flask, respectively, as follows. Immerse in an ice-bath and add, dropwise, with constant swirling, 10·0 ml of a reagent solution prepared by dissolving 125 mg of *p*-dimethylaminobenzaldehyde in a cooled mixture of 65 ml of concentrated sulphuric acid and 35 ml of water and adding 0·05 ml of N ferric chloride solution; the solution should be used within seven days. Allow to stand at room temperature for forty-five to sixty minutes with occasional mixing. Measure the extinction of each solution at 550 mμ, using as a reference blank a mixture prepared by adding 10·0 ml of reagent solution to 5·0 ml of 0·2N sulphuric acid.

Total alkaloid content as per cent ergotoxine $= 0{\cdot}150 \times E/S$

Water-soluble alkaloid content as per cent ergometrine $= 0{\cdot}01333 \times E_1/S$.

E = extinction of aliquot of assay preparation of total alkaloids,

E_1 = extinction of aliquot of assay preparation of water-soluble alkaloids

S = extinction of standard.

If further information is required about the constitution of the water-soluble alkaloids the ergometrine and ergometrinine may be separated by paper chromatography and a rough estimation of the respective alkaloid contents made by comparison of the intensity of fluorescence under an ultra-violet lamp of sample spots with standard spots.

ERGOMETRINE MALEATE, $C_{19}H_{23}O_2N_3,C_4H_4O_4$, Mol. Wt. 441·5

The acid maleate of an alkaloid obtained from ergot. It is officially assayed by the colorimetric method, given under Ergot, against a standard solution of ergometrine maleate. It can also be determined by the *U.S.P.* method.

Dissolve about 100 mg, accurately weighed, in 2 ml of ethanol and 3 ml of strong ammonia solution. Add 50 ml of saturated sodium chloride solution; extract with eight successive portions of ether. Evaporate the ether to 2 ml, add 25 ml of 0·02N hydrochloric acid, warm to remove traces of ether and titrate with 0·02N sodium hydroxide using bromophenol blue as indicator. 1 ml of 0·02N=0·00883 g $C_{19}H_{23}O_2N_3,C_4H_4O_4$.

Ergometrine exhibits a blue fluorescence in ultra-violet light. Advantage is taken of this to determine ergometrine quantitatively in official preparations. All solutions containing ergometrine should be kept in low actinic glassware.

Weigh accurately about 0·05 g and transfer to a 100-ml graduated flask with water. Dissolve and make up to volume with water. Pipette 4 ml of this solution into a 200-ml graduated flask, add 40 ml of a 1 per cent solution of tartaric acid and make up to volume with water.

Prepare a standard solution containing 10 μg per ml of ergometrine maleate in 0·2 per cent tartaric acid.

Pipette duplicate aliquots, each of 5 ml, of the sample solution into 25-ml graduated flasks, add 15 ml of 0·2M potassium dihydrogen phosphate solution and make up to volume with water.

Pipette triplicate aliquots, each of 5 ml, of the standard solution into 25-ml graduated flasks, add 15 ml of 0·2M potassium dihydrogen phosphate solution and make up to volume with water.

Using a primary filter OX1 and an OB2 in conjunction with an OY13 as a secondary filter calibrate the fluorimeter with one of the standard solutions. Measure the fluorescence of the sample solutions and the remaining standard solutions.

Calculate the percentage of ergometrine maleate in the sample.

Injection of Ergometrine Maleate, *B.P.* A sterile solution of ergometrine maleate in water for injection; it usually contains 0·5 mg in each ml. The official assay is colorimetric but the fluorimetric method is preferable.

Dilute the sample in 0·2 per cent tartaric acid to contain about 10 μg per ml of ergometrine maleate. Prepare a standard solution containing 10 μg per ml of ergometrine maleate in 0·2 per cent tartaric acid. Proceed as described under Ergometrine Maleate (above) commencing with the words 'Pipette duplicate aliquots, each of 5 ml, . . .' and calculate the ergometrine content of the injection.

Tablets of Ergometrine Maleate, *B.P.* Usually contain 0·5 mg in each tablet and can be assayed colorimetrically after solution in 1 per cent tartaric acid.

The fluorimetric assay is also applicable.

Weigh sufficient of the powdered tablets containing about 1 mg of ergometrine maleate, transfer to a 100-ml graduated flask with 20 ml of 1 per cent tartaric acid. Shake for thirty minutes and make up to volume with water. Prepare a standard solution containing 10 μg per ml of ergometrine maleate in 0·2 per cent tartaric acid. Proceed as described under Ergometrine Maleate (above) commencing with the words 'Pipette duplicate aliquots, each of 5 ml, . . .' and calculate the ergometrine maleate content of the tablets.

ERGOTAMINE TARTRATE, $(C_{33}H_{35}O_5N_5)_2,C_4H_6O_6$, Mol. Wt. 1313·5

The tartrate of an alkaloid obtainable from certain species of ergot. It is assayed colorimetrically by the dimethylaminobenzaldehyde method given under Ergot after solution in 1 per cent tartaric acid against a standard ergometrine maleate solution. 1 mg of ergometrine maleate = 1·488 mg of ergotamine tartrate.

Injection of Ergotamine Tartrate, *B.P.* A sterile solution of ergotamine tartrate in water for injection; it usually contains 0·5 mg in each ml. It is also assayed colorimetrically after dilution with 0·25 per cent tartaric acid solution.

Tablets of Ergotamine Tartrate, *B.P.* Usually contain 0·5 mg in each tablet and can be assayed colorimetrically after trituration with a small amount of 50 per cent ethanol and subsequent dilution with 1 per cent tartaric acid solution.

When ergotamine is to be determined in tablets containing other drugs (e.g. caffeine, phenacetin and phenobarbitone) the colorimetric method cannot be applied directly. Alexander[5] has described a column-chromatographic method of separation consisting of preliminary separation of the alkaloids from water-soluble excipients by means of a sodium bicarbonate column followed by retention of the ergotamine on a strongly acidic citric acid column from which the caffeine, phenacetin and phenobarbitone are eluted with ether followed by chloroform. The presence of water-soluble ergot alkaloids is detected by ultra-violet examination of an alum layer above the citric acid trap. The precision of the colorimetric method was improved by swirling the ergotamine solution in an ice-bath while adding the *p*-dimethylaminobenzaldehyde solution dropwise; addition of the reagent in this manner prevents charring of carbohydrate-type substances, with subsequent high extinction readings.

METHYLERGOMETRINE MALEATE, $C_{20}H_{25}O_2N_3,C_4H_4O_4$, Mol. Wt. 455·5.

The acid maleate of a partially synthetic homologue of ergometrine. It is officially assayed colorimetrically by the dimethylaminobenzaldehyde method given under Ergot against a standard ergometrine maleate solution. 1 mg of ergometrine maleate = 1·032 mg of methylergometrine maleate.

Injection of Methylergometrine Maleate, *B.P.* A sterile solution of methylergometrine maleate in water for injection; it usually contains 0·2 mg in each ml. It is also assayed colorimetrically.

1. Hampshire, C. H., and Page, G. R., *Quart. J. Pharm.*, 1936, **9**, 60.
2. Smith, M. I., *U.S. Public Health Reports*, 1930, **45** (26), 1466.
3. Foster, G. E., MacDonald, J., and Jones, T. S. G., *J. Pharm. Pharmacol.*, 1949, **1**, 802.
4. Alexander, T. G. and Banes, D., *J. Pharm. Sci.*, 1961, **50**, 201.
5. Alexander, T. G., *J.A.O.A.C.*, 1960, **43**, 224.

ETHER

$(C_2H_5)_2O$ Mol. Wt. 74·12

Owing to its inactivity there is no very satisfactory chemical method for the determination of ether either alone or in mixtures, and the usual methods of examination are concerned with the impurities present. Attempts to determine ether by oxidation with acid dichromate present so many possible errors that the method seems to be valueless. It is, however, interesting to note that the ether content in ether-air mixtures has been successfully determined with a considerable degree of accuracy by a modified Pregl micro-method of ultimate combustion (Coste and Chaplin[1]). The standard Pregl combustion apparatus was modified as follows:

Between the U-tube of the bubbler and the combustion tube proper insert a short length of capillary tubing from which a side capillary tube (sealed in) leads upwards for about 15 cm and then down nearly to bench level and finally up for about 25 cm. In order to decrease fluctuations in the rate of flow of gas through it, make a constriction in the capillary by drawing out close to the T-joint. Expand the open end somewhat, draw out finely and seal off (the expansion gives a drawn-out part which has thinner walls and is thus easily broken). Stand the long, narrow U-tube thus formed in a cylinder of mercury initially filled above the capillary end. Introduce the sample into a graduated and calibrated tube over mercury; measure at noted temperature and pressure and lower over the sealed end of the capillary as far as possible. Then remove mercury from the cylinder by means of a pump until the levels inside and outside the graduated tube are the same. Arrange a tap-funnel containing mercury above the cylinder and, when all is ready for combustion, depress the graduated tube sharply to break the sealed end of the capillary and then fix it in this lower position; then allow mercury to flow in from the funnel at such a rate as to cause the introduction of the sample at a suitable speed into the main oxygen stream.

An extensive literature on the examination of ether includes little on quantitative measurement of the impurities present, tests being devised mainly as limiting values. The impurities commonly present are water, ethanol, methyl ether, free acid, aldehyde, acetone and peroxides. The first four compounds are present from manufacture and the last three are formed by decomposition. Water and ethanol are not serious impurities and determine its weight per millilitre.

The presence of peroxide and aldehyde in ether is of more importance as they represent oxidation products, the aldehyde probably being formed by hydrolysis of the peroxide. King[2] in an investigation on the products of autoxidation considered the peroxide present to be probably monacetaldehyde hydrogen peroxide together with hydrogen peroxide, but the constitution is still in doubt. A rapid method was devised for the estimation of peroxide in deteriorated ethers.

Add 5 or 10 ml to 50 ml of approximately N sulphuric acid in a 200-ml bottle, followed by a few crystals of manganous sulphate. Run in 0·1N permanganate slowly with rotation of the contents to ensure extraction of peroxides by the aqueous layer. The end-point is taken when the pink colour produced has not completely faded in ten seconds.

The method is independent of the presence of acetaldehyde and formic acid, which both occur in ethers rich in peroxide, and gives a measure of the free hydrogen peroxide or that set free from labile compounds by the acid solution.

Middleton and Hymas[3] summarised all previous tests proposed for the detection of peroxides present in the quantities usually met with in anæsthetic ether and studied their relative values for experimental work. The sensitivities of twenty different methods were compared both for hydrogen peroxide and ether peroxide. As the best quantitative method would be that in which the intensity of colour is most nearly proportional to the amount of peroxide present, and observable over a wide range, the ferrous thiocyanate method (sensitive to 0·017 p.p.m. ether peroxide and 0·025 p.p.m. hydrogen peroxide) was eventually chosen as most suitable.

The red colour developed was also considered better for observation than the starch-potassium iodide method of the *B.P.* (sensitive to 0·025 p.p.m. ether peroxide and 0·05 p.p.m. hydrogen peroxide). The following test was used:

Place 30 ml of ether in a 35-ml stoppered bottle and fill to the neck with reagent. (For intermittent use the reagent is prepared as follows: Boil 30 ml of 10 per cent sulphuric acid and 100 ml of water for a few minutes in a flask through which passes a current of carbon dioxide. Add 5 g of ferrous sulphate heptahydrate and, after cooling, 30 ml of 10 per cent potassium thiocyanate solution. Decolorise the solution at 40° by the addition dropwise of 0·03N titanous chloride, taking care to avoid excess of reducing agent. The reagent is kept under carbon dioxide and should be decolorised, if necessary, immediately before use.) Shake and allow to stand in the dark for five minutes. Compare the colour developed with a solution of cobalt sulphate (0·15 g of crystalline cobalt sulphate and 2 ml of 10 per cent sulphuric acid in 100 ml of water).

It was considered that the colour should not be greater than an equal depth of the cobalt solution, which is equivalent to 0·15 p.p.m. The suggested standard is unnecessarily exacting (Coste and Garratt[4]).

1. Coste, J. H., and Chaplin, C. A., *Brit. J. Anæsthesia*, 1937, **14**, 115.
2. King, H., *J. Chem. Soc.*, 1929, 738.
3. Middleton, G., and Hymas, F. C., *Analyst*, 1928, **53**, 201.
4. Coste, J. H., and Garratt, D. C., *Analyst*, 1936, **61**, 459.

ETHYL ALCOHOL

C_2H_5OH Mol. Wt. 46·07

Ethyl alcohol is of such importance for fiscal purposes that the estimation has been standardised in detail. The only method of practical importance is by the determination of the specific gravity of its aqueous solution. Distillation and other methods of purification are necessary before the specific gravity can be taken, and the purity of the solution must be tested finally by its refractive index, which should agree closely with that of a pure alcohol solution of the same strength, as other substances such as acetone, higher alcohols and benzyl alcohol may not be wholly removed by the preliminary treatment. With the exception of methyl alcohol, which is also not removed, the other substances in solution give higher refractive indices than for an ethyl alcohol of the same specific gravity. Further details for estimating alcohol will be found in Appendix I. Ethyl alcohol may also be determined in aqueous mixtures by the following gas chromatographic method.

Dilute the sample in water so that the ethyl alcohol concentration is about 1 per cent. Add to this solution 1 per cent of *n*-propanol. Prepare a standard solution containing 1 per cent of ethanol and 1 per cent of *n*-propanol.

Chromatograph the standard and sample solutions on a suitable gas chromatographic apparatus using the following operating conditions:

Column length, 5 feet; column temperature, 98°; stationary phase, 30 per cent of Carbowax 1500 on 36- to 85-mesh Chromosorb; nitrogen flow rate, 20 ml per minute; flash-heater temperature, 145°; detector, thermal conductivity cell; detector current, 175 mA; sample size, 30 μl; recorder, Honeywell-Brown, 1 mV full-scale deflection, chart speed 12 inches per hour.

The order of elution is ethanol, *n*-propanol, water.

Calculate the ratios of the heights of the ethyl alcohol and propanol peaks of both standard and sample solutions.

per cent ethyl alcohol in sample =

$$\frac{\text{ratio of peak heights for sample}}{\text{ratio of peak heights for standard}} \times 1{\cdot}0 \times \text{dilution factor}$$

Small quantities of **methyl alcohol** in ethyl alcohol may be detected and estimated by a method based upon that of Georgia and Morales,[1] in which methyl alcohol is oxidised to formaldehyde and formic acid, ethyl alcohol to acetaldehyde; the method is as follows:

Potassium permanganate reagent: Dissolve 3 g of potassium permanganate in a mixture of 15 ml of concentrated phosphoric acid and 70 ml of water and dilute with water to 100 ml.

Oxalic acid reagent: This is a 5 per cent solution of oxalic acid in a cooled mixture of equal volumes of concentrated sulphuric acid and water.

Schiff's reagent: Dissolve 1 g of basic magenta in 600 ml of warm, not hot, water and cool in ice; add 20 g of sodium sulphite, $Na_2SO_3,7H_2O$, dissolved in 100 ml of water, cool in ice and add, slowly and with constant stirring, 10 ml of concentrated hydrochloric acid. Dilute to 1 litre with water. If the solution is turbid it should be filtered. If the solution is coloured brown, decolorise with 0·2 to 0·3 g of decolorising charcoal and filter immediately. Occasionally it is necessary to add 2 to 3 ml of concentrated hydrochloric acid and to shake, to remove a little residual pink colour. Allow to stand for twenty-four hours before use and store protected from light; the reagent will keep active for two months.

Dilute 0·5 ml of the sample to 5 ml with water, add 2·0 ml of the potassium permanganate reagent, allow to stand for ten minutes and add 2·0 ml of the oxalic acid reagent. To the colourless solution add 5 ml of Schiff's reagent, allow to stand at a temperature between 15° and 30° and examine after thirty minutes.

The phosphoric acid process was found to give higher yields of formaldehyde than the similar method of Simmonds.[2] The violet colour produced is matched against standards prepared with known amounts of methyl alcohol in ethyl alcohol. The best conditions for colour development are given with quantities of between 0·0001 and 0·001 ml of methyl alcohol in 5 ml of test solution. The original paper contains a comprehensive list of interfering substances, nearly all of which may be removed by one of the methods for alcohol determination (p. 778). Formaldehyde is removed by the following process:

To 1 g of pyrogallol dissolved in 10 ml of water, add 10 ml of the unknown solution, which has been diluted to contain 5 per cent alcohol by volume, followed by 5 ml of concentrated sulphuric acid. Stopper the flask, mix the solution and allow to stand for ten minutes. Distil 10 ml and use 5 ml for the test.

If insufficient pyrogallol has been added, the solution assumes a bright red colour instead of being colourless or pale green, and more reagent must be added. 1 g of pyrogallol will remove approximately 0·2 g of formaldehyde. Any preparation containing formaldehyde will also give the reaction for methyl alcohol after removing the formaldehyde, as commercial solutions contain a high percentage of the alcohol.

Acetaldehyde is removed by the addition of the sulphuric acid before Schiff's reagent. Adams and Nicholls[3] point out that propyl, amyl and benzyl alcohols, when present in sufficient proportions, give positive results in this test, hence it is not specific for methyl alcohol.

An unexpected phenomenon was observed by Ballard and Hersant[4] in this test for methyl in ethyl alcohol; if the decolorised solution of magenta is added at a temperature of 10° or less, an immediate violet colour is produced. This colour differs distinctly from the magenta colour obtained with small amounts of methyl alcohol and is probably due to interaction with acetaldehyde; a reaction temperature of 15° to 30° is necessary. Further, since a pale greenish-yellow colour is given in the official test by acetaldehyde and traces of formaldehyde produced from the ethyl alcohol itself, the authors recommend that an auxiliary solution should be used for compensation. By trial, an auxiliary containing 2·5 ml of 10 per cent ethyl alcohol, 2·5 ml of water and 0·20 mg of methyl alcohol was found to match the primary solution in the absence of methyl alcohol.

A more sensitive and specific test for the detection and determination of methyl alcohol has been developed by Boos[5] depending on the use of chromotropic acid. This reagent gives an intense violet-red colour with formaldehyde in the presence of sulphuric acid.

To 1 ml of test solution (a dilution of the distillate according to the expected methyl alcohol content) in a 10-ml graduated flask, add 3 drops of 5 per cent phosphoric acid and 5 drops of 5 per cent potassium permanganate solution. Allow to stand at room temperature for ten minutes with occasional swirling, then add a saturated solution of sodium bisulphite drop by drop to reduce the excess permanganate. Cool the solution in an ice-bath while adding 4 ml of concentrated sulphuric acid, followed by 4 drops of 2 per cent aqueous solution of chromotropic acid. Place the flask on a water-bath at 60° for fifteen minutes with occasional swirling, cool and make up to 10 ml.

Measure the extinction at 580 mμ against a blank prepared with 1 ml of distilled water. Compare the reading with a curve prepared by treating a series of methyl alcohol solutions, containing from 20 to 100 μg per ml, according to the above procedure.

The colour with chromotropic acid is only developed in the presence of high concentrations of sulphuric acid. Certain interfering organic compounds depress the full colour; this has been attributed to the fact that formaldehyde couples with these compounds in strong sulphuric acid, thereby preventing its colour development with the reagent. Bricker and Vail[6] found that chromotropic acid reacts with formaldehyde to give a non-volatile compound and evaporation of the reacting solution will eliminate volatile organic compounds such as acetone; when the sulphuric acid is added and the resulting solution is heated, the full dye colour is then developed.

For a pure mixture of ethyl and methyl alcohols in aqueous solution, the components may be estimated by determination of the density and refractive index of the solution and consultation of published tables.

Adams and Nicholls[3] state that if a distillate contains less than about 17 per cent of apparent proof spirit, the specific gravity and index of refraction for the low alcohols and acetone are very nearly a linear function of the quantities of each in solution. If the apparent proof spirit be found, then multiplying by the factor 0·585 for methyl alcohol and by 0·573 for ethyl alcohol, for each 1 per cent proof will give the percentage by volume, not differing by more than 0·1 per cent from the correct value.

The following table given by Adams and Nicholls shows the corresponding refractometer readings:

TABLE 18

Apparent proof spirit per cent	Immersion refractometer reading at 60° F	
	Methyl alcohol	Ethyl alcohol
0	15·4	15·4
1	15·7	16·1
2	16·0	16·8
3	16·2	17·5
4	16·5	18·2
5	16·8	18·9
6	17·1	19·7
7	17·4	20·5
8	17·7	21·2
9	17·9	22·0
10	18·2	22·8
11	18·5	23·6
12	18·8	24·4
13	19·1	25·3
14	19·3	26·1
15	19·6	26·9
16	19·9	27·8
17	20·2	28·7

In the presence of acetone and its homologues, where the specific gravity-refraction method would be inapplicable owing to the third constituent, Hoff and Macoun[7] have worked out a method for the determination of methyl and ethyl alcohols, based on the formation of non-volatile products when formaldehyde and acetone react in the presence of alkali.

For liquids free from volatile oils or any excessive proportion of acetone, dilute the sample, containing not more than 20 ml of alcohol, to a volume of about 100 ml in a spirit distillation flask. For each 1 ml of acetone expected to be present add 1·5 g of paraformaldehyde, followed by 50 ml of brine and 20 ml of N sodium hydroxide. Fit the flask to an efficient Liebig condenser and bring the mixture, slowly, just to the boiling-point, using an electric hot-plate as the most efficient source of heat. To the just-boiling mixture, add excess of Fehling's solution (usually 50 to 60 ml) through the top of the condenser and then cool the flask to room temperature; the supernatant liquid must remain distinctly blue. Rinse the condenser down with a little water, place an open glass tube, about 15 cm long, in the flask to facilitate gentle boiling during the ensuing distillation and distil the mixture as usual for spirit strength determination, care being taken to avoid undue frothing at the initial boiling. Determine the specific gravity and refractive index as usual.

Where the acetone content is high (*e.g.* wood spirit), or where volatile oils are present, the alcoholic liquid must first be treated by the Thorpe and Holmes method (process B) described in the Appendix. Paraformaldehyde of the usual medicinal grade contains small amounts of nitrogenous bases which are carried over into the distillate. Unless their absence is assured, the reagent must be purified before use by washing, first with dilute hydrochloric acid, then with water until the removal of acid is complete, and finally by air drying.

Hoskins[8] criticises the above method as giving rise to the formation of traces of methyl alcohol. If it is necessary to decide whether the alcohol present has been methylated or not, the formation of traces of methyl alcohol is, of course, inadmissible and a method based on the precipitation of the acetone as a complex mercury compound has been devised. By following the technique described below the loss of alcohol by oxidising action of the mercuric sulphate is made negligible.

The following solutions are necessary:

(*a*) Acid mercuric sulphate containing 50 g of mercuric oxide and 125 ml of concentrated sulphuric acid per litre.

(*b*) Potassium oxalate, approximately 300 g per litre.

(*c*) Sodium formate, approximately 100 g per litre.

Determine approximately the amount of acetone in the alcohol solution (see method of Adams and Nicholls, p. 7).

Introduce into a 750-ml flask an amount of alcohol solution containing not more than 1 ml of acetone. For each 0·1 ml of acetone to be removed, add 25 ml of solution (*a*) and 0·2 ml of solution (*c*). Heat the flask, with frequent agitation, under an efficient reflux at such a rate that clouding takes place in approximately ten minutes. The complex forms at about

80° and any appreciable rise above this should be avoided. Lower the flame under the flask so as to keep the solution at 80° for ten to twelve minutes. Pour a few ml of distilled water down the condenser to wash any acetone which may have condensed there into the flask. At the end of ten to twelve minutes add an excess [12 ml to each 100 ml of solution (*a*)] of solution (*b*) through the condenser to precipitate the excess of mercuric sulphate as mercuric oxalate. Cool the flask, again rinse the condenser with water, remove the flask and connect it to a distillation apparatus. Since the final volume of liquid may be as much as 400 to 500 ml it is advisable to collect at least 150 ml of distillate and to redistil this, preferably from an alkaline solution, to a smaller volume.

(*Cf.* Acetone and Isopropyl Alcohol.)

Surgical Spirit, *B.P.C.* Consists of industrial methylated spirit to which has been added 2·5 per cent of castor oil, 0·5 per cent of methyl salicylate and 2·0 per cent of ethyl phthalate.

The following method for determination of ethyl phthalate and methyl salicylate is based upon a two-point method and the formula given has been calculated from the following data:

	Wavelength	E (1 per cent, 1cm) v/v
Ethyl phthalate	306 mμ	zero
	227 mμ	419
Methyl salicylate	306 mμ	335
	227 mμ	432

Dilute 5 ml to 100 ml with dehydrated ethanol and then dilute 5 ml of the resulting solution to 100 ml with the same solvent (Solution A). Measure the extinction of a 1-cm layer of this solution at 306 mμ and calculate the E(1 per cent, 1 cm) of the original solution (X).

Dilute 10 ml of Solution A to 50 ml with dehydrated ethanol. Measure the extinction of a 1-cm layer of this solution at 227 mμ and calculate the E(1 per cent, 1 cm) of the original solution (Y).

The percentage of methyl salicylate (v/v) is $0{\cdot}299X$ and that of ethyl phthalate (v/v) is $0{\cdot}239Y - 0{\cdot}308X$.

1. Georgia, F. R., and Morales, Rita, *Ind. Eng. Chem.*, 1926, **18**, 304.
2. Simmonds, C., *Analyst*, 1912, **37**, 16.
3. Adams, C. A., and Nicholls, J. R., *Analyst*, 1929, **54**, 2.
4. Ballard, C. W., and Hersant, E. F., *Quart. J. Pharm.*, 1942, **15**, 97.
5. Boos, R. N., *Anal. Chem.*, 1948, **20**, 964.
6. Bricker, C. E., and Vail, W. A., *Anal. Chem.*, 1950, **22**, 720.
7. Hoff, R. W., and Macoun, J. M., *Analyst*, 1933, **58**, 749.
8. Hoskins, C. R., *Analyst*, 1937, **62**, 530.

FLAVINES

The medicinal flavines (acriflavine, euflavine and proflavine) are all derivatives of diaminoacridine or diaminomethylacridine and their quantitative assay has been the subject of considerable research. More recently other amino derivatives of acridine have been used similarly and their assay follows the same general procedure.

Except for elementary analysis for nitrogen and chlorine, the figures for which are of limited value as they possibly include impurities, the first attempt to determine the flavines either as pure chemicals, impregnations or solutions was by Udall,[1] depending on the titration of the amino grouping (only one reacting) by diazotisation with standard nitrite solution, using starch-iodide paper as an external indicator. Powell and Hall[2] found the method inapplicable and proposed another depending on the insolubility of the ferricyanides of the flavine dyes. In this method, the insoluble ferricyanide is removed by filtration and the excess of potassium ferricyanide remaining in solution is determined under suitable conditions by reduction to ferrocyanide with hydriodic acid, a zinc salt being added to remove the ferrocyanide from solution as formed. The iodine liberated is titrated with sodium thiosulphate solution. Suitable conditions for quantitative results were given in this paper, which also showed that one must adhere strictly to the experimental details. The general method evolved, applicable to all the medicinal flavines now in use, has been inserted in the *B.P.* for proflavine hemisulphate and in the *B.P.C.* for acriflavine.

> Dissolve 2 g in 250 ml of water, which may be hot if necessary. Dilute to 750 ml (to give a clear solution with proflavine; the dilution produces no appreciable effect due to solubility of acriflavine ferricyanide). Adjust the reaction at room temperature by the addition of N hydrochloric acid until faintly acid to congo red paper, and then add 5 g of sodium acetate. Add 50 ml of 0·1M potassium ferricyanide, stirring during the addition. Set aside for ten minutes, filter through a Büchner funnel and wash the precipitate with three successive quantities of 50 ml of water. Cool the combined filtrate and washings to below 10° (to avoid loss of iodine) and add 10 ml of concentrated hydrochloric acid, 10 g of sodium chloride, 1 g of potassium iodide and 3 g of zinc sulphate dissolved in 10 ml of water, mixing after each addition. Set aside for three minutes and titrate the liberated iodine with 0·1N sodium thiosulphate. When the end-point has nearly been reached, set aside for a further three minutes before completing the titration. Conduct a blank determination on 25 ml of the 0·1M ferricyanide.

The medicinal flavines are **acriflavine,** a mixture of the hydrochlorides of 2,8-diamino-10-methylacridinium chloride, $C_{14}H_{14}N_3Cl,HCl$, Mol. Wt. 296·2, 1 ml 0·1M = 0·08886 g, and 2,8-diaminoacridine, the latter being about one-third of the total; **euflavine,** neutral acriflavine, a mixture of 2,8-diamino-10-methylacridinium chloride, $C_{14}H_{14}N_3Cl$, Mol. Wt. 259·7, 1 ml 0·1M = 0·07792 g, and 2,8-diaminoacridine monohydrochloride; **proflavine hemisulphate,** 2,8-diaminoacridine neutral sulphate, $(C_{13}H_{11}N_3)_2,H_2SO_4,H_2O$, Mol. Wt. 534·6, 1 ml 0·1M = 0·07749 g $(C_{13}H_{11}N_3)_2,H_2SO_4$.

In 0·1N hydrochloric acid, proflavine hemisulphate has a maximum absorption at about 444 mμ, E(1 per cent, 1 cm) = 1,210.

It was shown by Gailliot[3] that commercial acriflavine actually consists of a mixture of the hydrochloride of 2,8-diamino-10-methylacridinium chloride with diaminoacridine hydrochloride, the pure methylated compound not satisfying the solubility requirements of the *B.P.C.*, but the ferricyanide estimation measures the total content of acridine derivatives. Hence methods have been evolved to determine the proportion of methylated and unmethylated compounds in the mixture.

Aminacrine hydrochloride, $C_{13}H_{10}N_2,HCl,H_2O$, Mol. Wt., 248·7. The hydrochloride of 5-aminoacridine. 1 ml 0·1M potassium ferricyanide = 0·06921 g $C_{13}H_{10}N_2,HCl$.

Hall and Powell[4] introduced the following procedure for the determination of unmethylated compounds in acriflavine and euflavine, depending on the difference in behaviour on treatment with alkali.

> Dissolve 0·5 g of sample in 20 ml of water (30 ml in the case of euflavine) and neutralise with 0·1N sodium hydroxide, using bromothymol blue as indicator. Dilute the solution with water to 35 ml, warm to about 60°, and then add exactly 25 ml of 0·1N sodium hydroxide. After the further addition of 20 g of pure sodium chloride, rotate the flask to mix the contents and allow to stand overnight, preferably at low temperature (about 5°). Filter through a sintered-glass crucible and wash with 5-ml quantities of saturated sodium chloride solution, previously cooled to 5°, three washings being usually sufficient. To the combined filtrate and washings add 26 ml of 0·1N sulphuric acid, boil, cool and titrate with 0·1N sodium hydroxide, using bromothymol blue as indicator. 1 ml 0·1N sodium hydroxide neutralised in the precipitation = 0·0282 g diaminoacridine dihydrochloride.

Reimers[5] introduced a colorimetric method for the separate determination of diaminoacridine which is apparently simpler and more rapid than that of Hall and Powell.[4] The colorimetric titration is done in an alcoholic medium, thus reducing the basicity of the diaminoacridine and shifting the end-point in the acid direction.

> Dissolve 0·5 to 0·7 g of euflavine in 10 ml of boiling water in a 250-ml conical flask with careful shaking so that the solution is not cooled too quickly. Add 90 ml of *iso*propyl alcohol (*cf.* Hall and Powell[6]) and 2 ml of thymol blue solution and titrate with 0·1N sodium hydroxide to a definite colour change, *i.e.* to a colour that may be approximately described as murky brownish, the titration being conducted in strong electric light on account of the greenish fluorescence of euflavine solutions. Titrate back with 0·1N hydrochloric acid, 0·1 ml being added at a time

until the colour no longer changes. The colour has then reverted from the dark murky brown to the original clear solution, 0·2 to 0·5 ml of hydrochloric acid generally being required. 1 ml 0·1N = 0·0282 g diaminoacridine dihydrochloride.

According to a criticism by Hall and Powell[6] the principal defect of the colorimetric method is the difficulty of determining the end-point; also differences are apparent in the titration figures with variation in *iso*propyl alcohol content. With considerably higher proportions of alcohol (250 to 400 ml) the end-point became sharper and results were more in accordance with those obtained by the titration method (above); correction for acidity is also necessary.

A procedure for estimating the total chlorine in acriflavine is given by Collins and Stasiak.[7]

Dissolve 0·25 g in 10 ml of water in a 250-ml flask. Add 10 ml of 5 per cent silver nitrate solution, 10 ml of concentrated sulphuric acid and 2 g of powdered potassium permanganate, in portions, whilst digesting on a water-bath for thirty minutes. Decolorise the mixture by warming with hydrogen peroxide solution, filter and weigh the silver chloride as usual.

Alternatively the total chlorine may be titrated electrometrically in buffer solution (0·2M to sodium acetate and 0·2M to acetic acid), with silver nitrate using a silver/silver chloride electrode and a mercurous sulphate reference electrode.

Ellis[8] published a method for the determination of acriflavine and euflavine, dependent on the precipitation of the picrate, which is particularly useful where smaller quantities are available. Details of this precipitation procedure are given in the method under Euflavine Lint.

Shaw and Wilkinson[9] described a colorimetric estimation of proflavine hemisulphate. A purple colour is developed with nitrous acid but it is not stable; if, however, excess of nitrous acid is removed and the quinone-imine is coupled in acid solution with *N*-(1-naphthyl)ethylenediamine dihydrochloride a stable purple colour is obtained which is more intense than that of the corresponding uncoupled quinone-imine.

Place in a 100-ml graduated flask an aqueous solution of the material under test containing up to 300 μg of anhydrous proflavine hemisulphate. Add 5·0 ml of 0·1N hydrochloric acid and make up to 50 ml with water. Cool the solution to 10° ± 2°, add 1·0 ml of freshly prepared 0·01N sodium nitrite, mix thoroughly and maintain at 10° ± 2° for forty minutes in a water-bath, protecting the solution from light throughout this period. Subsequent operations (until coupling has taken place) must be carried out in subdued light. After forty minutes add 1·0 ml of recently prepared 0·5 per cent sulphamic acid or ammonium sulphamate solution, mix thoroughly and allow to stand for one minute. Add 2·0 ml of 0·1 per cent *N*-(l-naphthyl)ethylenediamine dihydrochloride solution (which must be stored in a refrigerator and discarded when yellow), mix thoroughly and allow to stand for five minutes. Add 5·0 ml of 0·1N hydrochloric acid and make up to 100 ml with water. Prepare similarly a blank solution without the sample under test. Measure the extinction of the solution in a 1-cm cell by comparison with the blank, using a Spekker photoelectric absorptiometer and Ilford 605 filters, or another suitable combination of absorptiometer and filters. By the same method and with suitable dilutions of standard proflavine solution (0·02 per cent, stored in the dark) prepare a calibration graph covering the required range and read from the graph the amount of proflavine hemisulphate contained in the test solution.

The method can be applied directly to eye-drops, pessaries, solutions and solution-tablets; difficulty is sometimes experienced in recovering the last traces of proflavine in the presence of fatty matter. In such cases extraction with an immiscible solvent may be necessary and the authors described the following method for proflavine cream:

Weigh accurately 0·1 to 0·2 g of the sample into a boiling-tube provided with a lip. Warm on a water-bath, dissolve in 2 ml of ethylene dichloride, add 5·0 ml of 0·1N hydrochloric acid and maintain at about 50° for five minutes with occasional shaking. Transfer the contents to a 15-ml graduated centrifuge tube and add more ethylene dichloride if necessary; wash the boiling-tube with two successive 2-ml quantities of warm water and add the washings to the centrifuge tube. Close the tube by means of a well-fitting rubber stopper and shake vigorously for thirty to sixty seconds. Remove the stopper and rinse any adhering solution back into the original boiling-tube. Centrifuge at 2,500 r.p.m. for five to ten minutes or until a clear upper layer is obtained. By means of a Pasteur pipette, transfer the bulk of the aqueous layer to a 100-ml graduated flask, rinse the pipette with two portions of water and add the washings to the flask. Wash the lower layer remaining in the centrifuge tube with the rinsings from the boiling-tube, using a total of 8 ml of warm water. Shake, centrifuge, transfer the upper layer to the flask as before and repeat the washing procedure. Dilute the contents of the flask to 50 ml and complete the determination by the general method as described above.

FLAVINE PREPARATIONS AND DRESSINGS

Udall[1] claimed that a Kjeldahl nitrogen estimation was suitable for impregnations on medical gauzes by first extracting the impregnation with ethanol in a Soxhlet apparatus, evaporating the solvent and examining the residue. Control determinations on medical gauze gave negative results for nitrogen. Unless a micro-nitrogen technique were used large quantities of gauze would be needed for this estimation.

Hall and Powell[10] found that the nitrogen method is correct only for freshly prepared gauzes, free from decomposition products of euflavine, made from a textile material that does not itself yield a nitrogenous extract. They also stated that euflavine gauze, if exposed to light, gradually undergoes decomposition, and subsequent removal of euflavine leaves behind insoluble brown decomposition products.

Consequently these authors adapted their ferricyanide method to the determination of euflavine and other diaminoacridine derivatives in gauzes, and, with suitable preliminary treatment, in pessaries, emulsions and solutions. A modification of the original conditions (p. 255) was found by experiment to be generally applicable after preliminary treatment of the preparation (see below).

Dilute the solution derived from preliminary treatment, containing from 0·02 to 0·2 g of the diaminoacridine derivative, to approximately 200 ml and adjust the reaction until faintly acid to congo red paper. Add 1 g of sodium acetate, followed by excess of 0·02M potassium ferricyanide (10 to 30 ml according to the amount required for precipitation), stirring during the addition. Allow the mixture to stand for thirty minutes and then filter through a Büchner funnel. Wash the precipitate with three successive quantities of 10 ml of water, and to the combined filtrate and washings add, mixing after each addition, 5 ml of concentrated hydrochloric acid, 1 g of sodium chloride, 0·5 g of potassium iodide and 5 ml of 30 per cent zinc sulphate solution. After standing for three minutes, titrate the liberated iodine with 0·01N sodium thiosulphate. Conduct a blank experiment, using the same amount of 0·02M ferricyanide reagent. 1 ml 0·01N ferricyanide precipitated = 0·00889 g acriflavine, 0·00779 g euflavine, or 0·00775 g anhydrous proflavine hemisulphate.

The authors found that direct application of their process to the gauze is not possible as euflavine, adsorbed on the fabric, fails to react completely with ferricyanide solution. The following preliminary extraction of the flavine from the gauze is therefore necessary:

Extract 20 g or other convenient quantity, in a Soxhlet, with 95 per cent ethanol, slightly acidified with hydrochloric acid (250 ml of ethanol and 2 ml of dilute acid). Usually three hours are required. Transfer the extract to a beaker, add 50 ml of water, evaporate to remove the bulk of the ethanol, and whilst still hot, add 25 ml of chloroform. Mix thoroughly, cool, transfer to a separator, allow to separate and then complete the removal of fats by extraction with two 25-ml portions of chloroform. Wash these combined extracts with two successive quantities of 10 ml of water, acidified with 1 or 2 drops of dilute hydrochloric acid. Break any emulsions with a little ethanol. Evaporate the combined aqueous solutions to low volume to remove ethanol, dilute to about 200 ml, adjust the reaction with dilute sodium hydroxide solution, until slightly acid to congo red paper, and complete as the general method.

It is emphasised that experimental details must be adhered to. Ether extraction of fats cannot be used and the amount of hydrochloric acid must be small to avoid a high chloride content at the time of precipitation. Chambers[11] avoids emulsions in removal of fatty matter by extracting the hot aqueous solution with hot chloroform and then cooling; instantaneous separation is obtained.

The application of the general method of Hall and Powell for determination of the acriflavine content of fatty and oily preparations, involves extraction of the medicament from a chloroform solution of the base in a similar manner to that described for gauzes:

> Treat a suitable quantity of the preparation (generally 25 to 50 g) with about 50 ml of chloroform to dissolve the base. Transfer the solution to a separator and extract with 20 ml of water containing 2 ml of dilute hydrochloric acid, followed by two extractions with 10 ml of water containing 0·5 ml of dilute hydrochloric acid. Wash the combined acid-aqueous extracts with 25 ml of chloroform; re-extract any medicament taken into the chloroform with 10 ml of water containing 1 or 2 drops of dilute hydrochloric acid. If emulsions form, they can be broken by the addition of ethanol. Transfer the combined acid-aqueous extracts to a beaker, evaporate sufficiently to remove ethanol if present, cool and dilute to about 200 ml. Reduce the acidity by the addition of dilute sodium hydroxide solution until only slightly acid to congo red paper and complete the estimation by the general method.

This treatment is also suitable for acriflavine pessaries with a theobroma base. Pessaries made with a glyco-gelatin base, or glycerin preparations of acriflavine, cause errors in determination due to the action of glycerol, or impurities in the gelatin, on the ferricyanide reagent. Hall and Powell reduced the error to a minimum by the following preliminary treatment and modification of the general method:

> Dissolve about 15 to 30 g of the sample in 100 ml of warm water, and precipitate the gelatin by the addition of 200 ml of 95 per cent ethanol. Cool the mixture, coagulate the precipitate by stirring, remove by centrifugation, redissolve in 50 ml of water and reprecipitate with 100 ml of ethanol. Combine the clear alcoholic liquids, evaporate to remove the ethanol and dilute with water to a volume of 200 ml. After adjusting the reaction, if necessary, to congo red, follow the general method, with the modification of allowing the reacting mixture to stand in the dark in an ice-chest to minimise the reducing action of the glycerol.

Euflavine Gauze, *B.P.C.* Absorbent gauze impregnated with euflavine. Assayed by the picrate method of Chambers and Savage (below) using 20 g of gauze.

Euflavine Lint, *B.P.C.* Absorbent lint impregnated with euflavine. The *B.P.C.* method is based on removal of the fatty impurities by filtration, after extraction of the gauze with acidified ethanol and distillation of the ethanol, followed by determination of the euflavine by Ellis's method.

In an examination of euflavine gauze Chambers and Savage[12] found that the filtration process for removing the fatty impurities was often troublesome due to the formation of an almost impermeable mat, through which the liquid passed slowly and which sometimes defied washing, and preferred to use the purification process described by Hall and Powell. They further compared the ferricyanide method and the picrate precipitation method and favoured the latter method although their arguments for this are not strong and comparative determinations have shown closely similar results by both methods. Their modified technique for euflavine gauze, which is equally applicable to euflavine lint, is as follows:

Extract about 20 g accurately weighed, for four hours or until extraction is complete, in a continuous extraction apparatus, with 95 per cent ethanol acidified with hydrochloric acid (2 ml of dilute acid in 250 ml of ethanol). Distil the solution until the residue measures about 30 ml. Add 50 ml of water and heat to about 80° to 90°. Transfer to a separator, rinsing the flask with small quantities of water. Add 25 ml of chloroform and shake gently. Allow the chloroform to separate and complete the removal of fatty impurities by extracting with two further portions of 25 ml of chloroform. Wash the combined chloroform extracts with two successive quantities of 10 ml of water acidified with 1 or 2 drops of dilute hydrochloric acid, contained in a second and a third separator. Break any emulsions with 5 ml of ethanol. Evaporate the combined aqueous solutions to about 40 ml. If clear, and containing no more than a little insoluble matter and a few cotton threads, transfer to a graduated flask, dilute with water to 50 ml and allow impurities to settle. If necessary filter through a sintered-glass Gooch crucible before making up to volume. Transfer 25 ml to a 100-ml beaker, add 10 ml of a filtered saturated solution of picric acid, mix and place on ice for at least an hour. Transfer the precipitate to a sintered-glass crucible (A3) using dilute picric acid solution (5 ml of a saturated solution in 100 ml of water) followed by 10 ml of ice-cold water. Dry at 100°. The weight of the precipitate multiplied by 0·573 is the weight of euflavine taken, assuming this to be diamino-10-methylacridinium chloride.

Cream of Proflavine, *B.P.C.* Contains 0·104 per cent of proflavine hemisulphate in an emulsion base.

This may be assayed chemically either by the method of Hall and Powell or by that of Shaw and Wilkinson, both of which have been described above. Another method, and that which is preferred by the *B.P.C.*, is to dissolve 25 g in chloroform in a separator and extract four times with 0·1N hydrochloric acid; the aqueous extracts are neutralised to bromothymol blue and then precipitated with picric acid.

A direct physical assay can also be applied to this preparation:

Weigh 1 g into a 100-ml graduated flask, dissolve in a mixture of equal volumes of chloroform and 95 per cent ethanol and dilute to volume with the same solvent. Transfer a 5-ml aliquot of this solution to a 25-ml graduated flask, dilute to volume with the mixed solvent and, if necessary, filter. Measure the extinction of the resulting solution at the absorption maximum at about 458 mμ, using 1-cm cells with the mixed solvent in the comparison cell and calculate the proflavine hemisulphate content, assuming a value of 1700 for the E(1 per cent, 1 cm) of proflavine hemisulphate at 458 mμ.

1. Udall, P. J., *Analyst*, 1932, **57**, 295.
2. Powell, A. D., and Hall, G. F., *Quart. J. Pharm.*, 1933, **6**, 389.
3. Gailliot, M., *Quart. J. Pharm.*, 1934, **7**, 63.
4. Hall, G. F., and Powell, A. D., *Quart. J. Pharm.*, 1934, **7**, 522.
5. Reimers, F., *Quart. J. Pharm.*, 1935, **8**, 218.

6. Hall, G. F., and Powell, A. D., *Quart. J. Pharm.*, 1936, **9**, 510.
7. Collins, G. W., and Stasiak, A., *J. Amer. Pharm. Ass.*, 1929, 18, 659.
8. Ellis, B. A., *Analyst*, 1942, **67**, 226.
9. Shaw, W. H. C., and Wilkinson, G., *Analyst*, 1952, **77**, 127.
10. Hall, G. F., and Powell, A. D., *Quart. J. Pharm.*, 1937, **10**, 486.
11. Chambers, W. P., *Analyst*, 1943, **68**, 14.
12. Chambers, W. P., and Savage, R. M., *Quart. J. Pharm.*, 1945, **18**, 227.

FOLIC ACID

$C_{19}H_{19}O_6N_7$ Mol. Wt. 441·4

Folic acid is determined in the *B.P.* by a colorimetric method based upon diazotisation and coupling with *N*-(1-naphthyl)ethylenediamine after an initial reduction stage. *p*-Aminobenzoic acid has been used as a standard but this has been criticised since the production of diazotisable amino-groups by the reduction of folic acid may not be completely stoichiometric. The only solutions to this problem would be to use a purely empirical factor in conjunction with a *p*-aminobenzoic acid standard, which seems undesirable, or to use a reference standard sample of folic acid for comparative purposes. This latter course is adopted by the *U.S.P.* but as yet no suitable standard is available in Great Britain.

The method (making use of *p*-aminobenzoic acid for reference purposes) is given below. The factor of 3·22 is the stoichiometric one, but it has been suggested that the empirical use of a somewhat lower figure should be adopted.

Weigh 0·1 g into a 100-ml graduated flask, dissolve in 0·1N sodium hydroxide and dilute to volume with the same solvent (solution 'S').

Transfer a 10-ml aliquot of solution 'S' to a second 100-ml graduated flask, add 50 ml of N hydrochloric acid and dilute to volume with water. Shake 60 ml of this solution with 5 ml of zinc amalgam for thirty minutes and pipette 10 ml of the supernatant liquid into a 100-ml, amber-coloured graduated flask (A). Add 5 ml of N hydrochloric acid and 35 ml of water.

Transfer a further 10-ml aliquot of solution 'S' to a second 100-ml amber-coloured graduated flask (B) and add 10 ml of N hydrochloric acid and 30 ml of water.

To a third 100-ml, amber-coloured graduated flask (C) transfer 10 ml of 0·1N sodium hydroxide, 10 ml of N hydrochloric acid and 30 ml of water.

Treat the contents of flasks A, B and C as follows. Mixing after each addition, add 5 ml of freshly prepared 0·1 per cent sodium nitrite solution and allow to stand for two minutes; add 5 ml of 0·5 per cent ammonium sulphamate and allow to stand for three minutes; add 5 ml of freshly prepared 0·1 per. cent *N*-(1-naphthyl)ethylenediamine dihydrochloride solution and allow to stand for ten minutes. Dilute to volume with a mixture of equal volumes of 0·2N and 0·1N hydrochloric acid.

Measure the extinctions of the solutions in flasks A (D_1) and B (D_2) at 550 mμ, using 2·5-cm cells with the solution in flask C in the comparison cell in each case.

The corrected extinction of the sample = $D_1 - D_2/10$.

From a standard curve, prepared by carrying out the colour reaction with suitable amounts of *p*-aminobenzoic acid, read the g of *p*-aminobenzoic acid equivalent to the corrected extinction of the sample.

Each g of *p*-aminobenzoic acid = 3·22 g $C_{19}H_{19}O_6N_7$.

Tablets of Folic Acid, *B.P.* Usually contain 5 mg of folic acid per tablet.

Assayed as for folic acid, preparing solution 'S' by dissolving a weight of powdered tablets equivalent to 0·1 g of folic acid in 0·1N sodium hydroxide, filtering if necessary and diluting to exactly 100 ml with 0·1N sodium hydroxide.

FORMALDEHYDE

HCHO Mol. Wt. 30·03

Formaldehyde is used commercially either as its aqueous solution or in a solid polymerised form.

Many techniques have been devised for the estimation of formaldehyde; those most generally applied are:

(*a*) The *B.P.* method, due to Blank and Finkenbeiner,[1] based on the oxidation of formaldehyde to formic acid with hydrogen peroxide in alkaline solution, is least affected by impurities. The method is suitable in the presence of methanol, which is generally added to prevent polymerisation.

Add about 3 g of solution of formaldehyde (about 40 per cent) to a mixture of 50 ml of 3 per cent hydrogen peroxide solution and 50 ml of N sodium hydroxide. Warm on a water-bath until effervescence ceases; titrate the excess of alkali with N hydrochloric acid, using phenolphthalein as indicator. At the same time conduct a similar experiment without the formaldehyde and subtract the alkali used from that neutralised in the test experiment. 1 ml N = 0·03003 g HCHO.

If an excess of methanol over normal amounts is present, a high but proportionate figure is obtained by this method; 0·09 per cent should be deducted for every 10 per cent of methanol present.

With the above method effervescence continues for some time and the end-point is often not easily seen, but it can be improved by the addition of an excess of N acid about half an hour after the commencement of effervescence, allowing the renewed effervescence to subside and then titrating to neutrality with N sodium hydroxide. The *U.S.P.* employs bromothymol blue as an indicator.

(*b*) The British Standard method[2] uses neutral sulphite. The method is quicker and of general convenience but gives results about 0·06 per cent lower than the peroxide method.

Weigh an amount of solution containing about 1 g of formaldehyde into a conical flask containing 10 ml of water. Cover with a watch-glass, add two drops of thymolphthalein indicator then add 0·1N sodium hydroxide dropwise, until a faint blue colour is just perceptible. Measure 75 ml of a freshly prepared 12·6 per cent solution of anhydrous sodium sulphite into a second conical flask and add two drops of thymolphthalein indicator followed by 0·1N hydrochloric acid until the blue colour just disappears. Pour this solution into the prepared formaldehyde solution, mix carefully, set aside for two minutes and titrate with N hydrochloric acid until the blue colour just disappears. 1 ml N HCl = 0·03003 g.

Haslam and Squirrell[3] found that the change of indicator from blue to colourless occurs some five or six drops of N acid before the true end-point, which would account for low results reputed to be given by this method with thymolphthalein indicator, and they titrate to pH 8·95.

(*c*) Romijn's method[4] gives somewhat high results in the presence of acetone and more than 5 per cent of methanol but is widely used, being particularly suitable for the determination of small quantities.

To a solution containing about 0·03 g of formaldehyde (5 ml of Solution of Formaldehyde *B.P.* in 250 ml of water, 5 ml of dilution being taken) add 30 ml of 0·1N iodine and a few ml of 10 per cent sodium hydroxide solution. Allow to stand for ten minutes, acidify and titrate the excess of iodine with 0·1N sodium thiosulphate. 1 ml 0·1N = 0·001501 g.

(*d*) The cyanide method of the *A.O.A.C.*,[5] as in the case of (*c*), is suitable only for dilute solutions. The method is briefly:

Acidify 15 ml of 0·1N silver nitrate with 6 drops of 1 : 1 nitric acid in a 50-ml graduated flask. Add a quantity of formaldehyde solution (containing not more than 25 mg of formaldehyde) which has been previously mixed with 10 ml of a 0·62 per cent potassium cyanide solution. These solutions must be mixed together before adding to the silver nitrate as an addition compound is formed. Dilute to 50 ml shake and filter. Titrate 25 ml of the filtrate with 0·1N potassium thiocyanate, using iron alum as indicator. Repeat the experiment, omitting the formaldehyde solution. The difference between the two titrations, multiplied by 2, gives the number of ml of 0·1N solution corresponding to the cyanide combined with the formaldehyde. 1 ml 0·1N = 0·003003 g.

(*e*) The general reaction of aldehydes and ketones with hydroxylamine hydrochloride to form oximes can be used for formaldehyde, the liberated acid being titrated to methyl orange. Obviously this method is only applicable in the absence of other aldehydes or any ketones.

Kersey, Maddocks and Johnson[6] have examined Schryver's test for formaldehyde with a view to its quantitative application when the substance is present only in **traces.** The method evolved was for the determination of small amounts of formaldehyde in air but it would be useful generally for the determination of low concentrations. To extract formaldehyde, the authors aspirate a volume of the air through a phenylhydrazine hydrochloride solution as a fine gas spray by means of a fritted glass filter disc. The general assay is as follows:

To 10 ml of a 1 per cent phenylhydrazine hydrochloride solution (prepared by suspending 1 g of phenylhydrazine in about 5 ml of water, adding 2 ml of concentrated hydrochloric acid and 80 ml of water, filtering and diluting to 100 ml), add sufficient solution under test to contain between 0·05 and 0·25 mg of formaldehyde and dilute to 50 ml. To 10 ml of this solution add 1·0 ml of freshly prepared 5 per cent potassium ferricyanide solution and 4·0 ml of concentrated hydrochloric acid, dilute to 20 ml and allow to stand for ten minutes. Prepare simultaneously a series of standard comparison solutions using 2 ml of the phenylhydrazine solution, 7 ml of water, measured amounts of a solution of formaldehyde containing 1 mg of formaldehyde per litre (say, 1, 2, 5 ml), 1·0 ml of the ferricyanide solution and 4·0 ml of concentrated hydrochloric acid; dilute to 20 ml with water and allow to stand for ten minutes. Compare the colour of the test solution against those of the standard comparison solutions.

The determination of methanol in formaldehyde solution is described by Homer:[7]

To 50 ml of the formaldehyde solution add excess of strong ammonia solution, keeping the mixture well cooled. Allow to stand for six hours and then distil almost to dryness. Acidify the distillate, redistil and determine the specific gravity of the distillate in the usual manner.

A simple alternative method is to determine the formaldehyde content and the specific gravity of the solution at 25°/25°, reading the percentage by weight of methanol present from a three co-ordinate graph. The British Standard referred to above[2] has published such a graph based on information given by Skelding and Ashbolt.[8]

Since methanol is not oxidised by hydrogen peroxide in alkaline solution, it can be separated after such treatment by distillation and determined in the distillate.

Paraformaldehyde, $(CH_2O)_n$. A solid polymeride, soluble in sodium hydroxide solution is determined exactly as formaldehyde, by methods (*a*) or (*b*) above. 1 ml N = 0·03003 g.

Lozenge of Formaldehyde, *B.P.C.* Contains 9·7 mg of paraformaldehyde in each lozenge. Provided no inversion of the sucrose in the lozenge base has taken place, little loss in accuracy is involved in following a direct method of determination.

Dissolve a weighed portion of the sample, equivalent to about 0·05 g of paraformaldehyde, in water, add 50 ml 0·1N iodine and sufficient sodium hydroxide solution to remove the colour. Allow to stand for ten minutes, acidify with dilute hydrochloric acid and titrate the residual iodine with 0·1N sodium thiosulphate. 1 ml 0·1N = 0·0015 g CH_2O.

FORMALDEHYDE

For accurate determination distillation of the formaldehyde from the lozenge base is desirable. A quantity of powdered lozenge, equivalent to about 0·05 g of paraformaldehyde, is steam-distilled in the presence of dilute sulphuric acid into about 100 ml of water until the total volume collected is about 750 ml. The iodine absorption method given above is then used on the distillate. A considerable loss of formaldehyde is liable to occur during manufacture but loss on storage is slow.

HEXAMINE, $(CH_2)_6N_4$, Mol. Wt. 140·2

Hexamine is readily hydrolysed by acids to ammonia and formaldehyde, but the removal of the latter in order to titrate the excess of acid added is somewhat difficult. In the *B.P.C.* 1954 method the compound was boiled with excess of N acid until the odour of formaldehyde had disappeared and then titrated back to methyl red with N alkali, 1 ml N = 0·03505 g. The ammonia in the residual liquid after titration may be determined by alkaline distillation into excess acid as usual. The official method is now by Kjeldahl nitrogen. 1 ml 0·1N = 0·003505 g.

A nitrogen figure by Kjeldahl is also a useful means of estimating hexamine in medicines (N × 2·50 = hexamine). Hexamine may be extracted from aqueous solution by chloroform.

Methenamine mandelate (Hexamine mandelate), $C_6H_{12}N_4,C_8H_8O_3$, Mol. Wt. 292·3.

The *U.S.P.* has adopted the method recommended by Emery[9] for the assay of this salt:

> Weigh 1 g into a 250-ml flask and add 100 ml of water and 25 ml of dilute hydrochloric acid. Reflux gently for fifteen minutes, cool, wash down the condenser with water, transfer to a 250-ml graduated flask with water and dilute to volume with water.
>
> Prepare a modified Nessler's reagent as follows: Dissolve 10 g of mercuric chloride, 30 g of potassium iodide and 5 g of acacia in 200 ml of water and filter through cotton wool. Just before use, mix 20 ml of this solution with 10 ml of 15 per cent sodium hydroxide solution in a 250-ml flask, cool in an ice-bath and add a 10-ml aliquot of the sample solution. Wash down the neck of the flask with water and allow to stand for at least thirty minutes. Wash down the sides of the flask with 10 ml of a mixture of 2 volumes of glacial acetic acid and 3 volumes of water, mix quickly, add 40 ml of 0·1N iodine and titrate the excess iodine with 0·1N sodium thiosulphate using starch as indicator. 1 ml 0·1N iodine = 0·002436 g $C_6H_{12}N_4,C_8H_8O_3$.

ETHYLENE OXIDE RESIDUES

Ethylene oxide is extensively used for sterilisation of powders and it is sometimes necessary to determine residues. Methods which have been applied successfully depend on conversion of the residual ethylene oxide or glycol to formaldehyde and the determination of this product by the chromotropic acid method or the Hantzsch reaction. A method based on the chromotropic acid reaction has been applied by Critchfield and Johnson[10] to the determination of ethylene oxide residues in spices.

Weigh an amount of sample containing not more than 0·7 mg of ethylene oxide into a heat-resistant pressure bottle containing 20 ml of water and, at the same time, introduce 20 ml of water into a second, similar bottle for the blank. Pipette 1 ml of 0·5N sulphuric acid into each bottle and stopper the bottles, protecting the rubber gaskets on the stoppers with polyethylene film. Enclose the bottles securely in fabric bags and allow to stand, as close together as possible, in a water-bath (at 98° ± 2°) for sixty minutes. Remove the bottles from the bath, allow to cool to room temperature and then loosen the bags, uncap the bottles carefully to release excess pressure and remove the bags. Treat the contents of each bottle, respectively, as follows. Transfer quantitatively to a 100-ml graduated cylinder and add, by pipette, stoppering the cylinder and mixing after each addition, 1 ml of 0·5N sodium hydroxide followed by 2 ml of 0·1M sodium periodate (prepared from analytical-reagent grade sodium metaperiodate). Allow to stand for fifteen minutes at room temperature, add, by pipette, 2 ml of 5·5 per cent sodium sulphite solution (prepared not more than one week before use from analytical-reagent grade material), dilute to 100 ml with water, stopper the cylinder and mix. Transfer a 10-ml aliquot to another 100-ml glass-stoppered graduated cylinder, add about 0·05 g of chromotropic acid sodium salt and shake until dissolved. Dilute to 50 ml with concentrated sulphuric acid, added from an acid-burette, and allow the normal heat rise to occur. Bubble nitrogen through the solution, in a vigorous stream, for about ten minutes and then allow to cool to room temperature.

Measure the extinction of the sample solution at the absorption maximum at about 570 mμ using 1-cm cells with the blank solution in the comparison cell and read the concentration of ethylene oxide from a standard curve.

Prepare the standard curve as follows: Weigh a 100-ml graduated flask containing about 50 ml of water, introduce about 1·5 g of ethylene oxide, swirl and, when the ethylene oxide is dissolved, weigh again; calculate the weight of ethylene oxide added. Dilute to volume with water and mix. Transfer a 10-ml aliquot of this solution to a 1-litre graduated flask containing about 200 ml of water, dilute to volume with water and mix. Into three heat-resistant pressure bottles, each containing 20 ml of water, pipette, respectively, 1, 3 and 5 ml of the dilute ethylene oxide solution. Adjust with water so that the volume of liquid in each bottle is the same and prepare a blank by filling a fourth pressure bottle with water to the same level as the standards. Continue as described above from 'Pipette 1 ml of 0·5N sulphuric acid . . .' and prepare a curve by plotting extinction against weight of ethylene oxide.

If other materials that react with periodate to give formaldehyde are present they must first be removed. For this Critchfield and Johnson have detailed a method in which the sample is refluxed in a stream of air (from which interfering aldehydes have been removed if necessary) and the ethylene oxide carried over is collected in ice-cold water and transferred to the pressure flask. If this preliminary treatment is carried out a separate standard curve must be prepared since when ethylene oxide is evolved from boiling water only 86 per cent of it is recovered; the preliminary treatment is therefore carried out on the aliquots of standard solution before hydrolysing and developing the colour as above.

Bastow[11] attempted to apply a method of this type to the determination of ethylene oxide residues in samples of mineral origin (e.g. Heavy Kaolin and related materials) but experienced certain difficulties and developed the following procedure based on the method of Daniel and Gage[12] for formaldehyde. This method uses the Hantzsch reaction between formaldehyde, ammonia and acetylacetone to give the yellow 3,5-diacetyl-1,4-dihydrolutidine. Experimental applications of this reaction showed it to give a light extinction of only one-third of that obtained in the chromotropic acid method for a given amount of formaldehyde. However the blank solution has considerably less absorption than that with chromotropic acid and, hence, longer light paths are possible if greater sensitivity is required.

Weigh an amount of powder containing not more than 1,000 μg of total ethylene oxide plus glycol into a 50-ml, glass-stoppered cylinder, add 50 ml of water and shake for thirty minutes. Filter, pipette 10 ml of the filtrate into a glass-stoppered test-tube, add 1 ml of 0·2M periodic acid, stopper the tube and allow to stand for thirty minutes. Then add 2 ml of 0·5M sodium arsenite, mix and add 2 ml of a reagent prepared by dissolving 25 g of ammonium acetate, 3 ml of glacial acetic acid and 0·2 ml of redistilled acetylacetone in sufficient water to produce 100 ml. Stopper the tube loosely and heat in a water-bath for ten minutes. Cool, transfer to a 25-ml graduated flask with water and dilute to volume with water. Measure the extinction at the absorption maximum at about 412 mμ, using 1-cm cells with, in the comparison cell, a reagent blank prepared by repeating the operation described above using 10 ml of water instead of the 10 ml of filtrate. Read the ethylene glycol content from a standard curve prepared using known amounts of ethylene glycol, covering the range 0 to 200 μg.

For the determination of the larger amounts (of the order of 0·4 per cent of ethylene glycol) sometimes present in Heavy Kaolin the following titration method may be used.

Weigh 4 g into a 50-ml glass-stoppered cylinder, add 50 ml of water and shake for thirty minutes. Filter, pipette 25 ml of the filtrate into a 100-ml graduated flask and add 50 ml of freshly prepared 0·02N potassium periodate. Dilute to volume with water, mix and allow to stand for one hour. Then transfer a 50-ml aliquot to an iodine flask, add 1 g of sodium bicarbonate and 0·5 g of potassium iodide and titrate immediately with 0·02N sodium arsenite solution using 3 ml of starch solution, added towards the end of the titration, as indicator. Carry out a blank determination by pipetting 50 ml of 0·02M potassium periodate into a second 100-ml graduated flask, diluting to volume with water, allowing to stand for one hour and completing as above. 1 ml 0·02N sodium arsenite = 0·06207 g ethylene glycol.

1. Blank, O., and Finkenbeiner, H., *Ber.*, 1898, **31**, 2979.
2. B.S. 2942: 1957.
3. Haslam, J., and Squirrell, D. C. M., *Analyst*, 1957, **82**, 511.
4. Romijn, G., *Z. Anal. Chem.*, 1897, **36**, 18.
5. *A.O.A.C.*, 1960, p. 43.
6. Kersey, R. W., Maddocks, J. R., and Johnson, T. E., *Analyst*, 1940, **65**, 203.
7. Homer, H. W., *J. Soc. Chem. Ind.*, 1941, **60**, 213.
8. Skelding, A. A., and Ashbolt, R. F., *Chem. & Ind.*, 1959, 1204.
9. Emery, W. O., *J.A.O.A.C.*, 1920, **3**, 374.
10. Critchfield, F. E., and Johnson, J. B., *Anal. Chem.*, 1957, **29**, 797.
11. Bastow, R. A., private communication.
12. Daniel, J. W., and Gage, J. C., *Analyst*, 1956, **81**, 594.

GAMMA BENZENE HEXACHLORIDE

(Gammexane)

$C_6H_6Cl_6$ Mol. Wt. 290·9

Gammexane is the gamma isomer of 1,2,3,4,5,6-hexachloro*cyclo*hexane.

Gamma benzene hexachloride is readily decomposed with hot alcoholic alkali to give the trichloro-compound and determination of the total hexachloro*cyclo*hexane is based on this fact.

> To about 0·4 g add 25 ml of 95 per cent ethanol and warm on a water-bath until dissolved. Cool, add 10 ml of N alcoholic potassium hydroxide made with 95 per cent ethanol, swirl gently and allow to stand for ten minutes. Dilute to 150 ml with water, neutralise with dilute nitric acid and add 10 ml in excess, followed by 50 ml of 0·1N silver nitrate. Complete by Volhard's method (see under Halogen Acids, p. 290). Carry out a blank determination on about the same amount of sample as above ($\pm$10 mg), adding the same volume of all reagents in the order, dilute nitric acid, ethanol, potassium hydroxide solution and silver nitrate. 1 ml 0·1N = 0·009695 g of $C_6H_6Cl_6$. Alternatively the hydrolysed chlorine may be determined electrometrically.

The efficacy of the product as an insecticide rests almost entirely in the gamma-isomer and apart from differential refractometry[1] the most suitable method of ascertaining its purity is by a determination of the freezing-point. A convenient method, which gives the purity in terms of the gamma-isomer content to an accuracy of $\pm$0·1 per cent when the sample approaches 100 per cent purity, is that described by Handley.[2]

The apparatus (Fig. 5) consists of a bell-mouthed glass test-tube, to contain the sample, inside a larger test-tube which acts as an air-jacket. The sample tube is fitted with a cork through which pass a central thin-walled thermometer pocket and a reciprocating hand stirrer which serves also as a gas inlet tube. The stirrer, made of capillary tubing of 0·5 mm bore and 5 mm outside diameter, has a loop at the bottom with a pin-hole blown in the end of the capillary. The loop is made to encircle closely the thermometer pocket, which is positioned so that the bottom of the thermometer bulb is 10 mm above the bottom of the sample tube, and so that the

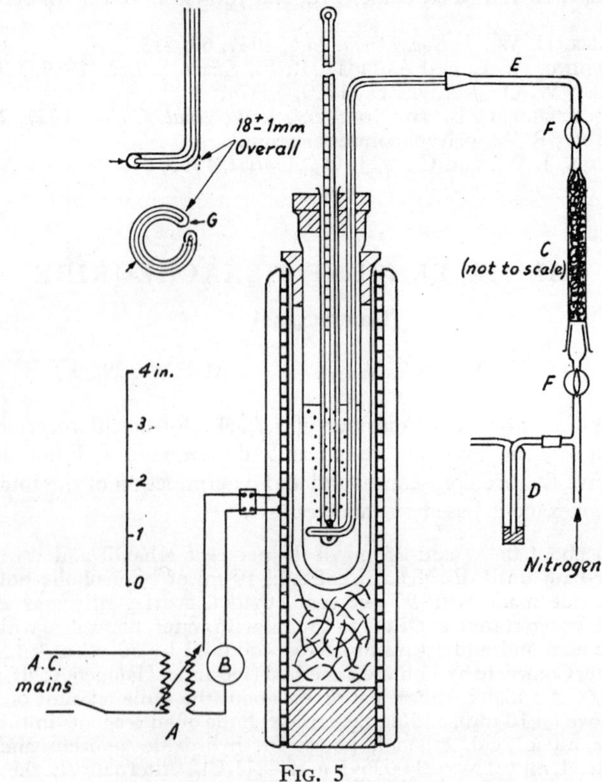

FIG. 5

Freezing-point apparatus showing structure of stirrer

A. Variable voltage-output transformer
B. 0–1 amp. meter
C. Drying tube containing magnesium perchlorate
D. Pressure release, $\frac{3}{4}$ in. depth of mercury
E. Flexible rubber tubing, approx. 3 mm bore
F. 2 mm tap
G. Capillary blown to give pin-hole orifice

immersion mark on the stem is level with, or slightly below, the bottom of the cork.

For the two essential operations in the determination, melting and freezing the sample, two heating jackets are required. First the sample is melted by placing the sample tube within a close-fitting metal cylinder, heated electrically to a controlled temperature within the range 120° to 125°, *i.e.* about 10° above the melting-point. For the freezing operation the sample is inserted in the wider glass air-jacket before being placed in a second metal cylinder which is maintained with close temperature control at 108° ± 1°, *i.e.* 5° below the freezing-point. At all times dry nitrogen is passed through the sample by means of the capillary stirrer connected to the gas supply with a narrow rubber tube. A gas cylinder, fitted with reducing valve, followed by a tube containing magnesium perchlorate, provides the source of dry nitrogen, while a small mercury bubbler is connected as shown to allow excess gas to escape.

The two metal heating jackets are made from 9-in. lengths of brass or copper tube with a wall thickness not less than $\frac{1}{16}$ in. and of internal diameter 1 and $1\frac{3}{4}$ in. respectively. The tubes are wrapped with a layer of asbestos tape for insulation. Bright ray wire 28 s.w.g. is wound spirally along the tubes at 5 turns per in. and then covered with two layers of asbestos tape or paper and the two leads, after being brought together over this last insulation, are inserted in a twin connector block. A final wrapping is made with asbestos rope or equivalent material to give a layer of at least $\frac{1}{2}$ in. thickness and each of the tubes is plugged at the lower end with asbestos rope or powder, held in place by a cork. The cylinders are heated by a controlled current passed through the spiral resistance winding and supplied from a mains transformer with variable voltage output. Both heating jackets should initially be calibrated by placing the sample tube, charged to a depth of $2\frac{1}{2}$ in. with dibutylphthalate, centrally in either of the jackets by means of a cork collar. The tube is inserted to a depth of 5 and $5\frac{1}{2}$ in. in the narrow and the wider jackets, respectively, and a reliable thermometer, range 0–250°, is held in a central position with the bulb immersed to within 10 mm of the bottom of the sample tube. By means of the voltage control a heating current is applied and the temperature is observed after at least thirty minutes. The voltage necessary to give the required temperature is then noted for each jacket.

For the measurement of freezing-points, a thermometer calibrated at the National Physical Laboratory and of the range 99·5°–130·5° Celsius as specified in B.S. 593 : 1954 (Laboratory Thermometers) under the schedule A.130/100, is used. To facilitate temperature readings, by interpolation, to ±0·02°, a magnifying device is attached to the thermometer.

Introduce 25 g of the sample, as a powder, into the sample tube, insert the cork fitted with thermometer pocket and combined stirrer/gas inlet and place the tube in the narrow heating jacket, which should already be at its steady temperature in the range 120° to 125°. When the sample has melted bubble dry nitrogen through it for one hour at such a rate that the gas bubbles emerge from the melt without producing splashing on the walls of the tube and no excess gas escapes through the mercury bubbler. At the end of this time, without interruption of the gas stream, remove the tube from its jacket, place it inside the air-jacket and insert the whole inside the wide metal cylinder at 108°. Stir immediately, by hand, with a steady movement approximating to 100 strokes per minute until when, in the later stages of the measurement, numerous small crystals of gamma benzene hexachloride have formed causing friction between stirrer and thermometer pocket and it is better to stir for only fifteen seconds in each minute. Note the temperature of the sample at one-minute intervals. A steady fall of temperature is observed until the liquid is supercooled by about 0·1° when spontaneous seeding usually takes place from the numerous small crystals formed by slight sublimation. (Occasionally more supercooling amounting to 0·3° occurs, probably due to failure to dislodge seeding crystals from the sides of the tube; in this case the results should be discounted and the determination repeated.) After spontaneous seeding has taken place the temperature rises quickly to a maximum and remains constant for several minutes, but when three consecutive readings at one-minute intervals agree within 0·02° this temperature may be regarded as the freezing-point.

Using this method the freezing-point of a pure sample of gamma-isomer, prepared by zone refining, was found to be 112·87 ± 0·2° which was in agreement with the value of 112·86 obtained by Toops and Riddick,[3] who used a rather elaborate method, and the purity of the sample may be calculated from the expression (due to Toops and Riddick), $\log_{10}$ (mole per cent purity) $= 2 - 0{\cdot}0148\Delta T/2{\cdot}30259$, where ΔT is the difference between the freezing-point of the sample and 112·86°. When the gamma-isomer content is greater than 99 per cent (as in the grade of gamma benzene hexachloride known as lindane) the purity can be calculated by assuming that 1 mole per cent impurity depresses the freezing-point by 0·7° giving: mole per cent purity $= 100 - (112{\cdot}86 - T)/0{\cdot}7$ where T is the initial freezing-point.

A number of polarographic methods have been described for the determination of the gamma-isomer in technical samples of benzene hexachloride. Although many refinements have been added by different workers to improve the accuracy, a procedure based upon that described by Ingram and Southern[4] gives reasonable results on samples containing 12 to 14 per cent although they may be a little on the high side, due to small amounts of interfering impurities.

Dissolve about 100 mg of sample in 52 ml of ethanol and add 40 ml of 2 per cent w/v aqueous solution of potassium iodide and 2 ml of a freshly prepared 0·25 per cent solution of gelatin. Mix, cool and make up to 100 ml with the 2 per cent potassium iodide. Remove the oxygen from a portion of the solution by passing through nitrogen previously passed through a solution of 50 per cent v/v ethanol in water.

Polarograph this solution in triplicate using a mercury pool anode over the range −0·2 to −1·7 volts maintaining the solution at a fixed temperature of about 25°. Polarograph also under the same conditions a solution containing 13 mg of gamma benzene hexachloride in 100 ml prepared as above.

The apparent half-wave potential of the gamma-isomer under these conditions is about −0·98 volts.

Draw a tangent through the point of greatest slope of the diffusion wave and measure the vertical distance between the points of intersection it makes with the production of the flat portions of the beginning and end-points of the curve. Calculate the concentration of the gamma-isomer in the sample by the direct comparison of wave heights obtained for the sample and standard solutions and the known concentrations of these solutions.

For the determination of gamma benzene hexachloride in formulations the active agent can be extracted by one of the methods given below and its purity then ascertained by melting-point, as indicated.

(*a*) For Dusts and Wettable Powders

Extract an amount of the sample containing about 0·5 g of gamma benzene hexachloride with light petroleum (b.p. 60° to 80°) in an apparatus for the continuous extraction of drugs, until at least 120 cycles have taken place. Cool and transfer the light-petroleum extract to a tared conical flask. Distil off most of the solvent and then evaporate to dryness and dry at 60° to constant weight.

(*b*) For Miscible Liquids

Introduce an amount of the sample containing about 0·5 g of gamma benzene hexachloride into one of the 25-ml flasks of the apparatus[5] (Fig. 6) and assemble the apparatus as shown.

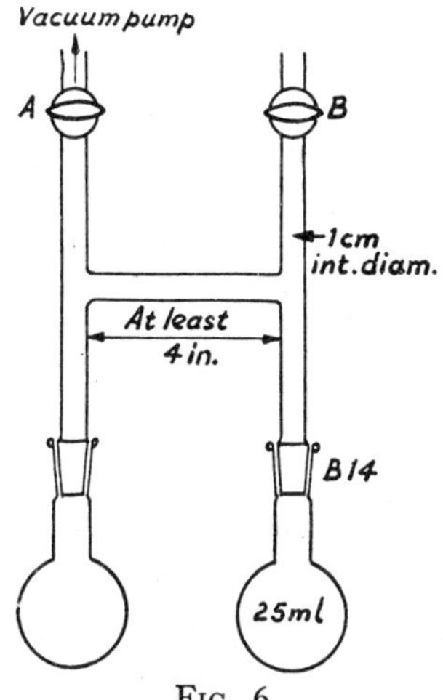

FIG. 6

Close both taps and immerse the bulbs of the flasks in solid carbon dioxide dissolved in trichloroethylene contained in wide-mouthed Dewar flasks. Open the tap to vacuum and evacuate to a pressure below 0·1 mm of mercury; the pressure should be maintained at this level. Close the tap to vacuum, remove the Dewar flask of refrigerant from the flask containing the sample and allow the latter to warm to room temperature. Leave until no further solvent passes into the cold trap.

Cool both flasks, evacuate again and repeat the process until all the solvent has distilled over. (It may be necessary to repeat this cycle four or five times and the whole operation may take up to thirty-six hours.) Remove both Dewar flasks, allow the apparatus to reach room temperature and release the vacuum by opening tap B. Disconnect the flask containing the residue of benzene hexachloride and wetting agents, wash this residue into a tared sintered-glass crucible (G.3) with water and continue washing until the residue is free from wetting agents. Dry the residue to constant weight *in vacuo* over phosphorus pentoxide.

Determine the melting-point of the residue from either (*a*) or (*b*) above by the *B.P.* method. If the melting-point of the extract is between 111° and 113° and a mixed melting-point with a specimen of pure gamma benzene hexachloride shows no depression the sample contains lindane. If the melting-point is outside the range quoted it can be concluded that either the original sample did not contain lindane or the formulation contains other pesticides.

For determination of the gamma-isomer content the *A.O.A.C.*[6] uses a partition chromatographic method. This depends upon separating the various isomers on a column of silicic acid and using a saturated solution of nitromethane in *n*-hexane as the mobile solvent. The gamma-isomer is recognisable by the typical crystal formation obtained when the eluate is evaporated. In our experience the success of the method depends upon rigid adherence to the specified grade of silicic acid.

Infra-red absorption measurement may be used when gamma benzene hexachloride is included either alone or with other insecticides in many different preparations. From a powder preparation it may be extracted with ether and a liquid preparation may be diluted with ether, then, after evaporation of the solvent, the residue may be dissolved in carbon disulphide to give a concentration of about 1 per cent. If the gamma benzene hexachloride is alone or with DDT a measurement on the band at 912 cm^{-1} using 1-mm cells can be used for its determination. If it is present with either aldrin or dieldrin, then the band at 952 cm^{-1} is preferred. Interfering absorption of solvents, wetters and emulsifiers may sometimes be removed by chromatography on oleum/kieselguhr or alumina as in the case of the determination of DDT.

Shaw[7] recommended the hydrolysable chlorine figure for the determination of gamma benzene hexachloride in galenicals and for the official *B.Vet.C.* preparations (**Cream of Gamma Benzene Hexachloride** containing 0·1 per cent; **Cream of Gamma Benzene Hexachloride and Proflavine** containing 0.1 per cent; **Dusting-Powder of Gamma Benzene Hexachloride and Pyrethrum** containing 0·5 per cent) this simpler method is satisfactory. A control titration is necessary to compensate for the presence of ionisable chlorine in sample and reagents. The official method is briefly:

Reflux 15 g (20 g of dusting powder) for one hour with 50 ml of 0·5N ethanolic potassium hydroxide, cool, acidify with dilute nitric acid and extract with ether. Wash the extracts with water, add the washings to the aqueous solution and neutralise with sodium hydroxide solution to methyl orange. Add 6 ml of dilute nitric acid, titrate electrometrically with 0·2N silver nitrate. Carry out a blank using, as nearly as possible, the same weight of sample but neutralising the 0·5N ethanolic potassium hydroxide with dilute nitric acid before adding the sample. 1 ml 0·02N $AgNO_3$ = 0·001939 g $C_6H_6Cl_6$.

1. HILL, R., and JONES, A. G., *Analyst*, 1955, **80**, 339.
2. HANDLEY, R., *J. Appl. Chem.*, 1960, **10**, 353.
3. TOOPS, E., and RIDDICK, J. A., *Anal. Chem.*, 1951, **23**, 1106.
4. INGRAM, G. B., and SOUTHERN, H. K., *Nature*, 1948, **161**, 437.
5. I.C.I. GENERAL CHEMICALS DIVISION, private communication.
6. *A.O.A.C.*, 1960, p. 53.
7. SHAW, W. H. C., *J. Pharm. Pharmacol.*, 1949, **1**, 813.

GELSEMIUM

Since an assay of gelsemium root was required for use with reference to the Poisons Regulations, 1935, the Analytical Methods Committee of the *S.A.C.* has recommended a method[1] for determination of the total alkaloids. It is acknowledged that the percentage of alkaloids obtained by the method may include non-alkaloidal coloured material which it was not found possible to eliminate without loss of alkaloid.

Introduce 10 g of the root and 5 g of acid-washed sand, both in No. 60 powder, into a pear-shaped separator of about 300 ml capacity, and add 100 ml of a mixture of three volumes of ether and one volume of chloroform, shake well and set aside for ten minutes; add 5 ml of dilute ammonia solution and shake for one minute at ten-minute intervals during one hour. Insert a plug of cotton wool into the stem of the separator and allow the liquid to percolate into another separator. When the liquid ceases to flow, pack the drug firmly and continue the percolation with further quantities of the solvent until complete extraction of the alkaloids is effected. Test the percolate for complete extraction by collecting separately about 2 ml in a dish, evaporating the solvent, dissolving the residue in a few drops of 0·1N sulphuric acid and adding 1 drop of 0·1N iodine. In the absence of alkaloids of gelsemium no precipitate or turbidity is formed.

To the percolate add 30 ml of N sulphuric acid, shake well, allow to separate and run off the lower layer. Continue the extraction with 10-ml portions of 0·1N sulphuric acid until extraction of the alkaloids is complete as shown by the iodine test. Wash the mixed acid solutions with about 10 ml of chloroform and run the latter into a second separator containing 20 ml of 0·1N sulphuric acid, shake, allow to separate and reject the chloroform. Repeat the washing of the liquid in the first separator with two further 5 ml quantities of chloroform, transfer each in turn to the second separator, wash with the same aqueous acid liquid, allow to separate and reject the chloroform layer as before. Transfer the acid liquid from the second separator to the first separator, make just alkaline with dilute ammonia solution and add 2 ml in excess; shake with successive portions of chloroform until complete extraction of the alkaloids is effected, washing each chloroform extract with the same 20 ml of water contained in another separator. Remove the chloroform by distillation, add to the residue 2 ml of dehydrated ethanol, evaporate, and dry at 60° for thirty minutes. Dissolve the residue in 2 ml of 95 per cent ethanol, warm until dissolved, add 2 ml of 0·1N sulphuric acid and 10 ml of water, cool and titrate with 0·1N sodium hydroxide from a micro-burette, using methyl red as indicator. 1 ml 0·1N acid = 0·0322 g of the alkaloids of gelsemium calculated as gelsemine.

Tincture of Gelsemium, *B.P.C.* Contains 0·032 per cent w/v of total alkaloids.

For assay evaporate 100 ml to about 20 ml, transfer to a separator with the aid of successive small portions of 0·1N sulphuric acid and chloroform; shake and allow to separate. Continue as under Gelsemium beginning with running the chloroform into a second separator containing 20 ml of 0·1N sulphuric acid.

1. *Analyst*, 1941, **66,** 108.

GLYCERIN

$CH_2OH.CHOH.CH_2OH$ Mol. Wt. 92·10

Considerable literature has been published on the determination of glycerol; oxidation methods are the most satisfactory but obviously they depend upon its separation in a fair state of purity. Any process which involves evaporation of aqueous or alcoholic solutions to low bulk gives rise to inaccuracies as concentration is difficult and glycerol is sensibly volatile at 100°, the amount of loss varying with the conditions and the apparatus used. The volatilisation may be prevented by the presence of an excess of lime with which glycerol forms a compound.

If glycerol can be isolated easily from the mixture either the periodate or 'acetin' method may be used (see below), but if the determination is only expected to give an approximation the following methods may be employed.

(*a*) A rapid method for mixtures where the glycerol can be extracted easily and in a fairly pure state (*cf.* Kaolin Poultice):

Accurately weigh sufficient of the material to contain about 5 to 10 g of glycerol, dilute with water, filter hot and wash the insoluble matter until all the glycerol is in the filtrate. Evaporate until the volume is below 50 ml and then transfer to a 50-ml graduated flask, washing in and making accurately up to the mark at 15·5°. Determine the specific gravity of the solution obtained and from the table given in Appendix XX, p. 890, calculate the glycerol content. Then

$$\text{glycerin } B.P. \text{ (per cent)} = \frac{\text{per cent found from table} \times 50}{\text{wt. taken} \times 98}.$$

(*b*) An approximate estimation (which was originally intended for wines but which may be adapted to drug mixtures by slight modifications) is summarised below from the *A.O.A.C.*:[1]

Evaporate a suitable quantity in a porcelain dish on a water-bath at 85° to 90° to a volume of about 10 ml. Treat the residue with about 5 g of fine sand and 4 to 5 ml of milk of lime (containing 15 g of CaO per 100 ml) for each g of extract present and evaporate almost to dryness. Treat the moist residue with 50 ml of 90 per cent ethanol and rub the whole into a paste. Heat to boiling with constant stirring, decant through a filter and wash the residue repeatedly with hot ethanol until the filtrate amounts to about 150 ml. Evaporate to a syrupy consistency in a porcelain dish on a hot, but not boiling, water-bath; transfer the residue to a small glass-stoppered, graduated cylinder with 20 ml of dehydrated ethanol, and add three 10-ml portions of anhydrous ether, shaking thoroughly after each addition. Allow to stand until clear, pour off through a filter, wash the cylinder and filter with a mixture of two parts of dehydrated ethanol to three parts of anhydrous ether, also pouring the wash solution through the filter. Evaporate the filtrate to a syrupy consistency, dry for an hour at 98° to 100°, weigh, ignite and weigh again. The loss on ignition gives the weight of glycerol.

(*c*) A method of interest, first devised by Shukoff and Schestakoff[2] and commendable in its simplicity, consists in mixing the glycerol solution with powdered anhydrous sodium sulphate, and extracting the mass so obtained with dry acetone. The method has been used successfully for the determination of glycerol in Ointment of Resorcinol.

To a solution containing a maximum of 1 g of glycerol add a slight excess of sulphuric acid, filter if necessary and then render slightly alkaline with potassium hydroxide solution. Concentrate the solution so obtained to a syrup at a temperature not exceeding 80° (evaporate solutions which precipitate salts on concentration to a semi-solid consistency). Mix the evaporated liquid with 20 g of anhydrous sodium sulphate and transfer the nearly dry powdery mass to an extraction thimble. Extract in an all-glass jointed Soxhlet apparatus with dry acetone for four hours. Evaporate and dry the extract at 75° to 80° to constant weight, taking care to protect the residue from atmospheric moisture during weighing, as anhydrous glycerol is very hygroscopic.

(*d*) A useful method for the determination of glycerol in galenical preparations depends upon the separation of interfering materials by adsorption chromatography[3] and the determination of the glycerol iodimetrically as its copper complex.[4] In our experience the conditions given in the literature for precipitation of the copper complex give rise to slightly low results but the following method is satisfactory and has given complete recovery on standard preparations containing sugars, colouring matter, flavouring agents and preservatives.

Preparation of chromatographic column. Weigh 2·5 g of Whatman coarse-grade cellulose into a beaker and work with acetone into a chromatographic tube about 20 cm long and 1·8 cm in internal diameter, plugged with a grade 0 sintered-glass disc and fitted with a tap. When all the cellulose has been transferred to the tube and has partially settled, add 5 g of alumina, allow to settle and press down gently with a glass packing-rod. Allow the acetone to pass through the column until the surface of the liquid is just above the top of the column and then wash with 100 ml of a mixture of 950 ml of pure, dry acetone, 50 ml of water and 0·5 ml of glacial acetic acid (solvent mixture).

Chromatographic separation. Weigh an amount of sample containing the equivalent of about 0·25 g of glycerol in a volume of about 5 to 10 ml into a porcelain dish and add 1·6 g of finely ground sodium sulphite heptahydrate (or 0·8 g of anhydrous sodium sulphite), 1 g of finely ground sodium acetate trihydrate (or 0·6 g of anhydrous sodium acetate) and, finally, 0·1 ml of glacial acetic acid. (If the sample is alkaline first neutralise with glacial acetic acid and then add 0·1 ml in excess.) Grind together, with a pestle, for five minutes, then add 15 g of alumina and grind again. Transfer this mixture to the column with 50 ml of solvent mixture (see above). The recommended method for this is as follows: Add 10 ml of solvent mixture to the column and then transfer the alumina, as completely as possible, to the column with a spatula and remove air from the column with a glass packing-rod. Remove the last traces of alumina mixture from the dish, pestle and spatula with a piece of cotton wool moistened with the solvent mixture and press the cotton wool gently onto the top of the column with the packing-rod. Use the remaining 40 ml of solvent mixture to rinse the dish, pestle, spatula and packing-rod before adding to the column. Add a further 200 ml of solvent mixture to the column and allow to pass through at a rate of about 1 ml per minute. When all the solvent mixture (250 ml) has passed through the column evaporate the eluate on a water-bath to a volume of 3 to 4 ml.

Determination of glycerol. Transfer the concentrated eluate to a 100-ml graduated flask with small portions of 95 per cent ethanol, using 50 ml of ethanol in all. Add 6 ml of 50 per cent sodium hydroxide solution, mix and cool to 20°. Add from a burette a 10 per cent solution of cupric chloride dihydrate in 95 per cent ethanol, in small portions at a time, with thorough shaking, until a clearly visible, permanent precipitate of cupric hydroxide is obtained and then add 0·5 ml in excess. (1 ml cupric chloride solution = 0·054 g glycerol.) Dilute to 100 ml with 95 per cent ethanol and shake vigorously for one minute. Centrifuge or filter the solution (Bertram and Rutgers[5] claimed that filtration caused low results; however, in our hands, if a Whatman No. 541 filter paper was used and the first 20 ml of filtrate discarded, satisfactory results were obtained). Pipette 50 ml of the clear liquid into a 500-ml flask and add 100 ml of water. Make just acid with glacial acetic acid (the end-point is indicated by a change in the colour of the solution from deep blue to light green) and add 2 ml of the acid in excess. Cool in an ice-bath for twenty minutes, add 10 g of potassium iodide and titrate with 0·1N sodium thiosulphate until white, using starch as indicator and adding 2 g of ammonium thiocyanate and shaking vigorously just before the end-point. Carry out a blank determination at the same time. 1 ml 0·1N thiosulphate = 0·009210 g $C_3H_8O_3$.

The 'acetin' process for the determination of glycerol may be used when the glycerol has been isolated in a reasonably pure state and is in fairly concentrated solution (but note the possibility of loss on evaporation); not more than 50 per cent of water should be present. The process is based on the conversion of glycerol into glyceryl triacetate by the action of acetic anhydride; after neutralisation of the free acid, the saponification value of the mixture is determined. An International Standard Method[6] based on this method was laid down, an abstract of which follows:

Weigh as rapidly as possible into an acetylation flask 1·25 to 1·5 g of the glycerol, add 3 g of anhydrous sodium acetate and 7·5 ml of acetic anhydride. Boil for one hour, cool the flask somewhat and through the condenser-tube add 50 ml of recently boiled warm water. When solution is complete, cool, wash down the condenser-tube, detach the flask and wash off from the ground-glass connection into the flask. Filter the contents of the flask through an acid-washed filter paper into a large flask and wash thoroughly with recently boiled cold water. Add 2 ml of phenolphthalein solution and N carbonate-free sodium hydroxide until the solution is nearly neutralised. Wash down the sides of the flask and then add the alkali drop by drop until a faint pinkish-yellow colour appears throughout the solution. This neutralisation must be done most carefully as an excess of alkali must be avoided, partial saponification of the acetin occurring in the presence of the slightest excess. Now add exactly 50 ml of N sodium hydroxide, boil gently for fifteen minutes under reflux, cool as quickly as possible and titrate the excess of sodium hydroxide with N acid. 1 ml N NaOH = 0·03070 g glycerol.

The reaction of periodic acid with polyalcohols was applied to the determination of glycerol by Allen, Charbonnier and Coleman.[7] Glycols also react but glycerol gives formaldehyde and a molecule of formic acid on oxidation, whereas ethylene glycol gives formaldehyde but not formic acid, hence acidimetric titration of the reaction gives a measure of the glycerol present. Subsequent iodometric titration of the excess periodic acid enables the joint percentage of glycerol and ethylene glycol to be determined in terms of glycerol; the ethylene glycol content is then 1·348 times the difference between the total apparent and true glycerol content. The acidimetric method for glycerol may be used in the presence of a variety of organic compounds, so long as these do not react with periodic acid to form an acid. Sorbitol and sugars would interfere. The field has been explored extensively. Erskine *et al.*[8] recommended the use of the soluble sodium salt and official methods are now based on this reaction.

Reagents: These should be of analytical reagent quality and water free from carbon dioxide should be used throughout.

Sodium periodate solution. Dissolve 60 g of sodium periodate in 500 ml of water, add 120 ml of 0·1N sulphuric acid and dilute to 1 litre. Do not heat to dissolve the sodium periodate; if the solution is not clear it should be filtered through a sintered-glass filter (No. 3). The solution should be kept from light.

Bromothymol blue indicator. Dissolve 0·1 g of dry indicator in 16 ml of 0·01N sodium hydroxide by grinding the indicator with the alkali in a mortar. Transfer to a 100-ml graduated flask, dilute to volume with water and mix.

Method: Weigh into a beaker an amount of well-mixed sample (the sample may be warmed to ensure uniform distribution of any separated salt, sediment or suspended matter; take care to avoid absorption or loss of water by the sample) within the limits given by the formula $\frac{41 \pm 9}{P}$ g, where P is the expected percentage of glycerol in the sample. Dilute to about 50 ml with water, add 5 to 7 drops of the bromothymol blue indicator and acidify with 0·2N sulphuric acid to a definite green or greenish-yellow colour. (If the sample contains more than 0·1 per cent of carbonate alkalinity, calculated as Na_2O, add 0·2N sulphuric acid until the pH is 3·0 or less, heat to boiling and cool to room temperature before neutralising with 0·05N sodium hydroxide to bromothymol blue.) Neutralise carefully with 0·05N sodium hydroxide to a blue free of green colour; if the colour of the solution interferes with the detection of the colour change of the indicator adjust by means of a pH meter to pH 8·1 ± 0·1. If the sample contains an appreciable amount of buffering material adjust the pH, by means of a pH meter, to the end-point to which the sample will be titrated. Add, by pipette, 50 ml of sodium periodate solution, swirl gently, cover the beaker with a watch-glass and allow to stand in the dark for thirty minutes at room temperature (not exceeding 35°). At the end of this time add 10 ml of a mixture of equal volumes of neutral ethylene glycol and water, swirl gently and allow to stand in the dark at room temperature for twenty minutes. Dilute to about 300 ml with water and titrate potentiometrically with carbonate-free 0·125N sodium hydroxide to pH 8·1 ± 0·1. Repeat the above operation omitting the sample and titrating to pH 6·5 ± 0·1. Deduct the blank titration from the sample titration and calculate the per cent glycerol. 1 ml 0·125N NaOH = 0·01151 g $C_3H_8O_3$.

Titration of the blank to pH 6·5 and of the test solution to pH 8·1 amounts to applying a correction of about 0·3 per cent glycerol expressed on 100 per cent glycerol.

The glycerol contents of certain pharmacopœial preparations are now standardised, based on the periodate oxidation after preliminary purification. For **Compound Tincture of Cardamom,** containing 5 per cent v/v of glycerin and **Elixir of Cascara,** containing 31·5 per cent v/v of glycerin the method is the same after initial dilutions of 20 to 100 and 2·5 to 100 respectively. It is unnecessary to heat to 40° for oxidation.

To 20 ml of dilution add 100 ml of water and 1 g of decolorising charcoal and boil under a reflux condenser for fifteen minutes. Filter and wash the filter and charcoal with water until the filtrate measures 150 ml. Add 5 drops of bromocresol purple indicator and neutralise with 0·1N acid or alkali to the blue colour of the indicator. Add 1·4 g of sodium periodate and allow to stand for fifteen minutes. Add 3 ml of propylene glycol, shake, and allow to stand for five minutes. Add 5 drops of bromocresol purple indicator and titrate with 0·1N sodium hydroxide to the same blue colour. 1 ml 0·1N NaOH = 0·009210 g $C_3H_8O_3$. Calculate the percentage v/v of glycerin, assuming the weight per ml of glycerin to be 1·260 g.

Injection of Insulin, *B.P.* (1·6 per cent glycerin w/w).

To 5 ml add 30 ml of water, a slight excess of 10 per cent sodium tungstate ($Na_2WO_4,2H_2O$) and slowly, with continuous stirring, 2 ml of N sulphuric acid. Filter, wash the residue with water and dilute the combined filtrate and washings to 200 ml with water. Add 2 drops of bromocresol purple indicator and neutralise with 0·1N sodium hydroxide to the blue colour of the indicator. Add 0·7 g of sodium periodate and allow to stand for fifteen minutes with occasional stirring. Add 3 ml of propylene glycol, mix, allow to stand for three to five minutes and titrate with 0·1N sodium hydroxide to the same blue colour. 1 ml 0·1N NaOH = 0·009210 g $C_3H_8O_3$.

Colorimetric methods for determination of small quantities of glycerol have been published based on oxidation and reaction with hydroxy-compounds, codeine being the most useful of those tested. Mikkelsen[9] describes a method suitable for colour matching of from 1 to 4 mg of glycerol.

To a solution containing glycerol add an equal volume of saturated bromine water. Heat the mixture in a water-bath for twenty minutes and then immediately boil to expel the excess of bromine completely. After cooling make up to a volume expected to contain about 0·1 to 0·5 per cent of glycerol.

To 1·0 ml of reagent (a 5 per cent solution of codeine in 96 per cent ethanol), add from 1·0 to 4·0 ml of the prepared glycerol dilution and water, if necessary, up to 5·0 ml. Add 20 ml of concentrated sulphuric acid (at least 95 per cent) cooling rapidly in running water. Heat the mixture in a water-bath for exactly two minutes, cool immediately to room temperature and make up to 25 ml with sulphuric acid. Allow to stand for thirty minutes and measure the extinction at 660 mμ using a standard curve constructed for known quantities of glycerol for comparison.

Solution of Glyceryl Trinitrate, *B.P.C.*

Nitroglycerin is rapidly hydrolysed by alkali and Solution of Glyceryl Trinitrate has been determined colorimetrically either as nitrate or nitrite, both being formed in the hydrolysis. Richmond[10] has shown, however, that the hydrolysis is a very complex reaction, oxidation products of glycerol also being obtained with other nitro-bodies, hence such methods must give erroneous results.

The *B.P.C.* method of determination, *i.e.* alkali saponification and measurement of the liberated nitric oxide with potassium iodide and sulphuric acid, is that due to Richmond.[10] From his observations the method must necessarily be empirical but it gives reasonably uniform results.

Mix 5 ml with 0·5 ml of 20 per cent sodium hydroxide solution and allow to stand for one hour. Transfer to a brine-charged nitrometer, rinsing in with 90 per cent ethanol. Add 5 ml of 10 per cent potassium iodide solution and 5 ml of 10 per cent sulphuric acid. Shake briskly for five minutes and measure the volume of nitric oxide produced. 1 ml NO at 15·5° and normal pressure = 0·00505 g of $C_3H_5(NO_3)_3$.

Many publications have described the successful use of methods involving saponification and reduction of the nitro-compounds formed with nascent hydrogen to ammonia. The *A.O.A.C.* includes official methods based on this reaction for the determination of glyceryl trinitrate, but it would appear from the work of Anderson[11] that they do not give accurate results. He describes a method based on the volatility of glyceryl trinitrate with steam.

Mix sufficient of the solution equal to 0·05 g of glyceryl trinitrate in an 800-ml Kjeldahl flask with 50 ml of saturated sodium sulphate solution, 150 ml of water and 5 to 10 drops of dilute sulphuric acid, or sufficient to give an acid reaction to litmus. Distil just to dryness, using a still-head, into a similar flask containing 30 ml of 5 per cent sodium hydroxide solution, keeping the outlet tube below the surface. The distillation should occupy about an hour. Wash the condenser with about 100 ml of water into the collecting flask. Add 2 g of Devarda's alloy, distil the ammonia into 25 ml of 0·02N sulphuric acid and titrate back the excess of acid with 0·02N alkali. 1 ml 0·02N = 0·001514 g. In order to obtain concordant results special attention must be given to details, especially with regard to the ammonia distillation where a Murray scrubber must be used as a splash trap. A blank experiment must be made, observing the same precautions as in the actual determination.

Shankster and Wilde[12] have found that glyceryl trinitrate is rapidly and quantitatively reduced by titanous chloride.

To a solution in ethanol, containing approximately 0·01 g of glyceryl trinitrate and through which is passing a current of carbon dioxide to expel air, add 25 ml of approximately 0·05N titanous chloride. Set aside for ten minutes, then boil for ten minutes and finally cool in ice for ten minutes. Titrate the excess of titanous chloride with 0·05N ferric alum using 5 ml of 5 per cent ammonium thiocyanate solution as indicator. Carry out a blank experiment simultaneously. 1 ml 0·05N = 0·000631 g of nitroglycerin.

Tablets of Glyceryl Trinitrate, *B.P.* For small quantities of glyceryl trinitrate such as are found in tablets colorimetric methods must be employed, unless sufficient tablets are available for the material to be extracted with ether or ethanol for the macro- or a semi-micro-method. A method is given in the *U.S.P.* where tablets equivalent to about 5 mg of glyceryl trinitrate are reduced with Devarda's alloy after ether extraction and saponification. Smith[13] adapted Anderson's method (above) to small quantities of material by using Nessler's reagent to determine the ammonia produced after reduction by reduced iron and acid; with this modification only five tablets are needed for the assay. The details are:

Place five tablets in a 500-ml Kjeldahl flask, add 25 ml of saturated sodium sulphate solution, 75 ml of water and sufficient sulphuric acid to make just acid to litmus paper (usually 0·3 ml of N sulphuric acid required). Distil just to dryness, using a still-head, into a flask containing 10 ml of 0·1N sodium hydroxide, keeping the outlet tube below the surface of the alkali. Wash down the condenser and outlet tube and evaporate the sodium hydroxide solution to dryness. Add 2 ml of water, 0·3 g

(±0·01 g) of reduced iron and 2 ml of 50 per cent v/v sulphuric acid, allow to stand for ten minutes and boil for two minutes. Transfer the acid solution to a steam-distillation apparatus, make alkaline with 4 ml of saturated sodium hydroxide solution and distil the liberated ammonia into a flask containing 10 ml of 0·1N sulphuric acid until the distillate measures 500 ml. Take 100 ml of the distillate, add 2 ml of Nessler's reagent and compare the colour with that produced by adding the same amount of reagent to 100 ml of a solution containing ammonium chloride equivalent to 0·1 mg of nitrogen. The colour of the unknown should not vary more than 20 per cent from that of the standard and a control experiment must always be carried out exactly as described, the distillate in this case being concentrated to 100 ml. N × 5·4 = glyceryl trinitrate.

Results are somewhat low, partly due to deterioration of the glyceryl trinitrate tablets with age, but also probably due to loss by reason of the complexity of the hydrolysis reaction as pointed out by Richmond. Experiments both with solution and tablets of glyceryl trinitrate have given low results by this method; it is tedious, the blank determination very high and frothing occurs in the alkaline distillation.

The method of Meek[14] is rapid and was found to be quite satisfactory with standard samples; this method is official in the *B.P.* and the following is a modification:

Weigh the equivalent of 4 mg of glyceryl trinitrate in the form of powdered tablets into a dry stoppered cylinder, add exactly 20 ml of glacial acetic acid and shake continuously for one hour. Filter through dry paper and pipette 2 ml of the filtrate into a dry 50-ml graduated flask. Add exactly 4 ml of phenoldisulphonic acid, mix by vigorous swirling and allow to stand for fifteen minutes. Place the flask in a cold water-bath and add 15·0 ml of water, slowly with swirling. Allow the reaction to subside and then dilute to volume at 20° with 30 per cent sodium hydroxide solution. Filter, if necessary to obtain a clear solution and measure the extinction at the wavelength of the maximum at about 430 mμ, using 1-cm cells.

Compare the extinction with that obtained by treating a 2-ml aliquot of a freshly prepared 0·02672 per cent solution of potassium nitrate as follows: Evaporate to dryness on a water-bath, dry in an oven and cool. Add exactly 2 ml of glacial acetic acid, exactly 4 ml of phenoldisulphonic acid and stir well with a glass rod to dissolve and mix the reagents and potassium nitrate residue. Allow to stand for fifteen minutes and add 15·0 ml of water, cooling during the addition. Transfer to a 50-ml graduated flask with the aid of small quantities of 30 per cent sodium hydroxide solution, dilute to volume with the sodium hydroxide solution at 20° and measure the extinction as for the sample. 1 mg of potassium nitrate = 0·7487 mg of glyceryl trinitrate.

Complete disintegration of the tablets is essential. Hora and Webber[15] found that in the presence of amounts of ammonium ion comparable with the amount of nitrate-nitrogen present, serious losses of nitrate-nitrogen occurred in the phenoldisulphonic acid method but prevented these by a preliminary evaporation of sample solution after adding one or more drops of 30 per cent potassium hydroxide solution and the authors recommend the use of this alkali (instead of ammonia) to develop the yellow colour.

Diluted Pentaerythritol Tetranitrate, *B.P.C.* This is a mixture of pentaerythritol tetranitrate with lactose, or with a mixture of three parts of lactose and one part of starch, containing about 20 per cent of $C_5H_8O_{12}N_4$, Mol. Wt. = 316·2. The content of pentaerythritol tetranitrate can be determined by direct extraction with acetone, cautious evaporation and drying *in vacuo*.

1. *A.O.A.C.*, 1960, p. 141.
2. SHUKOFF, A. A., and SCHESTAKOFF, P. J., *Z. Angew. Chem.*, 1905, **18**, 294.
3. SPOREK, K., and WILLIAMS, A. F., *Analyst*, 1954, **79**, 63.
4. THORPE, J. F., and WHITELY, M.A., Dictionary of Applied Chemistry, 4th Edn. London, Longmans Green, 1937–1956, Vol. VI, 57.
5. BERTRAM, S. H., and RUTGERS, R., *Rec. Trav. Chim.*, 1938, **57**, 681.
6. *Analyst*, 1911, **36**, 314.
7. ALLEN, N., CHARBONNIER, H. Y., and COLEMAN, R. M., *Ind. Eng. Chem., Anal. Edn.*, 1940, **12**, 384.
8. ERSKINE, J. W. B. *et al.*, *Analyst*, 1953, **78**, 630.
9. MIKKELSEN, V. H., *Analyst*, 1948, **73**, 447.
10. RICHMOND, H. D., *Analyst*, 1920, **45**, 260.
11. ANDERSON, E. L., *J.A.O.A.C.*, 1932, **15**, 140.
12. SHANKSTER, H., and WILDE, T. H., *J. Soc. Chem. Ind.*, 1938, **57**, 91.
13. SMITH, W., *Quart, J. Pharm.*, 1935, **8**, 370.
14. MEEK, H. O., *Quart. J. Pharm.*, 1935, **8**, 375.
15. HORA, F. B., and WEBBER, P. J., *Analyst*, 1960, **85**, 567.

GLYCEROPHOSPHORIC ACID

$C_3H_5(OH)_2.O.PO(OH)_2$ Mol. Wt. 172·1

Glycerophosphoric acid (a mixture of the asymmetrical α-acid and symmetrical β-acid) behaves towards methyl orange as a monobasic, and towards phenolphthalein as a dibasic acid. The *B.P.C.* assay is based upon this fact, although methyl orange is replaced by the more suitable indicator bromocresol green and phenolphthalein by thymol blue. After neutralisation of the free acid to bromocresol green, the titration to thymol blue should be the same volume for a given weight, but if alkali were present originally (as monobasic salt in acid solution) this will also titrate to thymol blue, so the excess of the second titration over the first equals the combined alkali. If free phosphate is present, when the solution is neutral to thymol blue it is in the form of disodium hydrogen phosphate, and if a large excess of calcium chloride is added to the neutralised solution, the reversible reaction, $2Na_2HPO_4 + 3CaCl_2 \rightleftharpoons Ca_3(PO_4)_2 + 2HCl + 4NaCl$, is almost completely to the right and the hydrochloric acid can be titrated, giving a measure of the free phosphate; hence the difference between the bromocresol green and thymol blue titrations, less the volume required for free phosphate, gives the titration due to glycerophosphoric acid. The details of the method are the following:

> Titrate 5 g after dilution with a little water, to pH 4·0 using bromocresol green with N alkali (*a* ml). Repeat the titration on another 5 g to thymol blue (*b* ml). To the latter neutralised solution add 40 ml of 30 per cent w/v calcium chloride solution (neutral to thymol blue), boil for five minutes, cool and titrate with N alkali (*c* ml).

Then glycerophosphoric acid $= b - c - a$, 1 ml N = 0·1721 g, combined alkali $= b - 2a$, 1 ml N = 0·031 g Na_2O, and free phosphate $= c$, 1 ml N = 0·0710 g P_2O_5.

GLYCEROPHOSPHATES

The medicinal salts of glycerophosphoric acid are all soluble in cold water and the glycerophosphate radical may be titrated direct to methyl orange or bromocresol green.

For potassium and sodium glycerophosphates a titration is used based on the reactions involved in the neutralisation of the free acid (above).

> Using 2·5 g of the glycerophosphate, neutralise to thymol blue with N acid (*a* ml). To the neutralised solution add 40 ml of 30 per cent w/v calcium chloride solution (neutral to thymol blue), boil for five minutes, cool and titrate with N alkali (*b* ml). Repeat the titration on 2·5 g with N acid to pH 4·0 using bromocresol green as indicator (*c* ml). Then alkali glycerophosphate $= c - a - b$ ml.

Potassium glycerophosphate, $C_3H_7O_6PK_2,3H_2O$, Mol. Wt. 302·3, potassium glycerophosphate $= c - a - b$, 1 ml N = 0·3023 g. **Sodium glycerophosphate,** $C_3H_7O_6PNa_2,5\frac{1}{2}H_2O$, Mol. Wt. 315·1, sodium glycerophosphate $= c - a - b$, 1 ml N = 0·3151 g. Free phosphate $= b$, 1 ml N = 0·0710 g P_2O_5. Free alkali $= a$, 1 ml N = 0·106 g Na_2CO_3 and 0·1382 g K_2CO_3.

The salts are also converted to pyrophosphates by strong ignition, preferably with an excess of ammonium nitrate, and the *B.P.C.* employs this method of assay for the calcium, magnesium and manganese salts as a standard of 'residue on ignition.' Since the residue may contain impurities in appreciable amounts, particularly in manganese glycerophosphate, commercial samples of which may contain from 1 to 3 per cent of calcium, calculation back to glycerophosphate may give misleading results. A minimum limit for glycerophosphate is included by titration to methyl orange after neutralising to phenolphthalein; this latter percentage is less than the minimum by ignition. **Calcium glycerophosphate,** consists largely of hydrated calcium α-glycerophosphate; the anhydrous material has the formula $C_3H_7O_6PCa$, Mol. Wt. 210·1, $Ca_2P_2O_7 \times 1{\cdot}654$, glycerophosphate,

GLYCEROPHOSPHORIC ACID

1 ml 0·5N = 0·1051 g; **magnesium glycerophosphate** is also a hydrated salt, the anhydrous material has the formula $C_3H_7O_6PMg$, Mol. Wt. 194·4, $Mg_2P_2O_7 \times 1{\cdot}747$, glycerophosphate, 1 ml 0·5N = 0·0972 g; **manganese glycerophosphate,** $C_3H_7O_6PMn$, Mol. Wt. 225·0, $Mn_2P_2O_7 \times 1{\cdot}586$, glycerophosphate, 1 ml 0·5N = 0·1125 g.

Read[1] proposes the following method for the determination of manganese in manganese glycerophosphate. The method is to dissolve the ash, after ignition, in dilute sulphuric acid, and to determine the manganese by a slight modification of the method of Willard and Thompson.[2]

> To an aliquot part of the ash, dissolved in dilute sulphuric acid and containing from 10 to 30 mg of manganese, add 1 to 2 ml of concentrated nitric acid, boil to remove nitrous fumes and dilute to 100 ml to give a sulphuric acid content of approximately 5 per cent w/v; add 0·3 g of potassium periodate, boil gently for fifteen minutes, dilute to 150 ml and cool to room temperature. Precipitate the excess of periodate by adding slowly with constant stirring, a precipitating reagent prepared by dissolving 2 to 3 g of mercuric nitrate in the minimum necessary quantity of dilute nitric acid and oxidising this solution with just sufficient permanganate. Filter immediately through a layer of asbestos or kieselguhr into a measured excess of ferrous sulphate solution containing 10 ml of 50 per cent sulphuric acid. Titrate the excess of ferrous sulphate with standard permanganate. 1 ml 0·1N ferrous sulphate = 0·001099 g Mn.

Sugar prevents rapid precipitation of phosphate and, for direct titration, addition of 20 ml of syrup before making alkaline with ammonia allows titration of calcium glycerophosphate with EDTA to a satisfactory end-point.

Compound Syrup of Glycerophosphates, *B.P.C.* A complex syrup containing the glycerophosphates of calcium, magnesium, iron, sodium and potassium, with caffeine and strychnine. It is coloured with a solution of amaranth.

For determination of caffeine and strychnine:

> Add 5 g of citric acid to 50 ml of the syrup in a separator, dilute somewhat and make alkaline with ammonia solution. Extract five times with chloroform, washing each extraction with the same 5 ml of water in a second separator. Evaporate the solvent in a tared flask, dry and weigh the anhydrous caffeine and strychnine.

To obtain the weight of anhydrous caffeine deduct the strychnine obtained in the separation given below. Caffeine and strychnine (as hydrochloride) can also be extracted from solution made strongly acid with hydrochloric acid, but, although separations are rapid and clean, eight or nine extractions are needed.

A good check on the percentage of caffeine present is a 'total nitrogen' figure on 10 ml of syrup by the usual Kjeldahl method. ($N \times 3{\cdot}466$ = anhydrous caffeine.)

For separation of strychnine (Garratt[3]):

> Dissolve the weighed caffeine and strychnine from 50 ml of syrup in 25 ml of water to which is added 1 ml of 25 per cent v/v sulphuric acid, warming if found necessary. Cool, add 1 ml of freshly prepared 5 per cent potassium ferrocyanide solution, stir to induce precipitation and allow to stand some hours, preferably overnight. Filter through a 7-cm No. 1 filter paper and wash well with water slightly acidified with sulphuric acid. Place the funnel in the neck of a separator, pierce the tip of the filter paper and wash in from the precipitating beaker successively with 10 ml of 10 per cent ammonia, water and chloroform. Extract three times with chloroform, evaporate with 5 ml of ethanol, dry at 105° and weigh.

This method of separation has been criticised by Dott[4] who asserts that with determinations on the syrup, high results are obtained. Repetition by the author confirmed the original findings, white residues of strychnine and theoretical results being obtained with *B.P.C.* syrups.

Ferrey[5] has adapted Pemberton's volumetric molybdate method for phosphorus in phosphate syrups to yield results close to those obtained by gravimetric means. The method is quick and, by following his recommendations in detail, gives good results for all the phosphate syrups and is described under Phosphoric Acid (see p. 530). For glycerophosphate syrups the following modification is necessary:

> To 1 to 1·5 g of syrup in a covered platinum dish add 0·5 g of light magnesium oxide, take to dryness on a water-bath and carefully ignite. Heat the white ash obtained for thirty minutes in the presence of 5 per cent nitric acid to ensure the whole of the phosphate being present as orthophosphate. Proceed by the method given on p. 530, but using 15 g of ammonium nitrate in precipitation and allowing the precipitated phosphomolybdate to stand for one hour before filtration.

A more rapid modification is to destroy the organic matter by wet oxidation. A considerable quantity of nitric acid should be added first and most of the sugar oxidised by cautious heating before adding the sulphuric acid; a large Kjeldahl flask is a good receptacle for the oxidation as considerable evolution of nitrous fumes occurs.

Middleton[6] obtained the iron directly from the syrup for estimation by titration.

> Dilute 50 ml of syrup to 400 ml, precipitate with sodium hydroxide and a little bromine water, to oxidise any iron in the ferrous state. Bring the mixture to the boil and allow the precipitate to settle. After filtration on paper in a Gooch crucible, dissolve the precipitate in hydrochloric acid, reprecipitate with sodium hydroxide and redissolve in hydrochloric acid. Add potassium iodide and titrate with 0·1N thiosulphate. 1 ml = 0·005585 g Fe.

Calcium may be determined by the method of the *B.P.C.* for Chemical Food.

1. READ, F. E., *Analyst*, 1939, **64**, 586.
2. WILLARD, H. H., and THOMPSON, J. J., *Ind. Eng. Chem., Anal. Edn.*, 1931, **3**, 399.
3. GARRATT, D. C., *Analyst*, 1937, **62**, 538.
4. DOTT, D. B., *Pharm. J.*, 1938, **140**, 357.
5. FERREY, G. J. W., *Quart. J. Pharm.*, 1934, **7**, 346.
6. MIDDLETON, G., *Y. B. Pharm.*, 1926, 421.

HALOGEN ACIDS AND SALTS

The free acidity of hydrochloric acid, HCl, Mol. Wt. 36·46, hydrobromic acid, HBr, Mol Wt. 80·92, and hydriodic acid, HI, Mol. Wt. 127·92, may be determined by titration with standard alkali to methyl orange or methyl red. More frequently these acids and their salts are determined by argentimetric methods.

For direct titration a number of alternative methods of end-point detection are possible. The oldest procedure, and still in use to a considerable extent for fairly pure samples, is Mohr's method.[1] In this method potassium chromate is added to the chloride solution which is then titrated with silver nitrate. Because it is so much more insoluble than silver chromate, silver chloride first precipitates in a colloidal form which tends to coagulate as the end-point is reached; immediately all the chloride is titrated silver chromate is formed as a brownish-red precipitate which gives a good indication of the end-point. It is important that the quantity of chromate added should not be too excessive or the red precipitate may form before all chloride is precipitated and so give a premature end-point. In very dilute or hot solution the end-point indication is poor, due to solubility of silver chromate. Mohr's method may be used for chlorides or bromides, but is unsatisfactory for iodides because (i) a mixed precipitate of iodide and chromate may be obtained and (ii) the colour of silver iodide masks that of the precipitating chromate. The following general procedure may be used:

> To a solution containing about 0·15 g of chloride ion in about 50 ml of water, add 1 ml of a 5 per cent aqueous solution of potassium chromate and titrate with 0·1N silver nitrate.

An alternative method of end-point detection in the direct titration of halides with silver nitrate is by the use of adsorption indicators. First described by Fajans,[2] these methods depend upon the fact that the colloidal precipitate of silver halide adsorbs ions from solution; before the end-point is reached a layer of negatively charged chloride ions is adsorbed but as soon as silver ions are present in excess these are adsorbed on to the precipitate and attract the negatively charged anion of indicators of the fluorescein type. When adsorbed on the precipitate the silver-dyestuff is coloured and gives a good indication of the end-point. Fluorescein itself was the first indicator of this type to be used, but it is not very satisfactory since the pH of the solution for titration is very critical. Eosin, dichlorofluorescein, phenosafranine and di-iododimethylfluorescein (said to be the most suitable for titration of iodides[3]) are among the indicators which have been used and phenosafranine is perhaps the most satisfactory. Large concentrations of salts must be avoided, since these cause coagulation of the colloidal precipitate and this leads to a poor end-point. A procedure based on the use of phenosafranine is given below, but adsorption indicator methods have not found general favour.

> To a quantity of sample containing about 0·1 g of halide add sufficient water to bring the volume to 100 ml and then add ten drops of a 0·25 per cent aqueous solution of phenosafranine. Titrate with 0·1N silver nitrate, shaking vigorously when nearing the end-point, until the colour of the precipitate changes from red to blue.

Detection of the end-point by potentiometric titration using a silver/silver chloride or silver/silver bromide indicator electrode and a platinum reference electrode is particularly valuable when highly coloured solutions are being titrated and also for titration of small quantities. The following procedure is generally applicable:

> To a quantity of sample containing about 0·1 g of chloride (or 0·15 g of bromide) add sufficient water to bring the volume to about 25 ml. Then add 75 ml of acetate buffer solution (prepared by dissolving 13·6 g of sodium acetate trihydrate and 6 ml of glacial acetic acid in sufficient water to produce 1 litre) and titrate with 0·1N silver nitrate using a freshly prepared silver/silver chloride (or silver/silver bromide) electrode and a platinum reference electrode.

Alternative electrode systems for the above titration are described in Appendix VIII.

For back-titration the method of Volhard[4] is used and is probably the most widely employed technique for determination of halide ions. The halide is precipitated from a nitric acid solution by addition of excess silver nitrate and the excess is back-titrated with ammonium thiocyanate using ferric alum as indicator; at the end-point the blood-red ferric thiocyanate is formed. Since silver thiocyanate is much less soluble than silver chloride, ammonium thiocyanate will attack the silver chloride precipitate and so cause erroneous results. For this reason the silver chloride must be removed or protected before titration of the excess silver nitrate is begun. This is best obtained by filtering off the precipitate before back-titration,

ic solvent

the silver

most satis-

a powerful

contact poison and care should be taken to avoid spilling it on the skin. Silver bromide and silver iodide are less soluble than silver thiocyanate and so in these cases there is no need to filter or add nitrobenzene. The following general procedure is satisfactory:

To a quantity of sample containing about 0·15 g of chloride (or 0·3 g of bromide) in about 35 ml (diluted with water and neutralised if necessary) add 15 ml of dilute nitric acid. Then add an excess of 0·1N silver nitrate and shake vigorously. Filter, wash the residue with water and titrate the excess silver nitrate in the combined filtrate and washings with 0·1N ammonium thiocyanate using as indicator 1 ml of a solution prepared by dissolving 0·2 g of ferric alum in 50 ml of water, adding 6 ml of dilute nitric acid and diluting with water to 100 ml. If, instead of filtering, nitrobenzene is to be used, add 1 ml for each 0·05 g of chloride and add not more than 5 ml of 0·1N silver nitrate in excess.

In most titrations where the Volhard method is specified, an electrometric end-point is applicable (see Appendix XIII).

For the titrimetric determination of **smaller quantities** of chloride or bromide the method of Vieböck[6] is useful. This depends on the liberation of alkali when mercuric oxycyanide is added to a halide solution. Belcher, Macdonald and Nutten[7] made modifications to the method which improve its accuracy, and their recommended procedure is as follows:

For chloride: To a solution containing up to 3 mg of chloride (acidified and boiled to expel carbon dioxide if necessary and subsequently cooled) add 5 to 8 drops of an indicator prepared by mixing, immediately before use, equal volumes of a 0·25 per cent solution of methyl red in 90 per cent ethanol and a 0·166 per cent solution of methylene blue in 90 per cent ethanol. Neutralise with 0·01N alkali until the colour of the solution is the same as that of a mixture of an equal volume of neutralised water containing the same volume of the indicator. If the test solution contains hydrogen peroxide it is usually necessary to adjust the colour of the test solution by adding extra aqueous indicator at this point. Add exactly 10 ml of a saturated solution of mercuric oxycyanide (prepared, without the aid of heat, by shaking 20 g of mercuric oxycyanide with 1 litre of water and stored, after filtration, in a brown bottle) and titrate with 0·01N sulphuric acid to match the colour of the comparison solution. Then add to the comparison solution exactly the same volumes of oxycyanide solution and of sulphuric acid as were added to the test solution and titrate the comparison solution with 0·01N sodium chloride until its colour matches that of the test solution. The amount of chloride added is exactly equivalent to the chloride present in the test solution.

For bromide: The reaction of bromide with mercuric oxycyanide goes more readily to completion and the back-titration given above for chloride is unnecessary. After the addition of mercuric oxycyanide titrate with 0·01N sulphuric acid using the mixed indicator and carry out a blank determination by diluting 10 ml of mercuric oxycyanide solution to the same volume as the final test solution and titrating with 0·01N sulphuric acid using the mixed indicator. 1 ml 0·01N = 0·0007916 g Br.

If more than 3 mg of halide is present in the initial test solution, more oxycyanide solution should be used.

An alternative and very satisfactory method for the determination of small amounts of chloride is by titration with mercuric nitrate. The conditions described by White (see p. 799) are suitable.

Bromides may be determined by the titrimetric method of Kolthoff and Yutzy[8] in which the bromide is oxidised to bromate with sodium hypochlorite in the presence of a sodium dihydrogen phosphate buffer; after destruction of the excess hypochlorite with sodium formate the bromate is determined iodometrically after adding ammonium molybdate as a catalyst to accelerate the liberation of iodine. The method, which is applicable in the presence of a considerable excess of chloride, has been critically examined by Haslam and Moses[9] who recommended the following procedure:

Prepare a hypochlorite solution to yield a reagent N in hypochlorite and 0·1N in hydroxide by diluting 14 to 15 per cent sodium hypochlorite liquor. Determine the hypochlorite strength by titration of a dilution against standard arsenious oxide solution in the presence of sodium bicarbonate and the hydroxide by titrating 10 ml of the strong hypochlorite liquor with 0·1N hydrochloric acid to phenolphthalein after adding 30 ml of neutral 6 per cent hydrogen peroxide and 5 ml of neutral 0·05M barium chloride.

Neutralise a suitable volume of test solution (50 ml of brine liquors) to methyl red with 0·1N sulphuric acid. Add 2 g of sodium dihydrogen phosphate dihydrate followed by 10 ml of the hypochlorite reagent and heat the solution just to boiling-point. Remove the source of heat and add 10 ml of sodium formate reagent (prepared by dissolving 30 g of sodium hydroxide in water, adding 32 ml of 90 per cent formic acid solution and diluting to 100 ml with water). Wash down the sides of the beaker and the cover-glass with water, allow the solution to stand for five minutes and then cool completely. Add 240 ml of water followed by 2·0 g of potassium iodide, 50 ml of 6N sulphuric acid and 1 drop of 3 per cent ammonium molybdate solution. Titrate the liberated iodine with 0·1N sodium thiosulphate using starch mucilage as indicator. Carry out a blank determination under identical conditions. 1 ml 0·1N = 0·001332 g Br.

This method is suitable for **small amounts** of bromide. Any organic matter must be completely destroyed and the following method is applicable:

Evaporate a suitable quantity of material with 5 ml of 10 per cent potassium hydroxide solution and dry in an air-oven at 150° for one hour. Ignite the dry solid in an electrically heated furnace at 480°, extract with water, filter and wash. Re-ignite the filter paper and insoluble residue in the presence of potassium hydroxide as before, extract with dilute hydrochloric acid, filter and add to the previous filtrate. Evaporate to low bulk and make just acid to methyl red with dilute hydrochloric acid, neutralise with potassium hydroxide solution and complete the assay as above, using one-third the quantities of reagents and titrating with 0·002N thiosulphate. 1 ml = 0·02664 mg of bromine. Correct for the blank on the reagents.

Iodide may be determined specifically by the method of Andrews.[10] This depends upon the fact that iodate quantitatively oxidises iodides to iodine, the latter reacting with more iodate in the presence of strong hydrochloric acid to form iodine monochloride. Hydrolysis of this is prevented by a high concentration of hydrochloric acid, at least 40 per cent of the final titration solution being strong acid. The original procedure employed an immiscible solvent such as chloroform or carbon tetrachloride for end-point detection; whilst free iodine is present the globule of solvent is an intense reddish-violet colour and titration is continued, with vigorous shaking in a glass-stoppered vessel, until the last trace of colour disappears. The end-point is extremely sharp, although some workers consider that the necessity to stopper and shake towards the end of the titration is tedious. This may be avoided by the use of a suitable dyestuff such as naphthol blue black, brilliant ponceau 5R or amaranth.[11] These dyes are irreversible and must be added to the titration liquid just before the end-point is reached. In considering the merits of the two methods it should be remembered that, when the solution to be titrated is highly coloured (as in the determination of iodide in Ammoniated Mixture of Potassium Iodide for example) the use of the chloroform method is applicable, whereas that of the dyestuff method is not. The following methods may be used:

(*a*) Using chloroform. To a solution containing about 0·15 g of iodide in about 50 ml add an equal volume of concentrated hydrochloric acid and about 5 ml of chloroform. Run in 0·05M potassium iodate (10·70 g per litre); the reacting solution becomes dark brown by liberation of iodine according to the first part of the reaction. Continue the titration until the colour fades to light brown and then stopper the flask and shake vigorously after each addition of potassium iodate until the violet colour of the iodine in the chloroform disappears. Note that the addition of the iodate has not been sufficient to dilute the reacting mixture far below the 50 per cent concentration of acid.

(*b*) Using amaranth. To a solution containing about 0·4 g of iodide in about 50 ml add 60 ml of concentrated hydrochloric acid and titrate with 0·05M potassium iodate until within about 1 ml of the end-point. Then add 1 ml of 0·2 per cent w/v amaranth solution and titrate slowly until the colour disappears.

Lang[12] introduced a modification of Andrews' method, using potassium cyanide, when the iodate similarly oxidises the iodine to iodine cyanide in the presence of acid, but the acidity required to prevent hydrolysis of the iodine cyanide is not so high in this method, titration in approximately 2N hydrochloric acid containing 0·6 g of potassium cyanide being suitable concentrations. The cyanide method has the advantage that the iodine cyanide end-point can be recognised by using starch as indicator, and the amount can be determined by adding excess of iodide and titrating the liberated iodine. It can be applied to the titration of iodine and potassium iodide solutions, but has the disadvantage of the objectionable nature of the reaction mixture, hydrocyanic acid being evolved. The general procedure is as follows:

To an amount of sample containing about 0·4 g of iodide in a long-necked flask add sufficient water to bring the volume to about 50 ml. Neutralise with concentrated hydrochloric acid and then add about 15 ml of the acid in excess followed by 6 ml of 10 per cent potassium cyanide solution, maintaining the temperature below 20°. Titrate with 0·05M potassium iodate until the dark brown solution becomes pale yellow, add 5 ml of starch mucilage and continue the titration until the liquid becomes colourless.

Although estimation of each halide in a mixture of the three is not a likely requirement in general pharmaceutical analysis the method of Berg[13] is included to meet occasions when it might be helpful. In presence of acetone, hydriodic acid is decomposed by iodic acid according to the equation: $2HI + HIO_3 + 3C_3H_6O = 3C_3H_5IO + 3H_2O$, while hydrobromic and hydrochloric acids are attacked but slowly or not at all.

To 50 ml of the solution, which must not contain more than 2 per cent of potassium bromide, add 20 to 30 ml of acetone, and sufficient dilute sulphuric acid to make the final volume 100 ml and the acid concentration 2N to 2·5N. Add starch indicator, and slowly run in 0·05M potassium iodate until the mixture is colourless. Then determine the chloride or bromide in the reaction mixture, with 0·1N silver nitrate.

In a mixture of the three halides, the iodide is first determined as above, the bromide destroyed with bromate (boil to free the solutions from bromine) and the chloride determined by Volhard's method. Bromide is obtained by difference after titration of the total halogen by Volhard's method. The process is said to give reasonably accurate results even for small amounts of bromide.

Leipert's method[14] for determination of iodide is widely used, especially on solutions derived from the combustion of organic compounds containing iodine. This method depends upon the oxidation of iodide to iodate with bromine water, removal of the excess bromine by addition of some suitable reagent (phenol is widely used—see under Chiniofon Sodium, p. 315—but formic acid is most convenient), addition of iodide and titration of the liberated iodine with thiosulphate. The method has the great advantage that it gives a six-fold increase in the quantity of iodine to be titrated. A detailed procedure for its application will be found in Appendix IV, p. 800.

Fluorides are usually determined by the lead chlorofluoride method. In the presence of an excess of chloride the double halide is precipitated from an acetate-buffered solution by addition of lead nitrate and heating on a water-bath for thirty minutes. After ageing overnight the precipitate is filtered off, washed with a saturated lead chlorofluoride solution and then either weighed after drying at 130° to 140° or, more usually, dissolved in nitric acid and the chloride titrated by Volhard's method. A detailed method for the volumetric procedure is given under sodium fluoride below.

A more rapid method, based upon titration of the lead in the precipitated lead chlorofluoride with EDTA at pH 10 using solochrome black as indicator, was suggested by Sakharova and Shishkina.[15] This procedure had a number of shortcomings and the following improved method was developed:[16]

Dissolve about 0·08 g of sodium fluoride, accurately weighed, in about 30 ml of water and add 15 ml of 0·2N sodium chloride followed by 20 ml of 95 per cent ethanol. Heat the solution until it is just boiling and then add, with stirring, exactly 50 ml of 0·05M lead nitrate solution; this addition should be made dropwise at first and then more rapidly. Heat further to coagulate the precipitate and allow the mixture to cool to room temperature. Filter the mixture and wash the precipitate three times with small quantities of 20 per cent ethanol. To the combined filtrate and washings add 1 g hexamine and a few drops of xylenol orange indicator solution and titrate with 0·05M EDTA to the yellow end-point; 1 ml 0·05M lead nitrate = 0·0021 g NaF.

Sulphate and phosphate both interfere giving high results.

Traces of bromide (0·004 to 0·020 mg) may be determined by the colori-etric method of Hahn and Ucko, with modification by Hardwick[17] which applicable in the presence of relatively large quantities of chloride. omine must first be fixed as bromide and organic matter suitably des-yed by ashing in the presence of alkali.

Pipette 0·5 to 2·0 ml of the neutral solution containing bromide into a 5-ml Nessler cylinder or small test-tube and add 0·5 ml of a sodium acetate and acetic acid buffer (pH 5·5 to 5·6. Mix 100 ml of N sodium acetate with 15 ml of N acetic acid). Then add 1 or 2 drops of 0·1 per cent fluorescein in 0·025N sodium hydroxide. Make the solution up to 3 ml with water, add 1 drop of 1 per cent solution of chloramine-T and mix immediately. After one minute stop the reaction by adding 2 drops of a 5 per cent solution of sodium hydroxide containing 0·5 per cent of sodium thiosulphate. Compare the colour developed with a series of standards prepared at the same time from 0·1 to 2·0 ml of a solution of potassium bromide (0·010 mg KBr per ml) viewing through the walls of the tube against a white background in daylight.

Traces of iodide may be determined by making use of the fact that the ide ion quantitatively catalyses the reduction of yellow ceric sulphate colourless cerous sulphate by arsenious oxide.[18] The method is so sensi-e that rigorous precautions must be taken to prevent contamination. e final solution for measurement should contain up to 0·06 μg of iodide. e following procedure is recommended by the Analytical Methods nmittee of the *S.A.C.*[19]

Reagents: All reagents should be iodide-free and of analytical reagent grade and redistilled water (or iodide-free distilled water) should be used in making up all solutions.

Redistilled water (for use if the distilled water available is not iodide-free). To 1,500 ml of distilled water in a 3-litre, round-bottomed distilling flask mounted on a shallow sand-bath, add 50 g of potassium carbonate and a few glass beads, connect the flask to a condenser with a ground-glass joint and distil. Discard the distillate until it is neutral to methyl red. If required successive 1,500-ml quantities can be distilled but the alkali should be replaced after 20 litres have been distilled.

Ceric sulphate. Wash 15 g of ceric sulphate (low in other rare earths) with 75 ml of boiling, redistilled 95 per cent ethanol. Allow to settle and decant the supernatant liquid. Repeat the washing twice and filter, with suction, through a Whatman No. 42 paper. Dry the residue at room temperature and store in a refrigerator (see Note 1).

0·1N ceric sulphate solution. Add 5 g of the ceric sulphate to 35 ml of 10N sulphuric acid and warm for ten minutes to effect solution. Dilute to 100 ml with redistilled water and filter through a Whatman No. 42 paper. Standardise by adding 0·5 ml of standard iodide solution B (≡ 0·5 mg iodide) to 10 ml of the ceric sulphate solution and titrating at 40° with 0·15N arsenious acid reagent (below) to a colourless end-point. Adjust the solution to 0·1N with 3·5N sulphuric acid.

0·15N arsenious acid reagent. Dissolve 3·71 g of arsenious oxide in 7 ml of 10N sodium hydroxide, add 300 ml of redistilled water and neutralise to methyl orange with 10N sulphuric acid (prepared from 18N acid, below). Add 21 ml of concentrated sulphuric acid and dilute to 500 ml with redistilled water.

Sulphuric acid, approximately 18N. Add 10 ml of concentrated hydrochloric acid to 2 litres of concentrated sulphuric acid and heat the mixture strongly for two hours to fume off halogens. Add 170 ml of this concentrated acid to 200 ml of water to produce 340 ml of 18N acid.

Standard iodide solutions:

A. Dissolve 6·541 g of analytical reagent grade potassium iodide in sufficient redistilled water to produce 500 ml (1 ml ≡ 10 mg iodide).

B. Dilute 5 ml of solution A to 50 ml with redistilled water (1 ml ≡ 1 mg iodide).

C. Dilute 5 ml of solution B to 50 ml with redistilled water (1 ml ≡ 100 μg iodide).

Prepare a series of dilutions in this manner, diluting each solution ten times with redistilled water, to give a series of solutions containing, respectively, 10 μg (D), 1 μg (E), 0·1 μg (F) and 0·01 μg (G) of iodide per ml. Prepare solutions A, B and C every four weeks, solutions D and E every week and solutions F and G immediately before use.

Determination. Weigh a suitable quantity of the sample, defatted if necessary, into the Kjeldahl reaction flask of the apparatus (Fig. 7), add 5 ml of 20 per cent sodium hydroxide solution and 15 ml of redistilled water and swirl until the sample is evenly dispersed. Add a piece of copper foil, ⅛ in. square (previously washed with concentrated hydrochloric acid, distilled water and redistilled water and dried at 100°), 10 mg of ceric sulphate and about twenty small glass beads. Add, carefully, 80 ml of 18N sulphuric acid, mix until homogeneous and then carefully add 5 g of potassium permanganate that has been recrystallised from redistilled water, dried at 100° and pulverised with an agate pestle and mortar to pass a 100-mesh B.S. sieve. Mix well with frequent shaking until the initial vigorous reaction has subsided and then heat gently in a fume cupboard, with occasional mixing to avoid excessive frothing. When the solution is golden-brown in colour heat it to 195° to 200°, checking the temperature with a thermometer. Allow to cool

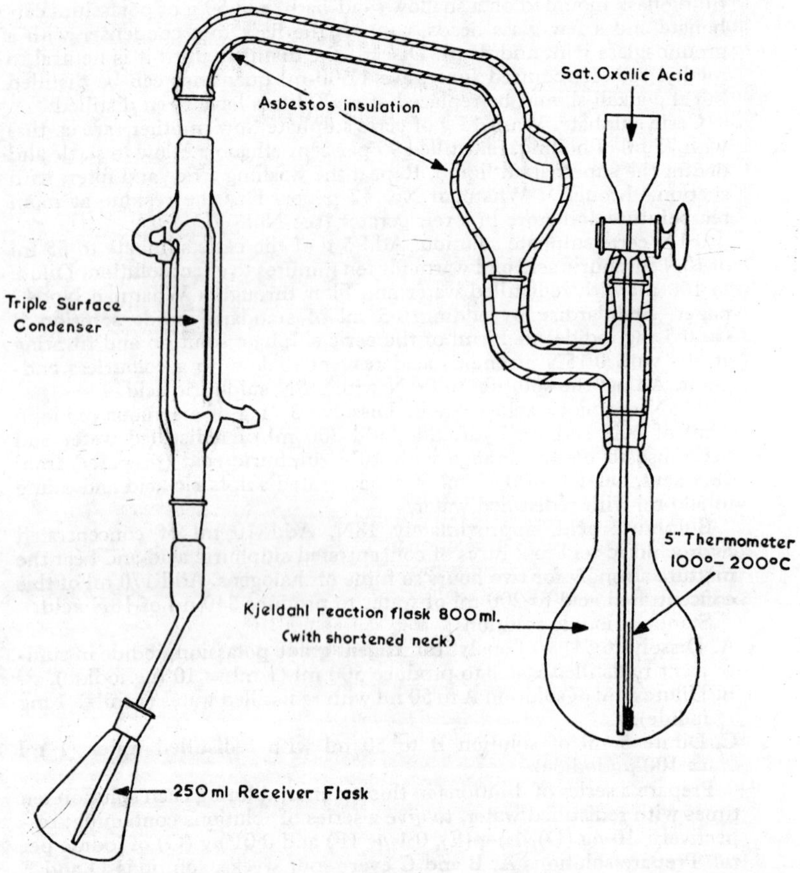

FIG. 7
Iodine Distillation Apparatus

to 90° and then carefully add exactly 25 ml of redistilled water, rinsing the thermometer and washing down the neck of the flask. Mix by swirling, connect the flask to the rest of the distillation apparatus as shown in Fig. 7 and fix in position the tap-funnel containing a saturated oxalic acid solution that has been stored in the dark. Measure into the receiver, by pipette, 2 ml of 1 per cent sodium hydroxide solution that has been prepared not more than a week before use, by diluting 10N sodium hydroxide in redistilled water. Heat the flask by means of an electric heating mantle, rocking the apparatus throughout to prevent settlement of manganese dioxide. When the temperature reaches 140° add the oxalic acid solution, dropwise from the tap-funnel, until the solution in the reaction flask becomes colourless, maintaining the temperature between 140° and 143°. (To prevent agglomeration the flask must be shaken continuously until reduction is complete and redistilled water may be added from time to time through the tap-funnel to keep the temperature within the specified limits.) Add a further 2 or 3 ml of saturated oxalic acid solution and continue distilling at 140° to 143° until about 75 ml of distillate has been collected. (Detach the reaction flask and wash out the contents while still hot to avoid solidification.) Add a few small glass beads to the distillate and evaporate on a hot plate to a volume of 10 to 15 ml. Cool, transfer the solution quantitatively to a 20-ml graduated flask and dilute to volume with redistilled water.

Into each of seven glass-stoppered tubes (6 in. × ½ in.) pipette 0·4 ml of 0·15N arsenious acid reagent. To the first tube add a suitable aliquot (0·1 to 1·0 ml) of the above distillate and to the remaining six tubes add, respectively, 0 ml, 1·0 ml, 2·0 ml, 3·0 ml, 4·0 ml and 5·0 ml of standard iodide solution, 0·01 μg iodide per ml. Adjust the contents of the tubes to equivalent volume with redistilled water. Place the tubes in a water-bath at 30° and at sixty-second intervals, timed by a stop-watch, add 0·3 ml of ceric sulphate solution to each tube in turn, mixing the contents of each tube by inversion. Exactly fifteen minutes (Note 2) from the time of addition of ceric sulphate remove each tube from the water-bath and measure the extinction at 440 mμ, using matched 1-cm cells with redistilled water in the comparison cell.

After allowing for any blank obtained by carrying out the oxidation, distillation and colour development procedures on the reagents alone, prepare a standard curve by plotting the extinctions of the standards against microgrammes of iodide and read the corresponding iodide content of the test solution.

Note 1. The double salt, ammonium ceric sulphate, should *not* be used for preparing the ceric sulphate reagent. It has been found that with this salt, the addition of chloride ion to the arsenious acid reagent appears to be necessary to obtain the full response, and this procedure can introduce a risk of iodine contamination.

Note 2. The timing is critical and must be identical for test and standards. If a turbidity occurs this can be overcome by the addition of a further 0·1 to 0·2 ml of arsenious acid reagent to the tubes initially.

Determination of **traces** of fluoride is of increasing importance. The majority of methods available depend upon non-specific reactions with dyestuff metal chelates in which the fluoride is estimated by its 'bleaching' reaction on the chelate. Such methods are capable of high sensitivity but suffer from the disadvantage that they do not distinguish between fluoride and other complex-forming ions such as phosphate, sulphate, citrate or oxalate. The Analytical Methods Committee of the *S.A.C.* standard procedure[20] is based on such a method and relies upon the decrease in colour of a thorium-alizarin S chelate when fluoride is present. The detailed procedure, applicable to foodstuffs, is as given below; for inorganic samples a simplified method of sample preparation can be used.

The distillation apparatus consists of a Claissen flask of 100- to 150-ml capacity, a large glass flask for generating steam and an efficient condenser. The main neck of the Claissen flask is fitted with a two-holed rubber stopper through which pass a thermometer and a glass tube for connecting with the steam supply, both the thermometer and the tube extending almost to the bottom of the flask. The side neck of the Claissen flask is closed with a solid rubber stopper and the side arm connected with the condenser. The steam is generated from water made alkaline with sodium hydroxide. Local overheating of the Claissen flask is avoided by use of an asbestos board with a hole which must fit closely to the lower surface of the flask, or by use of an asbestos gauze.

Mix a suitable quantity of the sample (10 g or less according to the amount of fluorine expected) in a platinum dish with about 1 g of fluorine-free lime and 50 ml of water, evaporate on a water-bath and thoroughly char at a temperature below visible red heat. Transfer to a muffle at about 600° (dull red heat) and ignite for one and a half to two hours.

Assemble the apparatus, introduce into the flask a number of fragments of Pyrex glass, 0·2 g of silver sulphate or sufficient to precipitate all the chloride in the portion of the sample being treated, 7 ml of water and 15 ml of 60 per cent w/w perchloric acid. Heat the flask until the temperature reaches 120° to 125°, connect the steam supply, regulate the gas and steam supplies so that the temperature of the distillation is maintained at 137° to 140° and distil 150 ml in twenty-five to thirty-five minutes, steaming out the condenser towards the end of the distillation; discard the distillate. Distil a further 150 ml and titrate an aliquot part by the method given below. Calculate the amount of fluorine in the whole fraction. (This figure, which should not exceed 1·5 μg, may be termed the 'apparatus blank' and should be approximately constant for any further 150-ml fractions.)

Cool the flask, transfer the acid contents to a suitable receptacle and rinse the flask and glass fragments with water, rejecting the rinsings. Introduce the bulk of the dry ash into the flask and wash in the remainder with about 5 ml of water containing a few drops of the acid. Add the remainder of the acid, whilst cooling the flask, and rinse down the neck of the flask with 1 to 2 ml of water. Connect up the apparatus and distil 150 ml as before.

Titrate 50 ml of the well-mixed distillate with 0·05N sodium hydroxide in a Nessler cylinder, using methyl orange as indicator, until the colour matches that of a comparison cylinder containing water and the same amount of methyl orange.

Transfer the remaining 100 ml of distillate to a Nessler cylinder and add an amount of 0·05N hydrochloric acid to make the total acidity equal to 5·0 ml of 0·05N acid. Prepare a 'control' cylinder containing 5·0 ml of 0·05N hydrochloric acid and water and add to both 'test' and 'control' cylinders 2 ml of 0·01 per cent alizarin S solution. From a burette which can be read to 0·02 ml add to the 'test' cylinder a solution of thorium nitrate (approximately 0·25 g per litre) until a slight pink colour persists as compared with the yellow of the 'control' cylinder. Add an exactly similar volume of the thorium nitrate solution to the 'control' cylinder, which then becomes more pink than the 'test' solution. Then add slowly, from a suitable burette, standard solution of sodium fluoride (0·0221 g of NaF per litre; 1 ml = 10 μg of fluorine) until the tints of 'test' and 'control' solutions match exactly. The volume of standard fluoride solution added corresponds to the amount present in the 'test' portion of the distillate. Calculate the amount of fluorine present in the 150 ml of distillate and subtract the 'apparatus blank.' Express the results as parts per million of the food.

The method requires some modification if a relatively large quantity of phosphate is present in the material being tested, since traces of phosphoric acid may then come over into the distillate and would be calculated as fluorine.

The results are satisfactory if the weight of sample taken is such that the amount of P_2O_5 in the flask does not exceed 0·5 g. When the method is applied to phosphates, or articles of food containing large proportions of phosphates, two successive 150-ml fractions of distillate should be collected and, if the second 150-ml fraction shows an appreciable apparent content, the first 150-ml fraction is evaporated to dryness in presence of 1 g of fluorine-free lime and redistilled to give 150 ml of distillate. The result of titration of this distillate will give the fluorine content of the sample.

The ashing temperature must be controlled; high temperatures such as uncontrolled red heat over Bunsen flames will cause loss of fluorine. A small quantity of carbon in the ash does not appear to affect the results. The silver sulphate added before distillation is to avoid production in the distillate of an excessive amount of free hydrochloric acid derived from chlorides; should the material contain a considerable proportion of chloride an excess of silver sulphate must be assured and more than the amount stated may be necessary.

A rapid method suitable for inorganic materials is based on that proposed by Milton *et al.*[21]

Transfer 1 g to the distillation apparatus described above. Add about 0·1 g of glass wool and 15 ml of 60 per cent w/w perchloric acid and steam distil at a temperature of 135° to 145° and a rate of about 2 ml per minute. Distil nearly 200 ml and dilute to volume; measure an aliquot containing less than 100 μg of fluorine and transfer to a Nessler cylinder. Into a similar cylinder introduce a volume of water equal to the volume of distillate taken. To both cylinders add one drop of phenolphthalein solution and 0·1N sodium hydroxide till pink then just discharge the pink colour with approximately 0·05N perchloric acid. Add 1 ml of a 0·02 per cent solution of chrome azurol S (colour index 43825) in water, 0·05N perchloric acid till just pink and 0·5 ml of chloracetic buffer. Prepare the latter by dissolving 22·7 g of chloracetic acid in water, diluting to 100 ml, neutralising 50 ml with 6N sodium hydroxide, mixing with the other 50 ml of solution and diluting to 1 litre. To the blank solution add 0·10 ml of 0·004N thorium nitrate. Titrate the sample solution with 0·004N thorium nitrate until the same colour is obtained. From this titration subtract 0·10 ml and refer the result to a calibration curve obtained by the above titration procedure using known amounts of sodium fluoride and 0·004N thorium nitrate. Deduct any apparatus blank and calculate the fluorine present in the sample.

A quite different kind of method is based on the specific and positive reaction between fluoride ions and the cerous chelate of the dyestuff alizarin complexan (3-aminomethylalizarin-*N*,*N*-diacetic acid). This was first described as a spot test by Belcher, Leonard and West[22] but was later applied to the determination of fluorine in organic compounds (see p. 800) and to the determination of trace quantities of fluoride. Johnson and Leonard[23] developed a method in which the coloured complex is extracted into an organic solvent consisting of a dilute solution of a hydrophobic amine in a higher alcohol and thus increased the sensitivity of the reaction so that it is ten times that of the thorium-alizarin procedure given above. For general work the older method is more rapid and as precise but, where only small quantities of sample are available, or where specificity is required, the alizarin-complexan extraction method is preferable. The detailed procedure is as follows:

Reagents:

0·0005M Alizarin complexan. Weigh 0·385 g of alizarin complexan and wash into a 2-litre graduated flask with 20 ml of freshly prepared 0·5N sodium hydroxide and allow to stand for five minutes with occasional swirling to ensure complete solution. Dilute to about 1,500 ml with water, add 0·2 g of sodium acetate trihydrate and adjust the pH to about 5 (thin layer of solution is pink) by the careful addition of N hydrochloric acid. Dilute to volume with water and filter into a brown glass bottle. This solution is stable for at least four months.

0·0005M Cerous nitrate. Standardise approximately 0·02M cerous nitrate by titration against standard EDTA at pH 6 (adding hexamine and a little nitric acid), using xylenol orange as indicator. To a suitable volume of this solution (about 50 ml) add 0·2 ml of concentrated nitric acid, 0·1 g of hydroxylamine hydrochloride and sufficient water to produce 2 litres; filter.

Acetate buffer solution, pH 4·3. Dissolve 75 g of sodium acetate trihydrate in about 600 ml of water, add 75 ml of glacial acetic acid, dilute to 1 litre with water and filter.

Standard fluoride solution, 1·00 μg per ml. Dissolve about 22 mg, accurately weighed, of dried, analytical-reagent grade sodium fluoride in water and dilute to 1 litre with water. Dilute an aliquot of this solution containing 1·00 mg of fluoride ion (approximately 100 ml) to 1 litre. Store in a polythene container.

Extraction solution. Mix together 600 ml of analytical-reagent grade *n*-pentanol and 1,400 ml of reagent-grade *sec.*-butyl alcohol. Weigh out 1·200 g of tribenzylamine (recrystallised from ethanol if necessary) and dissolve by gentle warming in about 100 ml of the alcohol mixture. Add the amine solution to the bulk of the alcohol mixture and mix well.

Determination: Weigh a suitable amount of sample, containing up to 5 μg of fluoride ion, into the inner bulb of the distillation apparatus (Fig. 8) and rinse down the walls of the entry tube with as small a volume of water as possible, followed by the rapid addition of 25 ml of 60 per cent w/v sulphuric acid. Connect the steam generator, already heated to a temperature of 60° to 80°, to the apparatus, replace the stopper and heat the liquid in the jacket (tetrachloroethane) until it boils with suffi-

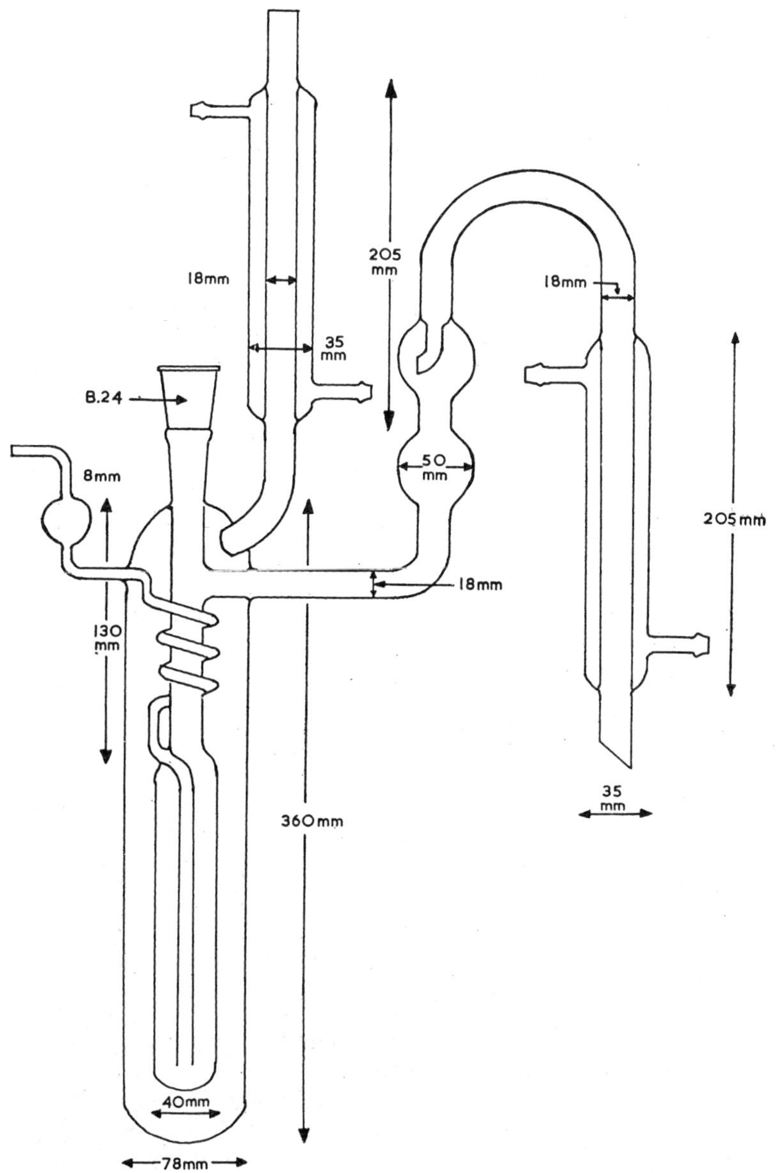
205
mm
18mm
35
mm
B.24
8mm
130
mm
360mm
40mm
78mm
50
mm
18mm
18mm
205mm
35
mm

Fig. 8

cient vigour to reflux in the condenser. Heat the steam generator to boiling and distil 150 ml of liquid.

Transfer the distillate to a 250-ml separator and add 10·00 ml of alizarin complexan solution and 2·00 ml of buffer solution, pH 4·3. Mix and immerse the separator almost completely in a water-bath, maintained at 25° ± 2°, for ten minutes, swirling periodically. Then add 10·00 ml of 0·0005M cerous nitrate, mix thoroughly and replace in the water-bath for a further ten minutes, again with occasional swirling. Add 40·0 ml of the extraction solution, previously adjusted to 25°, shake for fifteen seconds immediately after the addition and maintain at 25° for one hour, shaking for thirty seconds every ten minutes. At the end of this time, remove the separator from the bath and clamp in a position free from direct sunlight and draughts. Allow to stand for fifteen to twenty minutes and then run off and discard the aqueous layer, shaking the contents of the separator as little as possible while doing so. Swirl the organic layer round the interior surface of the separator and allow to stand for five minutes with occasional slight agitation. Run off any additional aqueous layer, at the same time bringing the liquid interface to the bottom of the stopcock bore. Place a small loosely packed, cotton-wool plug in the stem of the separator and pass the alcoholic solution into a 25-ml graduated flask. Rinse the walls of the separator with dehydrated ethanol and allow the rinsings to drain into the graduated flask until the mark is reached. Shake the flask well to dissolve any water droplets and measure the extinction at 580 mμ (the absorption maximum of the blue complex), using 4-cm cells with, in the comparison cell, a solution prepared by treating 150 ml of water exactly as above beginning with 'add 10·00 ml of alizarin complexan solution. . . .'. Read the amount of fluoride from a standard curve prepared by treating suitable volumes of standard fluoride solution, 1·00 μg per ml, covering the range 0 to 5 μg of fluoride ion, each diluted to 150 ml with water, exactly as described above beginning with 'add 10·00 ml of alizarin complexan solution. . . .' and plotting extinction against the quantity of fluoride ion present.

A linear calibration graph is obtainable over the range 0 to 5 μg of fluoride, and the extinction of a 1-cm layer increases by 0·13 unit for each μg of fluoride. Sulphuric acid is specified in the distillation procedure since perchlorate ions which may be carried over into the distillate cause a suppression of colour.

A third type of determination for traces of fluoride is based upon reaction with a metal chloranilate. Lanthanum chloranilate has been proposed for this purpose; the reagent is added to a solution of the fluoride at pH 4·6 when lanthanum fluoride is precipitated and an equivalent amount of coloured chloranilic acid is liberated; measurement of this colour against a blank gives a measure of the fluoride present. Beer's Law is obeyed over the range 2 to 200 μg per ml and the precision and accuracy of the method are said to be of the order of 1 per cent. Phosphate and molybdate both interfere with the method in a quantitative manner. The following procedure has been recommended by Fine and Wynne.[24]

Place a suitable aliquot of the solution in a 100-ml graduated flask.

Add 10 ml of a 0·1M sodium acetate-acetic acid buffer, pH 4·6. Adjust the volume to 100 ml using a mixture of equal parts of methyl cellosolve and distilled water. Add 0·2 g of lanthanum chloranilate, shake the flask immediately and then allow to stand for thirty minutes, shaking at frequent intervals. Filter or centrifuge to give a clear solution and measure the extinction in a 1-cm cell at 530 mμ against a blank prepared in the same way. For greater sensitivity (in the range 0·5 to 4·0 μg per ml), the extinction should be measured at 330 mμ.

SALTS OF HALOGEN ACIDS

The official methods of determining pharmaceutical salts of halogen acids are by the Volhard silver nitrate titration for chlorides and bromides and the Lang iodate method for iodides. The equivalents are given in Table 19:

TABLE 19

	BROMIDE (1 ml 0·1N $AgNO_3$)	CHLORIDE (1 ml 0·1N $AgNO_3$)	IODIDE (1 ml 0·05M iodate)
Ammonium	(*B.P.C.*) 0·009796 g	(*B.P.*) 0·005350 g	—
Potassium	(*B.P.*) 0·01190 g	(*B.P.*) 0·007455 g	(*B.P.*) 0·01660 g
Sodium	(*B.P.*) 0·01029 g	(*B.P.*) 0·005845 g	(*B.P.*) 0·01499 g

(for bismuth, calcium, iron, mercury and zinc halogen salts see the respective metals)

Sodium fluoride is determined in the *B.Vet.C.* by precipitation as lead chlorofluoride.

Dissolve 0·15 g in 200 ml of water and add dilute nitric acid until almost neutral to bromophenol blue. Heat to boiling-point and add 20 per cent sodium hydroxide solution, dropwise, until just alkaline. Then add a solution of 0·3 g of sodium chloride in 5 ml of water followed by 3 ml of dilute hydrochloric acid, 5 g of lead nitrate dissolved in 50 ml of hot water and finally 5 g of sodium acetate, stirring vigorously. Heat on a water-bath for thirty minutes with occasional stirring, cool and allow to stand for sixteen hours. Filter and wash the residue first with 10 ml of water and then with four quantities, each of 5 ml, of lead chlorofluoride solution (prepared as follows: dissolve 10 g of lead nitrate in 200 ml of water and add a solution of 1 g of sodium fluoride in 100 ml of water followed by 2 ml of concentrated hydrochloric acid. Mix, allow to settle, decant the supernatant liquid and wash the precipitate by decantation with successive quantities, each of 200 ml, of water. Add 1 litre of water to the precipitate, shake thoroughly, allow to stand for one hour and filter). Finally wash with 5 ml of water, transfer the residue to a beaker, add 70 ml of water and 30 ml of dilute nitric acid and complete by Volhard's method. 1 ml 0·1N silver nitrate = 0·0042 g NaF.

In the official assay of bromides a correction is made deducting the chloride found from the total halogen. The chloride content is determined by utilising the fact that bromides (and iodides) are more easily oxidised than chlorides.

Dissolve 1·0 g in a mixture of 75 ml of water and 25 ml of concentrated nitric acid in a 500-ml distillation flask fitted with a bung carrying a thermometer and a tapered air-inlet tube adjusted so that it is above the surface of the liquid. Pass a gentle stream of air, heat the solution to 105° to 106°, lower the inlet tube into the liquid and continue to heat for one minute, maintaining the temperature at 105° to 106°. Remove the source of heat and pass a brisk stream of air through the liquid for ten minutes. Determine the residual chloride by Volhard's method.

The following official preparations contain iodide, which is assayed by the Lang iodate method described above; equivalents are given for 1 ml of 0·05M potassium iodate:

Injection of Sodium Iodide, *B.Vet.C.*, 0·01499 g NaI.

Mixture of Belladonna and Ephedrine for Infants, *B.P.C.*, after evaporation to thick syrup and ignition with sodium carbonate, 0·01660 g KI.

Compound Mixture of Lobelia and Stramonium, *B.P.C.*, 0·01660 g KI.

Ammoniated Mixture of Potassium Iodide, *B.P.C.*, 0·01660 g KI.
Ammonium bicarbonate p. 454.

Mixture of Stramonium and Potassium Iodide, *B.P.C.*, 0·01660 g KI.

The following preparations are assayed for their content of halogen by the given method; equivalents are given for 1 ml 0·1N silver nitrate:

Injection of Potassium Chloride, Mohr 0·007455 g KCl.

Injection of Sodium Chloride, *B.P.*, Mohr 0·005845 g NaCl.

Compound Injection of Sodium Chloride, *B.P.C.*, Volhard 0·003546 g Cl.
Calcium chloride p. 153.

Injection of Sodium Chloride and Dextrose, *B.P.*, Mohr 0·005845 g NaCl.
Dextrose p. 605.

Injection of Sodium Chloride and Sodium Citrate, *B.Vet.C.*, Volhard 0·005845 g NaCl.
Sodium citrate p. 183.

Compound Injection of Sodium Lactate, *B.P.*, Volhard 0·003546 g total Cl.
Calcium chloride and lactic acid p. 368.

Mixture of Ammonium Chloride, *B.P.C.*, Potentiometric titration 0·005350 g NH_4Cl.

Mixture of Ammonium Chloride and Morphine, *B.P.C.*, Potentiometric titration 0·005350 g NH_4Cl.

Ammonium bicarbonate p. 454, morphine p. 493.

Mixture of Chloral and Potassium Bromide for Infants, *B.P.C.*, Volhard 0·01190 g KBr.

Chloral hydrate p. 166.

Compound Mixture of Gelsemium and Hyoscyamus, *B.P.C.*, Volhard 0·01190 g KBr.

Mixture of Potassium Bromide, *B.P.C.*, Potentiometric titration 0·01190 g KBr.

Mixture of Potassium Bromide for Infants, *B.P.C*, Potentiometric titration 0·01190 g KBr.

Mixture of Potassium Bromide and Chloral, *B.P.C.*, Volhard 0·01190 g KBr.

Chloral hydrate p. 166.

Mixture of Potassium Bromide and Nux Vomica, *B.P.C.*, Volhard 0·01190 g KBr.

Mixture of Potassium Bromide and Valerian, *B.P.C.*, Volhard 0·01190 g KBr.

Ammonium bicarbonate p. 454.

Compound Mixture of Sodium Chloride, *B.P.C.*, Volhard 0·005845 g NaCl.

Sodium bicarbonate p. 31.

Compound Mouthwash of Sodium Chloride, *B.P.C.*, Mohr 0·005845 g NaCl.

Sodium bicarbonate p. 31.

Compound Powder of Borax for Nasal Wash, *B.P.C.*, Volhard 0·005845 g NaCl.

Borax and sodium bicarbonate p. 137.

Solution of Ferrous Iodide, *B.P.C.*, Volhard 0·01548 g FeI_2.

Solution of Sodium Chloride, *B.P.C.*, Mohr 0·005845 g NaCl.

Syrup of Ferrous Iodide, *B.P.C.*, Volhard 0·01548 g FeI_2.

Tablets of Ammonium Chloride, *B.P.C.*, Volhard 0·005350 g NH_4Cl.

Tablets of Potassium Chloride, *B.P.*, Mohr 0·007455 g KCl.

Tablets of Sodium Chloride, *B.P.*, Mohr 0·005845 g NaCl.

CHLORINATED COMPOUNDS

Chlorinated compounds are all evaluated on their available chlorine content. For estimation the chlorine is liberated with acid in the presence of excess of potassium iodide, from which the chlorine displaces an equivalent of iodine; the liberated iodine is then titrated with thiosulphate.

Chlorinated Lime

For estimation, weigh about 0·2 g (or measure a 50-ml portion of a triturate of 4 g with 1 litre of water) into 20 ml of 10 per cent potassium iodide solution, acidify with acetic or hydrochloric acid and titrate with 0·1N thiosulphate. 1 ml 0·1N = 0·003546 g chlorine.

Solution of Chlorinated Lime with Boric Acid, *B.P.C.* (Eusol). Contains 1·25 per cent w/v boric acid.

For available chlorine titrate 25 ml as above, but acidify with a minimum excess of acid. (When fresh this preparation should contain about 0·4 per cent available chlorine, but it quickly loses strength.) Neutralise the titrated liquid to methyl orange, add glycerol or mannitol and titrate the boric acid to phenolphthalein with 0·5N sodium hydroxide (see p. 133).

Surgical Solution of Chlorinated Soda, *B.P.* (Dakin's Solution). Assayed similarly to the method for Eusol (above), but the boric acid is titrated with 0·1N alkali. The boric acid varies with the strength of the chlorinated lime originally used; the preparation should keep most of its strength for some time (Davis[25]).

Chloramine, $C_7H_7O_2NSClNa,3H_2O$, Mol. Wt. 281·7.

Chloramine, or toluene-*p*-sulphonsodiochloroamide, liberates iodine from potassium iodide in acid solution, one molecule giving two atoms of iodine.

Dissolve 0·4 g in 50 ml of water in a stoppered flask, add 1 g of potassium iodide and acidify with dilute sulphuric or acetic acid. Allow the mixture to stand for ten minutes and titrate the liberated iodine with 0·1N sodium thiosulphate. 1 ml 0·1N = 0·01409 g.

CHLORATES

Methods for the determination of chlorates invariably rely on their strong oxidising power with simultaneous reduction to chloride.

Oxidation of hydriodic or hydrobromic acid by chloric acid has received considerable attention, the latter reaction being the basis of the Rupp method[26] in which 10 ml of a 0·5 per cent potassium chlorate solution is allowed to stand for fifteen minutes with 1 g of potassium bromide and 15 ml of concentrated hydrochloric acid, after which 150 ml of 1 per cent potassium iodide solution is added and the liberated iodine titrated with 0·1N thiosulphate. Ferrey[27] obtained variable results by this method, apparently due to loss of bromine vapour when the potassium iodide solution was added; but he found that the similar reaction between chloric acid and hydriodic acid is very rapid provided the concentration of hydrochloric acid present is 7·5N or greater. To avoid appreciable error through the action of atmospheric oxygen on hydriodic acid, the time of reaction must be limited as far as possible:

Dissolve about 0·8 g of potassium chlorate in water and make up to 100 ml. To 10 ml in a stoppered bottle of about 300-ml capacity, add 1 g of potassium iodide, allow to dissolve and then add 30 ml of concentrated hydrochloric acid. Quickly replace the stopper (which should be moistened with a drop of potassium iodide solution) and allow to stand for one minute, during the last fifteen seconds of which slowly rotate the bottle under the tap to cool it slightly and prevent loss on removing the stopper. Add 120 ml of water and titrate with 0·1N thiosulphate. Starch may be used as indicator. 1 ml 0·1N = 0·002043 g.

The presence of as much as 5 per cent of potassium nitrate in potassium chlorate did not interfere with the accuracy of the assay.

The presence of ferrous sulphate in the reaction between chloric and hydriodic acid considerably accelerates the rate of reaction. Ferrey[28] found the following conditions gave quantitative results:

Dissolve about 0·8 g in 100 ml of water and heat 10 ml of the solution at about 50° for twenty minutes in a stoppered bottle with 25 ml of acid solution of ferrous sulphate (freshly prepared by dissolving 7 g of ferrous sulphate in 90 ml of boiled and cooled water, to which is added sufficient concentrated sulphuric acid to produce 100 ml) and 5 g of potassium iodide. Cool, add 50 ml of water and titrate the liberated iodine with 0·1N thiosulphate. Repeat the operation without the potassium chlorate and deduct the titration figure in the test from that in the control. 1 ml 0·1N = 0·002043 g $KClO_3$.

The chloride obtained by reduction with the acid ferrous sulphate solution may be determined gravimetrically as silver chloride, after reboiling with nitric acid (Harvey).[29]

The oxidation of nitrite in the presence of fairly strong nitric acid forms the basis of the *B.P.C.* assay for **potassium chlorate,** $KClO_3$, Mol. Wt. 122·6.

Dissolve about 0·3 g in 10 ml of water in a stoppered flask, add 1 g of sodium nitrite dissolved in 10 ml of water, followed by 20 ml of concentrated nitric acid. Allow to stand for ten minutes, add 100 ml of water and sufficient potassium permanganate solution to produce a permanent pink colour. Decolorise with a trace of ferrous sulphate, add 0·1 g of urea and complete by Volhard's method (see above). 1 ml 0·1N $AgNO_3$ = 0·01226 g $KClO_3$.

Gargle of Ferric Chloride, *B.P.C.* Contains 3·43 per cent of potassium chlorate and 0·47 per cent of ferric chloride.

Assay for potassium chlorate: To 2 ml add 8 ml of water, 1 g of potassium iodide and 30 ml of concentrated hydrochloric acid and allow to stand for three minutes. Then add 120 ml of water and titrate the liberated iodine with 0·1N sodium thiosulphate using starch as indicator. Deduct 0·12 ml for each 0·1 per cent of $FeCl_3$ found in the determination of ferric chloride. Each ml 0·1N thiosulphate represented by the difference = 0·002043 g of $KClO_3$.

Assay for ferric chloride: See under Iron, p. 356.

Gargle of Potassium Chlorate and Phenol, *B.P.C.* Contains 3·43 per cent of potassium chlorate and 1·32 per cent w/v of phenol.

Assay for potassium chlorate: Evaporate 5 ml to dryness on a water-bath, dissolve the residue in 10 ml of water, transfer to a stoppered flask and determine by the method given above for potassium chlorate.

Assay for phenol: See under Phenol, p. 517.

Lozenge of Potassium Chlorate, *B.P.C.* Contains 2 grains of potassium chlorate in a base of sugar and acacia.

A formalin or nitrite reduction method may be used with advantage for the determination of chlorate in this lozenge. Standard mixtures of potassium chlorate with sugar and acacia have given theoretical yields of potassium chlorate by the following method:

Dissolve the equivalent of one lozenge in 10 ml of hot water. Cool, add 25 ml of 0·1N silver nitrate, 10 ml of dilute nitric acid and 5 ml of formaldehyde solution. Heat just to boiling and leave on a water-bath until the precipitate has coagulated. Filter, wash the precipitate and titrate the filtrate and washings with 0·1N potassium thiocyanate, using iron alum as indicator. 1 ml 0·1N $AgNO_3$ = 0·01226 g $KClO_3$.

Tablets of Potassium Chlorate, *B.P.C.* Usually contain 5 grains of potassium chlorate.

The assay is the same as for lozenges, above.

Potassium perchlorate, $KClO_4$. Mol. Wt. 138·6. The official *B.P.* assay relies on reduction to chloride by heating in the presence of a large excess of ammonium chloride.

Mix 0·4 g with 2 g of ammonium chloride in a platinum crucible and heat carefully, without melting the residual chloride, until fuming has ceased. Allow to cool, add 2 g of ammonium chloride, mix, again heat carefully until fuming has ceased and then heat for a further one hour. Allow to cool, dissolve the residue in 50 ml of water and titrate with 0·1N silver nitrate by the Mohr method (p. 288). 1 ml 0·1N = 0·01386 g $KClO_4$.

Tablets of Potassium Perchlorate, *B.P.*

The official assay is as above, using a weight of powdered tablets equivalent to about 0·4 g of potassium perchlorate. However, sodium chloride is frequently used as a diluent in which case the following technique can be used.

Dissolve an amount of powdered tablets equivalent to 0·2 g of potassium perchlorate in sufficient water to produce 200 ml. To 50 ml add 10 ml concentrated hydrochloric acid, replace the air in the flask with carbon dioxide and maintain a stream of carbon dioxide throughout the determination. Add 50 ml of 0·1N titanous chloride, heat to boiling-point and boil gently for thirty minutes with occasional swirling. While still boiling, titrate the excess titanous chloride with 0·1N ferric ammonium sulphate using 5 ml of 10 per cent ammonium thiocyanate solution, added towards the end of the titration, as indicator. Carry out a blank determination omitting the sample. 1 ml 0·1N titanous chloride = 0·001732 g $KClO_4$.

1. MOHR, F., *Annalen*, 1856, **97,** 335.
2. FAJANS, K., and HASSEL, O., *Z. Elektrochem.*, 1923, **29,** 495.
3. FAJANS, K., and WOLFF, H., *Z. Anorg. Chem.*, 1924, **137,** 221.
4. VOLHARD, J., *Annalen*, 1878, **190,** 1.
5. CALDWELL, J. R., and MOYER, H. V., *Ind. Eng. Chem., Anal. Edn.*, 1935, **7,** 38.
6. VIEBÖCK, F., *Ber.*, 1932, **65B,** 586.
7. BELCHER, R., MACDONALD, A. M. G., and NUTTEN, A. J., *Mikrochim. Acta*, 1954, 104.
8. KOLTHOFF, I. M. and YUTZY, H., *Ind. Eng. Chem., Anal. Edn.*, 1937, **9,** 75.
9. HASLAM, J., and MOSES, G., *Analyst*, 1950, **75,** 343.
10. ANDREWS, L. M., *J. Amer. Chem. Soc.*, 1903, **25,** 756.
11. SMITH, G. F., and WILCOX, C. S., *Ind. Eng. Chem., Anal. Edn.*, 1942, **14,** 49.
12. LANG, R., *Z. Anorg. Chem.*, 1922, **122,** 332.
13. BERG, R., *Z. Anal. Chem.*, 1926, **69,** 369.
14. LEIPERT, T., *Mikrochemie Pregl Festschr.*, 1929, 266.
15. SAKHAROVA, Ya., and SHISHKINA, N. I., *Zavod. Lab.*, 1959, **25,** 1442.
16. LEONARD, M. A., private communication.
17. HARDWICK, P. J., *Analyst*, 1942, **67,** 223
18. RIGGS, E. D., and MAN, E. B., *J. Biol. Chem.*, 1940, **134,** 193.
19. Determination of Trace Elements, *S.A.C.*, p. 17.
20. *Analyst*, 1944, **69,** 243; 1945, **70,** 43.
21. MILTON, R. F., LIDDELL, H. F., and CHIVERS, J. E., *Analyst*, 1947, **72,** 43.
22. BELCHER, R., LEONARD, M. A., and WEST, T. S., *Talanta*, 1959, **2,** 92.
23. JOHNSON, C. A., and LEONARD, M. A., *J. Pharm. Pharmacol.*, 1961, **13,** 164 T.
24. FINE, L., and WYNNE, E. A., *Microchem. J.*, 1959, **3,** 515.
25. DAVIS, H., *Quart. J. Pharm.*, 1931, **4,** 360.
26. RUPP, E., *Z. Anal. Chem.*, 1917, **56,** 580.
27. FERREY, G. J. W., *Quart. J. Pharm.*, 1932, **5,** 409.
28. FERREY, G. J. W., *Quart. J. Pharm.*, 1932, **5,** 405.
29. HARVEY, C. O., *Analyst*, 1925, **50,** 538.

HALOGENS IN ORGANIC COMBINATION

This discussion is confined to those methods that are commonly employed in the determination of pharmaceutical substances and is not intended to be a comprehensive account of available methods. Each of the halogens is considered in turn although certain standard procedures are applicable in all cases.

CHLORINE IN ORGANIC COMBINATION

Choice of method depends to a large extent on how the chlorine is bound. In chloramines, for example, addition of potassium iodide in slightly acid solution is sufficient (see under Chlorinated Compounds, p. 305). In many cases simple hydrolysis with aqueous or alcoholic caustic alkali can be used (for example in the determination of hydrolysable chlorine in dicophane, p. 220). In the majority of cases, however, more vigorous treatment is necessary and a variety of methods is available:

(*a*) **Stepanow method.** In this method the halogen is removed as sodium halide by the action of metallic sodium and an alcohol. In Stepanow's original method[1] ethanol was used but in some instances this has been shown to lead to erratic results and higher boiling alcohols that do not react so readily with sodium have been proposed. Of these, the most commonly used are amyl alcohol[2] and *iso*propyl alcohol.[3] A significant advantage to be gained by using amyl alcohol is that the majority of the alcohol can be separated before titration of the halide.

*iso*Propyl alcohol is a better solvent than ethanol for a number of reasons, most of which are associated with its slower reaction with sodium:

(1) In ethanol the surface of the sodium is rapidly covered by nascent hydrogen which tends to impede the reaction.

(2) With *iso*propyl alcohol no interfering precipitate is formed during the reaction (sodium *iso*-propoxide starts to precipitate after three to four hours refluxing unlike sodium ethoxide which may precipitate quite rapidly).

(3) *iso*Propyl alcohol is a better solvent for many chlorinated hydrocarbons.

A procedure which is applicable to many chlorine-containing substances is as follows:

> Dissolve an accurately weighed quantity of the substance in a suitable organic solvent (Note 1) and dilute to exactly 100 ml with *iso*propyl alcohol. Transfer an aliquot of this solution, to contain about 60 to 70 mg of chlorine, to a round-bottomed flask of about 250-ml capacity and adjust the volume, if necessary, to about 25 ml with *iso*propyl alcohol. Add 2·5 g of sodium, in freshly cut small pieces, and boil gently under a reflux condenser for one hour (Note 2) shaking the flask occasionally. Destroy the excess of sodium by adding, cautiously and slowly, 10 ml of a mixture of equal volumes of *iso*propyl alcohol and water and boiling for ten minutes before adding 60 ml of water. Cool and neutralise with a mixture of equal parts of water and concentrated nitric acid, using phenolphthalein as indicator, then add a further 10 ml of the mixture. Cool, add an excess of standard silver nitrate and determine the halogen present by Volhard's method (see p. 290).

Note 1. The solvent used must be one in which the sample is readily soluble and which is miscible with *iso*propyl alcohol. For example, in the case of benzene hexachloride, benzene may be used and for hexachloro-ethane, *iso*propyl alcohol itself is suitable.

Note 2. In certain cases it may be necessary to extend this time; dieldrin, for example, must be refluxed for two hours after addition of the sodium.

A method in which amyl alcohol is used is as follows:

> Transfer a quantity of sample to contain 60 to 70 mg of chlorine to a round-bottomed flask and add 25 ml of amyl alcohol, followed by 2·5 g of sodium in freshly cut small pieces; warm under a condenser until evolution of hydrogen ceases and then boil for one hour (see Note). Cool to below 100° and add 50 ml of a mixture of equal parts of water and concentrated nitric acid, shaking well. Separate the aqueous layer and then extract the amyl alcohol with four quantities, each of 25 ml, of water. Combine the aqueous extracts and determine the chloride present by Volhard's method (see p. 290).

Note. It may be necessary to increase this time for particularly resistant compounds. For parachlorphenol the boiling should be continued for three hours, an additional 1 g of sodium being added in small pieces over this period.

In some cases, *e.g.* Chlorotrianisene, official methods still make use of the original Stepanow procedure using ethanol.

(*b*) **Raney nickel reduction.** This is a rapid and convenient method which is applicable to many substances, particularly chlorinated aromatic compounds. (Raney nickel is an alloy containing 50 per cent each of nickel and aluminium.) The following procedure is recommended but care should be taken at the stage of filtration through sintered glass; if air is allowed to suck through the drying residue for any length of time there is a danger of spontaneous ignition.

> Dissolve a quantity of sample equivalent to about 60 to 70 mg of chlorine in 1·5 ml of diethylamine, warming if necessary, and add 20 ml of water and 20 ml of 5N sodium hydroxide followed by 4 g of Raney nickel, added slowly and cautiously to avoid frothing. Reflux for one hour, cool, wash down the condenser with water and filter through a sintered-glass crucible, washing the residue well with water. Determine the halide in the combined filtrate and washings by Volhard's method (see p. 290).

(*c*) **Piria and Schiff's method.** This procedure, which is based on ignition of the sample with a mixture of 1 part of anhydrous sodium carbonate and 4 parts of lime, was first suggested by Piria[4] and slightly modified by Schiff.[5]

> Intimately mix the sample in a small nickel crucible with a little lime and sodium carbonate; pack more lime and sodium carbonate into the crucible until it is full; invert into a larger nickel crucible and seal the

junction between the crucibles with more of the lime mixture. Heat the crucibles for thirty minutes over a Bunsen flame so that the outer crucible is at a uniform dull red heat. Cool, leach out the mass with nitric acid and water and determine the chloride in the resulting solution by Volhard's method.

(*d*) **Parr bomb method.**[6] This method, which is of wide application, is used in certain cases in the *U.S.P.* The organic matter is oxidised by fusion with sodium peroxide in a bomb and the halogen present is converted to sodium halide which is subsequently determined by a suitable method.

The bomb, which should preferably be made of pure nickel, consists of a lower portion (the fusion cup), a lid fitted with a gasket and a union. Weigh a quantity of dried sample to contain about 100 to 150 mg of chlorine or bromine, or 150 to 200 mg of iodine directly into the fusion cup, followed by 0·5 g of sugar and about 15 g of sodium peroxide. Place the lid in position on the cup and screw the union tightly into place using a wrench. Mix the contents of the bomb by shaking thoroughly and then tap so that the entire charge is in the bottom of the fusion cup. Heat the bomb with a hot Bunsen flame for about three minutes (the exact amount of heating required will depend to some extent on the nature of the sample and will be decided by experience) and cool by placing the bomb in a bath of cold water. Dry the outside of the bomb, loosen the union without completely removing it, loosen the lid to release internal pressure and then remove both union and lid. Thoroughly wash the lid and fusion cup into a suitable vessel and determine the halide content of the liquid, which should be bright and almost free from carbon, by a suitable method.

After combustion chlorine is converted entirely to chloride, bromine occurs partly as bromide and partly as bromate and iodine is almost quantitatively converted to iodate.

Many modifications of the original bomb have been suggested and those suitable for semi-micro application, using a somewhat smaller charge than that described above, find wide application. It is important to carry out the fusion and the cooling stages behind an adequate screen and at no time should the face be brought near to the bomb without protection.

(*e*) **The oxygen-flask combustion method.** This elegant and useful technique is described in Appendix IV.

Hexachloroethane, CCl_3,CCl_3, Mol. Wt. 236·8. Assayed by the Stepanow method using ethanol as solvent. 1 ml 0·1N $AgNO_3$ = 0·003946 g.

Because of the volatility and high chlorine content of this material, the oxygen-flask combustion method is not applicable.

BROMINE IN ORGANIC COMBINATION

The methods given above for chlorine-containing substances are largely applicable to those containing bromine. Again, the choice of method depends to a large extent on the particular compound. Carbromal, for example, is readily decomposed by refluxing with alkali for a short time; dibromopropamidine isethionate requires more vigorous treatment and a Stepanow procedure is officially applied; mercurochrome is particularly resistant and requires fusion with a mixture of potassium nitrate, potassium carbonate and sodium carbonate. (The *N.F.* includes reduced iron in the fusion mixture.)

Dibromopropamidine isethionate, $C_{21}H_{30}O_{10}N_4S_2Br_2$, Mol. Wt. 722·5, is assayed in the *B.P.C.* by the Stepanow method given above using amyl alcohol as the solvent. 1 ml 0·1N $AgNO_3$ = 0·03612 g.

Sulphobromophthalein sodium, $C_{20}H_8O_{10}Br_4S_2Na_2$, Mol. Wt. 838·1 can be assayed for bromine and sulphur by the oxygen-flask combustion method (Appendix IV).

For bromine, use 0·2 g and, as absorbing liquid, 10 ml of 0·1N sodium hydroxide, 10 drops of hydrogen peroxide (100 vol.) and 10 ml of water. Complete by Volhard's method. 1 ml 0·1N $AgNO_3$ = 0·007991 g Br.

For sulphur, use 0·2 g and, as absorbing liquid, 30 ml of water and 0·5 ml of hydrogen peroxide (100 vol.). After combustion add 2 ml of concentrated hydrochloric acid, heat to boiling-point and precipitate and weigh as sulphate (see p. 618). $BaSO_4 \times 0{\cdot}1374 = S$.

IODINE IN ORGANIC COMBINATION

Many methods of determination have been published for the decomposition of compounds containing iodine in organic combination, their numbers suggesting that difficulties may be encountered in obtaining satisfactory results. They include:

(*a*) Charring with an excess of anhydrous sodium carbonate (see chiniofon sodium below). If the ignition is carried out by mixing with anhydrous carbonate and heating in an open crucible some loss of iodine may occur.

(*b*) Stepanow's method (see p. 310).

(*c*) Distillation from strong sulphuric acid and titration of the evolved hydriodic acid with silver nitrate in acid solution.

(*d*) Refluxing with glacial acetic acid and zinc filings and titrating the iodide solution with 0·05M iodate.

(*e*) Reduction with zinc in alkaline solution and titration of the iodide solution with iodate.

(*f*) Digestion with chloric acid (see below).

(*g*) By oxygen-flask combustion (see Appendix IV, p. 800).

Once the decomposition has been achieved, the iodide or iodate formed may be determined by any suitable method.

A rapid method for the determination of iodine in organic combination has been described by Zak and Boyle.[7] This method uses chloric acid as the oxidising digestion reagent and has been applied successfully to weights of iodine ranging from a fraction of a mg to 100 mg.

Prepare the chloric acid solution (approximately 28 per cent) as follows. Weigh 500 g of potassium chlorate into a 4-litre beaker, add 900 ml of water and heat the mixture until solution is effected. Add, with continuous stirring, 375 ml of 72 per cent w/w perchloric acid; potassium perchlorate will be present as a precipitate at this time. Cool, cover the beaker with a watch-glass, place in the freezing compartment of a refrigerator for two to three hours and then decant the supernatant liquid through a Whatman No. 41 H filter paper.

To a suitable amount of sample in a beaker add 10 to 25 ml of the chloric acid solution and evaporate on a low-temperature hot-plate until fumes of perchloric acid are evolved. The iodine, present in this solution as iodate, may then be determined volumetrically by titration with sodium thiosulphate using starch indicator, polarographically or spectrophotometrically.

Non-Staining Ointment of Iodine, *B.P.C.* Prepared to contain 5 per cent by weight of iodine in arachis oil and paraffin.

Considerable difficulty has been encountered with the analysis of this ointment. Results on submitted products are rarely close to the theoretical requirements of the formula. This may be partly due to the unsatisfactory nature of the preparation; some methods of manufacture produce a sludge, which evidently contains a considerable proportion of iodine, and sticks tenaciously to the sides of the containing vessel. But even allowing for this, results by different methods are generally not in agreement.

The official method for the determination of iodine in this ointment is the alkaline-fusion method given under Chiniofon Sodium, using 0·5 g.

Another method, which is satisfactory and rapid, is the oxygen-flask combustion method (Johnson and Vickers[8]). The method is described in detail in Appendix IV and for this determination 0·05 g of the sample should be used and the titration should be carried out with 0·01N sodium thiosulphate. 1 ml 0·01N = 0·0002115 g I.

Other methods that have previously been applied in official methods, *e.g.* refluxing with zinc powder and glacial acetic acid, gave low results in some workers' hands.

Non-Staining Ointment of Iodine with Methyl Salicylate, *B.P.C.* This is Non-Staining Ointment of Iodine containing 5 per cent v/w of methyl salicylate.

The iodine content may be determined by either of the methods given above under Non-Staining Ointment of Iodine. (For determination of methyl salicylate, see p. 432.)

Strong Ointment of Iodine, *B.Vet.C.* Prepared to contain 10 per cent of iodine and 7·5 per cent of potassium iodide in a wool fat and paraffin base. The total iodine content is determined by the method given under Chiniofon Sodium, using 1 g.

Injection of Iodised Oil, *B.P.C.*, is an iodine-addition product of poppy-seed oil and contains about 40 per cent of combined iodine. It can be assayed by the method of Cocking and Middleton[9] but the iodide is titrated by the Lang technique:

> Boil 1 g for one hour under a reflux condenser with 10 ml of glacial acetic acid and 1 g of zinc powder. Then add 30 ml of hot water down the condenser tube, filter the liquid through a plug of wet cotton wool and wash the flask and filter with two quantities, each of 20 ml, of water. Cool the filtrate, add 15 ml of concentrated hydrochloric acid and 5 ml of 10 per cent potassium iodide solution and titrate with 0·05M potassium iodate as described under Iodoxyl (below).

The iodine may also be determined by the oxygen-flask combustion method, using 8 mg and titrating with 0·01N thiosulphate. 1 ml 0·01N = 0·000423 g I.

Chiniofon Sodium, $C_9H_5O_4NISNa$, Mol. Wt. 373·1.

This is sodium 8-hydroxy-7-iodoquinoline-5-sulphonate. Details for the determination are useful as a general method for organically combined iodine.

> Intimately mix 0·2 g with 1 g of anhydrous sodium carbonate in a nickel crucible about 20 mm in diameter. Fill the crucible completely with anhydrous sodium carbonate, pressed well down, and invert into a larger crucible, about 25 mm in diameter, containing a layer of the sodium carbonate about 1 cm thick. Seal the junction between the two crucibles with more anhydrous sodium carbonate and then heat for thirty minutes over a Bunsen flame so that the outer crucible is at a uniform dull red heat. Allow to cool, transfer the crucibles and contents to a beaker, add 100 ml of water and boil gently for ten minutes. Filter through a small cotton-wool plug into a 1-litre flask and wash the residue with a little water. Boil the residue a second time with 100 ml of water for twenty minutes, again filter, and wash the residue with water until free from alkali. Cool the combined filtrate and washings and dilute with water to about 500 ml. Add three drops of 0·04 per cent w/v methyl orange solution and sufficient 50 per cent v/v sulphuric acid to neutralise the solution. Add 1 ml of the acid in excess and then add 0·2 ml or a slight excess of bromine and a small piece of marble (about 0·05 g) and boil briskly until the solution is colourless. Cool to about 20°, add 0·2 ml of a 25 per cent w/v solution of phenol in glacial acetic acid and allow to stand for two minutes. Add 5 ml of 10 per cent potassium iodide solution and titrate with 0·1N sodium thiosulphate using starch, added towards the end of the titration, as indicator. 1 ml 0·1N = 0·002115 g I, or 0·006219 g $C_9H_5O_4NISNa$.

Alternatively the material may be assayed by the oxygen-flask combustion method (Appendix IV) using 25 mg. 1 ml 0·02N thiosulphate = 0·0012449 g.

Tablets of Chiniofon Sodium, *B.P.* Usually contain 0·25 g in each tablet.

The tablets are assayed as Chiniofon Sodium using an amount of powdered tablets equivalent to about 0·2 g of Chiniofon Sodium.

However, if the oxygen-flask combustion method is to be used the tablet coating must first be removed and a 20-mg portion of the powdered cores used because, since these tablets are enteric coated, the small amount of sample required for this method might not be representative if the usual practice of powdering the coated tablets is followed.

Chiniofon, *N.F.*, is a mixture of 7-iodo-8-hydroxyquinoline-5-sulphonic acid, its sodium salt, and sodium bicarbonate.

The *N.F.* assay consists of three steps: (1) digestion with alkaline permanganate solution to decompose the material, (2) acidification and treatment with sodium bisulphite to reduce the manganese and iodine to their lower oxidation states and (3) titration with silver nitrate.

The details of the method are as follows:

> Dissolve 400 mg in 15 ml of N sodium hydroxide in a flask, warming gently to assist solution. Add 25 ml of potassium permanganate solution (1 in 15) then add several glass beads, place a small, short-stemmed funnel in the mouth of the flask and boil gently for ten minutes. Allow to cool to room temperature, wash the funnel and walls of the flask with 75 ml of water and add 10 ml of sulphuric acid (1 in 2). Decolorise by the addition, in one portion, of 15 ml of sodium bisulphite solution (1 in 5) and then add the permanganate solution, dropwise, until a yellow colour appears. At once add the sodium bisulphite solution, dropwise, until the yellow colour is again discharged. Now add, dropwise, a dilute solution of potassium permanganate, prepared by mixing 1 ml of the 1 in 15 solution with 49 ml of water, until a faint yellow colour appears. Add 1 ml of starch mucilage and titrate with 0·05N silver nitrate until the blue colour is just discharged, leaving a canary-yellow precipitate. 1 ml 0·05N = 0·006346 g I.

Di-iodohydroxyquinoline, $C_9H_5ONI_2$, Mol. Wt. 397·0.

This is 8-hydroxy-5,7-di-iodoquinoline. The easiest method of assay is by the flask-combustion technique, using about 12 mg, 1 ml 0·02N thiosulphate = 0·0006616 g $C_9H_5ONI_2$. It can also be determined by the general alkali-fusion method for organically combined iodine given under Chiniofon Sodium using 0·1 g of sample, 1 ml 0·1N thiosulphate = 0·003308 g. The *U.S.P.* uses the method for Chiniofon after heating the assay sample first with 1 ml of 95 per cent ethanol and then 15 ml of sodium hydroxide solution until the ethanol has been expelled, 1 ml 0·05N silver nitrate = 0·009924 g.

Tablets of Di-iodohydroxyquinoline, *B.P.* Usually contain 0·3 g and they can be assayed by the methods given above for the compound, using equivalent amounts of powdered tablets.

Injection of Diodone, *B.P.*

This is a sterile aqueous solution of the diethanolamine salt of 3,5-di-iodo-4-pyridone-*N*-acetic acid. The iodine is determined officially as for

Chiniofon Sodium using an amount of sample equivalent to about 0·1 g of the diethanolamine salt. The weight per ml is determined and the percentage w/v calculated. The iodine content can be checked either by the flask-combustion method (p. 800) or the Stepanow method (p. 310). The total solids are almost exactly double the iodine content.

Ethyl Iodophenylundecanoate, *B.P.C.* (Injection of Iophendylate, *U.S.P.*) $C_{19}H_{29}O_2I$, Mol. Wt. 416·4.

This is ethyl 10-(*p*-iodophenyl)undecanoate. It can be assayed by the flask-combustion method using 30 mg, 1 ml 0·02N thiosulphate = 0·001388 g or the alkali-fusion method given under Chiniofon Sodium. 1 ml 0·1N thiosulphate = 0·006939 g. In the *U.S.P.* the iodine is assayed as under Injection of Iodised Oil using 300 mg.

Iodoxyl, $C_8H_3O_5NI_2Na_2$, Mol. Wt. 492·9.

This is the disodium salt of 3,5-di-iodo-*N*-methyl-4-pyridone-2,6-dicarboxylic acid; it is mainly sold as a 20 per cent solution. It is assayed either by the flask combustion method on 16 mg, 1 ml 0·02N thiosulphate = 0·0008215 g, or as follows:

> Boil 1 g with 10 ml of glacial acetic acid and 1 g of zinc powder for one hour under a reflux condenser. Add 30 ml of hot water down the condenser tube, filter the liquid through a plug of wet cotton wool into a long-necked flask and wash the flask and filter with two quantities, each of 20 ml, of hot water. Cool the filtrate, add 15 ml of concentrated hydrochloric acid and 5 ml of 10 per cent potassium cyanide solution and titrate with 0·05M potassium iodate until the dark brown solution becomes light brown; add 5 ml of starch mucilage and continue the titration until the blue colour disappears. 1 ml 0·05M = 0·02465 g $C_8H_3O_5NI_2Na_2$.

Iopanoic Acid, $C_{11}H_{12}O_2NI_3$, Mol. Wt. 571·0.

This is α-(3-amino-2,4,6-tri-iodobenzyl) butyric acid. It can be assayed by the flask-combustion method using 12 mg, 1 ml 0·02N thiosulphate = 0·0006344 g. Semi-micro quantities for assay make it necessary for the sample to be finely powdered before weighing. The alkali-fusion method given under Chiniofon Sodium is also applicable, 1 ml 0·1N thiosulphate = 0·003172 g.

Tablets of Iopanoic Acid, *B.P.* Usually contain 0·5 g of substance. The iopanoic acid can be extracted directly by continuous extraction with acetone, solvent evaporation and drying at 105° before weighing. The *U.S.P.* method is preferable.

> Triturate an accurately weighed quantity of powdered tablets, equivalent to about 1 g of acid, with two successive quantities, each of 10 ml, of light petroleum (b.p. 40° to 60°), decanting, and filtering each extract through the same filter. Discard the filtrates. Warm the residue at 70°

with 10 ml of 95 per cent ethanol, previously neutralised to thymol blue, filter through the same filter and wash the residue with a further four quantities, each of 10 ml, of the neutralised ethanol, warmed to 70°. Cool the combined filtrate and washings to about 20° and titrate with 0·1N sodium hydroxide using thymol blue as indicator. 1 ml 0·1N = 0·05710 g $C_{11}H_{12}O_2NI_3$.

Pheniodol, $C_{15}H_{12}O_3I_2$, Mol. Wt. 494·1.

This is β-(4-hydroxy-3,5-di-iodophenyl)-α-phenylpropionic acid. Ballard and Spice[10] recommend reduction with zinc and alkali for reproducible and accurate results. This method is also applicable to the determination of iodoxyl and chiniofon.

Weigh an amount of material containing about 0·5 g of iodine into a 250-ml conical flask and dissolve in a mixture of 12 ml of sodium hydroxide solution and 20 ml of water, warming if necessary. Add 1 g of zinc powder, attach a condenser and reflux gently for thirty minutes. Cool, add through the condenser 20 ml of water, filter through cotton wool, wash the flask with two 15-ml quantities of water and pass the washings through the filter. To the filtrate add 25 ml of concentrated hydrochloric acid, cool, add 10 ml of 10 per cent potassium cyanide solution and titrate with 0·05M potassium iodate until the dark brown solution which is formed becomes light brown; add 5 ml of mucilage of starch and continue the titration until the solution is colourless. 1 ml of 0·05M potassium iodate = 0·02470 g $C_{15}H_{12}O_3I_2$.

The iodine content can also be determined as for Chiniofon Sodium, using 0·05 g of substance and titrating with 0·05N sodium thiosulphate, 1 ml 0·05N = 0·002059 g, or by the flask-combustion technique using 16 mg of substance, 1 ml 0·02N thiosulphate = 0·0008235 g of pheniodol.

Propyliodone, $C_{10}H_{11}O_3NI_2$, Mol. Wt. 447·0.

This is *n*-propyl 3,5-di-iodo-4-pyridone-*N*-acetate. The official assay is as given under Chiniofon Sodium, using about 50 mg and titrating with 0·05N sodium thiosulphate. 1 ml 0·05N thiosulphate = 0·001863 g of $C_{10}H_{11}O_3NI_2$.

The flask-combustion method is applicable using about 15 mg; 1 ml 0·02N thiosulphate = 0·0007450 g.

Injection of Propyliodone, *B.P.* A sterile, 50 per cent w/v suspension of propyliodone in water for injection containing suitable dispersing agents. It is assayed as under Chiniofon Sodium using 0·1 g of the well-mixed injection and titrating with 0·05N sodium thiosulphate.

Oily Injection of Propyliodone, *B.P.* A sterile, 60 per cent w/v suspension of propyliodone in arachis oil. It is assayed as the injection.

The flask-combustion method is unsuitable for these injections because, being suspensions, it would be difficult to ensure representative samples for the small quantities required for the assay.

Acetrizoic Acid, $C_9H_6O_3NI_3$, Mol. Wt. 556·9. This is 3-acetamido-2,4,6-tri-iodobenzoic acid and is assayed as under Iodoxyl, using about 0·7 g. 1 ml 0·05M KIO_3 = 0·01856 g $C_9H_6O_3NI_3$.

Sodium Diatrizoate, $C_{11}H_8O_4N_2I_3Na$, Mol. Wt. 635·9. This is sodium 3,5-diacetamido-2,4,6-tri-iodobenzoate and is assayed as under Iodoxyl using 0·6 g for the zinc reduction method, 1 ml 0·05M KIO_3 = 0·02120 g $C_{11}H_8O_4N_2I_3Na$, or 15 mg for the flask-combustion method, 1 ml 0·02N thiosulphate = 0·7066 mg.

FLUORINE IN ORGANIC COMBINATION

Fluorinated compounds are being used more extensively in medicine and the problem of determining fluorine in organic combination is becoming of increasing importance to the pharmaceutical analyst. A standard procedure which is applicable to many substances is based on fusion with sodium carbonate and subsequent precipitation of the fluoride as lead chlorofluoride (see p. 303) but this suffers from the disadvantage that a fairly large sample weight must be taken. Moreover, this form of decomposition may not be suitable for certain types of compound. A method which has wide applicability and which uses a modified precipitation procedure suitable for semi-micro work has been proposed by Belcher and Macdonald.[11] This depends upon fusion of the sample with sodium (or in the case of particularly resistant materials with potassium) in a nickel bomb (described by Belcher and Tatlow[12]). The detailed method is as follows:

Weigh into the cup of the nickel bomb an amount of sample containing 10 to 30 mg of fluoride ion (liquids should be weighed in gelatin capsules). Add 300 to 500 mg of sodium in small pellets (or potassium in the case of fluorocarbons, chlorofluorocarbons and compounds containing a fully fluorinated ring or long chain). Soften a copper, asbestos-packed gasket by heating to redness and dropping into ethanol, and place in position in the bomb. Close the bomb tightly and heat for one to one and a quarter hours in a muffle furnace at 600° to 650°. (Heating the bomb above 650° softens the nickel, shortens the life of the bomb and is not recommended.) Cool the bomb in a current of air, remove the lid and wash any material adhering to its under side into a 250-ml beaker with not more than 10 ml of water. Place the cup of the bomb in the beaker and fill it with ethanol. After several minutes stir the contents of the cup with a small nickel rod and add water, dropwise and at intervals to complete the destruction of the sodium without explosion. (If potassium has been used for the fusion it should be destroyed entirely with ethanol; water should not be added until the cup is ready to be rinsed.) Empty the contents of the cup into the beaker and rinse the cup with water; the volume of the solution should not exceed 30 ml at this stage, particularly if the zinc oxide separation is to be used.

(*a*) For compounds containing halogens and/or nitrogen. Remove carbon by filtration through a Pregl No. 1 filter, return the filtrate quantitatively to the beaker and neutralise with 5N nitric acid using methyl red as indicator.

(*b*) For compounds containing phosphorus or sulphur. Adjust the pH of the solution to 5 ± 0·3 with 5N nitric acid, using a pH meter. Rinse the electrodes with a volume of water not exceeding 10 to 15 ml and add 3 drops of 5N nitric acid, 3 drops of 30 per cent v/v acetic acid and about 0·8 g of solid zinc oxide. Heat the mixture almost to boiling-point and then allow to cool for twenty to thirty minutes, with occasional swirling (about every five minutes). Cool for a few minutes in a stream of cold water and filter off the zinc oxide and phosphate (or sulphide) on a pad of filter-paper pulp about 1 cm thick. Rinse the beaker with five quantities, each of 3 to 4 ml, of hot water, transferring most of the zinc oxide to the filter, and then rinse the filter paper and precipitate with five quantities, each of 2 to 3 ml, of hot water, allowing the filter to drain between all additions.

Precipitation of lead chlorofluoride. The volume of solution obtained from (*a*) or (*b*) above, must not exceed 80 ml and should preferably be less. Heat the solution almost to boiling-point and add 1 ml of 30 per cent v/v acetic acid. Then add, in a slow stream with continuous stirring until precipitation begins, 50 ml of hot lead chloronitrate solution (prepared as follows: dissolve 10·5 g of lead chloride and 13 g of lead nitrate by boiling with 1 litre of water. Some lead chloride may precipitate on standing; if heavy precipitation occurs, which may happen very readily in cold weather, the precipitated lead chloride must be redissolved by heating but a light scattering of crystals may be ignored if the solution is decanted before use). Cover the beaker and heat just to gentle boiling. Allow to cool overnight.

Filter through a tared sintered-glass crucible (No. 4) and transfer the precipitate quantitatively to the crucible with a saturated solution of lead chlorofluoride. Wash the precipitate, first with two quantities, each of 10 ml, of saturated lead chlorofluoride solution and then with two quantities, each of 10 ml, of acetone, dry at 110° for thirty minutes, allow to cool for thirty minutes and weigh.

Weight of precipitate × 0·07263 = weight of fluorine.

In some instances a Stepanow type of procedure is applicable as, for example, in the case of **Dyflos** $C_6H_{14}O_3PF$, Mol. Wt. 184·2.

Dissolve about 0·6 g in 10 ml of dehydrated ethanol, add and dissolve 0·5 g of sodium. Reflux gently for five minutes and then dilute with 100 ml of water. Make just acid to bromophenol blue with dilute nitric acid and then just alkaline with 5 per cent sodium hydroxide solution. Add 3 ml of 10 per cent sodium chloride solution, dilute to 250 ml with water, add 1 ml of concentrated hydrochloric acid and heat to about 80°. Add, with stirring, 5 g of finely powdered lead nitrate and when dissolved add, with vigorous stirring, 5 g of sodium acetate trihydrate. Filter, wash the residue first with water and then with four successive quantities of lead chlorofluoride solution (prepared as follows: dissolve 0·1 g of sodium fluoride in 100 ml of water and add 0·25 ml of bromophenol blue indicator, 3 ml of 10 per cent sodium chloride solution and 200 ml of water. Then add concentrated nitric acid, dropwise, until the solution turns yellow followed by 5 per cent sodium hydroxide solution until the solution turns faintly blue; add 1 ml of concentrated hydrochloric acid, maintain at 80° for ten minutes, add 5 g of finely powdered lead nitrate and stir gently for three minutes. Then add 5 g of finely powdered sodium acetate trihydrate and stir until the sodium acetate has dissolved and the colour of the solution has changed from yellow to blue. Heat on a water-bath for fifteen minutes, cool, allow the precipitate to settle, pour off the supernatant liquid and wash the precipitate repeatedly by decantation. Shake the precipitate with 1 litre of water for eight hours and filter). Finally wash the precipitate with water and add to the residue 50 ml of water, 50 ml of dilute nitric acid and 50 ml of 0·1N silver nitrate. Shake vigorously, heat on a water-bath for thirty minutes and complete by Volhard's method (see p. 290). 1 ml 0·1N = 0·01842 g $C_6H_{14}O_3PF$.

Application of the oxygen-flask combustion method to the determination of fluorine in organic combination has now been made by a number of workers. The fluoride in solution after combustion may be determined by thorium nitrate titration or colorimetrically as the alizarin complexan chelate[13] or with a chloranilate[14] (see Halogen Acids and Salts, p. 302). A method based upon the alizarin complexan chelate is given in Appendix IV.

Trifluoperazine Hydrochloride, $C_{21}H_{24}N_3SF_3,2HCl$. Mol. Wt. 480·4. This may be determined from its fluorine content by the flask-combustion method (see Appendix IV) or less specifically, by non-aqueous titration (see Appendix III) with 0·1N perchloric acid in glacial acetic acid. 1 ml 0·1N = 0·02402 g.

A number of fluorinated steroids can be determined by adaptation of the flask-combustion method in addition to their determination through the 17,21-dihydroxy-20-oxosteroid moiety (see p. 593).

Bendrofluazide and **Hydroflumethiazide** may also be determined from fluorine by the flask-combustion method but are more commonly determined by non-aqueous titration (see p. 702).

1. Stepanow, A., *Ber.*, 1906, **39**, 4056.
2. Palfray, L., and Sontag, D., *Bull. Soc. Chim. France*, 1930, **47**, 118.
3. Umhœffer, R. R., *Ind. Eng. Chem., Anal. Edn.*, 1943, **15**, 383.
4. Piria, R., *Lez. Chim. Org.*, 1857, 153.
5. Schiff, H., *Annalen*, 1879, **195**, 293.
6. Parr, S. W., *J. Amer. Chem. Soc.*, 1903, **30**, 767.
7. Zak, B., and Boyle, A. J., *J. Amer. Pharm. Ass., Sci. Edn.*, 1952, **41**, 260.
8. Johnson, C. A., and Vickers, C., *J. Pharm. Pharmacol.*, 1959, **11**, 218T.
9. Cocking, T. T., and Middleton, G., *Quart. J. Pharm.*, 1931, **4**, 175.
10. Ballard, C. W., and Spice, S., *J. Pharm. Pharmacol.*, 1952, **4**, 322.
11. Belcher, R., and Macdonald, A. M. G., *Mikrochim. Acta*, 1957, 510.
12. Belcher, R., and Tatlow, J. C., *Analyst*, 1951, **76**, 593.
13. Johnson, C. A., and Leonard, M. A., *Analyst*, 1961, **86**, 101.
14. Olson, E. C., and Shaw, S. R., *Microchem. J.*, 1961, **5**, 101.

HEPARIN

In the absence of a chemical method for the assay of heparin recourse must be made to comparison by biological ones against a standard preparation for which purpose the International Standard for Heparin (1957) containing 130 units/mg has been established.

The suggested *B.P.* method for the assay of heparin employs sulphated whole blood from oxen as the reagent; 50 per cent aqueous dilution of this reagent allows coagulation to proceed with proportional delays when the dilution is made with aqueous solutions of heparin. With the reagent alone times of coagulation are not easy to forecast and become longer as the blood ages but the addition of thrombokinase extracts enable the coagulation times to be shortened and controlled.

Reagents:

Sulphated Whole Blood: Collect four parts of ox blood from a freshly slaughtered beast into one part of a 7 per cent aqueous solution of anhydrous sodium sulphate. This should be stored in a refrigerator until required when it should be freed from any small clots which may have formed.

Thrombokinase Extract: Extract 1·5 g of acetone-dried ox brain with 60 ml of water for ten to fifteen minutes at 50°. Centrifuge for two minutes at 1500 r.p.m. The extract may be stored for several days in a refrigerator and a bacteriostat (0·3 per cent cresol) may be added if desired.

Acetone-dried Ox Brain: Pound fresh ox brain from which the vascular and connective tissues have been removed with successive quantities of acetone until a dry powder remains after filtration. Dry at 37° for two hours or until all traces of acetone are removed.

Method:

Prepare in water two dilutions of standard preparation containing 2·0 and 1·4 units per ml together with two similar dilutions of the unknown. Place 1 ml of each dilution into a $6'' \times \frac{1}{2}''$ test-tube followed by a quantity of thrombokinase solution (about 0·2 ml) sufficient to cause coagulation in the 2u/ml standard tube in about ten minutes after the addition of 1 ml of sulphated whole blood. Add 1 ml of sulphated whole blood to each tube, mix gently avoiding the formation of air bubbles. Record to the nearest fifteen seconds the time for the formation of a firm clot which remains in the bottom of the tube when it is inverted.

Repeat the observation four times for a complete assay and calculate the result by standard statistical methods accepting the linear relationship between log coagulation time and log concentration of heparin.

The onset of coagulation is shown by the change in fluidity observed during gentle tilting of the tube and by shortening the interval between examinations the operator can determine the end-point to within fifteen seconds and with practice avoid the breaking of the clot by premature inversion. If the tube is inverted before complete coagulation occurs the whole run of four tubes is repeated. The assay is conducted at room temperature.

Mechanical methods for the determination of the end-point of this method have been described (Randall,[1] Bryce[2]).

When the assays are being conducted regularly and fresh supplies of blood are easily obtained this method has much to commend it from the point of simplicity.

When assays are to be carried out intermittently or the blood is not easily obtained the method of the *U.S.P.* making use of citrated sheep plasma may be preferred.

Reagents:

Calcium Chloride Solution: 1 per cent in water.

Citrated Sheep Plasma. Prepare citrated sheep plasma by collecting 19 parts of blood from sheep directly into a vessel containing 1 part of 8 per cent sodium citrate solution. Promptly centrifuge the citrated blood after immediate and gentle mixing and pool the separated plasma.

Confirm the suitability of the plasma for use by adding 0·2 ml of calcium chloride solution to a 1-ml portion of the plasma and observing that coagulation is complete in five minutes. Store the plasma in portions not exceeding 100 ml by freezing at $-20°$ or below and holding at a temperature not exceeding $-8°$. For use in an assay thaw the plasma at a temperature not exceeding 37° and remove any particulate matter.

Method:

Prepare a solution of standard heparin in normal saline such that the quantity (usually between 1 and 1·5 units) contained in each 0·8 ml is the minimal amount to preserve fluidity in the plasma for one hour after the addition of 0·2 ml of calcium chloride solution. Make a similar solution of the unknown.

Clean hard glass test-tubes 13 × 100 mm by overnight immersion in chromic acid solution. To these tubes add graded amounts of the standard solution and of the unknown, so selected that the largest does not exceed 0·8 ml and the volumes correspond to a geometric series in which each concentration exceeds the lower by 5 per cent.

Add to each tube 1 ml of plasma together with sufficient normal saline to make the volume to 1·8 ml and follow this by the addition of 0·2 ml of calcium chloride solution. Stopper the tube and mix the contents by inversion three times in such a way that the entire inner surface of the tube is wetted. Note the time of addition of the calcium chloride and exactly one hour later record the extent of clotting in each tube noting three grades of clotting (0·25, 0·5, 0·75) between zero and full clotting (1·0). If the series does not contain two tubes graded more than 0·5 and two tubes graded less than 0·5 repeat the assay making suitable adjustments.

Assess the relative potency by comparing the concentrations of standard and unknown which produce a clotting of grade 0·5.

The *U.S.P.* prescribes that this be done by converting to logs the volumes used in the 5 or 6 tubes that bracket a grade of clotting of 0·5 including at least 2 tubes each with a larger and 2 tubes with a lower grading. The means of these logs are calculated for tubes 1, 2 and 3; 2, 3 and 4 etc., together with the corresponding mean of the clotting grading. The log concentration producing 0·5 grading is taken as that which corresponds exactly with a value of 0·5 or by interpolation between the two values which bracket it.

There is evidence that assays using these two methods do not always give precisely the same figures and that the deviation is not always one way. The difference is unlikely to exceed the tolerance allowed in the pharmacopœias and is certainly not of physiological importance. The difference may of course be of importance in the commercial transactions relating to heparin.

Jorpes[3] has made a critical comparison of methods for the assay of heparin and considers that only those employing whole blood yield results agreeing with those obtained by an *in vivo* method described by him and his colleagues.[4] His earlier observations (Jorpes[5]) suggested that only freshly shed blood was acceptable for this reason but his extended experience using the sulphated whole blood method of the *B.P.* has satisfied him that it is equally acceptable.

1. Randall, S. S., *Analyst*, 1952, **77**, 51.
2. Bryce, D. M., *J. Pharm. Pharmacol.*, 1952, **4**, 980.
3. Jorpes, J. E., Vrethammar, T., Öhman, B., and Blombäck, B., *J. Pharm. Pharmacol.*, 1958, **10**, 561.
4. Jorpes, J. E., Blombäck, M., and Blombäck, B., *J. Pharm. Pharmacol.*, 1954, **6**, 694.
5. Jorpes, J. E., *Acta Pharmacol. Toxicol.*, 1955, **11**, 367.

HYDRASTIS

Hydrastis contains the alkaloids hydrastine (about 2 to 3 per cent), berberine (about 2·5 to 4 per cent), and canadine (in traces), all present almost exclusively as the free alkaloids.

The value of the root is confined to the hydrastine content, berberine being physiologically less active, and methods of assay require separation of these constituents. This is effected either by precipitating the berberine with potassium iodide or by extracting the hydrastine with ether, berberine being only slightly soluble. The *N.F.*X method was briefly the following:

> Shake 10 g of hydrastis root in fine powder with 100 ml of ether and 10 ml of dilute ammonia solution, set aside overnight and decant 50 ml. Completely extract the alkaloids from 50 ml of the ether with weak sulphuric acid and, after making the bulked aqueous solutions ammoniacal, extract again with at least six portions of ether. Evaporate the ethereal solutions and weigh after drying at 105°.

The *B.P.C.* 1949 standardised hydrastis root by a method based on the above principle.

Another method of assay is to extract 10 g of finely powdered root with hot 90 per cent ethanol in a Soxhlet apparatus and make up to 100 ml, evaporate 50 ml to 10 ml and proceed as under Liquid Extract of Hydrastis.

If required, berberine may be determined by precipitation of its insoluble acid sulphate.

To 50 ml of extract obtained above and evaporated to 10 ml add 20 ml of 20 per cent sulphuric acid, allow to stand at low temperature overnight and filter through a Gooch crucible. Wash the precipitate with acidulated water and then with 10 ml of equal parts of ethanol and ether. Dry at 100° and weigh. $C_{20}H_{17}NO_4,H_2SO_4 \times 0{\cdot}8153$ = berberine.

Liquid Extract of Hydrastis, *B.P.C.* 1949. Contains 2·0 per cent w/v of hydrastine.

In the *B.P.C.* 1949 assay the berberine is first precipitated with potassium iodide. Briefly it is as follows:

Transfer 10 ml of liquid extract to a 100-ml graduated flask, add 20 ml of 10 per cent potassium iodide solution diluted with 60 ml of water, then make up to 100 ml. Shake for several minutes and filter. Make 50 ml of filtrate alkaline with ammonia and shake at intervals during several minutes with three successive portions, 30, 20 and 20 ml of ether. Evaporate the ether, dry the residue on a water-bath and weigh the hydrastine.

The ether solutions should be washed with water before evaporating.

The method is not very satisfactory; apparently the hydrastine content depends on the amount of extractive precipitated in the aqueous potassium iodide, the percentage of alkaloid found increasing considerably when smaller quantities of extract are used for assay.

Hydrastine hydrochloride, $C_{21}H_{21}O_6N,HCl$, Mol. Wt. 419·9, was official in the *B.P.C.* 1949. The base is obtained by the usual chloroform extraction in ammoniacal solution, washing, evaporating in the presence of ethanol and drying at 100°.

HYDROCYANIC ACID

HCN Mol. Wt. 27·03

Liebig's original method for estimation of alkali cyanides depends on the production of the soluble double cyanide of silver and the alkali. After the total formation of the double salt, the next addition of silver nitrate produces a precipitate of silver cyanide by decomposition of the double salt. In the titration of the free acid, after addition of ammonia the double silver ammonium cyanide is produced, but the silver cyanide precipitate is not formed owing to its solubility in the excess of ammonia, hence potassium iodide is added as an indicator, giving an immediate precipitation of silver iodide after formation of silver ammonium cyanide. Addition of ammonia and iodide also sharpens the end-point for the alkali cyanides, the iodide being more easily seen than the opalescence from silver cyanide. The *B.Vet.C.* method for hydrocyanic acid prescribes insufficient potassium iodide. A modification of the estimation is:

> Weigh about 5 g of acid into 5 ml of dilute ammonia solution and 20 ml of water; add 1 ml of 10 per cent potassium iodide solution, dilute and titrate with 0·1N silver nitrate to a permanent opalescence. 1 ml 0·1N = 0·005405 g.

Wellings[1] has shown that diphenylcarbazide can be used as an adsorption indicator for the estimation of cyanides by Liebig's method, and it gives a very sharp end-point especially for weak solutions (down to dilutions of 0·004M). By adding 2 or 3 drops of a 0·1 per cent ethanolic solution of diphenylcarbazide to the cyanide solution, the pink colour produced becomes pale violet at the end-point. The silver nitrate solution must be free from acid.

Ryan and Culshaw[2] claim a similar sensitivity by use of *p*-dimethylaminobenzilidene rhodanine which gives a sharp colour change from pale yellow to reddish-violet.

To estimate hydrocyanic acid in mixtures, especially where the percentage present is low, steam distillation is necessary in a neutral or slightly acid medium.

> Place a suitable quantity of sample in a distillation flask through which carbon dioxide may be passed and connect to a condenser dipping into 0·1N silver nitrate. After slightly acidifying with tartaric acid pass carbon dioxide through the solution and then carefully distil with steam. Either ignite the precipitated cyanide to silver and weigh (Ag × 0·2505 = HCN), or filter, wash the precipitate and acidify the filtrate with nitric acid, titrating the excess of silver with 0·1N thiocyanate. 1 ml 0·1N = 0·0027 g HCN.

Assays for hydrocyanic acid are almost invariably low compared with the amount added; it should be the first constituent determined immediately on opening the sample in order to avoid low results due to volatilisation. Monier-Williams[3] has also shown that hydrocyanic acid may form a cyanhydrin with lævulose which, in the presence of alkali, is hydrolysed to hydroxy-acids and ammonia. Hence, in mixtures containing invert sugar, hydrocyanic acid figures will be low.

CYANIDES

Commercial alkali cyanides are supplied in various strengths and both sodium cyanide and the double sodium-potassium salt are often referred to as **potassium cyanide,** KCN, Mol. Wt. 65·12, hence potassium cyanide 133 per cent would be the pure sodium salt. Alkali cyanides are assayed by the method given for hydrocyanic acid (above) using 0·5 g, 1 ml 0·1N = 0·01302 g KCN.

The *A.O.A.C.*[4] gives the following procedure for the determination of alkali cyanides.

> Break the sample into small lumps in a mortar (do not grind). Weigh quickly about 5 g in a weighing bottle and wash into a 500-ml volumetric flask containing about 200 ml of water. Add a little lead carbonate to precipitate any sulphides that may be present, dilute to the mark with water, mix thoroughly and filter through a dry filter. Transfer a 50-ml aliquot to a 400-ml beaker, add 200 ml of water, 5 ml of 10 per cent sodium hydroxide solution and a few crystals of potassium iodide. Titrate to a faint opalescence with 0·1N silver nitrate. 1 ml 0·1N = 0·01302 g KCN.
>
> In a liquid containing both alkali cyanide and free hydrocyanic acid, titrate first without addition of alkali hydroxide (= alkali cyanide), then add alkali and continue the titration (= free acid).

1. Wellings, A. W., *Analyst*, 1933, **58,** 331.
2. Ryan J. A., and Culshaw, G. W., *Analyst*, 1944, **69,** 370.
3. Monier-Williams, G. W., Ministry of Health Report on Public Health and Medical Subjects, No. 60; *Analyst*, 1931, **56,** 46.
4. *A.O.A.C.*, 1960, p. 38.

HYDROGEN PEROXIDE

H_2O_2 Mol. Wt. 34·02

The determination of hydrogen peroxide in solution can be made either gasometrically or volumetrically, the latter depending on the oxidising power of the peroxide.

Gasometric determination is less accurate than volumetric estimation but the former does definitely measure the available oxygen, whereas the latter may include impurities which react with the reagents used. The method of the *B.P.* 1914 was to shake 2 ml of the solution in a brine-charged nitrometer with 4 ml of a solution of copper ammonium sulphate, and the oxygen liberated catalytically was measured at 15·5° and normal pressure. 1 ml oxygen = 0·00304 g H_2O_2.

An excess of acidified potassium permanganate solution may also be employed for the liberation of the oxygen, but in this case 1 ml oxygen = 0·00152 g H_2O_2 as half the oxygen comes from the permanganate.

Volumetric determination is employed in the *B.P.* assay of Solution of Hydrogen Peroxide:

> Dilute 10 ml with 200 ml of water, to 20 ml of the dilution add 5 ml of 50 per cent sulphuric acid and titrate with 0·1N potassium perman-

ganate. 1 ml 0·1N = 0·001701 g H_2O_2 = 0·0056 volumes of oxygen per ml. Strong acidification is necessary to complete the titration.

The result may be affected by certain preservatives.

Other useful volumetric methods are available which are not influenced by the presence of organic preservatives.

Kingzett's iodimetric method:[1]

Dissolve approximately 2 g of potassium iodide in 200 ml of 5 per cent sulphuric acid in a stoppered bottle. To this solution add gradually, with constant shaking, an amount of hydrogen peroxide equivalent to 0·06 g (2 ml of 3 per cent solution). Allow the mixture to stand fifteen minutes and titrate the liberated iodine with 0·1N sodium thiosulphate. 1 ml 0·1N = 0·001701 g H_2O_2.

Jamieson's arsenious acid method:[2]

To a mixture of 25 ml of 0·2N sodium arsenite and 10 ml of 10 per cent sodium hydroxide solution in a stoppered bottle add a measured volume of solution containing about 0·06 g of hydrogen peroxide. After two minutes' standing, add 40 ml of concentrated hydrochloric acid and titrate the unoxidised arsenite with 0·05M potassium iodate, using chloroform as indicator (see Halogen Acids). 1 ml 0·2N As_2O_3=0·0034 g H_2O_2.

Small amounts of hydrogen peroxide in aqueous solution may be determined colorimetrically by the method of Eisenberg.[3] The reagent should be prepared by the method described and reliance on a commercial reagent is inadvisable.

Titanium sulphate reagent: Digest 1 g of anhydrous titanium dioxide with 100 ml of concentrated sulphuric acid for fifteen to sixteen hours on a sand-bath at 150°. Cool, dilute with four parts by volume of water and centrifuge to obtain a clear solution.

Mix 50 ml of the solution and 10 ml of the reagent. Transfer a portion to a colorimeter cell and measure the extinction using a violet filter (430 mμ). Compare with a curve prepared by treating standard hydrogen peroxide solutions containing between 200 and 5 p.p.m. in a similar manner. The curve is linear between limits 0 and 100 p.p.m.

Visual comparison using Nessler cylinders is satisfactory. A distinct yellow colour is obtained at a concentration of 5 p.p.m.

METALLIC PEROXIDES

Metallic peroxides are of little importance in pharmaceutical practice other than as ingredients of dentifrices. Their peroxide content may be determined either by permanganate titration in acid solution or by the iodide method given above.

Calcium peroxide, CaO_2, Mol. Wt. 72·08, is assayed by titration of 0·2 g in dilute hydrochloric acid with 0·1N potassium permanganate, 1 ml 0·1N = 0·003604 g. **Magnesium peroxide,** MgO_2, Mol. Wt. 56·32, is determined by adding 10 ml of water and 2·5 g of potassium iodide to 0·5 g of the material, then acidifying with 10 ml of 25 per cent sulphuric acid, allowing to stand for ten minutes and titrating the liberated iodine with 0·1N thiosulphate, 1 ml 0·1N = 0·002816 g.

Zinc peroxide, consists of a mixture of zinc peroxide, zinc oxide and zinc hydroxide and is assayed by titration in acid solution with 0·1N permanganate as given above. 1 ml 0·1N = 0·004869 g ZnO_2.

1. Kingzett, C. T., *J. Chem. Soc.*, 1880, 792.
2. Jamieson, G. S., *Amer. J. Sci.*, 1917, **44**, 150.
3. Eisenberg, G. M., *Ind. Eng. Chem., Anal. Edn.*, 1943, **15**, 327.

HYOSCYAMUS

Hyoscyamus consists of the dried leaves, or leaves and flowering tops, of *Hyoscyamus niger*, L. and contains from 0·04 to 0·14 per cent of alkaloids.

The *B.P.* method for the estimation of alkaloids in belladonna (see p. 107) can be used for hyoscyamus, although it is somewhat lengthy.

Since the leaf contains such a small quantity of alkaloids, more must be taken for assay (40 g) than with belladonna and the amount of percolating solvent is correspondingly larger. For hyoscyamus, distilling off some of the percolating ether is certainly an advantage. Foreign *Solanaceæ*, such as *Hyoscyamus muticus*, L. (containing up to 1·0 per cent of hyoscyamine), particularly need long-period drying of the isolated alkaloids before titration. No further comment is needed on the method other than reference to the remarks given under Belladonna.

Dry Extract of Hyoscyamus, *B.P.* Contains 0·3 per cent of the alkaloids of hyoscyamus, calculated as hyoscyamine.

This is probably the most difficult of the preparations of hyoscyamus, belladonna or stramonium to assay: the *B.P.* method is as follows:

> Mix about 10 g with 50 ml of 70 per cent ethanol, warm on a water-bath, and allow to stand for half an hour, shaking frequently. Transfer to a percolator and percolate slowly with warm 70 per cent ethanol until the alkaloids are completely extracted. Reduce the volume of the percolate to about 15 ml by evaporation at as low a temperature as possible, transfer to a separator with 40 ml of chloroform and a mixture of 15 ml of water and 5 ml of dilute ammonia solution, shake well, allow the layers to separate and run the lower layer into a second separator. Continue the extraction with further quantities of chloroform until the alkaloids are completely extracted, combining the extracts in the second separator. Extract the contents of the second separator, first with 25 ml of 0·2N sulphuric acid and then with successive quantities of 0·1N sulphuric acid until the alkaloids are completely extracted. Mix the acid liquids and wash with 10 ml, 5 ml and 5 ml of chloroform, washing

each chloroform solution with the same 20 ml of 0·1N sulphuric acid and rejecting the chloroform. Filter both the acid liquids through a tightly-packed, cotton-wool plug, previously moistened with water and wash the separators and plug with a little 0·1N sulphuric acid. Add an excess of dilute ammonia solution to the combined filtrate and washings and extract with successive quantities of chloroform until the alkaloids are completely extracted, washing each extract with the same 10 ml of water. Evaporate the chloroform, add 3 ml of 95 per cent ethanol, evaporate to dryness and dry at 80°, weighing at intervals of one hour until two successive weighings do not differ by more than 1 mg. Dissolve the residue in 2 ml of chloroform, add 10 ml of 0·05N sulphuric acid, warm to remove the chloroform, cool and titrate the excess acid with 0·05N sodium hydroxide using methyl red as indicator. 1 ml 0·05N H_2SO_4 = 0·01447 g of alkaloids, calculated as hyoscyamine.

The above method is slow and liable to emulsions and a modification, due to Ragg,[1] is given below:

To about 10 g in a conical flask, add 10 g of kieselguhr and 50 ml of 70 per cent ethanol; warm for thirty minutes on a water-bath and then filter through a Büchner funnel to dryness. Transfer the precipitate to a piece of paper and triturate with a spatula until powdery. Transfer the dry powder back to the flask and repeat the extraction four times from the beginning. Evaporate the ethanol *in vacuo* to 25 ml and transfer to a separator without filtering, washing in the residue from the dish with 50 ml of chloroform and finally with a few drops of ammonia solution. Extract twice with chloroform and evaporate the combined extracts to low volume. Add a little ethanol to the aqueous layer and extract twice more with chloroform, adding these extracts to the previous chloroform layer. Evaporate the chloroform until the total volume of the extracts is about 30 ml, transfer to a separator and continue as usual by extraction with acid as for Belladonna.

Almost identical results, as compared with those of the *B.P.* method, were obtained by Markwell[2] using the following procedure, which is much more rapidly carried out:

Reduce the extract to a No. 60 powder and transfer 10 g, together with a little ignited sand, to a long, pear-shaped separator. The separator is provided with a short outlet tube (about 2 in. long) below the stopcock; plug this tube with cotton wool. Add 50 ml of a mixture of 4 volumes of anæsthetic ether and 1 volume of 95 per cent ethanol. Stopper the separator, and after shaking during ten minutes, add 2 ml of dilute ammonia solution and shake the mixture at intervals during one hour, then allow the liquid to flow into another separator. When it ceases to flow, pack the contents of the first separator by means of a button-ended glass rod and percolate with another 25 ml of the menstruum, and subsequently with ether until exhausted. Shake the ethereal solution first with 20 ml of 0·5N hydrochloric acid and then with successive 10-ml portions of a mixture of 3 volumes of 0·1N hydrochloric acid and 1 volume of 95 per cent ethanol until the alkaloids are completely extracted. Continue the assay according to the *B.P.* method (above), commencing with the words 'Mix the acid liquids and wash . . .'. All the separations are quick and clean.

Liquid Extract of Hyoscyamus, *B.P.* Contains 0·05 per cent of the alkaloids of hyoscyamus.

The method of the *B.P.* is as follows:

> Evaporate 50 ml at a low temperature to about 15 ml and complete as described under Dry Extract of Hyoscyamus, beginning with the words 'transfer to a separator with 40 ml of chloroform . . .'.

Alternatively:

> Transfer 25 ml to a separator without previous evaporation, add 25 ml of water and 40 ml of chloroform, make just alkaline with dilute ammonia solution and shake out the alkaloids as rapidly as possible, continuing as in the *B.P.* method.

Tincture of Hyoscyamus, *B.P.* Contains 0·005 per cent of the alkaloids of hyoscyamus.

> Evaporate 250 ml to about 10 ml at a low temperature and transfer, with 30 ml of chloroform, to a separator containing a mixture of 10 ml of water and 3 ml of dilute ammonia solution, shake well, allow the layers to separate and run the lower layer into a second separator. Continue as described for Dry Extract of Hyoscyamus, beginning with the words 'Continue the extraction with further quantities of chloroform . . .'.

1. Ragg, L. W., private communication.
2. Markwell, W. A. N., *C. & D.*, 1936, **124,** 74.

HYPOPHOSPHOROUS ACID

H_3PO_2 Mol. Wt. 66·00

The total acidity, which includes other oxyacids of phosphorus (unlikely to be present in quantity, otherwise the acid would not pass the *B.P.C.* tests) can be titrated direct with alkali to methyl orange or bromophenol blue. 1 ml 0·5N = 0·03300 g. Hypophosphorous acid, after neutralisation may be determined by the methods described below for hypophosphites.

HYPOPHOSPHITES

The determination of hypophosphites is the method of Boyer and Bauzil,[1] based upon the fact that in acid solution hypophosphorous acid is oxidised by iodine to phosphorous acid, the latter not being oxidised further in acid solution; but if an alkali (sodium bicarbonate) is added, oxidation continues to phosphoric acid.

> For hypophosphites: Take 10 ml of a solution containing 0·1 g (insoluble salts may be dissolved in dilute sulphuric acid) in a stoppered flask, add 10 ml of 25 per cent w/v sulphuric acid and 30 ml of 0·1N

iodine. Keep the mixture in the dark for ten hours and titrate the excess of iodine with 0·1N thiosulphate. 1 ml 0·1N = 0·003300 g H_3PO_2.

For phosphites: Treat 10 ml of a solution containing 0·1 g with 10 ml of 5 per cent sodium bicarbonate solution and 20 ml of 0·1N iodine for two hours. Add 10 ml of 10 per cent acetic acid and titrate the excess of iodine with 0·1N thiosulphate. 1 ml 0·1N = 0·004100 g H_3PO_3.

Raquet and Pinte[2] proposed a rapid modification of the iodometric method which, in confirmatory experiments, has given good results with solutions of pure hypophosphites; but it has been found that more borax solution is required than is recommended by the authors. The amended method is:

For phosphites: Add 10 ml of a 1 per cent solution to 10 ml of 0·1N iodine and 20 ml of a warm 10 per cent borax solution. After ten minutes acidify with 2 to 3 ml of glacial acetic acid and titrate with 0·1N sodium thiosulphate. 1 ml 0·1N = 0·004100 g H_3PO_3.

For hypophosphites: Place 5 ml of a 1 per cent solution in a flask with a ground-glass stopper, add 25 ml of 0·1N iodine and 5 ml of 1 in 10 hydrochloric acid. Warm to 70° to 80° for fifteen minutes, cool and shake to dissolve iodine vapour. Add 20 ml of warm 10 per cent borax solution (additional borax does not affect the results), stand for fifteen minutes, acidify with glacial acetic acid and titrate with 0·1N thiosulphate. 1 ml 0·1N = 0·00165 g H_3PO_2.

In this method the hypophosphite is oxidised successively to phosphite and phosphate. If the metallic ion reacts with iodine, the alkali salt is first formed.

The *B.P.C.* hypophosphites, except that of iron, can all be estimated by the method of Boyer and Bauzil (above), after dissolving about 1 g in 100 ml of water, and taking 10 ml of the dilution for assay. **Calcium hypophosphite,** $Ca(H_2PO_2)_2$, Mol. Wt. 170·1, 1 ml 0·1N = 0·004252 g; **manganese hypophosphite,** $Mn(H_2PO_2)_2,H_2O$, Mol. Wt. 202·9, 1 ml 0·1N = 0·005073 g; **potassium hypophosphite,** KH_2PO_2, Mol Wt. 104·1, 1 ml 0·1N = 0·005205 g; **sodium hypophosphite,** NaH_2PO_2, Mol Wt. 87·98, 1 ml 0·1N = 0·00440 g.

The official *B.P.C.* method is by bromination.

Take 10 ml of a solution containing 0·05 g in a stoppered flask and immediately add 50 ml of 0·1N bromine and 20 ml of dilute sulphuric acid. Shake repeatedly during fifteen minutes, allow to stand for two hours at 20° to 25°, cool in ice, add 30 ml of 10 per cent potassium iodide solution and titrate with 0·1N sodium thiosulphate. Do a blank determination. 1 ml 0·1N bromine = 0·002126 g $Ca(H_2PO_2)_2$; 0·002537 g $Mn(H_2PO_2)_2,H_2O$; 0·002602 g KH_2PO_2 and 0·002200 g NaH_2PO_2.

Sugar prevents rapid precipitation of phosphate and, for direct titration, addition of 20 ml of syrup before making alkaline with ammonia allows titration of calcium hypophosphite with EDTA to a satisfactory end-point.

Compound Syrup of Hypophosphites, *B.P.C.* A complex mixture of calcium, manganese, potassium and iron hypophosphites and free hypophosphorous acid together with quinine and strychnine in syrup.

To determine the alkaloids quinine and strychnine, proceed as for Easton's Syrup (Nux Vomica, p. 469).

The total hypophosphorous acid may be determined by the iodometric method.

To 10 ml of syrup in a separator add 1 to 2 g of citric acid dissolved in 20 ml of water, make alkaline and extract the alkaloids with repeated small quantities of chloroform. Wash the chloroform extracts with water. Transfer the aqueous solution and washings to a 100-ml graduated flask, acidify with sulphuric acid, volatilise the dissolved chloroform, cool and make up to 100 ml. Estimate the hypophosphite in 20 ml of this solution by the method of Boyer and Bauzil given above.

The determination can be carried out without removal of alkaloids but the end-point in the titration is not so sharp.

Ferrey[3] has applied his method for total phosphate in syrups (see Phosphoric Acid, p. 530) to Compound Syrup of Hypophosphites. The following modification is necessary to oxidise the hypophosphite to phosphate and to destroy the alkaloids.

To 1 to 1·5 g of syrup weighed into a Kjeldahl flask, add 5 ml of water and 5 ml of concentrated nitric acid. Carefully boil down until the volume is 3 or 4 ml, then add 5 ml of water and 0·5 g of potassium permanganate and evaporate to about 3 ml. Wash the contents of the flask into a beaker, destroy any excess of permanganate with oxalic acid and proceed in the usual way.

1. Boyer, L., and Bauzil, L., *J. Pharm. Chim.*, 1918, **18**, 321.
2. Raquet, D., and Pinte, P., *J. Pharm. Chim.*, 1933, **125**, 5.
3. Ferrey, G. J. W., *Quart. J. Pharm.*, 1934, **7**, 346.

INSULIN

The assays required to standardise insulin preparations are those used to determine the absolute potency of the preparations and, where necessary, to assess the degree of delayed or prolonged activity and the completeness of any involved precipitation.

Official methods for the assessment of absolute activity depend on the production of hypoglycæmia in intact animals evidenced either by the incidence of hypoglycæmic convulsions in mice (a suggested *B.P.* method) or the measured hypoglycæmia in rabbits (prescribed by the *U.S.P.*) a comparison being made against a standard preparation for which purpose the International Standard for Insulin containing 24 units in each mg has been established.

INSULIN

Assay of insulin using mice

This method depends on equating the doses of standard and unknown which will cause 50 per cent of the mice to convulse (CD50). These doses are determined simultaneously in tests in which the standard and unknown are each injected at not less than two dose levels.

> Take at least 96 mice with weights not differing by more than 5 g which have been fed on an adequate diet and which have been deprived of food for not less than two hours nor for more than twenty hours preceding the test. Distribute into four groups and make subcutaneous injections respectively with two doses of standard and two of the unknown. Choose doses of standard which will be expected to cause convulsions on either side of 50 per cent and administer them in equal volumes using saline acidified to pH 2·5 with hydrochloric acid to make the solutions.
>
> Make dilutions of the unknown so that if the assumption of potency is correct concentrations of insulin equal to those of the standard will result. After injection keep the mice at a uniform temperature between 29° and 35° for one and a half hours and record the number that convulse or display symptoms of hypoglycæmic collapse. Calculate the results by standard statistical methods.

As a commercial practice it has been found convenient to arrange for the mouse colony to be fed at noon with a crumbled diet prepared from diet 41 bread soaked in water and oats and to consider the whole colony uniformly fasted on the next morning when those animals required for test are transferred to clean boxes. During the assay mice which convulse are injected with glucose and all surviving participants in the test used again after an interval of two days. Those comprising any one test are taken from mice of similar usage and in weight ranges of 17 to 20 g; 20 to 25 g; and 25 to 30 g.

Some adjustment in dosage may be required for the mice used on a further occasion, and for those used later in the day, but mice of either sex have been found to be equally sensitive. It has been found convenient to house the mice in battery jars (2 mice per jar) for the duration of the test during which time they have been kept in a glass fronted air incubator at 32°.

The use of angled wire screens fixed[1] or revolving[2] have also been described for this purpose. The mice fall from these screens when they exhibit a condition of hypoglycæmia prior to convulsion or hypoglycæmic collapse. In this condition it is claimed that they can partake of food presented to them and thus avoid the need for a therapeutic injection of glucose.

Test for prolongation of insulin effect

The *B.P.* prescribes a test for the prolongation of hypoglycæmic effect produced by modified insulin preparations compared with that produced by the Standard Preparation of Insulin in guinea pigs or rabbits.

> Distribute not fewer than 10 animals from a healthy colony at random into two equal groups. House the animals singly and deprive them of food from eighteen hours before to the completion of the test. At the beginning of the test determine the mean blood sugar level of each group and inject the animals in one group subcutaneously with the undiluted unknown preparation and those in the other group with a solution of the standard preparation in saline solution acidified with hydrochloric acid to pH 2·5 and prepared to have the nominal potency of the unknown. Use subconvulsive doses for the injections into each group and equivalent amounts corresponding to the body weights of the animals. At one, two, four and six hours determine the mean blood sugar of each group and express it as a percentage of the mean initial level for the group.

In practice it has been found convenient to examine more than one sample at a time and to use not less than 6 animals per group, permitting up to two convulsions in any group. Since convulsions remove the animals from the test some objection can be raised against the determination of the mean blood sugar level from a pooled blood sample. There can be little objection to this if the blood samples in any group are treated separately for the determination of the initial level but pooled for the subsequent readings.

Test for activity of the supernatant fluid from suspensions

It is required that the completeness of precipitation in the insulin zinc suspensions and in the suspensions with protamine be determined by showing that not more than 4 per cent of the total insulin activity is present in the supernatant fluid obtained by centrifuging. To establish this it is customary to carry out a biological assay on mice using at least 16 mice on each of one dose level of the standard preparations and on one of the supernatant fluid. The standard dose level is chosen to show a marked effect (to cause convulsions of the order 50 per cent, or more) and an equivalent amount of the supernatant fluid, assuming that the limiting potency is present, is used. The mice are observed for ninety minutes, and the incidence of hypoglycæmic reactions noted. It is unusual for these to occur with the test injection. On occasions, the conditions are such that an opalescent solution results even after prolonged centrifuging. It is pointless to continue with the test in these circumstances and a new sample in clean glassware should be obtained.

If the pH of the Insulin Zinc Suspension be correct then the insulin must be wholly precipitated and this is also true of the preparations with protamine providing the protamine level is as stated. It would seem therefore that assays of insulin content applied to the supernatant fluids are simply elaborate ways of checking pH.

If tests to limit the insulin activity are considered necessary biological assays could in any case be replaced by the simple process of applying spots of the solution to filter paper together with similar spots of suitable concentrations of insulin, allowing to dry, staining with bromocresol green and washing away excess stain with 1 per cent acetic acid. Such a process is quite capable of detecting the limiting concentrations of insulin which are specified (see below).

Assay of insulin using rabbits

This method depends on equating the doses of standard and unknown which will cause an equal fall in the measured blood sugar of rabbits.

A colony of rabbits is prepared for the assay by determining for each rabbit that volume of insulin solution containing 2 units/ml, which when injected subcutaneously under the test conditions will cause a marked but non-convulsive fall in blood sugar level. This volume, which may be expressed in terms of body weight of the animal or as a fixed dose per animal, is referred to as the 'standard volume'. As an alternative the same 'standard volume', suitably 0·3 to 0·5 ml, may be adopted for all rabbits, any abnormally sensitive or insensitive animals being discarded.

Deprive rabbits weighing between 1,800 and 3,000 g of food for the eighteen hours preceding their use and until the final blood sample is taken. Distribute them at random to four groups and inject on two occasions with their 'standard volumes' of the standard preparation at 2 units/ml (Standard High) or 1 unit/ml (Standard Low), or of equivalent concentrations of the test preparation, according to the following plan.

Group	*1st Day*	*2nd Day*
1	Standard (High)	Test (Low)
2	Standard (Low)	Test (High)
3	Test (High)	Standard (Low)
4	Test (Low)	Standard (High)

Response measurement: The earliest conception of the most informative measure of response called for a blood sugar determination to be made before injection and at hourly intervals after the injection for a period of five hours. The mean fall in blood sugar level was then expressed as a percentage of the initial level. Such a response is still retained in the method described in the *B.P.* but the *U.S.P.* method relies on the mean blood sugar level at one and two hours after injection without reference to the initial level. It is considered that a determination made ninety minutes after injection without reference to the initial level is an adequate measure of insulin effect.

Time interval between the halves of the test: The interval between the two parts of the test can be varied, but should not exceed seven days. If bleedings over five hours are avoided the feeding schedule can be arranged so that the test can be completed on the following day.

Chemical methods for the determination of insulin have been under investigation for several years. For simple solutions of crystalline insulin a gravimetric method, based upon precipitation by adjustment to pH 5·0, is possible, but this is obviously inapplicable when other protein material is present. Paper chromatographic methods of assay offer the greatest promise and a number of methods have been suggested. The first was that of Robinson and Fehr,[3] who determined insulin in protamine zinc insulin by streaking the solution across a paper and developing a chromatogram with the upper phase of *n*-butanol, glacial acetic acid and water (3 : 1 : 4). After the spots had been stained with bromocresol green the colour was intensified with ammonia vapour and then eluted with borate buffer; the solution so obtained was compared with a similarly treated insulin standard. Various developments of this type of method have been suggested, but in our opinion, the most satisfactory to date is that suggested by Fenton.[4] By this procedure high potency crystalline insulin may be assayed to give results which agree with those obtained biologically, but for crude or low potency insulin the method is inapplicable since the impurities tend to interfere and erroneously high results are obtained. Fenton later[5] described a method applicable to the various pharmacopœial insulin solutions; in this procedure Insulin Injection, *B.P.* and Insulin Zinc Suspension, *B.P.* give one compact spot on developing and staining; Protamine Zinc Insulin and Isophane Insulin give two spots—one of these being at the point of application, due to protamine. Globin Insulin cannot be assayed by Fenton's method owing to interference; results are high compared with those obtained biologically. Limited experience with gelled samples of Injection of Insulin has shown that the chromatograms from such samples exhibit an additional spot at the point of application, probably corresponding to the inactive fibril insulin present. This spot is appreciably smaller than those obtained in chromatograms of Protamine Zinc or Isophane Insulin. Bacteriostats such as phenol, cresol and the hydroxybenzoate esters do not interfere as they are removed at the picric acid precipitation stage before chromatography. It is unlikely that chromatographic methods will ever supersede biological assays of insulin, but they are of considerable value for production control and confirmatory purposes where the sample being examined is of known history. Fenton's procedures are as follows:

Apparatus:

Chromatography tanks. These are rectangular glass tanks of height 42 cm and base 27 cm × 9 cm, with ground tops and ⅛ in. plain glass lids. Each lid is drilled centrally to accommodate a rubber stopper through which passes a short length of glass tube, 7 mm in diameter. The tube is attached to the vertical member of an inverted T-piece of glass rod inside the tank, which forms a support rail from which the chromatograms may be suspended. Thus the position of the chromatograms within the sealed tank may be adjusted by external manipulation of the protruding vertical rod. A small circle of stiff sheet rubber with a central hole is pushed down over the protruding end of the vertical rod to retain the rod in the desired position.

Volumetric vessels. Since the method requires volumetric vessels of approximately 1 ml capacity that are not available commercially these must be made and calibrated as follows. Seal one end of a piece of glass tube 8 mm in diameter, form a constricted neck about 2 mm in diameter 5 cm from the sealed end and, with a diamond pencil, make a graduation mark in the centre of the neck. Calibrate the vessels by filling to the mark with water from a capillary pipette and weighing.

Reagents:

Developing solvent. Mix equal volumes of analytical-reagent grade butan-2-ol and 1 per cent acetic acid (prepared from analytical-reagent grade acid) in a large separator, shake vigorously for several minutes and allow to stand, at the temperature at which the assay is to be carried out, for twenty-four hours. Then discard the lower layer and transfer the upper, butanol layer to the chromatography tanks to give a layer 1·0 to 1·5 cm in depth.

Protein stain. Dissolve 0·425 g of bromocresol green in 125 ml of 0·1N sodium hydroxide by sprinkling the dye on the surface of the alkali and stirring. Add the solution to 2 litres of 0·1N acetic acid and filter; the pH of the mixture should be 3·6. The reagent is stable for some time but should be filtered at intervals.

Determination:

Weigh about 10 mg of the sample and of standard crystalline insulin into calibrated 1-ml vessels, using a semi-micro dispenser as described by Stock and Fill[6] and dry to constant weight (twenty-four to forty-eight hours) over phosphorus pentoxide *in vacuo*. Record the moisture content.

To each vessel add 0·05N hydrochloric acid from a capillary pipette and twirl between the palms of the hands for one minute to dissolve. Dilute to the mark with 0·05N hydrochloric acid and mix thoroughly by repeatedly drawing into and expelling from dry capillary pipettes fitted with rubber teats.

Apply 2 spots of the test solution and 2 spots of the standard solution to each of twelve sheets of Whatman No. 1 chromatography paper (28·5 cm long × 13 cm wide) at intervals of 2·5 cm on a line drawn 4 cm from the bottom of the paper; the volume of solution for each spot should be such that 40 to 60 μg of insulin is deposited per spot and the diameter of each spot should not exceed 1 cm. (Make the application with an Agla micrometer syringe and No. 20 Hypodermic needle, mounted vertically so that the needle point is in light contact with the surface of the paper; a thin film of petroleum jelly applied to the needle near the point prevents the solution from wetting the outside of the needle.) Dry the papers at room temperature for two to twenty-four hours, then make a fold 2·5 cm from the top edge of each paper, punch a hole centrally through the flap and paper with a paper punch and assemble the papers in the tanks, four or five papers per tank, with the rods retracted so that the papers are out of contact with the solvent; the folded tops of the papers form a series of corrugations serving to separate the papers from each other. Allow to equilibrate for four to sixteen hours in this position, then push the rods downwards until 2 to 4 mm of the bottom edge of each paper is immersed in the solvent and allow development to proceed until the solvent front has travelled at least 20 cm up the paper. (It has been found convenient to equilibrate overnight and then to allow development to proceed throughout the whole of the next day.) Carry out the chromatography at room temperature in a room reasonably free from draughts.

Remove the papers from the tanks, press between sheets of clean blotting paper to remove excess solvent and dry at 80° for ten minutes. Immerse in the protein stain for fifteen hours (overnight), wash four times, for three minutes each, in 1 per cent v/v acetic acid, with occasional agitation, and again press between sheets of clean blotting paper and dry at 80° for ten minutes. Then hold the papers over a beaker containing 5N ammonia, to intensify the dye colour, and mark the specific insulin spots (those with the highest R_F) by ringing with a hard pencil. Cut out the marked spots with sharp scissors and drop each one separately into a numbered test-tube (measuring about 12 cm × 1·5 cm). Cut out a blank, of size similar to the spots, from a point remote from the spots but within the solvent area and place in a separate tube. To each tube add 5 ml of eluent (a mixture of equal volumes of 0·1N sodium hydroxide and 95 per cent ethanol) and leave for thirty minutes, shaking at intervals.

Measure the extinction of each solution at 625 mμ, using 1-cm cells with the blank eluate in the comparison cell in each case.

$$\text{activity of test sample (units per mg)} = \frac{W_s \times V_s \times C_t \times \bar{M} \times U}{W_t \times V_t \times C_s}$$

W_s = weight of standard (mg) before drying.
V_s = volume of standard (ml) applied per spot.
C_t = capacity (ml) of volumetric vessel containing test sample.
U = units per mg of standard (not corrected for moisture content).
W_t = weight of test sample (mg) before drying.
V_t = volume of test solution (ml) applied per spot.
C_s = capacity (ml) of volumetric vessel containing standard.
$\bar{M}$ = geometric mean of the ratio of extinctions of test samples/extinctions of standards.

$\bar{M}$ is substituted into the above expression after its value has been calculated from the following equation:

$$\bar{M} = \sqrt[N]{\left[\left(\frac{X_t}{X_s}\right)_1 \cdot \left(\frac{X_t}{X_s}\right)_2 \cdots \left(\frac{X_t}{X_s}\right)_N\right]}$$

in which X_t is the extinction of the eluate from an inner or outer spot of test sample, X_s is the extinction of the eluate from the corresponding inner or outer spot of standard from the same paper and N is the number of observations.

For convenience of working the expression may be converted into logarithms to base 10, when

$$\bar{M} = \text{antilog}\left[\log\left(\frac{X_t}{X_s}\right)_1 + \log\left(\frac{X_t}{X_s}\right)_2 + \ldots \log\left(\frac{X_t}{X_s}\right)_N\right]\frac{1}{N}$$

If for any reason (breakages, etc.) a test observation is lost, the corresponding standard observation from the same paper should be omitted.

The values W_s and W_t are given in terms of insulin samples 'uncorrected for moisture content', since it is customary to express insulin potencies on this basis and to state the moisture contents with the assay results.

For application to injection solutions:[5]

Developing solvent, eluent, volumetric vessels and protein stain. These are as described in the above method.

Standards:

Distribute a stock of four-times recrystallised zinc insulin in approximately 20-mg amounts in hard glass tubes, dry *in vacuo* over phosphorus pentoxide to a moisture content of about 1·6 per cent, flame-seal the tubes and store at 2°. Determine the potency of the standard chromatographically, as described above, in terms of the Fourth International Standard for insulin.

Prepare, in duplicate, solutions of working standard of potency approximately 40 i.u. per ml, in sufficient quantity to last for one week's assays, by dissolving accurately weighed amounts of the crystalline insulin in 0·5N hydrochloric acid containing 0·3 per cent of *o*-cresol and 0·9 per cent of sodium chloride and store the solutions at 2°.

Determination:

Pipette two 5-ml quantities of standard solution (40 i.u. per ml) and two known volumes of sample into respective 100-ml centrifuge tubes; the volumes of sample should contain approximately 150 to 250 units. (For Insulin Zinc Suspensions and Protamine Zinc Insulins, dissolve by stirring rapidly with a glass rod wetted with a trace of 5N hydrochloric acid, and allow to stand for thirty minutes before sampling.) To each centrifuge tube add 2 volumes of a saturated aqueous solution of picric acid, mixing during the addition, and allow to stand for thirty minutes. Centrifuge for ten to fifteen minutes at 2,000 r.p.m. and discard the clear supernatant liquor. Dissolve the protein picrate precipitate in 1 to 1·5 ml of acidified acetone reagent (prepared by diluting 2 ml of concentrated hydrochloric acid to 1 litre with acetone) and reprecipitate the protein hydrochloride from the solution by the rapid addition of an excess (60 to 70 ml) of the acidified acetone reagent. Stir the suspensions thoroughly with glass rods to ensure complete flocculation; cover with cellophane caps and allow to stand for thirty minutes. Centrifuge for ten to fifteen minutes at 2,000 r.p.m., reject the supernatant liquid and evaporate the excess of acetone from the precipitates by directing a gentle stream of air from a glass jet into the centrifuge tubes. Dissolve the moist precipitates in about 0·3 ml of 0·05N hydrochloric acid and transfer each solution to a 1-ml volumetric vessel by means of a capillary transfer pipette. Wash the centrifuge tubes repeatedly with 0·15-ml quantities of 0·05N hydrochloric acid, transferring each washing to the corresponding volumetric vessel and allowing three to five minutes for the walls of the tubes to drain between transfers. Adjust the contents of each volumetric vessel to the calibration mark with 0·05N hydrochloric acid and mix thoroughly.

Cut, fold and mark out four sheets of Whatman No. 1 chromatographic paper, as described in the above method. Distribute 16 spots (applied with a micrometer syringe) between the four papers in the following Latin-square order:

Paper 1	S_1	T_1	S_2	T_2
Paper 2	T_1	S_2	T_2	S_1
Paper 3	S_2	T_2	S_1	T_1
Paper 4	T_2	S_1	T_1	S_2

where S_1 is the standard at low concentration level, S_2 is the standard at high concentration level, T_1 is the test at low concentration level and T_2 is the test at high concentration level. Calculate the exact volume to be expelled from the micrometer syringe so that about 1 unit of insulin per spot is delivered at each low level of test and standard and about twice this amount at each high level. Since the diameter of each spot should not exceed 1 cm (equivalent to about 10 μl) apply volumes in excess of this amount in portion and allow each portion to dry at room temperature between applications.

Place the four papers in one chromatography tank (of height 15 in. and base 11 in. × 8 in.) fitted with a retractable-rod assembly as described in the above method and containing a layer of eluent 1·0 to 1·5 cm deep. Allow to equilibrate for not less than sixteen hours (overnight) with the rods retracted and then continue as described in the above method from 'push the rods downwards until 2 to 4 mm . . .' down to the calculation of results, developing for seven and a half to eight hours.

Calculate the means of the extinctions of the two standard and two test series of spots and prepare a graph plotting the extinctions (E) as the ordinate and the microlitres of original solution applied to the paper (Z) as the abscissa.

$$Z = \text{microlitres of soln. applied to the paper} \times \frac{\text{volume of sample or standard taken}}{\text{volume of calibrated vessel}}$$

From the value of the potency of the standard solution and the values of Z given by a suitably selected value of E, the potency of the test solution may be calculated. Calculate the potency for 4 values of E (lying in the range of observations); the potency of the sample is the geometric mean of these values.

1. THOMPSON, R. E., *Endocrinology*, 1946, **39,** 62.
2. YOUNG, D. M., and LEWIS, A. H., *Science*, 1947, **105,** 368.
3. ROBINSON, F. A., and FEHR, K. L. A., *Biochem. J.*, 1952, **51,** 298.
4. FENTON, E. L., *Biochem. J.*, 1959, **71,** 507.
5. FENTON, E. L., *Biochem. J.*, 1961, **81,** 570.
6. STOCK, J. T., and FILL, M. A., *J. Chem. Educn.*, 1956, **33,** 345.

IODINE

I At. Wt. 126·90

Free iodine in solution may be determined by the usual volumetric methods of titration with sodium thiosulphate or sodium arsenite solution. The *B.P.* employs the former, after dissolving about 0·5 g of the solid in a concentrated solution of potassium iodide, in which it is freely soluble, then diluting and adding 1 ml of dilute acetic acid before titration. 1 ml 0·1N = 0·01269 g.

Titration of iodine with 0·1N sodium arsenite must be conducted in the presence of an excess of sodium bicarbonate to prevent reversal of the reaction.

In the titration of iodides with iodate by the method of Andrews (Halogen Acids, p. 292) quantitative oxidation of the iodide to iodine takes place first, with subsequent formation of iodine monochloride by further addition of iodate in the presence of hydrochloric acid. Consequently free iodine may be titrated by iodate in the presence of hydrochloric acid, only the second part of the reaction being involved. Hence with a mixture of free iodine and potassium iodide in solution, if the free iodine can be estimated by another method such as thiosulphate titration, the two components can be determined, the iodate required for the free iodine being half of that of the thiosulphate required. 1 ml 0·1N thiosulphate = 0·01269 g I, 1 ml 0·05M iodate = 0·0166 g KI. This method is adopted by the *B.P.* for solutions of iodine. With **Weak Solution of Iodine,** *B.P.* (Tincture of Iodine, containing 2·5 per cent w/v each of iodine and potassium iodide), and **Aqueous Solution of Iodine,** *B.P.* (Lugol's Solution, containing 5 per cent w/v of iodine and 10 per cent w/v of potassium iodide), 10 ml is used for titration. With **Strong Solution of Iodine,** *B.P.* (containing 10 per cent w/v of iodine and 6 per cent w/v of potassium iodide), the sample is diluted four times before proceeding as for the weak solution; ethanol should be used for dilution.

The proportion of iodine in **Simple Solution of Iodine**, *B.P.C.* (containing 9 per cent w/v of iodine), decreases rapidly on standing, owing to interaction of the iodine with the alcohol, and free hydriodic acid is formed. Equilibrium is reached in up to eight months and the mixture then contains about 80 per cent of the original iodine in the uncombined state (Page[1]). Even alcoholic solutions of iodine containing potassium iodide, if old or deficient in potassium iodide, develop hydriodic acid, and the apparent amount of potassium iodide as estimated by the official method is increased. All samples therefore, should be examined for the presence of hydriodic acid and the iodate titration corrected before the proportion of potassium iodide is calculated.

To correct for hydriodic acid one of the three following methods may be employed:

(*a*) Titrate 10 ml of the solution with 0·1N sodium thiosulphate, add methyl red and titrate with 0·1N sodium hydroxide. Percentage hydriodic acid = 10 × ml 0·1N alkali × 0·01279; ml 0·1N alkali × 10 × 0·0166 = percentage of potassium iodide to be subtracted from that found in the official process.

(*b*) Evaporate 10 ml of solution to dryness, treat it with water and re-evaporate. After drying, ignite the residue at a low temperature for a short time. Estimate the residue of potassium iodide by iodate as usual.

(*c*) Estimate free iodine (*A*) and potassium iodide (*B*) by the *B.P.* process. For hydriodic acid, after titration of free iodine, add neutral potassium iodide-iodate mixture and titrate the liberated iodine with

0·1N sodium thiosulphate (*C*). The percentages are obtained from the following equations: free iodine $= A \times 0{\cdot}1269$; hydriodic acid $= C \times 0{\cdot}1279$; potassium iodide $= (B - A/2 - C) \times 0{\cdot}166$; iodine originally used $= (A + C) \times 0{\cdot}1269$.

Another method for titration of iodine when iodide or other halogen salt is absent (as in Simple Solution of Iodine) is by keeping the solution in contact with zinc dust for a few minutes; interaction occurs and soluble zinc iodide is formed. After filtration from the excess of zinc the iodide may be titrated with 0·05M potassium iodate or 0·1N silver nitrate.

Compound Paint of Iodine, *B.P.C.* (Mandl's Paint). A mixture of iodine in strong potassium iodide solution diluted with glycerin; it also contains alcohol and peppermint oil. It contains 1·25 per cent w/v iodine and 2·50 per cent w/v potassium iodide.

Determination of iodine and potassium iodide follows the method for Solutions of Iodine. Weighed portions of the well-mixed sample are used (the oil separates). The probable formation of hydriodic acid should be noted and allowed for in the calculation (see above).

Experiments have proved that the peppermint oil absorbs practically none of the free iodine.

1. PAGE, G. R., *Quart. J. Pharm.*, 1935, **8,** 81.

IPECACUANHA

Ipecacuanha root of the *B.P.* consists of the dried root or the rhizome and root of either *Cephaëlis ipecacuanha* (Rio root) or *Cephaëlis acuminata* (Cartagena, Nicaragua, or Panama root). Good samples of the former variety contain between 2 and 2·5 per cent of total alkaloids, of which 60 to 70 per cent is non-phenolic (calculated as emetine) and about 25 per cent cephaëline with small quantities of other alkaloids such as psychotrine. *C. acuminata* may yield more total alkaloids and some samples have been examined which contain well over 3 per cent. The proportion of non-phenolic alkaloids is lower in this variety, however, being of the order of 20 to 40 per cent. At one time *C. ipecacuanha* was the only official variety of ipecacuanha and a requirement was, therefore, included for non-phenolic alkaloids. This standard no longer applies although the amount of non-phenolic alkaloids present in a sample is still required for some commercial transactions.

The *B.P.* method of assay is probably the most accurate available and presents few difficulties as little other extractive matter is obtained from the root.

Reduce a sufficient quantity to a No. 85 powder, weigh about 10 g of the powder into a flask and add 100 ml of a mixture of 3 volumes of ether and 1 volume of chloroform. Shake well and frequently during fifteen minutes and then allow to stand for ten minutes. Add 7·5 ml of dilute ammonia solution and shake continuously for two hours. Transfer the mixture to a small percolator plugged with cotton wool and, when the liquid ceases to flow, pack firmly and continue the percolation with more of the ether/chloroform mixture until the alkaloids are completely extracted. Heat the percolate on a water-bath until the volume is reduced to about 20 ml and then transfer to a separator with a little chloroform. Extract, first with 20 ml of N sulphuric acid, and then with successive quantities of a mixture of 3 volumes of 0·1N sulphuric acid and 1 volume of 95 per cent ethanol until the alkaloids are completely extracted. Combine the acid solutions and wash with 10 ml, 5 ml and 5 ml of chloroform, extracting each chloroform washing with the same 20 ml of 0·1N sulphuric acid; reject the chloroform. Combine the acid solutions, make distinctly alkaline with dilute ammonia solution and extract with successive quantities of chloroform until the alkaloids are completely extracted, washing each chloroform extract with the same 10 ml of water. Remove the chloroform, add to the residue 2 ml of 95 per cent ethanol, evaporate, and dry for about five minutes at 80° in a current of air. Dissolve the residue in 15 ml of 0·1N sulphuric acid and back-titrate with 0·1N sodium hydroxide using methyl red as indicator. 1 ml 0·1N H_2SO_4 = 0·02403 g of total alkaloids, calculated as emetine.

A few points on the method may be useful to note:

(*a*) The root must be ground to at least No. 60 powder to obtain efficient extraction, but it must be ground without drying as the alkaloids are susceptible to heat, especially in their natural state.

(*b*) To avoid agglomeration, careful attention must be given to the quantity of solution of ammonia added.

(*c*) It is not advisable to pack firmly in the separator, for it may slow down percolation too drastically.

(*d*) The isolated alkaloids, particularly the phenolic ones, are sensitive to heat; they should be only amber in colour and should not be dried above 80°. To redissolve the alkaloids for titration, either a little ethanol, say 0·5 ml, may be added to soften the residue before adding a slight excess of 0·1N acid, or it can be dissolved in a little ether, excess of 0·1N acid added and the ether evaporated off before titrating back to methyl red.

If it is required to determine the non-phenolic alkaloid content of the total alkaloids a suitable method is as follows:

Transfer the titrated liquid obtained in the assay of total alkaloids to a separator. Add 5 ml of 5N sodium hydroxide and 50 ml of ether, shake well and allow the layers to separate. Separate the ether layer and shake it with two successive quantities, of 10 ml and 5 ml respectively, of N sodium hydroxide. Combine the alkaline liquids and shake them with two successive quantities, each of 15 ml, of ether. Combine the ether layers and wash with successive quantities, each of about 5 ml, of water until free from alkali, shaking each washing with the same 10 ml of ether in a second separator.

Combine all the ether layers in a flask, evaporate the ether and dissolve the residue in 10 ml of 0·1N sulphuric acid. Titrate the excess acid with 0·1N sodium hydroxide using methyl red as indicator. 1 ml 0·1N H_2SO_4 = 0·02403 g of non-phenolic alkaloids, calculated as emetine.

Prepared Ipecacuanha, *B.P.* This is ipecacuanha reduced to a fine powder and adjusted, if necessary, by the admixture in suitable proportion of powdered exhausted ipecacuanha, or of powdered lactose, to contain 2·0 per cent of the total alkaloids, calculated as emetine. If lactose is used the residue of alkaloids is generally more discoloured.

The *B.P.* method is the following:

Weigh 10 g into a flask, add 100 ml of a mixture of 3 volumes of ether and 1 volume of chloroform and shake well and frequently during fifteen minutes. Allow to stand for ten minutes, add 2·5 ml of strong ammonia solution and 5 ml of 95 per cent ethanol and complete as for Ipecacuanha, above, beginning with the words 'shake continuously for two hours . . .'.

From the residual solutions in the assay for non-phenolic alkaloids the cephaëline and psychotrine may be separated.

Psychotrine is not soluble in ether, hence, after extraction of the emetine in sodium hydroxide solution, which retains phenolic bodies, acidify the aqueous residues with hydrochloric acid and then make alkaline with ammonia. Extract the cephaëline completely with ether and titrate as with emetine. 1 ml 0·1N = 0·0233 g. Finally, extract the ammoniacal residues with chloroform for psychotrine. 1 ml 0·02N = 0·00464 g.

Liquid Extract of Ipecacuanha, *B.P.* Contains 2·0 per cent of total alkaloids.

Transfer 5 ml to a separator, add 20 ml of water, 5 ml of dilute sulphuric acid and 10 ml of chloroform, shake thoroughly and allow the layers to separate. Run the chloroform layer into a second separator containing a mixture of 4 ml of 95 per cent ethanol and 20 ml of 0·1N sulphuric acid, shake, allow the layers to separate and reject the chloroform. Extract the contents of the first separator with two further 10-ml quantities of chloroform, running each chloroform extract into the second separator and washing, as before. Combine the acid solutions, make distinctly alkaline with dilute ammonia solution and extract with successive quantities of chloroform until the alkaloids are completely extracted, washing each extract with the same 10 ml of water. Combine the extracts, remove the chloroform, add to the residue 2 ml of 95 per cent ethanol, evaporate to dryness and dry for about five minutes at 80° in a current of air. Dissolve the residue in 10 ml of 0·1N hydrochloric acid and back titrate with 0·1N sodium hydroxide using methyl red as indicator. 1 ml 0·1N HCl = 0·02403 g of total alkaloids, calculated as emetine.

The extractions should be shaken vigorously. To prevent emulsions the acid washings are preferably kept separate from the main bulk of liquid, and, after making alkaline, the main bulk is then extracted with chloroform, each chloroform extraction being shaken successively with these alkaline washings and then with water.

Tincture of Ipecacuanha, *B.P.* Contains 0·2 per cent of total alkaloids. The *B.P.* assay follows that for the liquid extract, from which it is prepared. The method is quite satisfactory but as with the liquid extract, the acid washings are preferably extracted separately.

Transfer 50 ml to a separator, add 5 ml of dilute sulphuric acid and 10 ml of chloroform, shake thoroughly and allow the layers to separate. Complete as for Liquid Extract of Ipeçacuanha, beginning with the words 'Run the chloroform layer into a second separator . . .'.

Powder of Ipecacuanha and Opium, *B.P.*—see Opium (p. 488).
Tablets of Ipecacuanha and Opium, *B.P.*—see Opium (p. 489).

EMETINE HYDROCHLORIDE, $C_{29}H_{40}O_4N_2,2HCl,7H_2O$. Mol. Wt. 679·7

Evers and Smith[1] proposed the following method of assay:

For emetine. Dissolve 0·5 g in 50 ml of water, add 10 ml of 20 per cent sodium hydroxide solution and shake with separate quantities of chloroform until all the alkaloid is removed. Wash each chloroform extract in succession with the same two quantities of 10 ml of water, evaporate the solvent in a tared flask, add 2 ml of ethanol, evaporate, dry at 100° and weigh.

For cephaëline. Acidify the aqueous liquids from the assay for emetine with dilute hydrochloric acid, make just alkaline with ammonia, extract with chloroform and proceed as in the assay for emetine. Weigh the residue as cephaëline.

Emetine is sensitive to heat and is possibly decomposed during distillation of solvents, particularly chloroform, with loss of basicity.

Ashworth and Foster[2] found that when emetine hydrochloride is examined for cephaëline by extracting with chloroform, little if any cephaëline is found but its presence is nearly always indicated when ether is used. The *B.P.* uses the latter solvent in this test:

Dissolve 0·2 g in 20 ml of water and add 10 ml of 20 per cent sodium hydroxide solution. Extract the alkaloids completely by shaking with successive quantities, each of 50 ml, of ether. Combine the ether extracts and wash with successive quantities, each of 10 ml, of water until the washings, after extraction with a further 50 ml of ether, are neutral to litmus. Combine the ether solutions, add 20 ml of water and 10 ml of 0·1N hydrochloric acid, shake, allow to separate and collect the aqueous layer. Shake the ether layer with two further quantities, each of 20 ml, of water, mix the aqueous solutions and titrate the excess acid with 0·1N sodium hydroxide using methyl red as indicator. 1 ml 0·1N HCl = 0·02768 g of $C_{29}H_{40}O_4N_2,2HCl$.

Injection of Emetine, *B.P.* This is a sterile solution of emetine hydrochloride in water for injection and usually contains 60 mg in each ml. It is assayed as emetine hydrochloride using a measured volume equivalent to about 0·2 g of emetine hydrochloride diluted to 20 ml with water. 1 ml 0·1N HCl = 0·03398 g of $C_{29}H_{40}O_4N_2,2HCl,7H_2O$.

Emetine and bismuth iodide. The *B.P.* standardises this complex iodide on its emetine and bismuth contents.

For emetine: Transfer 0·5 g to a separator with the aid of a little 90 per cent ethanol, add 20 ml of water, 10 ml of 20 per cent sodium hydroxide solution and 75 ml of ether and shake at intervals during half an hour until no trace of red colour remains. Complete as under Emetine Hydrochloride, above, beginning with 'Extract the alkaloids completely . . .' 1 ml 0·1N HCl = 0·02403 g of $C_{29}H_{40}O_4N_2$.

For bismuth: To 0·5 g add 5 ml of concentrated nitric acid and boil vigorously until iodine vapour is no longer expelled. Cool, add a solution of 5 g of citric acid in 55 ml of water, then add strong ammonia solution until a slight permanent precipitate is obtained. Clear with 1 ml of concentrated nitric acid, heat to boiling-point and, while stirring vigorously, add slowly from a burette 30 ml of 10 per cent ammonium phosphate solution. Dilute to 400 ml with boiling water and allow to stand for at least one hour on a water-bath for the precipitate to settle. Filter through a layer of asbestos in a Gooch crucible and wash with hot 3 per cent ammonium nitrate solution made just acid with nitric acid. Dry, ignite gently and weigh. $BiPO_4 \times 0{\cdot}6875 = Bi$.

Evers and Smith[1] determined the emetine gravimetrically by extracting with chloroform from ammoniacal solution after dissolving in acetone and concentrated hydrochloric acid and preventing the precipitation of bismuth during the determination by converting it into bismuth citrate, which is soluble in ammonia.

The authors proposed an assay for iodine based on Volhard's method:

To about 0·5 g add 25 ml of 0·1N silver nitrate. After the addition of 10 ml of dilute nitric acid and heating on a water-bath for thirty minutes the salt is completely decomposed and the silver iodide precipitated. Titrate the excess of silver nitrate with 0·1N potassium thiocyanate solution, using ferric alum as indicator. 1 ml 0·1N = 0·01269 g I.

Titration with 0·05M iodate was found to be inaccurate owing to the yellow colour of the aqueous and chloroform solutions.

Tablets of Emetine and Bismuth Iodide, *B.P.* Usually contain 1 grain.

The assay is based on that for emetine hydrochloride. After complete extraction with ether from sodium hydroxide the extracts are washed free from alkali with a mixture of equal volumes of brine and water. The washings are extracted with ether, this extract is added to the main ether extracts and the mixture is then shaken first with 0·1N hydrochloric acid and then with water, combined acid and aqueous extracts are warmed to remove dissolved ether and the excess acid is titrated with 0·02N sodium hydroxide. 1 ml 0·02N HCl = 0·004807 g $C_{29}H_{40}O_4N_2$.

1. Evers, N., and Smith, W., *Quart. J. Pharm.*, 1938, **11**, 758.
2. Ashworth, F., and Foster, G. E., *J. Pharm. Pharmacol.*, 1950, **2**, 198.

IRON

Fe At. Wt. 55·85

The classical gravimetric determination of iron now finds little application in pharmaceutical work, partly because of the readiness with which other ions are adsorbed on to the precipitate but principally because of the variety of titrimetric methods which are available. Oxidising titrants are the most widely used and these may be applied directly to ferrous iron or, after suitable reduction, to ferric iron. Reducing titrants also find some application for the direct titration of ferric iron. Chelating titrants such as EDTA may be used but, because of the formation of a highly coloured complex and because other rapid titrimetric methods are already available, these are unlikely to find routine application.

Oxidising Titrants. (*a*) *Potassium permanganate.* This method is limited in its application to pharmaceuticals since organic matter must be completely absent. The titration is carried out in sulphuric acid solution; if hydrochloric acid is present high results may be obtained due to its oxidation by permanganate in the presence of iron. Low concentration of hydrochloric acid can be tolerated if the titration solution is very dilute and quite cold but if higher concentrations are present the titration can only be carried out after the addition of Zimmermann-Reinhardt solution (dissolve 50 g of manganous sulphate tetrahydrate in 250 ml of water and add a cooled mixture of 100 ml of concentrated sulphuric acid and 300 ml of water, followed by 100 ml of syrupy phosphoric acid) which inhibits the oxidation of hydrochloric acid by permanganate. The method is as follows:

Dissolve a quantity of sample to contain about 0·2 g of ferrous iron in 20 ml of dilute sulphuric acid and titrate with 0·1N potassium permanganate. 1 ml 0·1N = 0·005585 g Fe; 0·02780 g $FeSO_4,7H_2O$; 0·01519 g $FeSO_4$.

(*b*) *Potassium dichromate.* This reagent has many advantages over potassium permanganate; moderate amounts of chloride do not interfere and, since dichromate is not so strong an oxidising agent as permanganate, titrations can often be carried out in the presence of organic matter. The applicability is more restricted than was once believed, however, for carbohydrates have been shown to interfere considerably. Hartley and Linnell[1] first drew attention to the fact that high results are obtained for the percentage of ferrous carbonate in Saccharated Iron Carbonate when dichromate is used as titrant with diphenylamine as internal indicator; Morton and Harrod[2] showed that oxidation of iron and glucose by dichromate proceeds simultaneously so that no modification would be acceptable and recommended titration with iodate. Ferricyanide as an external indicator for this titration has long been superseded by internal indicators such as diphenylamine and related compounds. Diphenylamine sulphonic acid, obtainable commercially as its barium or sodium salt, is the best indicator available and should be used in a solution which is about N to 2N in hydrochloric or sulphuric acid. The addition of syrupy phosphoric acid is necessary for a sharp end-point, the colour change being from green to violet-blue. The amount of indicator used should be carefully controlled, otherwise a correction is necessary for the dichromate needed to oxidise the indicator. The following procedure is satisfactory:

Dissolve a quantity of sample to contain about 0·2 g of ferrous iron in 25 ml of water and dilute with about 60 ml of dilute sulphuric acid. Add 5 ml of syrupy phosphoric acid, 6 drops of a 0·2 per cent aqueous solution of barium diphenylamine sulphonate and titrate with 0·1N potassium dichromate. 1 ml 0·1N = 0·005585 g Fe; 0·01699 g $C_4H_2O_4Fe$.

For the determination of ferric salts the iron must first be reduced, stannous chloride being the best reagent for use prior to dichromate titration:

Heat to boiling a solution of ferric salt in moderately strong hydrochloric acid and gradually add a strong solution of stannous chloride until the colour, due to ferric iron, has disappeared. Cool rapidly, and add saturated mercuric chloride solution to oxidise the excess of stannous chloride.

A large excess of stannous chloride must be avoided otherwise a grey precipitate of mercury forms and upsets the determination.

(*c*) *Ceric sulphate.* Its powerful oxidising properties, freedom from interference by quite high concentrations of chloride and from moderate quantities of organic matter, including carbohydrates,[3] make this one of the best titrants for ferrous iron. The most convenient way in which to prepare a standard solution is to make use of commercially available ceric ammonium sulphate. This is not a primary standard, so that solutions must be standardised (against arsenious oxide, sodium oxalate or a ferrous salt) before use. The most satisfactory indicator is *o*-phenanthroline-ferrous sulphate complex, also known as ferroin (prepared by adding 1·5 g of *o*-phenanthroline to a solution of 0·7 g of ferrous sulphate heptahydrate in 70 ml of water and diluting to 100 ml with water).

Dissolve a quantity of sample to contain about 0·2 g of ferrous iron in a mixture of 75 ml of water and 25 ml of dilute sulphuric acid and immediately titrate with 0·1N ceric ammonium sulphate using *o*-phenanthroline-ferrous sulphate complex as indicator. 1 ml = 0·005585 g Fe; 0·04462 g $C_{12}H_{22}O_{14}Fe$; 0·04822 g $C_{12}H_{22}O_{14}Fe,2H_2O$.

For titration of ferric iron a convenient method of reduction is by use of zinc and sulphuric acid:

Dissolve a quantity of sample equivalent to about 0·2 g of total iron in 75 ml of water in a flask fitted with a Bunsen valve, add 15 ml of dilute sulphuric acid and 0·25 g of zinc powder. Allow to stand for twenty minutes, filter through an asbestos pad coated with a thin layer of zinc powder, wash the residue first with 10 ml of dilute sulphuric acid and then with 10 ml of water. Titrate the combined filtrate and washings with 0·1N ceric ammonium sulphate as above.

(*d*) *Potassium iodate.* This powerful oxidising agent is of considerable value for the titration of iron preparations which contain much organic matter. First applied to the determination of iron by Heisig[4] the reaction was later studied by Ferrey[5] who showed that ferrous iron may be accurately titrated in the presence of glucose, acacia, tragacanth, lactose, glycerol, lactic acid and citric acid. The method is, however, unsatisfactory in the presence of liquorice, marshmallow, quinine and aqueous extract of cochineal. Iodine is liberated from iodine monochloride in the presence of 5N hydrochloric acid and titrated with potassium iodate, the end-point being extremely sharp.

Dissolve a quantity of sample to contain about 0·25 g of ferrous iron in 20 ml of 25 per cent w/v sulphuric acid, add 6 ml of strong iodine monochloride solution and 60 ml of concentrated hydrochloric acid and titrate with 0·05M potassium iodate, using 5 ml of chloroform as indicator. 1 ml 0·05M potassium iodate = 0·01117 g Fe; 0·02317 g $FeCO_3$; 0·03038 g $FeSO_4$.

For tablets and pills digest 20 tablets with 50 ml of 25 per cent w/v sulphuric acid until not more than a small residue remains. Filter, wash the residue with sufficient of the dilute sulphuric acid to produce 100 ml and use a volume equivalent to about 0·5 g of $FeSO_4$, diluted to 20 ml with water if necessary, as above.

The strong iodine monochloride reagent is prepared as follows: dissolve 6·44 g of potassium iodate and 10 g of potassium iodide in 75 ml of water; add 75 ml of concentrated hydrochloric acid and shake until a clear solution is obtained; add 5 ml of chloroform and titrate with 0·05M iodate to the disappearance of the trace of liberated iodine.

Reducing Titrants. (*e*) *Titanous chloride.* Titration of ferric iron with titanous chloride, using ammonium thiocyanate as indicator, is not in general favour. The titrant must be kept in an inert atmosphere, it must be frequently standardised and a closed-flask system must be employed so that an inert atmosphere may be maintained during titration. Organic matter, phosphates and high concentrations of hydrochloric or sulphuric acids can be tolerated so that the method is particularly valuable for the titration of iron in phosphate syrups. Ferrous iron may be determined after first oxidising with a solution of potassium permanganate added drop by drop to a cold solution. When ferric chloride is to be determined in the presence of potassium chlorate, as for example in Gargle of Ferric Chloride *B.P.C.*, the chlorate is first destroyed by treatment with sulphur dioxide, the reduced iron being re-oxidised with permanganate prior to titration with titanous chloride.

To a quantity of sample containing about 0·1 g of iron add sufficient water to bring the volume to about 50 ml, and 0·2 ml of concentrated hydrochloric acid followed by 2 per cent potassium permanganate solution, dropwise, until a permanent pink colour is produced. Add 10 ml of concentrated hydrochloric acid and 3 ml of 10 per cent ammonium thiocyanate solution and titrate with 0·1N titanous chloride, maintaining a current of carbon dioxide through the flask during the titration. 1 ml 0·1N = 0·005585 g Fe; 0·02780 g $FeSO_4,7H_2O$; 0·01622 g $FeCl_3$.

(*f*) *Iodometric titration.* For the correct determination of ferric iron by the method of Mohr, in which the iron is reduced by digestion with hydriodic acid with consequent liberation of iodine, all the iron must be in the ionic condition. This is attained when the hydrogen ion concentration is high; if it is low, formation of unionised ferric hydroxide occurs and the reaction with iodide ions is incomplete. Hence in a sufficiently acid medium the reaction goes to completion rapidly. Ferrey[6] studied the reaction fully with regard to pharmaceutical salts and scale preparations and he showed that the practice of heating the reaction mixture to 40° and allowing it to stand at that temperature gave high results. He also showed that, in the presence of 6 molecules of potassium iodide per atom of ferric iron, reduction to ferrous iron occurs very rapidly if the concentration of the hydrochloric acid is sufficient; the required concentration of acid depends upon the radical associated with the ferric ions. For most preparations the modification of Jones and Glass[7], in which the sample is heated with sulphuric acid to bring all the iron into the ionic form, is used. As low results may be obtained with direct determination owing to the presence of small amounts of ferrous iron, oxidation with permanganate is necessary before titration. The general method is as follows (for values of (i), (ii), (iii), (iv) and (v) see Table 20).

Dissolve (i) g in (ii) ml of water and add 1 ml of concentrated sulphuric acid. Then add 0·1N potassium permanganate, dropwise, until a pink colour persists for five seconds. Add (iii) ml of concentrated hydrochloric acid and (iv) g of potassium iodide, set aside for three minutes, add (v) ml of water and titrate the liberated iodine with 0·1N sodium thiosulphate using starch as indicator. 1 ml 0·1N = 0·005585 g Fe; 0·01622 g $FeCl_3$.

Note I. Warm until the dark brown colour becomes pale yellow and cool to 15° before adding permanganate.

Note II. Iron is converted to the ionised condition by heating the solution to boiling-point after adding the hydrochloric acid, boiling for fifteen seconds and cooling before addition of potassium iodide (Ferrey[6]). The oxidation with permanganate and sulphuric acid is omitted.

Note III. For ferric hypophosphite, *B.P.C.* To 1 g add 10 ml of nitrohydrochloric acid (prepared by mixing cautiously 20 ml of concentrated nitric acid and 80 ml of concentrated hydrochloric acid, allowing to stand, or warming gently until no more gas is evolved, and remixing) and evaporate to dryness on a water-bath; add 5 ml of concentrated hydrochloric acid and again evaporate to dryness. Dissolve the residue in 25 ml of water and 5 ml of concentrated hydrochloric acid, add 4 g potassium iodide, allow to stand for fifteen minutes, add 50 ml of water and titrate the liberated iodine with 0·1N sodium thiosulphate using starch as indicator. Repeat the operation omitting the sample. 1 ml 0·1N = 0·005585 g Fe.

(*g*) *Mercurous nitrate.* This titrant for the direct determination of ferric iron, described by Bradbury and Edwards,[8] has advantages over many other reducing titrants in that it is stable and can be employed in the presence of nitric acid. Ferric iron is not quantitatively reduced by mercurous solutions unless an excess of thiocyanate is present.

Bradbury, Chatterjee and Edwards[9] and Chatterjee[10] have applied the method to a number of iron preparations, but it has not found much application in pharmaceutical work.

Chelating Titrants. (*h*) *EDTA.* Ferric iron forms a very stable complex with EDTA and may be titrated directly at a pH of about 2 and a temperature of about 50°. Tiron (blue to colourless), salicylic acid (violet to colourless) or thiocyanate (red to colourless) are all suitable indicators, although in the presence of a high concentration of iron the iron-EDTA complex is itself strongly coloured and will modify the end-point. In practice, so many other excellent titrants exist for iron that this method is unlikely to find wide application.

Physical Techniques. (*i*) *Spectrographic determination.* The arc emission spectrographic method for the determination of iron is particularly suitable for samples which are insoluble or available only in quantities of a few milligrams. The high sensitivity of the iron lines at 3720 A and 3020 A enables the metal to be detected in concentrations of the order of 1 p.p.m. For quantitative analysis an internal standard technique is used and the precision obtainable is about ± 5 per cent.

(*j*) *Flame photometric determination.* Iron has been estimated in aqueous solutions with an air-acetylene flame using the lines at 3860 A and 3720 A. Limitations are imposed, however, by weak molecular cyanogen background spectra in the region of the former wavelength and by MgO band emission from 3721 A to 3726 A, and such interference must be taken into consideration. Using an oxy-acetylene flame Dean and Burger[11] demonstrated the interference effects of several elements, including magnesium, manganese, aluminium, lithium, potassium and zinc, on the flame emission of iron at 3860 A. Dilute acids below 2M concentration were shown to have little effect. Dean and Lady[12] used a procedure involving extraction of the iron with acetylacetone followed by direct atomisation of the organic phase and obtained a six-fold increase in sensitivity compared with aqueous solutions. In general the concentration of iron required for quantitative determination is between 10 and 100 p.p.m. in the final solution.

(*k*) *Atomic absorption determination*. The absence of serious interference from background emission and other elements provides atomic absorption methods with considerable advantage over flame photometric techniques. David,[13] using the iron line at 3758 A found negligible interference from sodium, potassium, calcium, magnesium and aluminium, although sensitivity was not good. It is known, however, that the strongest emission lines are not necessarily the strongest absorption lines, and Allan,[14] using the line at 2483 A, obtained measurable absorption with a solution containing 2 p.p.m. of iron. It is possible to increase sensitivity by using a longer burner, thus increasing absorption, and also by atomising solutions of iron in organic solvents.

IRON AND REDUCED IRON

Iron *B.P.C.* is determined by dissolving in dilute sulphuric acid in a flask protected by a Bunsen valve, and then titrating with potassium permanganate.

In the *B.Vet.C.* method for determination of metallic iron in reduced iron, the copper is displaced from copper sulphate and the ferrous salt formed is titrated with 0·1N permanganate. 1 ml 0·1N = 0·005585 g. The process has been adversely criticised by Hartley, Linnell, Read and Rolfe.[15] Persistently high results were obtained and these were attributed to the hydrolysis of copper sulphate in hot solution, reaction between the acid formed and the mixed salts yielding products which react with permanganate. Preference was given to the Wilner-Merck[16] process using mercuric chloride. The modification of the method which was eventually adopted yielded consistent results which reflected the actual content of metallic iron in the sample:

> To approximately 0·5 g of sample, accurately weighed, in a clean, dry 100-ml graduated flask add 2·5 g of mercuric chloride and about 50 ml of recently boiled and cooled distilled water. Boil gently for twenty minutes (avoiding excessive frothing) with frequent shaking, make the volume up to 100 ml with recently boiled and cooled distilled water, cork the flask and cool. When cold, adjust the volume to 100 ml, shake well, allow the precipitate to settle and filter rapidly into a clean, dry, conical flask. Pipette 50 ml of the filtrate into 100 ml of dilute sulphuric acid, in which 2 g of manganese sulphate has been dissolved, and titrate with 0·1N potassium permanganate. 1 ml 0·1N = 0·005585 g.

IRON SALTS, SCALE PREPARATIONS AND GALENICALS

The iron salts, scale preparations and galenicals of the *B.P.*, *B.P.C.* and *B.Vet.C.* may be summarised conveniently in tabulated form. The letters in Table 20 denoting method of determination refer to those given above.

IRON

Traces of iron may be estimated colorimetrically with considerable accuracy. The formation of ferric thiocyanate, which was the basis of the *B.P.* 1932 method, is no longer used because of the many interferences which are possible. Strafford preferred the use of thioglycollic acid which produces a purple colour with traces of ferrous iron in ammoniacal solution (ferric salts also respond because the reagent has strongly reducing properties). Quantitative use of this reagent was described by Swank and

TABLE 20

SALTS AND SCALE PREPARATIONS OF IRON	METHOD OF DETERMINATION	IRON CALCULATED AS	NOTES ON DETERMINATION For method (*f*): (i) wt in g, (ii) H_2O for soln., (iii) HCl, (iv) KI, (v) H_2O before titration
Ferrous Carbonate, Saccharated, *B.P.C.*	(*d*)	Fe	
Ferrous Fumarate	(*b*)	Fe (Ferrous Iron)	
Ferrous Gluconate, *B.P.*	(*c*)	$C_{12}H_{22}O_{14}Fe$	
Ferrous Sulphate, *B.P.*	(*a*)	$FeSO_4,7H_2O$	
Ferrous Sulphate, Dried, *B.P.*	(*a*)	$FeSO_4$	
Ferric Ammonium Citrate, *B.P.*	(*f*) *Note I*	Fe	0·5 : 15 : 15 : 2 : 60
Ferric Chloride, Anhydrous, *B.Vet.C.*	(*f*)	$FeCl_3$	0·3 : 20 : 15 : 2 : 0
Ferric Glycerophosphate, *B.P.C.*	(*f*) *Note I*	Fe	1 : 15 : 15 : 2 : 60
Ferric Hypophosphite, *B.P.C.*	(*f*) *Note III*	Fe	*
Iron Phosphate, *B.P.C.*	(*a*)	Fe	Dissolve in 3 ml H_3PO_4 and 10 ml 25% w/v H_2SO_4 and dilute with 100 ml water before titrating
Iron Pyrophosphate, Soluble, *B.Vet.C.*	(*f*) *Note II*	Fe	1 : 14 : 6 : 3 : 0
Sodium Ironedetate	(*f*)	Fe	0·3 : 10 : 25 (dil. HCl) : 20 ml 10% soln. : 0 (omitting oxidation with H_2SO_4 and $KMnO_4$ but allowing to stand for 10 min before titration)

Mellon[17] and its application to pharmaceuticals by Strafford, Wyatt and Kershaw.[18] The colour is fully developed in five minutes and remains stable for several hours; comparatively small amounts of strong alkalies cause instability of colour, and oxidising agents should be avoided. Aluminium, if present, must be kept in solution with an excess of tartaric or citric acid. Cobalt and chromium seriously interfere and so does nickel if present in large quantity. The effect of small amounts of copper is negligible, and of the salts of common acids, chlorides, sulphates, fluorides and phosphates have no effect.

TABLE 20 (*contd.*)

SOLUTIONS OF IRON SALTS	METHOD OF DETERMINATION	IRON CALCULATED AS	NOTES ON DETERMINATION For method (*f*): (i) wt in g, (ii) H_2O for soln., (iii) HCl, (iv) KI, (v) H_2O before titration
Solution of Ferric Chloride, *B.P.C.*	(*f*)	$FeCl_3$	20 ml of 1 in 10 dilution : 0 : 15 : 2 : 50
Strong Solution of Ferric Chloride, *B.P.C.*	(*f*)	$FeCl_3$	0·7 : 20 : 15 : 2 : 0 Calculate % w/v from wt/ml
Solution of Ferric Hypophosphite, *B.P.C.*	—	$Fe(H_2PO_2)_3$	*
Solution of Ferric Sulphate, *B.P.C.*	(*f*)	Fe	1·5 : 25 : 7 : 3·5 : 0 (omitting oxidation with H_2SO_4 and $KMnO_4$). Calculate % w/v from wt/ml
Solution of Ferrous Iodide, *B.P.C.*	—	FeI_2	By Volhard's method (see Halogen Acids, p. 290)
Solution of Dialysed Iron, *B.Vet.C.*	(*f*) *Note II*	Fe	5 ml : 20 : 3 : 3 : 0
Compound Sclerosing Solution of Iron, *B.Vet.C.*	—	$FeCl_3$	To 10 ml of a 1 in 10 diln. add 40 ml H_2O, 5 g NH_4Cl and 0·5 ml conc. HNO_3; heat to boiling, add an excess of dil. NH_3 and filter. Wash ppt. with 1% NH_4NO_3 soln., dry, ignite and weigh 1 g residue = 2·032 g $FeCl_3$

TABLE 20 (*contd.*)

IRON GALENICALS	METHOD OF DETERMINATION	IRON CALCULATED AS	NOTES ON DETERMINATION For method (*f*): (i) wt in g, (ii) H_2O for soln., (iii) HCl, (iv) KI, (v) H_2O before titration
Gargle of Ferric Chloride, *B.P.C.*	(*e*)	$FeCl_3$	Previously treated with SO_2 to destroy $KClO_3$—see above. For potassium chlorate see p. 307
Mixture of Ferric Ammonium Citrate, *B.P.C.*	(*f*) *Note I*	Fe	5 ml : 10 : 15 : 2 : 60
Mixture of Ferric Ammonium Citrate for Infants, *B.P.C.*	(*e*)†	Fe	Use 5 ml
Mixture of Ferrous Sulphate, *B.P.C.*	(*e*)	$FeSO_4,7H_2O$	Calculate % w/v from wt/ml
Mixture of Ferrous Sulphate for Infants, *B.P.C.*	(*e*)	$FeSO_4,7H_2O$	Calculate % w/v from wt/ml
Mixture of Strychnine and Iron, *B.P.C.*	(*f*)	$FeCl_3$	30 ml : 0 : 15 : 2 : 50
Pills of Aloin, Compound, *B.P.C.* 1949	(*d*)†	$FeSO_4$	Use 10 pills and 20 ml 25% w/v H_2SO_4 for digestion
Pills of Ferrous Carbonate, *B.P.C.*	(*d*)	$FeCO_3$	Use 10 pills and 20 ml 25% w/v H_2SO_4 for digestion
Syrup of Ferrous Iodide, *B.P.C.*	—	FeI_2	By Volhard's method (see under Halogen Acids, p. 290)
Syrup of Ferrous Phosphate Compound, *B.P.C.* (Chemical Food)	(*e*)	Fe	Calculate % w/v from wt/ml. For calcium see p. 154
Syrup of Ferrous Phosphate with Quinine and Strychnine, *B.P.C.* (Easton's Syrup)	(*e*)	Fe	Calculate % w/v from wt/ml. For quinine see p. 467. For strychnine see p. 468. For phosphate see p. 530
Tablets of Ferrous Carbonate, *B.P.C.*	(*d*)	$FeCO_3$	Use amount of powdered tablets equivalent to 6 tablets

TABLE 20 (*contd.*)

IRON GALENICALS	METHOD OF DETERMINATION	IRON CALCULATED AS	NOTES ON DETERMINATION For method (*f*): (i) wt in g, (ii) H_2O for soln., (iii) HCl, (iv) KI, (v) H_2O before titration
Tablets of Ferrous Carbonate and Arsenic, *B.P.C.*	(*d*)	$FeCO_3$	Use amount of powdered tablets equivalent to 6 tablets. For arsenic see p. 85
Tablets of Ferrous Fumarate	(*b*)	$C_4H_2O_4Fe$	Dissolve powdered tablets equivalent to 4 tablets in 50 ml dilute H_2SO_4
Tablets of Ferrous Gluconate, *B.P.C.*	(*c*)	$C_{12}H_{22}O_{14}Fe$, $2H_2O$	Use wt of powdered tablets equivalent to 1 g Ferrous Gluconate dissolved as completely as possible in 30 ml H_2O + 20 ml dil. H_2SO_4
Tablets of Ferrous Phosphate with Quinine and Strychnine, *B.P.C.* (Easton's Tablets)	(*e*)	Fe	On 25-ml aliquot of 20 tablets in dilute H_2SO_4 to 150 ml. For quinine see p. 469. For strychnine see p. 469
Tablets of Ferrous Sulphate, *B.P.*	(*d*)	$FeSO_4$	*U.S.P.* uses method (*c*)
Tablets of Ferrous Sulphate Compound, *B.P.C.*	(*d*)	$FeSO_4$	
Tablets of Ferrous Sulphate with Quinine and Strychnine, *B.Vet.C.*	(*d*)	$FeSO_4$	Powder the tablets before digesting with H_2SO_4. For quinine see p. 469. For strychnine see p. 469

* This salt is better assayed through the hypophosphite radicle. To 10 ml of solution of about 1 g of the salt in hydrochloric acid diluted to 100 ml with water, add 20 ml of concentrated hydrochloric acid, 2 g of potassium iodide and 50 ml of 0·1N iodine; allow to stand in the dark for four hours and titrate the excess iodine with 0·1N sodium thiosulphate. Repeat the operation omitting the sample. 1 ml 0·1N = 0·005016 g $Fe(H_2PO_2)_3$.

Solution of Ferric Hypophosphite, *B.P.C.*, is assayed from the hypophosphite content, as above, using 10 ml of a 1 in 20 dilution and adding 10 ml of water before adding the potassium iodide.

† Method not official.

Add a drop of thioglycollic acid to 10 ml of a solution containing the iron salt, then add 0·5 ml of strong ammonia solution and dilute to 50 ml. Compare the colour produced with standard solutions containing known amounts of iron treated in exactly the same manner. The *B.P.* standard iron solution is a convenient strength for colorimetric comparison and contains 0·173 g of ferric ammonium sulphate per litre (1 ml = 0·00002 g Fe).

2,2′-Dipyridyl[19] gives a red colour with an absorption maximum at 522 mμ in the presence of ferrous iron.[20] The following method may be applied after suitably destroying organic matter (see Appendix XI).

Prepare a calibration graph by transferring suitable aliquots of standard iron solution (1 μg Fe per ml) containing between 0·2 and 8 μg of iron to a series of similar tubes. To each tube add 0·2 ml of a 0·5 per cent solution of 2,2′-dipyridyl in dehydrated ethanol, 1 ml of a freshly prepared 10 per cent solution of sodium sulphite in water and 0·1 ml of 5N hydrochloric acid. Adjust the volume in each tube to 10 ml and measure the extinction of a 1-cm layer at 522 mμ. Treat an aliquot of the solution under test in the same way and determine the amount of iron present by reference to the calibration graph.

Probably the best reagent for determination of traces of iron is *o*-phenanthroline. The red colour produced with ferrous iron is very stable over a wide range of pH and temperature, is unaffected by excess of reagent and obeys Beer's Law very closely.[21] Bismuth and silver produce precipitates with the reagent and coloured ions such as chromium, nickel and cobalt interfere. Cyanides and tungstates suppress the colour formation but most other commonly occurring ions have little or no effect. Hydroxylamine and hydroquinone are both satisfactory reducing agents for ferric iron, the latter being preferred if a citrate buffer is used; quantitative determination is best carried out in the pH range 3 to 3·5. The following method, which is of general applicability, has been recommended by the Analytical Methods Committee of the *S.A.C.*[22]

A suitable sample (containing up to 1,000 μg of iron) is treated to destroy organic matter (see Appendix XI, p. 851) and the iron determined spectrophotometrically.

To 5 ml of acid solution add a few drops of a 0·4 per cent solution of bromophenol blue in ethanol and titrate with 25 per cent sodium citrate solution until the yellow colour changes to blue.

Transfer a second 5-ml aliquot of the test solution to a 25-ml graduated flask, add 1 ml of 1 per cent hydroquinone solution, 3 ml of a 0·25 per cent solution of *o*-phenanthroline in 25 per cent ethanol and a volume of the sodium citrate solution equal to the volume required in the above titration. Dilute to volume with water and allow to stand for one hour.

Carry out a blank procedure on the reagents used.

Measure the extinctions at 510 mμ of the test and blank solutions, using matched 4-cm or 1-cm cells according to the depth of colour, with water in the comparison cell. Read the μg of iron equivalent to the extinctions from a standard curve and so obtain the iron content of the sample.

Preparation of standard curve: Into a series of 100-ml graduated flasks measure suitable volumes of a dilute standard iron solution (100 μg per ml) prepared by diluting a stock standard iron solution (see below) ten times with water immediately before use. Treat the contents of each flask, respectively, as follows. Add 40 ml of diluted hydrochloric acid (1 + 3) and dilute to volume with water. Using a 5-ml aliquot proceed as described above for the test solution beginning with the words 'add a few drops of a 0·4 per cent solution of bromothymol blue . . .'.

Measure the extinction of each solution at 510 mμ, using 4-cm or 1-cm cells, as appropriate, and prepare a curve by plotting extinctions against μg of iron.

Stock standard iron solution. Dissolve 0·8634 g of ferric alum, $Fe_2(SO_4)_3.(NH_4)_2SO_4,24H_2O$, in water containing 2 ml of 60 per cent w/w perchloric acid and dilute to 100 ml with water. (1 ml $\equiv$ 1 mg of iron—nominal.) Standardise this solution as follows. Pipette 20 ml into a 250-ml beaker containing 150 ml of water, add 1 ml of concentrated nitric acid and about 4 g of ammonium chloride and heat to boiling-point. Add slowly an excess of ammonia solution (strong ammonia solution diluted with an equal volume of water) and boil for one minute. Filter through a No. 41 Whatman paper, wash with hot 1 per cent ammonium nitrate solution, dry, ignite and weigh as Fe_2O_3. Wt of $Fe_2O_3 \times 0{\cdot}6994$ = wt of iron.

1. HARTLEY, F., and LINNELL, W. H., *Quart. J. Pharm.*, 1934, **7**, 549.
2. MORTON, C., and HARROD, D. C., *Quart. J. Pharm.*, 1936, **9**, 480.
3. LYONS, C. G., and APPLEYARD, F. N., *Quart. J. Pharm.*, 1936, **9**, 462.
4. HEISIG, G. B., *J. Amer. Chem. Soc.*, 1928, **50**, 1687.
5. FERREY, G. J. W., *Quart. J. Pharm.*, 1935, **8**, 344.
6. FERREY, G. J. W., *Quart. J. Pharm.*, 1930, **3**, 471.
7. JONES, A. J., and GLASS, N., *Quart. J. Pharm.*, 1930, **3**, 488.
8. BRADBURY, F. R., and EDWARDS, E. G., *J. Soc. Chem. Ind.*, 1940, **59**, 96.
9. BRADBURY, F. R., CHATTERJEE, K. C., and EDWARDS, E. G., *Quart. J. Pharm.*, 1940, **13**, 297.
10. CHATTERJEE, K. C., *Analyst*, 1942, **67**, 257.
11. DEAN, J. A., and BURGER, J. C., *Anal. Chem.*, 1955, **27**, 1052.
12. DEAN, J. A., and LADY, J. H., *Anal. Chem.*, 1955, **27**, 1533.
13. DAVID, D. J., *Analyst*, 1958, **83**, 655.
14. ALLAN, J. E., *Spectrochim. Acta*, 1959, **15**, 800.
15. HARTLEY, F., LINNELL, W. H., READ, F. E., and ROLFE, H.G., *Quart. J. Pharm.*, 1935, **8**, 100.
16. WILNER-MERCK, *Z. Anal. Chem.*, 1902, **41**, 710.
17. SWANK, H. W., and MELLON, M. G., *Ind. Eng. Chem., Anal. Edn.*, 1938, **10**, 7.
18. STRAFFORD, N., WYATT, P. F., and KERSHAW, F. G., *Analyst*, 1945, **70**, 232.
19. HILL, R., *Proc. Roy. Soc.* (*London*). **B**, 1930, **107**, 205.
20. MOSS, M. L. and MELLON, M. G., *Ind. Eng. Chem., Anal. Edn.*, 1942, **14**, 862.
21. FORTUNE, W. B., and MELLON, M. G., *Ind. Eng. Chem., Anal. Edn.*, 1938, **10**, 60.
22. Determination of Trace Elements, *S.A.C.*, p. 21.

ISONIAZID

$C_6H_7ON_3$ Mol. Wt. 137·1

The quantitative determination of isoniazid, *iso*nicotinohydrazide, has been the subject of considerable publication. Isoniazid reacts similarly to hydrazines in being oxidised in weakly alkaline solution with iodine but the method tends to give varying results, particularly with differences of temperature and time of reaction. This method is also unsuitable for determination in tablet mixtures where lactose is in the base, since iodine will oxidise sugars in alkaline media. Bromimetric assay provides a much better method and has been recommended by Haugas and Mitchell.[1]

Dissolve about 0·4 g in water and make up to 250 ml. Pipette 25 ml of this solution into a stoppered flask, add 25 ml of 0·1N bromine and 5 ml of concentrated hydrochloric acid. Shake the flask for one minute before allowing to stand for fifteen minutes, release the stopper carefully, since there is a slight pressure due to formation of nitrogen, add 2 g of potassium iodide and titrate with 0·1N sodium thiosulphate. 1 ml 0·1N bromine = 0·003429 g $C_6H_7ON_3$.

Other methods of determination, which are more specific, have been recommended by Scott,[2] all being applicable to tablets and to small quantities of isoniazid. The reaction with 1-chloro-2,4-dinitrobenzene to give a reddish-purple derivative is fairly specific and under the detailed conditions a straight line calibration curve is obtained.

To a dilution in dehydrated ethanol containing about 0·15 mg of isoniazid, add 0·1 g of borax and 5 ml of 5 per cent solution of 1-chloro-2,4-dinitrobenzene in dehydrated ethanol and evaporate by placing the tube in a water-bath for fifteen minutes, taking care to avoid mechanical loss of the ethanol. Cool the dry residue in ice for one minute, add 25·0 ml of methanol, shake and filter. Read the extinction of 1 cm of the filtrate at 530 mμ or, using a suitable filter, against a blank prepared as above omitting the sample and obtain the amount of isoniazid present from a calibration curve.

The colour developed should be read without delay as small decreases occur on exposure to daylight. The reproducibility is about $\pm$ 3 per cent.

Scott also observed the ultra-violet absorption of isoniazid in 0·01N hydrochloric acid at 266 mμ as about 430 calculated from the extinction of a 0·001 per cent solution.

Kühni, Jacob and Grossglauser[3] found that non-aqueous titration of isoniazid in acetic acid using perchloric acid in glacial acetic acid as titrant gave reproducible results only after acetylation of the isoniazid and recommended the following procedure.

Dissolve about 0·15 g of the sample, previously dried at 103° to 105°, in a mixture of 2 ml of acetic anhydride and 18 ml of glacial acetic acid, stirring to assist solution. Titrate with 0·1N perchloric acid in glacial acetic acid either potentiometrically, or visually to an emerald-green end-point using crystal violet as indicator. 1 ml 0·1N = 0·006857 g $C_6H_7ON_3$.

Buděšínský[4] proposed a method based on the quantitative reaction of isoniazid with cadmium thiocyanate at pH 6 to 7 to give the complex $[Cd(C_6H_7ON_3)] (SCN)_2$.

Dissolve 0·1 to 0·5 g in 15 ml of water, add 20 ml of 0·25M cadmium thiocyanate and dilute to volume with water. Mix well, filter and titrate the excess thiocyanate in 10 ml of the filtrate. 1 ml 0·25M cadmium thiocyanate = 0·03429 g $C_6H_7ON_3$.

The determination is not affected by temperature, time taken or the amount of thiocyanate added in excess.

Tablets of Isoniazid, *B.P.* Usually contain 50 mg of the active ingredient.

Bromimetric determination as described above can be carried out directly on the powdered tablets containing the usual diluents, otherwise a preliminary extraction by solvent is necessary.

For routine purposes direct spectrophotometric determination is satisfactory provided a blank is possible with the tablet excipients used.

Weigh an amount of powdered tablets, containing about 0·1 g of isoniazid, into a 100-ml flask. Add about 80 ml of water, shake for thirty minutes, dilute to 100 ml and filter. Dilute 10·0 ml to 100 ml with water and transfer 10·0 ml of this dilution to a 100-ml flask. Add 10·0 ml of 0·1N hydrochloric acid and dilute to 100 ml with water. Prepare a blank from the tablet excipients in an exactly similar manner. Measure the extinction of 1 cm at 266 mμ against the blank. E(1 per cent, 1 cm) at 266 mμ = 430.

The chlorodinitrobenzene method has also been applied to tablets by Scott[2] by first shaking an amount of finely ground tablet, containing about 0·06 g of isoniazid, with 100 ml of dehydrated ethanol and allowing to settle before continuing as in the method given above.

1. Haugas, E. A., and Mitchell, B. W., *J. Pharm. Pharmacol.*, 1952, **4,** 687.
2. Scott, P. G. W., *J. Pharm. Pharmacol.*, 1952, **4,** 681.
3. Kühni, E., Jacob, M., and Grossglauser, H., *Pharm. Acta Helv.*, 1954, **29,** 233.
4. Buděšínský, B., *Českosl. Farm.*, 1955, **4,** 185.

ISOPROPYL ALCOHOL

$(CH_3)_2CH.OH$ Mol. Wt. 60·10

*iso*Propyl alcohol is used in considerable quantities as a substitute for ethyl alcohol in cheap essences and perfumery products, and it has also been used for pharmaceutical preparations.

If the alcohol is present as the only volatile constituent in aqueous solution, the ordinary methods of alcohol determination may be applied, although Aiyar and Krishnan[1] have recommended the following modification of the Thorpe and Holmes separation (Process B; Appendix I) when the presence of *iso*propyl alcohol is suspected. They found that both *iso*-propyl alcohol and *n*-propanol are miscible with light petroleum, that they have only limited solubilities in saturated sodium chloride solution and that both alcohols can be removed from light petroleum by water to a much larger extent than by saturated brine.

> Saturate 100 ml of the alcoholic liquid (original sample or distillate), containing approximately 30 per cent of proof spirit, with common salt and shake with 50 ml of light petroleum (b.p. 40° to 60°) and allow to separate. Draw off the brine layer and wash the light petroleum extract with 10 ml of saturated brine, followed by five successive washings with 10 ml of water. Distil the combined brine and aqueous layers and collect 100 ml of distillate. When the specific gravity of the distillate has been determined the apparent proof spirit is read from the Official Specific Gravity Tables (see p. 780).

Adams and Nicholls[2] state that if a distillate contains less than about 17 per cent of apparent proof spirit, the specific gravity and refraction for the lower alcohols and acetone are very nearly linear functions of the quantity in solution, and if the apparent proof spirit be found, multiplying by 0·612 (the mean value for 1 per cent proof spirit) will give the percentage by volume of *iso*propyl alcohol, not differing by more than 0·1 per cent from the correct value.

Table 21, given by Adams and Nicholls,[2] shows the corresponding refractometer readings.

As at these dilutions the apparent proof strength and refraction of mixtures of the lower alcohols and acetone are practically the sum of those due to each of the ingredients, when two known substances only are present, the quantities of each can be calculated from these two figures. With more than two substances present, allowance can be made for any ingredients which can be separately determined. An instance cited in the paper is the estimation of mixtures of ethyl and *iso*propyl alcohols and acetone by regulated oxidation of the first two entirely to acetic acid and acetone respectively, the acetone being unappreciably affected under the selected conditions.

TABLE 21

APPARENT PROOF SPIRIT per cent	IMMERSION REFRACTOMETER READING AT 60° F
0	15·4
1	16·5
2	17·6
3	18·6
4	19·6
5	20·6
6	21·7
7	22·8
8	23·9
9	25·0
10	26·2
11	27·4
12	28·7
13	29·9
14	31·2
15	32·4
16	33·7
17	34·9

Place an aliquot part of the distillate to be tested, containing not more than 1·5 g ethyl alcohol or 3 g of *iso*propyl alcohol, in a distillation flask of about 800-ml capacity and dilute with water to about 100 ml. Add an equal volume of oxidising mixture (10 g of potassium dichromate and 25 ml of concentrated sulphuric acid per 100 ml), stopper the flask and allow to stand for twenty-five to thirty minutes. Add an excess of ferrous sulphate and steam-distil the solution, the contents of the flask being allowed to concentrate to about 100 ml. The concentration should not be carried further, or the distillate becomes yellowish and gives an acidity not due to acetic acid. The whole of the acetic acid should be in the distillate when about 500 to 600 ml have been collected. Titrate the distillate with N sodium hydroxide, using solid phenolphthalein as indicator. Add 10 to 20 g of common salt to make the end-point sharper. 1 ml N = 0·046 g ethyl alcohol = 0·058 ml ethyl alcohol = 0·101 ml proof spirit. Redistil the neutralised liquid, making the distillate up to a known volume, determining the acetone present from the specific gravity of the solution or by one of the methods described under Acetone (p. 7). The acetone found represents that originally present, together with that produced from the *iso*propyl alcohol; if the original acetone be estimated before oxidation, the difference can be calculated to *iso*propyl alcohol. 1 ml acetone = 1·043 ml *iso*propyl alcohol.

*iso*Propyl alcohol may be determined in various mixtures by a gas chromatographic method. The following procedure has been used for determination of *iso*propyl alcohol in a mixture with water and methyl *iso*butyl ketone.

ISOPROPYL ALCOHOL

Dilute the sample in acetone so that the expected concentration of *iso*propyl alcohol is about 1 per cent. To the acetone solution add an amount of *n*-butanol such that the final concentration of the latter is exactly 2·0 per cent.

Prepare a standard solution containing 1·0 per cent of *iso*propyl alcohol and 2·0 per cent of *n*-butanol in acetone.

Chromatograph the sample and standard solutions using the following operating conditions: column length, 6 ft.; column temperature, 80°; stationary phase, 30 per cent of glycerol on 100/120-mesh Celite; hydrogen flow rate, 45 ml per minute; flash heater temperature, 125°; detector, thermal conductivity cell; detector current, 180 mA; sample size, 30 μl; recorder, Honeywell-Brown with 1 mV full-scale deflection and chart speed of 12 inches per hour.

The order of elution is: acetone and methyl *iso*butyl ketone, *iso*propyl alcohol, *n*-butanol, water.

Calculate the ratios of the height of the *iso*propyl alcohol peak to that of the *n*-butanol peak for both sample and standard.

Per cent of *iso*propyl alcohol = (ratio of peak heights for sample/ratio of peak heights for standard) × dilution factor.

***n*-Propanol.** Mean value for 1 per cent apparent proof spirit (dilutions below 17 per cent proof) = 0·655 per cent by volume of *n*-propanol. The following table, given by Adams and Nicholls,[2] shows the corresponding refractometer readings.

TABLE 22

APPARENT PROOF SPIRIT per cent	IMMERSION REFRACTOMETER READING AT 60° F
0	15·4
1	16·5
2	17·7
3	18·9
4	20·1
5	21·3
6	22·6
7	23·9
8	25·2
9	26·6
10	28·0
11	29·4
12	30·8
13	32·2
14	33·6
15	35·0
16	36·4
17	37·8

When *n*-propanol is present in a mixture the above oxidation method of Adams and Nicholls can be used to determine *iso*propyl alcohol but not ethyl alcohol. Under the above specified conditions *n*-propanol gives about 70 per cent of propionic acid and 30 per cent of acetic acid; but as 1 mol. of alcohol gives 1 mol. of acid, the mixed acids can be titrated after steam distillation, and, with *n*-propanol alone present, 1 ml N alkali = 0·060 g *n*-propanol = 0·0743 ml *n*-propanol.

(*Cf.* Acetone and Ethyl Alcohol.)

1. Aiyar, S. S., and Krishnan, P. S., *Analyst*, 1935, **60,** 237.
2. Adams, C. A., and Nicholls, J. R., *Analyst*, 1929, **54,** 2.

JABORANDI

Jaborandi, as met with in commerce, consists of the dried leaflets of *Pilocarpus jaborandi* and other species of *Pilocarpus* and contains a number of associated alkaloids, among which are pilocarpine, *iso*pilocarpine and pilocarpidine. The method for the determination of total alkaloids described below is that recommended by the Analytical Methods Committee of the *S.A.C.*[1] and was official in the *B.P.C.* 1949.

To about 10 g, accurately weighed, in No. 40 powder and contained in a flask, add 50 ml of chloroform, shake well and allow to stand for ten minutes. Add 5 ml of dilute ammonia solution and shake continuously for one hour; transfer the mixture quantitatively, by means of further portions of chloroform, to a percolator plugged with cotton wool and continue percolation, using a total of 160 ml of chloroform or until complete extraction is effected as shown by evaporating 2 ml to dryness, dissolving the residue in 5 drops of 0·1N sulphuric acid and testing with Mayer's reagent. Mix the chloroform solutions and concentrate to a volume of about 40 ml. Transfer to a separator with a little chloroform, add 150 ml of ether and shake well with 20 ml of 0·5N sulphuric acid; allow to separate, run off the aqueous lower layer and continue the extraction with three 10-ml quantities of 0·1N sulphuric acid. Filter the combined acid extracts into another separator, make alkaline with dilute ammonia solution and shake with four successive 20-ml portions of chloroform, washing each extract with the same 10-ml portion of water. Combine the chloroform extracts, remove the solvent by distillation, add to the residue 2 ml of dehydrated ethanol and evaporate to dryness. Dry the alkaloidal residue for five minutes on a water-bath. Dissolve the residue in 1 or 2 ml of neutral ethanol, add 15 ml of 0·05N sulphuric acid and titrate with 0·05N sodium hydroxide, using methyl red as indicator. 1 ml 0·05N sulphuric acid = 0·0104 g of alkaloids calculated as pilocarpine.

PILOCARPINE, $C_{11}H_{16}O_2N_2$, Mol. Wt. 208·3

For a close approximation of the content of this physiologically important alkaloid, the following procedure is recommended:

Transfer the titrated liquid obtained in the assay for total alkaloids to a separator, render alkaline with dilute ammonia solution and shake with four successive 20-ml portions of chloroform, washing each extract with the same 10-ml portion of water. Combine the chloroform extracts, remove the solvent by distillation, add to the residue 2 ml of dehydrated ethanol and evaporate to dryness. Dry the residue for five minutes on a water-bath, then dissolve in about 10 ml of a saturated solution of pilocarpine nitrate in acetone of analytical purity. Add from a capillary tube a freshly prepared and well-cooled mixture of 9 volumes of acetone and 1 volume of concentrated nitric acid (sp. gr. 1·42) until the mixture is acid, as indicated by spotting on a piece of moistened congo red paper. Stir vigorously and leave overnight. Collect the crystals formed in a tared sintered-glass crucible of not less than No. 3 porosity. Wash with acetone previously saturated with pilocarpine nitrate, dry at 100° and weigh. The crystals should be nearly colourless and should not melt below 170°. If crystals do not form, the whole assay should be repeated.

Elvidge[2] developed the colorimetric method for the determination of small quantities of jaborandi alkaloids which, with the exception of apomorphine appeared to be specific for the glyoxaline group.

Into a 25-ml graduated flask place the pilocarpine solution containing from 1 to 4 mg of alkaloid in not more than 5 ml of 0·1N sulphuric acid. Add 1 ml of 2 per cent freshly prepared sodium nitroprusside solution and 1 ml of N sodium hydroxide and allow to stand for at least three minutes. Then add 5 ml of 0·01N potassium permanganate followed immediately by 3 ml of dilute sulphuric acid. Dilute to volume with water and measure the extinction at the maximum at about 520 mμ using matched 4-cm cells, with, in the comparison cell, a blank containing the reagents; the colour should be measured within five minutes. At the same time carry out the test on solutions containing 1, 2, 3, 4 and 5 mg of pilocarpine, together with a blank. The pilocarpine content of the sample is calculated from the calibration curve. The standard pilocarpine solution, 1 mg per ml, is prepared by making a 0·13 per cent solution of pilocarpine nitrate *B.P.*

The test was also carried out with other alkaloids of jaborandi, *iso*-pilocarpine, pilocarpidine and pilosine, to ascertain whether they are equally chromogenic with pilocarpine. With the exception of the pilosine, these were found to give the same colour as pilocarpine. Since the alkaloids present in jaborandi consist principally of pilocarpine and *iso*pilocarpine with smaller quantities of the other alkaloids, it would appear that the colorimetric method should be capable of giving reasonably accurate results in the determination of the total alkaloids of the drug calculated as pilocarpine.

Pilocarpine hydrochloride, $C_{11}H_{16}O_2N_2$,HCl, Mol. Wt. 244·7. This salt is assayed in the *U.S.P.* by non-aqueous titration.

Dissolve 0·5 g in a mixture of 20 ml of glacial acetic acid and 10 ml of a 6 per cent solution of mercuric acetate in glacial acetic acid, warming slightly to effect solution. Cool to room temperature and titrate with 0·1N perchloric acid in glacial acetic acid using crystal violet as indicator. Perform a blank titration making any necessary correction. 1 ml 0·1N = 0·02447 g.

Pilocarpine nitrate, $C_{11}H_{16}O_2N_2,HNO_3$, Mol. Wt. 271·3. There is no assay in the *B.P.* but the *U.S.P.* method is applicable.

Dissolve 0·6 g in 30 ml of glacial acetic acid, warming slightly to effect solution. Cool to room temperature and titrate potentiometrically with 0·1N perchloric acid in glacial acetic acid. 1 ml 0·1N = 0·02713 g $C_{11}H_{16}O_2N_2,HNO_3$.

Eye-drops of Pilocarpine, *B.P.C.* Contain 1·0 per cent of pilocarpine nitrate and sodium chloride in Solution for Eye-drops.

The tetraphenylboron method for determination of small quantities of bases given under Atropine (p. 116) can be applied to this preparation. To prepare the sample solution add 10 ml of buffer solution, pH 3·7, to 4 ml of sample in a 20-ml graduated flask and dilute to volume with water. 1 ml of cetylpyridinium chloride = 0·001870 g of pilocarpine nitrate.

1. *Analyst*, 1948, **73**, 311.
2. ELVIDGE, W. F., *Quart. J. Pharm.*, 1947, **20**, 234.

LACTIC ACID

$CH_3CHOH.COOH$ Mol. Wt. 90·08

The commercial quality consists of a mixture of lactic acid and its condensation products formed by loss of water on concentration. The condensation products slowly revert to lactic acid when diluted with water and easily to the lactate of the alkali when in contact with sodium hydroxide. Brindle[1] has shown that five minutes' boiling is ample to decompose the lactide, and that allowing the reaction to proceed for thirty minutes at room temperature will effect the same result. The simplest method of estimation is:

To 1 to 2 g of sample add 50 ml of 0·5N alkali, boil for five minutes and titrate the excess of alkali with 0·5N acid, using phenolphthalein as indicator. Carry out a control without the lactic acid. 1 ml 0·5N acid = 0·04504 g.

Boiling the mixture for twenty minutes as directed in the *U.S.P.* is unnecessary.

LACTATES

Only two salts of lactic acid are used to any considerable extent in pharmacy. **Calcium lactate,** $Ca(C_3H_5O_3)_2,5H_2O$, Mol. Wt. 308·3, can be assayed by a sulphated ash using 1 g, $CaSO_4 \times 2{\cdot}264$. An alternative and, in some respects, preferable method is by dissolving about 0·5 g in dilute hydrochloric acid, precipitating the calcium with ammonia after the addition of ammonium oxalate and titrating the washed precipitate with 0·1N permanganate in dilute sulphuric acid at 70°. 1 ml 0·1N = 0·01542 g; this is the *B.P.* method of assay. EDTA titration can also be used.

Dissolve 0·5 g in 50 ml of water, add 5 ml of diethylamine and sufficient methyl thymol blue mixture, prepared by grinding 0·1 g of indicator with 10 g of potassium nitrate, to impart a moderate blue colour to the solution. Titrate with 0·05M EDTA until the blue solution changes sharply to colourless. 1 ml 0·05M = 0·01542 g $C_6H_{10}O_6Ca,5H_2O$.

Calcium sodium lactate, $Ca(C_3H_5O_3)_2,2NaC_3H_5O_3,4H_2O$, Mol. Wt. 514·4, is standardised in the *B.P.C.* on its calcium and sodium contents. The calcium is determined as under calcium lactate above, 1 ml 0·1N = 0·002004 g Ca. For sodium, the ash from about 2 g is boiled with 50 ml of 0·5N hydrochloric acid, filtered, washed and back-titrated with 0·5N sodium hydroxide to methyl orange; a correction is made for the amount of 0·5N acid equivalent to the volume of 0·1N permanganate required by calcium in the weight of sample taken. 1 ml 0·5N = 0·0115 g Na.

Liversedge[2] applied Tabern and Shelberg's[3] magnesium uranyl acetate method for the determination of sodium in organic salts (see p. 28) to calcium sodium lactate, as a check on the ashing method, with good results.

Compound Injection of Sodium Lactate, *B.P.* A solution of lactic acid 0·25 per cent w/v neutralised with sodium hydroxide, containing sodium chloride 0·6 per cent, potassium chloride 0·04 per cent, and calcium chloride 0·04 per cent.

The lactic acid may be determined from the alkalinity of the ash, using bromophenol blue or, better, methyl orange, as indicator, 1 ml 0·1N = 0·009008 g $C_3H_6O_3$, calcium chloride by EDTA titration (see p. 145) and the total chlorine by the Volhard method (see p. 290).

Tablets of Calcium Lactate, *B.P.* Usually contain 5 grains. The calcium lactate can be determined by the method given above for the salt.

Tablets of Calcium Sodium Lactate, *B.P.C.* Usually contain $7\frac{1}{2}$ grains.

The calcium and sodium contents can be determined by the methods given above for the salt, preferably after removal of water-insoluble matter by filtration.

1. Brindle, H., *Quart. J. Pharm.*, 1931, **4**, 394.
2. Liversedge, S. G., *Quart. J. Pharm.*, 1937, **10**, 364.
3. Tabern, D. L., and Shelberg, E. F., *Ind. Eng. Chem., Anal. Edn.*, 1931, **3**, 278.

LEAD

Pb At. Wt. 207·19

As pharmaceutical salts, lead compounds are relatively unimportant but the estimation of traces of lead as an impurity or for toxicological work is of importance.

Lead as a major constituent may be determined gravimetrically as the sulphide or the chromate. More frequently it is determined titrimetrically, either by precipitation of lead oxalate which is then titrated with potassium permanganate or, better, by titration with EDTA. The oxalate method for lead acetate is as follows:

> Dissolve about 5 g of lead acetate in sufficient recently boiled distilled water to make exactly 100 ml. Mix 10 ml of this solution with 50 ml of 0·1N oxalic acid in a 200-ml graduated flask, shake for five minutes and make up to volume with water. Filter and collect exactly 100 ml of filtrate. To this add 10 ml of concentrated sulphuric acid and warm to about 60°, then titrate the residual oxalic acid with 0·1N potassium permanganate. 1 ml 0·1N = 0·01036 g Pb.

The end-point must be taken as the first excess of permanganate remaining for a minute or two without decolorisation, subsequent decolorisation probably being due to oxidisable impurities. Wetherell[1] preferred a smaller acid concentration to reduce the interfering action of the impurities in the liberated acetic acid and suggested the use of 25 ml of dilute sulphuric acid.

Lead may be titrated directly with EDTA at a pH of about 5 or 6 using xylenol orange as indicator. Under suitable conditions the end-point is very sharp but with materials such as lead monoxide where an excess of acid must be used to bring about solution, a rather sluggish end-point is obtained. Examples of the use of EDTA for titration of lead are given in the discussion of lead salts below.

Traces of lead were formerly invariably determined colorimetrically by precipitation of colloidal lead sulphide in alkaline solution. Since the determination is not truly colorimetric, the degree of accuracy attainable is subject to a probable error of about ± 10 per cent. Difficulty in matching is often experienced because different tints are shown by the solutions being matched when compared with a standard solution. The tint depends to a large extent on the size of the colloidal particles of lead sulphide and this is influenced by the nature and amount of salts in solution; hence this source of error is partially eliminated by making sure that the same salts are present in the comparison tube as in that under test or, better, by extracting the lead from interfering substances, particularly other metals in large amounts, by means of organic reagents.

Lead can conveniently be separated quantitatively from all other metals except bismuth, by the method of Allport and Skrimshire.[2] Diphenylthiocarbazone (dithizone) forms a metallic complex with lead, which is insoluble in water and can be extracted by organic solvents. Other metals can give a similar complex, but in most cases potassium cyanide prevents their formation. The method is of particular value in the presence of iron in quantity, which does not form a compound with the reagent.

If organic matter is present, destroy it in a suitable quantity of the material (to contain a maximum of 0·25 to 0·5 mg of lead) by wet oxidation (see Appendix XI) and free the residue from nitric acid as usual. Cool the mixture, dilute and, if free from insoluble matter, add 2 g of citric acid (which prevents precipitation of iron in ammonia and keeps lead sulphate in solution) and then make ammoniacal. Add 1 ml of 10 per cent potassium cyanide solution, transfer the liquid (100 to 150 ml) to a separator and extract three times with a solution of 0·1 per cent diphenylthiocarbazone in chloroform, using 10-, 5- and 5-ml portions. If the third extract is bright red (the lead complex gives a red chloroformic solution) continue the extraction until there is no further change in colour. Wash each of the chloroform extracts with water in another separator and evaporate. To the residue add 0·5 ml of concentrated sulphuric acid and destroy the organic matter by heating and adding a few drops of concentrated nitric acid, then dilute the solution. Add 2 g of ammonium acetate, make alkaline with ammonia and, after adding 1 ml of 10 per cent potassium cyanide solution, match an aliquot part by the sulphide method (below), using the same amount of ammonium acetate in the auxiliary solution as has been used in the aliquot of the main extraction solution.

This method is applicable in the presence of much iron and with appreciable quantities of copper, zinc, silver, mercury, manganese and chromium there is no interference. Special procedure is necessary if tin, aluminium, nickel or cobalt are present in appreciable amounts, and bismuth interferes.

The lead can be recovered from the dithizone-chloroform solution by extraction with 1 per cent nitric acid or the excess of dithizone in the extract may be removed by shaking with potassium cyanide solution and the red solution of lead complex finally compared colorimetrically with a standard.

The method outlined above is inaccurate if any insoluble matter such as calcium phosphate or calcium sulphate is present after wet oxidation, since the precipitate adsorbs the greater part of the lead; washing with ammonium acetate solution, which has been suggested, is inadequate. An important contribution was made by Roche Lynch, Slater and Osler,[3] who oppose ashing to destroy organic matter. They overcame the difficulty of adsorption of the lead in precipitates from wet oxidation by the following elegant modification:

Destroy organic matter in a suitable quantity of material by wet oxidation and free the residual liquid from nitric acid as usual. Transfer the contents of the Kjeldahl flask to a 250-ml beaker and wash out the flask with water and dilute ammonium acetate solution made faintly alkaline with ammonia solution, until the total volume reaches 50 ml. Add 25 ml of 90 per cent ethanol and allow the mixture to stand in a refrigerator overnight.

Filter the precipitate of calcium sulphate through a small Hirsch funnel and wash with a minimum volume of the acid-ethanol mixture (about 50 ml). Evaporate the filtrate to about 50 ml and reserve. Wash the precipitate back into the original beaker, using about 50 ml distilled water, heat to boiling and add 4 g of potassium carbonate in 50 ml of boiling water. After boiling the mixture, place on a water-bath for two to four hours, when conversion of calcium sulphate to calcium carbonate is complete, and the volume has been reduced to 25 to 50 ml. On cooling, filter off the calcium carbonate through the same Hirsch funnel and wash with a minimum volume of 0·5 per cent potassium carbonate solution.

Add the filtrate to the filtrate reserved above, and again evaporate to about 50 ml (*A*).

Wash back the calcium carbonate precipitate into the original beaker with distilled water, add sufficient glacial acetic acid to effect solution and drive off carbon dioxide by boiling (*B*).

Extract the two clear solutions, *A* and *B*, separately with the dithizone reagent by the Allport and Skrimshire method (above) and evaporate the chloroform extracts in the same flask.

Potassium sulphate was found to assist oxidation of the organic residue, but Roche Lynch *et al.*[3] frequently encountered difficulty in the colorimetric matching of the final solution after using nitric acid for oxidation of organic matter, a yellow colour developing in alkaline solution, which was probably due to the production of nitro-bodies which are resistant to further oxidation and which are extracted by the chloroform. Garratt[4] also experienced this difficulty, but developed the following technique to overcome it:

Warm the residues obtained after evaporation of the chloroform, with 2 ml of concentrated sulphuric acid on a water-bath for a few minutes to destroy the organic compound. Add 10 ml of 6 per cent hydrogen peroxide solution and boil the mixture until white fumes are evolved. After adding 2 g of pure ammonium persulphate, heat the flask on an asbestos gauze over a Bunsen burner for half an hour. The resulting solution is colourless and does not develop any yellow tint with ammonia.

Hamence[5] proposed a more rapid method than that of Allport and Skrimshire for the separation of traces of lead (up to 0·5 mg in 5 g of the salt) when the only interference is from iron in small quantities (say 25 mg), by removing the latter as ferric thiocyanate in an immiscible solvent:

For alkali and alkaline earth salts, dissolve 5 g of the salt in 30 ml of water in a separator. To this solution add 5 ml of 10 per cent nitric acid and 5 ml of saturated ammonium thiocyanate solution. Shake vigorously with a mixture of 15 ml of amyl alcohol and 15 ml of ether. Draw off the aqueous layer and determine the lead colorimetrically by the sulphide method. If the aqueous layer shows a pronounced red colour after extraction, it must be re-extracted with the solvent. A trace of red coloration may be ignored as it is discharged by potassium cyanide and ammonia.

In the presence of organic matter, after destruction by wet oxidation evaporate the solution until only 2 ml of acid is left. Dilute with 10 ml of water, add 2 g of lead-free ammonium acetate, make ammoniacal and then boil the solution until acid to litmus. Add concentrated nitric acid until the iron is redissolved, dilute with water to 30 ml and proceed as above.

Monier Williams[6] in an investigation on the determination of lead in foodstuffs, critically reviewed the methods available and suggested a combination of that by Allport and Skrimshire[2] using wet oxidation with sulphuric and nitric acids and that by Francis, Harvey and Buchan,[7] in which the dithizone-extracted lead is precipitated as sulphate. The latter procedure eliminates bismuth and the colour developed with ammonia from nitric acid digestion. Finally, the lead sulphate is dissolved in ammonium acetate and the lead determined colorimetrically as sulphide. The method is as follows:

After addition of citric acid to the colourless acid digestion mixture boil the solution and cool before filtering any small sediment of siliceous matter. In the presence of calcium sulphate follow the Roche Lynch, Slater and Osler technique (above). Wash the siliceous precipitate thoroughly with hot 1 : 1 hydrochloric acid and neutralise the total aqueous solutions to litmus paper with strong ammonia solution added from a burette in quantities of 0·5 ml at a time, and then add 0·5 ml in excess. Without delay follow the extraction method of Allport and Skrimshire until the colourless sulphuric acid digestion of the evaporated dithizone is obtained in about 0·5 ml of acid. Then reheat the acid with 5 ml of water until white fumes again appear, mix the residue with 15 ml of a mixture of 1 part of dehydrated ethanol and 2 parts of water and set the tube aside overnight. The next day, whether any precipitate is visible or not, filter the solution through a 5 cm Whatman filter (No. 44) which has been washed with hot 1 : 1 hydrochloric acid and hot water just before use. Wash the residue three times with a few ml of a mixture of 20 ml of water, 10 ml of ethanol and 1 ml of concentrated sulphuric acid. Dissolve the lead sulphate by boiling 10 ml of 10 per cent ammonium acetate solution in the tube in which the precipitation was carried out, and passing the hot solution through the filter. Repeat this operation, the same 10 ml of solution being again boiled and passed through the filter. Finally wash the filter three times with about 5 ml of hot water containing a little ammonium acetate. Continue with the colour matching as sulphide as given below using 10 ml of 10 per cent ammonium acetate solution in the control and 1·5 ml of strong ammonia solution and 1 ml of 10 per cent potassium cyanide solution in both the test and control.

If 0·02 mg of lead is present in 15 ml of ethanolic sulphuric acid a small but distinctly visible sediment of lead sulphate is produced on standing for twelve hours. There is a slight loss of lead owing to the solubility of lead sulphate in aqueous ethanol. Under the conditions of the experiment this is not more than about 1 p.p.m. working on 5 g, and is cancelled out when the control test colour is subtracted except in those rare cases in which the control test shows none.

A Sub-Committee of the Analytical Methods Committee of the *S.A.C.*[8] has recommended a method for the determination of lead. All the precautions against contamination normal in this type of work must be observed as follows:

(*a*) Borosilicate glass or silica should be used in the determination and the reagents must be stored in borosilicate glass or polythene bottles.

(*b*) The reagents must be free from lead. Nitric, sulphuric, hydrochloric and perchloric acids and ammonium hydroxide containing not more than 0·005 p.p.m. of lead are available commercially and potassium cyanide and citric acid containing not more than 0·5 p.p.m. of lead can be obtained. Some reagents can be freed from lead by washing with dithizone solution.

(*c*) Particular attention must be paid to the possibility of dust contamination during a determination.

(*d*) All water must be de-ionised or distilled and be free from lead.

The recommended method is as follows:

Destroy the organic matter in an amount of sample containing not more than 40 μg of lead by a suitable procedure (see Appendix XI). The methods generally suitable when lead is to be determined are:

(*a*) Dry ashing, with or without an ashing aid, at a temperature not exceeding 500°.

(*b*) Oxidation with nitric and perchloric acids.

(*c*) Oxidation with nitric and sulphuric acids. It should be noted that the use of sulphuric acid is to be avoided when appreciable amounts of calcium are present and dry ashing should be avoided in the presence of large amounts of chloride.

Preliminary treatment of sample

(*a*) If the organic matter has been destroyed by wet decomposition—Allow the contents of the Kjeldahl flask to cool, and add 5 ml of water.

If the solution is free from insoluble matter, transfer it to a 100-ml conical flask, rinsing with two 1-ml quantities of water. Place 10 ml of 5M hydrochloric acid in the Kjeldahl flask, boil gently for five minutes, swirl vigorously to wash the sides of the flask, and drain the acid into the conical flask. Finally, wash out the Kjeldahl flask with two 1-ml quantities of water.

If the contents of the Kjeldahl flask contain insoluble deposit or suspended matter, however small in amount, filter the solution and washings through a 7-cm Whatman No. 1 filter-paper. If possible, retain any deposit in the Kjeldahl flask until it has been boiled with 5M hydrochloric acid, and pass the hot acid also through the filter.

If the organic matter has been destroyed by an appropriate method, the amount of insoluble matter remaining should not be so great as to cause significant loss of lead through adsorption or occlusion. Any such difficulty is also minimised by restricting the amount of the sample.

(*b*) If the organic matter has been destroyed by dry ashing—Add 5 ml of water and 10 ml of 5M hydrochloric acid to the ash in the silica or platinum basin, and boil gently for five minutes. Transfer the solution to a 100-ml conical flask, and filter if insoluble matter is present, as described in (*a*) above.

Separation of Lead

Reagents:

I Chloroform. Shake 250 ml of chloroform with 25 ml of water containing 1 ml of 10 per cent potassium cyanide solution and about 20 drops of 5M ammonium hydroxide, separate and reject the aqueous layer, wash the chloroform with water and filter.

II Dithizone working solution. Shake 6 ml of a 0·1 per cent solution of diphenylthiocarbazone (dithizone) in chloroform (that has been filtered and stored in a refrigerator) with 9 ml of water and 1 ml of 5M ammonium hydroxide. Separate and reject the lower layer and spin the aqueous layer in a centrifuge until clear. Prepare this solution freshly on the day of use.

III Carbamate reagent. Dissolve 1 g of pure crystalline diethylammonium diethyldithiocarbamate in 100 ml of redistilled chloroform and store in an amber-coloured bottle. This solution is not stable and should be discarded after one week.

Method A (for samples in which the concentration of calcium, magnesium and phosphate are not high). Cool the solution and add 5 ml of 25 per cent ammonium citrate solution and 10 ml of 10 per cent sodium hexametaphosphate solution. Add a few drops of thymol blue indicator and sufficient strong ammonia solution to give the blue-green colour indicating pH 9·0 to 9·5. Cool, add 1 ml of 10 per cent potassium cyanide solution (prepared at least two days before use so that any traces of sulphide present may become oxidised) and, if much iron is present, add 1 ml of 20 per cent hydroxylamine hydrochloride solution. Transfer the solution to a 100-ml separator containing 10 ml of chloroform (I) and rinse with a few millilitres of water. The volume of the aqueous layer at this stage should be approximately 50 ml. Add 0·5 ml of dithizone working solution (II), shake vigorously for one minute and allow to separate. If the lower layer is red, add dithizone working solution until, after shaking, a purple, blue or green colour is obtained. Run the chloroform layer into a second separator and wash through with 1 or 2 ml of chloroform (I). Add to the liquid in the first separator 3 ml of chloroform (I) and 0·2 ml of dithizone working solution. Shake vigorously for thirty seconds, allow the chloroform layer to separate, and add it to the main chloroform extract. This last chloroform extract should be green. If it is not, further extractions with chloroform and dithizone must be made until the green colour of the final extract indicates that all the lead has been extracted. Reject the aqueous layer. Add 10 ml of a 1 per cent v/v solution of concentrated nitric acid in water to the combined chloroform extracts, and shake vigorously for one minute. Allow to separate and reject the chloroform layer as completely as possible.

Method B (for samples with a high content of calcium, magnesium and phosphate). To the solution obtained by one of the methods described under 'Preliminary treatment of sample' add 2 drops of methyl red indicator and make just alkaline with strong ammonia solution. Make the solution just acid with 5M hydrochloric acid, and add a further 10 ml. Warm the solution to 50° to 70°, add 2 ml of 20 per cent sodium iodide solution and reduce any liberated iodine with 2 ml of freshly prepared 1·25 per cent sodium metabisulphite solution, that has been filtered before use. Cool the solution, transfer it to a separator and adjust the volume to 50 to 75 ml in order to bring the acid concentration to N with respect to hydrochloric acid. Add 10 ml of carbamate reagent (III) by pipette and shake the separator vigorously for thirty seconds. Allow the layers to separate and transfer the chloroform layer to a 100-ml flask. Wash the aqueous layer twice with small amounts of chloroform (I) without mixing, and add these washings to the flask. Repeat the extraction with 10 ml of carbamate reagent (III) and add the second extract to the main extract. Reject the aqueous layer.

To the combined extracts add 2·0 ml of diluted sulphuric acid (1 + 1) and evaporate the chloroform. Add 0·5 ml of 60 per cent w/w perchloric acid to the residual solution, and heat until fumes are evolved and the fuming solution is clear and colourless. Cool the solution, add 10 ml of water and 5 ml of 5M hydrochloric acid, boil for one minute, cool, and then add 2 ml of 25 per cent ammonium citrate solution.

Continue as in Method A, beginning with 'Add a few drops of thymol blue indicator. . . .'.

Determination of Lead. To the nitric acid layer left in the separator add 30 ml of ammoniacal sulphite/cyanide solution (prepared by mixing 340 ml of strong ammonia solution, 75 ml of 2 per cent w/v anhydrous sodium sulphite solution, 30 ml of 10 per cent potassium cyanide solution and 605 ml of water; the concentrations of these reagents are critical). Then add exactly 10 ml of chloroform (I) and 0·5 ml of dithizone working solution (II), shake vigorously for one minute and allow to settle. Run off a little of the chloroform layer. Insert a plug of cotton wool into the dry stem of the separator and, after rejecting the first runnings, fill a 1-cm spectrophotometer cell with the chloroform solution.

At the same time carry out a blank determination on all the reagents, omitting only the sample.

Measure the extinctions at 520 mμ of the test and blank solutions against chloroform (I) (all in 1-cm cells). Read the number of microgrammes of lead equivalent to the observed extinctions from a standard curve and so obtain the net measure of lead in the sample.

Prepare the standard curve as follows: Measure, into separators, 0, 1·0, 2·0, 3·0 and 4·0 ml of standard lead solution [prepared by dissolving 1·60 g of lead nitrate in water and adding 10 ml of concentrated nitric acid and sufficient water to produce 1 litre (= 1·0 mg of lead per ml) and diluting this 100 times just before use so that 1 ml of diluted solution contains 10 μg of lead]. Dilute the contents of each separator to 10 ml with a 1 per cent v/v solution of concentrated nitric acid in water and proceed as described above under 'Determination of Lead'. Measure the extinctions with chloroform (I) in the comparison cell and prepare a curve relating the extinctions to the number of microgrammes of lead.

Bismuth is liable to interfere in the above method. An extinction measurement at 490 mμ as well as at 520 mμ may be useful in deciding whether bismuth interference is considerable. It has been found that, with a solution of pure lead dithizonate, the extinction at 490 mμ is approximately 0·84 times that at 520 mμ; with a solution of pure bismuth dithizonate, the extinction at 490 mμ is approximately 1·20 times that at 520 mμ. When considerable bismuth interference is indicated, the modified procedure given below should be used.

Prepare the digest from the wet decomposition or the ash in the silica or platinum basin, as described above under 'Preliminary treatment of sample'.

If the organic matter has been destroyed by wet decomposition—Add to the contents of the flask 6·0 ml of concentrated hydrochloric acid and transfer the solution to a 50-ml graduated separator. Rinse the conical flask with several 1-ml quantities of water and add the rinsings to the separator. The volume of the contents of the separator must not exceed 35 ml in order that the hydrochloric acid concentration may be not less than 3N (see Note).

Extract the acid solution directly in the cold first with 10 ml and then with 5 ml of carbamate reagent (III) shaking for thirty seconds each time; separate and discard the lower (chloroform) layer. Finally, shake the acid layer with 5 ml of chloroform (I) for ten to fifteen seconds, and discard the chloroform layer. Transfer the acid layer to a 100-ml conical flask, rinse the separator with a few millilitres of water, and add the rinsings to the conical flask.

Proceed as in Method A or Method B.

If the organic matter has been destroyed by dry ashing—Add 15 ml of concentrated hydrochloric acid, transfer to a 50-ml graduated separator and adjust the volume of the solution to a maximum of 35 ml in order that the hydrochloric acid concentration may be approximately 6N (see Note). Continue as described above from 'Extract the acid solution . . .'.

Note: After wet decomposition, the extraction solution consists of the residual sulphuric acid to which hydrochloric acid has been added; the acidity of the solution should not be less than 3N in sulphuric acid and 3N in hydrochloric acid.

When the organic matter has been destroyed by dry ashing, the extraction solution consists of hydrochloric acid alone, and the acidity must be raised to about 6N in hydrochloric acid to effect quantitative separation of bismuth and other elements from lead.

By whatever method the lead has been isolated, traces are generally determined for pharmaceutical purposes by matching the colour of the lead sulphide produced in alkaline solution by adding a few drops of a sodium sulphide solution. Iron and copper, even in traces, will interfere but the addition of potassium cyanide in ammoniacal solution inhibits the formation of the sulphides of these metals by converting them into complex cyanides. The iron present must be small in quantity and must be in the ferrous state (Wilkie[9]), obtained by boiling the acid solution with a crystal of potassium metabisulphite. It is essential that no precipitate or turbidity should develop in the solution being examined because lead salts are easily adsorbed (Roche Lynch, Slater and Osler[3]); filtration is not permissible if the turbidity is due to precipitation after solution, but clearing from particulate matter is necessary. The presence of aluminium salts, calcium and magnesium phosphates causes turbidity in alkaline solution, but calcium phosphate can be held in solution by the addition of ammonium citrate (Nicholls[10]). The disturbing effect of aluminium and magnesium salts in the absence of phosphate is also avoided by the addition of this reagent.

This method, elaborated by Hill,[11] is used by the *B.P.* (Appendix VII) as a limit test and is upset by only a few interfering substances; in many cases direct determination of the lead is possible after suitable solution in ammonia or ammonium acetate.

As previously noted, the same amounts of reagents used must be present in both solutions under comparison, not only to eliminate errors due to lead in the reagents but also to avoid errors from a difference in the tints of the solutions being matched. The standard lead solution is prepared by dissolving 0·16 g of pure lead nitrate in 5 ml of concentrated nitric acid, adding water to 100 ml (= 1·0 mg of lead per ml) and diluting this 100 times just before use so that 1 ml of diluted solution contains 0·01 mg of lead. The quantity of solution under test used for matching should, in order to obtain the most accurate comparison, be such that from 4 to 6 ml of standard lead solution is required. Although the standard lead solution may be added gradually to the control after the sulphide, until the colours are matched, the test should be repeated by adding the whole of the standard lead solution required before adding the sulphide.

LEAD SALTS

The determination of lead by chromate precipitation is usually adopted for official salts, but titration of the oxalate by the general method given on p. 369 can be used. For chromate precipitation:

> Dissolve about 0·25 g in a mixture of 1·5 ml of glacial acetic acid and 100 ml of water. Heat on a water-bath at 85° with 5 ml of 10 per cent potassium chromate solution for half an hour. Filter on a Gooch crucible, wash until colourless and dry at 120° to constant weight.

Lead acetate, $(CH_3COO)_2Pb,3H_2O$, Mol. Wt. 379·4, 1 g $PbCrO_4$ = 1·174 g, 1 ml 0·1N oxalic acid = 0·01897 g; **lead monoxide,** PbO, Mol. Wt. 223·2, 1 g $PbCrO_4$ = 0·6906 g, 1 ml 0·1N oxalic acid = 0·01116 g. For the oxalate precipitation method the lead monoxide is dissolved in 2 ml of acetic acid before diluting with 50 ml of water and proceeding as for lead acetate.

For EDTA titration:

> Dissolve 0·8 g of lead acetate in a mixture of 2 ml of 33 per cent w/w acetic acid and 100 ml of water. Add 5 g of hexamine and titrate with

0·05M EDTA, using 0·2 ml of a 0·1 per cent solution of xylenol orange as indicator until the colour becomes yellow. 1 ml 0·05M = 0·01897 g $C_4H_6O_4Pb,3H_2O$.

Dissolve 0·5 g of lead monoxide in 3 ml of 33 per cent acetic acid and 10 ml of water with gentle heat. Cool, dilute to 100 ml with water and complete as for lead acetate after adding 5 g of hexamine. 1 ml 0·05M = 0·01116 g PbO.

Lead arsenate, $PbHAsO_4$, Mol. Wt. 347·1, is officially assayed in the *B.Vet.C.* for lead content by precipitation as sulphate, which is appreciably less soluble in ethanolic sulphuric acid and is the basis of a method for the precipitation of traces of lead from solution described above.

Assay for PbO: Mix 0·5 g with 25 ml of a mixture of one volume of concentrated nitric acid and three volumes of water and digest on a water-bath until solution is complete. Filter and wash the filter with water until the washings are free from acid. To the combined filtrate and washings add 5 ml of concentrated sulphuric acid and evaporate on a sand-bath until white fumes are evolved. Cool, add 10 ml of water and again evaporate to fuming. Cool, add a mixture of 25 ml of 95 per cent ethanol and 25 ml of water and allow to stand for thirty minutes. Filter through a sintered-glass crucible (G4), wash the filter with 95 per cent ethanol until the washings are free from acid and dry the residue to constant weight at 105°. 1 g residue = 0·07360 g PbO.

The arsenic content is determined by the method of Fitzgibbon given under arsenic (p. 93).

Strong Solution of Lead Subacetate, *B.P.*

The total lead and alkalinity can be determined in a single procedure by a slight modification of the method of Berry:[12]

Place about 1 g in a 250-ml graduated flask, dilute with 50 ml of recently boiled distilled water and add 50 ml of 0·1N oxalic acid. Shake for five minutes, dilute to volume with water and filter.

To 100 ml of the filtrate, add 25 ml of dilute sulphuric acid, warm to 70° and titrate the residual oxalic acid with 0·1N potassium permanganate, maintaining the temperature at about 70° throughout the titration. 1 ml 0·1N = 0·01036 g total lead.

To another 100-ml aliquot of the filtrate, add 4 drops of 0·2 per cent phenolphthalein solution as indicator and titrate with 0·1N sodium hydroxide. Subtract the number of ml of 0·1N sodium hydroxide from 20. Each ml of the remainder = 0·01116 g of PbO.

For lead, the EDTA titration given under lead acetate is also satisfactory using about 2 g. 1 ml 0·05M = 0·01036 g Pb. The alkalinity must then be done on a separate portion of the sample by precipitation with oxalic acid as above.

Dilute Solution of Lead Subacetate, *B.P.* A 1 : 80 dilution of the strong solution with water.

Determine the lead and alkalinity as above, using 50 ml of the solution.

1. Wetherell, S., *Quart. J. Pharm.*, 1934, **7,** 459.
2. Allport, N. L., and Skrimshire, G. H., *Analyst*, 1932, **57,** 440.
3. Roche Lynch, G., Slater, R. H., and Osler, T. G., *Analyst*, 1934, **59,** 787.
4. Garratt, D. C., *Analyst*, 1935, **60,** 817.
5. Hamence, J. H., *Analyst*, 1932, **57,** 622.
6. Monier Williams, G. W., Public Health and Medical Subjects, No. 88. Lead in Food, H.M.S.O.
7. Francis, A. G., Harvey, C. O., and Buchan, J. L., *Analyst*, 1929, **54,** 725.
8. *Analyst*, 1959, **84,** 127.
9. Wilkie, J. M., *J. Soc. Chem. Ind.*, 1909, **28,** 636.
10. Nicholls, J. R., *Analyst*, 1931, **56,** 594.
11. Hill, C. A., *C. & D.*, 1905, **66,** 388.
12. Berry, P. A., *Chem. Eng. Mining Rev.*, 1930, **22,** 421.

LEPTAZOL

$C_6H_{10}N_4$ Mol. Wt. 138·2

Leptazol, or 1,5-pentamethylenetetrazole, can be extracted from aqueous solution saturated with ammonium sulphate by solvents such as chloroform or carbon tetrachloride but it has a low melting-point (57° to 60°) and is appreciably volatile at 100°, less so at room temperature. It forms complexes with many inorganic salts, some having relatively low solubilities. A method of assay for solutions using mercuric chloride has been proposed by Horsley;[1] as the solubility of the leptazol complex in 3·5 per cent mercuric chloride was found to be of the order of 0·01 per cent to 0·02 per cent and allowance for the precipitate is necessary, a method of using two dilutions is employed:

Into two 50-ml graduated flasks deliver respectively 2·0 and 0·5 ml of the unknown leptazol solution (5 to 15 per cent) at 20°, using a 2·0 ml microburette. To each flask add, from a burette, 35 ml of 5 per cent mercuric chloride solution. Make up each flask to the mark with distilled water, stopper, shake well and allow to stand with occasional shaking for at least three hours. Filter through dry 9-cm No. 30 Whatman filter papers into a 100-ml conical flasks, rejecting the first 5 to 10 ml of filtrate. From each filtrate pipette 10 ml into each of two iodine flasks of not less than 250 ml capacity, making four estimations in all.

Add 75 ml of distilled water and 10 ml of 10 per cent potassium iodide solution with swirling. The solution should give a precipitate redissolving in excess. Add 3 ml of formaldehyde solution followed, with swirling, by 15 ml of 20 per cent sodium hydroxide solution and continue to swirl for two minutes. Then add 10 ml of glacial acetic acid followed by 50 ml of 0·1N iodine from a pipette. Stopper and shake vigorously so that the mercury becomes well dispersed and dissolves rapidly. When all the mercury has dissolved, titrate the excess of iodine with 0·1N sodium thiosulphate, using starch solution as indicator. If *A* and *B* represent the titrations of a 2·0 ml and a 0·5 ml sample, respectively, then $A - B$ represents 1·5 ml of sample. 1 ml 0·1N I = 0·00691 g.

High concentrations of alkali halides interfere with this method. The mercuric chloride complex is not volatile at 100° and can be dried at this temperature without loss.

Sharp[2] employed the cuprous complex, which is more satisfactory because it is less soluble, and his method has been adopted in principle by the *B.P.* Further to Sharp's work, however, it has been shown that if analytical reagent grade cuprous chloride is used results are erratic and tend to be low but if freshly prepared cuprous chloride with a very low cupric content is employed results are much more reproducible. This effect cannot be ascribed solely to the presence of cupric ions and it is possible that some formation of oxychloride may affect the assay. It is essential that pure cuprous chloride which has been stored in sealed ampoules should be used, and that the reagent solution should be prepared immediately before use. The freshly prepared reagent solution is almost colourless and has a pH of about 3·3, but after only four hours' storage in a stoppered vessel the solution becomes straw coloured and the pH falls to about 2·0. The method of assay is as follows:

Dissolve 50 g of copper sulphate in 100 ml of water and add 200 ml of hydrochloric acid and 25 g of copper. Boil the mixture gently until the dark colour disappears and the liquid becomes clear. Pour into 2,000 ml of water containing sulphur dioxide, allow the white precipitate to settle and wash several times by decantation with water containing sulphur dioxide. Filter through a sintered-glass filter, wash with dehydrated ethanol and then with ether, taking care to draw only the minimum quantity of air through the solid. Dry the residue at 100° with frequent stirring until the ether is completely removed, transfer the product to ampoules and seal immediately.

Dissolve about 0·1 g of sample in 25 ml of water and add slowly with stirring, 25·0 ml of cuprous chloride solution (prepared by dissolving 1·25 g of cuprous chloride, removed from the sealed container immediately before use, in 100 ml of 10 per cent ammonium chloride solution containing 1 g of sodium metabisulphite). Stopper the flask and allow to stand for three hours with occasional shaking. Filter through a sintered-glass crucible (No. 3) and wash the precipitate and flask with 30 ml of water containing 1 per cent of glacial acetic acid. To the filtrate and washings add 10 ml of hydrogen peroxide solution and, if necessary, a few drops of dilute sulphuric acid to clarify the solution. After effervescence has ceased, boil for ten minutes to decompose the excess of hydrogen peroxide. Cool, add ammonia solution drop by drop to obtain an opalescence and clear by the addition, drop by drop, of acetic acid. Add 5 g of potassium iodide, titrate with 0·1N sodium thiosulphate until the liquid is pale brown, add mucilage of starch and 3 g of ammonium thiocyanate and continue the titration until the colour is discharged. Repeat the determination with 25·0 ml of cuprous chloride solution, omitting the sample. The difference between the two titrations is equivalent to the amount of copper present in the precipitate. 1 ml 0·1N sodium thiosulphate = 0·007891 g $C_6H_{10}N_4$.

The Kjeldahl nitrogen determination cannot be applied to leptazol. Low results (down to only 50 per cent) are obtained, presumably due to a loss of gaseous nitrogen when the tetrazole ring is broken open in the early stages of digestion.

Injection of Leptazol, *B.P.* Contains 10 per cent w/v of leptazol and 0·25 per cent of sodium phosphate in water for injection.

The above methods of assay are applicable to the injection.

1. Horsley, T. E. V., *Analyst*, 1946, **71**, 308.
2. Sharp, L. K., *J. Pharm. Pharmacol.*, 1952, **4**, 52.

LIQUORICE

Liquorice root contains a number of sugars, starch, gums and glycyrrhizin (the calcium and potassium salts of glycyrrhizic acid) in widely varying proportions. These proportions are too diverse for standards to be laid down, and the *B.P.* limits its quantitative requirements to water-soluble extractive, ash and acid-insoluble ash. For the water-soluble extractive the powdered root should be macerated for twenty-four hours with a measured volume of chloroform water before being filtered, and an aliquot part evaporated and dried.

A considerable amount of liquorice is sold as **liquorice juice,** which is an aqueous extract of the juice from the root, filtered and evaporated to a nearly solid consistency. Adulteration is frequent, mainly with starch and sugar, but it is difficult to judge sophistication as the constituents vary so widely according to the country of origin.

The following, mainly due to Parry,[1] is a combination of what are probably the most widely applied methods of analysis:

(*a*) Moisture. By drying at 100° to constant weight; varies up to 15 per cent.

(*b*) Mineral matter. By ashing, usually 4 to 7 per cent.

(*c*) Water-soluble matter.

Dissolve 5 g, after powdering, in hot water and transfer to a 500-ml graduated flask. Cool and make up to 500 ml, shake well and allow to stand for thirty-six hours. Pipette off an aliquot part (50 ml) of the clear supernatant liquid, evaporate in a tared dish and weigh.

About 70 to 75 per cent for Anatolian juices but somewhat less for Calabrian and Spanish.

(*d*) Gums and starches.

Weigh about 2·5 g in a 250-ml flask. Add 15 ml of hot water, cover with a watch-glass and stand the flask on a water-bath until the juice has dissolved, shaking frequently. Add 25 ml of 80 per cent ethanol, shake well and then add 50 ml of 95 per cent ethanol. Allow to settle and filter through a tared Gooch crucible containing a filter-paper mat, washing with 80 per cent ethanol until the washings are colourless; dry and weigh.

The figure obtained will include insoluble matter other than gums and starches. Block juice contains 20 to 30 per cent, but stick liquorice may contain considerably more.

(*e*) Crude glycyrrhizin. A large number of modifications have been published for the accurate determination of glycyrrhizin, but as the isolated substance is impure, since a little ammonium sulphate is present in the weighed residue and glycyrrhizic acid is appreciably soluble in water, an approximation is all that can be expected.

Transfer the filtrate and washings from (*d*) above to a dish and evaporate the ethanol. Evaporate further to a syrup and transfer to a 50-ml stoppered cylinder, washing in with water up to 30 ml. Add 3 ml of 10 per cent sulphuric acid slowly with constant shaking. Allow to stand overnight at a temperature of about 15° and then decant the supernatant liquid into a filter; wash the precipitate two or three times with ice-cold water and pass the washings through the filter. Dissolve the residue in the cylinder and on the filter in a little dilute ethanol, adding 2 or 3 drops of ammonia solution to neutralise the acid. Evaporate to dryness in a tared dish and weigh.

The glycyrrhizin may vary from 6 to 20 per cent.

(*f*) Sugars, before and after inversion.

To the filtrate and washings from (*e*) above, add 3 ml of basic lead acetate solution to precipitate sulphuric acid, colouring matter, etc., and remove the excess of lead by ammonium sulphate solution. Dilute to 100 ml after filtering and determine the sugars before and after inversion by Lane and Eynon's method (see Sugars).

For a normal edible juice the total sugars should not exceed 18 per cent, of which not more than 1 to 2 per cent should be cane sugar.

If added starch is suspected, the residue insoluble in cold water should be extracted with 3 per cent ammonia solution. The residual starch should not be more than 6 per cent and should not differ in appearance under the microscope from natural liquorice starch.

It should be noted that with preparations and prescriptions containing liquorice allowance must be made for the relatively high potassium and ammonia content of the extract.

1. Parry, E. J., *C. & D.*, 1910, **76**, 21; 1911, **78**, 625.

LOBELIA

Lobelia has a limited and decreasing use in pharmacy; it contains alkaloids, principally lobeline, but formerly it was not considered necessary to assay it for its alkaloidal content and consequently few methods have been published. However, the requirements of the Poisons Rules, by which the total alkaloid content of certain lobelia preparations has to be declared, re-awakened interest in its assay. Markwell[1] proposed a method which, with small modifications, was adopted by the Analytical Methods Committee of the *S.A.C.*[2] The method, which is essentially that official in the *B.P.C.*, is as follows:

Introduce 10 g of the lobelia in No. 60 powder and 10 g of ignited sand into a pear-shaped separator provided with a plug of cotton wool in the tube below the stopcock. Add 75 ml of a mixture of 4 volumes of ether and 1 volume of 95 per cent ethanol. Shake and set aside for fifteen minutes, add 5 ml of dilute ammonia solution and shake in a mechanical shaker for one hour or by hand for one minute at ten-minute intervals during one hour. Allow the liquid to percolate into another separating funnel. When the liquid ceases to flow, pack the drug firmly by means of a button-ended glass rod. Continue the percolation, first with 25 ml of the ether-95 per cent ethanol mixture and then with ether, until the alkaloid is completely extracted, as shown by testing in the usual manner.

To the percolate add 30 ml of N sulphuric acid; shake well and allow to separate. Run off the lower layer into another separator and repeat the extraction with a mixture of 25 ml of 0·5N sulphuric acid and 5 ml of ethanol. Run off the lower layer and repeat with three further quantities of 20 ml of the acid-ethanol mixture or until the alkaloids are completely extracted. Wash the mixed acid solutions, first with 10 ml and then with two successive quantities of 5 ml of chloroform, washing each chloroformic solution with the same 20 ml of 0·5N sulphuric acid contained in another separator. Reject the chloroform, transfer the acid liquid from the second separator to the first separator, neutralise to litmus with dilute ammonia solution and add a further 5 ml in excess.

Extract the alkaloids by shaking with successive quantities of 10 ml of chloroform. Combine the chloroform solutions and wash with 3 ml of water. Filter the chloroform solution through a 7-cm filter paper into a flask, wash the filter thoroughly with more chloroform and collect the washings in the flask. Distil the chloroform from a water-bath until about 2 ml remain, add 2 ml of dehydrated ethanol and continue the evaporation on the water-bath, using a gentle air-blast to complete the process. Repeat with two further portions of dehydrated ethanol, and heat the residue for one hour at 80°.

Add to the residue 2 ml of ethanol and warm until dissolved. Add 10 ml of 0·02N sulphuric acid, cool and titrate with 0·02N sodium hydroxide or sodium borate solution, using methyl red as indicator. 1 ml of 0·02N sulphuric acid = 0·00675 g of the alkaloids of lobelia calculated as lobeline.

Hydrochloric acid cannot be used in place of sulphuric acid, since lobeline hydrochloride is extracted from aqueous solution by chloroform.

Ethereal Tincture of Lobelia, *B.P.C.* This is prepared by percolation of lobelia with Spirit of Ether and the method of assay is the following:

To 50 ml add 50 ml of ether and extract with 15 ml of 0·5N sulphuric acid. Repeat the extraction with successive quantities, each of a mixture of 10 ml of 0·5N sulphuric acid and 5 ml of 95 per cent ethanol, until extraction is complete. Combine the extracts and wash with three successive 5 ml quantities of chloroform, washing each chloroform extract with the same 20 ml of 0·5N sulphuric acid. Discard the chloroform and make the combined acid extract and washings alkaline to litmus paper with dilute ammonia solution. Extract the alkaloids by shaking with successive quantities, each of 10 ml of chloroform. Combine the chloroform solutions and wash with 3 ml of water; discard the washing. Filter the chloroform solution, wash the filter with chloroform and evaporate the combined filtrate and washings on a water-bath until about 2 ml remain. Add three successive quantities, each of 2 ml, of dry ethanol, evaporating to dryness on the water-bath after each addition, and dry the residue for one hour at 80°. Dissolve the residue in 2 ml of warm neutral 95 per cent ethanol, add 5 ml of 0·05N hydrochloric acid and 10 ml of water, cool, and titrate the excess acid with 0·05N sodium hydroxide using methyl red and methylene blue solution as indicator. 1 ml 0·05N = 0·0169 g $C_{22}H_{27}O_2N$.

Although this assay can be improved by adding 5 ml of water during the first extraction, difficulty often occurs when washing the acid extracts with chloroform owing to the similarity in the weight per ml of the two layers and it not being apparent which is the wash layer. The following modification is recommended:

Pipette 50 ml into a separator, add 100 ml of ether and extract, first with 20 ml of 0·5N sulphuric acid and then with 15-ml quantities of a mixture of three volumes of 0·1N sulphuric acid and one volume of 95 per cent ethanol until extraction is complete. Combine the extracts and wash successively with 10, 5 and 5 ml of chloroform, extracting each washing with the same 20 ml of 0·1N sulphuric acid. Combine this acid layer with the acid extracts, make alkaline to litmus paper with dilute ammonia solution and complete as above from 'Extract the alkaloids . . .'.

Methyl red is a suitable indicator for the titration of the alkaloidal residue.

LOBELINE HYDROCHLORIDE, $C_{22}H_{27}O_2N,HCl$. Mol. Wt. 373·9

In water lobeline hydrochloride has an absorption maximum at 249 mμ, E(1 per cent, 1 cm) = 375. This maximum is suitable for use for its determination when mixed with various bacteriostats (see p. 519).

The base is volatile.

Injection of Lobeline Hydrochloride, *B.P.C.* This is a sterile solution of lobeline hydrochloride, usually 0·3 per cent, in water for injection.

The simplest method of assay is by ultra-violet absorption.

Dilute 4 ml of injection solution to 100 ml in water. Dilute 10 ml of this solution to 100 ml in water. Measure the maximum extinction of a 1-cm layer at about 249 mμ using water as blank. Calculate the amount of lobeline hydrochloride in each ml of injection.

A chemical method of assay is based on precipitation of the alkaloid with silicotungstic acid similar to the method for nicotine.

To 5 ml add 10 ml of a 5 per cent w/v solution of silicotungstic acid in water; allow to stand overnight. Collect the precipitate, wash with N hydrochloric acid until the washings yield no reaction with a 1 per cent w/v solution of quininc hydrochloride in water. Dry at 80° for one hour, ignite, cool, re-ignite with a few drops of nitric acid and weigh. 1 g of residue = 0·4598 g lobeline hydrochloride.

The tetraphenylboron method for determination of small quantities of bases given under Atropine (p. 116) can be applied to lobeline. For this preparation dilute 5 ml with 5 ml of buffer solution, pH 3·7, and use this solution to precipitate with the reagent. 1 ml of cetylpyridinium chloride = 0·001870 g.

1. Markwell, W. A. N., *Pharm. J.*, 1936, **136**, 617.
2. *Analyst*, 1939, **64**, 581.

LONCHOCARPUS

Lonchocarpus, or cubé root, is the dried roots of *Lonchocarpus utilis*, A. C. Smith, *L. uruca*, Killip and Smith, and possibly other species of *Lonchocarpus*. It contains a toxic substance, **rotenone,** $C_{23}H_{22}O_6$, Mol. Wt. 394·4 in varying amounts. Derris root, the original source of rotenone is no longer the article of commerce, little being available.

Although much published work tends to show that the uncrystallised resin from the root is almost as toxic as rotenone itself, the assay for the latter is generally undertaken.

The method for the determination of rotenone adopted as official by the *A.O.A.C.* was based on the work of Jones and Graham[1] and that included in the *B.Vet.C.* 1953 is a modification of the *A.O.A.C.* method proposed by Coomber, Martin and Harper.[2] These methods were in general use for some time, but widely divergent results were obtained in different laboratories. A joint committee of the Pharmaceutical Society and the Society for Analytical Chemistry[3] reviewed available methods and in particular considered the work of Martin[4] which had been overlooked for many years. Martin showed that the phenolic and emulsifying constituents of derris extract could be removed by washing with alkali. When this was done the subsequent crystallisation of rotenone from carbon tetrachloride was found to be much more satisfactory. The panel also examined an alternative procedure to the polarimetric method of determining the purity of the isolated rotenone. This alternative was a spectrophotometric method based on the work of Payfer.[5] Unsatisfactory results were obtained in collaborative trials, however, and the polarimetric method was adopted. The method finally recommended for ground lonchocarpus root is as follows:

Place 30 g of the well-mixed sample, ground to pass through a 30-mesh B.S. sieve, in a 500-ml flask fitted with a ground-glass stopper. Add 300 ml of chloroform, measured at a definite temperature, replace the stopper and shake mechanically for four to five hours. Set the flask aside overnight and shake it for thirty minutes next morning.

Filter the solution through a fluted fast filter paper, covering the top of the funnel to prevent loss of solvent, and collect 200 ml of filtrate (measured at the temperature at which the original 300 ml of chloroform were measured). Transfer the solution to a 500-ml flask, and evaporate to dryness. Dissolve the residue in 100 ml of a mixture of equal volumes of benzene and ether.

Transfer the solution to a pear-shaped 500-ml separator with a further 20 ml of the benzene-ether mixture and cautiously add 50 ml of 2 per cent potassium hydroxide solution, pouring the solution down the sides of the separator. Carefully turn the separator to a horizontal position, gently rotate it about six times, taking care to avoid emulsification, and carefully return the separator to the vertical position. Remove the alkaline layer as rapidly as possible by running it into a second separator containing 40 ml of the benzene-ether mixture. To carry out this separation rapidly it may be necessary to run off only the clear aqueous portion, leaving in the separator any trace of emulsion. The tendency to emulsify is markedly less in the later washings.

Carry out a second rapid extraction, with 50 ml of 5 per cent potassium hydroxide solution; use an increased degree of agitation, but still take care to avoid emulsification. Repeat the extraction with vigorous shaking, using a further 50 ml of 5 per cent potassium hydroxide solution, and run each alkaline layer into the second separator. Immediately after the third extraction, add 50 ml of water to the main benzene-ether solution and shake gently to reduce the concentration of any residual potassium hydroxide.

The whole extraction procedure should not take more than thirty minutes.

Gently shake the second separator, discard the aqueous liquid and transfer the benzene-ether layer to the first separator.

To the contents of the first separator add N hydrochloric acid, drop-wise, shaking after each addition, until the solution is just acid to litmus paper, allow to separate and discard the aqueous layer. Wash the benzene-ether solution with three successive quantities, each of 25 ml, of water, allowing effective drainage after each washing, and discard the washings. Run the benzene-ether solution into a flask through a layer of powdered, anhydrous sodium sulphate (about 10 to 15 g) supported in a filter funnel on a plug of cotton wool. Wash the separator and then the sodium sulphate with 25 to 30 ml of the benzene-ether mixture. Evaporate the solvent with the aid of gentle heat and reduced pressure. Dissolve the residue in 15 ml of hot carbon tetrachloride, evaporate under reduced pressure, again dissolve the residue in 15 ml of hot carbon tetrachloride, re-evaporate and dry the residue under reduced pressure for ten minutes.

Add 15 ml of carbon tetrachloride saturated with pure rotenone at 0° (see Note below), swirl the flask in ice-water to induce crystallisation and allow to stand at about 0° overnight.

Filter through a tared, sintered-glass filter (porosity No. 3) previously cooled to 0° and rapidly wash the crystals with three successive quantities, each of 5 ml, of ice-cold carbon tetrachloride saturated with pure rotenone at 0°. Maintain suction for about five minutes, dry the residue at 40° for one hour and weigh.

Remove the crystals from the crucible, mix well and prepare, accurately, a 4 per cent solution in benzene (analytical-reagent grade). Measure the optical rotation at 20° in a 1-dm tube.

Calculate the percentage of rotenone in the root from the formula, $(16{\cdot}26 \times W_1 \times \alpha)/W$, where W is the weight of sample taken, W_1 is the weight of residue and α is the observed optical rotation.

Note. Prepare the saturated solution of rotenone in carbon tetrachloride by dissolving 2·72 g of pure rotenone in hot carbon tetrachloride, cooling and making up to 1 litre at 0°. Prepare the pure rotenone by purifying a quantity of the carbon tetrachloride complex by first triturating it with cold dry ethanol, converting the rotenone thus liberated into complex again, dissolving in hot dry ethanol, and allowing the rotenone to crystallise out.

An empirical colorimetric method for the determination of rotenone in formulations when present in amounts of the order of 1 or 2 per cent has been standardised by the joint committee of the Pharmaceutical Society and the Society for Analytical Chemistry.[6] It can be of value for routine checking of manufacture but is not recommended for accurate assessment.

Standard Rotenone Solution. A 0·01 per cent w/v solution of purified rotenone in acetone. This should be prepared as required by suitable dilution of a 0·5 per cent w/v solution of purified rotenone in acetone which may be stored in the dark for not more than fourteen days.

Estimation of Extract Content. Dilute the sample with acetone so that the final solution contains about 0·01 per cent of extract. Run 1 ml of this solution into a 25-ml conical flask containing 10 ml of concentrated sulphuric acid containing 0·01 per cent of sodium nitrite at approximately 20°. Immediately place the flask in a water-bath maintained at 40° for fifteen minutes whereupon a reddish-purple colour develops. Transfer the flask to a water-bath at 20° for a period of five minutes and match the colour thirty minutes after the initial mixing of the acetone solution and the acid, against the colour developed by 1 ml of standard rotenone solution, which has been similarly treated. Prepare a 'blank' by heating and cooling 1 ml of acetone with 10 ml of the sulphuric/nitrous acid solution.

Record the extinctions of the standard (E) and sample solutions (E_1) at 540 mμ. The amount of extract (x) in the dilute solution is given by the expression:—

$$x = \frac{E_1}{E} \times 0{\cdot}01 \times 1{\cdot}1$$

From a knowledge of the dilution rates employed, the equivalent amount of extract (D) in the sample may readily be calculated.

Estimation of Rotenone Content. Dilute the sample with acetone so that the final solution contains about 0·02 per cent of extract. Pipette 1 ml of this solution into a dry 25-ml Erlenmeyer flask and add 1 ml of acetone. Add 2 ml of freshly prepared alkaline sodium nitrite solution, (one volume of 40 per cent w/v potassium hydroxide solution and seven volumes of 0·1 per cent sodium nitrite in 95 per cent ethanol), and place the flask in a water-bath at 20°. After seven minutes, add 5 ml of 25 per cent v/v sulphuric acid solution, stopper, shake sufficiently to mix, and return the flask at once to the water-bath. The bluish-red colour which develops reaches a maximum after fifteen minutes and is then stable for about one hour.

Similarly treat 1 ml of standard rotenone solution, and a 'blank' of 2 ml of acetone.

Record the extinctions of both the standard (E_2) and the sample (E_3) at 540 mμ. The measurements should be made within thirty minutes. The total rotenoids in the final dilution from the sample (y) is given by the expression:

$$y = \frac{E_3}{E_2} \times 0{\cdot}01$$

From a knowledge of the dilution rates employed, the quantity of total rotenoids in the original sample may readily be calculated. If this value be denoted by r, and D is the percentage of extract in the sample, then the percentage of true rotenone (R) in the sample is given by the formula:

$$R = r - \frac{23D}{100}$$

The flasks used in the test must be scrupulously clean before use, as both tests are very sensitive, and the slightest trace of organic matter will be detrimental to the development of the colours. The ethanolic solution of sodium nitrite is best prepared by dissolving it in a minimum of water before dilution with ethanol and should be kept in the dark. The mixing of the alkaline sodium nitrite solution can be done in a measuring cylinder.

1. Jones, H. A., and Graham, J. J. T., *J.A.O.A.C.*, 1938, **21,** 148.
2. Coomber, H. E., Martin, J. T., and Harper, S. H., *J. Soc. Chem. Ind.*, 1942, **61,** 110.
3. *Analyst*, 1959, **84,** 735.
4. Martin, J. T., *Ann. Appl. Biol.*, 1940, **27,** 274.
5. Payfer, R., *J.A.O.A.C.*, 1954, **37,** 630.
6. *Analyst*, 1961, **86,** 748.

MAGNESIUM

Mg At. Wt. 24·31

The classical method for the determination of magnesium by precipitation as magnesium ammonium phosphate and ignition to pyrophosphate has been largely replaced in pharmaceutical work by the use of EDTA. However, it is still of sufficient importance to justify inclusion. Epperson[1] showed that the optimum conditions for precipitation were obtained in cold solution and that the precipitation required exactly defined conditions. The following procedure was recommended.

To the weakly acid or neutral solution of magnesium chloride containing the equivalent of not more than 0·1 g of MgO, add 5 ml of concentrated hydrochloric acid and methyl red as indicator. Dilute the solution to 150 ml and add 10 ml (or a five or tenfold excess) of the precipitant, preferably as a saturated solution of diammonium hydrogen phosphate. Then add dilute ammonia solution slowly, while stirring, to neutralisation. Stir for about five minutes or until the precipitate of magnesium ammonium phosphate is well formed and then add 5 ml excess of ammonia water, stirring for ten minutes. Allow to stand for at least four hours (preferably overnight), filter and wash with water containing 3 to 5 per cent by volume of dilute ammonia solution. Dissolve the precipitate by washing the filter with warm 1 : 9 hydrochloric acid (sp. gr. 1·02). Add methyl red and about 1 ml of saturated ammonium phosphate solution and proceed as before, but in a volume of 100 to 150 ml. In this precipitation, standing for four hours is sufficient. Place the wet filter paper and precipitate in a platinum crucible and char without flaming, then ignite at a low temperature (approximately 500°) until the residue is white and finally at about 1,000° to constant weight.

If the residues for magnesium determination have been obtained during the course of separation of the alkaline earths, it is advisable to eliminate an excess of ammonium oxalate by evaporating the solution to dryness in the presence of nitric acid and heating to volatilise most of the ammonium salts, finally dissolving the residue in a minimum of hydrochloric acid and filtering before precipitating as above.

For work where extreme accuracy is not required the precipitate may be weighed as magnesium ammonium phosphate hexahydrate. In this modification, which provides a much more rapid result than the ignition method, the ammonia-washed precipitate, collected in a sintered-glass crucible, is washed with three 10-ml portions of 95 per cent ethanol followed by five portions, each of 5 ml, of ether. The precipitate is dried by drawing air through the crucible for ten minutes, followed by leaving for twenty minutes in a desiccator, and weighed as $MgNH_4PO_4,6H_2O$.

EDTA is now extensively used for the determination of magnesium in salts and preparations. The titration is usually carried out at pH 10 using solochrome black as indicator and a detailed method is given below for magnesium sulphate; when certain other elements are present, such as aluminium, a masking agent may be required to allow individual determination of the magnesium. The use of such masking agents is discussed in Appendix II. When calcium is also present it is not possible to determine the magnesium independently; the total magnesium and calcium is determined at pH 10 and the calcium alone is determined under more alkaline conditions (see p. 145). The magnesium is then calculated by difference.

Flame photometric determination cannot be recommended except for solutions containing upwards of 10 p.p.m. of magnesium because the resonance line occurs at 2852 A in the middle of an intense OH molecular band system and correction for this background is difficult even when a recording spectrophotometer is used. A hot flame is required and it has been reported by Knutson[2] that some increase in sensitivity is obtained if an oxy-acetylene flame containing 55 per cent by volume of acetylene is used instead of the stoichiometric level of 29 per cent by volume. The resonance line suffers no serious spectral interference from other elements present in the sample solution but aluminium, chromium and molybdenum cause varying degrees of depression. Silicate, phosphate and sulphur ions depress the emission seriously and other anions less seriously and so standards should be made up to contain the same acids in the same concentrations as the samples.

The atomic absorption technique provides one of the most sensitive and convenient methods of determining magnesium in solution. Allan,[3] David[4] and Willis[5] have shown that a sensitivity limit of about 0·1 p.p.m. can be reached and there is little difficulty in determining 1 p.p.m. or even less. The only serious interferences are from silicate, phosphate, aluminium and sulphate but these are eliminated according to David if calcium (or presumably any other alkaline earth element) is present in the solution.

The Analytical Methods Committee of the *S.A.C.*[6] has described a method for the determination of **traces** of magnesium, based on the method of Hunter.[7] In this method, after destruction of organic matter, the magnesium is complexed with Titan Yellow and the excess dye is extracted from the reaction mixture and determined spectrophotometrically. The method is generally applicable but zinc, if present in quantities greater than 10 per cent of the magnesium content, interferes and should be removed. Aluminium, cadmium, cobalt and nickel interfere also. The recommended procedure is as follows:

Reagents:

Calcium compensating reagent. Dissolve 0·5 g of analytical-reagent grade calcium carbonate in 1 litre of a 10 per cent v/v solution of concentrated hydrochloric acid in water.

Tartrate reagent. Dissolve, separately, 10 g of sodium hydrogen tartrate ($NaHC_4H_4O_6,H_2O$), 2·5 g of hydrazine sulphate and 10 g of mannitol, in water, mix the three solutions and dilute to 1 litre with water.

Titan Yellow solution. Dissolve 0·03 g of Titan Yellow (B.D.H. 'Spot Test' reagent) in 100 ml of water and add 1 drop of 15 per cent sodium hydroxide solution. The grade of dye is important—inferior dyes give limited light extinction ranges.

Method: Destroy the organic matter in the sample by a suitable method (see Appendix XI) and dilute the acid solution with a 10 per cent v/v solution of concentrated hydrochloric acid in water, so that 1 ml contains not more than 20 μg of magnesium. To 5 ml of the resultant solution add 5 ml of calcium compensating reagent and 5 ml of 1·5 per cent oxalic acid solution and then add 15 per cent sodium hydroxide solution until the pH is between 4 and 5. Mix well, allow to stand for one hour and then add 5 ml of tartrate reagent followed by 2·5 ml of Titan Yellow solution. Mix with vigorous shaking, make alkaline by the addition of 20 ml of 15 per cent sodium hydroxide solution, re-mix and allow to stand overnight. Extract the excess dye by shaking the mixture vigorously with 50 ml of a mixture of three volumes of *n*-butanol and two volumes of dehydrated ethanol, allow to stand for thirty minutes and then filter the alcoholic layer into a flask containing 0·5 ml of acetone. Mix the contents of the flask and measure the extinction relative to a blank solution at 495 mμ within thirty minutes.

Read the amount of magnesium equivalent to the extinction from a standard curve prepared by carrying out the entire operation described above on suitable aliquots of a standard magnesium solution covering the range 0 to 100 μg of magnesium. As a check, one or two standards should be taken through the procedure each time a sample is assayed.

MAGNESIUM SALTS

Magnesium oxide, MgO, Mol. Wt. 40·32. No assay is included in the *B.P.* but magnesium oxide may be determined by solution of a known weight in excess of 0·5N acid and back-titration to methyl orange. 1 ml 0·5N = 0·01008 g MgO. The *U.S.P.* requires the percentage of calcium oxide found by precipitation to be deducted from the total alkalinity.

The calcium may be determined approximately, but with sufficient accuracy for the purpose, by the method of Evers[8] who devised a roughly quantitative test for the determination of calcium in the presence of large proportions of magnesium such as in magnesium salts.

Dissolve 0·2 g to 0·4 g of the oxide in 25 ml of 25 per cent w/w sulphuric acid and 50 ml of 95 per cent ethanol. Allow to stand overnight, filter and wash the precipitate with a mixture of two volumes of ethanol and one volume of 25 per cent sulphuric acid, ignite and weigh as calcium sulphate.

The results are slightly low since calcium sulphate has a small solubility in the solution but a correction allowance of 3 mg for these quantities of reagents gives a more accurate determination.

Calcium may also be determined by flame photometry (see p. 146), or by using glyoxal-bis-hydroxyanil (see p. 152).

Magnesium carbonate, is a hydrated basic magnesium carbonate of indefinite composition; the light variety corresponds approximately with the formula, $3MgCO_3,Mg(OH)_2,3H_2O$, whilst the heavy carbonate is nearer $3MgCO_3,Mg(OH)_2,4H_2O$. It is assayed in the *B.P.* by direct ignition to oxide but often contains a somewhat smaller residue than the *B.P.* minimum allowance, and in calculating the proportion of magnesium carbonate in mixtures from the magnesium oxide figure, the lower limit should be used.

The equivalent total oxide may be determined by solution in excess of standard acid and back-titration to methyl orange. 1 ml N = 0·02016 g MgO.

Conformable with the assay of magnesium oxide, the *U.S.P.* directs the calcium oxide found to be deducted from the total alkalinity before calculating the magnesium oxide content. The calcium content may be determined by the methods discussed under magnesium oxide. For the Evers' method about 1 g of sample is used.

Magnesium sulphate, $MgSO_4,7H_2O$, Mol. Wt. 246·5. Assayed for its magnesium content either by precipitation as magnesium ammonium phosphate, followed by ignition of the precipitate, $Mg_2P_2O_7 \times 1{\cdot}082 = MgSO_4$, or by dissolving 0·4 g in 50 ml of water, adding 10 ml of ammonia buffer solution and titrating with 0·05M EDTA using solochrome black indicator, 1 ml 0·05M = 0·006019 g $MgSO_4$. **Dried magnesium sulphate** is assayed by the same methods using about half the amount of sample.

Magnesium hydroxide, $Mg(OH)_2$, Mol. Wt. 58·34. This can be assayed simply on its alkalinity by dissolving in excess of N acid and back-titrating to methyl orange. 1 ml N = 0·02917 g $Mg(OH)_2$.

Magnesium trisilicate. Hydrated magnesium silicate of approximate composition $2MgO,3SiO_2$, containing water of crystallisation. The *B.P.* assay is by classical methods.

For silica: Heat 0·5 g with concentrated hydrochloric acid for about three hours, maintaining the liquid just below the boiling-point and replacing the acid lost by evaporation. Evaporate to dryness, heat the residue for two hours at 105° and then on a water-bath for ten minutes with a mixture of 10 ml of concentrated hydrochloric acid and 10 ml of water. Dilute with an equal volume of water, filter, transfer the residue to the filter and wash with water until free from chloride. Recover any dissolved silica from the mixed filtrate and washings by evaporation to dryness on a water-bath, heating the residue for two hours at 105° and then on a water-bath for ten minutes with 20 ml of a mixture of equal volumes of concentrated hydrochloric acid and water, diluting with an equal volume of water, transferring the insoluble matter to a filter and washing with water until free from chloride. Dry and ignite the two filter papers and their contents to constant weight and weigh the residue of crude silica. Moisten the residue with five drops of concentrated sulphuric acid and 15 ml of 40 per cent w/w hydrofluoric acid, heat cautiously on a sand-bath until all the acid has been driven off and ignite to constant weight at a temperature not lower than 1,000°. Deduct the weight of the residue from the weight of crude silica; the difference is the weight of pure SiO_2.

For MgO: Adjust the volume of the combined filtrate and washings obtained in the assay for silica to 150 ml and complete by precipitation as magnesium ammonium phosphate, followed by ignition of the precipitate. $Mg_2P_2O_7 \times 0{\cdot}3623 = MgO$.

The following more rapid method was described by Hobson and Stephenson[9] and is very satisfactory.

Heat 0·5 g in a beaker with 5 ml of water and 10 ml of 60 per cent w/w perchloric acid until dense white fumes are evolved. Cover the beaker with a watch-glass and continue to heat for a further three hours. Allow to cool, add 30 ml of water, filter and wash the filter with 200 ml of hot water. Cool the filtrate and washings and dilute to 250 ml with water.

For SiO_2: Dry the filter paper and its contents and ignite to constant weight. Treat the residue (crude silica) by the procedure given in the method above.

For MgO: To a 100-ml aliquot of the filtrate and washings add 10 ml of ammonia buffer solution and titrate with 0·05M EDTA using solochrome black as indicator. 1 ml 0·05M = 0·002016 g MgO.

Magnesium stearate is a compound of magnesium with variable proportions of stearic and palmitic acids. The magnesium content may be determined by the following method:

Ignite 2 g in a silica dish, gently until all the fat has burned and then at about 800° to a white ash. Dissolve in 10 ml dilute hydrochloric acid, heating on a water-bath to assist solution. Dilute to 100 ml with water. To 20 ml add 10 ml of ammonia buffer solution and titrate immediately with 0·05M EDTA using solochrome black indicator. 1 ml 0·05M = 0·002016 g MgO.

Mixture of Kaolin, *B.P.C.* Contains approximately 13·7 per cent of light kaolin and 4·6 per cent each of magnesium carbonate and sodium bicarbonate in peppermint water.

For assay of the ingredients see under Compound Powder of Magnesium Carbonate, adjusting the quantities taken proportionately to the formula.

Mixture of Magnesium Carbonate, *B.P.C.* Contains approximately 4·6 per cent of magnesium carbonate and 6·9 per cent of sodium bicarbonate.

The sodium bicarbonate can be determined on 25 ml by the method given under Compound Powder of Magnesium Carbonate and the magnesium by solution of a portion of the mixture in dilute hydrochloric acid, completing as under that preparation.

A rapid determination of the magnesium carbonate is by direct ignition of the insoluble residue from the sodium bicarbonate assay to magnesium oxide.

Aromatic Mixture of Magnesium Carbonate, *B.P.C.* Contains approximately 2·3 per cent of magnesium carbonate and 4·6 per cent of sodium bicarbonate.

The assay follows the method given under Mixture of Magnesium Carbonate.

Mixture of Magnesium Hydroxide, *B.P.* (Cream of Magnesia). An aqueous suspension of hydrated magnesium oxide.

For assay:

To 40 ml of water in a 50-ml measuring cylinder, add 10 ml of suspension in such a manner that it is not allowed to touch the sides of the cylinder above the 50 ml mark. Wash into a flask, add 50 ml of N sulphuric acid or sufficient to dissolve the hydroxide completely. Titrate the excess of acid with N sodium hydroxide, using methyl orange as indicator. 1 ml N = 0·02917 g $Mg(OH)_2$.

Duplicate determinations should be made and the results averaged.

Although this preparation is made on a w/v basis, its standardisation would be more accurate if it were done w/w.

This preparation is subject to bacterial contamination, particularly of water-borne types including the genus *Pseudomonas*, and the growth of such organisms can give rise to off-odours and off-flavours. In order to avoid this, a preservative such as chloroform should be added.

Mixture of Magnesium Sulphate, *B.P.C.* (*Mist. Alba*). A suspension of light magnesium carbonate in a solution of magnesium sulphate in peppermint water.

This preparation is most conveniently standardised by weight and a rapid assay for both soluble and insoluble magnesium is as follows:

For magnesium sulphate: Boil 1·2 g with 25 ml of water and 25 ml of 95 per cent ethanol, cool, filter and wash with 50 per cent ethanol until the washings are free from sulphate. (Retain the residue for the determination of magnesium carbonate.) Determine the magnesium in the filtrate and washings by the EDTA method given under Magnesium Sulphate above, 1 ml 0·05M = 0·01232 g $MgSO_4,7H_2O$.

For magnesium carbonate: Dissolve the residue retained above in 10 ml N hydrochloric acid and wash the filter with successive small quantities of water until the washings are free from chloride. Titrate the combined filtrate and washings as above. 1 ml 0·05M = 0·001216 g Mg.

Compound Mixture of Rhubarb, *B.P.C.* Contains approximately 4·6 per cent each of magnesium carbonate and sodium bicarbonate.

For assay evaporate 25 ml of the mixture to dryness, ignite the residue and continue for sodium bicarbonate as under Compound Powder of Magnesium Carbonate. For magnesium a correction is necessary for the loss in the alkaline filtrate.

Dissolve the residue obtained in the determination of sodium bicarbonate in the minimum volume of dilute hydrochloric acid and dilute to 100 ml with water. To 10 ml add 200 ml of water and neutralise to methyl orange-xylene cyanol with dilute ammonia solution. Add 20 ml of ammonia buffer solution and titrate with 0·05M EDTA using solochrome black. The volume of 0·05M EDTA plus one tenth the volume of 0·05M EDTA required in the sodium bicarbonate determination represents the amount of Mg present. 1 ml 0·05M = 0·001216 g Mg.

Compound Mixture of Rhubarb for Infants, *B.P.C.* Contains approximately 2·3 per cent each of magnesium carbonate and sodium bicarbonate.

The assay is the same as given under Compound Mixture of Rhubarb using 50 ml of the mixture.

Paste of Magnesium Sulphate, *B.P.C.* Consists of 45 per cent of dried magnesium sulphate and 0·5 per cent of phenol in glycerin.

The magnesium sulphate can be determined directly by the EDTA method given under Magnesium Sulphate, taking 10 ml of a solution of 5 g of the sample in 100 ml of water.

For determination of phenol see p. 517.

Compound Powder of Kaolin, *B.P.C.* Consists of 3 parts of light kaolin, 2 parts of heavy magnesium carbonate and 1 part of sodium bicarbonate. For assay of the ingredients see Compound Powder of Magnesium Carbonate below, adjusting the quantities used proportionally to the formula.

Compound Powder of Magnesium Carbonate, *B.P.C.* Consists of 33·3 per cent each of magnesium carbonate and calcium carbonate and 25 per cent of sodium bicarbonate with light kaolin.

In such a mixture there is a tendency for some magnesium to go into solution as magnesium bicarbonate when the soluble alkali is being determined. The present official method tries to allow for this but an obviously better method is to determine the magnesium in solution and subtract it.

For sodium bicarbonate: To 1·5 g add 80 ml of water and boil for five minutes. Filter with the aid of suction, transfer the residue to a beaker, add 100 ml of water and again boil for five minutes. Filter and titrate the combined filtrates with 0·5N hydrochloric acid using methyl orange-xylene cyanol as indicator. To the titrated liquid add 10 ml of ammonia buffer solution and titrate with 0·05M EDTA using solochrome black as indicator. From the ml 0·5N hydrochloric acid required in the first titration, subtract one fifth of the ml 0·05M EDTA required in the second titration and calculate the sodium bicarbonate content from the difference. 1 ml 0·5N HCl = 0·04201 g $NaHCO_3$.

For kaolin: Heat about 2 g with 5 ml of water and an excess of dilute hydrochloric acid, filter through a Gooch or sintered-glass filter and wash, retaining the filtrate and washings for the determination of magnesium. Dry to constant weight at 105°. It is inadvisable to ignite kaolin as water of combination is lost and low results are obtained.

Calcium carbonate and magnesium can be determined complexometrically by the method given under Compound Mixture of Calcium Carbonate for Infants (p. 154) using 1 g of the sample.

Compound Powder of Magnesium Trisilicate, *B.P.C.* Consists of equal parts of magnesium trisilicate, magnesium carbonate, calcium carbonate and sodium bicarbonate.

The sodium bicarbonate can be determined by the method given under Compound Powder of Magnesium Carbonate using 25 g.

Since a variable amount of magnesium from magnesium trisilicate may be dissolved by dilute hydrochloric acid, the determination of both magnesium and calcium in preparations by titration with EDTA is not satisfactory. However, the calcium can be separately titrated (see p. 145).

MAGNESIUM

Compound Powder of Rhubarb, *B.P.* (Gregory's Powder). Contains 65 per cent of magnesium carbonate, 25 per cent of rhubarb and 10 per cent of ginger.

The magnesium carbonate is determined by igniting about 2 g in a silica dish, dissolving the residue in the minimum volume of dilute hydrochloric acid and diluting to 100 ml with water. 10 ml of this dilution is titrated with 0·05M EDTA as above.

The 45 per cent alcohol-soluble extract should be determined to show whether exhausted drugs have been used; it should be about 10 per cent.

Compound Tablets of Magnesium Carbonate, *B.P.C.* Each tablet contains 3 grains each of heavy magnesium carbonate and calcium carbonate, 2 grains of sodium bicarbonate and 1 grain each of light kaolin and ginger.

For sodium bicarbonate: To 1 g of powdered tablets, add 100 ml of water and heat at 50° for five minutes. Filter, transfer the residue to a beaker, add 100 ml of water and again heat at 50° for five minutes. Filter, cool and complete as for Compound Powder of Magnesium Carbonate above, beginning with the words 'titrate the combined filtrates . . .'.

The calcium and magnesium contents are determined as Compound Mixture of Calcium Carbonate for Infants, p. 154, using 1 g.

Compound Tablets of Magnesium Trisilicate, *B.P.C.* Each tablet contains 4 grains of magnesium trisilicate and 2 grains of dried aluminium hydroxide gel with peppermint oil.

Weigh and powder 20 tablets and determine the average weight per tablet. To an accurately weighed quantity of the powder equivalent to about 4 tablets add 7 ml of concentrated hydrochloric acid and dissolve as completely as possible by heating on a water-bath for about five minutes, avoiding excessive charring. Add 50 ml of water, filter, wash the residue with hot water and dilute the combined filtrate and washings to 100 ml with water. Use aliquot portions of this solution for the determination of aluminium and magnesium.

For aluminium: Neutralise 25 ml of the prepared solution to congo red paper with 20 per cent sodium hydroxide solution and add 75 ml of water and 50 ml of 0·05M EDTA. Mix, heat on a water-bath for thirty minutes and cool. Complete as given under Aluminium Hydroxide Gel (p. 33). 1 ml 0·05M = 0·002549 g Al_2O_3.

For magnesium: To 25 ml of the prepared solution add 1 g of ammonium chloride, swirl to dissolve and then add sufficient triethanolamine to dissolve the precipitate that first forms. Without delay, dilute to about 200 ml with water and add 5 ml of ammonia buffer solution and sufficient solochrome black indicator to give a good red colour. Titrate immediately with 0·05M EDTA to the formation of a full blue colour. 1 ml 0·05M = 0·002016 g MgO.

1. Epperson, A. W., *J. Amer. Chem. Soc.*, 1928, **50**, 321.
2. Knutson, K. E., *Analyst*, 1957, **82**, 241.
3. Allan, J. E., *Analyst*, 1958, **83**, 466.
4. David, D. J., *Analyst*, 1960, **85**, 495.

5. WILLIS, J. B., *Spectrochim. Acta* 1960, **16,** 259 and 273.
6. Determination of Trace Elements, *S.A.C.*, p. 24.
7. HUNTER, J. G., *Analyst,* 1950, **75,** 91.
8. EVERS, N., *Analyst,* 1931, **56,** 293.
9. HOBSON, F., and STEPHENSON, W. H., *Analyst,* 1959, **84,** 520.

MALE FERN

Male fern is standardised by exhaustion of the drug with ether and after evaporation to low bulk, continuing the assay on the extract. The proportion of oleoresin present may be determined by weighing the non-volatile residue from the percolate.

Extract of Male Fern, *B.P.* Contains 22 per cent of crude filicin. The *B.P.* determination is outlined below.

> Dissolve 1·0 g of well-mixed sample in 20 ml of ether and transfer to a separator with a further 20 ml of ether. Add 50 ml of 3 per cent barium hydroxide solution, shake vigorously for five minutes and allow to separate. Filter the aqueous layer, wash the ether layer with two 5-ml quantities of water and filter the washings through the same filter paper, adding them to the previous filtrate. Acidify with concentrated hydrochloric acid and extract with four successive quantities of 30, 20, 15 and 10 ml of chloroform. Combine the chloroform extracts, add 2 g of anhydrous sodium sulphate, shake and filter. Wash the sodium sulphate and filter with two 5-ml quantities of chloroform, adding the washings to the main chloroform solution. Evaporate the chloroform and dry the residue of filicin to constant weight at 100°.

The *U.S.P.* method is similar except that ether is used for the final extraction. The large amount taken, 3 g, may give rise to difficulties in manipulation and a limit of two hours drying at 105° is insufficient.

Capsules of Male Fern Extract, *B.P.* Usually contain 15 minims. The assay is as given under Extract of Male Fern, on material expressed from the shells.

EXTRACT OF MALT

Extract of malt is obtained by concentrating the aqueous extract of malted barley under reduced pressure; it may contain not more than 33 per cent of malted grain of wheat. It is a variable product containing maltose, dextrin, dextrose, other carbohydrates in small proportions and diastase.

The pharmacopœial material, used as a vehicle for cod-liver oil, must be prepared at such a temperature that the enzyme activity is destroyed.

For many commercial purposes a high diastatic activity is necessary. The minimum diastatic activity of a sample of malt extract may be measured by its ability to digest a definite minimum weight of starch to sugars in a prescribed time. A suitable method is described in the *N.F.*, the essential details of which are:

Determine the percentage of moisture in potato starch by drying about 0·5 g, accurately weighed, at 120° for four hours. Mix a quantity of the starch, equivalent to 5 g of dried starch, in a beaker with 10 ml of cold water. Add 140 ml of boiling water, and heat on a water-bath with constant stirring for two minutes, or until a translucent, uniform paste is obtained. Cool to 40°, add 20 ml of a fresh solution of extract of malt at 40°, prepared by dissolving 5 g of extract of malt in sufficient water to make 100 ml of solution at 40° (taking care not to heat the malt solution much above that temperature otherwise activity is destroyed). Mix well, and maintain at 40° for exactly thirty minutes, stirring frequently. A thin, nearly clear liquid should be produced. Add at once 0·1 ml of this liquid to a mixture of 0·2 ml of 0·1N iodine and 60 ml of water; no blue or red colour (the latter due to dextrins) develops in the mixture, showing that the extract of malt is capable of converting not less than five times its weight of starch into water-soluble sugars in thirty minutes.

For a more precise determination of diastatic activity the Lintner process modified by Ling[1] is probably the most widely applied method. This measures the amount of malt extract which, after acting on a starch solution under standard conditions, will exactly reduce a definite quantity of Fehling's solution.

It is very difficult to get concordant results between the various modifications suggested and even when using the same method serious discrepancies are observed unless the process under consideration is followed strictly in detail. In reporting the strengths of commercial samples the method used should always be stated.

Of the published methods that prescribed by the Agricultural Produce Regulations, 1933,[2] is recommended; only specially prepared soluble starch should be used for the test. Sufficient detail is given to eliminate the divergencies in results arising from the use of methods in which the conditions are less precisely standardised. It is essential that the following detailed instructions be *rigidly* followed:

Soluble Starch. Digest purified potato starch with dilute hydrochloric acid of sp. gr. 1·04 (in the proportion of 1 lb of starch to 1 litre of dilute acid) at a temperature not exceeding 20° for seven days, well shaking the mixture daily. Thoroughly wash the starch by decantation, first with tap water until the washings react only faintly acid, and then four times with distilled water. Weigh about 20 g of the well-mixed sludge, dissolve in 200 ml of boiling water and neutralise with 0·1N sodium hydroxide, using 2 or 3 drops of alizarin cream as indicator. Add to the remaining weighed starch sludge the calculated amount of 0·1N sodium hydroxide just to neutralise its acidity, shake thoroughly and set aside for twelve hours. Wash by decantation three times with distilled water, collect the soluble starch on a paper in a Büchner funnel and drain as far as possible by suction. Transfer to new unglazed porous plates and dry at a moderate temperature (40° to 45°) as quickly as possible. When the moisture content has been reduced to about 15 per cent, grind the soluble starch in a porcelain mortar and rub through a fine hair sieve.

Soluble Starch Solution. Rub 20 g of soluble starch into a cream with water and pour into about 700 ml of boiling water.

Bring to the boil, continue heating for a further two minutes, then cool to about 20°, shaking frequently to prevent the formation of a skin. Add 20 ml of acetate buffer solution (see below) and dilute to 1 litre with water. (10 ml of this solution should not reduce 0·1 ml of Fehling's solution.)

Fresh soluble starch solution is to be made for each day's determinations, uniform conditions of preparation being maintained as far as possible.

Acetate Buffer Solution. 1 litre to contain 68 g of sodium acetate ($CH_3COONa,3H_2O$) and 500 ml of N acetic acid.

Malt Extract (Syrup) Solution. 5 per cent solution. Weigh 10 g of extract in a porcelain basin and break down with cold water. (On no account must heat be used to assist in weighing or bringing into solution.) Transfer the solution to a 200-ml graduated flask, dilute to the mark at 15° and shake well. Weaker solutions, also made up at 15°, are prepared from this. The solutions must not be filtered and are to be used as soon as possible for starch conversion.

Malt Extract (Flour) Solution. 5 per cent solution. Weigh 10 g of flour into a beaker, add 200 ml of water at 15° and thoroughly stir the mixture. Cover and digest for three hours in a water-bath at 21°, stirring at intervals of half an hour. At the end of three hours filter through a good quality filter paper. Reject the first 25 ml of filtrate and, if the remainder of the filtrate is not quite bright, re-pass it through the paper. This solution, or weaker solutions prepared from it, is to be used as soon as possible for starch conversion.

Method of Starch Conversion. Measure 100 ml of soluble starch solution into a 200-ml graduated flask and immerse, suitably supported, in a water-bath maintained at 21°. Place a standardised thermometer in the flask and when the contents have reached 21° add, by means of a narrow-bore pipette (N.P.L. Standard), a definite volume of the malt extract solution, measured at 15°. The volume needed will depend upon the diastatic activity of the extract and will be about

$$\frac{80}{\text{diastatic activity of the sample}}$$ ml of 5 per cent solution and should not normally exceed 10 ml or correspondingly larger volumes of 2·5 or 1 per cent solutions. Mix well, maintain the contents of the flask at 21° for *exactly* one hour. Then add 20 ml of 0·1N sodium hydroxide and mix immediately, care being taken to wash down the thermometer and also to allow the alkali to flow over the inner surface of the neck of the flask. Cool the solution to 15°, dilute to 200 ml with water and shake well. This solution is referred to in the method of titration as *the conversion solution.*

Method of Titration. Measure from a burette into a 200-ml round-bottomed flask 5 ml of Fehling's solution (see below) and heat over a naked flame with continuous rotation of the flask until the solution boils.

Run from a burette into the boiling liquid 5 ml of the conversion liquid and subsequently further quantities. After each addition boil the liquid, the flask being continuously rotated. When the blue colour of the copper solution has nearly disappeared add 0·2 ml of 1 per cent aqueous solution of methylene blue. Continue the titration with small quantities of the conversion solution, say 0·05 to 0·1 ml, or drop by drop, until the blue colour of the indicator just disappears. (*Note.* The indicator is not added until the end-point is nearly reached as the final change is very rapid. The complete decolorisation of the methylene blue is indicated by the whole reaction liquid, in which the precipitated cuprous oxide is continually being churned up, becoming bright red or orange in colour. To ensure that the end-point has been reached, hold the flask against a sheet of white paper and if the indicator is completely decolorised there will be no blue tint at the edge of the liquid. The boiling process must be sufficiently continuous to prevent air obtaining access to the flask and so causing oxidation of the indicator with re-appearance of the blue colour.)

If the volume of the conversion solution used to reduce 5 ml of Fehling's solution is less than 20 ml or more than 25 ml, the conversion must be repeated, using less or greater quantities of the malt extract solution, in order to obtain a titration between these limits. If the extract solutions have become aerated in any way or subjected to warm conditions, it will be necessary to re-weigh and carry out the dilutions again.

A first titration to obtain approximate results is to be followed by a second, and third if necessary, to establish the end-point accurately. A confirmatory titration should be carried out in every case.

Fehling's Solution. Measure accurately into a dry flask equal quantities of the component solutions Nos. 1 and 2, and mix well.

Solution No. 1. 1 litre to contain 69·28 g of crystallised copper sulphate, $CuSO_4,5H_2O$.

Solution No. 2. 1 litre to contain 346 g of Rochelle salt and 150 g of sodium hydroxide.

Freshly mix the component solutions for each day's determinations.

Checked against 0·1 per cent standard invert sugar solution by the method of titration described above, 5 ml of Fehling's solution corresponds to 0·02533 g of invert sugar.

Method of Calculating Diastatic Activity (*Lintner Value*). Express the result according to the following equations:

(*a*) In the case of flour, Diastatic Activity (or Lintner Value)

$$= \frac{1000}{X \times Y}$$

(*b*) In the case of syrup, Diastatic Activity (or Lintner Value)

$$= \frac{1000}{X \times Y} - 9$$

X = number of ml of 5 per cent malt extract solution in 100 ml of the conversion solution.

Y = number of ml of conversion solution required to reduce 5 ml of Fehling's solution.

9 = a constant denoting the assumed equivalent of the reducing sugars present in the malt extract (syrup) used in making the determinations.

Note. 1. There is a tendency for a film to form on glassware used in starch conversions and all apparatus used for this purpose should be cleaned with warm concentrated sulphuric acid containing a little chromic acid and subsequently thoroughly washed.

2. Distilled water is to be used in making up all solutions and for rinsing apparatus.

3. When carrying out these determinations, it will be found advantageous to make control determinations simultaneously on a malt flour or syrup of known diastatic activity.

4. Standard invert sugar solution, 0·1 per cent, may be prepared by dissolving 0·9500 g of AnalaR saccharose in 150 ml of water, adding 30 ml of 0·5N hydrochloric acid, boiling sixty seconds, cooling, adding 30 ml of 0·5N sodium hydroxide and making up to 1 litre (Ling and Rendle).

Agreement between analysts to within 5° is amply sufficient commercially, and concordance of this order is readily obtained with a little practice if the official method is adhered to and the same starch used.

Extract of Malt with Cod-liver Oil, *B.P.* Contains 10 per cent w/w of cod-liver oil.

Several methods for the direct determination of oil in this preparation are known; they have mostly been evolved from general methods of fat determination. Their relative merits cannot be exactly assessed in any particular case because different brands of Extract of Malt with Cod-liver Oil vary considerably in their emulsifying properties. This is probably due to the practice of many manufacturers of introducing substances other than malt extract and oil, such as dextrin, glycerin, etc., into their products.

The methods available were critically examined by Garratt[3] with a view to accurate determination both of the oil and the vitamin A content. The Rose-Gottlieb and Gunn and Venables[4] methods were considered most suitable to satisfy both requirements provided the oil present has not hydrolysed. The Rose-Gottlieb method is as follows:

Disperse about 5 g of the preparation in 5 ml of water and transfer the mixture to a stoppered 100-ml tube by means of a further 5 ml of water. Add 1 ml of strong ammonia solution and 5 ml of ethanol followed by 25 ml of ether, using a portion of the ether to rinse in any oil possibly remaining in the original weighing vessel. Stopper and shake vigorously for two or three minutes, add 25 ml of light petroleum (b.p. 40° to 60°) and shake again. Allow the mixture to stand for at least half an hour to separate and siphon off the solvent layer into a tared flask. Repeat the shaking and extraction with the ether and light petroleum twice, using 15- to 20-ml portions of each for these extractions. Evaporate,* add a few ml of ethanol or acetone, re-evaporate, dry and weigh the oil.

* It is necessary to evaporate and dry all extracted oils in an atmosphere of nitrogen, not only for vitamin A determination, but also for oil assay. It is to be expected that a highly unsaturated oil, such as cod-liver oil, would easily gain in weight if heated in air.

Stokes' milk tubes (19 × 2·5 cm), specially made to fit a Gerber centrifuge and holding about 65 ml of liquid, have been successfully adapted for this determination; the quantities of ether and light petroleum are each reduced to 20 ml for the first extraction, with corresponding reduction in volumes for the second and third extractions. The tubes are centrifuged for two minutes at 1,000 r.p.m. and give sharp separations, so that the time is considerably reduced—a useful point in assaying vitamin A.

The Gunn and Venables method is based on different principles; the dextrin present is precipitated with ethanol and carries the oil down with it, leaving a clear supernatant aqueous-alcoholic layer. Kaolin is added to obtain a powdery precipitate which, after filtration, can be washed free from oil with ether.

> Weigh 5 to 10 g of extract into a beaker and mix thoroughly with water, using 3 ml for every g taken. Add ethanol in the ratio of 8 parts of dry ethanol to 5 parts of the above dilution, and 0·4 g of purified kaolin. Stir thoroughly and allow the precipitate to settle. Filter the clear supernatant liquid through filter paper of ordinary grade, and add to the precipitate about 50 ml of 70 per cent ethanol, stir again, and allow the precipitate to settle. Filter and collect the residue in the filter, washing out the beaker with 70 per cent ethanol. When the precipitate has drained, wash the residue with ether from a wash-bottle and collect the ether in a separator. Any precipitate adhering to the paper should be separated with a rounded glass rod. Continue washing with ether until a drop of the washings shows no film of oil on evaporation (about 150 ml is necessary). Wash the ether in the separator with three portions, each of 30 ml of water. Evaporate,* add a few ml of dry ethanol, re-evaporate, cool and weigh the residue.

In practice it has been found advisable to use an 11-cm filter paper and to wash the residue with a little strong ethanol before the ether. Extraction of the oil is usually almost complete after about 100 ml of ether has been used, but in this method of washing complete extraction is difficult.

A modification of this process is extraction of the oil by placing the wet filter paper and contents in a Soxhlet thimble, extracting as usual with ether for two or three hours, then transferring the extract to a separator and washing with water as directed above. Considerably less ether is used and complete extraction is more certain.

Extract of malt with cod-liver oil has been found to develop excessive acidity, probably by the action of lipase present in the malt extract. This acidity may be so great as to give discordant results with the Rose-Gottlieb method, the discrepancy being due to the formation of ammonium soaps, some proportion of which is extracted by the mixed ethers as acid soaps, the amount varying with the conditions. It has also been shown that low results are obtained with the Gunn and Venables method for such acid

* It is necessary to evaporate and dry all extracted oils in an atmosphere of nitrogen, not only for vitamin A determination, but also for oil assay. It is to be expected that a highly unsaturated oil, such as cod-liver oil, would easily gain in weight if heated in air.

preparations, due to the almost quantitative solubility of the fatty acids in the ethanol used, the figure for extracted oil being that of neutral oil only.

The total fatty matter may be determined by a modified Rose-Gottlieb method proposed by Bond and Druce.[5] The essential details are as follows:

> Weigh about 2·5 g into a stoppered tube, dissolve in 8 ml of water and add 5 ml of ethanol and 15 ml of ether. Shake vigorously for half a minute and either centrifuge or allow to stand until complete separation of the two layers is obtained. Siphon off the ethereal layer into a separator, add 5 ml of ether to the residue and, without shaking, transfer it to the separator. Repeat the extraction with 5 ml of ethanol and 15 ml of ether as before and make a third extraction with 15 ml of ether only (if an emulsion forms, add 2 ml of ethanol and reshake). Wash the bulked ethers with three 15-ml portions of water. Evaporate the ether in a weighed flask and dry the residue by evaporation with small successive quantities of acetone until the oil is clear. Cool and weigh.

This method was found to be applicable to Extract of Malt with Halibut-liver Oil.

It was concluded by Garratt and Woodhead[6] that, as extract of malt with vitaminised oil showed a similar development of free fatty acid, the cause pointed not to the relative ease of hydrolysis of cod-liver oil, but rather to the action of a general fat-splitting enzyme, such as lipase, in the extract of malt. The vitaminised oil had arachis oil as a diluent.

On spectrophotometric examination of the vitamin A activity of samples which had developed acidity up to 20 per cent of free fatty acids, normal curves without a shift of the peak from 325 mμ were obtained on the unsaponifiable matter of the extracted oils and, although the original vitamin A contents were not known, from the amounts found there was obviously little lost.

The conclusion reached on the cause of the development of acidity was supported by the experiments of Bond and Druce,[5] who have shown that bacterial action was not responsible for the increase, yet inactivation was obtained by heating the malt extract sufficiently to destroy the fat-splitting enzyme. The *B.P.* now recognises this and has imposed a limit for lipase activity in the malt extract and a maximum acid value for the extracted oil.

Powell[7] has drawn attention to the possibility of the extraction of a small quantity of oil from malt extract itself, present, in his opinion, to the extent of 0·2 to 0·3 per cent. By the method of Gunn and Venables, 0·09 per cent of oily residue has been obtained from a pharmaceutical malt extract.

For the determination of vitamin A in galenicals containing cod-liver oil and halibut-liver oil see p. 667.

Extract of malt with or without cod-liver oil is liable occasionally to ferment owing to the presence of osmophilic yeasts. The yeasts are naturally present in the original raw materials and some growth can take place during the malting stages. As a result of the subsequent concentration process the growth is suppressed and finally stopped in the majority of cases but this still leaves viable cells in the final product. Occasionally, however, growth will continue at a much reduced rate giving rise to fermentation.

Dissolve 10 g of bacteriological peptone, 500 g of glucose, 1 g of sodium acid phosphate and 1 g of citric acid in water and make up to 1 litre. Distribute in 12- to 15-ml amounts in 1-oz screw-capped bottles and sterilise at 115° (10 lb steam pressure) for twenty minutes.

Weigh about 1 g of the extract of malt and disperse into 9 ml of sterile saline. From this first dilution prepare further ten-fold serial dilutions in saline and inoculate 1 ml of each (representing 0·1 g, 0·01 g and so on of the original sample) into a bottle of the sterilised medium. Incubate at about 25° for seven days. Each bottle of inoculated medium showing gas production (easily observed on swirling gently) indicates growth of an osmophilic yeast.

Material can be considered satisfactory if there is fermentation from 0·001 g (*i.e.* the 1/1,000 dilution) but not thereafter. Fermentation as far as the 1/10,000 dilution indicates that the material should be regarded with suspicion.

1. Ling, A. R., *J. Fed. Insts. Brewing*, 1900, **6**, 355.
2. Statutory Rules and Orders, 1933, No. 540, H.M. Stationery Office.
3. Garratt, D. C., *Analyst*, 1939, **64**, 795.
4. Gunn, C., and Venables, P. F. R., *Quart. J. Pharm.*, 1936, **9**, 430.
5. Bond, C. R., and Druce, S., *Analyst*, 1942, **67**, 379.
6. Garratt, D. C., and Woodhead, J. E., *Analyst*, 1942, **67**, 194.
7. Powell, A. D., *Quart. J. Pharm.*, 1936, **9**, 542.

MENAPHTHONE

$C_{11}H_8O_2$ Mol. Wt. 172·2

The chemical assay of menaphthone was devised by Pinder and Singer,[1] who showed that under suitable conditions the quinone could be quantitatively reduced to hydroquinone with titanous chloride, the end-point of the reduction being shown by the use of an internal oxidation-reduction indicator.

Weigh out accurately about 0·2 g of the substance, and transfer to a 200-ml conical flask. Dissolve it in a mixture of 10 ml of 95 per cent ethanol and 15 ml of glacial acetic acid. Add 4 g of anhydrous sodium carbonate and 25 ml of 10 per cent sodium potassium tartrate solution. Titrate with 0·1N titanous chloride, using 3 drops of 0·1 per cent indigo carmine solution as indicator. A sharp end-point is obtained, the blue dye being changed to the colourless leuco base by the addition of 1 drop of the titanous chloride solution in excess. Phenosafranine is also a suitable indicator. During the titration pass a steady stream of carbon dioxide through the solution. 1 ml 0·1N = 0·008609 g $C_{11}H_8O_2$.

The quantities of carbonate and tartrate should be correct as they control the pH of the solution and prevent it becoming too acid during the titration.

In the *U.S.P.* assay the quinone is first reduced before titration with ceric sulphate.

Weigh about 0·15 g dried sample into a 150-ml flask, add 15 ml of glacial acetic acid and 15 ml of dilute hydrochloric acid and rotate the flask until the sample is dissolved. Add about 3 g of zinc dust, close the flask with a stopper bearing a Bunsen valve, shake well and allow to stand in the dark for one hour, shaking frequently. Rapidly decant the solution through a cotton-wool plug into a second flask, wash the first flask immediately with three quantities, each of 10 ml, of freshly boiled and cooled water, add 0·1 ml of *o*-phenanthroline-ferrous complex to the combined filtrate and washings and titrate immediately with 0·1N ceric sulphate. Carry out a blank determination. 1 ml 0·1N = 0·008609 g $C_{11}H_8O_2$.

Pinder and Singer[1] also proposed a method for the estimation of small quantities such as are found in tablets and ampoules.

For tablets; grind in a mortar and extract in the cold with ethanol, adjusting the volume and taking suitable aliquots for assay. For solutions in oil; shake a suitable weighed quantity with ethanol and proceed with the determination on the resulting emulsion; the ethanol extracts the quinone from the oily solution and any undissolved oil is removed after the final dilution with water by shaking with ether.

To 1 to 5 ml of ethanolic solution containing 0·4 to 0·8 mg of the quinone, add 3 ml of a mixture of equal volumes of 95 per cent ethanol and strong ammonia solution. Add 3 to 5 drops of ethyl cyanacetate and allow the mixture to stand for exactly half a minute. Add 5 ml of 6N potassium hydroxide, mix, and leave for fifteen minutes, preferably out of direct sunlight. Dilute to 50 ml and measure the extinction at 445 mμ. Read off the quantity of quinone from a previously prepared graph.

Menaphthone sodium bisulphite, $C_{11}H_9O_5SNa,3H_2O$. Mol. Wt. 330·3. Both the *B.P.* and the *U.S.P.* extract the menaphthone by the same method and then determine it by their individual methods given above.

For extraction:

Dissolve 0·3 g in 20 ml of water, add 5 ml of N sodium hydroxide and extract with three quantities, each of 20 ml, of chloroform. Combine the extracts, wash with 10 ml of water, filter through a filter paper rinsed with chloroform and wash the filter with 5 ml of chloroform. Evaporate the chloroform on a water-bath under a jet of air. 1 ml 0·1N = 0·01381 g $C_{11}H_9O_5SNa$.

Injection of Menaphthone Sodium Bisulphite, *B.P.* A sterile solution of menaphthone sodium bisulphite (usually 10 mg per ml) in water for injection containing 0·2 per cent w/v of sodium metabisulphite. The assay is the same as for menaphthone sodium bisulphite using a volume containing about 75 mg of the substance and titrating with 0·05N titanous chloride. 1 ml 0·05N = 0·008257 g $C_{11}H_9O_5SNa,3H_2O$.

ACETOMENAPHTHONE, $C_{15}H_{14}O_4$, Mol. Wt. 258·3.

Acetomenaphthone is prepared by reducing menaphthone with zinc and acetic acid in the presence of acetic anhydride. No direct method of assay has been applied but hydrolysis to the quinol and oxidation of this to the quinone is the best method.

> To approximately 0·2 g acetomenaphthone add 15 ml of glacial acetic acid and 15 ml of dilute hydrochloric acid and boil under reflux condenser for at least fifteen minutes. Cool, protecting against aerial oxidation, and titrate with 0·05N ceric ammonium sulphate using 0·1 ml of *o*-phenanthroline-ferrous complex as indicator. Carry out a blank determination using exactly the same amount of indicator. 1 ml 0·05N = 0·006457 g.

During hydrolysis a red colour is developed, which is partially discharged during oxidation and does not interfere with the end-point.

Tablets of Acetomenaphthone, *B.P.* Contain 5 mg of the drug. The assay given above for acetomenaphthone can be applied to the tablets by extracting a quantity of the powder in a Soxhlet apparatus with chloroform for two hours and removing the solvent.

Menadiol sodium diphosphate, $C_{11}H_8O_8P_2Na_4,6H_2O$, Mol. Wt. 530·2, is assayed in the *U.S.P.* with a potentiometric end-point.

> Dissolve about 0·1 g in 25 ml of water, add 25 ml of glacial acetic acid and 25 ml of dilute hydrochloric acid and titrate with 0·02N ceric ammonium sulphate, determining the end-point potentiometrically using a platinum/calomel electrode system. 1 ml 0·02N = 0·004221 g $C_{11}H_8O_8P_2Na_4$.

1. PINDER, J. L., and SINGER, J. H., *Analyst*, 1940, **65**, 7.

MERCURY

Hg At. Wt. 200·6

Many methods have been suggested for the determination of mercury, whether in inorganic or organic combination; it is only possible here to review those which have been found to be of value in pharmaceutical work.

The principal methods for the determination of mercury are as follows:

(i) Thiocyanate titration. This method is applicable to solutions in which all the mercury is in the mercuric state and from which halides are absent. Nitrous acid must also be absent as it masks the end-point by forming a red compound with thiocyanate in acid solution; it may be removed from solution by boiling or, better, by the dropwise addition of potassium permanganate solution until the latter is present in slight excess. The method may be applied to metallic mercury as follows:

To about 0·4 g of mercury add 20 ml of 1 : 1 nitric acid, boil until the solution is colourless, cool and dilute. Add potassium permanganate solution until no further decolorisation occurs, removing any excess with a trace of ferrous sulphate and titrate with 0·1N ammonium thiocyanate, at a temperature not exceeding 20°, using iron alum as indicator. 1 ml 0·1N = 0·01003 g Hg.

Mercuric oxide, HgO, Mol. Wt. 216·6, in either the yellow or red variety may be determined as follows:

Dissolve about 0·4 g in 5 ml of concentrated nitric acid and 10 ml of water. Dilute to about 150 ml with water and titrate with 0·1N ammonium thiocyanate as above. 1 ml 0·1N = 0·01083 g.

(ii) Sulphide precipitation. Although much used in the past there is little application for this classical procedure today (but see Allport's method p. 413). The precipitate from hydrochloric acid is easily filtered but may be contaminated with sulphur; to avoid errors from this source the precipitate should be washed with ethanol and then allowed to stand for about half an hour with carbon disulphide and finally washed with carbon disulphide and dried at 110°.

(iii) In the mercurous state, mercury may be determined with iodine and thiosulphate after conversion into calomel (by the addition of excess sodium chloride followed by filtration). As applied to **mercurous chloride,** HgCl, Mol. Wt. 236·1, the method is as follows:

Disperse about 0·7 g in 10 ml of water contained in a stoppered flask, add 50 ml of 0·1N iodine and 5 g of potassium iodide dissolved in 10 ml of water. Stopper the flask and shake frequently until the solid matter has completely dissolved. Titrate the excess of iodine with 0·1N sodium thiosulphate. 1 ml 0·1N = 0·02361 g.

(iv) Rupp's iodimetric method.[1] In this method, applicable to all mercuric compounds, the sample is dissolved in a solution of potassium iodide to form the double iodide, which is then treated with alkaline formaldehyde to reduce the mercury to the metallic state. The solution is then acidified and the mercury dissolved in standard iodine solution, excess of which is determined by back-titration with sodium thiosulphate.

Many modifications of the original procedure have been published from time to time and it seems clear from the conflicting reports that the precision of the method has not been good in everyone's hands. Modifications have been particularly directed to increasing the speed of solution of the precipitated mercury in iodine solution. The recommendation by Brindle and Waterhouse[2] to add 10 ml of calcium chloride solution before the alkaline formaldehyde is effective, its efficiency being probably due to the precipitation of mercury in a fine state of division simultaneously with the calcium hydroxide. The method is of value because it can be applied to halide-containing mercuric salts, the following procedure being applicable to **mercuric chloride,** $HgCl_2$, Mol. Wt. 271·5.

Dissolve about 0·3 g in 100 ml of water, add 10 ml of a 10 per cent solution of calcium chloride, followed by 1 g of potassium iodide, 3 ml of formaldehyde solution and 15 ml of sodium hydroxide solution. Shake and allow to stand for two minutes. Add 20 ml of acetic acid and 40 ml of 0·1N iodine, shake until the precipitate has redissolved and titrate the excess of iodine with 0·1N sodium thiosulphate. 1 ml 0·1N = 0·01358 g $HgCl_2$.

(v) EDTA titration. Many procedures may be used for the complexometric titration of mercury but undoubtedly the most suitable for pharmaceutical work is that which depends upon the release of free EDTA from a mercury-EDTA complex by addition of potassium iodide. This method is unaffected by the presence of chloride (though not, of course, of iodide), is highly specific and is capable of a high degree of precision. Details of the method are as follows:

Dissolve about 0·3 g of mercuric chloride, accurately weighed, in 100 ml of water, add about 40 ml of 0·05M EDTA (this solution need not be accurately standardised), 5 ml of ammonia buffer solution and 0·5 ml of solochrome black indicator and titrate with 0·05M zinc solution until the blue colour changes to purple (do not overshoot the end-point); add 3 g of potassium iodide, swirl to dissolve, allow to stand for two minutes and then continue the titration with zinc solution to the same end-point as before. Each ml of zinc solution required after addition of the potassium iodide = 0·01358 g $HgCl_2$.

A modification of this method, applicable to solutions resulting from the flask combustion of mercury-containing organic materials, is described in Appendix IV.

(vi) A modification of the thiocyanate titration method given above consists in amalgamating the mercury, obtained by reduction with nascent hydrogen, with zinc, washing the amalgam free from impurities, dissolving in nitric acid and titrating as usual with thiocyanate. For further details see Mercuric Iodide Solution-tablets. The principle of this method is also used for the assay of red **mercuric iodide,** HgI_2, Mol. Wt. 454·4, where direct replacement of the mercury by 1 g of zinc powder in intimate contact with 0·5 g of the iodide for ten minutes, produces soluble zinc iodide quantitatively; this is filtered from the amalgam and the iodide titrated by Volhard's method (see p. 290), 1 ml 0·1N $AgNO_3$ = 0·02272 g.

(vii) Precipitation as zinc mercuric thiocyanate. This method, originally due to Jamieson[3] is discussed more fully under Zinc (see p. 688). The method given there is applicable except that the precipitating reagent contains 39 g of ammonium thiocyanate and 29 g of zinc sulphate per litre.

Traces of mercury in organic matter may be determined by the process, detailed by Strafford and Wyatt,[4] which involves destruction of organic matter, precipitation and decomposition of mercuric sulphide, electrolysis and final colorimetric determination of the isolated mercury. Electrolysis is necessary as the final colorimetric determination cannot be carried out in a solution containing even traces of sulphate or halogen ions, and sulphate is certain to be present after solution of the sulphide precipitate. The detailed method is somewhat involved and too long to include here in full; but the final colorimetric procedure may be useful when suitable conditions arise. *p*-Dimethylaminobenzylidine-rhodanine gives with small amounts of mercuric ion a brick-red colour, the intensity of which is proportional to the amount of mercury present. The colour may be developed in neutral or acetic acid solution to which a carefully controlled amount of nitric acid is added to discharge the yellow colour due to the excess of reagent. The best gradation of colour is obtained with amounts of mercury ranging from 0·01 to 0·20 mg in 100 ml of solution. The only common metals other than mercury which give a positive reaction under the conditions described are silver and cuprous copper; cupric copper does not interfere.

To 90 ml of a suitable concentration of mercury in neutral or acetic acid solution add 5·0 ml of N nitric acid from a pipette, mix thoroughly, add 3·0 ml of *p*-dimethylaminobenzylidine-rhodanine reagent (0·04 g shaken with 200 ml of ethanol, left overnight and filtered), adjust the volume to 100 ml and mix. Compare with standards prepared by adding suitable known amounts of standard mercuric nitrate solution (0·5 g mercury in 5 ml of concentrated nitric acid, dilute, boil to remove nitrous fumes and dilute to 250 ml; make further dilutions so that 1 ml = 0·0001 g Hg) to similar amounts of nitric acid and reagents as used in the test solution. Develop the colour in both test solution and standards simultaneously, allow to stand for five minutes and compare.

A Sub-committee of the Analytical Methods Committee of the *S.A.C.*[5] has recommended the following methods for the destruction of organic matter when mercury is to be determined.

Method A—Destruction with Sulphuric, Nitric and Perchloric Acids. Weigh accurately about 2·5 g of the well-mixed sample into the Kjeldahl flask (A) of the apparatus (Fig. 9) and place the reflux head (B) and the condenser (C) in position.

Maintain a steady flow of water through the condenser. Add, through the side-arm of the Kjeldahl flask, 4 to 5 ml of concentrated sulphuric acid and heat the contents of the flask gently until the sample is charred; add concentrated nitric acid, slowly in small portions (0·25 to 0·5 ml at a time) until the solution darkens between additions. Continue this procedure until the liquid is colourless or pale yellow on prolonged boiling (about fifteen minutes) after the last addition of nitric acid. When, during this procedure, the reflux head becomes filled with condensate (which may contain some solidified volatile organic matter), run off the liquid into a 5-ml cylinder, and reserve it. When the wet oxidation is apparently complete, gradually add the contents of the cylinder to the

Kjeldahl flask via the side-arm, and boil to fuming, running off the condensate and collecting it as required. If necessary, again pass the condensate through the apparatus until the solution is colourless. Add concentrated nitric acid to the Kjeldahl flask until no further darkening occurs. Then add gradually 0·5 ml of 60 per cent w/w perchloric acid and heat strongly for ten minutes. Allow the mixture to cool, wash out

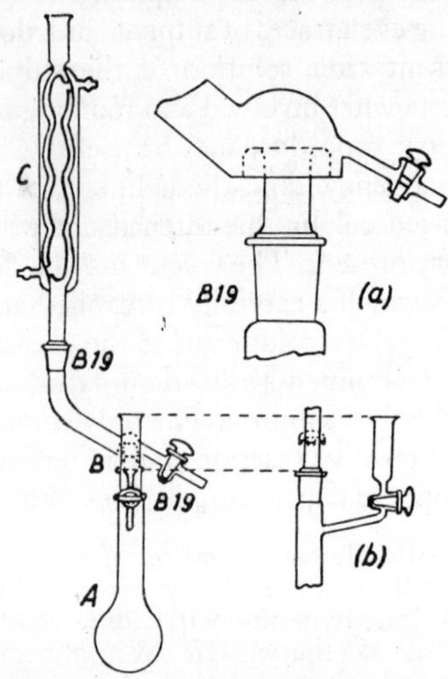

FIG. 9

Arrangement and details of apparatus for the destruction of organic matter in preparation for the determination of mercury. (*a*) Detail of reflux head. (*b*) Side view of top part of Kjeldahl flask.

A, Kjeldahl flask fitted with side-arm; B, reflux head; C, double-surface condenser.

the reflux head with the minimum amount of distilled water, and add the washings and separated condensate to the contents of the Kjeldahl flask. Disconnect the apparatus and boil the contents of the flask for about fifteen minutes. The volume at this stage should be about 40 to 50 ml.

Instead of concentrated nitric acid, analytical-reagent grade 100 volume hydrogen peroxide may be used to effect decomposition of the sample. After each small addition of peroxide, most of the water formed should be driven off so that the digest does not become diluted and the condensate should be drawn off as it accumulates.

Mercury is then determined in the contents of the Kjeldahl flask by an appropriate method.

Method B—Destruction with Potassium Permanganate and Nitric and Sulphuric Acids.

Ammoniacal hydroxylamine solution. Dissolve 25 g of hydroxylamine hydrochloride in about 60 ml of water, add 0·2 ml of a 0·02 per cent solution of phenol red in 20 per cent ethanol and make alkaline with strong ammonia solution to the full red colour of the indicator. Cool the solution and extract it with 5 ml portions of a 0·01 per cent solution of dithizone in chloroform until the last extract remains green; wash the solution free from excess of dithizone by repeated extraction with 10-ml portions of chloroform. Warm the solution until the excess of chloroform has been removed; cool, filter and dilute the solution with water to 250 ml.

This solution should be freshly prepared on the day of use.

Transfer 100 ml of the liquid sample to a 500-ml round-bottomed flask fitted by means of a standard ground joint to a long water-cooled reflux condenser. Add 40 ml of concentrated nitric acid and 3 g of potassium permanganate. Insert the stopper in the condenser, using a thread to prevent an air-tight fit. Boil gently under reflux for two hours (avoiding overheating, with resultant volatilisation of mercury); and then cool thoroughly. Remove the thread. Shake the flask carefully so that the solution comes into contact with the vapour. Rinse down the condenser.

If necessary, add potassium permanganate until an excess is present after two minutes' standing. (A further 1 to 2 g may be added.) Add ammoniacal hydroxylamine solution until the solution is colourless. Add several drops of a 0·02 per cent solution of phenol red in 20 per cent ethanol and then strong ammonia solution until the solution attains the full red colour of the indicator, keeping the solution cool during the addition of the ammonia. Add 18 ml of a mixture of equal volumes of concentrated sulphuric acid and water and 10 ml of ammoniacal hydroxylamine solution, cool, mix and allow to stand for at least three hours, or preferably overnight.

The solution is now ready for treatment with dithizone.

Applicability:

Method A—Slight losses of mercury occur when organic matter is completely oxidised by this method but the loss is of an order generally acceptable when the mercury content of the sample is in excess of 5 p.p.m. and for some purposes the method can be useful at lower levels of mercury content.

Method B—This is suitable for the partial oxidation of liquids containing relatively small amounts of organic matter and for the determination of mercury in urine.

A method for the determination of mercury in amounts up to 100 μg has been recommended by the joint *A.B.C.M.–S.A.C.* Committee on Methods for the Analysis of Trade Effluents.[6]

After destruction of organic matter by *Method B* (above) any iron present is first suppressed by hydroxylamine and the solution is made acid to eliminate other heavy metals; the mercury is then extracted with toluene as the golden-brown dithizonate, which is determined colorimetrically. The detailed method is as follows:

Reagents:

Toluene. This should be redistilled sulphur-free toluene.

Dithizone extraction solution. Extract 20 ml of a 0·1 per cent solution of diphenylthiocarbazone in toluene with two 50-ml portions of dilute ammonium hydroxide (50 ml of water containing 1 ml of strong ammonia solution), rejecting the toluene layer each time. Acidify the aqueous layer with diluted hydrochloric acid (1 + 1) and extract the precipitated dithizone with 100 ml of toluene. Wash the extract with two quantities, each of 10 ml, of water and filter the toluene layer through a dry filter paper. This solution should be freshly prepared on the day it is to be used.

Sodium hydroxide/hydroxylamine solution. Dissolve 20 g of sodium hydroxide in 500 ml of water and add 20 ml of ammoniacal hydroxylamine solution (see above under *Method B* for destruction of organic matter). Dilute to 1 litre with water and mix.

Procedure: Transfer a suitable aliquot of the prepared solution containing not more than 100 μg of mercury to a 250-ml, pear-shaped separator, add 3 ml of dithizone extraction solution and 7 ml of toluene and shake vigorously for thirty seconds. Allow the layers to separate and observe the colour of the dithizone in the toluene layer; excess of dithizone is indicated by a green or brownish-green colour. If the colour of the toluene layer is golden brown, continue the addition of the dithizone extraction solution, 0·5 ml at a time, with shaking, as directed above, until an excess is present as indicated by the appearance of a green tint. Note the volume of dithizone extraction solution used. Allow the layers to separate, discard the aqueous (lower) layer, wash the toluene layer with 10 ml of water without mixing and reject the washings.

Add 10 ml of diluted hydrochloric acid (1 + 1) and shake the mixture vigorously for half a minute. Allow the layers to separate, run the lower layer into a second separator and wash the toluene/dithizone layer twice without shaking, using 50 ml of water for each washing. Add the washings to the acid extract in the second separator and reject the toluene layer.

To the acid extract and washings add 5 ml of ammoniacal hydroxylamine hydrochloride solution (see above), a volume of dithizone extraction solution equal to that used in the initial extraction and 7 ml of toluene and shake the mixture vigorously for half a minute. Allow the layers to separate and reject the aqueous layer. Wash the toluene/dithizone layer once with 10 ml of water without shaking and reject the washings.

Remove excess of dithizone by the addition of 10 ml of the sodium hydroxide/hydroxylamine solution, shake for half a minute and allow the layers to separate. Reject the aqueous layer. Repeat the sodium hydroxide/hydroxylamine extraction twice more, rejecting the aqueous layer each time. The toluene layer is golden brown in colour when mercury is present. Separate the last aqueous layer as completely as possible, discard it and dry the bore of the stem of the separator with a strip of filter paper. Filter the toluene/mercury dithizonate solution through a dry 9-cm Whatman No. 41 filter paper containing about 0·5 g of anhydrous sodium sulphate, and collect the dry filtrate in a 25-ml graduated flask. Rinse the separator several times with small volumes of toluene and pass the rinsings through the same filter paper, collecting them in the flask. Dilute to volume with toluene and mix.

Carry out a blank procedure on all the reagents used.

Measure the extinctions at 480 mμ of the test and blank solutions, using 4-cm or 1-cm cells according to the depth of colour, with toluene in the comparison cell in either case. Read the μg of mercury equivalent to the observed extinctions of the test and blank solutions from a calibration graph and so obtain the net measure of mercury in the sample.

Preparation of calibration graph: First prepare a standard mercury solution as follows. Weigh 0·4 to 0·5 g of pure dry mercury into a 100-ml beaker, add 10 ml of water, cover the beaker with a watch-glass and gradually add 10 ml of concentrated nitric acid. Warm until the mercury is completely dissolved, add 25 ml of diluted sulphuric acid (1 + 1) and evaporate until white fumes are evolved. Cool, dilute, cautiously, with 50 ml of water, boil for one minute and then cool. Transfer the solution to a 500-ml graduated flask, dilute to volume with water and mix. Immediately before use, measure from a 25-ml burette a volume of this solution that will contain 0·0100 g of mercury into a 1-litre graduated flask. Add 5 ml of diluted sulphuric acid (1 + 1), dilute to volume with water and mix. (1 ml ≡ 10 μg of mercury). Measure appropriate amounts of this solution, covering the range 0 to 100 μg of mercury, into a series of 250-ml, pear-shaped separators. To each add 7 ml of diluted sulphuric acid (1 + 1) and dilute each solution to 100 ml; then add 5 ml of ammoniacal hydroxylamine hydrochloride solution and extract the mercury with toluene-dithizone solution as described above, beginning with 'add 3 ml of dithizone extraction solution . . .'. Measure the extinctions at 480 mμ, using 4-cm cells to cover the range 0 to 30 μg of mercury and a 1-cm cell to cover the range 30 to 100 μg, and construct a graph relating extinctions to μg of mercury.

The Food and Agriculture Organization of the United Nations[7] has recommended methods for the determination of mercury in pesticides. The method selected depends on the other constituents of the formulation and in the presence of copper the method of Brookes and Solomon[8] (see p. 419) is most suitable. In the presence of most other constituents the selected method is one in which the sample is refluxed with concentrated sulphuric acid and potassium nitrate before determining the mercury volumetrically with thiocyanate. When large amounts of calcium carbonate or highly chlorinated compounds (*e.g.* benzene hexachloride) are present, the mercury is isolated as a sulphide before conversion to the ionic form with strong acid.

The preparations in Table 23 are all assayed on their mercury content by the thiocyanate method [(i) p. 407] with the modifications given.

Oleated mercury, *B.P.C.* contains 21 per cent of mercuric oxide in a fatty base in combination as oleate.

Allport[9] has developed a useful method for the assay of mercury in the presence of fatty matter, in which it is precipitated as sulphide *in situ* from a mixture of organic solvents. Sulphur is not precipitated and the method may be used for most ointments containing wool fat. It is very rapid and to be recommended provided the filtrations are done with solutions as hot as possible.

Dissolve about 0·75 g of oleated mercury by warming to 50° with 100 ml of a mixture by volume of 13 parts benzene, 2 parts glacial acetic acid and 5 parts 90 per cent ethanol. Whilst keeping the mixture at 50°

MERCURY

TABLE 23

PREPARATION	MERCURY CONTENT PER CENT	MODIFICATION
*Ointment of Mercury, Strong, *B.P.C.*	30	1 g, 30 ml 1 : 1 nitric acid, boil for ten minutes, decant through wet filter, wash with 20 ml 1 : 1 nitric acid.
Ointment of Mercury, Dilute, *B.P.C.*	10	3 g as for Strong Ointment of Mercury.
*Ointment of Mercury, Compound, *B.P.C.*	12	3 g as for Strong Ointment of Mercury.
Ointment of Mercuric Nitrate, Strong, *B.P.C.*	6·7	4 g in 25 ml benzene and 2 ml glacial acetic acid. Add 1 g zinc powder, shake for ten minutes, wash amalgam with benzene, dissolve in nitric acid under reflux.
†Pill of Digitalis, Compound, *B.P.C.*	0·0214 g per pill	16 pills as for Pill-Mass of Mercury.
*Pill-Mass of Mercury, *B.P.C.*	33	1 g, boil under reflux with 10 ml nitric acid and 25 ml water, dilute and filter.
Powder of Mercury with Chalk, *B.Vet.C.*	33	1 g as for Pill-Mass of Mercury, without filtration.
Tablets of Digitalis, Compound, *B.P.C.*	0·0216 g per tablet	16 tablets as for Pill-Mass of Mercury.

* Can also be assayed, rapidly and accurately, by the oxygen-flask method (see p. 801).

† Also by the oxygen-flask method after preliminary treatment: Since it is not practicable to grind the pills directly to give a uniform sample they must first be dried for one hour at 105° and then ground in a mortar; there is no evidence of significant loss when this drying is carried out. Dry twenty pills and use an amount of powder approximately equivalent to one pill for the flask-combustion method, as described in Appendix IV. In calculating the weight of mercury per pill, allowance must be made for the loss in weight on drying.

pass hydrogen sulphide through it to precipitate mercuric sulphide completely. Warm at 50° to 60° until the precipitate has coagulated and filter through a sintered-glass filter or a Gooch crucible, which has been previously warmed with some of the hot solvent. Wash free from fat with a mixture of hot benzene and ethanol or with more of the hot prepared solvent. Wash with ethanol and finally with ether. Dry at 120° and weigh, $HgS \times 0{\cdot}9309 = HgO$.

The *N.F.* method uses digestion with sulphuric and nitric acids to obtain the mercury in the inorganic form before titrating with 0·1N thiocyanate as usual in the presence of nitric acid.

Mercuric oxycyanide, $HgO.3Hg(CN)_2$, Mol. Wt. 974·5 is an unionised salt. It may be assayed in one solution for both oxide and cyanide radicals by the method of Tagliavini.[10]

Dissolve about 0·5 g in 50 ml of water. For mercuric oxide, add 1 g of sodium chloride and neutralise with 0·1N hydrochloric acid to methyl orange, thus forming the neutral salt $HgCl_2,2NaCl$. 1 ml 0·1N = 0·01083 g HgO. For mercuric cyanide, add an excess (3 g) of potassium iodide, which forms unionised $HgI_2,2KI$ and liberates an equivalent of ionised KCN. Titrate the alkalinity of the potassium cyanide by additional 0·1N hydrochloric acid to the same indicator. 1 ml 0·1N = 0·01263 g $Hg(CN)_2$.

Mercuric cyanide, $Hg(CN)_2$, Mol. Wt. 252·6, is determined similarly:

To about 0·4 g in solution add 1 g of sodium chloride to liberate the potassium cyanide, then add 2 or 3 g of potassium iodide to convert the mercuric chloride formed to non-ionised $HgI_2,2KI$ before titrating the alkalinity of the cyanide with 0·1N hydrochloric acid to methyl orange. 1 ml 0·1N = 0·01263 g.

Ammoniated mercury, $NH_2.HgCl$, Mol. Wt. 252·1, is assayed acidimetrically after addition of an excess of potassium iodide. The following directions for determination are preferable to those of the *B.P.*

Triturate about 0·25 g in a glass mortar with a few drops of water until uniformly dispersed, wash into a flask quantitatively with about 40 ml of water, finally rinsing the mortar with a solution of 3 g of potassium iodide in 10 ml of water and adding the washings to the contents of the flask. After the solution of the mercuric iodide formed is complete, titrate the ammonia and potassium hydroxide liberated in the reaction with 0·1N hydrochloric acid to methyl orange. 1 ml 0·1N = 0·01260 g.

The *U.S.P.* determines ammoniated mercury by a zinc amalgam method:

Heat 0·4 g with 5 ml of water and 5 ml of acetic acid (6N) on a water-bath, with frequent agitation, until dissolved. Add 4 to 5 g of zinc (10–40 mesh), cover the flask and heat on a water-bath for fifteen minutes, with frequent shaking. Decant the supernatant liquid without loss of zinc and wash the zinc by decantation with 25-ml quantities of water until the last washing is free from chloride. Add 30 ml of dilute nitric acid (1 in 2) in portions, through a funnel inserted in the neck of the flask, allowing the reaction to subside before each successive portion is added. Heat gently until complete solution is effected and rinse the funnel and stem with water, collecting the rinsings in the flask. Dilute with 15 to 20 ml of water and then add 0·1N potassium permanganate, in small quantities, until a permanent pink colour is obtained. Decolorise by the dropwise addition of N oxalic acid, cool, add 50 ml of water and titrate with 0·1N ammonium thiocyanate, using ferric alum as indicator. 1 ml 0·1N = 0·01260 g $NH_2.HgCl$.

Eye Lotion of Mercuric Oxycyanide, *B.N.F.* Contains 0·03 per cent of mercuric oxycyanide and 3·2 per cent of potassium nitrate.

The mercuric oxycyanide is determined on 100 ml by the method given above for the salt, *i.e.*, adding 1 g of potassium iodide to 100 ml and titrating to methyl red with 0·02N hydrochloric acid, 1 ml = 0·002006 g Hg.

Eye Ointment of Mercuric Oxide, *B.P.* Contains 1·0 per cent of yellow mercuric oxide in a paraffin base.

The official assay is as follows:

Weigh an amount equivalent to 0·1 g of yellow mercuric oxide into a stoppered flask with the aid of 20 ml of chloroform, add 10 ml of dilute nitric acid and 20 ml of water and shake until the mercuric oxide is dissolved. Add 50 ml of water and titrate with 0·1N ammonium thiocyanate, at a temperature not exceeding 20°, using ferric alum as indicator. 1 ml 0·1N = 0·01083 g.

However, efficient extraction of mercuric oxide from fats with dilute acids is difficult, especially in the presence of wool, fat and Allport's method (p. 413) using 5 g is satisfactory.

Eye Ointment of Atropine with Mercuric Oxide, *B.P.C.* Usually contains 1 per cent each of yellow mercuric oxide and atropine sulphate.

Allport's method (p. 413) using 5 g of ointment is satisfactory for determining the mercuric oxide in this preparation.

The atropine can be determined by the method for Eye Ointment of Atropine (p. 117).

Lotion of Salicylic Acid and Mercuric Chloride, *B.P.C.* Contains 0·114 per cent of mercuric chloride and 2·29 per cent of salicylic acid in a solvent mixture.

For mercury: Heat 100 ml with 5 ml of glacial acetic acid to a temperature not exceeding 55°, pass hydrogen sulphide through the hot solution for ten minutes and filter; wash the residue with hydrogen sulphide solution, with 95 per cent ethanol and finally with carbon disulphide and dry to constant weight at 105°. Each g of residue = 1·167 g $HgCl_2$.

For salicylic acid, see p. 559.

Ointment of Ammoniated Mercury, *B.P.* Contains 2·5 per cent of white precipitate in a simple ointment base.

Methods of assay using filtration of the active ingredient from solutions of the base in solvents usually give low results from loss of finely divided ammoniated mercury which passes through the filter.

The *B.P.* assay is improved by using a screened methyl orange:

To 5 g of ointment in a stoppered flask, add 25 ml of ether, 25 ml of light petroleum, 2 g of potassium iodide and 50 ml of water. Shake until the fats dissolve and titrate with 0·1N hydrochloric acid using methyl orange-xylene cyanol FF as indicator and shaking vigorously during the titration. 1 ml 0·1N = 0·01260 g $NH_2.HgCl$.

Allport's method for determination of this ointment, given under Oleated Mercury, requires the solvent used to contain different proportions to effect solution of the constituents of the ointment. The solvent described below is satisfactory for dissolving, at 70°, ointment made with paraffin, but not more than 3 g will dissolve in 100 ml of this solvent.

Dissolve 2·5 g of the ointment at 70° in 100 ml of a mixture by volume of 9 parts benzene, 10 parts glacial acetic acid and 1 part 90 per cent ethanol. Precipitate the mercury with sulphuretted hydrogen as given under Oleated Mercury. $HgS \times 1{\cdot}0837 = NH_2.HgCl$.

The *U.S.P.* assay of this ointment is by shaking about 3 g, dissolved in 50 ml of ether, in a separator with a mixture of equal volumes of concentrated hydrochloric acid and water until the ammoniated mercury has dissolved, filtering the aqueous layer into a beaker, repeating the extraction and filtration with successive portions of water and precipitating the mercury as sulphide.

Ointment of Ammoniated Mercury and Coal Tar, *B.P.C.* The assay for ammoniated mercury in this preparation follows that for Ointment of Ammoniated Mercury given above.

Ointment of Ammoniated Mercury, Coal Tar and Salicylic Acid, *B.N.F.* Contains about 2·5 per cent of ammoniated mercury.

The most satisfactory assay for ammoniated mercury is the following:

Disperse 10 g in 80 ml of a mixture of ether and light petroleum (b.p. 60° to 80°) with the aid of gentle heat and extract with four 25-ml quantities of warm 33 per cent w/w acetic acid. Combine the extracts in the flask of an ammonia-distillation apparatus, cool and add 50 ml of 50 per cent sodium hydroxide solution and 2 g of sodium thiosulphate. Immediately connect the apparatus and distil the liberated ammonia into an excess of 0·1N sulphuric acid. Titrate the excess acid in the receiver with 0·1N sodium hydroxide using methyl red as indicator. 1 ml 0·1N H_2SO_4 = 0·02521 g ammoniated mercury.

For salicylic acid, disperse 2 g in 50 ml of light petroleum and follow the method given under Ointment of Salicylic Acid and Sulphur, p. 560.

Solution of Mercuric Chloride, *B.Vet.C.* A 0·1 per cent solution in water. This is assayed officially by the Rupp method, using 200 ml of solution, but it is better estimated gravimetrically by precipitation with hydrogen sulphide, $HgS \times 1{\cdot}167 = HgCl_2$, or by EDTA titration.

Solution-tablets of Mercuric Chloride, *B.Vet.C.* Contain 8·75 grains each of mercuric chloride and sodium chloride, tinted with methylene blue.

The official method for mercury is the modified Rupp method described earlier but gravimetric estimation as sulphide ($HgS \times 1{\cdot}167 = HgCl_2$) or the EDTA titration may be used.

Solution-tablets of Mercuric Iodide, *B.Vet.C.* A mixture of mercuric iodide (8·75 grains) with potassium iodide (8·75 grains) tinted with eosin.

The total analysis is obtained by the method of Sage and Stevens[11] which has yielded consistently trustworthy results for this preparation. The procedure is the following:

(*a*) For mercury. Boil a known weight of tablet with an excess (2 g) of pure zinc filings in 50 per cent acetic acid for thirty minutes under reflux. After cooling, pour off from the amalgam and wash thoroughly with water (the aqueous portion being kept for iodine determination).

Dissolve the amalgam in 40 ml of a hot mixture of equal volumes of nitric acid and water; boil to remove nitrous fumes. Oxidise with permanganate and titrate with 0·1N ammonium thiocyanate as usual. 1 ml 0·1N = 0·01003 g Hg.

(*b*) For iodine. Transfer the acetic acid and aqueous washings from the above experiment to a stoppered bottle, add an equal volume of concentrated hydrochloric acid and 5 ml of chloroform. Titrate with 0·05M iodate to the disappearance of colour in the chloroform. 1 ml 0·05M = 0·0127 g I_2. Potassium iodide is obtained by subtracting the iodine due to mercury from the total iodine found in (*b*). The following factors are necessary: Hg × 1·265 = I; Hg × 2·265 = HgI_2; I × 1·308 = KI.

The tablets are extremely hygroscopic and all precautions against contamination with atmospheric moisture must be taken; for estimation a number of tablets should be dissolved in water and an aliquot part, equivalent to about one tablet, taken for determination. Complete solution of the tablets, free from a deposit of undissolved mercuric iodide, is effected by adding only a few ml of water until solution is complete and then diluting.

ORGANIC MERCURY COMPOUNDS

A number of methods are available for the conversion of organically bound mercury to the ionic form.

(i) By wet digestion with a mixture of nitric and sulphuric acids. This type of assay is used officially by the *U.S.P.*, details being as follows:

Weigh 0·3 to 0·5 g into a Kjeldahl flask and add 10 ml of concentrated sulphuric acid. Insert a small, short-stemmed funnel into the neck of the flask and add 10 ml of concentrated nitric acid. Heat the mixture, at first gently and then more strongly, until copious fumes of sulphur trioxide are evolved and the solution is colourless or only slightly yellow, adding more nitric acid if necessary and keeping the funnel in the neck of the flask during the heating. Allow to cool and then add 50 ml of cold water through the funnel. Rinse the funnel and the neck of the flask with a few millilitres of water, collecting the rinsings in the flask, and then add 0·1N potassium permanganate until a pink colour persists. Remove the excess of permanganate with a trace of hydrogen peroxide solution, cool, add 3 ml of concentrated nitric acid and titrate with 0·1N ammonium thiocyanate using ferric alum as indicator. 1 ml 0·1N = 0·01003 g Hg.

(ii) By formation of a zinc-mercury amalgam, following the method of Pierce.[12]

Weigh 0·3 to 0·5 g of the sample into a 100-ml flask, add 5 ml of 85 per cent formic acid, 15 ml of water and 1 g of zinc dust, and heat under reflux for thirty minutes. Filter off the amalgam, wash until the washings are not acid to litmus, and dissolve in a mixture of 20 ml of concentrated nitric acid and 20 ml of water. Leave on the water-bath for 3 minutes and then add 0·5 g of urea and sufficient 0·1N potassium permanganate to give a permanent pink colour. Cool, decolorise with a few drops of hydrogen peroxide solution, and titrate with 0·1N ammonium thiocyanate, using ferric alum as indicator; 1 ml 0·1N = 0·01003 g of Hg.

Stross and Stuckey[13] pointed out that under the conditions of assay, mercury being to some extent volatile, vigorous boiling causes condensation of the metal on the cold part of the reflux condenser, mercury in such a form often being difficult to wash off. It was suggested, therefore, that glass jointed apparatus be used, and that after the reduction, the condenser should be washed with water and the precipitate transferred to the filter paper as directed. 20 ml of concentrated nitric acid and 10 ml of water are then placed in the flask and refluxed in the apparatus for ten minutes. The condenser is finally washed with 10 ml of water, and the acid, after cooling, used to dissolve the zinc amalgam in the usual way, the assay then being completed in accordance with the directions given. This modification is recommended.

The formic acid may be replaced by acetic acid according to Chambers,[14] with the advantage that phenylmercuric nitrate is soluble in the latter and hydrolysis is rapid. Two volumes of glacial acetic acid and 1 volume of water is a suitable solvent and zinc filings are preferable to the powder.

(iii) By dry distillation of the mercury. A convenient method has been proposed by Brookes and Solomon[8] which has the advantage that it is applicable to a wide range of compounds and preparations. The mercury is isolated, free from interfering substances, by a distillation process and the metal is then dissolved in nitric acid and titrated with ammonium thiocyanate solution. It can be applied to a wide range of preparations with a small, constant and determinable error.

Procedure for decomposition of powders—Weigh a suitable amount of the sample, mix with 2 g of powdered sucrose, if necessary (see Note), and transfer to the flask (Fig. 10) with a funnel. (A small amount of calcium oxide mixed with the powder helps it to flow more freely.) Fill the flask to the neck with iron filings, and fill the neck to the bottom of the cone with a mixture of equal parts by volume of iron filings and calcium oxide. Fit the cone with a tight plug of steel wool (grade 0 Supreme, obtained from the Brillo Manufacturing Co. Ltd., was used). Plug the end of receiver *b* with zinc wool. Prepare the glass-wool trap by plugging the bulbous portion with glass wool that has been washed with acid and then dried; keep in place by means of zinc wool. Attach the trap to the receiver, and fix by a spring.

Lubricate the B14 joint with silicone grease, attach the receiver to the flask, and secure by tying iron wire round the lugs provided. Clamp the flask vertically with the U-bend of the receiver immersed in water in a 100-ml beaker.

If the semi-micro receiver, *c*, is used, charge the flask in the way just described but use a weight of sample equivalent to less than 50 mg of mercury.

Heat the neck of the flask to a dull red for five minutes with burner A. (A piece of wire gauze over the standard joint protects it from the direct heat of the flame.) Heat the bulb of the flask with burner B; use an extremely small flame, so that evolution of gas is not too rapid (five to ten minutes). Adjust burner B so that a steady stream of gas is evolved for a total time of fifteen minutes. When evolution of gas has considerably reduced, heat for another two minutes with the full heat of burner B. (Owing to great dissimilarity in mercury-containing preparations, it is not possible to state exact heating periods for the whole range of preparations but a total heating period of fifteen to twenty minutes was generally ample.) Pass the evolved gases into a flask containing carbon tetrachloride by means of a length of narrow rubber tubing attached to

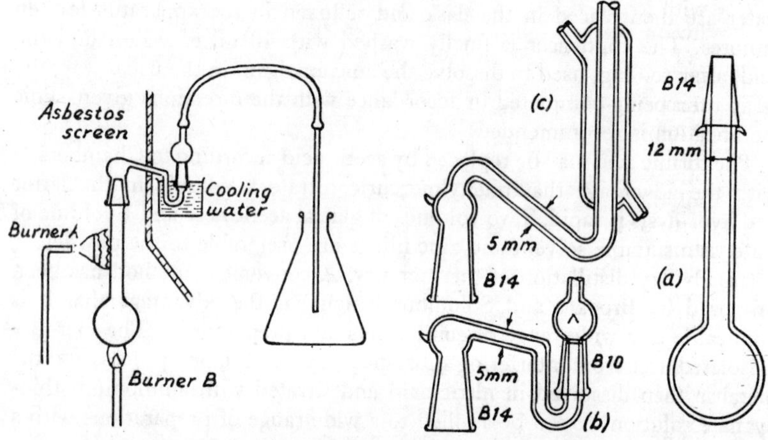

FIG. 10

Distillation apparatus

(*a*) Fused-silica flask
(*b*) Pyrex-glass receiver
(*c*) Pyrex-glass semi-micro receiver

the outlet of the receiver. A good indication of the rate of evolution of gas can be obtained from the position of the 'ring' of condensing mercury globules in the receiver, which should pass about 1 inch beyond the upper bend of the receiver.

At the end of the heating period, turn off burner A, cut the iron wire and detach the receiver. Turn off burner B and allow the receiver to cool (about five minutes).

Note. Organic mercurials, except the most volatile (such as methylmercuric chloride), decompose when heated, and sucrose need not be added to preparations containing these mercurials, e.g., seed dressings, or to those containing a large proportion of vegetable matter. Sucrose must be added to preparations that are more difficult to decompose and to inorganic mercury compounds. When ignited with mercurous chloride, a 2-g portion of sucrose produces enough gas to clear the flask of mercury in about twenty minutes, a fairly steady flow of gas being evolved.

Procedure for decomposition of tablets—Crush twenty tablets to a powder, transfer a suitable amount to the flask, and add powdered sucrose until the total weight of sample is about 2 g. Charge the flask with iron filings and calcium oxide, and then continue in the way described for decomposition of powders.

Procedure for decomposition of ointments—Accurately weigh 1 or 2 g of ointment on a piece of grease-proof paper. With the ointment spread fairly evenly, roll the paper into a 2½- to 3-inch roll. Place the roll in the flask, and press it against the bottom of the bulb with a glass tube. Add 1 g of powdered sulphur, charge the flask with iron filings and calcium oxide, and then continue in the way described for decomposition of powders. (In our experience, the periods for which the bulb of the flask is heated are approximately the same for most ointments—six minutes with an extremely low flame, six minutes with a slightly higher flame and five minutes at full heat.)

Procedure for titrating mercury—Amounts of mercury greater than 50 mg—Wash the receiver free from tarry matter by adding acetone through the B14 socket, and then wash several times with water to remove acetone. Detach the glass-wool trap, and transfer the receiver to a wide-necked 500-ml conical flask. Add 15 ml of water and then 15 ml of concentrated nitric acid, slowly at first, until most of the zinc dissolves. Warm on a water-bath to dissolve the mercury, and then boil to remove nitrous fumes. Add 5 per cent potassium permanganate solution, dropwise, until a permanent pink colour is obtained, cool and decolorise with a trace of ferrous sulphate. Dilute with water to about 120 ml, cool to below 15°, and titrate with 0·1N ammonium thiocyanate using ferric alum as indicator. 1 ml 0·1N = 0·01003 g Hg.

Amounts of mercury less than 50 mg—Invert the receiver, and fix it in the neck of a flask by means of a cork that has a second hole through which a glass tube passes so that suction may be applied. Wash with acetone until free from tarry matter. (Slight suction is necessary to draw liquid through at first; it then percolates through by siphon action.) Wash the receiver thoroughly with water to remove acetone.

Transfer the receiver and cork attachment to the neck of a 100-ml conical flask. Dissolve the mercury by allowing three 2-ml quantities of concentrated nitric acid to percolate through, wash with six 3-ml quantities of water, and remove the receiver. Place the flask on a water-bath for a few minutes, and add 5 per cent potassium permanganate solution until a permanent pink colour is obtained. Cool, and decolorise by adding a freshly prepared 2 per cent solution of ferrous sulphate. Cool to below 15°, add 0·5 ml of 10 per cent ferric alum solution, and titrate with 0·01, 0·02 or 0·05N ammonium thiocyanate until the solution has a distinct brown tinge (the titre should be between 5 and 10 ml).

(iv) By oxygen-flask combustion. This very convenient method, described by Vickers and Wilkinson[15] is given in full in Appendix IV (p. 801). It has been applied with excellent results to a large number of organic mercurials including phenylmercuric nitrate, mersalyl sodium, mercurochrome, chlormerodrin, tolylmercuric acetate and ethylmercuric phosphate.

All these methods are suitable for assaying official organic mercurials, method (i) being used by the *U.S.P.* and *N.F.* and method (ii) by the *B.P.* and *B.P.C.* Substances for which they are applicable are the following:

TABLE 24

SUBSTANCE	FORMULA	MOL. WT.	1 ML 0·1N
Chlormerodrin, *B.P.C.*	$C_5H_{11}O_2N_2ClHg$	367·2	0·01836 g
Meralluride, *B.P.C.* and *U.S.P.*	$C_9H_{16}O_6N_2Hg$*	448·9	0·02244 g
Mercaptomerin Sodium, *U.S.P.*	$C_{16}H_{25}O_6NSHgNa_2$	606·0	0·03030 g
Mercurophylline, *N.F.*	$C_{14}H_{24}O_5NHgNa$*	510·0	0·02550 g
Mersalyl Acid, *B.P.*	$C_{13}H_{17}O_6NHg$	483·9	0·02419 g
Mersalyl Sodium, *B.P.C.*, and *N.F.*	$C_{13}H_{16}O_6NHgNa$	505·9	0·02529 g
Phenylmercuric Acetate, *B.P.C.*	$C_8H_8O_2Hg$	336·8	0·01684 g
Phenylmercuric Nitrate, *B.P.* and *N.F.*	$C_{12}H_{11}O_4NHg_2$	634·4	0·01586 g

* With theopylline in approximate molecular proportions; for determination, see p. 143.

Certain mercurials are officially determined by slight modifications of the procedures given above.

Thiomersal, $C_9H_9O_2HgSNa$, Mol. Wt. 404·8, is assayed as follows:

> Weigh 0·5 g into a 100-ml Kjeldahl flask, add 5 ml of concentrated sulphuric acid and heat gently until charred. Continue to heat and add strong hydrogen peroxide solution, dropwise, until colourless. Dilute, evaporate until slight fuming occurs, dilute to 10 ml with water and titrate with 0·1N ammonium thiocyanate using ferric alum as indicator. 1 ml 0·1N = 0·02024 g.

Nitromersol, $C_7H_5O_3NHg$, Mol. Wt. 351·7, is assayed as follows:

> Weigh 0·2 g into a 500-ml Kjeldahl flask, add 15 ml of concentrated sulphuric acid and heat gently for fifteen to twenty minutes. Cool, decolorise by the dropwise addition of 30 per cent hydrogen peroxide solution, digest for a further two to three minutes and add more hydrogen peroxide if necessary to produce a colourless solution. Cool, dilute to about 100 ml, add sufficient 0·1N potassium permanganate to give a permanent pink colour on heating and then decolorise with a few drops of hydrogen peroxide solution. Cool, add a mixture of 5 ml of concentrated nitric acid and 10 ml of water and titrate with 0·1N ammonium thiocyanate using ferric alum as indicator. 1 ml 0·1N = 0·01759 g.

At the concentrations at which organic mercurials such as phenylmercuric nitrate, thiomersal, etc., are used as preservatives in pharmaceutical and cosmetic preparations microbiological methods of assay are frequently more reliable than are chemical ones.[16] Either the plate-diffusion or the tube-dilution technique, as described on pp. 814 to 826 for the assay of antibiotics, can be used. The former is probably the method of choice although the latter is the more sensitive, being able to detect the organic mercurials down to 0·05 p.p.m. against about 1 p.p.m. by the plate-diffusion method. For both methods, the standard, or control, material should preferably be of a similar basic formulation to that of the test material, but with sufficient of the mercurial under assay added, in as small a volume as possible, to give the theoretical amount in the final formulation. If a simple aqueous solution of the standard is used, invalid assays will frequently result due to interference by other constituents of the formulation.

By plate-diffusion: The assay medium contains Oxoid peptone 10 g, Lab-Lemco 15 g and agar powder 15 g made up to 1 litre with water and adjusted to pH 7·2. For seeding the medium use about 0·4 ml of a sensitive strain of *Staphylococcus aureus* (the Heatley penicillin assay strain is suitable) grown for twenty-four hours in nutrient broth to each 100 ml of agar medium.

Satisfactory zones of response can be expected from concentrations of 10 and 2 p.p.m. of the mercurials.

By tube-dilution: Basically, the method is that described on p. 815 for the assay of antibiotics, the test organism being *Escherichia coli* (NCTC 5934) grown for twenty-four hours at 37° in nutrient broth. Transfer 5 ml of each dilution to each of 4 tubes and then add 5 ml of a sterile medium containing Oxoid peptone 1 g, glucose 2 g, sodium phosphate 5·5 g, solution of bromocresol purple *B.P.* 5 ml in 1 litre water. Add one drop of the test culture to each tube and transfer them to a water-bath at 37° for four hours. The end-point is the greatest dilution at which there is marked inhibition of growth as shown by a significant decrease in turbidity. With preparations which are initially turbid, the end-point can be read after a slightly longer incubation period by the colour change. Calculate the mercurial content of the test sample by comparing the mean end-point with that of the control preparation.

Injection of Mersalyl, *B.P.* Contains 10 per cent of mersalyl sodium and 5 per cent of theophylline in pH-adjusted solution.

Mersalyl may be determined directly on 5 ml either by the acid reduction method of Pierce or by hydrolysis and sulphide precipitation, as follows:

Dilute 5 ml to 100 ml with water; add 15 ml of concentrated hydrochloric acid. Boil under a reflux condenser for three hours, add 200 ml of hot water and pass in hydrogen sulphide for fifteen minutes. Filter while hot through a Gooch crucible, wash the precipitate first with solution of hydrogen sulphide, then with ethanol and finally with carbon disulphide. Dry at 110° and weigh. 1 g = 0·8622 g Hg.

Although criticism has been made that the method gives high results, provided the details are followed closely, comparable figures are possible.

For the determination of theophylline, see p. 143.

1. Rupp, E., *Arch. Pharm.*, 1905, **243,** 300.
2. Brindle, H., and Waterhouse, C. E., *Quart. J. Pharm.*, 1936, **9,** 519.
3. Jamieson, G. S., *J. Ind. Eng. Chem.*, 1919, **11,** 296.
4. Strafford, N., and Wyatt, P. F., *Analyst,* 1936, **61,** 528.
5. *Analyst,* 1960, **85,** 651.
6. *Analyst,* 1956, **81,** 176.

7. FAO Plant Protection Bulletin, 1960, **9** (2), 19.
8. Brookes, H. E., and Solomon, L. E., *Analyst*, 1959, **84**, 622.
9. Allport, N. L., *Quart. J. Pharm.*, 1928, **1**, 23.
10. Tagliavini, A., *Boll. Chim. Farm.*, 1917, **56**, 297.
11. Sage, C. E., and Stevens, S. G., *C. & D.*, 1932, **116**, 84.
12. Pierce, J. S., *Quart. J. Pharm.*, 1942, **15**, 367.
13. Stross, P. S., and Stuckey, R. E., *J. Pharm. Pharmacol.*, 1949, **1**, 421.
14. Chambers, W. P., *Quart. J. Pharm.*, 1943, **16**, 6.
15. Vickers, C., and Wilkinson, J. V., *J. Pharm. Pharmacol.*, 1961, **13**, 156T.
16. Carter, D. V., and Sykes, G., *Analyst*, 1958, **83**, 536.

MISCELLANEOUS METALLIC COMPOUNDS

A few metals find occasional use in pharmaceutical practice but are not sufficiently important to merit separate monographs. Others are sometimes required to be determined in trace amounts. This section will discuss macro-methods for gold, manganese and titanium and trace-methods for cobalt, nickel and manganese.

GOLD

Gold is used pharmaceutically in organic combination and is almost always determined gravimetrically as the metal. The organic compound is first mineralised by heating with sulphuric acid and the gold is then precipitated by boiling with nitric acid. Alternatively the sulphuric acid solution may be heated to fuming and then diluted with water, when the gold precipitates. Variations on these basic methods exist and some are given below.

Sodium aurothiomalate, $C_4H_3O_4SAuNa_2,H_2O$, Mol. Wt. 408·1. This contains about 45 per cent of gold and is assayed as follows:

For Au. Weigh about 0·2 g into a Kjeldahl flask, add 10 ml of concentrated sulphuric acid and heat to boiling-point. Continue to boil gently until a clear, pale yellow liquid is produced, allow to cool, add about 1 ml of concentrated nitric acid, dropwise, and then boil for one hour. Cool, add 70 ml of water, boil for a further five minutes and filter. Wash the residue of gold with hot water (retaining the filtrate and washings for the assay for sodium), dry and ignite to constant weight.

For Na. Evaporate the filtrate and washings, retained above, to dryness, moisten with concentrated sulphuric acid and ignite to constant weight. $Na_2SO_4 \times 0{\cdot}3237 = Na$.

Injection of Sodium Aurothiomalate, ***B.P.*** This usually contains 10 mg per ml in water for injection. Assay as follows:

To a volume of sample equivalent to about 0·1 g of sodium aurothiomalate add 2 g of potassium bromide and 25 ml of concentrated nitric acid. Evaporate slowly to dryness and then continue to heat until fumes cease to be evolved. Allow to cool, add 50 ml of water, warm and filter. Wash the residue of gold with hot water, dry and ignite to constant weight.

Aurothioglucose, $C_6H_{11}O_5SAu$, Mol. Wt. 392·2. This may be determined by the method given above for sodium aurothiomalate but the following simple alternative has also been used:

Dissolve 1 g in 100 ml of water and add, slowly, 10 ml of concentrated nitric acid. When the reaction has subsided boil for five minutes, filter, wash the residue of gold with hot water, dry, and ignite to constant weight. Au × 1·9909 = $C_6H_{11}O_5SAu$.

MANGANESE

Manganese is commonly determined by oxidation with sodium bismuthate in nitric acid solution when permanganic acid is formed to give a fairly specific method. This is the *B.P.C.* method for **manganese sulphate,** $MnSO_4,4H_2O$, Mol. Wt. 223·1.

Weigh 0·15 g into a flask, dissolve in 40 ml of water and add 8 ml of concentrated nitric acid that has been freshly boiled and cooled. Cool, add 1·5 g of sodium bismuthate, stopper the flask and shake for two minutes. Then add 25 ml of a mixture of three volumes of the nitric acid and 97 volumes of water, filter and wash the filter and flask with 40 ml of the diluted acid, collecting the filtrate and washings in 50 ml of 0·1N ferrous ammonium sulphate. Immediately titrate the excess ferrous ammonium sulphate with 0·1N potassium permanganate. Repeat the operation omitting the sample; the difference between the two titrations represents the amount of ferrous ammonium sulphate required by the sample. 1 ml 0·1N = 0·003021 g $MnSO_4$.

Manganese can also be determined by titration with EDTA. The following method, due to Malát, Suk and Jeníčková,[1] is suitable:

To 100 ml of a neutral solution containing about 20 mg of manganese add a small amount of hydroxylamine hydrochloride to prevent oxidation of the manganese. Then add 10 ml of ammonia buffer solution followed by 3 to 5 drops of catechol violet indicator and titrate immediately with 0·01M EDTA until the colour changes from greenish-blue to reddish-purple. 1 ml 0·01M EDTA = 0·0005493 g manganese.

Another method for the determination of manganese is by precipitation with 8-hydroxyquinoline at pH 6 to 10.

TITANIUM

This metal is usually determined gravimetrically as TiO_2 by precipitation as an organic complex which is then ignited. A number of organic precipitants are suitable, the method given below for **titanium dioxide** (TiO_2, Mol. Wt. 79·90) being based upon the use of cupferron.

Heat 0·15 g with 10 ml of concentrated sulphuric acid and 5 g of anhydrous sodium sulphate until dissolved, cool and pour into 100 ml of water. Add 2 g of tartaric acid, make just alkaline to litmus paper with dilute ammonia solution and then add dilute sulphuric acid until just acid and add 10 ml of the acid in excess. Cool, add 20 ml of a 6 per cent aqueous solution of ammonium nitrosophenylhydroxylamine, stirring during the addition; allow to stand for ten minutes and filter. Wash the residue with dilute sulphuric acid containing a trace of ammonium nitrosophenylhydroxylamine and then with dilute ammonia solution, dry, and ignite the residue of titanium dioxide to constant weight.

SOME TRACE DETERMINATIONS

In addition to the elements for which methods of determination of small amounts have been given in other monographs, cobalt, nickel and manganese may occur in small amounts, in particular in fertilisers and feeding stuffs but also in pharmaceutical products, and the following methods are satisfactory for their determination.[2] All the reagents used in the determinations should be substantially free from the element being determined.

First it is necessary to prepare a solution of the sample in which the element can conveniently be determined and this is best done as follows:

For organic materials: Destroy the organic matter by dry ashing, method A (see Appendix XI), using a suitable quantity of the sample. When all the organic matter has been destroyed, cool the basin and contents, add 10 ml of hydrochloric acid (1 + 1 v/v) and evaporate to dryness on a water-bath. Extract the soluble salts with two 10-ml quantities of boiling hydrochloric acid (1 + 5 v/v), decanting the solution each time through the same Whatman No. 541 filter paper into a 50-ml graduated flask. Add 5 ml of hydrochloric acid (1 + 1 v/v) and about 5 ml of nitric acid (1 + 2 v/v) to the residue in the basin and evaporate to dryness on a hot-plate at low heat to remove all the nitric acid. Finally extract the residue with a further 10 ml of boiling hydrochloric acid (1 + 5 v/v) and filter into the flask through the same paper as before. Dilute the combined extracts to volume with water, washing the filter paper in the process. This final solution should be approximately normal with respect to hydrochloric acid.

For inorganic materials: Extract a suitable amount of sample directly with acid as described above for organic materials beginning with the words 'add 10 ml of hydrochloric acid (1 + 1 v/v) . . .'.

Cobalt. In this method, based on the method of Claasen and Daamen,[3] the cobalt, with other trace metals, is extracted with hydrochloric acid in the presence of citrate which prevents precipitation of iron and phosphate. The cobalt is then determined by measuring the extinction, at 367 mμ, of a toluene solution of the complex formed between cobalt and 2-nitroso-1-naphthol. Claasen and Daamen used a chloroform solution and measured at 530 mμ; the conditions given below result in a more sensitive method which is less susceptible to interference from other elements, particularly copper.[2]

Standard cobalt solution. Dissolve 0·494 g of cobaltous nitrate, $Co(NO_3)_2,6H_2O$, in sufficient water to produce exactly 100 ml; this solution contains 1 mg of cobalt per ml. Dilute this solution freshly as required to give a solution containing 1 μg of cobalt per ml.

Method: Pipette a volume of the acid solution containing not more than 15 μg of cobalt into a 100-ml beaker and add 15 ml of 40 per cent sodium citrate solution. Dilute with water to about 50 ml and adjust the pH to between 3 and 4 with 2N hydrochloric acid and 2N sodium hydroxide, using pH test paper. If a precipitate of ferric hydroxide forms it can be destroyed by heating the solution. Cool to room temperature and add 10 ml of hydrogen peroxide solution (10 volumes). After five minutes add 1 ml of 2-nitroso-1-naphthol reagent (prepared by dissolving 1 g of 2-nitroso-1-naphthol in 100 ml of glacial acetic acid and adding 1 g of activated carbon; shake before use and filter the required amount), heat to about 90° and then allow to stand at room temperature for at least thirty minutes.

Transfer the solution to a 125-ml separator, add exactly 10 ml of redistilled toluene and shake vigorously for two minutes. Discard the lower, aqueous layer, add 20 ml of 2N hydrochloric acid to the toluene extract and shake for one minute. Run off the lower layer and discard. Then wash the toluene layer with two 20-ml quantities of 2N sodium hydroxide, shaking for one minute each time, discard the washings and filter the toluene layer through a little anhydrous sodium sulphate and a cotton-wool plug into a glass-stoppered tube. At the same time prepare a blank solution by carrying out the entire operation omitting the sample and prepare two internal standards using, instead of the sample, 5 and 10 ml of standard cobalt solution, 1 μg per ml.

Measure the extinctions of the sample and blank solutions at the absorption maximum at about 367 mμ, using 1-cm cells with redistilled toluene in the comparison cell in each case. Read the μg of cobalt equivalent to the extinctions from a standard curve (checked against the two standards) and so obtain the net amount of cobalt in the sample.

Prepare the standard curve as follows. Into a series of 100-ml beakers, pipette suitable volumes of standard cobalt solution, 1 μg per ml, covering the range 0 to 15 μg of cobalt, treat each standard exactly as described above beginning with the words 'Dilute with water to about 50 ml . . .' and prepare a curve by plotting extinction against μg of cobalt.

Manganese. In this method the manganese is oxidised with periodate in acid solution and the resulting permanganate solution is measured colorimetrically.

Standard manganese solution. Dissolve 0·288 g of potassium permanganate in 100 to 200 ml of water, add 5 ml of diluted sulphuric acid (1 + 3 v/v) and dilute to 1 litre with water. This solution contains approximately 100 μg of manganese per ml. Standardise by titration with oxalate and dilute with water just before use to give a solution containing 10 μg of manganese per ml.

Method: Pipette a volume of the acid solution containing not more than 70 μg of manganese into a small beaker and evaporate to dryness at low temperature on a hot-plate. Cool, add 3 ml of orthophosphoric acid and warm until the residue is dissolved. Cool, carefully add 3 ml of water, warm again and transfer the solution to a 10-ml, glass-stoppered, calibrated tube, washing the beaker with 3 ml of warm water and adding the washing to the tube. Add 0·5 g of analytical-reagent grade potassium periodate and dilute with water to just above the 10-ml mark. Stopper the tube loosely, heat in a water-bath for thirty minutes, cool and adjust the volume to 10 ml with water.

At the same time prepare a blank solution by repeating the entire operation omitting the sample.

Measure the extinctions of the sample and blank solutions at the absorption maximum at about 526 mμ using 1-cm cells with water in the comparison cell in each case, read the μg manganese equivalent to the extinctions from a standard curve and so obtain the net manganese content of the sample.

Prepare the standard curve as follows. Into a series of 10-ml, glass-stoppered, calibrated tubes pipette suitable volumes of standard manganese solution, 10 μg per ml, covering the range 0 to 70 μg of manganese. To each of the tubes add 3 ml of orthophosphoric acid and 0·5 g of analytical reagent grade potassium periodate and continue as described above beginning with the words 'dilute with water to just above the 10-ml mark . . .'. Prepare a curve by plotting extinctions against μg of Mn.

Nickel. In this method nickel is extracted from an ammoniacal solution as its dimethylglyoxime complex and then determined spectrophotometrically as the nickelic complex.

Standard nickel solution. Dissolve 1·002 g of pure metallic nickel in concentrated nitric acid, boiling to effect solution, add 2 ml of concentrated sulphuric acid and evaporate until white fumes are evolved. Cool, transfer to a 1-litre graduated flask and dilute to volume with water. Transfer a 5-ml aliquot of this solution to a 500-ml graduated flask and dilute to volume with water to give a solution containing 10 μg of nickel per ml.

Method: Pipette a volume of acid solution containing not more than 100 μg of nickel into a beaker, dilute to 100 ml with water and add 10 ml of 25 per cent sodium citrate solution. Then add strong ammonia solution, with mixing, until just alkaline to litmus paper and add ten drops of the ammonia in excess. Transfer the solution to a 250-ml separator, add 10 ml of a 0·2 per cent solution of sodium dimethylglyoxime in dilute ammonia solution (1 + 19), shake for one minute and allow to stand for ten minutes. Add 10 ml of chloroform, shake for one minute and run the chloroform layer into a second separator, rinsing the stem of the first separator with about 3 ml of chloroform and adding the rinsings to the second separator. Extract the aqueous layer with a further 10 ml of chloroform, again shaking for one minute, and add this extract to the first, rinsing the stem of the separator as before. Extract the combined chloroform extracts first with 15 ml and then with 5 ml of diluted hydrochloric acid (1 + 19), shaking vigorously for one minute each time, and discard the chloroform layer. Combine the acid extracts in a 100-ml beaker, rinsing the two separators with a few millilitres of water and adding the rinsings to the acid extract. Heat the solution very carefully over a low Bunsen flame to remove any chloroform and then boil gently until the volume of the solution is about 25 ml. Cool, transfer to a 50-ml graduated flask with two 5-ml quantities of water and add 2 ml of 25 per cent sodium citrate solution followed by 2 ml of saturated bromine water, mixing after each addition. Then add just enough strong ammonia solution to destroy the bromine colour and to give a 1-ml excess and, finally, 4 ml of the 0·2 per cent solution of sodium dimethylglyoxime in dilute ammonia solution (1 + 19). Mix, dilute to volume with water and again mix.

Repeat the entire operation omitting the sample to obtain a reagent blank solution.

Measure the extinction of the sample and blank solutions at the absorption maximum at about 480 mμ using 4-cm cells with water in the comparison cell in each case, read the μg of nickel equivalent to the extinctions from a standard curve and calculate the net amount of nickel in the sample.

Prepare the standard curve as follows. Into a series of 50-ml graduated flasks measure suitable volumes, covering the range 0 to 100 μg of nickel, of standard nickel solution containing 10 μg of nickel per ml. To each flask add 20 ml of diluted hydrochloric acid (1 + 19) and complete as described above from the words 'add 2 ml of 25 per cent sodium citrate solution . . .'. Prepare a curve by plotting extinction against μg of nickel.

1. Malát, M., Suk, V., and Jeníčková, A., *Chem. Listy*, 1954, **48**, 663.
2. Determination of Trace Elements, *S.A.C.*, pp. 3, 12, 27 and 29.
3. Claasen, A., and Daamen, A., *Anal. Chim. Acta*, 1955, **12**, 547.

METHADONE HYDROCHLORIDE

$C_{21}H_{27}ON,HCl$ Mol. Wt. 345·9

Methadone hydrochloride is assayed by extraction of the base and titration of the latter after removal of the solvent.

To 0·25 g in 25 ml of water in a separator add a few drops of sodium hydroxide solution and extract with four portions of ether. Wash each extract with the same 10-ml portion of water, evaporate, dissolve the residue in 3 ml of neutral ethanol, add 10 ml of 0·1N hydrochloric acid and titrate back to methyl red with 0·02N sodium hydroxide. 1 ml 0·02N = 0·006918 g.

In ethanol, methadone hydrochloride has an extinction maximum at 294 mμ, E(1 per cent, 1 cm) = 13·2.

Injection of Methadone Hydrochloride, *B.P.* This preparation is assayed as for the tablets, given below, using a volume of injection containing about 0·1 g of methadone hydrochloride, diluted to 20 ml with water.

Linctus of Methadone Hydrochloride, *B.P.C.* Contains 0·057 per cent w/v of methadone hydrochloride in a base of glycerin and syrup of tolu, coloured with tartrazine.

Dilute 15 g with an equal quantity of water, acidify with dilute sulphuric acid and extract with 10 ml of light petroleum. Wash the extract with two successive 5-ml quantities of water, add the washings to the aqueous solution and reject the light petroleum extract. Make just alkaline to litmus paper with 20 per cent sodium hydroxide solution, add 2 g of sodium chloride and extract with three successive quantities of 30, 15 and 15 ml of anæsthetic ether. Wash the combined ether extracts with two 5-ml quantities of water, combine the washings and wash with 5 ml of anæsthetic ether. Add the ether washing to the combined ether extracts and extract with two quantities, each of 10 ml, of 0·02N hydrochloric acid. Combine the acid extracts, add a small piece of porous pot and warm to remove any dissolved ether. Cool, dilute to 25 ml with water and measure the extinction at the maximum at about 293 mμ, using 1-cm cells. Per cent methadone hydrochloride = E(1 per cent, 1 cm) × 6·49. Calculate the per cent w/v from the weight per ml.

Tablets of Methadone Hydrochloride, *B.P.* Usually contain 5 mg of methadone hydrochloride.

The assay follows the method given above by the extraction of the base. Sufficient powdered tablets to contain about 0·1 g are transferred to a separator containing 20 ml of water and extracted in alkaline solution with ether. The ether extracts should be washed twice with 20 per cent sodium chloride solution, the washings being again extracted with ether. The bulked ethers are then extracted with 20 ml of 0·02N acid followed by water washing. The bulked aqueous solutions after removal of ether on a water-bath are back titrated with 0·02N alkali to methyl red.

A simple spectrophotometric assay is also possible.

Weigh accurately a quantity of powdered tablet material equivalent to about 25 mg of methadone hydrochloride and transfer to a 50-ml graduated flask. Add about 30 ml of ethanol, warm on a water-bath until boiling occurs, cool immediately and shake for thirty minutes. Make up to volume with ethanol, mix, centrifuge a portion of the solution and measure the maximum extinction of a 1-cm layer at about 294 mμ, using ethanol as the blank. Calculate the amount of methadone hydrochloride in each tablet.

METHYL SALICYLATE

$C_6H_4(OH).COOCH_3$ Mol. Wt. 152·2

Methyl salicylate, if free from interfering substances, may be determined by the general method for esters by direct saponification with 0·5N ethanolic potash, and back-titration with 0·5N acid, using phenolphthalein as indicator. 1 ml 0·5N = 0·07608 g.

Being phenolic in nature, methyl salicylate may be extracted from solvent solution by aqueous potassium hydroxide, practically no hydrolysis occurring in the cold if the alkali solution is weak. Other methods of determination can be more advantageously discussed in the analysis of the preparations containing methyl salicylate, which are described below.

In *cyclo*hexane, methyl salicylate has an extinction maximum at 308 mμ, E(1 per cent, 1 cm) v/v = 357.

Liniment of Methyl Salicylate, *B.P.C.* Contains 25 per cent v/v of methyl salicylate in arachis or cottonseed oil.

Assuming methyl salicylate to be the only volatile matter present, a determination of loss of weight when about 5 g is heated in a flat-bottomed metal dish on a hot-plate at about 120°, will give a satisfactory result providing the heating is not prolonged (one hour should be sufficient) otherwise oxidation of the oil may occur. To obtain the proportion by volume of methyl salicylate a weight per ml is necessary and an average weight per ml of methyl salicylate of 1·182 may be assumed.

For a direct determination of methyl salicylate, the methods given under Ointment of Methyl Salicylate are applicable.

A rapid physical assay can also be used:

> Dilute 5 ml of liniment to 100 ml in *cyclo*hexane. Make further dilutions as follows: 5 ml to 50 ml, then 5 ml to 50 ml, then 5 ml to 50 ml, all in *cyclo*hexane. Measure the maximum extinction of a 1-cm layer of this final solution at about 308 mμ using *cyclo*hexane as the blank. Calculate the methyl salicylate content of the liniment.

Ointment of Methyl Salicylate, *B.P.C.* Contains 50 per cent by weight of methyl salicylate in a base of equal parts of beeswax and hydrous wool fat.

The total loss on evaporation by the method given above for the liniment, less the water found by a Dean and Stark distillation (p. 803), is a measure of the methyl salicylate.

For a direct determination the obvious method of steam distillation into excess of 0·5N alkali, boiling the distillate to saponify and back-titration has inexplicably yielded low results. Hatfull,[1] however, obtained good recovery by steam distillation in the presence of mineral acid but a large volume of distillate (300 ml) must be collected.

For routine control, it has been found that hydrolysis in dilute ethanol does not appreciably saponify the fats and a close approximation of the methyl salicylate content is possible:

> To about 5 g of ointment add 30 ml of N aqueous sodium hydroxide and 10 ml of ethanol. Boil until all the ethanol has been evaporated. Titrate while hot with N hydrochloric acid using phenol red as indicator. 1 ml N = 0·1522 g.

Non-aqueous titration of methyl salicylate using lithium methoxide with quinaldine red as indicator or with tetrabutylammonium hydroxide and a potentiometric finish (see p. 794) has been applied by Allen.[2] This method is applicable to the ester itself and to the liniment, but with ointments the end-point tends to be somewhat sluggish although probably adequate for routine laboratory control.

METHYL SALICYLATE

A determination of methyl salicylate by isolation of the salicylic acid can be applied, eliminating fatty acids as barium soaps.[3] The *B.P.C.* method is a modification:

To 0·3 g add 10 ml of ether and 10 ml of 0·5N ethanolic potassium hydroxide and boil under a reflux condenser for one and a half hours, shaking well during the first fifteen minutes. Evaporate the solvents, add 30 ml of water and warm to melt the waxy matter. Add 10 ml of 10 per cent barium chloride solution, mix well, heat to boiling-point, cool and filter. Add a further 10 ml of the barium chloride solution to the residue and again mix well, heat to boiling-point, cool and filter; repeat the operation with a third 10-ml quantity of the barium chloride solution. Combine the filtrates, add 10 ml of dilute hydrochloric acid and extract with four or more successive quantities, each of 40 ml, of ether until extraction is complete.

Combine the extracts, wash with two successive 10-ml quantities of water and evaporate the ether at a temperature not exceeding 40°. Either dissolve the residue in 10 ml of neutral 95 per cent ethanol and titrate with 0·1N sodium hydroxide using phenol red as indicator, 1 ml 0·1N = 0·01522 g, or determine the salicylic acid by one of the methods given in that monograph (p. 557).

The determination of methyl salicylate in **Compound Ointment of Methyl Salicylate,** *B.P.C.* (which contains 50 per cent with aromatics in beeswax and hydrous wool fat) and **Non-Staining Ointment of Iodine with Methyl Salicylate,** *B.P.C.* (see also p. 314) is the same as given above using 0·3 g and 3·0 g respectively.

The method of determining phenols based upon coupling with 4-amino-phenazone (see Phenol p. 514) has been applied to the determination of methyl salicylate in ointments by Johnson and Savidge.[4] Because of the possibility of hydrolysis of methyl salicylate to the free acid, which gives no reaction (see Note below under Non-Staining Ointment of Iodine), it has not been possible to quote an E(1 per cent, 1 cm) value for the final solution and calculations should always be made from a standard or a calibration curve prepared at the same time as the assay is being carried out. The method for Ointment of Methyl Salicylate, *B.P.C.*, and Compound Ointment of Methyl Salicylate, *B.P.C.*, is as follows:

Weigh 0·5 g into a 100-ml round-bottomed flask, add 20 ml of 95 per cent ethanol and two glass beads and reflux on a water-bath for thirty minutes using a straight-bore water-condenser. Allow to cool somewhat, wash down the condenser with 10 ml of 95 per cent ethanol and cool thoroughly. Filter through a fast filter paper into a 100-ml graduated flask and wash the original flask and the filter paper with 95 per cent ethanol, collecting the washings in the graduated flask, until the volume of filtrate and washings is exactly 100 ml. Transfer a 10-ml aliquot to a 1-litre graduated flask containing 800 ml of water and 2 ml of strong ammonia buffer solution (see p. 514). Dilute to volume with water and mix thoroughly. Immediately (see Note, below) transfer a 10-ml aliquot to a 150-ml separator and continue by the general method (chloroform extraction procedure) described under Phenol, p. 514, beginning with 'Add 1 ml of 4-aminophenazone . . .', measuring the extinction at the maximum at about 470 mμ and using 0·5-cm cells. Read the mg of methyl salicylate equivalent to the extinction from a standard curve prepared as follows:

Dissolve 0·2 g of methyl salicylate in sufficient acetone to produce exactly 100 ml. Transfer a 10-ml aliquot of this solution to a 1-litre graduated flask containing 800 ml of water and 2 ml of strong ammonia buffer solution (see above) and dilute to volume with water (standard methyl salicylate solution). Continue by the general method, as above, using measured quantities of standard methyl salicylate solution, covering the range 0·1 to 0·4 mg of methyl salicylate and plot the mg of methyl salicylate against extinction.

For Non-Staining Ointment of Iodine with Methyl Salicylate an additional heating with ethanol has been prescribed since with a single treatment a somewhat intractable residue is formed from which it is difficult to extract all the methyl salicylate.

Proceed as described above to the words 'filter through a fast filter paper into a 100-ml graduated flask,' but during this filtration retain the bulk of the residue in the flask and wash the flask and filter two or three times with 95 per cent ethanol. Add 20 ml of 95 per cent ethanol to the residue in the flask and reflux again for thirty minutes. Cool, filter through the same paper and wash the flask and filter with 95 per cent ethanol until exactly 100 ml of filtrate and washings have been collected. Transfer a 10-ml aliquot to a 1-litre graduated flask containing 800 ml of water and 2 ml of strong ammonia buffer solution (see above), dilute to volume with water and mix thoroughly. Immediately (see Note below) transfer a 50-ml aliquot to a 150-ml separator and continue by the general method (chloroform extraction procedure) described under Phenol, p. 514, beginning with 'Add 1 ml of 4-aminophenazone . . .', measuring the extinction at the maximum at about 470 mμ and using 0·5-cm cells. Read the mg of methyl salicylate equivalent to the extinction from the standard curve.

Note: If the alkaline solution is allowed to stand before colour development, progressive hydrolysis of the ester occurs and low results are obtained since salicylic acid does not give a colour. It is important that not more than five minutes elapses between preparing the alkaline solution and completion of colour development.

In conclusion it might be said that no really satisfactory method for the determination of methyl salicylate in ointments has yet been described. Each of the methods given above has its advantages and its drawbacks.

1. HATFULL, R. S., *Analyst*, 1948, **73**, 559.
2. ALLEN, J., private communication.
3. GARRATT, D. C., *Quart. J. Pharm.*, 1935, **8**, 472.
4. JOHNSON, C. A., and SAVIDGE, R. A., *J. Pharm. Pharmacol.*, 1958, **10**, 171T.

METHYLCELLULOSE

A number of compounds of this type are in use and they consist of methyl (and in some cases ethyl or hydroxypropyl) ethers of cellulose; they are characterised by their alkoxyl content. A general method for the determination of methoxyl groups is as follows:

Apparatus: This consists essentially of a 50-ml round-bottomed flask (A) with a ground-glass joint, an air condenser (E) and scrubber (B) and two receivers (C) and (D). Into the flask (A) is sealed a capillary side arm, of 1 mm diameter, to provide an inlet for a stream of carbon dioxide. The condenser, which should be about 25 cm in height and about 9 mm in diameter, is bent through 180° at the top and terminates in a glass capillary, 2 mm in diameter, dipping into the scrubber (B). The outlet from the scrubber is a tube of about 7 mm diameter terminating in a removable tube of 4 mm diameter which passes through a one-holed rubber stopper and dips below the surface of the liquid in the first of the two receivers; the receivers are connected in series. The apparatus must be dried before use.

Reagents:

Potassium acetate in glacial acetic acid. Weigh 100 g of anhydrous potassium acetate into a 1-litre graduated flask, dissolve in a mixture of 9 volumes of glacial acetic acid and 1 volume of acetic anhydride and make up to volume with the acetic acid/acetic anhydride mixture.

Bromine in acetic acid. Dissolve about 5 ml of bromine in 145 ml of the potassium acetate in glacial acetic acid. This solution must be freshly prepared.

Redistilled hydriodic acid. This is 55 per cent w/w hydriodic acid redistilled, in an atmosphere of carbon dioxide, over red phosphorus. It is stabilised by the addition of 5 ml of 30 per cent w/w hypophosphorous acid to each 100 ml of the hydriodic acid. Store in a cool, dark place in small, brown glass-stoppered bottles, previously swept out with carbon dioxide and sealed with paraffin wax. If the colour of the reagent is more than pale yellow it should be redistilled before use.

Determination: Weigh into the flask (A) an amount of sample approximately equivalent to 50 mg of methyl iodide and add a few small pieces of porous pot (not less than $\frac{1}{8}$ in. in diameter). Half-fill the scrubber (B) with a 25 per cent solution of sodium acetate trihydrate in water and introduce 6 ml of bromine in acetic acid into receiver (C) and 4 ml of bromine in acetic acid into receiver (D). Connect up the condenser, scrubber and receivers and connect the side arm of flask (A) to a source of carbon dioxide (a Kipp's apparatus is suitable) from which the gas is being supplied, at the rate of two bubbles a second, through a wash-bottle containing saturated sodium bicarbonate solution. Add to the contents of the flask about 2·5 ml of melted phenol, *B.P.*, taking care that none remains on the ground-glass joint, and 6·0 ml of redistilled hydriodic acid. Connect the flask with the condenser, securing it by means of rubber bands. Clamp in position on a small sand-bath such as might be contained in a silica dish 9 cm in diameter and heat the sand-bath until the contents of the flask begin to boil. Adjust the rate of heating so that the vapours condense about half-way up the condenser (a piece of wet cotton wool wrapped round the upper part of the condenser will assist this) and continue to heat for forty minutes; for most substances this is long enough to complete the reaction and sweep out the apparatus. Transfer the contents of the two receivers to a 500-ml iodine flask containing 10 ml of a 25 per cent solution of sodium acetate trihydrate in water, washing the receivers, the connecting tube and the end of the apparatus dipping into receiver (C) with water and transferring the washings to the iodine flask. Add formic acid (containing not less than 90 per cent w/w of CH_2O_2), dropwise, with swirling, until the colour of the bromine is discharged, add six drops in excess and allow to stand for two minutes. Add 2 g of potassium iodide and 25 ml of dilute sulphuric acid and immediately titrate the liberated iodine with 0·1N sodium thiosulphate using starch as indicator. Carry out a blank determination by repeating the entire operation omitting the sample. 1 ml 0·1N sodium thiosulphate = 0·0005172 g of methoxyl ($—OCH_3$).

The above method is applicable to the determination of methoxyl groups in **methylcellulose 20,** *B.P.C.* (which contains about 28 per cent of $—OCH_3$), and to the determination of ethoxyl groups in **ethylcellulose,** *N.F.* In the latter case 1 ml 0·1N sodium thiosulphate = 0·0007510 g of ethoxyl ($—OC_2H_5$).

The sodium salts of polycarboxymethylcelluloses are also used, **sodium carboxymethylcellulose,** *U.S.P.*, being a typical example. For compounds of this type the degree of substitution is a criterion of the particular compound in the series and this may be assessed by determining the sodium content. In the *U.S.P.* this is done by a non-aqueous titration as follows:

Weigh 0·5 g into a beaker, add 80 ml of glacial acetic acid and heat on a water-bath for twenty minutes. Cool to room temperature and titrate potentiometrically with 0·1N perchloric acid. 1 ml 0·1N = 0·002299 g Na.

Alternatively, the sample may be ashed to convert to sodium carbonate and the residue titrated with acid.

Pectin, *N.F.*, consists chiefly of partially methoxylated polygalacturonic acids and may be assayed for methoxyl groups and for galacturonic acid as follows:

Weigh exactly 5 g into a beaker, add a mixture of 5 ml of concentrated hydrochloric acid and 100 ml of 60 per cent ethanol and stir for ten minutes. Transfer to a coarse, sintered-glass filter of 30- to 60-ml capacity, and wash, first with six 15-ml quantities of the acid/ethanol mixture and then with 60 per cent ethanol until the filtrate is free from chlorides. Finally wash with 20 ml of 95 per cent ethanol, dry for one hour at 105°, cool and weigh. Transfer exactly one-tenth of the total net weight of dried sample (representing 0·5 g of the original sample) to a 250-ml flask and moisten with 2 ml of 95 per cent ethanol. Add 100 ml of water that has recently been boiled and cooled, stopper the flask and swirl occasionally until solution is effected. Add 5 drops of phenolphthalein indicator and titrate with 0·5N sodium hydroxide ('*a*' ml). Add exactly 20 ml of 0·5N sodium hydroxide, shake vigorously, and allow to stand for fifteen minutes. Add exactly 20 ml of 0·5N hydrochloric acid and shake until the pink colour disappears. Add a further 3 drops of phenolphthalein indicator and titrate with 0·5N sodium hydroxide until a faint pink colour persists after vigorous shaking ('*b*' ml). Each ml of 0·5N sodium hydroxide ('*b*') is equivalent to 0·01552 g of $—OCH_3$ with reference to the undried material. Each ml of sodium hydroxide $(a + b) = 0{\cdot}09707$ g $C_5H_9O_5COOH$ with reference to the undried material.

METHYLENE BLUE

$C_{16}H_{18}N_3ClS,2H_2O$ Mol. Wt. 355·9

Methylene blue, tetramethylthionine chloride, may be determined by the following methods:

(*a*) The *B.P.* method:

Dissolve 0·5 g in 100 ml of water, add 10 ml of concentrated hydrochloric acid and heat to boiling. Replace the air in the flask by a stream of carbon dioxide and titrate with 0·1N titanous chloride until the blue colour disappears leaving the solution reddish-grey. 1 ml 0·1N = 0·01599 g $C_{16}H_{18}N_3ClS$.

This method determines the total reducing substances and is not specific for methylthionine chloride.

Gravimetric methods based on the insolubility of the perchlorate and dichromate are more satisfactory. The small solubility of the compounds in water is made negligible by washing with a weak solution of the precipitating reagent or, better, a saturated solution of the precipitate.

(*b*) A slight modification of the perchlorate method of Maurina and Deahl[1] is official in the *U.S.P.* (Moisture must be determined on a separate portion dried for eighteen hours at 105°; some decomposition occurs on heating at this temperature.)

Dissolve about 0·1 g of undried methylene blue, accurately weighed, in 70 ml of water in a 250-ml beaker, using gentle heat to complete the solution if necessary. Add to this 30 ml of saturated potassium perchlorate solution and stir the mixture intermittently for about ten minutes in order to complete the precipitation. Filter through a prepared Gooch crucible which has previously been dried at 105° and weighed. With the aid of a rubber-tipped glass rod transfer the last traces of precipitate from the sides of the beaker to the crucible, using 50 ml of methylthionine perchlorate solution (prepared as follows: to 500 ml of 0·1 per cent potassium perchlorate solution add, dropwise with constant shaking, 1 per cent methylene blue solution until a slight permanent turbidity results; allow to settle, decant the supernatant liquid through paper and use only the clear solution). Finally, wash the precipitate with an additional 50 ml of wash solution, dry the crucible and precipitate for one hour at 105°, cool and weigh. 1 g of methylene blue perchlorate is equivalent to 0·8333 g of methylene blue.

Correct the weight of the sample for the moisture content, determined on a separate portion of methylene blue by heating at 105° for eighteen hours.

(*c*) Ferrey[2] has studied the reaction with dichromate which is applicable to pills and tablets. If precipitation is effected in the cold, pill excipients do not interfere with a volumetric determination of the excess dichromate after filtration but gravimetric assay is preferable. Coating should be removed and the methylene blue extracted with 5 per cent acetic acid.

Dissolve 0·1 to 0·4 g of methylene blue in 100 ml of water or extract pills with 5 per cent acetic acid, filter the acid extracts hot, cool and shake with carbon tetrachloride to remove traces of paraffin or fatty matter. Add 50 ml of 0·1N potassium dichromate, heat the mixture to 75° for five minutes, cool and filter through a tared No. 3 sintered-glass filter or a Gooch crucible. Wash with 0·1N dichromate, then with 0·02N dichromate and finally with a few ml of water, dry at 105°, cool and weigh. Each g of precipitate is equivalent to 0·8151 g of anhydrous methylene blue.

(*d*) By precipitation as picrate (François and Seguin[3]):

Dissolve 1 g in water, taking care to obtain complete solution, and make up to 100 ml. To 10 ml in a 125-ml flask, add 20 ml of 0·5 per cent picric acid solution. Filter the precipitate, wash carefully with 10 ml of water to remove the excess of picric acid and press lightly between filter papers. Dry over sulphuric acid in a desiccator and weigh. Weight of precipitate × 0·6483 = $C_{16}H_{18}N_3ClS, 2H_2O$.

A determination of small amounts of methylene blue based on this precipitation has been devised by Bollinger,[4] in which the methylene blue solution is placed in a separator with 100 ml of chloroform and titrated with 0·01N picric acid, with shaking. The methylene blue picrate is chloroform-soluble and the end-point is reached when the aqueous layer becomes colourless. The chloroform should be renewed just before the end-point, which is stated to be very sharp.

MEDICINAL DYESTUFFS

A method of assay, applicable to most medicinal dyestuffs, depends upon their reduction with titanous chloride. The procedure has to be modified in detail for dissolving the dyestuff and for some dyes the end-point is not indicated by a sharp decolorisation and an excess of titrant must be added, the excess being back titrated with ferric ammonium sulphate.

After solution and addition of 10 g of sodium potassium tartrate, heat to boiling, maintain a current of carbon dioxide through the flask and titrate the hot solution with 0·1N titanous chloride.

TABLE 25

	FORMULA	MOL. WT.	FACTOR	ASSAY		
				Weight g	H_2O ml	Other solvent ml
Amaranth, *B.P.C.* 1954	$C_{20}H_{11}O_{10}N_2S_3Na_3$	604·5	0·01511	0·4	150	*
Brilliant Green, *B.P.*	$C_{27}H_{34}O_4N_2S$	482·7	0·02413	0·6	25	20% sod. citrate soln. 30†
Congo Red, *B.P.C.*	$C_{32}H_{22}O_6N_6S_2Na_2$	696·7	0·008709	0·25	150	
Crystal Violet, *B.P.*	$C_{25}H_{30}N_3Cl$	408·0	0·02040	0·4	25	‡
Indigo Carmine, *B.P.*	$C_{16}H_8O_8N_2S_2Na_2$	466·4	0·02332	0·5	100	Dil. H_2SO_4, 10
Magenta, *B.P.C.*	$C_{20}H_{20}N_3Cl$	—	0·01689	0·3	50	95% ethanol, 75 (25 ml 30% sod. pot. tartrate soln.)
Methylene Blue, *B.P.*	$C_{16}H_{18}N_3ClS,2H_2O$	355·9	0·01599	0·5	100	HCl, 10
Orange G., *B.P.C.* 1954	$C_{16}H_{10}O_7N_2S_2Na_2$	452·4	0·01131	0·4	150	§
Scarlet Red, *B.P.C.*	$C_{24}H_{20}ON_4$	380·5	0·004755	0·15		Glacial acetic 30 ‡ (but boil 15 min) Assay *B.P.C.* 1949
Sulphan Blue, *B.P.C.* 1954	$C_{27}H_{31}O_6N_2S_2Na$	566·7	0·02833	0·5	150	§
Tartrazine, *B.P.C.* 1954	$C_{16}H_9O_9N_4S_2Na_3$	534·4	0·01336	0·4	150	§
Trypan Blue, *B.P.C.* 1954	$C_{34}H_{24}O_{14}N_6S_4Na_4$	960·8	0·01201	0·4	150	

* 15 g Sodium citrate.

† Add about 0·1 g $NaHCO_3$ and 50 ml 0·1N $TiCl_3$, boil ten minutes, acidify with 20 ml HCl, dilute to 150 ml and titrate with 0·1N ferric ammonium sulphate, methylene blue indicator. Repeat operation without sample.

‡ Add 10 ml HCl, 50 ml 0·1N $TiCl_3$, boil ten minutes and titrate with 0·1N ferric ammonium sulphate, ammonium thiocyanate indicator. Repeat operation without sample.

§ 15 g Sodium acid tartrate.

Table 25 summarises the modifications required for individual products. Of the dyestuffs used medicinally the following important ones are determined by other methods.

Azovan Blue, $C_{34}H_{24}O_{14}N_6S_4Na_4$, Mol. Wt. 960·8.

Dissolve 10 mg in sufficient water to produce 200 ml and dilute 10 ml of this solution to 100 ml with water. Measure the extinction of the final solution at 612 mμ, using 1-cm cells. E(1 per cent, 1 cm) at 612 mμ = 1,046.

Eosin, $C_{20}H_6O_5Br_4Na_2$, Mol. Wt. 691·9.

For total acid dye. Dissolve about 0·5 g in 50 ml of boiling water, add 25 ml of 0·2N hydrochloric acid and heat on a water-bath for sixteen hours. Cool, filter, wash the residue with 0·05N hydrochloric acid and finally with water. Dry for three hours at 130° and weigh; residue × 1·068 = $C_{20}H_6O_5Br_4Na_2$.

For organically combined bromine in acid dye. Mix about 0·2 g of the residue obtained above with 1 g of potassium nitrate and 4 g of fusion mixture; cover with fusion mixture and heat to dull red heat until fused. Complete by the Volhard method (p. 290). 1 ml 0·1N = 0·007992 g Br.

The acid dye theoretically contains 49·3 per cent of bromine.

Fluorescein Sodium, $C_{20}H_{10}O_5Na_2$, Mol. Wt. 376·3.

Dissolve 0·5 g in 20 ml of water, add 5 ml of dilute hydrochloric acid and extract with four quantities, each of 20 ml, of a mixture of equal volumes of *iso*butyl alcohol and chloroform. Combine the extracts, wash with 10 ml of water, extract the washing with 5 ml of the *iso*butyl alcohol/chloroform mixture and add this extract to the combined extracts. Evaporate the organic solvents on a water-bath under a jet of air, dissolve the residue in 10 ml of 95 per cent ethanol, evaporate the ethanol and dry to constant weight at 105°. Each g of residue = 1·132 g of fluorescein sodium.

Phenolsulphonphthalein, $C_{19}H_{14}O_5S$, Mol. Wt. 354·4.

The following method is official but, as often with bromination methods, it is liable to give erratic results unless conditions are rigidly controlled and a blank is run at the same time.

Dissolve 0·15 g in 30 ml of 0·1N sodium hydroxide and dilute with water to 200 ml in a glass-stoppered flask. Add 50 ml of 0·1N bromine and 10 ml of concentrated hydrochloric acid and shake for five minutes. Then add 1 g of potassium iodide and titrate the liberated iodine with 0·1N sodium thiosulphate using starch as indicator. 1 ml 0·1N bromine = 0·004430 g.

1. Maurina, F. A., and Deahl, N., *J. Amer. Pharm. Ass., Sci. Edn.*, 1943, **32**, 301.
2. Ferrey, G. J. W., *Quart. J. Pharm.*, 1943, **16**, 208.
3. François, M., and Seguin, L., *J. Pharm. Chim.*, 1929, **10**, (viii), 5.
4. Bollinger, A., *J. Roy. Soc., N.S.W.*, 1934, **47**, 240, 411.

NICOTINE

$C_{10}H_{14}N_2$ Mol. Wt. 162·2

The determination of nicotine in tobacco leaves (1 to 8 per cent present) and insecticides may be required.

Pizer[1] investigated Chapin's silicotungstate process for nicotine determination, which has been adopted as an official method in the *A.O.A.C.*[2] and confirmed its accuracy. The method is given below with slight modifications to include Pizer's findings:

> Weigh a quantity of the preparation, preferably to contain between 0·1 g and 1·0 g of nicotine; wash with water into a 500-ml round-bottomed distillation flask, add a little paraffin to prevent frothing, some pumice and a slight excess of 40 per cent sodium hydroxide solution, using phenolphthalein as indicator. Steam-distil rapidly through a well-cooled condenser, connected by means of an adapter with a suitable flask containing 10 ml of dilute hydrochloric acid (1 + 4). When distillation is well under way, heat the flask to reduce the volume of the liquid as far as practicable without bumping or undue separation of insoluble matter. After complete distillation of volatile matter, make the distillate, which may amount to 1,000 to 1,500 ml, to a convenient volume (the solution may be concentrated on a water-bath without loss of nicotine); mix well and filter if not clear. Test a portion with methyl orange to confirm its acidity. To an aliquot portion, containing about 0·1 g of nicotine (if the sample contains a very small quantity of nicotine, a portion containing as little as 0·01 g may be used), add for each 100 ml of liquid 3 ml of dilute hydrochloric acid (1 + 4), or more if the necessity is indicated by the test with methyl orange, and 1 ml of silicotungstic acid solution (containing 12 per cent of $4H_2O,SiO_2,12WO_3,22H_2O$ in water; it is important to note that the correct silicotungstic acid is used) for each 0·01 g of nicotine supposed to be present. Stir thoroughly and allow to stand overnight. Before filtering, stir the precipitate to see that it settles quickly and is in crystalline form; filter through an ashless filter paper and wash with cold hydrochloric acid (1 in 1,000). After washing, take the filter paper and contents to apparent dryness in a steam-oven. This point must be carefully watched as the brittle condition of the paper that results on further drying is to be avoided. Transfer the paper and precipitate to a porcelain crucible and ignite directly at 1,000° to constant weight. Weight of residue × 0·1141 = nicotine.

The precipitate may be collected in a Gooch crucible with an asbestos mat, washed repeatedly with dilute hydrochloric acid (1 + 1,000) until the filtrate shows no opalescence when added to fresh nicotine distillate and then dried for three hours at 105° and weighed.[3] Weight of residue × 0·1012 = nicotine. The dried precipitate is somewhat hygroscopic.

Ammonium salts retard the precipitation.[4] For amounts of nicotine above 50 mg per 100 ml, a concentration of ammonium chloride below 5 per cent will not interfere but smaller amounts of nicotine require longer standing for precipitation of the silicotungstate; appropriate dilutions can be made to within these limiting conditions.

If nicotine extracts are being examined, distillation is unnecessary and a suitable amount of material is weighed directly into a stoppered flask containing dilute hydrochloric acid.

Solution of Nicotine Sulphate, *B.Vet.C.* Contains 40·0 per cent of the alkaloids of tobacco.

The official assay requires distillation and precipitation of a portion of the distillate with silicotungstic acid similar to the method given above. By its method of preparation, the distillation does seem unnecessary and direct precipitation of about 0·25 g of the sample would be adequate. This latter method has been considered satisfactory for the compounded preparation following.

Solution of Copper and Nicotine Sulphates, *B.Vet.C.* Contains 5 per cent w/v of copper sulphate and 5 per cent v/v of nicotine sulphate solution.

For nicotine a direct precipitation of 5 ml with silicotungstic acid as above can be used.

For copper 10 ml of solution is made alkaline with sodium carbonate solution, reduced by saturating with sulphur dioxide and precipitated with a measured excess of 0·1N ammonium thiocyanate solution at boiling-point. After filtration, the filtrate is acidified with dilute nitric acid and the excess titrated with 0·1N silver nitrate. 1 ml 0·1N = 0·02497 g $CuSO_4$, $5H_2O$.

1. PIZER, N. H., *J. Soc. Chem. Ind.*, 1934, **53,** 356T.
2. *A.O.A.C.*, 1960, p. 40.
3. RAPP, K. E., WOODMANSEE, C. W., and MCHARGUE, J. S., *J.A.O.A.C.*, 1942, **25,** 760.
4. OGG, C. L., WILLITS, C. O., and RICCIUTI, C., *Anal. Chem.*, 1950, **22,** 335.

NICOTINIC ACID

$C_6H_5O_2N$ Mol. Wt. 123·1

Nicotinic acid is pyridine-3-carboxylic acid and can be determined by direct titration with carbonate-free 0·1N sodium hydroxide using phenol red or phenolphthalein as indicator. 1 ml 0·1N = 0·01231 g.

Chemical methods for the determination of small amounts of nicotinic acid are based on the development of a colour when treated with cyanogen bromide in the presence of an aromatic amine; the aromatic amines used include metol, aniline, procaine, orthoform and *p*-aminoacetophenone;

the choice of amine is important for the development of colour. The reaction is not specific for nicotinic acid since it is given by pyridine and other compounds containing the pyridine nucleus, hence the figure given is a maximum. The pyridine impurity is negligible in the small quantities of extract used in good quality material but where only traces are to be determined in the presence of much interfering matter the method becomes inaccurate unless procedures are adopted for removing or correcting for the presence of interfering substance. Methods used include adsorption techniques and corrections for different blanks. Dennis and Rees[1] used a modification of Bandier's acetone method on all materials that have a low nicotinic acid content and yield highly coloured solutions after hydrolysis and neutralisation; this is rapid and sufficiently accurate for all routine purposes. It is more generally accepted that the pH should be maintained between 6·2 and 7·0 although the authors use a pH of 4·5.

Weigh sufficient material to contain between 250 and 500 mg of nicotinic acid and digest with 25 ml of 4N sodium hydroxide or 15 ml of concentrated hydrochloric acid; yeast products are best hydrolysed with alkali but acid is preferable for cereal products. After hydrolysis, cool, neutralise to pH 6·5 and make up to 50 ml. To 5-ml aliquots in 50-ml centrifuge tubes add 1 g of kieselguhr (Supercel) and mix thoroughly. Run in 10 volumes of dry acetone from a burette with constant stirring, close each tube with a rubber bung and shake. The precipitate should be of a light, fluffy nature; if it is not, insufficient kieselguhr has been used. Centrifuge and decant the supernatant liquid into a 150-ml narrow-necked flask and evaporate the acetone under vacuum to a volume of about 5 ml. To the residue in the centrifuge tube, add a further 10 volumes of acetone, re-extract, centrifuge, transfer to the flask and re-evaporate until free from the odour of acetone. Transfer the contents to a 25-ml graduated flask with successive small portions of a buffer solution of standard pH 6·2. Make up to volume and filter through a sintered-glass funnel to obtain a bright test solution containing between 1 and 2 mg of nicotinic acid per ml.

The purified extract or a prepared solution of the original material if of high nicotinic acid content or a simple galenical is then assayed colorimetrically. Hydrolysis of the amide, in which form the natural vitamin is usually present, is a necessary preliminary and a suitable technique is the following:

Dissolve a quantity of the material, containing about 1 mg of nicotinamide, in 10 ml of water, add 2·5 ml of concentrated hydrochloric acid and heat on a water-bath under a reflux condenser for one hour. Cool, adjust the pH of the liquid to 6·5 with 7·5N sodium hydroxide, using bromothymol blue solution as external indicator, add 25 ml of solution of standard pH 6·2 and dilute to 100 ml with water. Transfer 5 ml of this solution to each of two 25-ml flasks and heat at 80° in the dark for ten minutes. Cool, add to one flask 2 ml of cyanogen bromide solution (prepared by just decolorising freshly prepared saturated bromine water by the gradual addition of 10 per cent potassium cyanide solution; the reagent remains stable in a stoppered bottle for several days) and re-heat both flasks for a further four minutes. Cool in ice for five minutes, add 1 ml of 10 per cent procaine hydrochloride solution to each flask, allow to stand in the dark for ten minutes, dilute to 25 ml with water, mix, and measure the extinction in a 4-cm cell at the maximum at about 425 mμ. Calculate the content of nicotinamide in the sample from the calibration curve.

Repeat the determination using an equal quantity of the material dissolved in a quantity of standard 0·01 per cent nicotinamide and sufficient water to produce 10 ml. Calculate the percentage of added nicotinamide recovered; it should be not less than 85 per cent. The calibration curve is prepared by carrying out the determination on 5, 10 and 15 ml of standard nicotinamide solution.

The final intensity of the colour depends on the amine concentration, hence when the colour is too intense it is inadvisable to dilute the solution, a fresh test on a similar quantity of prepared solution being necessary.

For the microbiological assay of nicotinic acid and nicotinamide:

Weigh 1 to 5 g of the sample, finely ground, transfer to a conical flask with 50 ml of N hydrochloric acid, cover the flask with a small beaker and autoclave at 121° (15 lb steam pressure) for fifteen minutes. Cool, add 2 ml of 2·5M sodium acetate solution and adjust to pH 4·5 using bromocresol green as external indicator. Dilute to 100 ml with water, filter and extract an aliquot with anæsthetic ether. Adjust to pH 6·8 using bromothymol blue as external indicator and dilute as required so that the final solution contains about 0·1 mg nicotinic acid per ml. Proceed with the assay as described in Appendix VII on Microbiological Assays (p. 813).

Note. Materials with a high fat content should have a preliminary extraction with light petroleum (b.p. 40° to 60°) for sixteen to eighteen hours.

Tablets of Nicotinic Acid, *B.P.* Usually contain 50 mg of nicotinic acid.

Although the *B.P.* directs that the nicotinic acid should be extracted with hot neutral ethanol and the extract diluted with water and titrated, this procedure is not necessary for tablets with normal excipients and a direct titration on the powdered tablets with 0·1N alkali to phenol red is satisfactory. 1 ml 0·1N = 0·01231 g $C_6H_5O_2N$.

Dried Yeast, *B.P.C.*, and **Tablets of Yeast,** *B.P.C.* (containing 5 grains of dried yeast), are assayed for nicotinic acid by the microbiological method given above.

Nicotinamide, $C_6H_6ON_2$, Mol. Wt. 122·1, is pyridine-3-carboxylic acid amide and is determined by hydrolysis with sodium hydroxide, distilling the ammonia formed into standard hydrochloric acid. It is not necessary to perform the preliminary boiling given in the *B.P.* assay; it is easily hydrolysed and a direct distillation can be used. 1 ml 0·1N = 0·01221 g.

The *U.S.P.* assays nicotinamide by non-aqueous titration, in benzene and glacial acetic acid, with 0·1N perchloric acid using crystal violet as indicator (see p. 792), 1 ml 0·1N = 0·01221 g $C_6H_6ON_2$.

Injection of Nicotinamide, *B.P.* Usually contains 50 mg of nicotinamide in each ml of water for injection.

It is assayed as for nicotinamide above, using a volume equivalent to about 0·3 g of nicotinamide.

Tablets of Nicotinamide, *B.P.* Contain 50 mg of nicotinamide.

Direct hydrolysis of the powdered tablets by the method given for nicotinamide is satisfactory for assay.

Capsules of Vitamins, *B.P.C.*, are assayed for nicotinamide by the microbiological method given above under Nicotinic Acid. **Compound Tablets of Aneurine,** *B.P.C.*, and **Strong Compound Tablets of Aneurine,** *B.P.C.*, are assayed for nicotinamide by direct hydrolysis as given above under Nicotinamide using the equivalent of 20 and 15 tablets respectively.

Nikethamide, $C_{10}H_{14}ON_2$, Mol. Wt. 178·2, is the diethylamide of nicotinic acid. Acid hydrolysis is necessary to hydrolyse this compound and for assay it is necessary to hydrolyse about 0·3 g with 50 per cent sulphuric acid for two hours before distilling the liberated diethylamine in the presence of excess of sodium hydroxide into standard acid and titrating the excess acid using methyl red as indicator. 1 ml 0·1N = 0·01782 g.

Small quantities of nikethamide may be determined by the cyanogen bromide method for nicotinic acid using standards prepared by diluting a 0·1 per cent aqueous solution of nikethamide.

For the determination of nicotinamide in the presence of nicotinic acid the following method described by Lisboa,[2] in which nicotinamide is coupled with barbituric acid in the presence of cyanogen bromide, is claimed to have advantages over other methods in that the nicotinamide is measured directly and the determination is independent of the concentration of nicotinic acid.

Dissolve the mixture of nicotinamide and nicotinic acid in 3 ml of phosphate buffer solution, pH 7·2, and add 1 ml of a 1 per cent aqueous barbituric acid solution and 1 ml of cyanogen bromide solution (see above). Allow to stand for thirty minutes at 20° to 22° and measure the extinction at 513 mμ. (Nicotinic acid shows no extinction at this wavelength.)

The method is sensitive for quantities of nicotinamide down to about 3 μg per ml.

A method for the separation and independent determination of nicotinic acid and nicotinamide, by which the analysis of mixtures containing only 1 part of one form of the vitamin in the presence of 100 parts of the other, has been described by Sweeney and Hall.[3] In this method solutions containing the two forms of the vitamin, buffered at pH 5, are added to ion-exchange tubes containing IRA-400 in the basic form. The nicotinamide is eluted with water and subsequently the nicotinic acid is eluted with hot N hydrochloric acid. The two substances may then be determined separately by the cyanogen bromide method for nicotinic acid.

Injection of Nikethamide, *B.P.* Contains 25 per cent of nikethamide in water for injection. The assay is exactly that given under nikethamide using a volume of solution equivalent to about 0·3 g of nikethamide.

NICOTINATES

Various esters (*e.g.* benzyl, ethyl and phenyl) of nicotinic acid are met with in pharmaceutical products and they can be determined in ointments by non-aqueous titration after extraction from the basis.

Weigh into a 250-ml separator an amount of sample containing about 0·5 g of the nicotinate, add 100 ml of a mixture of 3 volumes of ether and 2 volumes of toluene, warm and shake to disperse the sample and allow the layers to separate. Run the aqueous layer into a second separator and extract with further quantities of 50, 25 and 25 ml, of the ether/toluene mixture. Combine the solvent extracts, wash with 5 ml of water and discard the washings. Transfer the ether/toluene solution to a 250-ml flask and evaporate the solvent until the volume of solution is about 50 ml. Rinse the separator with a further 25 ml of the solvent mixture and, after washing with 5 ml of water, add this rinsing to the concentrated extracts and again evaporate until the volume is about 50 ml. Add 50 ml of glacial acetic acid and titrate with 0·1N perchloric acid to the green colour of crystal violet indicator. 1 ml 0·1N = 0·0123 g of nicotinate, calculated as nicotinic acid.

1. Dennis, P. O., and Rees, H. G., *Analyst,* 1949, **74,** 481.
2. Lisboa, B. P., *Naturwissenschaften,* 1957, **44,** 617.
3. Sweeney, J. P., and Hall, L., *J.A.O.A.C.*, 1953, **36,** 1018.

NITRIC ACID

HNO_3 Mol. Wt. 63·02

The free acid is estimated by the usual direct titration method with standard alkali, using methyl orange or methyl red as indicator. 1 ml N = 0·06302 g HNO_3.

NITRATES

Potassium nitrate, KNO_3, Mol. Wt. 101·1, is assayed in the *B.P.* by reduction with Devarda's alloy.

Weigh 0·3 g into the flask of an ammonia-distillation apparatus, dissolve in 300 ml of water and add 3 g of Devarda's alloy and 10 ml of

20 per cent sodium hydroxide solution. Connect the apparatus, distil into 50 ml of 0·1N hydrochloric acid and titrate the excess of acid with 0·1N sodium hydroxide using methyl red as indicator. Repeat the operation omitting the sample. 1 ml 0·1N acid = 0·01011 g KNO_3.

The simplest method for the estimation of nitrates is that of Foerster,[1] but it is only applicable if other substances attacked by hydrochloric acid are absent, and it is not accurate in the presence of organic matter.

Evaporate to dryness a solution containing about 0·2 g of nitrate with 10 ml of concentrated hydrochloric acid in a porcelain dish, repeat the process with a further 10 ml of acid, heating until all free acid has been driven off. Dissolve the residue in water and determine the chloride formed by Volhard's method (see p. 296). 1 ml 0·1N $AgNO_3$ = 0·01011 g KNO_3.

The *N.F.* method for potassium nitrate is that of Foerster, given above, using 0·4 g.

A method applicable in the presence of organic matter, such as in asthma powders, depends on the reduction of the nitrate to ammonia by nascent hydrogen but in some cases this may give rise to substantial blanks. The reduction method is included below under Determination of Nitrogen Method D (*a*) but an alternative method which has also been used for preparations of this type is as follows:

Weigh an amount of sample containing about 1 g of potassium nitrate into a flask, add exactly 100 ml of water, stopper the flask and shake continuously for thirty minutes. Filter and pipette 10 ml of the filtrate into a beaker. Dilute with 70 ml of water, add 1 ml of glacial acetic acid and heat to boiling-point. Then add 7 ml of a 10 per cent solution of nitron (1,4-diphenyl-3,5-endanilo-4,5-dihydro-1,2,4-triazole) in dilute acetic acid, stir well, cool and allow to stand in ice-water for two hours. Filter through a No. 2 sintered-glass crucible, transferring to the filter any precipitate remaining in the beaker with small quantities of the filtrate, and wash the precipitate with two 5-ml quantities of ice-cold water. Dry for one hour at 105°, cool and weigh. 1 g of residue ($C_{20}H_{14}N_4,HNO_3$) = 0·2693 g KNO_3.

This method does not give any appreciable blank value with the ingredients likely to be encountered in asthma powders.

Small quantities of nitrate may be estimated colorimetrically either with (*a*) phenoldisulphonic acid or (*b*) 2,4-xylenol. Reduction with Devarda alloy or aluminium foil can also be used (see under Determination of Nitrogen) and the ammonia produced determined with Nessler's reagent.

In the phenoldisulphonic acid method chlorides must be eliminated.

To a quantity of sample containing 0·05 mg or less of nitrogen, add a 0·44 per cent solution of silver sulphate (1 ml = 1 mg Cl) to precipitate all but about 0·5 mg of chloride. Heat to boiling, allow to settle and filter. Evaporate the filtrate to dryness in a porcelain dish, cool, treat with 2 ml of phenoldisulphonic acid solution (prepared by dissolving 25 g of phenol in 150 ml of concentrated sulphuric acid, adding 75 ml of fuming sulphuric acid and heating at 100° for two hours), rubbing with a glass rod to ensure intimate contact. Dilute with water and slowly add strong ammonia solution until the maximum colour is developed. Compare with standards in the usual way; these are prepared by evaporating quantities of a standard solution containing 0·01 mg per ml of nitrogen (0·607 g of pure $NaNO_3$ per litre) and treating with the reagent as above.

Hora and Webber[2] have drawn attention to a possible source of error in this method. They reported that a serious loss of nitrate nitrogen may occur if the determination is carried out in the presence of ammonium ions, possibly due to the formation of nitramide. This error may be avoided by using potassium hydroxide rather than ammonium hydroxide for making alkaline, although potassium hydroxide is liable to produce an undesirable tint with residual silver ions if silver sulphate has been used for removal of chloride.

A distillation method for determination of traces of nitrate is of value where it is necessary to remove interfering material. The nitro-derivative of 2,4-xylenol is steam volatile and this compound has been used successfully.[3]

To 5 ml of a solution containing not more than 0·3 mg of nitrate nitrogen add 15 ml of 85 per cent w/w sulphuric acid and 1 ml of a 5 per cent solution of 2,4-xylenol in glacial acetic acid. Stir well, cool to 35° and maintain at this temperature for thirty minutes. Transfer to a distillation flask with 100 ml of water and distil 40 ml into 10 ml of 2N sodium hydroxide in a 50-ml Nessler cylinder, maintaining the temperature of the distillate at 20°; the rate of distillation should be such that the 40 ml of distillate is collected in about fifteen minutes. Measure the extinction of the resulting solution at the absorption maximum at about 437 mμ, using cells of dimensions suitable to the nitrate concentration of the sample, with, in the comparison cell, a solution prepared by carrying out a blank determination on the reagents. Read the concentration from a standard curve prepared using standard sodium nitrate solutions.

Holler and Huch[4] studied the reaction using all the six isomeric xylenols and preferred the 3,4-xylenol, mainly because the nitration product formed with this isomer gave a high molecular extinction (at about 432 mμ) and because their results using this isomer indicated a more constant nitration yield than with other isomers.

There is serious interference with this method by chloride but it has been reported that this can be suppressed by the addition of mercury.

DETERMINATION OF NITROGEN

The determination of nitrogen by the Kjeldahl[5] method using boiling sulphuric acid to destroy organic matter has been the subject of a large volume of published work and of much controversy. Gunning[6] recommended the addition of potassium sulphate to increase the boiling temperature and a very large number of catalysts have been suggested, although only three (copper, mercury and selenium) have found general application. Selenium has been shown by many workers to cause loss of ammonia while mercury has been proved far superior to copper by the work of Osborn and Krasnitz,[7] Milbauer[8] and many others.

In order to standardise the method, Middleton and Stuckey[9] studied the optimum conditions required for satisfactory analysis. They showed that the residual acid after digestion should be such that the final ratio of sulphuric acid to sodium sulphate is kept constant and a volume of 6 ml is recommended with 3 g of sodium sulphate. The additional acid consumed in the destruction of the compound under test is obtained from the formula of the substance by calculation. A constant amount of alkali can then be added before the distillation. The catalyst prescribed was mercuric oxide and a two hour 'after-boil' was considered necessary. For those compounds which fail to char on treatment with sulphuric acid, *e.g.*, nicotinic acid, 0·1 g of dextrose was added and a three hour 'after-boil' recommended. The constant amount of alkali proposed is 15 ml of a solution containing 10 g of sodium hydroxide and 2 g of sodium thiosulphate. Calculated amounts are used in the *B.P.* and *B.P.C.* In the *B.P.* the amount of sulphuric acid to be added has been calculated to the nearest 0·1 ml but this is clearly unnecessary. Firstly, it is extremely difficult to measure concentrated sulphuric acid so accurately and, secondly, neither the size of flask nor the rate of boiling is stipulated, leading to loss of different amounts of sulphuric acid in practice. Savidge[10] has shown, for example, that 15 ml of concentrated sulphuric acid and 10 g of potassium sulphate, when maintained at a rolling boil in a 100-ml Kjeldahl flask lost 0·4 g per hour, whereas the same amount treated in the same way in a 300-ml Kjeldahl flask lost over 1·2 g per hour. Bradstreet[11] has also studied the acid requirements of the Kjeldahl method and favours the use of potassium sulphate in place of sodium sulphate because of the smaller amount of acid required to obtain a liquid digest. He showed that wherever a solid digest remained at the final stage after cooling, a loss of nitrogen occurred.

Further modifications were introduced by Jodlbauer[12] to deal with nitrate nitrogen. In this method a solution of salicylic acid in sulphuric acid is added to the compound to be assayed and nitrosalicylic acid is formed. This is then reduced by zinc or thiosulphate to an amino compound and the usual Kjeldahl method used to complete the digestion. Dyer and Hamence,[13] however, pointed out that the result by the Jodlbauer method is inaccurate if a substantial quantity of chloride is present. More recently Dickinson[14] has proposed a method for nitro and refractory nitrogen compounds in which a preliminary reduction in formic acid with zinc and iron is followed by the Kjeldahl digestion. One of Dickinson's most important observations was that although nitrosalicylic acid is quantitatively reduced by zinc or thiosulphate, many other nitro compounds are not, so that the common use of Jodlbauer's method for nitro-compounds is contra-indicated.

The methods described in the Fertilisers and Feeding Stuffs Regulations, 1960[15] for determination of nitrogen form a very useful basis for application to much pharmaceutical work. The presence or absence of nitrates in the sample is first ascertained by use of the indigo-carmine test.

Standard indigo solution: Weigh 1 g of indigo carmine *B.P.* into a beaker, cautiously add 40 ml of concentrated sulphuric acid and stir until dissolved. Pour the solution into 800 ml of water, cool and dilute to 1 litre with water. Adjust the strength of the solution so that when 20 ml is added to a solution of 4 mg of potassium nitrate in 20 ml of water, 40 ml of concentrated sulphuric acid is rapidly added and the mixture is heated to the boiling-point, the blue colour is just discharged in one minute.

Test. Shake 5 g of the sample with 80 ml of water in a 100-ml graduated flask, add 1 g of ferric alum, dilute to volume with water, mix and filter into a dry beaker. Dilute 1 ml of the filtrate to 8 ml with water, add 1 ml of the standard indigo solution followed by 10 ml of concentrated sulphuric acid and heat to the boiling-point; if the blue colour is not discharged the sample may be regarded as free from nitrates.

The following methods are then applied:

A. Nitrogen (organic and ammoniacal) in absence of nitrates

(*a*) Weigh into a Kjeldahl digestion flask 2 g of sample (or an amount equivalent to not more than 250 mg of nitrogen) and add 25 ml of nitrogen-free concentrated sulphuric acid. Then add two small globules of mercury (equivalent to about 400 mg) or about 0·5 g of mercuric oxide, followed by 10 g of anhydrous sodium sulphate or potassium sulphate. Heat the flask gently until frothing ceases (if necessary add about 0·5 g of paraffin wax to reduce frothing) and the liquid is practically colourless. Continue the digestion for two hours thereafter to ensure complete oxidation of the organic matter; avoid local overheating. (Care is necessary to prevent loss of acid sufficient to concentrate the mixture approximately to the composition of potassium bisulphate, otherwise, as shown by Self,[16] there is danger of loss of ammonium sulphate by volatilisation at the high temperature reached.

(*b*) To determine the quantity of ammonia present in the liquid, dissolve the cooled digest in sufficient water to produce about 250 ml and, taking precautions against loss of ammonia, add sufficient 50 per cent sodium hydroxide solution to neutralise the acid and give 10 ml in excess. Then add 5 g of sodium thiosulphate, mix well and connect the flask immediately to an ammonia-distillation apparatus. Distil into an excess of 0·2N acid, controlling the rate of distillation so that not less than 150 ml distil in thirty minutes, and titrate the excess of acid with carbonate-free 0·2N sodium hydroxide, using methyl red indicator. (If desired a screened methyl red may be used.) Carry out a blank on the reagents using 2 g of sucrose in place of the sample. 1 ml 0·2N acid = 0·002802 g N.

B. Nitrogen (total) when nitrates are present

The apparatus employed consists of a 500-ml Kjeldahl flask having a doubly perforated rubber bung fitted with a tap-funnel and a U-tube with bulbs. Before commencing a determination charge the U-tube with 10 ml of 10 per cent v/v sulphuric acid and place a small plug of filter paper in the top of the tube in order to catch any spray that might be produced during the bubbling of gas through the dilute sulphuric acid. Transfer 2 g of the sample (or an amount equivalent to not more than 250 mg of nitrogen) and 3 g of finely powdered Devarda alloy to the Kjeldahl flask and wash the sides down with 50 ml of water. Close the flask with the rubber bung fitted with tap-funnel and tube, and add, through the tap-funnel, 5 ml of 50 per cent sodium hydroxide solution. Allow to stand for thirty minutes, then heat at just below the boiling-point for a further one hour, shaking gently at intervals. Cool, add 20 ml of 50 per cent v/v sulphuric acid through the tap-funnel in such a manner that the sides of the Kjeldahl flask are well washed by the acid. Again allow to cool, then remove the bung and rinse into the flask, into which also wash the contents of the U-tube. Add 25 ml of concentrated sulphuric acid, boil off the water and proceed with the determination by the Kjeldahl method in the usual way.

C. Nitrogen in the form of ammonium salts in the presence of organic matter

Weigh about 5 g of the sample into a 250-ml graduated flask, add 200 ml of water and shake thoroughly to ensure solution of all the water-soluble matter. Dilute to volume with water, filter and pipette 50 ml (or a volume equivalent to not more than 250 mg of nitrogen) into the flask of an ammonia-distillation apparatus. Add about 300 ml of water followed by 20 ml of 50 per cent sodium hydroxide solution. (If urea is known to be present add 10 g of light magnesium oxide instead of the sodium hydroxide solution.) Determine the ammonia by distillation into standard acid, distilling at the rate of 250 to 300 ml in thirty minutes. Carry out a blank determination on the reagents and water used, omitting only the sample.

Wilson[17] has questioned the value of the use of magnesium oxide since the pH of a suspension of magnesium oxide is about 11 to 11·5 and this is quite high enough to decompose urea and some other types of organic matter.

D. Nitrogen in nitrates

(*a*) Weigh about 3 g into a 250-ml graduated flask with 200 ml of water, shake to dissolve, dilute to volume with water, and if necessary, filter. Pipette 50 ml of the solution or filtrate (or a volume equivalent to not more than 250 mg of nitrogen) into the flask of an ammonia-distillation apparatus, add 10 g of finely powdered Devarda's alloy, 250 ml of water and 15 ml of 50 per cent sodium hydroxide. Connect the apparatus immediately and allow to stand in the cold for fifteen minutes. Warm gently for a further thirty minutes, slowly increasing the temperature, and then distil into an excess of standard acid at a rate of not less than 150 ml in thirty minutes. (The residual bulk should be small.) Titrate the excess acid with 0·2N sodium hydroxide using methyl red as indicator. Carry out a blank determination on the reagents used, omitting only the aqueous solution of the sample.

Note: This method determines the ammoniacal and nitric nitrogen together. To obtain the nitric nitrogen content, determine the ammoniacal nitrogen by method C and deduct this from the total.

Frey[18] has pointed out that a disadvantage of the Devarda method is the fine spray which is produced and which must be prevented from being carried over into the standard acid. He has designed a distillation apparatus which obviates this difficulty.

The following method (not included in the Fertilisers and Feeding Stuffs Regulations) is based on that of Cotte and Kahane[19] and has proved very useful in practice, being preferred by some workers to Devarda's method:

(*b*) Weigh an amount of sample containing not more than 300 mg of nitrogen into a 500-ml Kjeldahl digestion flask and wash the sides of the flask down with 25 ml of water. Add a solution of 40 g of reagent-grade ferrous sulphate heptahydrate in 100 ml of water followed by 25 ml of 0·5 per cent silver sulphate solution and connect the flask with a distillation apparatus. Distil at the rate of 100 ml in twenty to thirty minutes, into an excess of N acid after liberation of the ammonia with alkali (100 ml of 30 per cent sodium hydroxide solution) and back titrate with N sodium hydroxide. 1 ml N acid = 0·014008 g N.

(*c*) Applicable in the presence of urea.[20]

First determine the total nitrogen: Weigh 0·7 to 2·2 g of sample into a 500-ml Kjeldahl digestion flask, add 40 ml of nitrogen-free concentrated sulphuric acid containing 2 g of salicylic acid, mix thoroughly and allow to stand with occasional shaking for at least thirty minutes. Then add either 5 g of sodium thiosulphate pentahydrate or 2 g of zinc dust (as impalpable powder, not granulated zinc or filings), shake, allow to stand for five minutes and heat over a low flame until frothing ceases. Then add potassium sulphate and mercury and digest as in method A(*a*) and complete by method A(*b*). Secondly, weigh 0·5 g of the sample into a Kjeldahl flask. Add 50 ml of water and mix; then add 2 g of ferrous sulphate heptahydrate and shake. Add 20 ml of concentrated sulphuric acid and digest, heating strongly. When the water is evaporated and white fumes appear, continue the digestion followed by distillation as in A. The total nitrogen less the nitrogen thus found gives the nitrate nitrogen.

In addition to the above methods it will be useful to detail Dickinson's method,[14] already referred to, for application to nitro compounds and to refractory nitrogen compounds:

Weigh 0·35 g of the sample into a 500-ml Kjeldahl flask and add a mixture of 5 ml of 88 per cent w/w formic acid and 2 ml of concentrated hydrochloric acid, washing down the neck of the flask with the mixture. Heat on a water-bath until most of the sample has dissolved and then, while swirling the flask, add 2 g of zinc dust (nitrogen-free) and continue to swirl for two minutes. Allow to stand on a water-bath for five minutes, add 1 g of reduced iron and swirl for two minutes. Then add 2 ml of concentrated hydrochloric acid and 5 ml of 95 per cent ethanol and heat on the water-bath for five minutes. Continue to add 2-ml quantities of concentrated hydrochloric acid, heating on the water-bath for five minutes between each addition, until the iron has almost completely dissolved and then transfer the flask to an efficient fume cupboard and add 25 ml of concentrated sulphuric acid in very small portions with swirling. Swirl the flask in a Bunsen flame until the reaction has subsided, add 12 g of potassium sulphate or anhydrous sodium sulphate and heat gently over a small flame until frothing ceases and the liquid is practically colourless. Continue to heat for a further one hour and then distil in the usual way into an excess of 0·1N acid after liberation of the ammonia with alkali.

Occasionally a substance may be encountered which will neither melt nor go into solution in the prescribed quantities of formic acid and hydrochloric acid, and in such cases, 5 ml of acetic acid or 5 ml of 85 per cent phosphoric acid may be substituted for the formic acid.

AMMONIA, NH_3, Mol. Wt. 17·03

Solutions of ammonia. For determination weigh directly into excess of N acid and titrate back to methyl red with N alkali.

An indirect method, of limited application, is given under Acetates.

If the ammonium salt being determined is fairly pure, an excess of N sodium hydroxide may be added to a known weight, the solution boiled until all ammonia is evolved and the excess of alkali titrated back with N acid to methyl orange. 1 ml N = 0·01703 g NH_3.

Traces of ammonia are determined colorimetrically by comparison with standards after adding Nessler's reagent (see *B.P.* for its preparation). The reaction is extremely delicate and precautions must be taken to prevent extraneous ammonia interfering with the estimation, *e.g.* ammonia should not have been used in the laboratory for some hours previous to the determination. The solution containing the ammonia should preferably be distilled (after cleaning the apparatus free from ammonia by continuous distillation of water through it until the distillate gives no reaction with Nessler's reagent). The standard solution for comparison contains 0·0314 g of ammonium chloride per litre in ammonia-free distilled water (1 ml = 0·01 mg NH_3) and a convenient quantity of this solution for use is 2 ml, diluted with ammonia-free water to 50 ml before adding the Nessler's reagent.

The two solutions should be as nearly as possible at the same temperature and the reagent should be added to the test and comparison cylinders at the same time. If the colour in the test cylinder is more intense than that of the darkest standard, a smaller volume of test solution is measured out; dilution should not be made once the Nessler's reagent has been added. Direct determination is preferable in some cases particularly in that it avoids errors arising from the hydrolysis of urea and other organic compounds during distillation. Some interfering ions cause turbidity in the alkaline mixture and thus render accurate colour matching impossible;

these can be held in solution by the use of sodium hexametaphosphate (Calgon),[21] 1 ml of a 10 per cent solution being added to test and controls before the Nessler reagent.

AMMONIUM SALTS

The general method for determination of ammonium salts consists in boiling with an excess of sodium hydroxide and distilling the liberated ammonia into a measured volume of 0·1N acid; the excess acid is then titrated to methyl red with 0·1N alkali.

Some workers prefer to distil the ammonia into a 4 per cent solution of boric acid, in which it may then be titrated directly with standard acid using methyl red as indicator. This is the method used in the *B.P.* for Kjeldahl determinations and has the obvious advantage that only one standard solution is used. However, in our experience this method sometimes leads to unsatisfactory end-points and we prefer to recommend the reliable back-titration procedure.

Ammonium bicarbonate, NH_4HCO_3, Mol. Wt. 79·06, is weighed for determination by difference from a weighing bottle into excess of N acid; the solution may be titrated back direct to methyl orange, or, preferably, after boiling off the carbon dioxide, titrated back with N alkali to methyl red. 1 ml N = 0·07906 g.

Ammonium carbonate, being a variable mixture of ammonium bicarbonate and ammonium carbamate, $NH_4NH_2CO_2$, is standardised in the *U.S.P.* on its ammonia content, determined as for the bicarbonate. 1 ml N = 0·01703 g NH_3.

Ammonium bicarbonate is a common ingredient of dispensed medicines and the method used to determine it will depend upon the other ingredients present. Where no interfering substances are present Method I, given below, is adequate, but in the presence of certain materials (notably extract of liquorice) which may decompose on boiling with sodium hydroxide, Method II is to be preferred. In this procedure mildly alkaline conditions are used but even so some degradation of liquorice may occur and the method still tends to give results which are somewhat high. As an alternative to the use of magnesium oxide a phosphate buffer, pH 7·6, has been used by some workers but this may give rise to incomplete recoveries.

Method I. Pipette a suitable volume of the mixture into the flask of an ammonia-distillation apparatus, dilute to 200 ml with water and add 5 ml of 20 per cent sodium hydroxide solution. Connect the apparatus immediately and distil into 50 ml of 0·1N sulphuric acid. Back titrate with 0·1N sodium hydroxide using methyl red as indicator. Carry out a blank determination on the reagents, omitting only the sample. 1 ml 0·1N acid = 0·007906 g NH_4HCO_3.

Method II. Pipette a suitable volume of the mixture into the flask of an ammonia-distillation apparatus, dilute to 200 ml with water and add a suspension of 1 g of heavy magnesium oxide in 10 ml of water. Connect the apparatus and distil into 50 ml of 0·1N sulphuric acid. Boil to remove carbon dioxide, cool and back titrate with 0·1N sodium hydroxide using methyl red as indicator. Carry out a blank determination on the reagents, omitting only the sample. 1 ml 0·1N acid = 0·007906 g NH_4HCO_3.

Some commonly occurring mixtures are:

TABLE 26

	NH_4HCO_3 PER CENT W/V	METHOD	VOL. OF SOLN. TAKEN	
Mixture of Ammonia and Ipecacuanha, *B.P.C.*	1·37	II	20 ml	
Mixture of Ammonium Chloride and Morphine, *B.P.C.*	1·37	II*	5 ml	For ammonium chloride, see p. 305.
Mixture of Ipecacuanha, Alkaline, *B.P.C.*	1·37	I	20 ml	For sodium bicarbonate, see p. 31.
Mixture of Ipecacuanha and Ammonia for Infants, *B.P.C.*	0·91	I	20 ml	For sodium bicarbonate, see p. 31.
Mixture of Potassium Iodide, Ammoniated, *B.P.C.*	1·14	II	20 ml	For potassium iodide, see p. 304.
Mixture of Rhubarb and Soda, Ammoniated, *B.P.C.*	1·37	I	20 ml	For sodium bicarbonate, see p. 31.

* Volume of 0·1N acid must be corrected by deducting the volume of 0·1N silver nitrate required in the determination of ammonium chloride.

Aromatic Spirit of Ammonia, *B.P.C.* A mixture of ammonium bicarbonate and ammonia with volatile oils in diluted alcohol.

The content of free ammonia in this product is obtained from the total ammonia determined as above for ammonium bicarbonate, using 20 ml of the spirit and 50 ml of N acid, and deducting the equivalent of combined ammonia. The ammonium carbonate is determined by precipitating it as barium carbonate from 20 ml with 25 ml of N sodium hydroxide and an excess of barium chloride solution at 70°, adding, after cooling, neutral formaldehyde to fix the ammonia and titrating the excess of alkali with N acid to the grey colour of thymol blue indicator. 1 ml N = 0·04805 g $(NH_4)_2CO_3$.

The *U.S.P.* method of assay for the normal carbonate content follows the method given for carbonate in caustic alkali (see Alkali Metals). After boiling with a known excess of 0·5N alkali until all the ammonia has been evolved, the residue is well diluted with cold carbon dioxide-free water and titrated, first to phenolphthalein and then to methyl orange. 1 ml

0·5N acid neutralised in the methyl orange titration = 0·04805 g $(NH_4)_2CO_3$ = 0·0220 g CO_2.

Aromatic Solution of Ammonia, *B.P.C.*, is prepared from the same ingredients as the Aromatic Spirit of Ammonia other than the proportion of alcohol. The assay for free and combined ammonia is the same as above.

UREA, $CO(NH_2)_2$, Mol. Wt. 60·06

Although of less interest in pharmaceutical practice the determination of urea in blood and urine is of importance and the methods may be adapted for other purposes.

The measurement, in a nitrometer, of the nitrogen liberated by urea when acted upon by a strong solution of sodium hypobromite (carbon dioxide formed in the decomposition being absorbed in the alkali) is somewhat empirical. Only approximately 92 per cent of the nitrogen (measured at N.T.P.) is evolved from normal urine, but the increase in the volume of the gas at room temperature and the aqueous vapour tension in the nitrometer approximately compensate for this difference and volumes are read without correction; in urine containing sugar nearly all the nitrogen is evolved.

Fit a brine-charged nitrometer, by a side connection, to a bottle containing 5 ml of urine in a short upright glass tube and a solution of sodium hypobromite (take 23 ml of a solution of 100 g of sodium hydroxide and 250 ml of water; add 2·2 ml of bromine) in the bottom. Shake to mix the solutions and measure the nitrogen evolved. 1 ml = 0·0027 g urea.

This hypobromite method has largely been replaced by the more accurate and specific urease process. Urease will rapidly hydrolyse urea into ammonium carbonate and fairly stable preparations of the enzyme are available in the form of tablets. The method for the estimation of urea in urine due to Dunning[22] is applicable using these tablets:

Crush one urease tablet under 50 ml of water in a 150-ml stoppered flask, add a few drops of toluene to prevent frothing and then exactly 2 ml of the urine to be examined. Place the same amounts of materials, but omitting the urease, in a similar flask. Allow to stand for three hours at room temperature or for one hour at 40°. Add methyl orange to each flask and titrate with 0·1N hydrochloric acid. Subtract the control titration, which represents pre-formed ammonia in the urine, from the titration of the test and multiply by 0·15 to give the percentage of urea in the sample.

1. Foerster, O., *Chemiker-Ztg.* 1890, **14,** 509.
2. Hora, F. B., and Webber, P. J., *Analyst,* 1960, **85,** 507.
3. Swain, J. S., *Chem. & Ind.*, 1957, 479.
4. Holler, A. C., and Huch, R. V., *Anal. Chem.*, 1949, **21,** 1385.
5. Kjeldahl, J., *Z. Anal. Chem.*, 1883, **22,** 366.
6. Gunning, J. W., *Z. Anal. Chem.*, 1889, **28,** 188.

7. Osborn, R. A., and Krasnitz, A., *J. A. O. A. C.*, 1933, **16,** 107; 1934, **17,** 339.
8. Milbauer, J., *Z. Anal. Chem.*, 1938, **111,** 397.
9. Middleton, G., and Stuckey, R. E., *J. Pharm. Pharmacol.*, 1951, **3,** 829.
10. Savidge, R. A., private communication.
11. Bradstreet, R. B., *Anal. Chem.*, 1957, **29,** 944.
12. Jodlbauer, M., *Z. Anal. Chem.*, 1888, **27,** 92.
13. Dyer, B., and Hamence, J. H., *Analyst*, 1938, **63,** 866.
14. Dickinson, W. E., *Anal. Chem.*, 1958, **30,** 992.
15. Ministry of Agriculture, Fisheries and Food, Fertilisers and Feeding Stuffs Regulations, 1960, S.I. No. 1165.
16. Self, P. A. W., *Pharm. J.*, 1912, **88,** 384.
17. Wilson, H. N., Paper read at Symposium on Fertiliser Analysis, London, April, 1960.
18. Frey, M., *Chim. et Ind. (Paris)*, 1953, **70,** 213.
19. Cotte, J., and Kahane, E., *Bull. Soc. Chim. France*, 1946, 542.
20. *A.O.A.C.*, 1960, 14.
21. Houlihan, J. E., *Analyst*, 1949, **74,** 511.
22. Dunning, H. A. B., *J. Amer. Pharm. Ass.*, 1916, **5,** 809.

NITROUS ACID

NITRITES

Sodium nitrite, $NaNO_2$, Mol. Wt. 69·00. This is the only inorganic nitrite used pharmaceutically. The assay of alkali nitrites by means of permanganate is not possible by direct titration in acid solution owing to the decomposition of nitrite by the acid and loss of oxides of nitrogen by volatilisation. Corfield and Self[1] pointed out that this method is only accurate when the nitrite solution is added slowly to the warm dilute acidified solution of permanganate so that the liberated nitrous acid is oxidised before any loss occurs. This form of assay is now used by the *B.P.C.*

> Dissolve about 0·5 g in water and make up to 100 ml. Warm a mixture of 50 ml of 0·1N potassium permanganate, 5 ml of concentrated sulphuric acid and 100 ml of water to about 40° and slowly titrate with the nitrite solution until the colour of the permanganate is destroyed. 1 ml 0·1N = 0·003450 g $NaNO_2$.

Alternatively:

> Add a known weight of nitrite, after solution in water, to an excess of warm 0·1N potassium permanganate and dilute sulphuric acid, allow to stand for five minutes and titrate the excess of permanganate with 0·1N oxalic acid.

The latter method is official in the *U.S.P.* except that excess of 0·1N oxalic acid is added and this is back titrated with 0·1N permanganate.

Stempel[2] describes an acidimetric determination of alkali nitrites which he claims will give results identical with those furnished by oxidation with permanganate; this has been confirmed to be accurate when dealing with pure nitrites. Hydrazine sulphate may be regarded as the diammonium salt of sulphuric acid, *i.e.* $OH.SO_2.O.NH_2NH_3$, and so if mixed with neutral formaldehyde solution and titrated with sodium hydroxide, one molecule of hydrazine sulphate requires two molecules of the alkali when phenolphthalein is used as indicator. In neutral solution, nitrites are reduced by hydrazine sulphate to alkali ammonium salts; hence if the titre of the hydrazine sulphate solution is determined by formaldehyde titration and the excess remaining after reaction with the nitrite is similarly titrated with sodium hydroxide to phenolphthalein, the hydrazine required to reduce the nitrite used may be calculated. Since the alkali ammonium sulphate has a formol titration value of one molecule per molecule of alkali, and hydrazine sulphate a formol titration value of one molecule per two molecules of alkali, it follows that one molecule of nitrite corresponds to one molecule of the alkali. The procedure is as follows:

Dissolve about 0·65 g of hydrazine sulphate in water and make up to 100 ml. To about 0·15 g of nitrite dissolved in 20 ml of water in a conical flask add 40·0 ml of the hydrazine solution, heat the mixture for twenty minutes on a water-bath, cool, add 15 ml of 40 per cent formaldehyde solution (previously neutralised to phenolphthalein) and titrate with 0·1N sodium hydroxide to phenolphthalein. Meanwhile, repeat the titration with 40·0 ml of the hydrazine solution and 15 ml of neutral formaldehyde without the nitrite. The difference is the hydrazine required to reduce the nitrite. 1 ml 0·1N = 0·006900 g $NaNO_2$.

If the original nitrite solution is alkaline to neutral red, it must be neutralised with 0·1N acid, the hydrazine sulphate solution required as above being diminished by an amount equivalent to the volume of acid added.

The use of chloramine-T, which acts as a hypochlorite in solution and yet is far more stable, is the basis of a method for estimating nitrites by van Eck.[3]

To a nitrite in solution add a known excess of 0·1N chloramine-T and then a slight excess of acetic acid; allow to stand for a few minutes then titrate the excess of chloramine with 0·1N thiosulphate after addition of potassium iodide. Standardise the chloramine-T solution by the same method. 1 ml 0·1N = 0·00345 g $NaNO_2$.

Small amounts of nitrite may be determined colorimetrically by the well-known Griess-Ilosvay method which is briefly the following:

To 50 ml of prepared solution containing nitrite add 1 ml of sulphanilic acid reagent (0·33 per cent in 20 per cent acetic acid) mix well, allow to stand five minutes for completion of diazotisation, then add 1 ml of α-naphthylamine reagent (5 g of 1-naphthylamine in 60 ml of 1 : 1 acetic acid, warming if necessary and diluting with water to 100 ml), mix and allow to stand fifteen minutes in diffused light. Similarly and at the same time treat 50 ml of water containing a known amount of standard nitrite solution. Match the pink colours produced by comparing depths of liquid in the test and standard solutions in a colorimeter or at 546 mμ if a spectrophotometer is used for measurement.

Standard nitrite solution: 0·493 g of sodium nitrite per litre, preserved with chloroform, diluted ten times immediately before use. 1 ml diluted solution = 0·01 mg nitrous nitrogen.

The temperature of the sample and controls should be approximately the same, preferably about 20°, since the velocity of diazotisation in acetic acid solution decreases rapidly at low temperatures.

Amyl nitrite, $C_5H_{11}O_2N$, Mol. Wt. 117·2, is a mixture of isomeric amyl nitrites with a small proportion of homologues. It is estimated by diluting about 5 g with 95 per cent ethanol to 100 ml and then proceeding gasometrically as under ethyl nitrite (below) using 2 ml of the dilution. 1 ml moist nitric oxide at 15·5° and normal pressure = 0·0049 g amyl nitrite. It can also be assayed by the argentiometric method using the above dilution, 1 ml 0·1N $AgNO_3$ = 0·0351 g but erratic results are obtained due to the presence of other oxidisable compounds.

Vitrellæ of Amyl Nitrite. Amyl nitrite is often used in muslin-wrapped glass capsules containing 3 or 5 minims each.

For analysis crush three capsules, after weighing, in a beaker containing 15 to 20 ml of ethanol. Make the ethanol accurately up to 50 ml and, using 10 ml of this dilution, proceed as above to determine the percentage content of amyl nitrite. Weigh the beaker and glass from the capsules, after drying, to obtain the weight of the contents in the capsules.

Ethyl nitrite, $C_2H_5O_2N$, Mol. Wt. 75·07. This is contained in the *B.P.C.* preparation of **Spirit of Nitrous Ether,** which is an alcoholic solution containing ethyl nitrite together with decomposition products such as acetaldehyde, nitrous, nitric and acetic acids. If possible, original bottles filled to the neck should be used for analysis as the decomposition is fairly rapid in less favourable conditions of storage, especially with free access of air such as would be occasioned by the repeated opening of a bottle to extract portions.

Gasometric assay is the usual form of determination.

Introduce 2 ml into a nitrometer charged with brine, wash in with 5 ml of ethanol, followed successively by 2 ml of 10 per cent potassium iodide solution and 2 ml of dilute sulphuric acid. Invert the closed tube a number of times to mix the contents thoroughly, taking care that no gas escapes into the open tube. Allow to stand to regain room temperature and measure the volume of nitric oxide produced.

The volume must be corrected to normal pressure at 15·5° from the observed values. A handy nomogram for this purpose was described by Coste.[4] 1 ml of moist nitric oxide at 15·5° and 760 mm pressure = 0·0032 g $C_2H_5O_2N$.

The volumetric assay of ethyl nitrite in Spirit of Nitrous Ether was devised by Smith,[5] the nitrite reducing chlorate to chloride. It has been improved by Andrews[6] in the following way:

Mix 15 ml of a saturated aqueous solution of potassium chlorate with 5 ml of dilute nitric acid in a 100-ml graduated flask and weigh. Add 10 ml of the spirit of nitrous ether from a pipette, shake and reweigh. Set aside in a moderately warm place for one hour and shake occasionally. Then add 20 ml of 0·1N silver nitrate, shake well and make up to volume with water. Filter, rejecting the first 20 ml of filtrate. To 50 ml of the remainder add 10 drops of iron alum solution and titrate the excess of silver nitrate with 0·1N potassium thiocyanate. 1 ml 0·1N $AgNO_3$ = 0·0225 g ethyl nitrite.

Although by this method reproducible results have been obtained which were comparable with the nitrometer method for sodium nitrite, Spirit of Nitrous Ether and amyl nitrite, some workers have reported a considerable divergence between various methods and have generally attributed the variability to volatility of the nitrite and the presence of other oxidising substances.

Octyl nitrite. $C_8H_{17}O_2N$, Mol. Wt. 159·2, is determined either gasometrically as under ethyl nitrite above, using 3 ml of a dilution of 5 ml to 100 ml with 90 per cent ethanol (1 ml moist nitric oxide at 15·5° and normal pressure = 0·0066 g $C_8H_{17}O_2N$) or by the argentiometric method on about 0·5 g of sample in 10 ml of 90 per cent ethanol in a stoppered flask (1 ml 0·1N nitric acid = 0·04777 g).

1. Corfield, C. E., and Self, P. A. W., *Pharm. J.*, 1923, **110**, 359.
2. Stempel, B., *Z. Anal. Chem.*, 1933, **91**, 413.
3. Van Eck, *Pharm. Weekblad.*, 1926, **63**, 1117.
4. Coste, J. H., *Analyst*, 1929, **54**, 656.
5. Smith, C. E., *Amer. J. Pharm.*, 1898, **70**, 273.
6. Andrews, M. J., *J. Amer. Pharm. Ass.*, 1932, **21**, 886.

NUX VOMICA

Good quality nux vomica (the dried ripe seeds of *Strychnos nux vomica*, Linn.) usually yields from 2·5 to 3·0 per cent of total alkaloids, about one half of which is strychnine and the rest mainly brucine, although the proportion is subject to some variation (the ratio of strychnine to brucine is generally between the limits of 1 : 1 to 1 : 1·2).

The *B.P.* method is the following:

Reduce a sufficient quantity to a No. 85 powder, weigh about 10 g of the powder into a flask, add 66 ml of ether and 33 ml of chloroform, shake, and allow to stand for ten minutes. Add 5 ml of dilute ammonia solution and shake continuously for six hours. Transfer the suspension to an apparatus for the continuous extraction of drugs with more of the ether/chloroform mixture and extract for two hours. Filter the solvent extract, washing the filter with ether, and extract, first with 20 ml of N sulphuric acid and then with successive 10-ml quantities of N sulphuric acid until the alkaloids are completely extracted. Combine the acid extracts, make alkaline with strong ammonia solution and extract with two 20-ml quantities of chloroform. Continue the extraction with successive 10-ml quantities of chloroform until the alkaloids are completely extracted. Combine the chloroform extracts, evaporate almost to dryness, add 5 ml of 95 per cent ethanol and complete the evaporation to dryness. Dissolve the residue in a mixture of 15 ml of a 3 per cent w/v solution of concentrated sulphuric acid in water and 2 ml of concentrated nitric acid, add a few crystals of sodium nitrite and allow to stand at a temperature between 15° and 20° for thirty minutes. Transfer to a separator containing 20 ml of 20 per cent sodium hydroxide solution, shake for two minutes and then shake with 20 ml of chloroform. Allow the layers to separate, run off the chloroform layer and wash it, first with 5 ml of 20 per cent sodium hydroxide solution and then with two 10-ml quantities of water. Continue the extraction with successive 10-ml quantities of chloroform until the alkaloids are completely extracted, washing each chloroform extract separately with the sodium hydroxide solution followed by each of the two quantities of water used for washing the first chloroform extract. Titrate the second wash water with 0·1N sulphuric acid using methyl orange as indicator; if more than 0·1 ml of acid is required, wash the combined chloroform extracts with further 10-ml quantities of water until the last washing requires not more than 0·1 ml of 0·1N sulphuric acid for neutralisation to methyl orange. Remove the chloroform, add 5 ml of 95 per cent ethanol, evaporate, and dry for half an hour at 100°. Dissolve the residue in 10 ml of 0·1N sulphuric acid and back-titrate with 0·1N sodium hydroxide, using methyl red as indicator. 1 ml 0·1N sulphuric acid = 0·03344 g of strychnine. Multiply the result by 1·02 to correct for loss of strychnine.

The procedure needs little comment other than emphasising the necessity for carrying out certain parts of the method strictly to detail. Some explanatory notes and comments on these particular operations are:

(*a*) Nux vomica seeds cannot be ground to powder without drying and it is best to chop them up, dry in a water-oven at 100° until they are friable (taking note of the moisture content) and then grind.

(*b*) Considerable controversy has centred round the nitric acid method for destroying the brucine without appreciable loss of strychnine. Many modifications of the original Keller method have been published, but those introducing the application of heat to the sulphuric-nitric acid mixture give low results for strychnine owing to appreciable decomposition of the alkaloid, which commences as low as about 35°. Complete destruction of the brucine is obtained at ordinary temperatures (15° to 20°). A small loss of strychnine was believed to occur even under these conditions and a correction factor of 1·02, obtained experimentally, for the weight of strychnine obtained in the assay is used in the *B.P.* method. However, the work of Elvidge and Proctor[1] has tended to throw doubt on the need for the correction factor. The *B.P.* directs that the acids are to be mixed before they are added to the alkaloidal residue followed by a crystal of sodium nitrite; if the nitric acid is free from nitrous acid the reaction often does not commence, but if the strong nitric acid is added to the solution of alkaloids in the dilute sulphuric acid immediate oxidation results. This observation is in agreement with the conclusion of Reynolds and Sutcliffe[2] that the nitric acid should be added in a strength of sp. gr. 1·42 and not more diluted, otherwise it may be necessary to add a trace of nitrite to start the reaction. Local concentration of nitric acid apparently causes production of a trace of nitrite by reaction with the organic matter.

(*c*) The decomposition of the strychnine nitrate solution by shaking with sodium hydroxide for two minutes before adding the chloroform is important since strychnine nitrate is appreciably soluble in chloroform and otherwise would be extracted as such and give low results on titration. The washing of the chloroform extracts with dilute sodium hydroxide solution is for the same object.

(*d*) Towards the end of the evaporation of the final chloroform extractions, a few ml of ethanol containing 2 per cent of amyl alcohol should be added to remove the last traces of chloroform and also prevent loss of strychnine by decrepitation.

The determination of strychnine in nux vomica and its preparations may be carried out by solvent extraction and ion exchange isolation of the alkaloids followed by a 2-point spectrophotometric method. Oxycellulose[1] can be used or, preferably, treated alginic acid[3] which can replace it in all cases, is more stable and less difficult to prepare.

For preparation of alginic acid columns:

Preparation of Alginic Acid Ion-Exchanger—Dust alginic acid (40 g) slowly on to a solution of sodium hydroxide (12 g) in water (450 ml) with vigorous stirring. Continue stirring until a glutinous, homogenous solution results. Add this dropwise through a nozzle approximately 1·5 mm internal diameter to 10 per cent w/w hydrochloric acid, stirring continuously during and for fifteen minutes after addition. Decant the liquid from the precipitate through a muslin filter over the mouth of the vessel and wash the precipitate until the washings are neutral to litmus and chloride-free. Wash the alginic acid three times with acetone, steep in the same solvent overnight and dry at a temperature not exceeding 50°.

Powder the product (a rotary-blade coffee mill is useful for this purpose) and select a suitable mesh fraction for use.

Preparation of Column—Use Pyrex tubes of 2-cm internal diameter. Soak the prepared alginic acid (4 g 50–100 mesh B.S. per column) in water until swelling is complete (about four hours), then pack in suspension into the tubes previously plugged with cotton wool. Allow the alginic acid to settle and place a second plug on top. Wash the columns with 2N hydrochloric acid until the washings have no measurable extinction at the wavelengths subsequently to be employed and then with water until the effluent is neutral to litmus. Several hundred millilitres of wash liquid may be required.

When not in use, leave the columns saturated with water.

For determination of strychnine:

Weigh accurately about 1 g of powdered nux vomica into a Soxhlet thimble and extract with 80 ml of 70 per cent ethanol for two hours. Cool and transfer the extract to a 100-ml graduated flask, make up to volume and pipette 5 ml of this solution on to the alginic acid column. Wash the column with successive quantities of 10 ml of ethanol, 50 ml of chloroform, 20 ml of ethanol and 50 ml of water. Elute the alkaloids with 50 ml of N sulphuric acid, collecting the eluate in a 50-ml graduated flask, and adjust to volume. Measure the extinctions of this solution at 262 mμ and 300 mμ in a 1-cm cell using N sulphuric acid as the blank. Calculate the percentage of strychnine in the sample using the following formula:

$$\text{per cent strychnine} = \frac{1{,}000}{W} \times \frac{(a \times E_4 - b \times E_2)}{(E_1 \times E_4 - E_2 \times E_3)}$$

W = weight of sample in g
a = extinction of sample solution at 262 mμ
b = extinction of sample solution at 300 mμ
E_1 = E(1 per cent, 1 cm) at 262 mμ for strychnine in N sulphuric acid
E_2 = E(1 per cent, 1 cm) at 262 mμ for brucine in N sulphuric acid
E_3 = E(1 per cent, 1 cm) at 300 mμ for strychnine in N sulphuric acid
E_4 = E(1 per cent, 1 cm) at 300 mμ for brucine in N sulphuric acid

The E(1 per cent, 1 cm) values for strychnine and brucine at 262 mμ and 300 mμ are as follows:

	Strychnine	Brucine
262 mμ	318	314
300 mμ	4·59	216

It can be shown that, for a solution containing only strychnine and brucine, if the extinction coefficients (*i.e.* observed reading/concentration) are 'a' and 'b' at 262 mμ and 300 mμ respectively, it follows that $x = 0{\cdot}321a - 0{\cdot}467b$ where 'x' is the percentage concentration of strychnine.

Dry Extract of Nux Vomica, *B.P.C.* Contains 5 per cent of strychnine.

The *B.P.* assay for nux vomica is satisfactory and the notes (*b*) to (*d*) given above are applicable to this preparation.

The process of extraction may be expedited by adding about 5 g of kieselguhr to the ethanolic solution, then filtering through a Büchner funnel to dryness, transferring the residue back to the flask and repeating until all the alkaloids are in the filtrate.

This preparation can be assayed spectrophotometrically after separation on an alginic acid column, exactly as given under nux vomica, dissolving 0·1 g of sample in 100 ml of 70 per cent ethanol and taking 10 ml of this dilution for chromatography.

Liquid Extract of Nux Vomica, *B.P.* Contains 1·5 per cent of strychnine.

The following method should give clean separations. If emulsions are formed a modification, adding 0·5 ml of 6N sulphuric acid and no water at the commencement of the assay, may be effective.

To 10 ml of extract add 10 ml of N sulphuric acid, extract with 30 and 20 ml of chloroform, washing each extract with three portions each of 10 ml of 0·1N sulphuric acid. Make the acid layer and washings alkaline with dilute ammonia solution, extract with four portions each of 50 ml of a mixture of 4 volumes of chloroform and 1 volume of 95 per cent ethanol, washing each extract with the same 10 ml of water. Mix the extracts, remove the solvent, add 5 ml of 95 per cent ethanol and evaporate to dryness. Complete as under Nux Vomica for the destruction of brucine.

For the spectrophotometric assay given under Nux Vomica, a sample dilution of 5 ml to 100 ml with 70 per cent ethanol and a further 1 in 10 dilution with the same solvent is all that is necessary before placing 10 ml of the dilution directly on the alginic acid column.

Tincture of Nux Vomica, *B.P.* Contains 0·125 per cent of strychnine.

For assay by the *B.P.* method, evaporate 100 ml to about 10 ml, transfer to a separator with a mixture of 20 ml of N sulphuric acid and 5 ml of ethanol and complete as for Liquid Extract of Nux Vomica.

For spectrophotometric assay, dilute 5 ml of sample to 100 ml with 95 per cent ethanol, place 10 ml of this dilution on an alginic acid column and complete as given under Nux Vomica.

Mixture of Potassium Bromide and Nux Vomica, *B.P.C.* Contains 4·57 per cent of potassium bromide and 4·17 per cent of Tincture of Nux Vomica with amaranth.

In the presence of the dye-stuff a preliminary purification by solvent extraction is necessary before applying the alginic acid isolation of the alkaloids described above.

Pipette 10 ml into a 100-ml separating funnel, make alkaline with a few drops of dilute ammonia and extract with 20 ml of chloroform for two minutes. Transfer the chloroform layer into a second separating funnel and wash with 10 ml of water. Run off the washed extract into a flask, and extract the original sample in a similar manner with three further portions of 20 ml of chloroform. Wash these further extracts with the same 10 ml of water and add to the original extract. Transfer the bulked chloroform extracts to an alginic acid column and complete as under Nux Vomica.

Pills of Aloes and Nux Vomica, *B.P.C.* Each pill contains $\frac{1}{4}$ grain of Dry Extract of Nux Vomica.

For spectrophotometric determination this preparation cannot be purified sufficiently by alginic acid alone, because of the high proportion of interfering materials, which also occasionally prevent the repeated use of the column. Preliminary purification by treatment with alumina is satisfactory.[1]

Prepare an alumina column as follows: Mix 20 g of alumina (chromatographic grade) with sufficient 70 per cent ethanol to form a thin slurry and transfer to a glass tube 1 in. in diameter fitted with a tap at the lower end and which has previously been plugged with glass wool. Allow the alumina to settle and drain the tube until the level of liquid is just above the surface of the alumina. Do not allow the column to become dry.

Weigh an amount of powdered tablet material containing about 10 mg of strychnine and transfer to a 50-ml conical flask. Add about 20 ml of 70 per cent ethanol and heat to boiling on a water-bath. Cool and allow the solid powder to settle and decant the liquid through a filter paper (No. 1 porosity) on to the alumina column. Allow the liquid to percolate through the alumina and collect the eluate in a 100-ml graduated flask. Repeat the extraction and chromatography with three further quantities each of 20 ml of 70 per cent ethanol. Adjust the volume of the bulked extracts to 100 ml with 70 per cent ethanol, pipette 5 ml of this solution on to an alginic acid column and proceed as described under Nux Vomica.

Tablets of Aloes and Nux Vomica, *B.P.C.* Each tablet contains $\frac{1}{4}$ grain of Dry Extract of Nux Vomica.

This preparation is assayed for strychnine exactly as given under Pills of Aloes and Nux Vomica.

STRYCHNINE, $C_{21}H_{22}O_2N_2$, Mol. Wt. 334·4

Small amounts of strychnine may be determined colorimetrically by applying Malaquin's colour test as modified by Deniges.[4] In this test the alkaloid, dissolved in dilute hydrochloric acid, is reduced with zinc amalgam and then treated with sodium nitrite. The red colour produced is then matched against a series of standards prepared by application of the test to solutions of strychnine sulphate of known concentration.

The reaction was critically studied by Allen and Allport[5] with the object of using it in the colorimetric determination of strychnine in nux vomica and its preparations. They showed that while the colour produced is quite satisfactory when applied to solutions of pure strychnine salts, it is altered by the presence of brucine, which itself produces an orange colour; in this case, precipitation as ferrocyanide is recommended, details of which are given on p. 468. The colour produced by a solution of strychnine ferrocyanide in hydrochloric acid is slightly less intense than that due to an equivalent quantity of strychnine alkaloid dissolved in the same mineral acid, hence appropriate curves must be obtained for each condition of test.

Beer's Law is obeyed provided not more than 0·10 mg of the alkaloid is present.

To 5 ml of solution in a test-tube containing from 0·02 to 0·10 mg of strychnine and 10 per cent w/w of hydrochloric acid, add 0·2 g of zinc amalgam (in 20 mesh and containing 40 per cent of mercury, recently treated by momentary immersion in a 5 per cent aqueous solution of mercuric chloride followed by a brief wash with water). Immerse the tube in a water-bath for seven minutes, cool under the tap and add 0·05 ml of a freshly prepared, approximately 0·1 per cent, aqueous solution of sodium nitrite. Transfer a portion of the red liquid to a 0·5-cm cell and determine the maximum extinction at about 525 mμ. Prepare a calibration graph under identical conditions.

In order to convert the values obtained for the content of anhydrous strychnine base into strychnine hydrochloride ($2H_2O$), multiply by the factor 1·217 and to convert into strychnine sulphate ($5H_2O$) multiply by 1·281.

The time of heating with zinc amalgam is not critical and may vary from five to ten minutes, but heating for any time outside these limits results in weak colours.

Another colorimetric method is that of Rasmussen[6] which is easily applied to simple solutions of strychnine; chlorides interfere and the reagent must be matured for some days before use.

To 1 ml of solution containing about 0·75 mg of strychnine, add 5 ml of ammonium vanadate solution (0·5 g of ammonium vanadate in 100 ml of 65 per cent by volume sulphuric acid), allow to stand for two minutes and dilute to nearly 50 ml with water, cool and adjust the volume to 50 ml. Determine the maximum extinction at about 496 mμ.

Prepare a calibration graph by dissolving 0·1281 g of strychnine sulphate ($5H_2O$) in 0·2N sulphuric acid to produce 100 ml; each ml of solution contains 1 mg of strychnine alkaloid. 0·1, 0·2, 0·3 . . . to 1·0 ml is treated in the same manner as the sample.

Beer's Law is obeyed between 0·4 mg and 1·0 mg, the colour is fairly stable but the reproducibility is not so good as might be desired.

Strychnine hydrochloride, $C_{21}H_{22}O_2N_2,HCl,2H_2O$, Mol. Wt. 406·9, **strychnine phosphate,** $C_{21}H_{22}O_2N_2$, H_3PO_4, $2H_2O$, Mol. Wt. 468·5 and **strychnine sulphate,** $(C_{21}H_{22}O_2N_2)_2$, H_2SO_4, $5H_2O$, Mol. Wt. 857·0 are assayed by the general method for the determination of alkaloids in solution, *i.e.* extraction with chloroform in ammoniacal solution, washing the extracts, evaporation and drying after the addition of ethanol, and back-titration with 0·1N alkali to methyl red after dissolving by boiling with an excess of 0·1N sulphuric acid. 1 ml 0·1N = 0·03344 g of strychnine base, $C_{21}H_{22}O_2N_2$. A modification is to add an excess of 0·1N sulphuric acid after removing most of the chloroform, warming to remove the remainder of the solvent and titrating with 0·1N sodium hydroxide to methyl red.

Strychnine can also be assayed by non-aqueous titration; the dried extracted alkaloid is dissolved in glacial acetic acid and titrated with 0·1N perchloric acid using crystal violet as indicator.

Strychnine hydrochloride has an absorption maximum in N hydrochloric or sulphuric acid at about 254 mμ. E(1 per cent, 1 cm) = 310.

It is interesting to note that strychnine hydrochloride is much less soluble in water containing hydrochloric acid and this is of importance in the distribution of strychnine hydrochloride between hydrochloric acid and immiscible solvents such as chloroform. Obviously the proportion of hydrochloride present in the chloroform phase at equilibrium increases with increase in the concentration of hydrochloric acid in the aqueous phase (Driver and Thompson[7]) and by a sufficient number of extractions with chloroform from solution in 2N hydrochloric acid, the hydrochloride may be obtained completely in solution in the organic solvent. This property can be used for the separation of strychnine in acid solution from other alkaloids.

Caws and Foster[8] have drawn attention to a source of error which may arise in the assay of strychnine salts. These authors observed that a discrepancy exists between results obtained when the recovered alkaloid is weighed as strychnine and when it is titrated with standard acid. This was found to be due to the formation of a compound (at first thought to be between chloroform and strychnine but later shown to be strychnine chloromethobromide, resulting from the presence of chlorobromomethane as an impurity in samples of chloroform *B.P.*). The error can be avoided by extracting the chloroform solution obtained in the official assay with standard acid and back-titrating the acid extracts, rather than by evaporating the chloroform solutions to dryness, when compound formation is likely to occur. An alternative procedure which overcomes the difficulty is to carry out the *B.P.* assay, but to titrate the final alkaloidal residue in glacial acetic acid with 0·1N perchloric acid (see Appendix III).

Injection of Strychnine, *B.P.C.* Usually contains 0·4 per cent of strychnine hydrochloride in water for injection. It may contain a bacteriostat.

In the absence of a bacteriostat absorbing at 254 mμ a direct spectrophotometric assay in N sulphuric acid can be used. In the presence of a bacteriostat which interferes at this wavelength, it is separated on an alginic acid column.

The column is prepared as instructed on p. 461 but using N sulphuric acid instead of hydrochloric acid.

Dilute an accurately measured volume with water to give a final concentration of about 0·015 per cent of strychnine hydrochloride; pass 10 ml of this solution through the column and wash with water until the washings are free from bacteriostat. Elute the column with 50 ml of N sulphuric acid, dilute to 100 ml with N sulphuric acid and measure the extinction at the maximum at about 254 mμ. E(1 per cent, 1 cm) of strychnine hydrochloride = 310.

The direct colorimetric method of Rasmussen given above can also be used after extraction of the alkaloid.

Make a volume of solution, containing about 0·01 g of strychnine hydrochloride, alkaline with ammonia solution and extract with six 10-ml portions of chloroform, washing each extract with the same 10 ml of water. Evaporate to low bulk, add 5 ml of N sulphuric acid, evaporate the remainder of the solvent and dilute to 25 ml with water. Use 1 ml of this solution.

Mixture of Strychnine, *B.P.C.* A dilution of solution of strychnine hydrochloride with hydrochloric acid and chloroform water; it contains approximately 0·02 per cent of strychnine hydrochloride.

The content of strychnine hydrochloride can be determined either by a direct spectrophotometric measurement at 254 mμ on a 1 in 10 dilution in N hydrochloric acid, E(1 per cent, 1 cm) = 310 or by the colorimetric method of Rasmussen given above after extraction of the alkaloid from 20 ml, as given under Injection of Strychnine, and diluting to 10 ml before using the general method.

Mixture of Strychnine and Iron, *B.P.C.* Contains 0·0125 per cent of strychnine hydrochloride.

The assay for strychnine is the same as given under Injection of Strychnine after extracting the alkaloid with chloroform from sodium hydroxide solution.

Solution of Strychnine Hydrochloride, *B.P.* A solution of strychnine hydrochloride, 1 per cent, in alcohol and water.

Assayed by the method for strychnine hydrochloride using 20 ml of solution, 1 ml 0·1N = 0·04069 g $C_{21}H_{22}O_2N_2,HCl,2H_2O$. The alkaloid should be weighed after drying as a check on the titration figure.

The possible error arising from reaction of strychnine with impurities in the chloroform may be avoided by using the following alternative method:

Evaporate 25 ml to dryness, avoiding loss by decrepitation, and determine the strychnine hydrochloride in the residue by the general method for non-aqueous titration with perchloric acid (Appendix III). 1 ml 0·1N perchloric acid = 0·04069 g $C_{21}H_{22}O_2N_2,HCl,2H_2O$.

Syrup of Ferrous Phosphate with Quinine and Strychnine, *B.P.C.* The official method for the determination of strychnine is by precipitation of its insoluble ferrocyanide by the method of Simmonds,[9] re-precipitation being necessary in the presence of the large excess of quinine.

For quinine. Mix 50 ml with 5 g of sodium citrate in 100 ml of water, make alkaline with sodium hydroxide solution and extract with chloroform, washing each extract with the same 20 ml of water. Evaporate, add

5 ml of ethanol, re-evaporate and dry at 105°. Deduct the weight of strychnine obtained in the assay below to obtain the anhydrous quinine.

For strychnine. Dissolve the total alkaloids in 50 ml of 10 per cent sulphuric acid in a beaker. Run in 5 ml of 4 per cent freshly prepared potassium ferrocyanide solution drop by drop from a burette, stir well, scraping the side of the beaker with a glass rod and set the mixture aside for a few hours. Filter the precipitate through a 7-cm filter, and wash lightly three times with about 3 ml of 5 per cent sulphuric acid. Wash the precipitate into a small separator with the aid of about 10 ml of dilute ammonia solution and a fine jet of water. Extract with three portions of chloroform, each of 10 ml. Extract the alkaloids from the bulked chloroform solutions with 20 ml of 10 per cent sulphuric acid, using 10 ml, 5 ml and 5 ml. Repeat the precipitation with 1 ml of potassium ferrocyanide solution and other operations as before until the chloroform extracts are again obtained. Evaporate the chloroform, adding a little ethanol towards the end and weigh the residue of strychnine after drying for an hour or two at 105°.

Allen and Allport[5] confirmed the observation by Hibbard[10] that for precipitation of strychnine ferrocyanide in very low concentrations the addition of oxalic acid to a solution of the alkaloid in dilute sulphuric acid made the precipitation quantitative. Best conditions are obtained when potassium ferrocyanide is added to an acid solution of strychnine which is approximately 0·1N with respect to sulphuric acid and 0·33N to oxalic acid and is effective in the presence of only a fraction of a mg of alkaloid.

A more rapid determination of both quinine and strychnine can be made by physical methods:[11,12]

For quinine, dilute about 2 g of syrup to 100 ml with 0·1N sulphuric acid. Dilute this solution suitably and compare the fluorescence with that of a standard solution of quinine as given on p. 179. Determine the weight per ml at 20° to calculate the volume of syrup taken.

For strychnine. Plug the bottom of a clear glass chromatographic column 30 cm long and 2 cm in internal diameter with cotton wool and mount vertically.

Stir 1·0 g of Celite 545 with exactly 1 ml of water until fluffy and uniform. Transfer the mixture to the chromatographic tube and press down firmly and uniformly with a flat-ended glass packing-rod. Mix thoroughly 3·0 g of Celite 545 with exactly 3 ml of N hydrochloric acid. Transfer to the tube and press firmly and uniformly as before.

Stir about 1 g of sample with 5·0 g of Celite 545, exactly 2 ml of 6N hydrochloric acid and exactly 1 ml of water. Transfer the mixture to the top of a suitably prepared chromatographic column and clean the beaker with 1 g of Celite 545, transferring it to the top of the column and press down. Wipe the inside of the beaker with a plug of cotton wool and then push the plug slowly down the chromatographic column on to the top of the sample layer ensuring that any particles of Celite adhering to the sides of the tube are retained by the cotton wool. Wash the prepared column with 50 ml and four successive quantities of 25 ml of water-saturated anæsthetic ether, applying a slight air pressure to the top of the tube. Elute the strychnine with six successive quantities, each of 25 ml of water-saturated chloroform, combining the eluate. Remove the chloroform by heating on a water-bath under a stream of air. Add successive quantities of a few ml of 0·1N hydrochloric acid, warming to aid solution, until the residue is completely dissolved, combining the 0·1N hydrochloric acid solutions. Dilute to 25 ml with 0·1N hydrochloric acid. Measure the extinctions at 247 mμ, 254 mμ and 262 mμ, comparing the solution with 0·1N hydrochloric acid in matched 1-cm cells.

The extinction at 254 mμ corrected for irrelevant absorption is given by

$$6{\cdot}9(\text{E}254\ \text{m}\mu - 0{\cdot}533\ \text{E}247\ \text{m}\mu - 0{\cdot}467\ \text{E}262\ \text{m}\mu)$$

The E(1 per cent, 1 cm) at 254 mμ of strychnine is 375.

Determine the weight per ml at 20° and calculate the percentage of strychnine w/v.

For iron, see p. 356.

Compound Syrup of Hypophosphites, *B.P.C.*

Both quinine and strychnine can be determined by the methods given above under Syrup of Ferrous Phosphate with Quinine and Strychnine using 10 g for the quinine and 2 g for the strychnine determination.

Tablets of Ferrous Phosphate with Quinine and Strychnine, *B.P.C.*

Quinine and strychnine are determined by the methods given above for the syrup after preliminary treatment.

For total alkaloids and precipitation of strychnine as ferrocyanide, digest 20 tablets after powdering, with 30 ml of dilute sulphuric acid until completely disintegrated and only a white residue remains. Filter, wash and make the combined filtrate and washings up to 150 ml with water. Extract the alkaloids from 100 ml with chloroform after adding 2 g of citric acid and an excess of ammonia or sodium hydroxide solution.

For quinine by the fluorimetric method, transfer about 0·06 g of powdered tablets to a 100-ml graduated flask, add 50 ml of 0·1N sulphuric acid and shake continuously for thirty minutes. Make up to volume with 0·1N acid, mix and allow to stand until the insoluble matter has deposited before taking an aliquot for dilution.

For strychnine by the spectrophotometric method, powder 5 tablets very finely and mix thoroughly 0·1 g of the powder with 5·0 g of Celite 545, exactly 2 ml of 6N hydrochloric acid and exactly 2 ml of water in a beaker. Continue as for the syrup, transferring the mixture to the top of the prepared chromatographic column.

For iron, see p. 357.

1. Elvidge, D. A., and Proctor, K. A., *J. Pharm. Pharmacol.*, 1957, **9**, 974.
2. Reynolds, W. C., and Sutcliffe, R., *J. Soc. Chem. Ind.*, 1906, **25**, 512.
3. Foster, J. S., and Murfin, J. W., *Analyst*, 1961, **86**, 32.
4. Deniges, M. G., *Bull. Soc. Chim. France*, 1911, **9**, 537.
5. Allen, J., and Allport, N. L., *Quart. J. Pharm.*, 1940, **13**, 252.
6. Rasmussen, S. K., *Dansk Tidsskr. Farm.*, 1942, **16**, 11; 1943, **17**, 1.
7. Driver, J. E., and Thompson, S. P., *Quart. J. Pharm.*, 1928, **1**, 37.
8. Caws, A. C., and Foster, G. E., *J. Pharm. Pharmacol.*, 1956, **8**, 790; 1957, **9**, 824.
9. Simmonds, C., *Analyst*, 1914, **39**, 81.
10. Hibbard, P. L., *Ind. Eng. Chem., Anal. Edn.*, 1934, **6**, 423.

11. Banes, D., *J. Amer. Pharm. Ass., Sci. Edn.*, 1954, **43**, 580.
12. Brealey, L., private communication.

SYNTHETIC ŒSTROGENS

Synthetic œstrogens containing a reactive hydroxyl group can be assayed chemically by quantitative esterification. This method is suitable for **dienœstrol,** $C_{18}H_{18}O_2$, Mol. Wt. 266·3, **hexœstrol,** $C_{18}H_{22}O_2$, Mol. Wt. 270·4, and **stilbœstrol,** $C_{18}H_{20}O_2$, Mol. Wt. 268·4.

> Weigh 1·5 g into a flask, add exactly 10 ml of a 15 per cent v/v solution of acetic anhydride in pyridine, connect the flask to a reflux condenser and heat on a water-bath for two hours. Cool, add 50 ml of ice-cold water through the condenser and filter through a No. 2 sintered-glass crucible. Wash the flask and crystals with three 15-ml quantities of ice-cold water and titrate the combined filtrate and washings, slowly and with vigorous shaking, with carbonate-free 0·5N sodium hydroxide, using phenolphthalein as indicator, until a red colour persists for ten seconds. Repeat the operation omitting the sample. The difference between the two titrations represents the amount of acetic acid required for acetylation. 1 ml 0·5N = 0·06709 g $C_{18}H_{20}O_2$; 0·06659 g $C_{18}H_{18}O_2$; 0·06759 g $C_{18}H_{22}O_2$.

The di-acetates may also be weighed as follows:

> Mix about 0·5 g, previously dried, with 2 ml of acetic anhydride and 4 ml of dry pyridine. Boil under reflux for fifteen minutes, cool and shake with 50 ml of water. Bring the mixture to 50°, filter, wash with four quantities each of 15 ml of water, dry at 105° and weigh. Wt. × 0·7600 = $C_{18}H_{18}O_2$, × 0·7628 = $C_{18}H_{22}O_2$ and × 0·7614 = $C_{18}H_{20}O_2$.

The *U.S.P.* method for stilbœstrol which is more specific than the above is based on a method proposed by Goodyear, Hatfield and Marsh.[1] 25 ml of a solution of the sample in 95 per cent ethanol, prepared to contain about 20 μg per ml, is mixed with an equal volume of dibasic potassium phosphate solution (1 in 55) and the solution, in a quartz cell or tube, is then irradiated in ultra-violet light and its extinction measured at the maximum at about 418 mμ, when the maximum yellow colour has been developed. The optimum conditions (time of irradiation, distance from source of light and quality of quartz container) for maximum colour development are determined prior to making the determination, using a standard solution of stilbœstrol in 95 per cent ethanol, containing 20 μg per ml, and the stilbœstrol content of the sample is determined from a comparison of the extinction of the sample solution with that of the standard solution determined at the same time under these conditions. This method has been adapted by the Analytical Methods Committee of the *S.A.C.*[2] for determination of small amounts of stilbœstrol (about 5 mg per pound) in complex mixtures such as animal feeding-stuffs.

Apparatus:

Extraction apparatus. Any apparatus that permits the uniform percolation of the powdered sample with the extracting solvent and a regular flow of the solvent vapour round the percolator may be used. A suitable form consists of a glass tube 15 cm long and 4 cm in internal diameter with a piece of coarse filter paper covered with fine calico tied firmly over its lower, flanged end. This percolator rests on a glass spiral inside an outer tube 25 cm long and 6 cm in internal diameter, the spiral being supported on the shoulder of a B24 standard joint sealed to the lower end of the outer tube. The joint fits into a flask of suitable size to contain the solvent and a reflux condenser is attached to the top of the tube. Alternatively, an alundum crucible of medium porosity and suitable size may be used as the percolator.

Irradiation equipment.* This consists of a mercury-discharge tube, mounted in a suitable reflector to give a horizontal beam, and a holder capable of containing four silica cells, so arranged that the cells are perpendicular to the light beam and fixed at 6 in. from the light source. The holder is also positioned so that a line through the liquid centres in the cells is level with the centre of the discharge tube and the cells themselves, spaced about 1 cm apart, are centrally located relative to the ends of the discharge tube.

Determination: Crush about 1 kg of the sample, mix and grind about 100 g of the crushed material until at least 95 per cent passes a 30-mesh sieve. Weigh about 40 g of the ground material into a flask and add about 10 g of washed sand followed by 100 ml of chloroform (the chloroform used throughout the determination should be of analytical-reagent grade and should comply with the following test. Shake 35 ml with 70 ml of water and allow the layers to separate. Mix 10 ml of the aqueous extract with 40 ml of water and 2 ml of Nessler's reagent and allow to stand in the dark for fifteen minutes; no colour or turbidity is produced). Stopper the flask, shake vigorously and allow to stand overnight. Transfer the contents of the flask to the extraction apparatus and extract for six hours, using more chloroform if necessary. When extraction is complete, filter the extract through a pad of cotton wool into a 200-ml graduated flask, washing the extraction flask and filter with chloroform, and dilute the combined filtrate and washings to 200 ml with chloroform.

Transfer a 25-ml aliquot of this solution to each of two separators, add 25 ml of chloroform to each separator and then, to one of the separators, add 1 ml of a standard solution containing 55 μg of stilbœstrol per ml (prepared by diluting 10 ml of a stock solution in chloroform, containing exactly 55 mg of stilbœstrol per 100 ml, to 100 ml with chloroform). Treat the contents of each separator, respectively, as follows. Add 25 ml of N sulphuric acid, shake vigorously for thirty seconds, avoiding the formation of emulsions as far as possible, allow to separate for ten minutes and run the chloroform phase into another separator. (If emulsions are formed at this stage, it may be helpful to centrifuge the mixture.) Add 10 ml of chloroform to the acid phase, shake for ten seconds, allow to separate and add the chloroform phase to the previous chloroform solution. Repeat this last operation with two further 10-ml quantities of chloroform and then reject the acid phase.

* The Phillips Germicidal tube TuV (15 watt), together with a trough fitting, A 7003, with the grill removed, is a suitable source of radiation.

Extract the combined chloroform extracts carefully with two 10-ml quantities of N sodium hydroxide, shaking for thirty seconds each time and allowing to stand for ten minutes before running off the chloroform. Reject the chloroform. Combine the alkaline extracts, add 5 ml of chloroform, shake for five seconds and run the chloroform layer into the separator that previously held the second sodium hydroxide extract. Repeat this procedure two or three times in a similar manner until the last chloroform washing is colourless, combining all the chloroform washings in the separator. To the combined washings add 5 ml of water, shake and then discard the chloroform. Combine the washed alkaline extract and the water used for washing the chloroform in a 50-ml beaker, and rinse the empty separator with small quantities of water until free from all alkalinity, adding the rinsings to the beaker.

Add 4 ml of 2N phosphoric acid to the alkaline solution and adjust to pH 9·0 to 9·5 with 2N phosphoric acid, using a pH-meter. Return the adjusted solution to the separator, rinsing the beaker first with two 2-ml quantities of water and then with 15 ml of chloroform and adding the rinsings to the separator. Shake carefully for thirty seconds with a rotary motion to avoid forming an emulsion and allow the layers to separate. Run the chloroform into a separator containing 25 ml of water, shake for five seconds and, after separation, filter the chloroform layer through a 1-in. layer of anhydrous sodium sulphate in a sintered-glass crucible into a 50-ml graduated flask. Extract the pH 9·0 to 9·5 solution with two further 15-ml quantities of chloroform, washing and filtering the extracts as before. Shake the wash water with successive small portions of chloroform and use these to rinse the crucible and sodium sulphate before adding to the graduated flask. Continue this process until the flask contains exactly 50 ml of solution.

Transfer a 25-ml aliquot of this solution to a 100-ml beaker that has previously been rinsed out with chloroform and evaporate the solvent on a water-bath under a current of air until only the last traces remain.

Dissolve the residue in 5 ml of dehydrated ethanol, warming gently to assist solution if necessary, add 5 ml of a 1·8 per cent solution of dipotassium hydrogen phosphate and mix.

Measure the extinction of the solution at 418 mμ, using 1-cm cells with water in the comparison cell.

Transfer about 3 ml of the solution to a silica cell and irradiate with ultra-violet light for ten minutes, using the apparatus described above. Measure the extinction at 418 mμ, using 1-cm cells with water in the comparison cell. Irradiate for further one-minute periods until a peak extinction reading is obtained and then perform a duplicate determination on a further 3 ml of the solution, irradiating for the optimum period found previously.

Let the extinction of the sample solution before irradiation be 'e' and the extinction of the solution containing sample plus added stilbœstrol before irradiation be 'e_1'. Let the extinction of the sample solution after irradiation be 'E' and the extinction of the solution containing sample plus added stilbœstrol after irradiation be 'E_1'. Then,

$$\text{p.p.m. stilbœstrol} = \frac{E - e}{(E_1 - e_1) - (E - e)} \times \frac{27{\cdot}5 \times 8}{\text{weight of sample taken}}$$

Hexœstrol may be similarly extracted from animal feeding-stuffs (containing about 5 mg per pound) for a colorimetric finish to the determination.

Chromatographic tube. This is a glass tube about 15 cm long and 1 cm in internal diameter, drawn out at the bottom for a length of about 2 cm to terminate in a jet of about 3 mm internal diameter.

Preparation of chromatographic column. Plug the bottom of the tube with cotton wool and mount in a vertical position.

To 2 g of cellulose powder add 6 ml of a 5 per cent solution of arachis oil, *B.P.*, in redistilled ether, then add more of the ether, mix thoroughly and evaporate off the ether while still mixing. Mix the residual oleated cellulose into a thin slurry with THF-TEA solvent (a mixture of 5 volumes of triethylamine, 25 volumes of tetrahydrofuran and 70 volumes of water), transfer to the chromatographic tube and allow to drain.

Determination: Crush about 1 kg of the sample; mix and grind about 100 g of the crushed material until at least 95 per cent passes a 30-mesh sieve. Weigh about 40 g of the ground material into a flask and add about 10 g of washed sand followed by 100 ml of reagent-grade chloroform. Stopper the flask, shake vigorously and allow to stand overnight. Transfer the contents of the flask to an extraction apparatus (the apparatus described above under determination of stilbœstrol is suitable) and extract for six hours, using more chloroform if necessary. Filter the extract through a pad of cotton wool into a 200-ml graduated flask, wash the extraction flask and filter with chloroform and dilute the combined filtrate and washings to 200 ml with chloroform.

Transfer a 50-ml aliquot of this solution to a separator and continue as described above under the determination of stilbœstrol beginning with the words 'Add 25 ml of N sulphuric acid . . .' and ending with the words '. . . until the flask contains exactly 50 ml of solution.'

Evaporate a 25-ml aliquot of the chloroform solution to dryness, dissolve the residue in the minimum amount of THF-TEA solvent and transfer the solution to the prepared chromatographic column. Allow the solution to drain into the column until the liquid surface just disappears below the top of the column, stopper the end of the tube and allow to stand for one hour. Add 10 ml of the THF-TEA solvent to the column and allow the solvent to pass through the column to remove impurities. When the flow has ceased, remove residual solvent from the column by applying gentle suction to the bottom of the tube.

Extrude the column containing the sample into a separator, wash out the tube with a little freshly redistilled anæsthetic ether and add the washing to the separator. Add 1 ml of N sulphuric acid and extract with three 20-ml quantities of the ether. Combine the ether extracts and extract successively with 10, 10, 5, 5 and 5 ml of N sodium hydroxide, washing each alkaline extract with the same 5 ml of ether. Combine the alkaline extracts, acidify with dilute sulphuric acid and extract successively with 10, 10, 5, 5 and 5 ml of the freshly redistilled anæsthetic ether, washing each ether extract with the same 5 ml of water. Combine the extracts and filter through a 1-cm layer of fine sand, washing the filter with several small quantities of ether. Evaporate the ether, by gentle warming, to a volume of about 5 ml, transfer quantitatively to a 14-ml centrifuge tube with more ether and carefully evaporate the remainder of the ether.

Dissolve the residue in 0·5 ml of ethanol and add 0·5 ml of water followed by 0·4 ml of dilute hydrochloric acid, 0·8 ml of Folin and Denis' reagent (see below) and 5 ml of water. Mix thoroughly, allow to stand for ten minutes and add 3 ml of 10 per cent sodium carbonate solution and sufficient water to produce 12 ml. Mix, allow to stand for one hour, centrifuge for fifteen to twenty minutes and measure the extinction of the clear supernatant liquid at 750 mμ using 1-cm cells with, in the comparison cell, a solution prepared by treating 1 ml of 50 per cent ethanol as above from the addition of 0·4 ml of dilute hydrochloric acid.

Compare the extinction with one of those obtained by treating 0·8, 1·0 and 1·2 ml of a standard solution containing 50 μg of hexœstrol per ml (prepared by diluting 5 ml of a stock solution in equal volumes of ethanol and water, containing exactly 50 μg of hexœstrol per 100 ml, to 50 ml with the diluted ethanol) exactly as described above from the addition of 0·4 ml of dilute hydrochloric acid. The extinctions of the test solution and the chosen standard solution should not differ by more than 10 per cent.

Other more recently introduced synthetic œstrogens are less reactive analytically. Of these, **methallenœstril,** $C_{18}H_{22}O_3$, Mol. Wt. 286·4, and **chlorotrianisene,** $C_{23}H_{21}O_3Cl$, Mol. Wt. 380·9, are of pharmacological importance. The former can be assayed by non-aqueous titration in butylamine, with tetrabutylammonium hydroxide, using azo-violet in benzene as indicator and the latter by Stepanow's method (p. 310) using 0·5 g, 1 ml 0·1N silver nitrate = 0·03809 g $C_{23}H_{21}O_3Cl$.

Tablets of Stilbœstrol, *B.P.* Usually contain 0·5 mg.

A further colorimetric determination of stilbœstrol depends on the reduction of Folin and Denis' reagent by the phenolic groups of the stilbœstrol molecule; the method is applicable to tablets and the following details are modifications of those originally published by Tubis and Bloom.[3]

Macerate a quantity of powdered tablets, equivalent to about 5 mg of stilbœstrol, with successive quantities of ether until completely extracted. Filter the ethereal solution, wash the filter with ether and evaporate off the solvent. Dissolve the residue in 50 ml of 95 per cent ethanol and add water to 100 ml in a graduated flask. Transfer a 10-ml aliquot to a second 100-ml graduated flask and add 2 ml of dilute hydrochloric acid followed by 4 ml of Folin and Denis' reagent [prepared by refluxing for two hours a mixture of 350 ml of water, 50 g of sodium tungstate ($Na_2WO_4,2H_2O$), 12 g phosphomolybdic acid ($H_3PO_4,12MoO_3,24H_2O$), and 25 ml of concentrated phosphoric acid, cooling and diluting to 500 ml with water]. Then add 50 ml of water, allow to stand for ten minutes, add 10 ml of a 25 per cent solution of anhydrous sodium carbonate and dilute to volume (100 ml) with water. Mix thoroughly and allow to stand for one hour; if the solution is hazy or contains a precipitate, mix a suitable volume with a quarter of its volume of ether in a stoppered centrifuge tube, shake, centrifuge and reject the upper layer, including any precipitate that has collected at the interface.

Repeat the operation using, instead of the 10-ml aliquot of sample solution, 10 ml of a solution of 5 mg of stilbœstrol in 50 ml of 95 per cent ethanol and sufficient water to produce 100 ml, and beginning with the words 'add 2 ml of dilute hydrochloric acid . . .'. Measure the extinction of each solution at 780 mμ using 1-cm cells with, in the comparison cell, a solution prepared as above but omitting the sample.

The assay is applicable to **Tablets of Dienœstrol,** *B.P.*, and **Tablets of Hexœstrol,** *B.P.C.*, using a standard solution of dienœstrol or hexœstrol for comparison in place of the stilbœstrol used in the assay given above.

Another colorimetric method for the determination of stilbœstrol, described by Duerr and Pappas[4] depends on the colour produced when sulphuric acid and ferric chloride are added to ethanolic solutions of stilbœstrol and the method is as follows:

Pipette 3 ml of an ethanolic solution, containing about 0·5 mg of stilbœstrol per ml, into a 25-ml graduated flask and dilute to 5 ml with ethanol. Then add, in 1-ml portions, with continuous swirling, 4 ml of ferric chloride/sulphuric acid reagent, prepared by adding 40 ml of concentrated sulphuric acid to 1 ml of a 10 per cent solution of ferric chloride hexahydrate; the reagent should be covered and allowed to cool to room temperature before use. Allow to stand in a water-bath at 20° for five minutes, dilute almost to volume with ethanol and replace in the water-bath. Allow the colour to develop for a further ten minutes, diluting to volume with ethanol and mixing after the first five minutes and replacing in the water-bath. After the full ten minutes measure the extinction at the absorption maximum at about 558 mμ using 2-cm cells with, in the comparison cell, a solution prepared in exactly the same way as described above using 3 ml of ethanol in place of the sample solution. Read the stilbœstrol content from a standard curve prepared by carrying out the procedure on suitable volumes, covering the range 1·0 to 2·0 mg, of a standard solution of stilbœstrol made to contain 0·5 mg per ml.

Esters of œstrogens may be determined by the usual saponification with 0·5N ethanolic potassium hydroxide as given under Oils and Fats (p. 755). **Stilbœstrol dipropionate,** $C_{24}H_{28}O_4$, Mol. Wt. 380·5, 1 ml 0·5N = 0·09512 g is the only one of pharmaceutical interest.

Injection of Stilbœstrol Dipropionate, *B.Vet.C.* A solution, usually 10 mg per ml, in ethyl oleate or a suitable fixed oil.

The assay of solutions of stilbœstrol dipropionate in oil presents difficulties; direct spectrophotometric determination is unreliable as the oil used contributes a high general absorption and extraction after saponification is unsatisfactory. The following technique is due to Dracass and Foster[5] and was found suitable when arachis oil was the solvent.

To 1 ml of the sample, containing 1 to 10 mg of stilbœstrol dipropionate per ml, add 10 ml of 95 per cent ethanol containing 2 to 3 drops of concentrated sulphuric acid and boil the mixture under reflux for two hours. Allow to cool, wash the reaction mixture into a separator with about 50 ml of ether and extract the solution three times with 10-ml portions of N sodium hydroxide, care being taken to ensure that an excess of alkali is present during the first shake. Wash the combined alkaline extracts with about 25 ml of ether and, after separating, shake the ethereal layer with 5 ml of N sodium hydroxide. Discard the separated ether, mix the alkaline liquids, acidify with dilute sulphuric acid and extract the stilbœstrol with two 25-ml portions of ether. Wash the separated ethereal extracts successively with the same 5-ml portion of water then transfer to a flask and remove the ether by evaporation. Dissolve the residue in sufficient 0·4 per cent sodium hydroxide solution to make a solution expected to contain approximately 10 mg of stilbœstrol dipropionate in 100 ml. To 5 ml of this solution add 3 ml of Folin and Ciocalteu's reagent, then 2 ml of a 20 per cent anhydrous sodium carbonate solution. Heat the mixture in a water-bath for five minutes, allow to cool, dilute with water to 25 ml and filter or centrifuge. Compare the intensity of the blue colour thus produced by means of a colorimeter with a standard made by dissolving 7 mg of stilbœstrol (equivalent to 10 mg of stilbœstrol dipropionate) in 2 ml of 20 per cent sodium hydroxide solution, diluting to 100 ml with water and treating 5 ml of this solution with Folin and Ciocalteu's reagent and sodium carbonate as above.

The stock solution of Folin and Ciocalteu's reagent is prepared as follows: Dissolve 100 g of sodium tungstate, $Na_2WO_4,2H_2O$, and 25 g of sodium molybdate, $Na_2MoO_4,2H_2O$, in 800 ml of water in a 1,500-ml flask, add 50 ml of concentrated phosphoric acid and 100 ml of concentrated hydrochloric acid and reflux for ten hours. Cool, add 150 g of lithium sulphate, 50 ml of water and 4 to 6 drops of bromine and allow to stand for two hours. Boil for fifteen minutes to expel excess bromine, cool, filter and dilute to 1 litre with water. Store at a temperature below 4° and use within four months of preparation; do not use if any trace of green colour is present.

Dilute 1 volume of this stock solution with 2 volumes of water before use.

Sesame oil contains sufficient naturally occurring phenolic bodies to interfere and a correction must be applied to the colorimetric reading for the colour due to the oil. The method is liable to give low results but increasing the time of saponification improves the recovery.

1. Goodyear, J. M., Hatfield, L. S., and Marsh, M. M., *J. Amer. Pharm. Ass., Sci. Edn.*, 1954, **43,** 605.
2. *Analyst*, 1963, **88,** in the press.
3. Tubis, M., and Bloom, A., *Ind. Eng. Chem., Anal. Edn.*, 1942, **14,** 309.
4. Duerr, J. D., and Pappas, B. A., *J. Amer. Pharm. Ass., Sci. Edn.*, 1959, **48,** 13.
5. Dracass, W. R., and Foster, G. E., *Analyst*, 1943, **68,** 181.

OPIUM

Opium is the partly dried latex obtained from the unripe capsules of *Papaver somniferum* Linn. and it is collected mainly in Turkey, the Indian subcontinent, China and parts of south-eastern Europe (Yugoslavia, Greece and Bulgaria). The British Pharmacopœia still mentions four commercial varieties of opium (Turkish, Persian, Indian and European) although in practice the Persian variety is no longer met. Opium contains a considerable number of alkaloids, mostly in small proportions, but the principal ones are morphine, narcotine, codeine and papaverine, present both free and combined with meconic, sulphuric, lactic and acetic acids. The proportion in which these alkaloids occur varies from species to species; Indian opium usually contains 9 to 12 per cent of morphine and about 2·5 to 3 per cent of codeine whilst Turkish opium may contain 14 to 18 per cent of morphine and only 1 per cent or less of codeine. Some samples, particularly those of European origin (Yugoslavian) contain 21 per cent or more of morphine. In addition to variations in alkaloid content there is also a considerable difference in appearance and texture. Turkish and European opiums are light in colour and are easily worked whilst Indian opium, containing more gummy and resinous matter, is dark and difficult to mix to a uniform consistency. These differences affect the ease with which assay processes may be applied and it is still true to say that, despite the very considerable amount of work which has been devoted to the analysis of opium, no one method has been devised which may be applied with confidence to all samples.

A number of types of method have been used for the determination of morphine in opium but only two of these, the lime and the dinitrophenylether method can be recommended and they will be dealt with in detail. The earliest methods depended upon precipitation of the morphine with ammonia after prior removal of many of the other alkaloids but this type of assay, though rapid, is very inaccurate due mainly to (*a*) incomplete extraction, (*b*) co-precipitation of morphine with other alkaloids when these are being removed and (*c*) incomplete crystallisation of morphine. The many errors to which this type of method is subject have been discussed by Vollmer,[1] but despite its unsatisfactory nature it is still the basis of the official procedure in some foreign pharmacopœias, *e.g. D.A.B.* VI. Methods based on solvent extraction, which are of value in separating alkaloids from other drugs of natural origin, are of little use for the determination of morphine in opium because morphine is amphoteric and poorly soluble in most organic solvents. The classical method is by extraction with hot amyl alcohol but objections to this solvent are obvious. Morphine is appreciably soluble in ethanol and methods employing a mixture of ethanol and chloroform as extracting solvent are published; Nicholls[2] determined the best proportions for extracting morphine completely in the shortest time. Since the base is more soluble in ethanol than in water, it is desirable to add the ethanol to the morphine solution before freeing the base with ammonia. The best method for separation was found to be:

> If present, nearly all alkaloids other than morphine can first be removed without loss of morphine by making alkaline with sodium, potassium or calcium hydroxides and extracting successively with ether and alcohol-free chloroform, the extracts being washed once with fixed alkali and the washings added to the main bulk.

To an aqueous solution thus suitably prepared add an equal volume of 95 per cent ethanol. Make the liquid ammoniacal with 1 ml of 4N ammonia if alkali has not been previously used, or with an excess of ammonium sulphate if alkaline extraction has been employed (if ammonium chloride is used, extracts may contain traces of chloride; in fact, ethanol present much above 50 per cent removes an appreciable quantity). Shake with one volume of chloroform. After running off the separated lower layer, add one half volume of ethanol and shake with one volume of chloroform. Separate and repeat the process for a third extraction and, if quantities of morphine above 0·1 g are present, a fourth extraction will be necessary.

Wash the extracts separately with the same mixture of 5 ml ethanol and 10 ml water. Evaporate the combined extracts; dissolve in standard acid, make up to a definite volume and estimate by an appropriate method (see below).

(i) **Lime Methods.** The successful use of lime in the assay of opium for morphine was first made by Hager in the 1870's. In 1882 Portes and Langlois[3] described a method from which modern procedures, as exemplified by those of the *B.P.* and the *Ph.I.*, have developed largely through the investigations of Debourdeaux.[4] Lime assists in the complete extraction of morphine as a soluble salt and at the same time eliminates much alkaloidal and other extractive matter (including the meconic acid which forms an insoluble salt with calcium). The result obtained for the morphine content of a given sample of opium will depend to a large extent on the particular version of the assay which is used; it is essential to adhere to the conditions laid down and to state the method used when quoting results.

Official lime methods depend upon the complete extraction of the opium by a single maceration with lime water and the quantitative precipitation of the morphine directly from the lime with ammonium chloride. Since some of the water used for extraction is retained by the marc it is never possible to examine the entire extract and so the morphine must be determined in an aliquot portion of it. In the case of the *B.P.* it is assumed that 52 ml will contain five-eighths of the morphine from the entire sample of opium, but this can only be an approximation since the increase in volume of the opium extract due to moisture and extractives from the opium will vary from sample to sample. Some methods, including that prescribed by the *Ph.I.*, allow for these variations by determining extractive matter and moisture at the same time as morphine on a given sample of opium.

Büchi, Huber and Schumacher[5] have carried out an extensive examination of various methods of opium determination using paper chromatographic examination of the various stages of the assays to check their validity. They concluded that some morphine is lost in both the ether and the aqueous mother liquor and that the morphine finally obtained contains 'considerable quantities of side alkaloids, particularly codeine, and traces of thebaine, papaverine and narcotine.'

Lime methods are used in the majority of pharmacopœias at the present time, but variations in detail occur from one to another. As stressed before, it is essential to carry out the determination precisely as laid down for comparative results to be obtained. The *U.S.P.* method differs from all others in that the initial extraction is carried out by repeated treatment with water and only after concentration of the aqueous extraction is the lime added.

The method of the *B.P.*, which exemplifies the classical lime procedure and has continued the same in principle through six revisions, is as follows:

> Weigh 8 g into a mortar and triturate with 10 ml of water until a homogeneous mixture is obtained. Then add a further 20 ml of water and 2·0 g of calcium hydroxide and mix well. Transfer the mixture to a tared flask, washing in with water, added in small quantities, until the total weight of the mixture is 90 g. Stopper the flask and allow to stand for thirty minutes, shaking occasionally. Filter, transfer 52 ml of the filtrate (equivalent to 5 g of the sample) to a small conical flask and add 5 ml of 90 per cent ethanol, 25 ml of ether and, after shaking, 2·0 g of ammonium chloride. Stopper the flask and shake continuously for five minutes and then occasionally during about half an hour; the mixture should be shaken for about fifteen minutes in all. Allow to stand overnight and then decant the ether layer as completely as possible into a funnel plugged with tightly packed cotton wool. Rinse the flask and contents with a further 10 ml of ether, decant the rinsings through the filter and then wash the filter with 5 ml of ether, added slowly in small portions. Pour the aqueous liquid on to the filter, without attempting to remove the crystals from the flask and when all the liquid has passed through wash the flask and filter with a saturated solution of morphine in chloroform water, filtered from undissolved morphine immediately before use, until the washings are free from chloride. Wash the crystals on the filter back into the flask, add 30 ml of 0·1N sulphuric acid, boil, cool and titrate the excess acid with 0·1N sodium hydroxide using methyl red as indicator. 1 ml 0·1N H_2SO_4 = 0·02853 g of anhydrous morphine. To correct for loss of morphine due to its solubility, add 0·052 g to the weight of anhydrous morphine indicated by the titration.

Certain points of detail of technique should be noted:

(*a*) The mixing of the original sample to a uniform paste with slaked lime is very important and some workers have added fine washed sand at this stage to assist in completely disintegrating the opium. In general, Indian and Persian opiums present more difficulties than Turkish or European.

(*b*) It is convenient to use a Büchner funnel or sintered-glass filter when the lime and opium mixture is filtered.

(*c*) After precipitation of the morphine, the mixture should be allowed to stand overnight at a temperature close to normal. Experiments carried out on two portions of the same lime extract, one kept at 5° overnight and the other at 25°, showed that the weight of morphine obtained might vary by as much as 0·7 mg for each degree difference.

(*d*) The *B.P.* method directs that the total morphine obtained in the assay is to be titrated and so this must be done when testing to the official requirements. However, the alkaloid obtained inevitably contains some lime salts and the following procedure gives greater accuracy. Weigh the total alkaloids after drying and then (i) dissolve a portion of the residue in excess 0·1N acid by boiling and determine the total alkalinity by back-titration and (ii) ash a further portion of the residue and determine the alkalinity of ash. The morphine content may then be calculated after subtracting the alkalinity of ash from the total alkalinity.

(*e*) The correction for the loss of morphine in the assay is largely due to the dilute ethanol medium from which it is precipitated, the ethanol being necessary to keep resinous matter in solution and give better crystallisation of the morphine. The value of 0·001 g per ml of filtrate used is quite accurate provided the quantities of reagents used are strictly as directed in the *B.P.* As an example of the necessity for adhering closely to the details of the method, higher figures can be obtained for the morphine content of tincture of opium by using only two-thirds of the amount of ammonium chloride prescribed by the *B.P.*

(*f*) A convenient apparatus in which the whole of the determination, after lime filtration, can be conducted consists of a 100-ml cylindrical separator made with a wide-bore tap at the lower end and a wide ground-in stopper. A plug of cotton wool is firmly inserted in the lower part of the cylinder just above the tap. After shaking the lime filtrate with the solvents and reagents and allowing it to stand overnight, the aqueous layer is filtered through the wool by inserting the tap-tube into the bung of a Büchner flask and applying slight suction. The ether layer is then removed by pouring it out at the top, the ether washings removed similarly (or the ether may be drawn off by suction) and then the residue is washed with morphinated water and this is removed as before by suction. Finally, the wool is dislodged from the base with a thin glass rod and, after addition of an excess of 0·1N acid, the cylinder is washed out carefully, the wool being squeezed out repeatedly by rolling it against the sides with the glass rod, and the solution boiled and titrated as usual.

(ii) **Dinitrophenylether methods.** Mannich[6] proposed a method for the determination of morphine based on the formation of an insoluble dinitrophenylether by reaction with 1-chloro-2,4-dinitrobenzene in alkaline aqueous methanol.

Various modifications, notably by Van Pinxteren and Smeets,[7] have improved the method. These authors modified the procedure so as to include a lime-manganous chloride extraction and by so doing were able to obtain a precipitate which gave a purity of 98 to 99 per cent on titration and which was relatively free from methoxyl groups, indicating a low contamination with other opium alkaloids.

Methods based upon precipitation with chlorodinitrobenzene are official in the Dutch, Finnish, Polish and Swedish pharmacopœias.

However, a notable advance was made with the introduction of 1-fluoro-2,4-dinitrobenzene by Dann and Wippern.[8] This reagent is much more reactive than the chloro-derivative and quantitative precipitation of morphine is obtained from an aqueous ethanol solution within two to four hours, instead of the eighteen to twenty-four hours which was previously necessary. Coupled with this, a method of extraction was proposed by Svendsen and Aarnes,[9] which involved triturating the opium or opium preparation with ammonia and then with alumina until a free-flowing powder was produced. This powder was packed into a column and the morphine eluted and precipitated as the dinitrophenylether. The method was critically examined by Garratt, Johnson and Lloyd[10] who recommended procedures both for Turkish and Indian opiums. These authors examined the precipitation of the dinitrophenylether in some detail and in particular the washing conditions necessary. Morphine dinitrophenylether precipitates simultaneously with 2,4-dinitroaniline, which is formed by interaction of the excess fluorodinitrobenzene with ammonia. When the filtered precipitate is washed with acetone it is necessary to use sufficient to remove all the dinitroaniline but not so much that loss of the morphine dinitrophenylether is incurred.

The method recommended by Garratt, Johnson and Lloyd is as follows:

For Turkish Opium. Weigh about 1 g of powdered sample into a small porcelain dish and triturate with 4 ml of a mixture of 3 volumes of 95 per cent ethanol and 1 volume of dilute ammonia solution until a smooth cream is obtained. Then add chromatographic aluminium oxide, gradually with stirring, until sufficient has been added to give a free-flowing powder. Transfer the powder to a chromatographic tube about 40 cm long and 1·5 cm in diameter, previously lightly plugged with cotton wool just above the tap. Wipe the dish and pestle with a piece of cotton wool moistened with ethanol, to remove any residual powder, and push the cotton wool down the tube. Insert the lower end of the tube into a separator provided with a side-arm assembly so that gentle suction may be applied to the tube. Elute the morphine with 100 ml to 150 ml of a mixture of 3 volumes of chloroform and 1 volume of *iso*propyl alcohol, adjusting the flow rate to about 1·5 ml per minute by means of gentle suction. Extract the eluate with 20 ml of 0·1N sodium hydroxide and transfer the organic layer to a second separator. Filter the aqueous layer through a cotton-wool plug into a 150-ml beaker and extract the organic layer with two further quantities, each of 15 ml, of 0·1N sodium hydroxide, filtering the extracts into the beaker. Make the aqueous extracts just acid to litmus paper with N hydrochloric acid and concentrate on a water-bath to a volume of about 30 ml. Cool, add 30 ml of a 0·8 per cent solution of 1-fluoro-2,4-dinitrobenzene in acetone followed by 5 ml of dilute ammonia solution, stir gently, cover the beaker and allow to stand for four hours at a temperature of 15° to 20°. At the end of this time filter through a sintered-glass filter (porosity No. 3), using the filtrate in portions of 2 to 3 ml to transfer the dinitrophenylether quantitatively to the filter. Rinse the beaker with 2 ml of acetone and transfer to the filter. After several seconds' contact with the crystals remove the acetone by applying gentle suction. Repeat this washing procedure with three further 2-ml quantities of acetone, dry the residue for one hour at 80° and weigh. Morphine dinitrophenylether × 0·6321 = anhydrous morphine.

For Indian Opium. Proceed by the method described for Turkish opium, above, to the words 'Elute the morphine with 100 ml . . .'. Wash the eluate in the separator by shaking gently with four 20-ml quantities of saturated sodium bicarbonate solution. Combine the washings and extract with two 10-ml portions of the chloroform/*iso*propyl alcohol mixture. Reject the aqueous layer, add the washings to the original washed eluate and continue by the method for Turkish opium from the words 'Extract the eluate with 20 ml of 0·1N sodium hydroxide . . .'.

The use of four portions, each of 2 ml, of acetone used to purify the precipitated complex, was reported to give a yield of 100 per cent of morphine in a gravimetric determination, the morphine dinitrophenylether being of 100 per cent purity when titrated non-aqueously. Subsequent to the publication of this work, Moss and Handisyde[11] reported recoveries of between 101 and 102 per cent by this method when applied to pure morphine (the purity of the dinitrophenylether by titration being of the order of 98 per cent), and results of this order were also obtained in the authors' laboratory. More recently still, Büchi, Huber and Schumacher[5] in a lengthy paper which for this method is mainly repetitive work confirming results already published by other workers, reported that the use of 4 × 2 ml of acetone gave them a 100 per cent yield of 100 per cent purity. It is clear, therefore, that disagreement remains on this point but, for practical application to opium and its galenical preparations, this possible error of 1 or 2 per cent is within acceptable limits. The value of this method has been recognised by its adoption without modification by the Austrian pharmacopœia.

Occasionally analysts require an assay of opium for alkaloids other than morphine. Space does not permit of the inclusion of methods here but the following references may be of value. Total alkaloids (Rakshit[12]); codeine and narcotine (Rakshit[13]); narcotine and papaverine (Annett and Bose[14]); separation of all principal alkaloids (United Nations method[15]); paper chromatographic separation of various alkaloids (Büchi, Huber and Schumacher[5]).

When the amount of opium present in a preparation is low, a colorimetric method must be used. The fluorodinitrobenzene method is applicable to most preparations containing 0·1 per cent or more of morphine, but not less since the sample size required becomes too large. Two colorimetric methods are of sufficient importance to discuss here:

(i) **The nitrosomorphine reaction.** The interaction of morphine with nitrite to form a nitroso-compound, the colour of which is intensified on making the solution alkaline, was introduced by Radulescu;[16] this has been modified from time to time.

Garratt[17] reported interference in the official method of the *B.P.* 1932 from some extracted non-morphine material in galenicals to which the method was applied. The extraneous material not only gave a brown colour with ammonia in the absence of nitrite, but this colour was a different tint from that of nitrosomorphine. In order to make the determination more accurate and a matching of the colours easier he proposed a method of compensating the blank solution, after making ammoniacal, with a quantity of test solution equal to that used in the test.

Adamson and Handisyde[18] investigated the reaction and critically reviewed the conditions for production of the colour. They found that the colour of the final solution was significantly affected by the time of reaction with nitrous acid and also by the relative amounts of nitrite and hydrochloric acid present. They proposed the following procedure:

> Dilute an aliquot of a 0·1N hydrochloric acid solution of morphine, containing not more than 1 mg of morphine, to 20 ml with 0·1N hydrochloric acid in a 50-ml graduated flask, add 8 ml of freshly prepared, 1 per cent sodium nitrite solution and mix well. After exactly fifteen minutes add 12 ml of dilute ammonia solution, dilute to volume and remix. Measure the extinction at the absorption maximum at about 442 mμ, using 4-cm cells, with, in the comparison cell, a solution prepared exactly as above but substituting 20 ml of 0·1N hydrochloric acid for the sample solution. Read the morphine content from a standard curve prepared by carrying out the procedure on suitable volumes of a standard solution of morphine in 0·1N hydrochloric acid, covering the range 0 to 1 mg of morphine.

Stephens[19] investigated the reaction in some detail. He concluded that the following points were critical:

(*a*) the pH of the solution during reaction with nitrite, since small differences in the concentration of hydrochloric acid led to significant changes in the extinction.

(*b*) nitrite concentration. This must be carefully controlled because of its effect in raising the pH.

(*c*) temperature; control within the limits 15·5° to 18·5° was found necessary for a precision of ± 1 per cent.

(*d*) time of reaction; within the temperature range given above maximum extinction is reached between fifteen and seventeen minutes.

(*e*) effect of light during the nitrite reaction. The reaction is sensitive to light, greater extinction values being obtained when the reaction is carried out in the dark.

The difference in colour between galenical extracts and pure morphine solutions is not entirely eliminated by the matching-technique referred to above and the colorimetric determination of morphine in galenicals by this reaction always tends to give high results. Tunstall and Taylor[20] found the interfering substance to be one which gives a red colour on boiling with dilute hydrochloric acid; they suggested that the alkaloid rhœdine, present in opium, might be responsible, and succeeded in reducing the interference somewhat by a preliminary extraction with benzene. Considerable difficulty with emulsions was met with when this modification was used, however.

The version of the nitrosomorphine method at present used for many official assay procedures is as follows:

Dilute an aliquot of a 0·1N hydrochloric acid solution of morphine, containing not more than 1 mg of morphine, to 20 ml with 0·1N hydrochloric acid in a 50-ml Nessler cylinder. Add 8 ml of freshly prepared 1 per cent sodium nitrite solution and mix well. After exactly fifteen minutes add 12 ml of dilute ammonia solution, dilute to 50 ml with water and remix. Transfer an equal amount of test solution to a second Nessler cylinder, dilute to 20 ml with 0·1N hydrochloric acid, add 5 ml of dilute ammonia solution and then add freshly prepared morphine and nitrite reagent until the colour matches the colour in the first cylinder. Repeat the colour matching after preliminary dilution of the comparison solution to give approximately the same volume at the match point.

Morphine and nitrite reagent is prepared as follows. Dissolve 10 mg of anhydrous morphine in sufficient 0·2N hydrochloric acid to produce 100 ml. To 10 ml add 10 ml of water and 8 ml of freshly prepared 1 per cent sodium nitrite solution, followed after fifteen minutes by 12 ml of dilute ammonia solution and dilute to 50 ml with water. 1 ml of the reagent is equivalent to 0·02 mg of anhydrous morphine.

(ii) **The iodic acid-nickel chloride reaction.** In 1906 Georges and Gascard[21] described a method for determination of morphine based on the action of iodic acid followed by ammonia to give a brown colour. Although many reducing substances do, morphine is one of the few alkaloids to react. Various authors have modified the method by complexing with a metal. Pride and Stern[22] investigated the procedure using nickel and described its quantitative application to opium and to poppy capsules. Johnson and Lloyd[23] extended the investigation of the method and applied it to a wide range of galenical preparations.

The method is much more specific than the nitrosomorphine reaction but it is not so sensitive. The detailed procedure is as follows:

Nickel chloride/ammonia solution. Transfer to a 100-ml graduated flask 8·0 g of ammonium bicarbonate that has been dried over silica gel at room temperature and stored in the same manner. Add exactly 25 ml of 4M ammonium chloride solution, exactly 20 ml of N ammonia solution and exactly 10 ml of a 1 per cent aqueous solution of nickel chloride hexahydrate and dilute to about 90 ml with water. Stopper the flask, shake vigorously until the ammonium bicarbonate has dissolved and dilute to volume with water.

Method: Pipette 10 ml of a prepared solution containing 0·4 to 4 mg of anhydrous morphine in 0·05N hydrochloric acid into each of two 25-ml graduated flasks. To the first flask add exactly 2 ml of a 4·5 per cent solution of reagent-grade iodic acid, with thorough mixing. After exactly two minutes add, by pipette, 10 ml of freshly prepared nickel chloride/ammonia solution, again mix and dilute to volume with water (solution A). To the second graduated flask add exactly 5 ml of 0·1N hydrochloric acid and exactly 10 ml of nickel chloride/ammonia solution, and mix (solution B). Leave to stand for ninety minutes to allow the green colour to develop. Measure the extinction of solution A at 670 mμ, using 1-cm cells with solution B in the comparison cell, and read the weight of anhydrous morphine equivalent to the extinction from a standard curve prepared by carrying out the entire process described above on suitable amounts of a standard morphine solution.

Tincture of Opium, *B.P.* Standardised to contain 1·0 per cent of morphine.

It is assayed by the *B.P.* method for opium after evaporating 80 ml nearly to dryness and using 5 ml of water for trituration, except that the total weight is made up to 86 g (52 ml of the filtrate represents 50 ml of the tincture of opium being assayed).

Comparable results are obtainable by application of the fluorodinitrobenzene precipitation method of Garratt, Johnson and Lloyd.[10] Evaporate 10 ml in a porcelain dish to dryness on a water-bath and continue by the method for raw opium.

Camphorated Tincture of Opium, *B.P.* (Paregoric). A compound tincture composed of benzoic acid, camphor, anise oil and tincture of opium, in alcohol. It contains 0·05 per cent w/v of anhydrous morphine.

Benzoic acid is determined as follows:

Make 20 ml of tincture distinctly alkaline with sodium hydroxide and evaporate to a low bulk to remove the alcohol. Then extract the alkaline solution with ether, wash the ether with water and add it to the other aqueous portion. Acidify the alkaline liquid and extract the benzoic acid with portions of ether. Wash the mixed ethers with water until free from mineral acid and either dry the ether and evaporate, or titrate the ether layer by the method given under Benzoic Acid.

For routine purposes a direct determination of benzoic acid can be made by titrating to phenol red. The acidity contributed by the tincture of opium is equivalent to approximately 0·04 per cent benzoic acid.

For morphine assay, the *B.P.* extraction is essentially that due to Nicholls, described above.

Evaporate 5 ml to dryness, extract the residue with 10 ml of lime water and filter into a separator, washing the dish and filter with a further 10 ml of lime water. To the filtrate add 0·1 g of ammonium sulphate and extract with two quantities of 10 ml of alcohol-free chloroform, washing each extract with the same 10 ml of water. Reject the chloroform and extract the mixed extracts and washings first with 30 ml of 95 per cent ethanol and 30 ml of chloroform and then with two quantities of a mixture of 15 ml of 95 per cent ethanol and 30 ml of chloroform. Wash each of these extracts with the same mixture of 5 ml of 95 per cent ethanol and 10 ml of water. Evaporate the mixed ethanol-chloroform solutions to dryness, dissolve the residue in 10 ml of N hydrochloric acid, filter and wash the residue on the filter with sufficient water to produce 50 ml.

Continue the nitrosomorphine colorimetric assay using 10 ml of this solution diluted with 10 ml of water.

The *U.S.P.* method of morphine assay is somewhat cumbersome but the alkaloid is finally titrated; if sufficient sample (100 ml) is available the *B.P.* method may be followed until evaporation of the chloroform-ethanol mixture and then the alkaloids determined by solution in excess of 0·02N acid and back-titration after boiling the solution, using methyl red as indicator (1 ml 0·02N = 0·005707 g anhydrous morphine).

For application of the fluorodinitrobenzene method to this preparation, transfer 100 ml to a porcelain dish and evaporate to a volume of about 10 ml on a water-bath. Add about 5 g of chromatographic aluminium oxide and continue the evaporation to dryness. Continue by the appropriate method for raw opium.

The iodic acid-nickel chloride colorimetric method may also be applied as follows:

Transfer 10 ml to a small dish and evaporate to dryness on a water-bath. Triturate the residue with 1 ml of dilute ammonia solution and then add chromatographic aluminium oxide gradually, with stirring, until sufficient has been added to give a free-flowing powder. Transfer the powder to a dry chromatographic tube about 40 cm in length and 1·5 cm in diameter, previously lightly plugged with cotton wool just above the tap. Remove any adhering powder from the dish and pestle with cotton wool moistened with *iso*butyl alcohol and push the cotton wool down the tube. Insert the lower end of the tube into a separator provided with a side-arm assembly so that gentle suction may be applied to the tube and elute the morphine with 50 ml of a mixture of 3 volumes of chloroform and 1 volume of *iso*butyl alcohol, adjusting the flow rate to about 1·5 ml per minute by means of gentle suction. Wash the eluate with 10 ml of water, allow to separate and filter the organic layer through cotton wool moistened with solvent into a 150-ml beaker. Shake the aqueous layer with 10 ml of the chloroform/*iso*butyl alcohol mixture and after separation filter the organic layer into the beaker. Wash the filter with a little more of the solvent mixture, evaporate the solvent on a water-bath under a gentle current of air and leave the residue on the water-bath for five minutes after all the solvent has evaporated. Dissolve the residue in exactly 5 ml of 0·5N hydrochloric acid, warming on the water-bath for a few seconds if necessary. Filter through a Whatman No. 41 filter paper into a 50-ml graduated flask, washing the beaker and filter with small quantities of water and collecting the washings in the flask. Cool to room temperature if necessary and dilute to volume with water. Use 10 ml of this solution for application of the iodic acid-nickel chloride reaction (see above).

Concentrated Camphorated Tincture of Opium, *B.P.C.* Eight times the strength of the camphorated tincture. For assay it is diluted eight times with 60 per cent ethanol and one of the above methods employed.

Opiate Linctus of Squill, *B.P.C.* (Gee's Linctus). Consists of equal volumes of camphorated tincture of opium, oxymel of squill and syrup of tolu.

Squill contains substances which interfere with the morphine assay but they can be removed by extraction with alcohol-free chloroform.

Transfer 12 g to a separator with 5 ml of water, add 1 ml of dilute ammonia solution and extract with 15 ml of ethanol and 15 ml of chloroform. Continue the extraction with two quantities of a mixture of 7·5 ml of ethanol and 15 ml of chloroform and wash each extract with the same mixture of 10 ml of ethanol and 10 ml of water. Evaporate the mixed solutions, extract the residue with 10 ml of lime water and filter into a separator, washing the flask with 10 ml of lime water. To the filtrate and washings add 0·1 g of ammonium sulphate and extract with two portions of 10 ml of alcohol-free chloroform, washing the mixed chloroform solutions with 10 ml of water and then rejecting the chloroform. To the mixed alkaline liquids add 10 ml of N hydrochloric acid and heat on a water-bath to remove the chloroform, cool and dilute with water to 100 ml. Continue with the colorimetric assay using 20 ml of solution.

For the iodic acid-nickel chloride method prepare the solution as follows:

Transfer 30 ml to a separator, add 1 ml of dilute ammonia solution and mix. Continue as given under Mixture of Ammonium Chloride and Morphine from the words 'shake vigorously for two to three minutes . . .', but dissolve the residue in exactly 5 ml of 0·5N hydrochloric acid and dilute with water to 50 ml. Use 10 ml of this solution for application of the iodic acid-nickel chloride reaction (see above).

Opiate Linctus of Squill for Infants, *B.P.C.* A similar preparation to the above, diluted with glycerin and syrup.

The assay of this preparation follows that for Opiate Linctus of Squill but using three times the weight of sample and diluting to 50 ml before taking a 20-ml aliquot for colorimetric assay.

Ointment of Gall and Opium, *B.P.C.* Consists of opium and gall in a lard base. It contains 0·75 per cent of morphine.

Although numerous attempts have been made to obtain a satisfactory assay of this preparation, none has yet been successful. A determination by first extracting the fat with light petroleum and then using the method given under Powder of Ipecacuanha and Opium will give an approximation but it cannot be used for standardisation.

Pastilles of Opiate Linctus of Squill, *B.P.C.* (Gee's Linctus Pastilles). Pastilles containing active ingredients equivalent to 30 minims of Gee's Linctus are prepared either with a glyco-gelatin or acacia and sucrose basis. For the nitrosomorphine assay a double extraction is necessary.

Take 20 pastilles and determine the average weight. Dissolve two pastilles, accurately weighed, in 20 ml of warm water, cool and add 0·5 g of sodium bicarbonate. Extract with four 30-ml portions of a mixture of 3 volumes of chloroform and 1 volume of ethanol, shaking gently for two minutes at each extraction. Wash each extract with the same

10 ml of water and evaporate to dryness. Warm the residue with 20 ml of lime water, filter and wash with 20 ml of water. Shake with two 5-ml portions of ether and wash the ethers with 5 ml of lime water. To the combined aqueous solutions add 0·25 g of ammonium sulphate and extract with four 20-ml portions of the chloroform-ethanol mixture. Evaporate the extracts to dryness, dissolve in 25 ml of warm 0·1N hydrochloric acid, cool and dilute to 50 ml with 0·1N acid. Determine the morphine in 20 ml of this dilution colorimetrically and calculate the weight of anhydrous morphine in each pastille of average weight.

The theoretical content of morphine is approximately 0·00032 g per pastille.

To prepare pastilles for application of the iodic acid-nickel chloride method:

Weigh 20 pastilles and determine the average weight per pastille. Cut up some of the pastilles and weigh into a separator an amount equivalent to about 5 pastilles. Add 30 ml of water, stopper the separator and shake vigorously to dissolve. Make alkaline with dilute ammonia solution and extract with three 30-ml quantities of a mixture of 3 volumes of chloroform and 1 volume of *iso*butyl alcohol, shaking well for two to three minutes at each extraction. Combine the extracts in a second separator, reject the aqueous phase and extract the solvent mixture with 10, 10 and 5 ml of 2 per cent w/v sulphuric acid solution, combining the extracts in a separator. Make ammoniacal and continue as described below for Mixture of Ammonium Chloride and Morphine from the words 'shake vigorously for two to three minutes . . .' but dissolve the residue in exactly 5 ml of 0·5N hydrochloric acid, dilute with water to 50 ml and use 4-cm cells for the measurement of the extinction.

Powder of Ipecacuanha and Opium, *B.P.* (Dover's Powder). Contains prepared ipecacuanha and powdered opium, of each 10 per cent, with lactose.

The ipecacuanha in this preparation does not interefere with the morphine determination:[17]

Mix intimately 1 g of sample with 0·25 g of slaked lime in a glass mortar. Add water gradually and transfer quantitatively to a 100-ml graduated flask. Shake the mixture (approximately 90 ml) frequently during thirty minutes, make up to 100 ml, shake and filter. To 10 ml of filtrate add 0·15 g of ammonium sulphate and continue the nitrosomorphine colorimetric assay as given under Camphorated Tincture of Opium except that the residue is dissolved in 5 ml of N hydrochloric acid and diluted to 50 ml. 20 ml of this solution is used for the colorimetric assay.

The iodic acid-nickel chloride colorimetric assay or the fluorodinitrobenzene method can be used using 5 g of powder by the appropriate method of raw opium, above.

Aromatic Powder of Chalk with Opium, *B.P.C.* Contains 0·25 per cent of powdered opium in aromatic powder of chalk.

This preparation can be assayed by the method for Powder of

Ipecacuanha and Opium using 4 g of sample, but there is a tendency for low results to be obtained, probably due to adsorption on the chalk.

Tablets of Aspirin with Dover's Powder, *B.P.C.* Contain a mixture of equal parts of aspirin with ipecacuanha and opium powder. The anhydrous morphine content is 1·62 mg per tablet.

The assay for morphine follows that for Powder of Ipecacuanha and Opium using 2 g of powdered tablets but 0·75 g of lime.

The aspirin may be determined directly by boiling a quantity of powder equivalent to about 5 tablets with 20 ml of water and 2 g of sodium citrate for thirty minutes and titrating with 0·5N sodium hydroxide using phenolphthalein as indicator. 1 ml 0·5N = 0·04505 g $C_9H_8O_4$.

Compound Tablets of Aspirin with Dover's Powder, *B.P.C.* Contain 3 grains of aspirin, 1¼ grains of phenacetin and 1 grain of ipecacuanha and opium powder. The anhydrous morphine content is 0·65 mg per tablet.

In this complex mixture the general method of preparation for the colorimetric nitrosomorphine assay given under Powder of Ipecacuanha and Opium requires considerable modification. For this preparation:

> Mix intimately 2 g of the powdered sample with 0·5 g of calcium hydroxide. Add water gradually and transfer to a 100-ml graduated flask and dilute with water to 90 ml. Shake frequently during thirty minutes, dilute to 100 ml and filter. Extract 25 ml of filtrate twice with 10-ml portions of ether and wash the extracts with 5 ml of lime water. To the combined aqueous solutions add 0·15 g of ammonium sulphate and extract with 70 ml of equal volumes of 95 per cent ethanol and chloroform, followed by two portions of 45 ml of a mixture of one volume of ethanol and two volumes of chloroform and wash each solvent extract with a mixture of 5 ml of ethanol and 10 ml of water.
>
> Evaporate the solvent, dissolve the residue in 25 ml of N hydrochloric acid, make slightly alkaline with sodium hydroxide and extract three times with 5-ml portions of chloroform. Wash the chloroform twice with 5-ml portions of water. To the combined alkaline liquid and washings add 5 ml of N hydrochloric acid and dilute to 50 ml with water. Using 20 ml of this solution continue the determination by the nitrosomorphine reaction given above.

Tablets of Ipecacuanha and Opium, *B.P.* Usually contain 5 grains of the powder.

The powdered tablets are assayed by the method for Powder of Ipecacuanha and Opium.

PAPAVERETUM

Consists of either the hydrochlorides of the total alkaloids of opium standardised to the required proportion of alkaloids or a mixture of the hydrochlorides of morphine, codeine, narcotine and papaverine.

The assay for morphine follows that of the *B.P.* for the assay of opium after a preliminary washing with ether in alkaline solution instead of lime treatment:

> Dissolve 1 g in 20 ml of water in a separator, add 5 ml N sodium hydroxide and extract with two portions of 50 ml and 25 ml of ether. Filter the aqueous layer through a cotton-wool plug into a 50-ml graduated flask; wash the ether successively with a mixture of 2·5 ml N sodium hydroxide and 5 ml of water, followed by small portions of water passed through the filter until 50 ml have been collected. Continue the *B.P.* assay for opium beginning with the transference to a small conical flask. In this assay the correction for loss of morphine due to its solubility is 0·025 g.

Adamson, Handisyde and Hodgson[24] found it necessary to use a rather elaborate technique for determination of codeine, narcotine and papaverine if the assay were to be suitable for a mixture composed of the total alkaloid hydrochlorides of opium. Exposure to direct sunlight should be avoided during the assay and preferably subdued light should be used. The method recommended was the following:

> Dissolve 1 g of sample in 20 ml of water in a separator and add 40 ml of chloroform. Add 1 drop of dilute hydrochloric acid and shake vigorously for thirty to forty seconds. After separation, wash the chloroform first with 10 ml of N sodium hydroxide and then with 10 ml water. Repeat the extraction with four 20-ml portions of chloroform, washing each extract as before with the sodium hydroxide and water and reserving the aqueous layer, the sodium hydroxide and the water washings for the determination of codeine. Filter the washed chloroform extracts into a dry flask, recover the chloroform, add 2 ml of dehydrated ethanol and evaporate on a water-bath in a current of air with constant rotation of the flask, avoiding undue heating.
>
> Dissolve the crude narcotine and papaverine in 6 ml of benzene, add 3 ml of a 10 per cent w/v solution of potassium hydroxide in dehydrated ethanol, and place in a water-bath at 20° for forty minutes. Transfer to a separator, washing in with three quantities of 5 ml of benzene and then with 10 ml of N sodium hydroxide. Shake well, separate; wash the aqueous layer with 10 ml benzene and transfer to a small conical flask. Wash the benzene layers with two 5-ml quantities of N sodium hydroxide and finally with two 5-ml quantities of water, adding all washings to the first aqueous layer and retaining the benzene layers for the determination of papaverine.
>
> To the combined aqueous extracts add 6·5 ml of concentrated hydrochloric acid and place in a water-bath until the temperature of the solution reaches 95°. Cool and transfer to a separator, washing in with three quantities, each of 3 ml, of water; add 7 ml of strong ammonia solution and extract the alkaloid with 20, 10, 10 and 10 ml of chloroform, washing each extract with the same 10 ml of water in a second separator. Filter into a tared flask, recover the chloroform, add 2 ml of ethanol and heat in a current of air, with rotation. Finally, dry at 100° to 105° for ten minutes, cool and weigh as narcotine.
>
> Transfer the aqueous layer and washings remaining after the extraction of the crude narcotine and papaverine to a 100-ml beaker, washing in with 10 ml of water, passed in turn through the separators. Warm the

contents of the beaker to remove chloroform, cool and add 3 ml of 5 per cent sodium hydroxide solution; stir and set aside for thirty minutes. Filter through a small paper into a separator, washing the beaker and filter with two quantities, each of 5 ml, of water. Extract the combined filtrate and washings with three quantities, each of 20 ml of benzene, washing each extract with the same 10 ml of water. Filter the benzene extracts into a separator, washing with 10 ml of benzene, and extract with 25 ml of dilute sulphuric acid, shaking vigorously for five minutes. Transfer the acid solution to a 100-ml beaker, washing the benzene layer once with 20 ml of water and adding the washings to the acid extract. Make the combined extract and washings alkaline with strong ammonia solution and boil until the volume has been reduced to 20 to 30 ml. Check the pH of the solution, which should be between 4·0 and 3·6 (yellowish-green to bromocresol green paper), and filter into a separator, washing with two quantities, each of 5 ml, of water. Extract the combined filtrate and washings three times with 20 ml of chloroform, washing each extract in turn with the same 10 ml of water. Discard the chloroform extracts. Combine the aqueous layers, making alkaline with 2 ml of dilute ammonia solution and extract the codeine three times with 20 ml of chloroform, washing each extract with the same 10 ml of water. Filter the chloroform extracts into a tared flask, recover the chloroform and dry in the manner already described above. Cool and weigh as codeine.

The purity of the product may be checked, if required, by dissolving in 10 ml of dehydrated ethanol and obtaining the specific rotation at 20°; the rotation should not be less than −130°.

Filter the benzene layers into a dry flask, washing with 5 ml of benzene. Evaporate and dry, with the addition of 2 ml of ethanol as previously described. Moisten the residue with 1 ml of concentrated hydrochloric acid, cover, and allow to stand for fifteen minutes. Wash into a separator with 20 ml of water and extract the papaverine with 20, 10, 10 and 10 ml of chloroform, washing each extract with 10 ml of N sodium hydroxide and then with 10 ml of water. Filter the chloroform extracts into a tared flask, evaporate and dry in the manner described above. Cool and weigh as papaverine.

The fluorodinitrobenzene assay given above can be applied for morphine. If papaveretum has been prepared from the total alkaloids of opium the full procedure for determination of morphine in raw opium must be used. Since codeine, narcotine and papaverine have been shown to cause no interference in the precipitation of morphine as the dinitrophenylether, however, it is unnecessary to adopt the column procedure where the papaveretum is a mixture of pure alkaloids.

For material prepared from the total alkaloids of opium. Take 0·2 g and proceed by the method for raw opium.

For material prepared by mixing the hydrochlorides of morphine, codeine, narcotine and papaverine. To 0·2 g in a 150-ml beaker, add 30 ml of water and stir to dissolve. Continue by the method for raw opium from the words 'add 30 ml of a 0·8 per cent solution of 1-fluoro-2,4-dinitrobenzene in acetone . . .'.

Injection of Papaveretum, *B.P.C.* Contains 2 per cent of papaveretum.

The proportion of morphine in the solids is so high that interference is negligible and a direct nitrosomorphine colorimetric assay is applicable. A dilution of 1 in 500 is made with 0·1N hydrochloric acid and 20 ml of the dilution taken for the colorimetric assay.

For the fluorodinitrobenzene assay morphine may be determined on 10 ml, with or without column treatment, according to the type of papaveretum used.

Tablets of Papaveretum, *B.P.C.* The proportion of morphine is sufficiently high to neglect interference from other alkaloids or impurities in the nitrosomorphine colorimetric assay. The equivalent of one tablet is dissolved as completely as possible in warm 0·1N hydrochloric acid, diluted to 250 ml with 0·1N acid and 20 ml of the dilution taken for direct colorimetric assay.

For the fluorodinitrobenzene assay apply the method for raw opium using a weight of powdered tablets equivalent to 0·2 g of papaveretum.

MORPHINE AND ITS SALTS

Morphine, $C_{17}H_{19}O_3N,H_2O$, Mol. Wt. 303·4, is not used to any extent in pharmaceutical practice. The official salts, **morphine hydrochloride,** $C_{17}H_{19}O_3N,HCl,3H_2O$, Mol. Wt. 375·9, **morphine sulphate,** $(C_{17}H_{19}O_3N)_2,H_2SO_4,5H_2O$, Mol. Wt. 758·9 and **morphine tartrate,** $(C_{17}H_{19}O_3N)_2,C_4H_6O_6,3H_2O$, Mol. Wt. 774·8, are all assayed by the ethanol-chloroform method of Nicholls after a preliminary cleaning from other alkaloids in sodium hydroxide solution with chloroform. The assay is completed by titration.

In N sulphuric acid, morphine hydrochloride and morphine sulphate have absorption maxima at 285 mμ, E(1 per cent, 1 cm) = 40.

Injection of Morphine and Atropine, *B.P.C.* A sterile solution of morphine sulphate, 1 per cent, atropine sulphate, 0·06 per cent and sodium metabisulphite in water for injection.

The determination of both atropine and morphine in a single 10-ml portion of the sample can be made by (*a*) extracting the atropine with chloroform in the presence of excess of sodium hydroxide, washing the extracts, evaporating, dissolving in excess of 0·05N acid and titrating with 0·05N alkali, 1 ml 0·05N = 0·01737 g of $(C_{17}H_{23}O_3N)_2,H_2SO_4,H_2O$ and (*b*) adding 1 g of ammonium chloride to the residual aqueous solution and washings and extracting with mixed ethanol-chloroform by Nicholls' method above, evaporating and titrating as for the atropine, 1 ml 0·1N = 0·03794 g of $(C_{17}H_{19}O_3N)_2,H_2SO_4,5H_2O$.

A direct spectrophotometric assay can be used for morphine, proceeding as directed under Injection of Morphine Sulphate, using 10 ml diluted to 100 ml, then 10 ml diluted to 100 ml, both in N sulphuric acid.

Atropine does not interfere with the colorimetric assay of morphine so that the direct determination can be employed, with modifications, after suitable dilutions.

Morphine interferes with the colorimetric assay of atropine; Allport and Jones[25] oxidised the morphine with ferric chloride and then extracted the atropine in the normal way after adding sodium citrate and ammonia.

Transfer a measured quantity of the injection expected to contain approximately 1 mg of atropine into a small separator, dilute with water until the volume of the liquid approximates to 5 ml, add 0·5 ml of a solution of ferric chloride (5 per cent w/v $FeCl_3$ in water) and allow to stand for two minutes. Add 2 g of sodium citrate, shake until dissolved, render the mixture alkaline by adding 0·5 ml of dilute ammonia solution and proceed with the extraction and colorimetric determination of atropine as described on p. 113.

Injection of Morphine Sulphate, *B.P.* A sterile solution of morphine sulphate with sodium metabisulphite in water for injection.

A direct colorimetric assay is used after suitable dilution with 0·1N hydrochloric acid. Anhydrous morphine × 1·330 = morphine sulphate.

For spectrophotometric assay:

Dilute the injection with N sulphuric acid so that the final concentration of morphine sulphate is about 0·01 per cent. Measure the maximum extinction of a 1-cm layer of this solution at about 285 mμ using N sulphuric acid as the blank. Calculate the amount of morphine sulphate in each ml of injection solution.

Note. If phenol or any other bacteriostat exhibiting ultra-violet absorption which interferes with the determination of morphine is present the latter may be determined after isolation on an oxycellulose or alginic acid column (see p. 519).

The tetraphenylboron method for the determination of small quantities of bases given under Atropine (p. 116) can be applied to simple morphine preparations. For this preparation dilute 2 ml of the $\frac{1}{2}$ grain per ml strength to 20 ml with equal volumes of buffer solution, pH 3·7, and water and take 10 ml for the assay. 1 ml of cetylpyridinium chloride = 0·001897 g.

Mixture of Ammonium Chloride and Morphine, *B.P.C.* A complex mixture containing chlorodyne.

It may be assayed for morphine by the iodic acid-nickel chloride method described above after preliminary treatment to eliminate interference, particularly from the liquorice present. The solution is prepared as follows:

Transfer 100 ml of the sample to a continuous extraction apparatus containing a suitable volume of a mixture of 3 volumes of chloroform and 1 volume of *iso*butyl alcohol. Make the aqueous layer distinctly alkaline with strong ammonia solution, add a little sodium metabisulphite to the aqueous layer and to the flask of the apparatus, which should also contain about 50 ml of the chloroform/*iso*butyl alcohol mixture, and reflux for two hours or until the morphine is completely extracted. Cool the solution, filter into a separator through a cotton-wool plug and wash the flask and filter with small volumes of the chloroform/*iso*butyl alcohol mixture, adding the washings to the separator.

Extract with 10, 10 and 5 ml of 2 per cent w/v sulphuric acid and combine the acid extracts. Make alkaline to litmus paper with dilute ammonia solution and shake vigorously for two to three minutes with 30 ml of the chloroform/*iso*butyl alcohol mixture. Allow to separate and run the solvent layer into another separator containing 10 ml of water. Shake well, allow to separate and filter the solvent layer through a small filter paper into a beaker. Repeat the extraction in the first separator with two further quantities, each of 30 ml, of the chloroform/*iso*butyl alcohol mixture, washing each extract with the same 10 ml of water as before and filtering into the beaker. Wash with a little of the solvent, evaporate to dryness on a water-bath under a current of air and leave the residue on the water-bath for five minutes after all the solvent has evaporated. Cool, dissolve the residue in exactly 2·5 ml of 0·5N hydrochloric acid, warming slightly if necessary. Filter through a Whatman No. 41 filter paper into a 25-ml graduated flask and wash the beaker and filter paper with small quantities of water, collecting the washings in the flask. Adjust to room temperature and dilute to volume with water. Use 10 ml of this solution for application of the iodic acid-nickel chloride reaction (see above).

Solution of Morphine Hydrochloride, *B.P.* A 1 per cent solution in acidified aqueous alcohol.

The assay of this preparation follows the general method of Nicholls given above, but the extraction is made in presence of sodium bicarbonate instead of ammonia. It is not clear why this departure from the normal method has been used although Nicholls has shown that local anæsthetics of the procaine type are not extracted by solvents at this pH.

For spectrophotometric assay:

Dilute 10 ml of sample to 100 ml in N sulphuric acid and dilute 10 ml of this solution to 100 ml in N sulphuric acid. Measure the maximum absorption at about 285 mμ in a 1-cm cell using N sulphuric acid as the blank. Calculate the amount of morphine hydrochloride in each ml of sample.

Suppositories of Morphine, *B.P.C.* Contain $\frac{1}{4}$ grain of morphine hydrochloride in oil of theobroma basis.

Dissolve the equivalent of one suppository in 20 ml chloroform. Extract with four portions each of 30 ml 0·1N hydrochloric acid, washing each extract separately with the same portion of 10 ml chloroform. Make the washed aqueous extracts up to 200 ml with 0·1N acid. Dilute an aliquot five times with 0·1N acid and continue by the usual nitrosomorphine colorimetric assay.

The tetraphenylboron method for the determination of bases given under Atropine (p. 116) has been successfully applied to this preparation. The equivalent of 4 suppositories is dissolved in 10 ml of light petroleum (b.p. 40° to 60°), with warming, and extracted first with 10 ml of 2N acetic acid and then with three 5-ml quantities of buffer solutin, pH 3·7, filtering each extract in turn through a small plug of cotton wool to remove traces of solvent and diluted to 25 ml with the buffer solution. 10 ml of this solution is taken for assay. 1 ml of cetylpyridinium chloride = 0·00188 g morphine hydrochloride.

Tablets of Morphine Sulphate, *B.P.*

For assay by base extraction shake a quantity of powdered tablets containing about 0·1 g of morphine sulphate in a separator with 25 ml of water and 5 ml of N sodium hydroxide. Continue by the Nicholls extraction method given above, after addition of 1 g of ammonium sulphate and titrate the residue of morphine.

For spectrophotometric assay:

> Weigh an amount of finely powdered tablet material containing about 100 mg of morphine sulphate, transfer to a 250-ml graduated flask, add about 100 ml of N sulphuric acid and shake for thirty minutes. Make up to volume with N sulphuric acid, mix and filter a portion of the solution, rejecting the first 30 ml. Dilute 25 ml of the filtrate to 100 ml in N sulphuric acid and measure the maximum extinction at about 285 mμ in a 1-cm cell using N sulphuric acid as the blank. Calculate the amount of morphine sulphate in each tablet.

Tincture of Chloroform and Morphine, *B.P.C.* (Chlorodyne). This tincture is a complex mixture of chloroform, ether, alcohol, morphine hydrochloride, peppermint oil, extract of liquorice, treacle, and syrup. It is liable to separate and should be thoroughly shaken before assay.

> Transfer about 13 g, accurately weighed in a stoppered weighing bottle after thorough shaking, to a separator with the aid of 1 ml of dilute ammonia solution, 4 ml of water, 15 ml of ethanol and 15 ml of chloroform. Shake, separate and run off the lower layer into a second separator and wash it with 20 ml of a mixture of equal volumes of ethanol and water. Continue the extraction in the first separator with two successive quantities of a mixture of 15 ml of chloroform and 7·5 ml of ethanol, washing each ethanol-chloroform solution with the same liquid as before. Evaporate the mixed ethanol-chloroform solutions to dryness and dissolve the residue in 100 ml of approximately N hydrochloric acid and dilute with water to 500 ml. To 10 ml add 10 ml of water and complete the assay by the nitrosomorphine colorimetric method.

The nitroso-phenol reaction, when applied to extractives of chlorodyne, is subject to interference from substances other than morphine present in the residue. Garratt[26] drew attention to apparent 'morphine' contents of treacle. McLachlan[27] reported the interference from liquorice as being due to the colour which develops with ammonia and glycyrrhizin and some of its hydrolysis products. The apparent morphine contents of both treacle and liquid extract of liquorice were also reported on in 1956.[28] By the extraction procedure detailed below morphine can be separated from the substances present in liquorice which give a yellow colour with ammonia and the iodic acid-nickel chloride reaction may then be applied.

Weigh 4 g into a small dish and evaporate the volatile solvents on a water-bath. Triturate the residue with 1 ml of dilute ammonia solution until a smooth cream is obtained and continue as described above for Camphorated Tincture of Opium beginning with the words 'add chromatographic aluminium oxide . . .' and ending with the words '. . . to about 1·5 ml per minute by means of gentle suction.' Extract the morphine from the eluate with 10, 10 and 5 ml of 2 per cent w/v sulphuric acid solution, combine the extracts in another separator and make alkaline to litmus paper with dilute ammonia solution. Complete by the method for Mixture of Ammonium Chloride and Morphine from the words 'shake vigorously for two to three minutes . . .', but dissolve the residue in exactly 5 ml of 0·5N hydrochloric acid and dilute with water to 50 ml. Use 10 ml of this solution for application of the iodic acid-nickel chloride reaction described above.

Chloroform can be determined by the direct hydrolysis method given on p. 168 using 0·4 g of sample, or by gas chromatography. The weight per ml at 20° must be determined to calculate the percentage w/v.

CODEINE, $C_{18}H_{21}O_3N,H_2O$, Mol. Wt. 317·4

Codeine is extracted from alkaline solution by chloroform and assay of its salt and galenicals is effected by normal alkaloidal extraction technique. **Codeine phosphate,** $C_{18}H_{21}O_3N,H_3PO_4,1\frac{1}{2}H_2O$, Mol. Wt. 424·4, is official in the *B.P.*, but the *U.S.P.* salt is a hemihydrate, Mol. Wt. 406·4, and this is the more usual commercial product. It may be determined by non-aqueous titration (see p. 792). 1 ml 0·1N perchloric acid = 0·03974 g $C_{18}H_{21}O_3N,H_3PO_4$ or 0·02994 g $C_{18}H_{21}O_3N$.

Linctus of Codeine, *B.P.C.* Consists of syrup of codeine phosphate with wild cherry and tolu. For assay the method used for Syrup of Codeine Phosphate is applicable, using 20 g.

Mixture of Codeine for Infants, *B.P.C.* A complex mixture containing Syrup of Codeine Phosphate. The assay for codeine requires modification to eliminate traces of volatile oils before extraction of the base.

To 20 ml in a separator, add 2 ml of dilute sulphuric acid and shake with 20 ml of chloroform. Allow the layers to separate, reject the chloroform and make the aqueous liquid alkaline to litmus with dilute ammonia solution. Extract with three 20-ml quantities of chloroform, or until complete extraction is effected, washing each extract with the same 10 ml of water. Combine the extracts, evaporate the solvent, add 5 ml of 95 per cent ethanol and re-evaporate. Dissolve the residue in 5 ml of 0·02N hydrochloric acid and titrate the excess acid with 0·02N sodium hydroxide using methyl red as indicator. 1 ml 0·02N HCl = 0·008488 g $C_{18}H_{21}O_3N,H_3PO_4,1\frac{1}{2}H_2O$.

Syrup of Codeine Phosphate, *B.P.C.* A simple solution of codeine phosphate in syrup with spirit of chloroform.

The codeine is determined on 10 g of the syrup by extraction with chloroform in presence of ammonia, dissolving the residue in excess 0·05N acid and titrating back to methyl red. 1 ml 0·05N = 0·02077 g $C_{18}H_{21}O_3N,H_3PO_4,H_2O$.

Tablets of Codeine Phosphate, *B.P.* Contain ½ grain of codeine phosphate.

Assayed by dissolving the powdered tablets in dilute acid, filtering, washing and extracting the alkaloid in ammoniacal solution with chloroform. After adding ethanol and re-evaporating, the alkaloid can be dried and weighed, or titrated using methyl red as indicator. 1 ml 0·1N = 0·02994 g codeine or 0·04244 g codeine phosphate.

The tetraphenylboron method for the determination of small quantities of bases given under Atropine (p. 116) can be applied to codeine. For this preparation, powder and dissolve the equivalent of 2 tablets, with gentle warming in 12·5 ml of buffer solution, pH 3·7, and dilute to 25 ml with water. Centrifuge if necessary and take 10 ml of clear solution for the assay. 1 ml cetylpyridinium chloride solution = 0·002122 g.

Compound Tablets of Codeine, *B.P.* See under Acetylsalicylic Acid, p. 13.

PAPAVERINE, $C_{20}H_{21}O_4N$, Mol. Wt. 339·4

Papaverine in N hydrochloric acid has an absorption maximum at 250 mμ, E(1 per cent, 1 cm) = 1,840.

Papaverine hydrochloride, $C_{20}H_{21}O_4N,HCl$, Mol. Wt. 375·9 and **papaverine sulphate,** $(C_{20}H_{21}O_4N)_2,H_2SO_4,5H_2O$, Mol. Wt. 867·0, can be assayed by non-aqueous titration (see p. 792); the base may be also extracted by chloroform or carbon tetrachloride from alkaline solution and weighed after drying at 105°. 1 g residue = 1·107 g of $C_{20}H_{21}O_4N,HCl$, 1·144 g of $(C_{20}H_{21}O_4N)_2,H_2SO_4$ or 1·277 g of $(C_{20}H_{21}O_4N)_2,H_2SO_4,5H_2O$.

Papaverine hydrochloride and sulphate are soluble in chloroform and can be isolated from complex mixtures in acid solution by this characteristic, before extraction of the base as above.

APOMORPHINE HYDROCHLORIDE, $C_{17}H_{17}O_2N,HCl,\frac{1}{2}H_2O$, Mol. Wt. 312·8

Apomorphine hydrochloride is a synthetic alkaloidal salt obtained by heating morphine with concentrated hydrochloric acid under pressure. It is unstable in solution in the absence of hydrochloric acid.

The *B.P.* assay is by base extraction and titration, taking precautions against oxidation.

> To 0·1 g in a separator add 25 ml of freshly boiled and cooled water, and 25 ml anæsthetic ether and rotate until dissolved. Add 2 ml of freshly prepared, saturated sodium carbonate solution and shake. Allow to separate, run the lower layer into a second separator and transfer the

ether layer to a third separator. Extract the aqueous layer with four 15-ml quantities of anæsthetic ether, using the first and second separator alternately, and combine the ether layers in the third separator. Wash the ether solution with three 5-ml quantities of water, extract the combined washings with 10 ml of anæsthetic ether and add the ether to the main ether extracts. Shake the ether solution with 20 ml of 0·02N hydrochloric acid, allow to separate and run off the aqueous layer. Wash the ether layer with two 5-ml quantities of water, add the washings to the aqueous layer and titrate with 0·02N sodium hydroxide using methyl red as indicator. 1 ml 0·02N HCl = 0·006076 g $C_{17}H_{17}O_2N,HCl$.

Apomorphine in 0·1N hydrochloric acid has an absorption maximum at 273 mμ, E(1 per cent, 1 cm) = 550.

Apomorphine hydrochloride can be assayed by non-aqueous titration (see p. 792).

Injection of Apomorphine Hydrochloride, *B.P.* A 0·3 per cent solution of apomorphine hydrochloride; it contains sodium metabisulphite.

It is assayed spectrophotometrically after dilution to a 0·001 per cent solution with 0·1N hydrochloric acid.

DIAMORPHINE, $C_{21}H_{23}O_5N$, Mol. Wt. 369·4

Like morphine, diamorphine is not extracted from aqueous solution by ether or chloroform but may be completely extracted by the ethanol-chloroform technique.

Allport and Jones[25] observed that the alkaloid can be hydrolysed to morphine quantitatively with boiling dilute hydrochloric acid. The alkaloidal residue is boiled under a reflux condenser for ten minutes with 10 ml of 5 per cent hydrochloric acid and the morphine so produced then determined colorimetrically. The indicated morphine content is multiplied by 1·486 to convert it into equivalent of **diamorphine hydrochloride,** $C_{21}H_{23}O_5N,HCl,H_2O$, Mol. Wt. 423·9.

Diamorphine hydrochloride can be assayed by non-aqueous titration (see p. 792).

Elixir of Diamorphine and Terpin, *B.P.C.* Diamorphine hydrochloride 0·1 per cent, with terpin hydrate in a mixture with alcohol, glycerin and syrup of wild cherry. It is assayed by the method given below for Linctus of Diamorphine.

In the determination of diamorphine, terpin hydrate cannot be eliminated by preliminary extraction with solvent or by hydrolysis with acid; however, it is mainly volatilised in the evaporation of the solvent extracts.

Linctus of Diamorphine, *B.P.C.* Diamorphine hydrochloride 0·1 per cent, in a mixture of oxymel, glycerin, colouring matter and syrup.

Assayed by extracting about 5 g in ammoniacal solution with chloroform and ethanol by Nicholls' method, evaporating to a viscous residue (as some glycerol is extracted) and hydrolysing to morphine with dilute hydrochloric acid as given above. During the acid boiling the solution darkens, but the decomposition products are extracted with chloroform from the acid solution.

Transfer 5 g to a separator with 25 ml of water, add 2 ml dilute ammonia solution and extract with 30 ml of ethanol and 30 ml of chloroform, washing with a mixture of 5 ml of ethanol and 10 ml of water. Continue the extraction with two portions of a mixture of 15 ml of ethanol and 30 ml of chloroform. Evaporate the mixed solutions, dissolve the residue in 5 ml water and 5 ml 4N hydrochloric acid and boil for ten minutes under a reflux condenser. Cool and transfer to a separator, add 15 ml water and extract with two 15-ml portions of chloroform, washing with the same 10 ml of water and rejecting the chloroform. Heat the mixed aqueous solutions on a water-bath, cool and dilute to 200 ml with water. Continue with the nitrosomorphine colorimetric assay using 20 ml of solution.

ETHYLMORPHINE

Like codeine and unlike morphine and diamorphine, ethylmorphine is extracted from alkaline solution by chloroform and assay of its salts and preparations is effected by normal alkaloidal extraction technique. **Ethylmorphine hydrochloride,** $C_{19}H_{23}O_3N,HCl,2H_2O$, Mol. Wt. 385·9. 1 ml 0·1N = 0·03498 g anhydrous salt, or 0·03859 g $C_{19}H_{23}O_3N,HCl,2H_2O$.

PHOLCODINE, $C_{23}H_{30}O_4N_2,H_2O$, Mol. Wt. 416·5

The base is assayed by solution in excess of standard acid and back-titration of the excess with bromocresol green as indicator, 1 ml 0·01N = 0·01992 g $C_{23}H_{30}O_4N_2$. It can also be determined by non-aqueous titration (p. 792).

Pholcodine is extracted from alkaline solution by chloroform and assay of its salts and preparations follows normal alkaloidal extraction procedure.

Pholcodine tartrate, $C_{23}H_{30}O_4N_2,2C_4H_6O_6,3H_2O$, Mol. Wt. 752·7, 1 ml 0·1N HCl = 0·03493 g anhyd. The correct titration end-point is at pH 4·8 and is given by using as indicator a solution containing 0·1 per cent of bromocresol green and 0·025 per cent of methyl red in 95 per cent ethanol.

Linctus of Pholcodine, *B.P.C.* Contains 1 per cent of pholcodine. For assay:

Weigh about 50 g into a separator, make alkaline to litmus with dilute ammonia solution and extract with four 25-ml quantities of chloroform, washing each extract with the same 5 ml of water. Combine the extracts and evaporate the chloroform until the volume is reduced to about 15 ml. Add 30 ml of glacial acetic acid and titrate with 0·02N perchloric acid using quinaldine red as indicator. Repeat the operation omitting the sample. 1 ml 0·02N = 0·00417 g $C_{23}H_{30}O_4N_2,H_2O$.

Syrup of Pholcodine Citrate, *B.P.C.* Contains 2 per cent of pholcodine.

It can be assayed by the method given above for Linctus of Pholcodine using about 25 g of sample.

SYNTHETIC NARCOTICS

Little analytical chemistry has been applied to these compounds. The bases can be extracted with solvent and titrated with standard acid. They can also be assayed by non-aqueous titration after extraction (see p. 792).

Dextromethorphan hydrobromide, $C_{18}H_{25}ON,HBr,H_2O$, Mol. Wt. 370·3, is assayed in the *B.P.C.* by extracting about 0·3 g with chloroform from sodium hydroxide solution and titrating the extracts directly with 0·02N perchloric acid using methyl red as indicator, 1 ml 0·02N = 0·007047 g of $C_{18}H_{25}ON,HBr$.

Dihydrocodeinone bitartrate, $C_{18}H_{21}O_3N,C_4H_6O_6,2\frac{1}{2}H_2O$, Mol. Wt. 494·5, is assayed in the *N.F.* by extraction with chloroform from ammoniacal solution and titration, after solution in excess acid. 1 ml 0·02N = 0·00989 g. It should be noted that the conditions specified in the *N.F.* may lead to high results. Satisfactory results are obtained if the chloroform extracts are taken to dryness twice with 2-ml portions of acetone and then dried for ten minutes in a steam-oven before continuing.

Levorphanol tartrate, $C_{17}H_{23}ON,C_4H_6O_6,2H_2O$, Mol. Wt. 443·5. The official *B.P.C.* method of assay is the following:

> Dissolve 0·2 g in 20 ml of water in a separator, add 1 g of sodium bicarbonate, shake and extract with successive 25-ml portions of a mixture of 3 volumes of ether and 1 volume of chloroform until extraction is complete. Combine the extracts, wash with three 5-ml quantities of water, combine the washings and extract with two 10-ml portions of the ether/chloroform mixture. Combine the extracts and extract with 20 ml of 0·05N hydrochloric acid. Wash the ether/chloroform layer with successive 10-ml quantities of water until the washings are no longer acid to litmus paper, combine the aqueous extract and washings and titrate the excess acid with 0·05N sodium hydroxide using methyl red as indicator. 1 ml 0·05N = 0·02037 g $C_{21}H_{29}O_7N$.

NARCOTIC ANTAGONISTS

The analytical chemistry of these compounds follows that for the synthetic narcotics. The bases can be extracted with solvent and either titrated with standard acid or assayed by non-aqueous titration.

Levallorphan tartrate, $C_{19}H_{25}ON,C_4H_6O_6$, Mol. Wt. 433·5, is assayed in the *B.P.C.* by non-aqueous titration of the extracted base:

> Dissolve 0·5 g in 30 ml of hot water, add 10 ml of a 10 per cent solution of sodium carbonate decahydrate, cool and extract with 35, 25 and 25 ml of ether, washing each extract with the same two quantities, each of 5 ml, of water. Combine the extracts, dry over anhydrous sodium

sulphate, filter and wash the residue with two 5-ml quantities of ether. Combine the filtrate and washings, evaporate the ether, dissolve the residue in 20 ml of glacial acetic acid and titrate with 0·05N perchloric acid using oracet blue B as indicator. 1 ml 0·05N = 0·02168 g.

Nalorphine hydrobromide, $C_{19}H_{21}O_3N,HBr$, Mol. Wt. 392·3. The *B.P.* extracts the base with a mixture of chloroform and *iso*propyl alcohol and titrates it with acid.

Dissolve about 0·5 g in 15 ml of water, add 5 ml of dilute ammonia solution and extract with four portions of about 20 ml of a mixture of 3 volumes of chloroform and 1 volume of *iso*propyl alcohol, washing each extract with the same 10 ml of water. Evaporate the extracts to dryness and re-evaporate with two 5-ml quantities of 95 per cent ethanol. Dissolve the residue in 1 ml of ethanol, add 20 ml of 0·1N hydrochloric acid and titrate with 0·1N sodium hydroxide to methyl red, 1 ml 0·1N HCl = 0·03923 g $C_{19}H_{21}O_3N,HBr$.

Injection of Nalorphine Hydrobromide, *B.P.* Usually contains 10 mg in 1 ml of water for injection.

The assay is the same as for nalorphine hydrobromide above using an amount of injection equivalent to about 0·2 g.

Nalorphine hydrochloride, $C_{19}H_{21}O_3N,HCl$, Mol. Wt. 347·9, can be assayed as for the hydrobromide. The *U.S.P.* assay is spectrophotometric. Nalorphine hydrochloride has an absorption maximum at about 285 mμ, E(1 per cent, 1 cm) = 44.

1. Vollmer, K., *Dtsch. Apoth.-Ztg.*, 1955, **95,** 258.
2. Nicholls, J. R., *Analyst*, 1937, **62,** 440.
3. Portes and Langlois, *J. Pharm. Chim.*, 1881, **4** [v], 560.
4. Debourdeaux, L., *J. Pharm. Chim.*, 1911, **4** [vii], 105.
5. Büchi, J., Huber, R., and Schumacher, H., *Bull. Narcotics*, 1960, **12,** 25.
6. Mannich, C., *Arch. Pharm.*, 1935, **273,** 97; 1942, **280,** 386.
7. Van Pinxteren, J. A. C., and Smeets, M. A. G., *Pharm. Weekblad.*, 1950, **85,** 48.
8. Dann, O., and Wippern, F., *Dtsch. Apoth.-Ztg.*, 1951, **91,** 905.
9. Svendsen, A. B., and Aarnes, E. P., *Sci. Pharm.*, 1955, **23,** 18.
10. Garratt, D. C., Johnson, C. A., and Lloyd, C. J., *J. Pharm. Pharmacol.*, 1957, **9,** 914.
11. Moss, A. R., and Handisyde, F. P., private communication.
12. Rakshit, J. N., *Analyst*, 1926, **51,** 491
13. Rakshit, J. N., *Analyst*, 1921, **46,** 481.
14. Annett, H. E., and Bose, M. N., *Analyst*, 1923, **48,** 53.
15. United Nations Secretariat, ST/SOA/Ser.K/34. Unified Analysis of Opium for Alkaloids.
16. Radulescu, D., *Bul. Soc. Sţi. Bucureşti*, 1905, **14,** 602.
17. Garratt, D. C., *Quart. J. Pharm.*, 1937, **10,** 466.
18. Adamson, D. C. M., and Handisyde, F. P., *Quart. J. Pharm.*, 1946, **19,** 350.
19. Stephens, R. L., *J. Pharm. Pharmacol.*, 1951, **3,** 815.

20. Tunstall, G., and Taylor, M. P., *J. Pharm, Pharmacol.*, 1953, **5**, 737.
21. Georges, L., and Gascard, *J. Pharm. Chim.*, 1906, **23** [vi], 513.
22. Pride, R. R. A., and Stern, E. S., *J. Pharm. Pharmacol.*, 1954, **6**, 590.
23. Johnson, C. A., and Lloyd, C. J., *J. Pharm. Pharmacol.*, 1958, **10**, 60T.
24. Adamson, D. C. M., Handisyde, F. P., and HODGSON, F. W., *Quart. J. Pharm.*, 1947, **20**, 218.
25. Allport, N. L., and Jones, N. R., *Quart. J. Pharm.*, 1942, **15**, 238.
26. Garratt, D. C., *Quart. J. Pharm.*, 1946, **19**, 419.
27. McLachlan, T., *Pharm. J.*, 1951, **167**, 24.
28. Pharmaceutical Society Laboratory Reports, *Pharm. J.*, 1956, **176**, 384.

PANCREATIN

In the chemical assay of pancreatin and other enzyme-containing preparations the end-points often leave much to be desired.

The *B.P.* method of assay for trypsin in pancreatin is based on the fact that amino-acids are formed by hydrolysis of protein by trypsin; formaldehyde forms methylene compounds with the amino-groups, the carbonyl groups being free for titration with alkali. This method, due to Evers and Smith,[1] uses purified casein adjusted to pH 7 before the addition of formaldehyde and then titration to pH 8·7. A slightly modified method is the following:

Casein Solution. Dissolve 4 g of Hammarsten's casein in 90 ml of water containing 3 ml of N sodium hydroxide, adjust to pH 8·7, using phenolphthalein as external indicator, and make up the volume to 100 ml.

Neutral Standard. Take 10 ml of the *B.P.* phosphate buffer solution at pH 7·0 and add 1 drop of 0·1 per cent solution of neutral red in 50 per cent ethanol.

Alkaline Standard. Take 10 ml of the *B.P.* boric acid-potassium chloride-sodium hydroxide buffer solution at pH 8·7 and add 1 drop of 0·1 per cent solution of neutral red in 50 per cent ethanol and 3 drops of 0·1 per cent solution of phenolphthalein in 50 per cent ethanol.

Preparation of the Enzyme Solution. Triturate 0·5 g of the sample with a little chloroform water in a small mortar, wash into a 300-ml graduated flask and make up to volume with chloroform water. The liquid should not be filtered but should be used as a suspension if insoluble matter is present.

Digestion. Dilute 30 ml of the casein solution to 90 ml with chloroform water and place 45 ml of the solution in each of two flasks. To one flask add 10 ml of the pancreatin solution, previously boiled and cooled, and adjust the temperature to 55°. Adjust the temperature of the other flask to 55°, place in an incubator at that temperature and add another 10-ml portion of the pancreatin solution. Keep both flasks at this temperature for twenty minutes. Cool rapidly to laboratory temperature. Add 5 drops of neutral red solution to both liquids and 0·1N acid or alkali to both until each colour matches the neutral standard. (This is most easily done by pouring 10 ml into a test-tube and comparing with the standard in a similar tube.) Add 15 drops of 0·1 per cent phenolphthalein solution and 10 ml of formaldehyde solution (*B.P.*) previously neutralised to phenolphthalein, to both liquids. Titrate with 0·1N alkali until the colour matches the alkaline standard. The difference between the two titrations represents the amino-acids formed. The result is preferably expressed as a volume of standard alkali for a definite weight of the enzyme preparation. A convenient method of expression is as the number of ml of N sodium hydroxide for 1 g of the sample.

As the value of the titration is not directly proportional to the amount of trypsin used, the quantity of trypsin taken must be adjusted so as to give approximately the same titration in every case.

It is important to note that in the final titration the neutral red changes from pink to yellow before the pink of the phenolphthalein appears. Consequently there is a point in the first colour change at which the tint matches that of the alkaline standard. This must be disregarded; the end-point is reached during the change from yellow to pink.

It is suggested in this paper that a standard for pancreatin be that 1 g by the above method should give a titration of not less than 15 ml of N sodium hydroxide, whereas the *B.P.* requirement is a minimum of 18 ml N sodium hydroxide for 1 g.

The *B.P.* test for amylase in pancreatin is equivalent to a digestion of 300 times its weight of starch at 40° in one hour.

Prepare a 1 per cent solution of soluble starch in 5 per cent sodium chloride, dilute ten times and to 5-ml portions of the dilution add a solution of 10 mg of the pancreatin in 300 ml of water in amounts of from 0·35 to 0·60 ml and incubate at 40° for one hour. Cool rapidly and add 1 drop of 0·02N iodine to each; the tubes containing 0·5 ml and upwards of the solution should show no blue colour, indicating complete digestion of the starch.

The estimation of lipase activity depends upon the measurement of the rate at which it is capable of bringing about the hydrolysis of a glyceride or simple ester and the acid liberated by the lipase in a given time is titrated with standard alkali. Bullock[2] proposed an assay process using triacetin as substrate which takes only thirty minutes; the acid liberated by the lipase is neutralised by dropwise addition of dilute alkali so as to maintain an approximately constant pH.

Add 6·5 ml of triacetin and 0·2 ml of bromocresol purple solution to 95 ml of water in a stoppered measuring cylinder. Shake, neutralise with 0·05N sodium hydroxide and make up to 110 ml. Place 50 ml of the mixture into each of two large (3 × 20 cm) test-tubes A and B in a water-bath at 30°. Insert in each a rubber stopper having two holes, one for the drawn-out tip of a burette and the other for a short glass tube through which passes a silk or cotton thread operating a glass stirring coil. Stir the contents of the tubes until they attain the temperature of the bath. To tube A add 1 ml of the enzyme solution (0·1 g pancreatin made up to 10 ml with water) and to tube B add 1 ml of the enzyme solution previously boiled. Bring the contents of both tubes to a pH between 6·2 and 6·4 by dropwise addition of 0·05N sodium hydroxide. This is done by comparing the colour of the two tubes with two standard tubes each containing 0·18 ml of bromocresol purple solution and 15 ml of *B.P.* buffer solution, in the one case of pH 6·2 and in the other of pH 6·4, and in both cases made up to 50 ml with water. When this has been done note the time and read the burettes. Continue to maintain the pH of the digestion mixture between 6·2 and 6·4 by dropwise addition of 0·05N sodium hydroxide, stirring as required, and note the burette readings after ten, twenty and thirty minutes. Ascertain the amount of acid liberated by the enzyme at ten-minute intervals by subtracting the readings for tube B from those for tube A.

As a standard it is suggested that a 1 per cent suspension of pancreatin should, under the conditions of the test, liberate acid at a rate equivalent to 1 ml of 0·05N sodium hydroxide in thirty minutes. Since the amount of alkali liberated is approximately proportional to the time, it is not necessary to continue the test beyond ten minutes if three times the alkali then added is definitely more than 1 ml. Only if an accurate assay is required, or if the activity of the sample of pancreatin being assayed is on the borderline, is it necessary to continue the test for the full thirty minutes. Variation of the pH by 0·1 units has no appreciable effect on the result; variation of the temperature by 1° either way has an effect of less than 0·1 ml on a result of 1·0 ml.

A more precise assay of pancreatin can be made by an adaptation of the plate-diffusion method[3] as used in the microbiological assay of antibiotics (see p. 814). The four point assay procedure is employed, that is, two dilutions of the standard preparation are compared with two equivalent dilutions of the test preparation, the stronger dilution in each case being four times that of the weaker. Large, flat-bottomed plates or trays are preferred, thus allowing an 8 × 8 Latin square design to be used, but petri dishes are also satisfactory.

The diffusion medium is a gel of washed agar (1·2 per cent of Davis New Zealand agar is satisfactory) to which has been added a buffer solution and a suitable concentration of a substrate appropriate for the enzyme to be assayed. The depth of agar gel in the plates is about 0·1 in. (2·5 mm) and the cups, cut out with a No. 5 cork borer, are about 7 mm in diameter. A stock concentrate of the agar in water can be prepared (see below) which for storage purposes must be sterilised; asepsis in the assay is not necessary.

For trypsin and amylase. To 90 ml of 2·4 per cent agar gel in water, previously melted and cooled not below 75°, add 45 ml of double-strength McIlvaine buffer at pH 6, 22 ml of an 8 per cent solution of light soluble casein, 22 ml of a 4 per cent starch gel in water and about 1·8 g of sodium chloride, pour on a levelled plate, and allow to cool and solidify. Cut out the cups and fill them according to design with the standard and test preparations diluted as required with half-strength

McIlvaine buffer at pH 6. The standards should preferably be of the pure enzymes, although a selected batch of pancreatin, previously standardised, may be used, and the most suitable dilutions are:—for pure trypsin 1 : 10,000 and 1 : 40,000 (freshly prepared*), for pure amylase (α-amylase derived from pancreatic extract must be used) 1 : 2,000 and 1 : 8,000 and for pancreatin 1 : 200 and 1 : 800.

After incubating at 37° for sixteen to twenty hours, measure the diameters of the *outer* edges of the white haloes to estimate the trypsin content, then flood the plate with 0·1 per cent iodine solution and measure the clear zone diameters on the blue background to estimate the amylase content. The usual linear relationship holds between log concentration of enzyme and zone diameter.

For lipase. To 90 ml of a 5 per cent agar gel in water, previously melted and cooled not below 75°, add 18 ml Solution of Standard pH 8·5 *B.P.*, 27 ml water and 45 ml bromocresol purple solution *B.P.* Then add 5 ml tributyrin, shake vigorously to give as fine a dispersion as possible and pour immediately on a levelled plate. Proceed as in the assay for trypsin and amylase above, measuring the zones of colour change after incubation.

PAPAIN

The proteolytic enzyme of papain is active in both acid and alkaline media. Bullock and Sen[4] recommended casein as substrate for formol titrations. The importance of activation, preferably with cysteine hydrochloride, was established and the following assay proposed.

Dissolve 4 g of light white soluble casein by shaking with 90 ml of water. Adjust the pH to 7·0, using bromothymol blue as external indicator, and make up the volume to 100 ml. Dissolve 0·5 g of cysteine hydrochloride in 10 ml of water and adjust the pH to 7·0. Triturate 0·5 g of papain with the solution of cysteine hydrochloride and make up to 100 ml.

In each of two flasks place 15 ml of casein solution and 30 ml of water, adjust the temperature to 60° and place in a water-bath at 60°. To one flask add 5 ml of the solution of papain and cysteine hydrochloride and to the other add 5 ml of a portion of the same activated enzyme solution previously boiled for three minutes and cooled. Maintain both at 60° for thirty minutes. Cool rapidly to room temperature and to each flask add 0·75 ml of 0·1 per cent phenolphthalein solution and 10 ml of formaldehyde solution previously neutralised to phenolphthalein. Titrate both liquids with 0·1N sodium hydroxide to a definite pink colour (pH 8·7). The difference between the two titrations should not be less than 4·5 ml or more than 6·0 ml.

The plate-diffusion method can also be applied in the assay of papain. The method is similar to that described above for the assay of pancreatin.

To 90 ml of 2·4 per cent agar gel in water, previously melted and cooled not below 75°, add 45 ml of double-strength McIlvaine buffer at pH 6 and 45 ml of 4 per cent light soluble casein solution and pour on a levelled plate. Proceed as in the assay of pancreatin, measuring the

* Pure trypsin is not stable for long periods in McIlvaine buffer.

outer edges of the white haloes produced after incubation. Pure papain is not available for use as a standard, therefore a selected commercial preparation must be used. The recommended dilutions for the assay are 1 : 100 and 1 : 400.

PEPSIN

The digestive action of the proteolytic enzyme in pepsin only takes place in acid solution.

The *B.P.C.* assay is only a limiting test and does not distinguish between samples of different activity.

The official assay is based on the recommendations of Bullock[5] who made a critical survey of various methods official in different pharmacopœias. Too strict an interpretation of the tolerated amount of undigested albumen at the end of the assay is not justified as the condition of the undigested albumen will vary in repeat assays. The age of the egg used in the assay can have a considerable effect on the results; it is to be noticed that the official test prescribes a fresh egg and an egg from two to six days old should be used.

> Triturate 0·25 g with 1 g of sodium chloride, slowly add acidified water containing 65 ml of N hydrochloric acid per litre, dilute to 1 litre with the acidified water and shake for fifteen minutes. Prepare coagulated egg albumen by boiling fresh eggs for fifteen minutes, cooling and immediately rubbing the separated whites through a No. 40 sieve; reduce 12·5 g to uniform granules by triturating with 50 ml of the acidified water, add a further 50 ml and completely immerse in a water-bath at 50° to 52° until the mixture has attained this temperature; add 20 ml of the solution of the sample, digest for four hours, shaking at intervals of fifteen minutes, centrifuge, decant, rejecting the liquid, transfer the residue to a 10-ml cylinder, and allow to stand for thirty minutes; the volume of undissolved albumen is not greater than 2 ml. This is equivalent to the pepsin dissolving not less than 2,500 times its weight of coagulated egg albumen.

A quantitative assay can be obtained by using the plate-diffusion method. It is similar to that described above for the assay of pancreatin.

> To 90 ml of 2·4 per cent agar gel in water, previously melted and cooled not below 75°, add 45 ml of 1 per cent light soluble casein solution and then 45 ml of McIlvaine buffer at pH 3·5. By this means the casein is obtained as a finely dispersed suspension in the agar base. Pour immediately on a levelled plate and proceed as in the assay of pancreatin, measuring the zones of clearing after incubation. The recommended dilutions for the standard pure pepsin are 1 : 1,600 and 1 : 6,400; for *B.P.C.* '2,500' material they are 1 : 50 and 1 : 200 and for *B.P.C.* '10,000' material 1 : 200 and 1 : 800. A 1 per cent solution of pepsin in acidified chloroform water is a convenient stock supply for this standard.

1. EVERS, N., and SMITH, W., *Quart. J. Pharm.*, 1936, **9**, 392.
2. BULLOCK, K., *Quart. J. Pharm.*, 1945, **18**, 234.

3. CARTER, D. V., and SYKES, G., *J. Pharm. Pharmacol.*, 1961, **13**, 195 T.
4. BULLOCK, K., and SEN, J. K., *J. Pharm. Pharmacol.*, 1951, **3**, 476.
5. BULLOCK, K., *Quart. J. Pharm.*, 1935, **8**, 13.

PARAFFINS

Because of the inert chemical nature of the paraffins, their quantitative analytical chemistry, as far as pharmaceutical requirements are concerned, is limited to extraction from mixtures; this is comparatively easy as paraffin is unaffected by most reagents.

Pharmaceutical preparations containing paraffin are generally ointments and emulsions. The estimation of paraffin in the former follows the determination of unsaponifiable matter described in the section on Oils and Fats. Strong hydrochloric acid will clear paraffin emulsions rapidly.

To about 2 g of the emulsion add 10 ml of concentrated hydrochloric acid and 5 ml of water and heat on a water-bath for a few minutes until the mixture is light brown in colour. Transfer to a separator, cool and extract with four portions, each of 25 ml, of a mixture of equal volumes of light petroleum (b.p. 40° to 60°) and ether, washing each extract with 10 ml of dilute ammonia solution followed by two 5-ml quantities of water. Combine the extracts in an unweighed flask and evaporate the solvents. Add 3 ml of acetone to the residue, evaporate and then repeat this process with two further 3-ml quantities of acetone. Dry the residue at 105° for fifteen minutes and weigh. Wash out the residue with light petroleum (b.p. 40° to 60°), again dry the flask at 105° for fifteen minutes and reweigh for the tare.

Bond and Druce[1] were able to apply their method (p. 403) successfully for determination of oil in emulsions to paraffin preparations. In the presence of phenolphthalein the second water wash is replaced by 15 ml of 0·5N sodium hydroxide.

The ethanol coagulation technique (p. 402) is particularly suitable for paraffin emulsions since fatty acids are absent and no portion of the oil is lost by solubility in the ethanol; the coagulated gums absorb the oil which can be recovered by extraction with ether. To prevent the coagulum becoming horny during filtration and difficult to extract, kaolin is added. Washing of the ethereal extract from impurities is not necessary unless phenolphthalein is present but it avoids evaporation of a quantity of aqueous ethanol extracted by the ether.

To about 2·5 g, accurately weighed, in a beaker add 0·5 g of kaolin and mix. Add 5 ml of 70 per cent ethanol and stir thoroughly; add a further 45 ml of ethanol and stir again. Filter through a fluted open-texture filter paper, transferring the precipitate to the filter with the aid of further portions of ethanol. Place the filter paper and precipitate in an extraction thimble, transfer to an apparatus for continuous extraction and exhaust with ether, the extraction being continued for about two hours. Transfer the ethereal extract to a separator and wash with two 15-ml portions of water. Transfer the ether solution to a weighed flask, remove the solvent, add 5 ml of acetone and evaporate. Repeat the addition and evaporation of acetone until the residue is free from water. Dry at 105° for fifteen minutes and weigh.

Emulsion of Liquid Paraffin, *B.P.* An emulsion of liquid paraffin, 50 per cent v/v, with glycerin, gums, sodium benzoate and flavouring matter.

Any of the above methods is suitable for determination of the liquid paraffin.

Emulsion of Liquid Paraffin with Cascara, *B.P.C.* Liquid Paraffin Emulsion to which has been added a small proportion of Elixir of Cascara.

The liquid paraffin in this preparation is best determined by the coagulation method given above.

Emulsion of Liquid Paraffin with Magnesia, *B.P.C.* Contains 3 parts of Mixture of Magnesium Hydroxide with 1 part of liquid paraffin.

The assay for oil is the same as above, although the paraffin can be extracted directly from an acidified solution with ether or a mixture of ether and light petroleum, completing as given above. The alkali may be titrated directly to methyl orange after dilution with water, the benzoic acid not interfering with this indicator. 1 ml 0·5N = 0·01458 g $Mg(OH)_2$.

Emulsion of Liquid Paraffin and Phenolphthalein, *B.P.C.* Contains 50 per cent of liquid paraffin, emulsifying agent, flavouring, and 0·34 per cent w/v of phenolphthalein. The assay for liquid paraffin is the same as above except that the ethereal extracts are washed first with 15 ml 0·5N sodium hydroxide and then with 15 ml water. 1 to 2 mg of phenolphthalein may be absorbed in the coagulated solids.

For phenolphthalein, see p. 525.

1. BOND, C. R., and DRUCE, S., *Analyst*, 1942, **67**, 379.

BALSAM OF PERU

Balsam of Peru is frequently adulterated as it is an expensive product, and if possible the source of supply should be ascertained as a reliable criterion of purity. Bennett[1] summarised the analysis of balsam of Peru and in his opinion the best guide to value is the content of 'cinnamein' (which name was originally used for benzyl cinnamate but is now employed for esters soluble in ether but insoluble in caustic soda and might better be termed 'balsamic esters'). This may, however, be deliberately increased by the addition of benzoic esters, benzyl benzoate being commonly used. The extreme limits of cinnamein for genuine balsam lie between 51 and 66 per cent. The refractive index of the balsam at 25° was found to be 1·5886 to 1·5952 and that of the extracted cinnamein, 1·5750 to 1·5820; the refractive index of cinnamein from synthetic balsams is generally below 1·5650.

The acid and ester values of the balsam, 56 to 84 and 170 to 190, respectively, are only of value as control tests and are of little use as a guide to purity; but the saponification value of the extracted cinnamein is of importance and is included in the *B.P.C.* requirements with a minimum of 230 and for the *N.F.* it should be between 230 and 240. The *B.P.C.* figure for the saponification value of the balsamic esters (8·2 ml per g of residue) corresponds approximately to that required for benzyl cinnamate. The volume of 0·5N ethanolic potash required per gram of benzyl benzoate would be approximately 9·4 ml with a saponification value of 264, hence the fact that only a minimum figure is given in the *B.P.C.* would allow addition of a considerable proportion of this adulterant. Another helpful figure would appear to be the iodine value of the balsamic esters (20 to 30, Bennett[1]) or of the alcohols obtained after saponification of the cinnamein (38 to 51, Rosenthaler[2]), the iodine value of the products obtained from synthetic balsams being much lower; only a few genuine specimens have been examined on these lines.

Smelt[3] has compared many of the qualitative tests for adulteration, which should be used in conjunction with quantitative tests, since it is probable that other substances would be added to a synthetic mixture to imitate the characteristics of the natural drug and detection of these substances by qualitative tests would be indicative of such adulteration; the original paper should be consulted for details of the proposed tests.

1. BENNETT, C. T., *P.E.O.R.*, 1920, **11,** 131; 1928, **19,** 428.
2. ROSENTHALER, L., *Pharm. Ztg.*, 1928, **73,** 837.
3. SMELT, E. M., *Quart, J. Pharm.*, 1932, **5,** 378.

PETHIDINE HYDROCHLORIDE

$C_{15}H_{21}O_2N,HCl$ Mol. Wt. 283·8

Pethidine hydrochloride can be determined by direct non-aqueous titration and is assayed in the *U.S.P.* by this method.

Dissolve about 0·5 g in a mixture of 10 ml of glacial acetic acid and 10 ml of a 6 per cent solution of mercuric acetate in glacial acetic acid, warming slightly if necessary to effect solution. Titrate with 0·1N perchloric acid using crystal violet as indicator. Carry out a blank determination and make any necessary correction. 1 ml 0·1N = 0·02838 g $C_{15}H_{21}O_2N,HCl$.

The official *B.P.* method, however, first extracts the base with chloroform and titrates the chloroform solution, since this technique is applicable to the preparations. Pethidine base is slightly volatile at 105° but can be dried in a desiccator (wt. × 1·147 = $C_{15}H_{21}O_2N,HCl$).

Dissolve about 0·5 g in 40 ml of water in a separator, add 2 ml of 20 per cent sodium hydroxide solution and extract immediately with successive quantities of 25, 10 and 10 ml of chloroform. Wash each extract with the same 15 ml of water and filter into a dry flask. Titrate the combined filtrates, which should be clear and free from droplets of water, with 0·05N perchloric acid using 0·15 ml of oracet blue B solution as indicator. 1 ml 0·05N = 0·01419 g $C_{15}H_{21}O_2N,HCl$.

The hydrochloride can be titrated with 0·1N silver nitrate using phenosafranine as an adsorption indicator (1 ml 0·1N = 0·02838 g).

Injection of Pethidine Hydrochloride, *B.P.* A sterile solution of pethidine hydrochloride in water for injection.

Dilute a volume of the injection equivalent to about 0·15 g of pethidine hydrochloride with 40 ml of water in a separator and add 1 ml of 20 per cent sodium hydroxide solution. Complete as above by the *B.P.* method but titrating with 0·02N perchloric acid. 1 ml 0·02N = 0·005676 g $C_{15}H_{21}O_2N,HCl$.

The tetraphenylboron method for the determination of small quantities of bases given under Atropine (p. 116) can be applied to pethidine.

For this preparation dilute 1 ml of a 5 per cent injection or equivalent amount of other strength to 20 ml with equal volumes of buffer solution, pH 3·7, and water, taking 10 ml of this for the assay, 1 ml of cetylpyridinium chloride = 0·001419 g.

Tablets of Pethidine Hydrochloride, *B.P.* Usually contain 50 mg of pethidine hydrochloride.

The assay of the tablets follows the method given above using a quantity of powdered tablets equivalent to about 0·5 g of pethidine hydrochloride for the extraction method and the equivalent of 1 tablet in 25 ml of the diluted buffer solution for the tetraphenylboron method.

PHENACETIN

$C_2H_5O.C_6H_4NH.COCH_3$ Mol. Wt. 179·2

Phenacetin, or aceto-*p*-phenetidide, can be readily and completely extracted with ether, or preferably with chloroform from aqueous solution, in which it is not very soluble. As it is easily hydrolysed by acids to salts of *p*-phenetidine, the latter not being extracted by chloroform, phenacetin is generally determined in mixtures by first hydrolysing a solution with acid, then extracting interfering substances with chloroform, finally re-acetylating to phenacetin with acetic anhydride in alkaline solution and extracting it with chloroform.

In the presence of acetanilide, phenacetin cannot be separated by acid hydrolysis and a method for separation of phenacetin from acetanilide as well as from caffeine and phenazone (other substances likely to be found in admixture with it) was devised by Emery.[1] The method depends upon the fact that when phenacetin is added to a solution of iodine in potassium iodide containing a mineral acid, an iodine addition compound separates, whilst the corresponding product of acetanilide remains soluble. The details of the method are briefly:

Dissolve 0·2 g of the mixture in 2 ml of glacial acetic acid and 40 ml of water by warming. Pour into 25 ml of 0·2N iodine in a 100-ml graduated flask, previously warmed to 40°. Add 3 ml of concentrated hydrochloric acid, shake until a crystalline precipitate appears and then cool. Dilute nearly to 100 ml and allow to stand overnight. Adjust the volume of the liquid to 100 ml, filter and titrate 50 ml of filtrate with 0·1N thiosulphate. 1 ml 0·2N = 0·01792 g phenacetin. The phenacetin may be determined gravimetrically if desired; filter off the precipitate of periodide, $(C_2H_5O.C_6H_4NH.COCH_3)_2HI.I_4$, through a Gooch crucible, wash it with the standard iodine solution and transfer it to a separator. Add an excess of sodium sulphite to remove the iodine, and extract the phenacetin with chloroform.

For the determination of acetanilide, to an aliquot part of the filtrate from the iodide precipitation add sodium sulphite and sodium bicarbonate in slight excess; add 2 drops of acetic anhydride and extract with three 60-ml portions of chloroform. Evaporate the chloroform to low bulk, add 10 ml of dilute sulphuric acid and evaporate the rest of the chloroform. Add 20 ml of water and digest on a water-bath for one hour. Add 10 ml of concentrated hydrochloric acid and titrate with 0·1N potassium bromate-bromide, adding the volumetric solution very slowly to the well-shaken mixture until a faint yellow colour remains. Standardise the bromate-bromide solution against pure acetanilide.

If caffeine and phenazone are present, digest the mixture with dilute sulphuric acid to convert phenacetin and acetanilide to *p*-phenetidine sulphate and aniline sulphate respectively. Extract the phenazone and caffeine with chloroform and regenerate the others in the aqueous residues by adding an excess of sodium bicarbonate and a few drops of acetic anhydride and extracting with chloroform before proceeding to separate the phenacetin and acetanilide as above.

Tablets of Phenacetin, *B.P.C.* Each tablet contains 5 grains of phenacetin.

The lengthy *B.P.C.* method which is designed to eliminate impurities is, in the writers' opinion, unnecessary with modern formulation and direct extraction of the phenacetin in a Soxhlet apparatus with ether or chloroform will give a sufficiently close approximation for normal control purposes.

Tablets of Phenacetin and Caffeine, *B.P.C.* Each tablet contains 4 grains of phenacetin and 1 grain of caffeine.

Assayed by the method given under Compound Tablets of Aspirin using 0·25 g of powdered tablets (p. 12), without extracting for salicylic acid, *i.e.* hydrolyse the mixture in acid solution, extract the caffeine with chloroform, reconvert the *p*-phenetidine into phenacetin, extract and weigh.

Compound Tablets of Aspirin and Opium, *B.P.C.*, Tablets of Aspirin and Phenacetin, *B.P.C.*, Compound Tablets of Codeine, *B.P.* and Soluble Compound Tablets of Codeine, *B.P.*, see under Acetysalicylic Acid, p. 13.

1. Emery, W. O., *J. Ind. Eng. Chem.*, 1914, **6**, 665.

PHENAZONE

$C_{11}H_{12}ON_2$ Mol. Wt. 188·2

Phenazone is very soluble in water but chloroform will extract it completely from neutral or alkaline solutions.

According to Brindle,[1] Kolthoff's iodine method[2] of determination, suitably modified, is the most satisfactory. The original method was found to give results 0·3 to 1·0 per cent too high, mainly due to the absorption of iodine by the reagents. The following process offers advantages both in convenience and accuracy:

Dissolve 0·2 g of phenazone and 2 g of sodium acetate in 20 ml of water in a stoppered flask and add 30 ml of 0·1N iodine. Allow the flask and contents to stand with occasional shaking for twenty minutes, then dissolve the precipitate by adding 10 ml of chloroform and shaking; titrate the excess of iodine with 0·1N sodium thiosulphate. Repeat the process omitting the phenazone as a blank. 1 ml 0·1N = 0·009412 g.

The iodo-phenazone may be extracted with successive portions of chloroform, the solvent solution washed with water, filtered and evaporated and the residue, dried for half an hour at 110°, wt. × 0·5992 = phenazone (Emery and Palkin[3]). In the presence of caffeine this method may be extended.[4]

A method of assay applicable to other pyrazolone derivatives (*e.g.* amidopyrine) is by the precipitation of the picrate:[5]

To 10 ml of an approximately 5 per cent solution of phenazone add 90 ml of approximately 0·05N picric acid. Shake the mixture, leave overnight, filter and titrate 50 ml of the filtrate with 0·1N sodium hydroxide. Titrate 90 ml of the original picric acid solution with 0·1N sodium hydroxide, then subtract twice the former titration from this and multiply by 0·0188 for the phenazone in the amount of solution taken for assay.

Difficulty is experienced in separating phenazone from amidopyrine. According to Sinton and Rotondaro,[6] amidopyrine can be separated from phenazone (and caffeine) by first extracting the latter with chloroform from an aqueous solution containing from 3·5 to 5 per cent by weight of sulphuric acid and then extracting the amidopyrine with chloroform after making the solution ammoniacal. Patein[7] found that on treating the mixture with hydrochloric acid and formaldehyde, amidopyrine is unaffected but phenazone gives a compound precipitated by ammonia, which is collected and weighed. Wt. × 0·9345 = phenazone. Amidopyrine is then shaken out with chloroform.

Amidopyrine also acts as a monobasic substance and can be titrated with 0·1N acid to methyl orange, phenazone being neutral; the end-point is not very sharp.

1. Brindle, H., *Quart. J. Pharm.*, 1934, **7**, 453.
2. Kolthoff, I. M., *Pharm. Weekblad*, 1923, **60**, 164.
3. Emery, W. O., and Palkin, S., *J. Ind. Eng. Chem.*, 1914, **6**, 751.
4. Emery, W. O., and Palkin, S., *J. Ind. Eng. Chem.*, 1915, **7**, 519.
5. Lemaire, P., *Ann. Chim. Anal. et Chim. Appl.*, 1904, **9**, 433.
6. Sinton, F. C., and Rotondaro, F. A., *J.A.O.A.C.*, 1939, **22**, 678.
7. Patein, G., *J. Pharm. Chim.*, 1904, **21** [vi], 611.

PHENOL

C_6H_5OH Mol. Wt. 94·11

For the determination of phenol, Koppeschaar's method[1] is frequently used; it is based on the formation of a mixture of tribromphenol and tribromphenyl hypobromite by the addition of an excess of bromine; the labile bromine atom of tribromphenyl hypobromite is displaced on the addition of potassium iodide and the final product of the reaction is tribromphenol. The method is capable of considerable accuracy and is the official one for the determination of phenol. It is not necessary for the mixture to stand for as long as directed in the *B.P.*:

Transfer an aliquot part, containing from 0·03 to 0·04 g, of phenol in solution to a stoppered bottle. Add 30 ml of 0·1N bromine (2·784 g potassium bromate and 15 g potassium bromide per litre) and 5 ml of concentrated hydrochloric acid. Allow to stand with occasional shaking for fifteen minutes, add 5 to 10 ml of 20 per cent potassium iodide solution quickly to avoid loss of bromine and titrate the liberated iodine with 0·1N sodium thiosulphate. Carry out a blank determination. 1 ml 0·1N = 0·001569 g. Starch indicator need not be used.

The *U.S.P.* modifies the method by adding 1 ml of chloroform before the final titration; this dissolves tribromphenol and prevents occlusion of free iodine in the precipitate.

The method is unaffected by sucrose or invert sugar provided the bromine is added to a neutral or slightly acid solution; under these conditions they showed no absorption of bromine.

Another method for the determination of many phenolic substances, which has found wide application although it has not yet been officially adopted, is that based on the use of 4-aminophenazone first described by Emerson.[2] The method has been examined by Johnson and Savidge[3] who recommended the following general procedure:

Reagents:

4-aminophenazone solution. Dissolve 0·5 g of 4-aminophenazone in 25 ml of water, shake and filter. This solution is stable for two to three days if stored protected from light.

Strong ammonia buffer. Dissolve 67·5 g of ammonium chloride in 570 ml of strong ammonia solution and dilute to 1 litre with water.

Dilute ammonia buffer. Dilute 2 ml of strong ammonia buffer to 1 litre with water.

Method:

For phenols giving aminophenazone dyes soluble in chloroform. Transfer a suitable aliquot of a prepared solution containing 0·2 to 0·4 mg of the phenol to a 150-ml separator. Add 1 ml of 4-aminophenazone solution and wash in with sufficient dilute ammonia buffer to give a volume of about 50 ml. Add 1 ml of a freshly prepared, 8 per cent solution of potassium ferricyanide and mix. Extract with successive quantities, of 25, 10 and 10 ml, of chloroform, passing each extract into a dry, 50-ml graduated flask through a small cotton-wool plug, previously rinsed with chloroform. Dilute to volume with chloroform, mix and measure the extinction at the absorption maximum* using 1-cm cells with chloroform in the comparison cell. (For phenol use 0·5-cm cells.)

For phenols giving aminophenazone dyes insoluble in chloroform. Transfer a suitable aliquot of a prepared solution containing 0·2 to 0·4 mg of the phenol to a 50-ml graduated flask and add 1 ml of 4-aminophenazone solution. Wash in with dilute ammonia buffer to give a volume of about 45 ml, mix, add 1 ml of a freshly prepared 8 per cent solution of potassium ferricyanide and dilute to volume with the dilute buffer. Mix and measure the extinction, as rapidly as possible, at the absorption maximum,* using 1-cm cells with, in the comparison cell, a suitable aliquot of the prepared solution, diluted to 50 ml with dilute ammonia buffer.

The amount of a particular phenol equivalent to the extinction found is read from a standard curve prepared for that substance by carrying out the general procedure on suitable aliquots of a standard solution, suitably buffered, covering the range 0·1 to 0·4 mg, and plotting the extinction against the quantity of the phenol present.

* For most phenols this occurs at 450 mμ.

Usually the above method may be applied to substances with a free phenolic hydroxyl group and a free para position or a para position that is substituted by a halogen, hydroxyl or alkoxyl, sulphonic acid or carboxylic acid group since in general these substances give a positive reaction.

The bathochromic shift which occurs in the spectra of many phenolic compounds with change of pH may be used as the basis of a simple spectrophotometric assay (ΔE method) when they are present in complex formulations. A pre-requisite of the method is the absence of spectral changes of the other constituents under the same conditions. The method has been adapted by Elvidge and Peutrell[4] for the determination of hexachlorophane and other phenols (phenol, resorcinol, cresol and methyl hydroxybenzoate) in various pharmaceutical products.

The spectral changes used for measurement occur at different pH values for different phenols, hexachlorophane from pH 3 to pH 8 but phenol, resorcinol and cresol are not ionised at pH 8 and a more alkaline solution is used for these compounds. This consists of a 0·2M solution of potassium hydroxide in 90 per cent methanol; the pH of this solution is 13·4.

Methyl *p*-hydroxybenzoate does not appear to show changes in spectral characteristics in the presence of large amounts of methanol but differences are observed in aqueous solutions. In phosphate buffer at pH 7·5 methyl hydroxybenzoate shows maximum absorption at 257 mμ and in 0·1N sodium hydroxide at 296 mμ.

The appropriate buffer, differential E(1 per cent, 1 cm) values and wavelength criteria are given in Table 27 below. The buffers are prepared as follows:

A. Solution pH 8·0—Dissolve 6·07 g of tris-(hydroxymethyl)aminomethane in 900 ml of methanol. Add 50 ml of 0·5N hydrochloric acid and make up to 1 litre with water.

B. Solution pH 1·4—Add 18 ml of glacial acetic acid and 3 ml of concentrated hydrochloric acid to 900 ml of methanol and make up to 1 litre with water.

C. Potassium hydroxide 0·2N in methanol—Dissolve 11·2 g of potassium hydroxide pellets in about 50 ml of water, add 900 ml of methanol and make up to 1 litre with water.

TABLE 27

COMPOUND	SAMPLE BUFFER	BLANK BUFFER	ΔE(1 PER CENT, 1 CM)	$\lambda_{max.}$ Mμ
Hexachlorophane	A	B	144	312
Phenol	C	A	280	289
Resorcinol	C	A	305	291
Cresol *B.P.*	C	A	266	293
Methyl *p*-hydroxybenzoate	E	D	1,290	296

D. Solution pH 7·5—Dissolve 22·2 g of potassium dihydrogen phosphate and 178 g of dipotassium hydrogen phosphate in 1 litre of water.

Three general methods of extraction are used.

(*a*) Direct dilution or extraction with the appropriate buffer solution. Applicable to liquid preparations.

Weigh or pipette a suitable amount into a 100-ml stoppered conical flask, add about 50 ml of buffer solution appropriate to the phenol being examined (Table 27). Shake or warm until the sample is completely dispersed, then filter through a Whatman No. 42 filter paper. Wash the conical flask and filter paper with three portions, each of 10 ml, of buffer solution and transfer the filtrate quantitatively to a 100-ml graduated flask. Make up to volume with buffer solution.

(*b*) Extraction with chloroform. Applicable to samples in powder form.

Weigh a suitable amount into a sintered-glass funnel (No. 3 porosity). Extract the powder with five successive portions, each of about 20 ml, of chloroform, drawing each extract through the sinter with gentle suction and collecting the extract in a Buchner flask. Remove the chloroform on a water-bath, taking care to avoid volatilisation of the phenol, and dissolve the residue in a suitable volume of the appropriate buffer solution.

(*c*) Extraction with light petroleum-methanol mixtures. Suitable for ointments.

Weigh a suitable amount into a small beaker, add 20 ml of light petroleum and disperse the sample as far as possible with a glass rod. Allow to settle and decant the supernatant liquid into a 150-ml separator. Wash the beaker successively with the following solutions, transferring each in turn to the separator. (1) Three portions, each of 20 ml, of light petroleum-methanol (1 : 1). (2) Two portions, each of 10 ml, of methanol. (3) One portion of 10 ml of light petroleum-methanol (1 : 1). Finally add 15 ml of water to the separator, stopper and shake gently for one minute. Allow the layers to separate, filter the lower layer through a small plug of cotton wool into a 100-ml graduated flask, wash the light petroleum layer in the separator with 10 ml of methanol-water (1 : 1) and add these washings to the graduated flask through the cotton-wool plug. Make up to volume with methanol.

For spectrophotometric determination—Dilute a suitable aliquot of the extracted phenolic compound with the 'sample' buffer solution and a second aliquot in the appropriate 'blank' buffer solution (listed in Table 27). It is important that the concentration of the phenolic compound is the same in both 'sample' and 'blank' buffer solutions. For all the samples examined the final dilution with the appropriate buffer solution should be at least tenfold. Under these conditions the pH value of the final solution should be within 0·1 units of that of the diluent buffer.

Measure the extinction of the more alkaline solution in a 1-cm cell at the appropriate wavelength (see Table 27) using the more acid solution in the reference cell. Calculate the content of phenolic compound in the sample using the ΔE(1 per cent, 1 cm) value found for the pure phenol in the same pair of buffer solutions. The figures quoted in Table 27 are only intended as a guide.

Thus phenol may be determined in Calamine Lotion, *B.P.*, by the following method.

Weigh about 4 g of sample into a 100-ml stoppered conical flask, add 50 ml 0·2N potassium hydroxide in methanol and shake for ten minutes. Transfer the contents of the flask to a Buchner funnel containing a Whatman No. 42 filter paper and apply gentle suction. Rinse the flask and filter paper with three portions, each of 10 ml, of potassium hydroxide in methanol. Transfer the filtrate to a 100-ml graduated flask, make up to volume with potassium hydroxide in methanol and mix. Pipette 3 ml of this solution into a 50-ml graduated flask and make up to volume with 0·2N potassium hydroxide in methanol. Pipette a further 3 ml of the original extract into a second 50-ml graduated flask and make up to volume with pH 8·0 buffer solution.

Measure the extinction of the final 0·2N potassium hydroxide in methanol solution at 289 mμ in a 1-cm cell, using the pH 8·0 buffer solution of the sample in the reference cell.

Calculate the phenol content of the lotion as follows:

$$\text{per cent phenol (w/w)} = \frac{\Delta E}{\Delta S} \times \frac{50}{3} \times \frac{100}{W}$$

ΔE = the extinction of the sample at 289 mμ
ΔS = the difference in E(1 per cent, 1 cm) at 289 mμ of pure phenol in 0·2N potassium hydroxide in methanol and in pH 8·0 buffer solution
W = the weight of sample taken.

Mixtures of phenols may be assayed by the method of White and Vaughan[5] in which the phenols are separated by partition chromatography between *cyclo*hexane and sodium carbonate or sodium silicate, the resultant fractions being assayed by a spectrophotometric procedure. This technique is particularly useful for substances such as cresols and xylenols which are mainly isomeric mixtures.

The method for the determination of phenol in galenicals that is official at the present time is Koppeschaar's method. For many preparations in which no ingredient that interferes with the reaction is present, this method can be applied directly:

Liquefied Phenol, *B.P.*, containing 80 per cent w/w, **Ear-drops of Phenol,** *B.P.C.*, a 37·5 per cent v/v solution of Glycerin of Phenol in glycerin (using 0·7 g), **Gargle of Phenol,** *B.P.C.*, a 5 per cent v/v solution of Glycerin of Phenol (5 ml), **Glycerin of Phenol,** *B.P.*, containing 16 per cent w/w of phenol (0·3 g), **Alkaline Mouth-wash of Phenol,** *B.P.C.*, containing 3·13 per cent v/v of liquefied phenol (2 ml), **Paste of Magnesium Sulphate,** *B.P.C.*, containing 0·5 per cent of phenol (5 g).

Preparations of phenol that contain ingredients which will interfere with the Koppeschaar determination require special treatment, generally involving distillation.

Gargle of Potassium Chlorate and Phenol, *B.P.C.* Contains 1·56 per cent v/v of phenol with potassium chlorate and dye.

To 2 ml add 20 ml of water and steam-distil into 5 ml of 20 per cent sodium hydroxide solution in a glass-stoppered flask, at such a rate that

100 ml of distillate is collected in thirty minutes, maintaining the volume in the distillation flask at 20 to 30 ml. Wash down the condenser with 20 ml of water and complete by Koppeschaar's method given above.

Providing the acidification is kept to a minimum and the hydrochloric acid is diluted before addition, the chlorate does not interfere and a direct determination without distillation is possible.

The 4-aminophenazone method has been successfully applied to this preparation by direct application on a 2-ml portion.

Oily Injection of Phenol, *B.P.C.* Contains 5 per cent w/v phenol in almond oil.

The phenol in this preparation can be assayed after extraction with alkali.

Dissolve 10 g in 50 ml of ether and extract with successive quantities, each of 10 ml, of 20 per cent sodium hydroxide solution until extraction is complete. Combine the extracts, dilute to 250 ml with water and complete by the Koppeschaar method given above.

Determination of phenolic bacteriostats in injection solutions.

A number of possible methods is available:

(1) Steam distillation, followed by application of Koppeschaar's method. This method is lengthy and requires an amount of sample which is frequently not available when individual samples are being examined. A satisfactory distillation procedure is as follows:

The apparatus consists of a 250-ml distillation flask connected to a condenser through a still-head, ground-glass joints being used throughout. Sealed into the bulb of the still-head is the stem of a separator, so that liquid can be introduced into the distillation flask without disconnecting the apparatus.

Pipette 10 ml of the sample into the distillation flask, add 20 ml of water and sufficient dilute hydrochloric acid to ensure acidity and distil into an iodine flask until about 20 ml of distillate has been collected. By means of the separator introduce a further 20 ml of water into the distillation flask and again distil about 20 ml of distillate.

Determine the phenol in the bulked distillates by Koppeschaar's bromine method given above.

(2) 4-Aminophenazone method. This method is applicable to the determination of most phenolic substances used as bacteriostats. It is unaffected by the presence of most active ingredients likely to be found in injection solutions and hence may be applied directly. The general procedure (which takes no more than fifteen to twenty minutes to complete) is given above.

(3) Spectrophotometric methods also offer a very convenient method for determining phenolic substances, especially if the differences in their spectral character at different pH values are used. The complexity of many modern pharmaceuticals often precludes the direct spectrophoto-

metric determination of phenols and various techniques have been described to overcome the effect of extraneous absorbing substances. These may involve separation of the phenol by chromatography, two-point methods of calculation or differential spectrophotometry.

(*a*) Direct spectrophotometric methods.

Brealey and Proctor[6] showed that chlorocresol could be determined in Injection of Pethidine Hydrochloride, *B.P.*, by measurement of the extinction of a diluted sample at 279 mμ, the wavelength of maximum absorption of chlorocresol. Pethidine has zero absorption at this wavelength and does not interfere.

(*b*) Two-point correction methods.

Where the active ingredient of an injection exhibits absorption at the wavelength of maximum absorption of the bacteriostat a two-point method is sometimes applicable. Thus phenol may be determined in Injection of Lobeline, *B.P.C.*, by the following procedure.

Dilute a suitable aliquot of the injection solution in water to contain about 0·002 per cent of phenol. Measure the extinctions of this solution at 249 mμ and 269 mμ in a 1-cm cell. Calculate the phenol content of the injection as follows:

$$\text{per cent phenol (w/v)} = \frac{100(a \times E_3 - b \times E_1)}{E_2 \times E_3 - E_1 \times E_4}$$

a = observed E(1 per cent, 1 cm) of the sample at 249 mμ
b = observed E(1 per cent, 1 cm) of the sample at 269 mμ
E_1 = E(1 per cent, 1 cm) of lobeline hydrochloride at 249 mμ
E_2 = E(1 per cent, 1 cm) of phenol at 249 mμ
E_3 = E(1 per cent, 1 cm) of lobeline hydrochloride at 269 mμ
E_4 = E(1 per cent, 1 cm) of phenol at 269 mμ

Glenn[7] has extended the theoretical considerations of two-point methods with reference to injection solutions containing bacteriostats and has evolved criteria which enable the analyst to select optimum pairs of wavelengths and concentrations for satisfactory precision. Although few specific examples are quoted the mathematical treatment is useful in deciding whether or not a particular mixture can be assayed by a two-point method.

(*c*) By preliminary separation on an ion-exchange column.

The use of oxycellulose as an ion-exchange medium for separating phenolic bacteriostats from the active ingredients of certain official injections was described by Elvidge, Proctor and Baines.[8] The method is of value when it is necessary to separate the bacteriostat in order to determine the active ingredient of a mixture, otherwise the 4-aminophenazone method above is preferable.

Procedure for Preparing Columns

Slurry one gram of oxidised cellulose with 50 ml of N sulphuric acid and transfer to a column, shown in Fig. 11, plugged with glass wool. After the cellulose has settled place a small plug of glass wool on top to avoid disturbance of its upper surface. Then wash the column with water (about 200 ml) until the eluate is free from acid, slight air pressure being applied to give a flow rate of about 3 ml per minute. Check the final few millilitres of eluate on a spectrophotometer to ensure that they are free from impurities absorbing between 220 and 280 mμ.

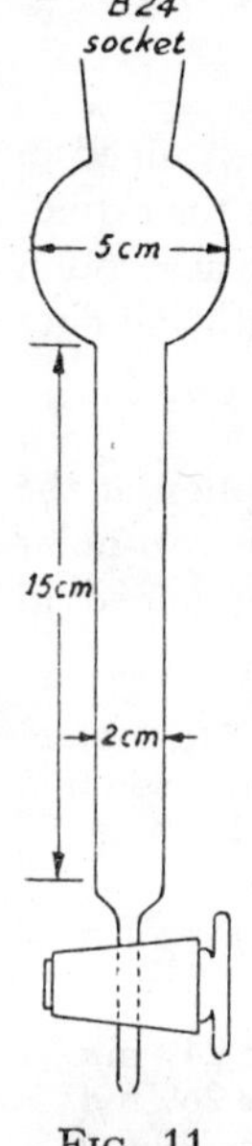

FIG. 11
Apparatus for the cellulose column

Procedure for Determining the Bacteriostatic Agent

Transfer a volume of injection solution to the column so that the amount of active ingredient when eluted with a minimum volume of 25 ml of N sulphuric acid can be determined spectrophotometrically. Wash the column with at least 50 ml of water (two 25-ml portions) under pressure and dilute the eluate containing the bacteriostatic agent to a suitable volume so as to permit its determination by measuring the maximum extinction at about 269 mμ for phenol or 279 mμ for chlorocresol. When 0·5 per cent of phenol is used as the bacteriostatic agent, it is necessary to dilute the initial aliquot 100 to 200 times to obtain a suitable concentration in the eluate; when 0·3 per cent of chlorocresol is used the dilution is 50 to 100 times.

In calculating the amount of bacteriostatic agent, the E(1 per cent, 1 cm) value at 269 mμ of phenol is taken as 164 and the E(1 per cent, 1 cm) value at 279 mμ of chlorocresol as 105.

After elution of the bacteriostatic agent as described above, the active ingredient can be eluted under pressure with N sulphuric acid, a minimum volume of 25 ml being used. The eluate is adjusted to a suitable volume and the active ingredient is determined spectrophotometrically.

A modification of this method using alginic acid is proposed by Murfin and Foster[9] (see p. 461).

TRINITROPHENOL (Picric Acid), $C_6H_2(OH)(NO_2)_3$, Mol. Wt. 229·1

Picric acid can be titrated with alkali using phenolphthalein as indicator. 1 ml 0·5N = 0·1146 g. The end-point is quite sharp.

Picric acid may also be extracted directly from aqueous solution by chloroform in the presence of mineral acids. The solution in chloroform is colourless and four extractions should be sufficient unless an unduly large quantity of picric acid is present; the aqueous portion will retain some yellow colour but the amount of picric acid left is negligible. The chloroform is evaporated and the picric acid dried and weighed.

Picric acid forms insoluble molecular compounds with many substances. This property may be utilised if necessary for its estimation, the compound with phenazone being particularly useful.

SALOL, $C_6H_4OH.COOC_6H_5$, Mol. Wt. 214·2

Salol (phenyl salicylate) is phenolic, hence it can be removed from solution in chloroform or ether by extracting with cold sodium hydroxide solutions, but not with sodium bicarbonate; fatty acids may be separated from salol solutions with the latter.

A method of determination by bromination is due to Emery *et al.*:[10]

To the residue obtained after eliminating interfering substances by extraction as above, or to a weighed portion of a mixture, containing not more than 0·05 g salol, add 10 ml of 2·5 per cent sodium hydroxide solution and heat on a water-bath for five minutes to hydrolyse the salol to sodium salicylate and sodium phenate. Cool the solution and transfer it to a stoppered bottle; dilute with water to about 200 ml. Add a considerable excess (50 ml) of 0·1N potassium bromate-bromide solution and 10 ml of concentrated hydrochloric acid. Shake the mixture frequently during half an hour, then add 15 ml of 10 per cent potassium iodide solution and shake the mixture frequently during a further fifteen minutes. Titrate the excess of iodine with 0·1N sodium thiosulphate. Tribromphenol and tribromsalicylic acid are first formed, the latter then loses its carboxyl group and the final product is tribromphenol; hence 12 atoms of bromine are equivalent to 1 molecule of phenol and 1 ml 0·1N = 0·001785 g.

Various excipients, such as tragacanth, acacia, starch and dextrin, cause no interference but lactose does, and if this is present the salol must first be extracted by ether.

Salol may be determined by the 4-aminophenazone method (chloroform extraction procedure), the maximum extinction occurring at about 470 mμ.

A mixture of salol and phenacetin may be separated by extracting the latter from the alkaline hydrolysis products with chloroform.

β-NAPHTHOL, $C_{10}H_7OH$, Mol. Wt. 144·2

Chemically β-naphthol behaves as a phenol; hence it is soluble in alkalies and is precipitated by acids or carbon dioxide. Other properties of β-naphthol, which should be of value for devising means of estimation under varying conditions, are that it is steam volatile and can be extracted easily from acid solutions by ether and chloroform. When ether is used the solution must be dried with anhydrous sodium sulphate and the ether only just completely evaporated before drying the residue over concentrated sulphuric acid, as the moist substance volatilises on heating.

For the determination of small quantities of β-naphthol Patterson and Lerrigo[11] have used the red colour obtained on making a solution containing β-naphthol, naphthionic acid and sodium nitrite alkaline. A convenient range, where the depth of colour is proportional to the amount of β-naphthol present, is obtained between 1 and 5 p.p.m. of the substance:

Pipette 4 ml of an ethanolic solution containing β-naphthol into a 50-ml graduated flask and add 2 ml of a freshly prepared 0·1 per cent solution of 1-naphthylamine-4-sulphonic acid sodium salt (sodium naphthionate) in water, 1 ml of a freshly prepared 0·1 per cent solution of sodium nitrite and 1 ml of N hydrochloric acid. Mix well and then add 1·5 ml of 10 per cent w/w ammonia solution, making the volume up to 50 ml with ethanol. A blank determination should be carried out on the reagents made up to 50 ml in the same way. The resultant red colour develops in the solution immediately after the ammonia has been added and is stable for several hours.

The intensity was measured on a Hilger 'Spekker' absorptiometer, using a Chance glass filter OB2 (blue-green), but it can equally well be compared visually with standards prepared at the same time. The paper deals with the determination of β-naphthol in gelatin capsules, in which it is used to prevent mould growth, where some remains in the gelatin and some is extracted in the oil.

HEXACHLOROPHANE, $C_{13}H_6O_2Cl_6$, Mol. Wt. 406·9

The pure substance may be assayed by dissolving 1 g in 25 ml of 95 per cent ethanol, previously adjusted to pH 9·0, and titrating potentiometrically to pH 9·0, with 0·1N sodium hydroxide. 1 ml 0·1N = 0·04069 g.

For determination of small quantities of hexachlorophane the 4-aminophenazone method (above) is satisfactory but, since the aminophenazone dye produced is insoluble in chloroform, the general method (aqueous procedure) must be used. The differential spectrophotometric method is also applicable.

Hexachlorophane and dichlorophen in soaps, pharmaceutical and cosmetic preparations, etc., can be determined microbiologically by the plate-diffusion method given on pp. 814 to 826. The standard, or control, preparation should be of a similar basic formulation to that of the test material but with sufficient of the hexachlorophane or dichlorophen added to give the theoretical amount in the final formulation.

If the preparation is soluble in water dissolve 1 to 2 g, accurately weighed, in 100 ml of water. If the preparation is not soluble in water, suspend a weighed amount in acetone and then add about four volumes of water. From these solutions prepare final dilutions for use in the assay of 1 in 100,000 and 1 in 400,000 of hexachlorophane, or of 1 in 10,000 and 1 in 40,000 of dichlorophen with phosphated buffer at pH 8. The assay medium is a peptone Lemco agar at pH 8, and the test organism a suspension of spores of *Bacillus pumilus* (*B. subtilis*) as used in the assay of streptomycin.

DICHLOROPHEN, $C_{13}H_{10}O_2Cl_2$, Mol. Wt. 269·1

Small quantities of dichlorophen may be determined by the 4-aminophenzone method or microbiologically as described above under hexachlorophane.

1. KOPPESCHAAR, W. F., *Z. Anal. Chem.*, 1876, **15**, 232.
2. EMERSON, E., *J. Org. Chem.*, 1943, **8**, 417.
3. JOHNSON, C. A., and SAVIDGE, R. A., *J. Pharm. Pharmacol.*, 1958, **10**, 171T.
4. ELVIDGE, D. A., and PEUTRELL, B., *J. Pharm. Pharmacol.*, 1961, **13**, 111T.
5. WHITE, D., and VAUGHAN, G. A., *Anal. Chim. Acta.*, 1957, **16**, 439.
6. BREALEY, L., and PROCTOR, K. A., *J. Pharm. Pharmacol.*, 1955, **7**, 830.
7. GLENN, A. L., *J. Pharm. Pharmacol.*, 1960, **12**, 595.
8. ELVIDGE, D. A., PROCTOR, K. A., and BAINES, C. B., *Analyst*, 1957, **82**, 367.
9. MURFIN, J. W., and FOSTER, J. S., *Analyst*, 1961, **86**, 32.
10. EMERY, W. O., *et al.*, *J. Ind. Eng. Chem.*, 1915, **7**, 681.
11. PATTERSON, Stella J., and LERRIGO, A. F., *Quart. J. Pharm.*, 1947, **20**, 83.

PHENOLPHTHALEIN

$C_{20}H_{14}O_4$ Mol. Wt. 318·3

Phenolphthalein is soluble in alkali hydroxide solution and is extracted in acid solution by immiscible solvents, preferably ether. It is only sparingly soluble in light petroleum or carbon tetrachloride, and fats may be removed with a minimum of these solvents.

Many impurities can be removed by extraction with ether from alkaline solution before acidifying and extracting the phenolphthalein; moreover phenolphthalein is extracted by ether in the presence of sodium bicarbonate and can thus be separated from benzoic acid.

A precipitation method suitable for chocolate preparations and depending on the formation of the tetra-iodide is official in the *A.O.A.C.*[1] Briefly the method is the following:

> To prepare the ethanolic extract, finely grate the chilled sample, mix well and weigh an amount containing about 0·1 g of phenolphthalein into a Gooch crucible. Remove the fat by extracting with successive quantities of 5, 4 and 3 ml of carbon tetrachloride and then extract the phenolphthalein from the sample with successive quantities of hot 95 per cent ethanol, collecting the filtrate in a tall, 300-ml beaker. Wash the under side of the crucible free from phenolphthalein with hot ethanol; 50 ml of ethanol should be sufficient for extraction and washing. Evaporate the combined extracts and washings to dryness on a water-bath.
>
> Dissolve the residue at room temperature in 1 to 1·5 ml of 5N potassium hydroxide (see *Note* below) and add a piece of ice (about 40 g). Then add 7 to 8 ml of iodine solution (prepared by dissolving 12·7 g of potassium iodide in 10 ml of water, adding and dissolving 6·35 g of iodine and finally adding 12 ml of 5N potassium hydroxide before diluting to 100 ml with water). Add concentrated hydrochloric acid from a burette, stirring the solution, to complete precipitation. If sufficient iodine has been added, the precipitate as well as the supernatant liquid

will be brown; if not, add more iodine to ensure excess, and then add the potassium hydroxide solution dropwise, with stirring, to dissolve the precipitate completely and consume all excess iodine. Repeat the precipitation and re-solution process three or four times, adding small pieces of ice, if necessary, to keep the solution cold. Then, to the clear blue or bluish-purple alkaline solution, add 1 to 1·5 ml of 12·6 per cent sodium sulphite solution and filter the cold mixture through a Gooch crucible into a tall 250-ml beaker, washing several times with water. Acidify the filtrate with hydrochloric acid, using a slight excess, and heat on a water-bath for twenty to thirty minutes, stirring occasionally. Decant the hot supernatant liquid through a weighed Gooch crucible and wash the precipitate in the beaker several times by decantation with hot water. Transfer the precipitate completely to the crucible and wash with hot water until the washings are clear and free from chloride. When the apparatus has cooled and the precipitate has been sucked fairly dry, wash the precipitate several times with light petroleum, using suction towards the end. Dry the precipitate to constant weight at 110° to 130°. Weight of precipitate × 0·3872 = weight of phenolphthalein.

Note: Alkaline phenolphthalein solution is unstable in air and the phenolphthalein should be converted to the tetraiodide within one hour.

The *A.O.A.C.* applies this method to the determination of phenolphthalein in emulsions after preliminary treatment.

Weigh an amount of well-mixed sample containing about 0·1 g of phenolphthalein into a centrifuge bottle, add 100 ml of a mixture of 1 volume of 95 per cent ethanol and 3 volumes of ether, shake vigorously and then centrifuge until clear. Decant the clear supernatant liquid into a separator and wash the residue in the bottle with two quantities, each of 10 ml, of the solvent mixture, adding the washings to the separator. Dissolve the residue in the bottle in a few millilitres of water and re-precipitate the gums with 50 ml of the solvent mixture. Again shake and centrifuge, as before, decanting into the separator. Wash the residue and the bottle with three quantities, each of 10 ml, of the solvent mixture and add these washings to the separator. Dissolve the residue in a few millilitres of water and test for complete extraction with sodium hydroxide. Shake the contents of the separator with successive 10-ml quantities of 0·1N sodium hydroxide until the phenolphthalein is completely extracted, as indicated by absence of colour. Combine the alkaline extracts in a second separator and acidify with dilute sulphuric acid. Extract the phenolphthalein with successive quantities, each of 10 ml, of ether, again testing for complete extraction with sodium hydroxide. Combine the ether extracts in a 150-ml beaker, evaporate to dryness and determine the phenolphthalein as described above for chocolate preparations, omitting filtration of the alkaline solution.

A method for the determination of phenolphthalein in chocolate preparations by non-aqueous titration has been described by Doernberg, Hubacher and Lysyj.[2]

Most published methods for the colorimetric determination of phenolphthalein depend upon formation of the red colour in alkaline solution. Earlier procedures, such as that of Frederick and Koff,[3] made use of a strong alkali but in our hands this has given variable results. Phenolphthalein exists in coloured and leuco forms and the equilibrium depends very considerably on the pH. This led Allen, Gartside and Johnson[4] to propose the use of a buffered system for colour formation; using glycine-sodium hydroxide buffers they showed that the highest and most reproducible extinction values were obtained within the pH range 10·9 to 11·7. For practical purposes a buffer solution pH 11·1 was chosen, and at the wavelength of maximum absorption at about 555 mμ the E(1 per cent, 1 cm) = 1,055. To obtain this maximum intensity of colour some pre-treatment of the phenolphthalein is necessary; either the phenolphthalein must be dissolved in buffer solution and the solution then heated on a water-bath or, more conveniently, a portion of a solution of phenolphthalein in a suitable organic solvent, such as ethanol or acetone, should be evaporated to dryness and the residue then taken up in buffer solution. The methods given below depend on evaporation of an ethanolic solution to give full colour development. The same authors have shown that no ethanol must be allowed to remain in the final solution since even small proportions markedly reduce the colour intensity. The colour is stable for fifteen minutes from the time of first addition of buffer solution to the phenolphthalein residue but if a solution has faded on standing the full intensity can be restored by heating in a water-bath for five to ten minutes.

Recommended methods for phenolphthalein itself and a number of preparations are as follows:

Buffer solution, pH 11·1. Mix a solution containing 7·51 g of aminoacetic acid and 5·85 g of sodium chloride per litre with an equal volume of 0·1N sodium hydroxide. The pH of this solution should be checked electrometrically and, if necessary, adjusted to 11·1.

In the determination given below industrial methylated spirit may be used instead of 95 per cent ethanol.

Transfer a solution in 95 per cent ethanol containing about 0·5 mg of phenolphthalein to a small beaker and evaporate the ethanol on a water-bath. Dissolve the residue in buffer solution pH 11·1, and transfer to a 100-ml graduated flask, rinsing the beaker with successive quantities of the buffer solution and adding the washings to the flask until a volume of 100 ml is obtained. Measure the extinction of this solution at the absorption maximum at about 555 mμ using 1-cm cells. This measurement must be completed within ten minutes of the first addition of buffer solution to the residue of phenolphthalein. For the purposes of calculation, assume the E(1 per cent, 1 cm) of phenolphthalein under these conditions to be 1,055.

For **Emulsion of Liquid Paraffin and Phenolphthalein,** *B.P.C.* (containing 0·343 per cent w/v), the following method of extraction has been found to be satisfactory:

Weigh 3 g into a 100-ml evaporating dish and mix to a stiff paste with about 1 g of Filtercel.* Add 95 per cent ethanol in small quantities,

* Johns-Manville Co. Ltd.

continuing the stirring to maintain a uniform smooth paste, until the volume of the mixture is about 25 ml. Transfer with the aid of 95 per cent ethanol to a 40-ml centrifuge tube and centrifuge at 2,500 r.p.m. for ten minutes. Decant the clear supernatant liquid into a 100-ml graduated flask and wash the dish, centrifuge tube and residue by repeating this procedure with 10-ml portions of 95 per cent ethanol until complete extraction is effected. Add the washings to the 100-ml flask and dilute to volume with ethanol. Apply the general method for colour development to 5 ml of this solution.

For routine purposes the more rapid method given below has proved useful, although it occasionally yields a cloudy solution.

Disperse about 3 g of the sample in 40 ml of 95 per cent ethanol and centrifuge at 2,500 r.p.m. for ten minutes. Decant the supernatant liquid into a 100-ml graduated flask, wash the residue with 40 ml of 95 per cent ethanol by dispersing and centrifuging as before and dilute the combined ethanol solution and washing to volume with 95 per cent ethanol. Apply the general method for colour development to 5 ml of this solution.

Tablets and pills, such as **Compound Pills of Phenolphthalein,** *B.P.C.* (containing $\frac{1}{2}$ grain); **Compound Tablets of Phenolphthalein,** *B.P.C.* (containing $\frac{1}{2}$ grain); and **Tablets of Phenolphthalein,** *B.P.* (usually containing 2 grains), are rapidly prepared for colour development as follows:

Dissolve as completely as possible a quantity of powdered pills or tablets expected to contain about 10 mg of phenolphthalein in 100 ml of 95 per cent ethanol. Allow any insoluble matter to settle and apply the general method for colour development to 5 ml of the clear supernatant liquid.

The method is also directly applicable to chocolate preparations as given below. Grinding of the sample is conveniently done by adding solid Drikold to the mortar.

Reduce the sample to coarse granules and chill by immersing in a freezing mixture until brittle. Grind the sample to a fine powder with a chilled pestle and mortar, weigh an amount of the powder, expected to contain about 20 mg of phenolphthalein into a prepared Gooch crucible and extract the fat with three 5-ml quantities of carbon tetrachloride, using slight suction, if necessary, towards the end of the extraction. Extract the phenolphthalein with about 100 ml of hot 95 per cent ethanol, applied in successive portions, until complete extraction is effected; transfer the mixed extracts to a 200-ml graduated flask, cool and dilute to volume with 95 per cent ethanol. Apply the general method for colour development to 5 ml of this solution.

A volumetric determination of phenolphthalein in mineral oil emulsion has been developed by Warren, Logun and Thatcher[5] based on the iodination of phenolphthalein in an alkaline medium. The emulsion is broken by the addition of acidified solution of sodium chloride, the coagulum made alkaline and the phenolphthalein iodinated, excess of iodine being titrated:

Pour approximately 10 ml of the emulsion into a 125-ml separator from a tared weighing bottle, the weight of sample being obtained by difference. Add 30 ml of 25 per cent sodium chloride solution containing 0·25 per cent hydrochloric acid and shake continuously for five minutes. Allow to separate and draw off the aqueous layer on to a 12·5-cm filter paper which has been moistened with distilled water and which contains 1 g of Hyflo Super Cel. Repeat the extraction with 30 ml of the sodium chloride solution and then with four 20-ml portions, filtering in each case and discarding the clear filtrate. Finally wash the filter paper with two 20-ml portions of the sodium chloride solution, and then place the paper in a 500-ml glass-stoppered Erlenmeyer flask. Add 30 ml of 5 per cent sodium hydroxide to the material in the separator and shake for one minute, then transfer the contents to the flask containing the filter paper, rinsing the separator with about 50 ml water; the total volume of liquid should not exceed 125 ml. Add 50 ml of 0·1N iodine, stopper the flask and shake occasionally until the pink colour has been discharged and the mixture is a white colour with a greenish-yellow tint. Add 15 ml of concentrated hydrochloric acid and immediately titrate the excess iodine with 0·1N sodium thiosulphate using starch as indicator. Prepare a blank by mixing 30 ml of 5 per cent sodium hydroxide solution, 15 ml of concentrated hydrochloric acid, 75 ml of water, one 12·5-cm filter paper, 1 g of Hyflo Super Cel, and 25 ml of 0·1N iodine solution in a 500-ml flask. 1 ml 0·1N sodium thiosulphate = 0·003979 g phenolphthalein.

Tablets of Phenolphthalein, *B.P.* The tablets usually contain 2 grains of phenolphthalein and are made with a chocolate base.

For assay, advantage is taken of the insolubility of phenolphthalein in light petroleum, which removes cocoa fat, before extraction with ether.

Triturate a weight of powdered tablets equivalent to about 0·25 g of phenolphthalein with ten times its weight of anhydrous sodium sulphate and extract with six quantities, each of 20 ml, of light petroleum (b.p. 40° to 60°). Reject the petroleum extracts and extract the residue with six quantities, each of 20 ml, of ether. Combine the ether extracts, evaporate the ether and dry the residue of phenolphthalein to constant weight at 105°.

The method of Allen, Johnson and Gartside (above) is also very satisfactory for this preparation.

1. *A.O.A.C.*, 1960, p. 533.
2. Doernberg, S., Hubacher, M., and Lysyj, I., *J. Amer. Pharm. Ass., Sci. Edn.*, 1954, **43,** 418.
3. Frederick, M., and Koff, A., *J. Amer. Pharm. Ass., Sci. Edn.*, 1946, **35,** 158.
4. Allen, J., Gartside, B., and Johnson, C. A., *J. Pharm. Pharmacol.*, 1962, **14,** 73T.
5. Warren, A. T., Logun, J. E., and Thatcher, K. L., *J. Amer. Pharm. Ass., Sci. Edn.*, 1950, **39,** 10.

PHOSPHORIC ACID

H_3PO_4 Mol. Wt. 98·00

Phosphoric acid may be titrated with alkali, in the presence of methyl orange, to the acid phosphate stage (end-point pH 4·4) and then to the dibasic salt (end-point pH 9·2) with phenolphthalein, but the end-point of the latter is obscured by partial hydrolysis of the Na_2HPO_4; this hydrolysis can be prevented by the addition of a large excess of sodium chloride, the titration being effected in a cold concentrated solution of the latter. The procedure is to mix about 2 g of sample with 10 g of sodium chloride and 30 ml of water and titrate in the cold with N sodium hydroxide. Only a few drops of indicator should be added and the titration continued to a decided pink colour. 1 ml N = 0·04900 g. Mixed indicators with narrowed pH range must be used with caution as the accuracy will depend on more precise conditions of temperature and foreign salt content; they are more advantageous with solutions of pure substances.

PHOSPHATES

The methods which have been evolved for the accurate determination of phosphate have been the subject of a great deal of research, but a discussion of their respective merits is scarcely within the scope of this book. A summary of the principal ones is, however, stated somewhat briefly. If strict attention is given to detail, accurate results should be obtained.

(*a*) Direct precipitation of phosphate as magnesium ammonium phosphate may be used in the absence of organic matter or of metals whose phosphates are insoluble in ammonia.

To a neutral or slightly acid solution (50 to 100 ml) of the phosphate, containing not more than 0·1 g of P_2O_5, add 3 ml of concentrated nitric acid, a few drops of methyl red indicator and 25 ml of magnesia mixture. Then add strong ammonia solution, slowly with vigorous stirring but without scratching the sides of the container, until the indicator turns yellow. Continue to stir for five minutes, adding ammonia solution, dropwise, to keep the solution yellow and finally add 5 ml of the ammonia solution in excess. Allow to stand in a cool place for at least four hours before filtering. Wash with cold 1·5M ammonia solution until the washings are free from chloride, dry at 100° to 150° for one hour and then heat at 1,000° to 1,100° to constant weight. $Mg_2P_2O_7 \times 0{\cdot}6379 = P_2O_5$.

Magnesia mixture is prepared as follows: Dissolve 25 g of magnesium chloride hexahydrate and 50 g of ammonium chloride in 250 ml of water, add a slight excess of ammonia solution and allow to stand overnight. Filter if any precipitate is present, just acidify with dilute hydrochloric acid and then add 2 ml of concentrated hydrochloric acid and dilute to 500 ml with water.

If other salts are present in solution the precipitate will be contaminated by co-precipitation of their phosphates and, in this case, the precipitate should be dissolved in dilute hydrochloric acid and reprecipitated before conversion to pyrophosphate.

(*b*) In the presence of interfering metals such as calcium and iron, precipitation of the phosphate is first made with ammonium molybdate.

To a neutral solution (about 100 ml) of the phosphate containing not more than 0·1 g of P_2O_5 in a 250-ml conical flask, add 12 g of ammonium nitrate and shake to dissolve. Then add 75 ml of molybdate reagent previously warmed to 40° to 45°, slowly, from a tap funnel, with continuous shaking. (There is some discrepancy over the temperature at which precipitation should be carried out—some authorities heat to 65° to 70° whereas others maintain that in order to avoid contamination of the precipitate with molybdic anhydride the temperature must not rise above 45°.) Stopper the flask, shake vigorously for ten minutes, allow to stand for thirty minutes at that temperature and filter.

The molybdate reagent is prepared as follows: Dissolve 118 g of reagent-grade molybdic acid (about 85 per cent MoO_3) in a mixture of 400 ml of water and 80 ml of strong ammonia solution; filter if necessary. Add the solution so obtained, slowly and with constant stirring, to a mixture of 400 ml of concentrated nitric acid and 600 ml of water; the molybdate solution should be added through a tube, the end of which dips below the surface of the dilute nitric acid. Allow to stand in a warm place for several days or until a portion heated to 40° to 45° deposits no yellow precipitate. Decant the solution from any sediment and store in glass-stoppered bottles.

The precipitate may then be titrated with alkali. Wash the flask and filter with 1 per cent ammonium nitrate solution until the washings are free from acid, return the precipitate and filter paper to the original flask and dissolve the precipitate in the smallest possible excess of 0·5N sodium hydroxide. According to Richards and Godden:[1]

Dilute to 250 ml and boil for twenty minutes to eliminate ammonia; while the solution is still warm titrate back with 0·5N acid to phenolphthalein, adding 1 or 2 ml of acid in excess. Repeat the boiling for fifteen minutes and after cooling titrate again with 0·5N alkali, taking the end-point as the first definite pink obtained. The total alkali less the acid used gives the volume of alkali equivalent to the phosphate, and under the conditions of the titration above, whereby the ammonia in the phosphomolybdate precipitate is eliminated, one atom of phosphorus is equivalent to 26 mols. of sodium hydroxide, hence 1 ml 0·5N = 0·001365 g P_2O_5.

If the solution of phosphomolybdate in standard alkali is titrated back directly with 0·5N acid without boiling the solution, as in the original Pemberton method, the ammonia in the phosphomolybdate is not eliminated and one atom of phosphorus is equivalent to 23 mols. of sodium hydroxide, hence in these circumstances 1 ml 0·5N = 0·001544 g P_2O_5.

The determination of phosphorus in phosphate syrups has been the subject of investigation by Ferrey.[2] When followed in detail the process evolved has provided trustworthy results over the years although there is no reason to suppose that the more recent citro-molybdate method (below) would not be satisfactory. Ferrey's general method is:

> Dissolve an amount of material, corresponding to 15 to 20 mg of P_2O_5, in 70 ml of water, add 5 ml of concentrated nitric acid and 10 g of ammonium nitrate and raise the temperature to 65°. Add gradually to the stirred solution 35 ml of nitric acid solution of ammonium molybdate. (Nitric acid solution of ammonium molybdate is prepared by mixing 125 g of molybdic acid with 100 ml of water and adding 300 ml of 8 per cent ammonia while the flask is shaken; then 400 g of ammonium nitrate is introduced and the whole made up to 1 litre; to this is added an equal volume of nitric acid of sp. gr. 1·19 and the mixture kept for seven days in a warm place before use.) Stir the mixture for a further thirty seconds, allow to stand at 65° to 70° for fifteen minutes and then cool for a further fifteen minutes. Filter the supernatant liquid through asbestos in a Gooch crucible. Wash the precipitate, as far as possible by decantation, with two 20-ml portions of 5 per cent nitric acid, then with five 20-ml portions of 5 per cent ammonium nitrate solution, and finally with small quantities of water. Wash the precipitate into the original beaker, add 50 ml of 0·2N sodium hydroxide and, after solution of the precipitate, titrate the excess of alkali with 0·2N acid, using thymol blue or phenol violet as indicator, titrating to the yellowish-green tint (phenolphthalein at colourless point is stated to give low results). 1 ml 0·2N = 0·0002693 g P; $P \times 2{\cdot}291 = P_2O_5$.

The method may be applied directly to the *B.P.C.* Compound Syrup of Ferrous Phosphate, none of the ingredients of which interferes; take about 0·4 g of the syrup (calculated 2·35 to 2·40 per cent w/v phosphorus).

The alkaloids must be removed from Easton's Syrup:

> Dilute about 0·5 g of syrup with 20 ml of water, and add 1 g of sodium citrate before making distinctly alkaline with ammonia. Extract the alkaloids with chloroform as usual. Slightly acidify the residual aqueous liquid with nitric acid and warm on the water-bath to remove chloroform, adjust the temperature to 65° and proceed with the assay as above.

Wilson[3] critically surveyed the present methods of determining P_2O_5 and has shown that by precipitating as quinoline phosphomolybdate and completing volumetrically, accurate results can be obtained. Calcium, iron, magnesium, alkali metals, citrates and nitrates do not interfere but ammonium salts must be destroyed and a high concentration of sulphuric acid must be avoided.

Later, however, it was pointed out that soluble silica interferes to an unknown extent and this method has been superseded by a further method of Wilson[4] in which citric acid is added; this forms a complex with molybdic acid of such stability that its reaction with silicic acid is prevented, whereas the reaction with phosphoric acid proceeds normally. Further, in this method it is no longer necessary to destroy ammonium salts before precipitating quinolinium phosphomolybdate.

Reagents:

Citric-molybdic acid reagent. Add 54 g of reagent-grade molybdic anhydride (MoO_3) to 200 ml of water. Stir and add 11 g of sodium hydroxide pellets, heating to produce a clear solution. Dissolve 60 g of citric acid in a further 250 ml of water and 140 ml of concentrated hydrochloric acid. Pour the first solution into the second solution, stirring continuously, cool, filter if necessary and dilute to 1 litre with water. Add, dropwise, 1 per cent potassium bromate solution until the green colour is just discharged. Store in the dark.

Quinoline solution. To 60 ml of concentrated hydrochloric acid and 300 ml of water in a beaker, warmed to 70° to 80°, add 50 ml of synthetic quinoline, stirring continuously. When the quinoline has dissolved, cool and dilute to 1 litre with water. Filter through paper pulp to yield a clear filtrate.

Mixed phenolphthalein/thymol blue indicator. Mix 3 volumes of a 0·1 per cent solution of thymol blue (dissolve 0·1 g in 2·2 ml of 0·1N sodium hydroxide and 50 ml of 95 per cent ethanol and dilute to 100 ml with water) with 2 volumes of a 0·1 per cent solution of phenolphthalein in 60 per cent ethanol.

Method:

Weigh 10 g of the sample into a 500-ml graduated flask, add 400 ml of water at 20° and shake mechanically for exactly thirty minutes. Dilute to volume, mix and filter. Take a volume of the filtrate containing not more than 70 mg of P_2O_5 (and preferably about 50 mg) in a 500-ml conical flask marked at 150 ml. Dilute to 150 ml with water, add 50 ml of citric-molybdic acid reagent and heat the liquid to incipient boiling. Maintain it at this temperature for three minutes and then heat to boiling-point and add 25 ml of quinoline solution. This should be added from a burette with a coarse jet, dropwise for the first few ml and then in a slow stream, swirling continuously throughout to ensure a precipitate of the maximum particle size. Immerse the flask in boiling water for five minutes, cool to 15° and filter through paper pulp. Wash the precipitate with cold water until free from acid, transfer the pulp-pad and precipitate to the original flask with not more than 100 ml of water and shake vigorously until the pulp and precipitate are completely dispersed. Add a slight excess of 0·5N sodium hydroxide (carbonate-free) and shake until the precipitate is completely dissolved. To assist the dispersal of the precipitate at this stage a few drops of 0·5 per cent solution of sodium dodecyl benzene sulphonate may be added if necessary. Titrate the excess alkali with 0·5N hydrochloric acid using mixed phenolphthalein/thymol blue indicator. The end-point is very sharp; the solution becomes pale green and at the end-point suddenly changes to pale yellow. Run a blank on all reagents, excluding only the aliquot of sample solution but use 0·1N acid and alkali solutions for the titration and calculate it to 0·5N sodium hydroxide used. Subtract this blank from the volume neutralised by the original precipitate. 1 ml of 0·5N sodium hydroxide ≡ 1·365 mg of P_2O_5.

(*c*) Another rapid method for the determination of phosphate has been evolved by Taylor and Hobson.[5] This method involves the precipitation of the phosphate by the addition of an excess of bismuth nitrate, filtration, and the titration of excess bismuth with standard EDTA.

To a solution (about 70 ml) of phosphate, containing the equivalent of about 70 mg of P_2O_5, in a 400-ml beaker, add 5 ml of dilute nitric acid. Heat to boiling-point and add, by pipette, 50 ml of a solution of 9 g of bismuth subnitrate in 80 ml of concentrated nitric acid diluted with water to 1 litre, stirring during the addition. Allow to stand on a water-bath for five minutes, stirring occasionally. Filter while hot, wash the residue with two 10-ml quantities of hot water and cool the filtrate and washings. Add 0·5 g of urea and 4 to 8 drops of catechol violet indicator and then add dilute ammonia solution, dropwise, until a purplish-blue colour is obtained. Titrate with 0·05M EDTA until the solution is pinkish-violet, add 200 ml of water (and more indicator if necessary) and complete the titration to the full yellow end-point. Carry out a blank titration omitting the sample (the titre should not be less than 30 ml). 1 ml 0·05M EDTA = 0·003549 g P_2O_5.

In the presence of calcium, low results were obtained, due presumably to the co-precipitation of calcium phosphate, and it is necessary to modify the method as follows:

Weigh an amount of sample containing the equivalent of about 4 g of P_2O_5, add 50 ml of dilute nitric acid, heat to boiling-point and cool. Transfer to a 500-ml graduated flask and dilute to volume with water. Pipette 50 ml of the bismuth nitrate solution (see above) into a 400-ml beaker, add 10 ml of dilute nitric acid and 50 ml of water, heat to boiling-point and add, by pipette, 10 ml of sample solution, stirring occasionally. Complete as above from 'Allow to stand on a water-bath . . .'.

This method is to be preferred in the presence of magnesium. Chloride and sulphate ions interfere also and must be removed by boiling with excess silver nitrate and/or barium hydroxide prior to the addition of the bismuth nitrate solution, after which the mixed chloride/sulphate/phosphate precipitate can be filtered off.

A rapid colorimetric method for the determination of phosphate has been described by Donald, Schwehr and Wilson[6] which is suitable for **traces.** This method has also been adopted in principle by the Fertilisers and Feeding Stuffs Regulations (1960) as a standard method:

Reagents:

Standard phosphate solution. Dissolve 0·9587 g of reagent-grade potassium dihydrogen phosphate (previously dried for one hour at 105°) in water and dilute to 500 ml in a graduated flask. Dilute a 50-ml aliquot of this solution to 250 ml with water and mix. 1 ml of the solution contains 0·2 mg P_2O_5.

Vanadomolybdate reagent. Dissolve, separately, 20 g of ammonium molybdate, $(NH_4)_6Mo_7O_{24},4H_2O$, and 1 g of ammonium vanadate, NH_4VO_3, in warm water, filtering if necessary. Mix the two solutions, acidify with 140 ml of concentrated nitric acid and dilute to 1 litre with water. The reagent is stable for at least three months.

Preparation of standard curve. Into a series of 100-ml graduated flasks measure volumes of standard phosphate solution covering the range 5·0 to 6·2 mg of P_2O_5 in increments of 0·2 mg. Add 25 ml of vanadomolybdate reagent to each flask and dilute to volume with water, ensuring that the temperature of reagent and water is 20°. Shake, and allow to stand for ten minutes. Fill two 1-cm cells with the 5·0 mg solution and check the identity of the cells by measuring the extinction at 420 mμ of the two solutions. If there is a small difference select the cell with the smaller reading as the standard reference cell. Measure the apparent extinction at 20° (corrected for cell differences) of the other standard solutions, each referred to the 5·0 mg P_2O_5 solution as standard, and prepare a curve by plotting readings against P_2O_5 content.

Determination: Weigh 10 g of sample into a 500-ml graduated flask, add 400 ml of water at 20° and shake mechanically for thirty minutes. Dilute to volume, mix well and filter. To 25 ml of the filtrate add 1 ml of concentrated nitric acid, heat to incipient boiling on a hot-plate and maintain at this temperature for ten minutes. Cool, neutralise with N sodium hydroxide and then successively dilute until a final volume of about 25 ml contains between 5·5 and 6·2 mg of P_2O_5, taking care that the water used for dilution is at a temperature of 20°. Transfer this volume to a 100-ml graduated flask, add 25 ml of vanadomolybdate reagent (at 20°), dilute to volume, mix and allow to stand for ten minutes. At the same time pipette 25 ml of standard phosphate solution (at 20°) into a second 100-ml graduated flask, add 25 ml of the vanadomolybdate reagent (at 20°), dilute to volume, mix and allow to stand for ten minutes. Measure the difference in extinction at 420 mμ between the two solutions and estimate the P_2O_5 content of the volume of sample solution from the standard curve. (*Note:* Prepare a fresh standard for each series of readings.)

This method has been applied to the determination of phosphate in mineral supplements by Pentelow.[7] The phosphate is dissolved by boiling with a nitric acid/water mixture and, after filtering, the solution is diluted to a suitable volume with water. The phosphate may then be determined as above.

The alkali phosphates in the pure state can be simply assayed by titration. **Potassium phosphate,** K_2HPO_4, Mol. Wt. 174·2, and **sodium phosphate,** $Na_2HPO_4,12H_2O$, Mol. Wt. 358·2, represent the second stage in the titration of phosphoric acid; hence they are alkaline to methyl orange and may be titrated with 0·5N acid to this indicator, bromocresol green or, better, a mixture of 4 volumes of bromocresol green and 1 volume of methyl red (pH 4·4). 1 ml 0·5N = 0·08709 g K_2HPO_4 and 0·07098 g Na_2HPO_4. **Potassium acid phosphate,** KH_2PO_4, Mol. Wt. 136·1, and **sodium acid phosphate,** $NaH_2PO_4,2H_2O$, Mol. Wt. 156·0, represent the first stage in the titration of phosphoric acid; hence they are titrated, as in the case of the acid, to phenolphthalein, which titration is only accurate in the presence of sodium chloride. 1 ml 0·5N $\doteq$ 0·06805 g KH_2PO_4 and 0·07801 g $NaH_2PO_4,2H_2O$.

Sodium polymetaphosphate consists mainly of $(NaPO_3)_x$ but to which sufficient disodium hydrogen phosphate to give a product containing about 10 per cent of tetrasodium pyrophosphate, $Na_4P_2O_7$, has been added; this increases the pH to about 7.

The polymetaphosphate can be determined by the above method for acid phosphates after converting to orthophosphate by boiling with standard acid. Each ml of N alkali in excess of the volume of standard acid used = 0·1020 g $(NaPO_3)_x$.

The pyrophosphate reacts as normal phosphate in solution and is titrated to methyl orange. 1 ml N HCl = 0·1330 g $Na_4P_2O_7$.

Considerable attention has been directed to the contamination of phosphates with fluorine owing to the possible manufacture of the phosphate from phosphatic rocks or bones contaminated with fluorine. Suitable methods are fully discussed on pp. 297 to 303.

1. Richards, M. B., and Godden, W., *Analyst*, 1924, **49**, 565.
2. Ferrey, G. J. W., *Quart. J. Pharm.*, 1934, **7**, 346.
3. Wilson, H. N., *Analyst*, 1951, **76**, 65.
4. Wilson, H. N., *Analyst*, 1954, **79**, 535.
5. Taylor, H., and Hobson, F., private communication.
6. Donald, R., Schwehr, E. W., and Wilson, H. N., *J. Sci. Food Agric.*, 1956, **7**, 677.
7. Pentelow, J. E., private communication.

PHYSOSTIGMINE SALICYLATE

$C_{22}H_{27}O_5N_3$ Mol. Wt. 413·5

Physostigmine salicylate is official in both the *B.P.* and the *U.S.P.* but no official method of assay is given. However, a non-aqueous titration would be applicable.

In preparations, especially where the concentration is low, the determination of physostigmine presents some problems for there is no reliable colorimetric method of assay. According to the nature of the preparation, use can be made of the light absorption characteristics or of the tetraphenylboron method. Examples of the application of each of these are given below.

Eye-drops of Physostigmine, *B.P.C.* Contain 0·5 per cent physostigmine salicylate, 0·8 per cent sodium chloride and 0·4 per cent sodium metabisulphite in solution for eye-drops. The tetraphenylboron method given under Atropine (p. 116) can be applied, using 10 ml of a solution prepared by mixing 5 ml of the eye-drops with 5 ml of buffer solution, pH 3·7. 1 ml of cetylpyridinium chloride = 0·002068 g physostigmine salicylate. The precipitated tetraphenylborate, after washing with five portions, each of 20 ml, of water and drying in vacuo over phosphorus pentoxide, melts at about 109°, and this may be used to add a degree of specificity to the determination.

Oily Eye-drops of Physostigmine, *B.N.F.* Contain 1 per cent of physostigmine in sterile castor oil. The tetraphenylboron method may be applied to the preparation as follows:

Weigh 5 g of sample into a separator, add 5 ml of ether and extract, first with 5 ml of 2N acetic acid and then with three 5-ml quantities of buffer solution, pH 3·7. Filter each extract through the same cotton-wool plug into a 20-ml graduated flask, warm to remove traces of ether, cool, and dilute to volume with buffer solution. Transfer a 10-ml aliquot to a clean, dry beaker and proceed as described on p. 116 beginning with the words 'add 15 ml of 0·01M sodium tetraphenylboron . . .'. 1 ml cetylpyridinium chloride = 0·001377 g $C_{15}H_{21}O_2N_3$.

Eye Ointment of Physostigmine, *B.N.F.* This contains 0·125 per cent of physostigmine salicylate in eye ointment basis and the ratio of alkaloid to ointment base makes application of the tetraphenylboron assay somewhat difficult. A spectrophotometric method can be applied as follows:

Weigh 2·5 g into a separator containing 40 ml of light petroleum and mix to disperse the sample. Extract with six 10-ml quantities of water, combine the extracts in a 100-ml graduated flask, dilute to volume with water and mix.

Measure the extinction of the resulting solution at the maximum at about 298 mμ, using 1-cm cells with water in the comparison cell, and calculate the percentage physostigmine salicylate in the sample, assuming a value of 150 for the E(1 per cent, 1 cm) of physostigmine salicylate at 298 mμ.

PHYTOMENADIONE

$C_{31}H_{46}O_2$ Mol. Wt. 450·7

Phytomenadione, vitamin K_1, is 2-methyl-3-phytyl-1,4-naphthaquinone. In trimethylpentane it has an absorption maximum at 249 mμ, E(1 per cent, 1 cm) = 420 which is used for its assay. However, an assay based on a direct determination of the extinction is unsatisfactory because the absorption characteristics of the decomposition products of phytomenadione closely resemble those of the pure compound and chromatographic separation is necessary. All operations in the assay of phytomenadione should be carried out in subdued light or by use of amber-tinted glassware.

Dissolve 0·1 g in sufficient trimethylpentane to produce 200 ml. Prepare a chromatographic column by filling a glass chromatographic tube, 5 mm in internal diameter, with trimethylpentane, adding 4·5 g of alumina containing 7 per cent water (see below), allowing to settle and reducing the depth of the layer of solvent above the column to about 2 mm. Transfer a 2-ml aliquot of the sample solution to the top of the column and carry out the chromatographic procedure with 20 ml of a mixture of 1 volume of anæsthetic ether and 49 volumes of trimethylpentane. Dilute the eluate to 50 ml with trimethylpentane and measure the extinction of the solution at the maximum at about 249 mμ. E(1 per cent, 1 cm) of phytomenadione is 420.

The E(1 per cent, 1 cm) at 249 mμ of the trimethylpentane used in the above assay should not exceed 0·10 and should not show a significant change after passage through a column of alumina (7 per cent water).

Alumina (7 per cent water). Sift aluminium oxide trihydrate through a 150-mesh sieve and then through a 300-mesh sieve. Mix nine parts of the material retained by the 300-mesh sieve with one part of the material that passes through it, heat the mixture at 780° to 820° for seven hours, cool and store with careful exclusion of moisture. Partially de-activate the anhydrous alumina before use by the addition of 7 per cent of water in a well closed container with ample head space; mix by tumbling and allow to stand for equilibration for not less than twelve hours, with further occasional mixing.

Capsules of Phytomenadione, *B.P.* These are flexible capsules containing an emulsion of phytomenadione with suitable dispersing and stabilising agents; the shells are coloured to protect the contents from light.

Mix the contents of 10 capsules. Weigh accurately an amount of the mixture equivalent to about 7 mg of phytomenadione and mix with about 5 g, accurately weighed, of alumina (7 per cent water). Prepare a chromatographic column by filling a glass chromatographic tube, 5 mm in internal diameter, with trimethylpentane, adding 4 g of alumina (7 per cent water), allowing to settle and reducing the depth of the layer of solvent above the alumina to about 4 cm. Transfer about 0·4 g, accurately weighed, of the sample/alumina mixture to the top of the chromatographic column, so as to form a compact cylinder and complete as described above for phytomenadione, beginning with 'carry out the chromatographic procedure . . .'.

Injection of Phytomenadione, *B.P.* This is a sterile preparation of phytomenadione in water for injection containing suitable dispersing and stabilising agents.

Mix an accurately weighed quantity equivalent to not more than 7 mg of phytomenadione and containing not more than 0·3 g of water with about 5 g, accurately weighed, of alumina (4 per cent water)—prepared in the same way as alumina (7 per cent water). Complete the assay described above for phytomenadione capsules, using about 0·75 g, accurately weighed, of the sample/alumina mixture.

Tablets of Phytomenadione. The method of assay given above for capsules is suitable without modification.

PIPERAZINE

$C_4H_{10}N_2,6H_2O$ Mol. Wt. 194·2

Piperazine itself can be titrated in aqueous solution using screened methyl orange as indicator, but the titration curve is not sharp and this method is not to be recommended. Non-aqueous titration with perchloric acid in glacial acetic acid usually gives a sharp end-point when crystal violet is used as indicator, but in some cases precipitation occurs during titration and the end-point is rather obscured; this method is used by the *U.S.P.* for piperazine citrate and is applied also to the syrup and tablets (1 ml 0·1M = 0·01071 g).

A more specific titration method than either of the above is based upon formation of a dithiocarbamic acid. The method given below follows that of Critchfield and Johnson[1] for the titration of secondary aliphatic amines, but results may vary within a range of about 0·5 per cent. The precipitate which forms on addition of the carbon disulphide dissolves as the titration proceeds:

Dissolve about 1·5 g, accurately weighed, in 25 ml of water, add 50 ml of pyridine, 50 ml of *iso*propyl alcohol and 5 ml of carbon disulphide, and titrate with 0·5N sodium hydroxide using a 1 per cent solution of thymolphthalein in pyridine as indicator. 1 ml 0·5N = 0·04855 g $C_4H_{10}N_2,6H_2O$.

A gravimetric procedure based upon precipitation with carbon disulphide is possible, but the precipitate must be dried in a vacuum desiccator; any method involving the use of heat, however mild, results in a continuing loss.

Probably the most satisfactory method for determination of piperazine, although it lacks the specificity of the carbon disulphide methods, is by precipitation as the picrate. If picric acid is added slowly to a solution of piperazine the precipitate which at first forms (probably a monopicrate) redissolves; on continued addition of picric acid the dipicrate precipitates. If, however, the piperazine solution is first neutralised with a theoretical quantity of mineral acid precipitation is instantaneous and complete. The reproducibility of this method is very good.

Weigh about 0·2 g into a beaker, dissolve in a mixture of 3·5 ml of N sulphuric acid and 10 ml of water and add 100 ml of a reagent prepared by adding 0·5 ml of 20 per cent sodium hydroxide solution to 100 ml of a saturated solution of trinitrophenol in water. Heat on a water-bath for fifteen minutes, allow to stand for one hour and filter through a tared No. 4, sintered-glass crucible. Wash the precipitate with a saturated solution of piperazine dipicrate in water until the washings are free from sulphate and dry to constant weight at 105°. Each g of residue = 0·4267 g $C_4H_{10}N_2,C_6H_{10}O_4$; 0·3935 g $(C_4H_{10}N_2)_3,2C_6H_8O_7$; 0·3567 g $C_4H_{10}N_2$, $6H_2O$; 0·3383 g $C_4H_{10}N_2,H_3PO_4$.

The principal salts used pharmaceutically are **piperazine adipate,** $C_4H_{10}N_2,C_6H_{10}O_4$, Mol. Wt. 232·3, **piperazine citrate,** $(C_4H_{10}N_2)_3$, $2C_6H_8O_7$, containing variable amounts of water of crystallisation equivalent to $5H_2O$ or $6H_2O$, Mol. Wt. (anhyd.) 642·7, **piperazine hydrate,** $C_4H_{10}N_2,6H_2O$, Mol. Wt. 194·2, and **piperazine phosphate,** $C_4H_{10}N_2,H_3PO_4,H_2O$, Mol. Wt. 202·2.

Tablets of Piperazine Adipate, *B.P.*, **Tablets of Piperazine Citrate** and **Tablets of Piperazine Phosphate,** *B.P.*, can all be determined by the picric acid precipitation method given above after dissolving an amount of powdered tablets equivalent to about 0·2 g of the salt, as completely as possible, in 10 ml of water, filtering, washing and precipitating the combined filtrate and washings as directed after adding 3·5 ml of N sulphuric acid. **Elixir of Piperazine Citrate,** *B.P.C.*, can also be assayed by the general method, using 1·5 g and calculating the percentage w/v of anhydrous piperazine citrate from the weight per ml.

1. CRITCHFIELD, F. E., and JOHNSON, J. B., *Anal. Chem.*, 1956, **28**, 430.

POTASSIUM HYDROXYQUINOLINE SULPHATE

It was shown by Hartley and Linnell[1] that potassium hydroxyquinoline sulphate is almost certainly a simple mixture of potassium sulphate and 8-hydroxyquinoline sulphate. This is substantiated by extraction of the 'compound' with ethanol, when complete separation of the two components results.

Hartley and Linnell proposed standardisation on the hydroxyquinoline content. They found the volumetric determination of Berg[2] gave both consistent and accurate results:

> Dissolve about 0·35 g of the sample in 50 ml of water. Add 20 ml of concentrated hydrochloric acid and 50 ml of 0·1N bromate-bromide solution and, after shaking repeatedly during fifteen minutes and allowing to stand for a further fifteen minutes, dilute the mixture to 200 ml with water. Then add 1 g of potassium iodide and titrate the liberated iodine with 0·1N sodium thiosulphate, starch mucilage being added near the end-point. 1 ml 0·1N = 0·003629 g C_9H_7ON.

The 4-aminophenazone method (see under Phenol, p. 514) has been applied by Savidge[3] to a cream containing 7·5 per cent of zinc oxide and 0·1 per cent of potassium hydroxyquinoline sulphate.

The recommended method is as follows:

> Weigh 5 g of the sample into a 250-ml separator, add 25 ml of dilute hydrochloric acid, 15 ml of 95 per cent ethanol and 30 ml of chloroform and shake until solution is effected. Allow the layers to separate, run the lower (chloroform) layer into a second separator and extract it with two 10-ml quantities of water. Combine the aqueous phases and wash with two 20-ml quantities of chloroform. Reject the chloroform. Decant the aqueous phase into a 1-litre graduated flask, wash in with water and make just alkaline to litmus paper with dilute ammonia solution. Add 10 ml of strong ammonia buffer solution and dilute to volume with water. Transfer a 50-ml aliquot to a 150-ml separator and add and dissolve 0·1 g of the disodium salt of EDTA. Continue as described in the general

method (p. 514), beginning with the words 'add 1 ml of 4-aminophenazone solution. . . .'.

1. HARTLEY, F., and LINNELL, W. H., *Quart. J. Pharm.*, 1935, **8,** 674.
2. BERG, R., *Pharm. Ztg.*, 1926, **71,** 1542.
3. SAVIDGE, R. A., private communication.

PROPAMIDINE ISETHIONATE

$C_{21}H_{32}O_{10}N_4S_2$ Mol. Wt. 564·7

The substance is standardised on a nitrogen content. It is used in a jelly or cream.

Ballard[1] examined the application of the colorimetric determination of aromatic di-amidines to propamidine in the presence of other constituents of pharmaceutical preparations. The effect of esters of *p*-hydroxybenzoic acid, alginate and methyl cellulose was slight but not negligible; neglecting to take them into account in the proportions likely to be present would lead to errors of up to about 4 per cent.

Reagents: Borate buffer—Boric acid, 2·76 g, N sodium hydroxide, 23·4 ml, water to 100 ml. Glyoxal solution (freshly prepared)—A 0·22 per cent solution of glyoxal sodium bisulphite in water. Gelatin solution (freshly prepared)—To 100 ml of hot water add 1 g of gelatin *B.P.*, previously broken into small pieces, shake until dissolved and cool.

Prepare a solution of the sample to contain about 0·6 mg of propamidine isethionate in 5 ml. To 5 ml add 2 ml of glyoxal solution, 10 ml of borate buffer and 5 ml of gelatin solution and mix. Heat in a water-bath for ten minutes and cool in ice-water for five minutes. Transfer to a 25-ml graduated flask and dilute to 25 ml with water. Measure the extinction at the maximum at about 520 mμ, using 4-cm cells and correct for the value of a blank carried out as above but omitting the heating. Read off the corresponding amount of propamidine isethionate from a calibration curve derived from an amidine-free preparation of the same strength with known amounts of amidine added.

The glyoxal is added before the buffer to minimise risk of hydrolysis of the amidine and the buffer is added before the gelatin to avoid precipitation which occurs with some preparations. The method is not specific.

Propamidine can be extracted from water-immiscible creams by boiling with very dilute hydrochloric acid but full recovery was not obtained by Ballard, without obtaining a solution too dilute for colorimetric examination, since repeated extractions were necessary.

Dibromopropamidine isethionate, $C_{21}H_{30}O_{10}N_4S_2Br_2$, Mol. Wt. 722·5. This substance can be assayed through its bromine content using the Stepanow method (p. 310) with amyl alcohol and sodium and completing by the Volhard method. 1 ml 0·1N $AgNO_3$ = 0·03612 g.

1. BALLARD, C. W., *Quart. J. Pharm.*, 1948, **21,** 376.

PROTAMINE SULPHATE INJECTION

The *B.P.C.* includes a method for the determination of protamine sulphate on its capacity to neutralise heparin in which the end-point is determined biochemically.

Reagents:

Citrated plasma of such quality that when 0·2 ml of a 1·5 per cent solution of calcium chloride is added to 1 ml, coagulation occurs in five minutes.

Thrombokinase extract prepared by extracting 1·5 g of acetone-dried ox brain with 60 ml of water for fifteen minutes at 60°, centrifuging and filtering; 0·3 per cent of cresol may be added as a bacteriostat. Acetone-dried ox brain can be prepared by cutting fresh ox brain into small pieces which are first placed in acetone; dehydration is completed by pounding this material with successive quantities of acetone until a dry powder remains after filtration. It is finally dried at 37° to remove traces of acetone.

Calcium chloride-thrombokinase solution is a 3 per cent w/v solution of calcium chloride and water containing a sufficient quantity of thrombokinase extract so that when 0·1 ml is added to 0·5 ml of plasma diluted with 0·4 ml of saline coagulation occurs in about thirty-five minutes.

Heparin solution containing 86 units per ml in saline solution.

Method:

Make a solution of the protamine sulphate in saline containing 1 mg per ml. To each of ten tubes add 2·5 ml of plasma, maintain at 37° and to the first nine tubes add 0·5 ml of diluted sample. To the tenth tube add 2·0 ml of saline and 0·5 ml of calcium chloride-thrombokinase solution. Determine the time for fibrin threads to appear on a wire loop drawn through the mixture.

To the remaining tubes add respectively 0·43, 0·45, 0·47, 0·49, 0·50, 0·51, 0·53, 0·55 and 0·57 ml of heparin solution diluted in each case to 1·5 ml with saline. Add to each tube 0·5 ml of calcium chloride-thrombokinase solution and record the coagulation time. The percentage of protamine sulphate is given by the formula $a/0{\cdot}5 \times 100$ where '*a*' is the maximum volume of heparin solution which does not prolong clotting time.

The *B.P.C.* determination is based on the assumption that 1 mg protamine sulphate neutralises 86 units of heparin. There is little foundation for this assumption and in fact the amount of heparin neutralised depends on the sample of heparin used. For this reason simultaneous comparison should be made using a standard preparation of protamine sulphate.

In a test of this kind it is not essential to assess the presence of excess heparin by means of its biological activity; any other property of heparin, *e.g.* its ability to combine with toluidine blue, would serve equally well. Birkinshaw and Smith[1] showed that when the protamine sulphate is in excess the spots made on paper (Whatman No. 1) and stained with bromocresol green remain small and compact well within the area of the paper wetted. When heparin is in excess the whole wetted area stains. This method has been applied to the assay of protamine sulphate. The amounts of heparin recorded as being neutralised by this method and that of the *B.P.C.* are of the same order but not identical, but the relative potencies determined by both methods, through a standard preparation of protamine sulphate, agree satisfactorily with one another.

Make an aqueous solution of protamine sulphate standard containing 1 mg per ml and similar solutions of the sample under test. Into two series of tubes pipette 1 ml of these solutions and to successive tubes add quantities of heparin in amounts differing by 2 units and contained in 1 ml water. Spot approximately 0·01 ml from each tube on Whatman No. 1 paper pencilling the outline of the wetted area. Allow to dry and stain for five minutes in a 0·02 per cent solution of bromocresol green. Wash three times for five minutes in 2 per cent w/v acetic acid solution. Allow to dry and observe the activity of the sample in terms of the standard. This is proportional to the respective maximal concentrations of heparin which still permit the production of a compact stained spot.

1. BIRKINSHAW, V. K., and SMITH, K. L., *J. Pharm. Pharmacol.*, 1962, **14**, 95T.

PYRETHRUM

Pyrethrum flower consists of the dried flowerhead of *Chrysanthemum cinerariæfolium* Vis. and it owes its insecticidal properties to two types of ketoesters. One group consists of pyrethrin I and cinerin I, both of which have chrysanthemum monocarboxylic acid (chrysanthemic acid) as their acid component. The assay given below for pyrethrin I, which is based on the determination of total chrysanthemic acid, will therefore include cinerin I. The second group of esters consists of pyrethrin II and cinerin II, both of which have the monomethyl ester of chrysanthemum dicarboxylic acid (pyrethric acid) as their acid component; since the assay given below for pyrethrin II is based on the determination of total pyrethric acid it will therefore include cinerin II. The keto-alcohol component of the pyrethrins is pyrethrolone and that of the cinerins is cinerolone.

Apparently the biological activity of pyrethrum is not correlated with a definite entity or group and it has been asserted that a mixture of the pyrethrins is more toxic than the isolated principles (Ripert and Gaudin[1]). Many methods have been devised for the evaluation of pyrethrum. They are all open to criticism and there is considerable controversy as to their accuracy, conflicting results being obtained by different workers.

The most commonly used method of analysis of pyrethrum is the so-called Mercury Reduction Method, a version of which is given below. Formerly, a method due to Seil[2] was in common use but this has now been largely replaced. In Seil's method the powdered flowers are extracted with light petroleum and after evaporation of the solvent the pyrethrins and cinerins are hydrolysed with ethanolic sodium hydroxide to give the chrysanthemum acids. The reaction solution is then treated with barium chloride and after filtration of extraneous material the chrysanthemum acids are liberated by the addition of sulphuric acid and the mixture steam-distilled, when the volatile monocarboxylic acid derived from pyrethrin I in the distillate may be titrated with standard alkali. The dicarboxylic acid, derived from pyrethrin II remaining in the residue after distillation, is then extracted and determined separately by titration.

A number of versions of the Mercury Reduction Method are available. There is a significant difference between the method given in the *B.Vet.C.* and that given by the *A.O.A.C.*[3] This difference concerns the acid used for neutralisation of the aqueous solution obtained after removal of the barium salts of the fatty acids. The American version uses sulphuric acid, whilst the British favours hydrochloric acid. Mitchell[4] has published results showing that the *A.O.A.C.* procedure gives lower results for pyrethrin I (by about 10 to 15 per cent) and he isolated chrysanthemum monocarboxylic acid from the barium sulphate precipitate arising from the use of sulphuric acid. Other workers have confirmed this finding but Kelsey[5] considered that the point was not proved and although he agreed that the use of hydrochloric acid gave higher results he was not convinced that the chrysanthemum monocarboxylic acid adsorbed on to the barium sulphate precipitate arose from insecticidally active esters. Consequently, the *A.O.A.C.* method still recommends the use of sulphuric acid.

More recently Byrne, Mitchell and Tresadern[6] have described a method that depends upon infra-red measurement at about 9·0 $m\mu$ of a carbon tetrachloride extract for determination of pyrethrin I. This gives results that compare closely with those obtained by the *A.O.A.C.* method and the authors conclude that the results obtained by the latter method are approximately correct, though resulting from a summation of positive and negative errors. It seems likely that, although it is a rather unsatisfactory compromise, the *A.O.A.C.* method will be used as a basis for commercial transactions for some time to come; support for this has been afforded by recent work published by Brierley and Brown.[7] The *A.O.A.C.* method is given in detail below for both **Pyrethrum flowers** and **Extract of Pyrethrum.** It cannot be too strongly stressed that the conditions set down must be strictly adhered to; the factors given are empirical ones, resulting from a collaborative trial undertaken by several laboratories.

Reagents:

Denigès reagent: Mix 5 g of yellow mercuric oxide with 40 ml of water, add, slowly while stirring, 20 ml of concentrated sulphuric acid followed by 40 ml of water and stir until all the mercuric oxide has dissolved. Test for the absence of mercurous mercury as follows: To 10 ml add a few drops of iodine monochloride solution, 50 ml of cooled dilute hydrochloric acid (3 + 2), 5 ml of chloroform or carbon tetrachloride and 1 ml of freshly adjusted iodine monochloride solution. Titrate with 0·01M potassium iodate, shaking vigorously for at least thirty seconds after each addition, until no iodine colour remains in the chloroform or carbon tetrachloride layer. (The end-point is taken when the red colour disappears from the solvent layer and does not return within one to three minutes.) Record the ml 0·01M potassium iodate required.

Iodine monochloride solution: Dissolve 10 g of potassium iodide and 6·44 g of potassium iodate in 75 ml of water in a glass-stoppered bottle, add 75 ml of concentrated hydrochloric acid and 5 ml of chloroform and then adjust to a faint iodine colour in the chloroform by adding dilute potassium iodide or potassium iodate solution. If much iodine is liberated, use a stronger solution of potassium iodate than 0·01M at first and make the final adjustment with 0·01M solution. Store in a cool dark place and readjust with potassium iodide or potassium iodate solution when necessary.

0·01M Potassium iodate: Dissolve 2·14 g of pure potassium iodate, previously dried at 105°, in water and dilute to 1 litre with water.

Light petroleum: This is aromatic-free material of b.p. 30° to 60°.

Ether: Use analytical-reagent grade peroxide-free material.

Preparation of Sample:

(*a*) Pyrethrum flowers. Extract an amount of sample equivalent to 40 to 150 mg of total pyrethrins in a Soxhlet or other efficient extraction apparatus for seven hours with light petroleum. After extraction is complete, concentrate the extract to a volume of about 40 ml and leave it in a stoppered flask in a refrigerator at 0° ± 0·5° overnight. Filter the cold extract through a plug of cotton wool (previously saturated with ice-cold light petroleum) in a glass funnel, collecting the filtrate in a 250-ml Erlenmeyer flask. Wash the flask and filter with three 15-ml quantities of ice-cold light petroleum, combine the filtrate and washings and evaporate on a water-bath in a current of air until less than 1 ml of solvent remains.

Add 15 to 20 ml of 0·5N ethanolic sodium hydroxide to the flask containing the extract, connect to a reflux condenser and boil gently for one to one and a half hours. Transfer to a 600-ml beaker and dilute with water to about 200 ml. Add a few glass beads, or, preferably, use a boiling-tube and boil gently until the volume is reduced to 150 ml. Transfer to a 250-ml graduated flask, and add 1 g of filtercel and 10 ml of a 10 per cent solution of barium chloride dihydrate. Do not shake before diluting to volume. Dilute to volume with water, mix thoroughly, filter off 200 ml (measured in a graduated flask), neutralise with sulphuric acid (1 + 4), using 1 drop of phenolphthalein as indicator, and add 1 ml of the acid in excess. (If it is necessary to leave the solution overnight before continuing the assay, leave in an alkaline condition.)

(*b*) Pyrethrum Extracts in Mineral Oil: Weigh an amount of sample equivalent to 40 to 150 mg of total pyrethrins into a flask and add 50 ml of light petroleum and 1 g of filtercel. Allow to stand in a refrigerator at 0° ± 0·5° overnight. Filter through a Gooch crucible into a 300-ml Erlenmeyer flask and wash with three 15-ml quantities of cold light petroleum. Evaporate the combined filtrate and washings on a water-bath under a current of air until the volume is reduced to less than 1 ml.

Add 20 ml of N ethanolic sodium hydroxide (or more if necessary, see

Note below), connect the flask to a reflux condenser and boil gently for one to one and a half hours. Transfer to a 600-ml beaker and add sufficient water to make the aqueous layer 200 ml. (If more than 20 ml of ethanolic sodium hydroxide was used add enough water so that all the ethanol is removed when the volume is reduced to 150 ml.) Add a few glass beads or, preferably, use a boiling-tube, and boil gently until the volume of the aqueous layer is reduced to 150 ml. Transfer to a 500-ml separator and drain the aqueous layer into a 250-ml graduated flask. Wash the oily layer once with water and add the washing to the aqueous layer. If, at this stage, a slight emulsion still persists, add 2 to 3 ml of a 10 per cent solution of barium chloride dihydrate and swirl gently. (Vigorous shaking at this stage may cause the formation of a reversed emulsion, difficult to separate.) To the contents of the graduated flask add 1 g of filtercel and 10 ml or more of the barium chloride solution, swirl gently and allow to stand for thirty minutes. Dilute to volume with water, mix thoroughly and filter off 200 ml (measured in a graduated flask). Test the filtrate with barium chloride solution to see if enough has been added to obtain a clear solution. Add 1 drop of phenolphthalein indicator, neutralise with sulphuric acid (1 + 4) and add 1 ml of the acid in excess. (If it is necessary to leave the solution overnight before continuing the assay, leave in an alkaline condition.)

Determination of pyrethrin I: Filter the acid solution from *(a)* or *(b)* above, through a 7-cm filter paper, coated lightly with a suspension of filtercel in water, in a Büchner funnel and wash with three 15-ml quantities of water. Transfer to a 500-ml glass-stoppered separator and extract with two 50-ml quantities of light petroleum, shaking for at least one minute each time and inverting the separator and releasing excess pressure through the stopcock if necessary; allow the layers to separate for at least five minutes, or until the aqueous layer is clear, between the extractions. Retain the aqueous layer for the determination of pyrethrin II. Do not combine the light-petroleum extracts but wash each, in turn, with the same three 10-ml quantities of water before filtering through a small cotton-wool plug into a clean 250-ml separator. Wash the separators and cotton-wool plug, in turn, with 5 ml of light petroleum. Extract the combined light-petroleum solutions with 5 ml of 0·1N sodium hydroxide, shaking vigorously for at least one minute and allowing the layers to separate for at least five minutes before running the aqueous layer into a 100-ml beaker. Wash the light petroleum solution with a further 5 ml of 0·1N sodium hydroxide and then with 5 ml of water, adding the washings to the beaker. Add 10 ml of Denigès reagent and allow to stand in complete darkness for one hour at 25° ± 2°.

Add 20 ml of 95 per cent ethanol and precipitate the mercurous chloride with 3 ml of brine. Warm to about 60° and allow to stand for several minutes until the precipitate coagulates and settles. Filter through a small filter paper, transferring all the precipitate to the paper, and wash with 10 ml, or more of hot 95 per cent ethanol. Wash with two or more 10-ml quantities of hot chloroform (see Note below) and place the paper and its contents in a 250-ml glass-stoppered Erlenmeyer flask. Add 50 ml of cooled dilute hydrochloric acid (3 + 2) followed by 5 ml of chloroform or carbon tetrachloride and 1 ml of freshly-adjusted iodine monochloride solution. Titrate with 0·01M potassium iodate, shaking vigorously for at least thirty seconds after each addition, until no iodine colour remains in the solvent layer. (The end-point is taken when the red colour disappears from the solvent layer and does not return within one to three minutes.) From the ml 0·01M potassium iodate solution required subtract the blank obtained on the Denigès reagent. 1 ml 0·01M potassium iodate = 0·0057 g pyrethrin I.

Note: With samples containing perfume or other saponifiable ingredients, it may be necessary to add as much as 50 ml of N ethanolic sodium hydroxide. When lethanes are present, after washing the mercurous chloride precipitate with 95 per cent ethanol and chloroform, wash once more with 95 per cent ethanol and then several times with hot water.

Determination of pyrethrin II: If necessary, filter the aqueous layer, retained above for the determination of pyrethrin II, through a Gooch crucible. Concentrate the filtrate to about 50 ml and transfer to a 500-ml glass-stoppered separator. Wash the beaker with three 15-ml quantities of water and add the washings to the separator. Acidify with concentrated hydrochloric acid and saturate with sodium chloride. (The acidified aqueous layer must contain visible sodium chloride crystals throughout the following extractions.)

Extract successively with 50, 50, 35 and 35 ml of ether, shaking for at least one minute each time and allowing the layers to separate for at least five minutes, or until the aqueous layer is clear, after each extraction. Combine the ether extracts, drain, and wash with three 10-ml quantities of brine. Filter the washed ether extracts through a cotton-wool plug into a 500-ml Erlenmeyer flask and wash the separator and cotton-wool plug with 10 ml of ether. Evaporate the ether on a water-bath and remove any fumes of hydrochloric acid with a current of air and continued heating for not more than five minutes. Dry the residue for ten minutes at 100°, treat with 75 ml of boiling water and filter through a Whatman No. 1 paper, washing with 20-ml quantities of boiling water until the last washing is neutral to litmus. Add one or two drops of phenolphthalein indicator and titrate with 0·02N sodium hydroxide that has been standardised on the same day that the sample is titrated. 1 ml 0·02N = 0·00374 g pyrethrin II.

Several other approaches have been made to the analysis of pyrethrum but a discussion of these does not fall within the scope of this book. The interested reader is recommended to a review article by Phipers.[8]

Dusting-powder of Gamma Benzene Hexachloride and Pyrethrum, *B.P.C.* Contains 2 per cent of extract and is assayed for pyrethrins by the method given below for Dusting-powder of Pyrethrum.

Dusting-powder of Pyrethrum, *B.Vet.C.* Contains 2 per cent of extract in a mixture of diatomite and talc.

For assay extract about 40 g with hexane for eight hours in a Soxhlet apparatus, repeat the extraction for a further four hours with a fresh quantity of solvent and evaporate the solvent from the combined extracts before applying the above method for pyrethrum extract.

1. RIPERT, J., and GAUDIN, O., *Compt. Rend.*, 1935, **200,** 2219.
2. Imperial Institute Consultative Committee on Insecticide Materials of Vegetable Origin, Report, London, 1950, p. 40.
3. *A.O.A.C.*, 1960, p. 42.

4. Mitchell, W., *J. Sci. Food Agric.*, 1953, **4,** 278.
5. Kelsey, D., *J.A.O.A.C.*, 1953, **36**, 369; 1954, **37**, 628.
6. Byrne, J. H. N., Mitchell, W., and Tresadern, F. H., *Analyst*, 1963, **88**, 538.
7. Brierley, A., and Brown, N. C., *Soap, Sanit. Chemicals*, 1962, **38**, 105.
8. Phipers, R. F., *Pyrethrum Post*, 1958, **4**, 3.

RADIOACTIVE SUBSTANCES

A number of radioactive substances are now in medical use, mainly as diagnostic agents. A full discussion of methods applicable to the assessment of these materials is outside the scope of this book and, indeed, their application is outside the scope of most laboratories. For information the reader is referred to Modern Radiochemical Practice.[1] However, it may be of interest to give some indication of the type of specification which is applicable to such radioactive materials.

The worker with radioactive substances is fortunate in that, by their very nature, the materials he has to examine possess characteristic and specific properties. For identification purposes use is made of the radiation characteristics and of the half-life. Substances which give rise to gamma radiation exhibit characteristic gamma ray spectra which may be determined in a suitable spectrometer and compared with standardised solutions (obtainable from the Radiochemical Centre, Amersham, Bucks). Beta ray emitters may be characterised by comparing the beta ray absorption curve with that of a standardised solution; the curve is constructed by placing a prepared sample under a Geiger-Muller counter having a thin end-window and making measurements of the counts obtained when aluminium foils of increasing thickness (about ten in all) are successively interposed between the sample and the counter. Naturally, when carrying out a determination of this type the counts obtained as the experiment proceeds must be corrected for the decay which occurs. The radiation energies and half-life periods of a number of isotopes used in medicine are given in Table 28.

Assay of radioactive isotopes is made by comparing the activity of the material under test with that of a standardised solution, using suitable counting equipment. Alternatively instruments are available which have been calibrated with standardised solutions (N.P.L. Reference Ionisation Chamber No. 1383, for example).

Having identified the isotope and measured the total count a test of radiochemical purity should be carried out, wherever possible, to confirm that the radioactivity of the sample is due to the one species only. In many cases this may be done by diluting the sample until the activity is of the order of about 20,000 counts per minute and then carrying out a suitable paper chromatographic separation. The radioactivity, as identified by scan-

TABLE 28

ISOTOPE	RADIATION (IN MeV)		HALF-LIFE (DAYS)
	Beta	*Gamma*	
Chromium-51 (^{51}Cr)	—	0·32	27·8
Gold-198 (^{198}Au)	0·96	0·41	2·7
Iodine-131 (^{131}I)	0·61	0·36	8
Iron-59 (^{59}Fe)	0·27 (46 per cent)	1·10 (57 per cent)	45·1
	0·46 (54 per cent)	1·29 (43 per cent)	
Phosphorus-32 (^{32}P)	1·71	—	14·2

ning with a collimated Geiger-Muller counter, should appear in one spot only.

In addition to the tests of radioactivity discussed above purely chemical tests to determine the total amount of, say, chromate or phosphate may also be carried out. Typical preparations, controlled on the principles outlined above, are sodium iodide (^{131}I) injection and solution, sodium phosphate (^{32}P) injection and solution, sodium chromate (^{51}Cr) injection and ferric citrate (^{59}Fe) injection.

1. COOK, G. P., and DUNCAN, J. F., Oxford, Oxford University Press, 1952.

RAUWOLFIA

A considerable volume of literature has been devoted to the analysis of rauwolfia since the renewal of interest in this drug a few years ago. In general, the main approaches to the problem have been:

(i) by determination of total alkaloids, as given in the *B.P.C.* Such methods are quite unsatisfactory, since the principal anti-hypertensive alkaloids, reserpine and rescinnamine, form only a small proportion of the total amount.

(ii) by separation and determination of the weakly basic alkaloids, reserpine and rescinnamine (present in Rauwolfia species which are imported commonly into Great Britain) as a group; this has been carried out fluorimetrically, by dye extraction, by reaction with vanillin or by reaction with sodium nitrite and sulphuric acid. The last method forms the basis of the procedure recommended by the Joint Pharmaceutical Society/*S.A.C.* Committee[1] on the assay of crude drugs, which is given in detail below.

(iii) by complete separation of the reserpine. This has been effected by liquid-liquid partition chromatography, by counter-current extraction, by paper chromatography and by paper ionophoresis. In general, methods of these types are somewhat tedious and are to be avoided for routine work if other acceptable methods are available.

The method given below is that recommended by the Joint Committee mentioned above. The colour development conditions advised involve heating solutions at 55° for thirty minutes; in some published versions of the method the solutions are maintained at room temperature for periods of up to three hours, but such conditions may be inadequate and result in incomplete colour development. The entire assay procedure should be carried out protected from light as much as possible and the alkaloids should be allowed to remain in chloroform for the minimum possible time. The use of grease as a lubricant for taps should be avoided.

Weigh accurately a suitable amount of sample ground to pass through a 60-mesh B.S. sieve and triturate with 10 ml of a 5 per cent v/v solution of analytical-reagent grade glacial acetic acid in 95 per cent ethanol (use analytical-reagent grade 95 per cent ethanol throughout); the amounts to take are as follows: for whole-root samples of *R. serpentina* and *R. vomitoria*, which contain between 0·10 and 0·40 per cent of reserpine-like alkaloids, use 2·5 g: for root-bark samples of *R. vomitoria*, which may contain more than 1 per cent of reserpine-like alkaloids, use 1·0 g (if the extinction values of the final coloured solutions are too great, test smaller aliquots of the chloroform solution, without delay, or extract a smaller portion of the ethanolic solution with trichloroethane).

Allow to stand for two hours, stirring from time to time. Transfer to a Soxhlet apparatus with 95 per cent ethanol and extract for four hours with the ethanol, shielding the apparatus from light during the extraction. Cool the extract, concentrate to below 100 ml if necessary, transfer to a 100-ml graduated flask and dilute to volume with 95 per cent ethanol.

Transfer a 20-ml aliquot of this solution to a separator containing 200 ml of 0·05N sulphuric acid and extract with three 25-ml quantities of 1,1,1-trichloroethane. Wash each successive extract with the same 50 ml of 0·5N sulphuric acid in a second separator and discard the organic layers. Extract the weakly basic alkaloids from the aqueous acid solution in the first separator first with 20 ml, and then with five 15-ml quantities, of analytical-reagent grade chloroform. Wash each chloroform extract, first with the acid in the second separator and then with two 10-ml quantities of a freshly prepared 2 per cent solution of analytical-reagent grade sodium bicarbonate, in two further separators. Filter the chloroform extracts through a small cotton-wool plug into a 100-ml graduated flask, dilute to volume with analytical-reagent grade chloroform and mix thoroughly.

Transfer duplicate 20-ml aliquots of the solution to boiling-tubes and evaporate to dryness on a water-bath in a current of warm air, protecting the tubes from light. Dissolve the contents of each tube in a mixture of 10 ml of 95 per cent ethanol and 2 ml of 0·5N sulphuric acid, warming to assist solution.

To one tube, the test solution, add 2 ml of a freshly prepared 0·3 per cent solution of analytical-reagent grade sodium nitrite, mix and treat the contents of each tube, respectively, as follows. Heat in a water-bath at 55° for thirty minutes, protecting the solutions from light, cool and add 1·0 ml of a freshly prepared 5 per cent solution of sulphamic acid. Transfer to a 20-ml graduated flask, rinsing the tube with small portions of 95 per cent ethanol and using the rinsings to dilute the contents of the graduated flask to volume.

Measure the extinction of the test solution at 390 mμ, using 1-cm cells with the blank solution (the solution from the second tube) in the comparison cell, and read the amount of reserpine-like alkaloids equivalent to this extinction from a standard curve prepared as described below at the same time as the test.

Preparation of standard curve

Standard reserpine solution. Moisten 25·0 mg of reserpine, *B.P.*, with 2 ml of 95 per cent ethanol, add 2 ml of 0·5N sulphuric acid followed by 10 ml of 95 per cent ethanol and warm gently to effect solution. Cool and dilute to 100 ml with 95 per cent ethanol in a graduated flask; when this solution is subjected to the procedure for colour development described above the value of E(1 per cent, 1 cm) of the reserpine should not be less than 390, calculated on the dried material.

Dilute the standard solution with 95 per cent ethanol to give standards containing, respectively, 100 μg, 200 μg and 300 μg of reserpine in 10 ml.

Pipette 10 ml of each solution into boiling-tubes and add to each 2 ml of 0·5N sulphuric acid and 2 ml of the 0·3 per cent sodium nitrite solution. Mix and heat in a water-bath at 55° for thirty minutes, protecting the tubes from light. Cool, add 1·0 ml of the 5 per cent sulphamic acid solution to each tube and transfer to 20-ml graduated flasks, rinsing the tubes with small quantities of 95 per cent ethanol and using the rinsings to dilute to volume.

Measure the extinction of each solution at 390 mμ, using 1-cm cells with, in the comparison cell, a solution prepared in a similar manner using 10 ml of 95 per cent ethanol instead of the standard reserpine solution. Prepare a curve by plotting extinction against concentration of reserpine.

Extracts of rauwolfia may be determined by dissolving a suitable amount, dependent on the concentration, in 100 ml of 95 per cent ethanol and proceeding as above from 'Transfer a 20-ml aliquot of this solution to a separator . . .'.

RESERPINE, $C_{33}H_{40}O_9N_2$, Mol. Wt. 608·7

The pure material is conveniently determined by non-aqueous titration, dissolving 0·5 g in 30 ml of warm glacial acetic acid, cooling and titrating with 0·05N perchloric acid using quinaldine red as indicator. 1 ml 0·05N = 0·03043 g (see p. 792).

Such a method would not detect contamination with 11-desmethoxyreserpine (deserpidine) which occurs with reserpine in certain species of rauwolfia. However, deserpidine gives a negligible response with the nitrite colour reaction given above and this method may be used to give a more specific, though somewhat less precise, measure of the reserpine content of a sample. The E(1 per cent, 1 cm) of reserpine developed by the conditions for colour formation given above is 403 at the maximum at about 390 mμ.

Tablets of Reserpine, *B.P.* Usually contain 0·25 mg of reserpine. These may be assayed by the recommended method as follows:

Shake a weight of powdered tablets equivalent to about 2 mg of reserpine with 50 ml of chloroform for thirty minutes and centrifuge into a stoppered tube. Pipette 5 ml of the clear supernatant liquid into a boiling-tube and evaporate to dryness on a water-bath, protecting the tube from light. Dissolve the residue in 10 ml of analytical-reagent grade 95 per cent ethanol and 2 ml of 0·5N sulphuric acid, warming gently to assist solution, and complete by the above method from the addition of sodium nitrite. Calculate the reserpine content of the tablets using a value of 403 for the E(1 per cent, 1 cm) of reserpine at 390 mμ.

RESCINNAMINE, $C_{35}H_{42}O_9N_2$, Mol. Wt. 634·7

This alkaloid is similar to reserpine except that the reserpic acid moiety of the molecule is esterified with trimethoxycinnamic acid rather than with trimethoxybenzoic acid. A non-aqueous titration similar to that given above is applicable (1 ml 0·05N = 0·03174 g), or the colorimetric nitrite procedure may be applied. If the sample is thought to be contaminated with some of the other alkaloids of rauwolfia (less weakly basic), an extraction procedure can be applied followed by colour development as in the recommended method above. An aliquot of a suitable extract is diluted with 0·5N sulphuric acid and the aqueous ethanol is then extracted with trichloroethane which is discarded. The rescinnamine is then separated from other alkaloids by extracting the acid solution with chloroform and a suitable aliquot of the chloroform solution, containing 100 to 300 μg of rescinnamine is evaporated and used for the colour development stage. The rescinnamine content is obtained from a standard curve prepared using a solution of rescinnamine in 95 per cent ethanol.

1. *Analyst*, 1960, **85**, 755.

RESORCINOL

$C_6H_4(OH)_2$ Mol. Wt. 110·1

Resorcinol, being phenolic, may be extracted in acid solution with ether and is re-extracted from ethereal solution by shaking with dilute caustic alkali.

Resorcinol is slowly volatilised in steam and after extraction in aqueous alkaline solution is best determined bromometrically, as it readily produces tribromoresorcinol. The method is very similar to that for phenol but it requires less time; it may be recapitulated here for convenience:

Dissolve about 1·5 g in water and make up to 500 ml. Transfer a 25-ml aliquot to an iodine flask, add 50 ml of 0·1N bromine, 50 ml of water and 5 ml of concentrated hydrochloric acid and immediately stopper the flask. Shake for one minute, allow to stand for two minutes and then add 5 ml of N potassium iodide, taking care to avoid loss of bromine vapour. Shake thoroughly, allow to stand for five minutes and remove the stopper, rinsing it and the neck of the flask with 20 ml of water into the flask. Titrate the liberated iodine, equivalent to the excess of bromine, with 0·1N thiosulphate using starch as indicator. 1 ml 0·1N = 0·001835 g.

Compound Ointment of Resorcinol, *B.P.C.* A very complex ointment containing 4 per cent of resorcinol, 8 per cent of bismuth subnitrate and 4 per cent of zinc oxide with other ingredients.

For water-soluble phenols, shake about 0·4 g with 20 ml of light petroleum (b.p. 100° to 120°) and extract with four 20-ml quantities of warm water. Filter the extracts and wash the filter with water, combining the filtrates and washings in an iodine flask. Continue the assay as given above. 1 ml 0·1N bromine = 0·001835 g $C_6H_6O_2$.

For bismuth and zinc, destroy the organic matter by ignition and either determine the bismuth by precipitation as phosphate (see p. 128) and the zinc gravimetrically as zinc mercuric thiocyanate (see p. 689) or both bismuth and zinc by EDTA titration as given on p. 698.

The water-soluble phenols from birch-tar oil may increase the apparent resorcinol content by about 0·2 per cent.

Paste of Resorcinol and Sulphur, *B.P.C.* Contains 6·25 per cent each of resorcinol and sulphur and 37·5 per cent of zinc oxide in emulsifying ointment.

For resorcinol: Disperse about 0·8 g in 20 ml of warm light petroleum (b.p. 60° to 80°) and extract with three 20-ml quantities of warm water, filtering the extracts through a moistened filter paper. Wash the filter paper and transfer the mixed filtrates and washings to a stoppered flask and determine bromometrically as above.

Determine the sulphur by the sulphite method (p. 614) or by flask-combustion (p. 801).

For zinc oxide: see p. 699.

Zinc oxide may also be determined by direct ignition in a porcelain crucible.

HEXYLRESORCINOL, $C_{12}H_{18}O_2$, Mol. Wt. 194·3

Hexylresorcinol may be determined by bromination and the following method is that given in the *B.P.*

Weigh 1·2 g into a 100-ml graduated flask, dissolve in methanol and dilute to volume with the same solvent. Transfer a 10-ml aliquot to an iodine flask, add 50 ml of 0·1N bromine and 10 ml of concentrated hydrochloric acid, stopper the flask, swirl occasionally during fifteen minutes and allow to stand for fifteen minutes. Add 10 ml of 10 per cent potassium iodide solution and titrate with 0·1N thiosulphate until only a faint yellow colour remains. Add a few drops of starch mucilage and 10 ml of chloroform and complete the titration with vigorous shaking. Carry out a blank determination with the same quantities of the same reagents and make any necessary correction. 1 ml 0·1N bromine = 0·004857 g $C_{12}H_{18}O_2$.

A similar method is official in the *U.S.P.* Some workers have replaced methanol by glacial acetic acid and it has been stated that if the reaction be allowed to proceed at room temperature overnight it avoids a difficulty in detecting the end-point due to reappearance of colour.

RIBOFLAVINE

$C_{17}H_{20}O_6N_4$ Mol. Wt. 376·4

Riboflavine has absorption maxima in pH 4·0 buffer at 267 mμ, 375 mμ and 444 mμ, E(1 per cent, 1 cm) = 850, 275 and 320 respectively. The *B.P.* assay is based on the extinction at 267 mμ. All determinations should be made in subdued light, preferably by use of amber-coloured glassware.

The determination of riboflavine in most pharmaceutical materials does not require the complicated procedure necessary for its extraction from natural products (where the extraction is the cause of most error). A microbiological method is, however, necessary for yeast preparations and is official for vitamin capsules.

Although the measurement of the fluorescence of riboflavine solutions at known pH values has been widely used for assay and forms the basis of the *U.S.P.* method, riboflavine is best determined in simple formulations by extraction and measurement of the extinction at 444 mμ.

Tablets of Riboflavine, ***B.P.*** Usually contain 1 mg of riboflavine.

Weigh accurately an amount of powdered tablet material containing about 15 mg of riboflavine and transfer to a 250-ml graduated flask. Add about 50 ml of buffer solution pH 4·0 (prepared by diluting 250 ml of 0·2M potassium dihydrogen phosphate and 3·6 ml of a 1 per cent v/v solution of phosphoric acid to 1 litre with water), and warm on a water-bath for fifteen minutes. Cool and make up to volume with pH 4·0 buffer solution. Dilute 25 ml of this solution to 100 ml in pH 4·0 buffer solution, filter a portion, discarding the first 20 ml and measure the maximum extinction of the clear filtrate at about 444 mμ in a 1-cm cell using pH 4·0 buffer solution as the blank. Calculate the amount of riboflavine in each tablet.

The riboflavine in Compound Tablets of Aneurine and Strong Compound Tablets of Aneurine can be determined by the above method.

In more complex formulations riboflavine may be determined after reduction with sodium dithionite and subsequent re-oxidation.[1] Many coloured materials, such as some pharmaceutical dyestuffs, are simultaneously reduced but not re-oxidised under the conditions used in the assay.

Capsules of Vitamins, *B.P.C.*, may be assayed for riboflavine either by the microbiological method given below for dried yeast using 5 capsules or by the method of Brealey and Elvidge.[1]

Place 3 capsules in a 150-ml round-bottomed amber flask, add 50 ml of pH 4·0 phosphate buffer solution and boil under reflux for thirty minutes. Cool, transfer the solution to a 100-ml graduated flask and make up to volume with pH 4·0 buffer solution. Filter a portion, discarding the first 20 ml, and to about 50 ml of the clear filtrate add about 10 mg of sodium dithionite ($Na_2S_2O_4,2H_2O$). Dissolve by shaking gently and allow the solution to stand for about one minute. During this time the yellow colour should have changed to a pale straw colour. Reserve a portion of this solution as a blank and pass a rapid stream of air bubbles through the remainder for two minutes. During this time the colour should have returned to a distinct yellow. Measure the extinction of this solution at 444 mμ in a 1-cm cell against the blank. Determine the riboflavine content of the capsules by reference to a solution of riboflavine in the buffer solution, reduced and re-oxidised in the same manner as the sample solution.

Although this method was applied to **dried yeast** with results fairly comparable with those obtained microbiologically the chemical properties of the non-riboflavine pigments are unknown and the effect of reduction and re-oxidation on these pigments cannot be properly assessed. Hence microbiological assay is necessary.[2]

Weigh 1 to 5 g of finely ground sample and transfer to a conical flask with 50 ml of 0·1N hydrochloric acid. Cover the flask with a small beaker and autoclave at 121° (15 lb steam pressure) for fifteen minutes. Cool, add 2 ml of 2·5M sodium acetate, adjust to pH 4·5 using bromocresol green as external indicator. Dilute to 100 ml with distilled water, filter, and extract an aliquot with anæsthetic ether. Adjust to pH 6·8 using bromothymol blue as external indicator and dilute as required so that the final concentration of riboflavine is about 0·1μg per ml and carry out the microbiological assay (see p. 813).

Notes. (1) Material with high fat content should have a preliminary extraction with light petroleum (b.p. 40° to 60°) for sixteen to eighteen hours. (2) All operations should be carried out in a dim light or with a red 'safe' light.

1. Brealey, L., and Elvidge, D. A., *J. Pharm. Pharmacol.*, 1956, **8,** 885.
2. *Analyst*, 1946, **71,** 397.

SACCHARIN

$C_7H_5O_3NS$ Mol. Wt. 183·2

The evaluation of saccharin by the method of Richmond and Hill[1] has provided consistently trustworthy results. The process depends on preliminary hydrolysis of the saccharin (*o*-benzoicsulphimide) to *o*-sulphaminobenzoic acid by caustic alkali and then further to the ammonium salt of sulphobenzoic acid by hydrochloric acid. Under the conditions recommended, hydrolysis of common impurities is stated to be negligible:

Boil about 0·5 g of saccharin with 10 ml of 30 per cent w/v sodium hydroxide solution for two minutes, care being taken not to concentrate the liquid appreciably. To the product add 15 ml of concentrated hydrochloric acid and boil for fifty minutes under a reflux condenser; sodium chloride should not be deposited whilst the liquid is boiling. Cool, dilute with 75 ml of water, removing any acid vapours with a current of air. Add 20 ml of 30 per cent sodium hydroxide solution, distil the ammonia (preferably in steam) into excess of 0·1N acid, titrating back to methyl red with 0·1N alkali. 1 ml 0·1N = 0·01832 g.

Saccharin can be titrated directly with sodium hydroxide to phenolphthalein. This is the basis of the *U.S.P.* assay in which 0·5 g is dissolved in 75 ml of hot water, cooled quickly and titrated with 0·1N alkali. 1 ml 0·1N = 0·01832 g.

Saccharin sodium, $C_7H_4O_3NSNa,2H_2O$, Mol. Wt. 241·2, is determined in the *B.P.* by the method given above for saccharin using about 0·7 g. 1 ml 0·1N = 0·02412 g or 0·02052 g anhydrous.

Saccharin calcium, $C_{14}H_8O_6N_2S_2Ca, 3\frac{1}{2}H_2O$, Mol. Wt. 467·5, is assayed in the *U.S.P.* by extraction and direct titration of the residue of saccharin.

Weigh 0·5 g into a separator with 10 ml of water, add 2 ml of dilute hydrochloric acid and extract the precipitated saccharin with 30, 20, 20, 20 and 20 ml of a mixture of 9 volumes of chloroform and 1 volume of 95 per cent ethanol, filtering each extract through a small filter paper rinsed with the solvent. Evaporate the filtrates to dryness, on a water-bath under a current of air, and dissolve the residue in 75 ml of hot water. Cool and titrate with 0·1N sodium hydroxide using phenolphthalein as indicator. 1 ml 0·1N = 0·02022 g $C_{14}H_8O_6N_2S_2Ca$.

The hydrolysis of saccharin into the acid ammonium salt of sulphobenzoic acid is effected directly with hydrochloric acid but the time required for completion is somewhat longer.

After acid hydrolysis to ammonia, distillation of even small amounts (20 mg) gives accurate determinations provided conditions are rigorously standardised. All-glass distillation apparatus is necessary and after hydrolysis a current of air should be passed through the flask to remove acid vapour; direct distillation is carried on until salt commences to separate and 0·02N acid is used for absorption of the distillate and titration with Kjeldahl indicator (methyl red solution to which sufficient 1 per cent methylene blue has been added to give a green colour; the end-point is sharp from pink through colourless to green). A blank, carried out exactly as the test, must be done.

Lerrigo and Williams[2] studied the reactions of saccharin for the determination of **small amounts.** They recommended the method of conversion into ammonia by acid hydrolysis. The following was the procedure finally adopted:

Evaporate the ethereal extract from an acidified sample (see below) in a 100-ml flask and weigh. Weigh a quantity of pure saccharin rather less than the weight of the ethereal extract into another 100-ml flask. Add 25 ml of approximately 3N hydrochloric acid to each, cover the flasks with watch-glasses and place on a water-bath for two hours. Cool, make alkaline to litmus paper with approximately 3N sodium hydroxide and make up to 100 ml.

Nesslerise aliquot parts of these two solutions. A quantity equivalent to between 0·5 to 1·0 mg is most convenient. Comparison against a known amount of saccharin is necessary as the colour produced by a solution of hydrolysed saccharin differs in tint from that given by a standard solution of ammonium chloride. All reagents and dilutions should be made with ammonia-free water.

Saccharin is more easily extracted by ether from aqueous solutions if they are rendered strongly acid (0·7N) with hydrochloric acid and saturated with salt. It is almost insoluble in light petroleum or carbon tetrachloride and solutions may be freed from fat by a preliminary extraction with either of these solvents.

A determination of sulphur content may be used for the assay of saccharin.

To the residue from ether extraction add, in a platinum dish, sufficient sodium carbonate solution to make the mixture alkaline and evaporate to dryness; add about 5 g of fusion mixture (equal parts of anhydrous sodium carbonate and potassium carbonate) and heat to complete fusion for thirty minutes. Dissolve the cooled melt in water, add 5 ml of bromine water, acidify carefully with hydrochloric acid, boil free from bromine and filter if necessary. Precipitate the sulphate as barium sulphate. $BaSO_4 \times 0{\cdot}7848$ = saccharin.

Saccharin may be separated from benzoic acid by extraction of the latter in strongly buffered solution of pH 4·0.[3]

Benzoic acid: To a suitable volume of sample add 20 ml of buffer solution (10 per cent sodium citrate and 6·5 per cent citric acid adjusted to pH 4·0) and extract three times with 25 ml of ether, washing each extract with a few millilitres of water and reserving the washings. Filter through a dry paper, remove the ether at a low temperature, the last few millilitres at room temperature. To the residue add 3 ml of pure acetone and remove cautiously. Dissolve the residue in a further 2 ml of acetone, add 2 ml of water and titrate with 0·05N sodium hydroxide using phenol red as indicator. 1 ml 0·05N = 0·0061 g benzoic acid.

Saccharin: To the aqueous residues and washing add 10 ml of concentrated hydrochloric acid and extract with three 25-ml quantities of ether. Wash the bulked ether with two portions each of 10 ml of water; wash the bulked aqueous washings once with ether. Filter the total ether extracts and washings through a dry paper and remove the ether, add 3 ml of acetone, evaporate, add 2 ml of water and titrate with 0·05N sodium hydroxide using bromothymol blue as indicator. 1 ml 0·05N = 0·00916 g saccharin.

A check on the result is easily made by Kjeldahl nitrogen determination on the recovered saccharin as indicated above; this is often desirable when the saccharin content is higher than the expected amount.

Parikh and Mukherji[4] have described a volumetric method for the determination of saccharin by quantitative precipitation of its silver salt with subsequent titration of excess silver nitrate. In our hands, however, low results were obtained when this method was applied to saccharin and saccharin sodium; these were shown by experiment to be due to the solubility of the silver saccharinate.

Tablets of Saccharin, *B.P.C.* Made to contain the equivalent of $\frac{1}{5}$ grain of saccharin sodium per tablet, or a mixture of saccharin with an excess of sodium bicarbonate.

The saccharin may be determined exactly as above, using 25 tablets, but Richmond *et al.*[5] preferred direct hydrolysis if theobroma emulsion or saponaceous material has been used for granulation, because frothing may be troublesome in alkaline solution:

To determine the alkalinity, dissolve a known weight of tablets in 0·1N hydrochloric acid, boil to eliminate carbon dioxide and titrate back to phenolphthalein.

To 20 tablets in a 200-ml Kjeldahl flask, add approximately 4N hydrochloric acid equivalent to the alkalinity, then 25 ml of 4N hydrochloric acid and water to make the volume up to 50 ml. Boil under reflux for an hour and a half, then, after adding a little pumice and paraffin wax, make alkaline with sodium hydroxide and distil the ammonia produced into excess of 0·1N acid as usual.

Addition of barium or calcium hydroxide before the alkaline distillation of the ammonia will also eliminate frothing.

Calcium cyclamate may be present with saccharin salts in pharmaceutical preparations; the latter may be determined, after preliminary extraction of interference with chloroform, by ultra-violet absorption at 266 mμ or by extraction with ether from an acidified solution and then using one of the methods given above, such as fusion and barium sulphate precipitation.

Calcium cyclamate, $C_{12}H_{24}O_6N_2S_2Ca,2H_2O$, Mol. Wt. 432·6. This material is officially assayed in the *U.S.P.* by a Kjeldahl determination of nitrogen but it may be determined through its organic sulphur content, a method particularly useful in compounded preparations. To an appropriate amount of sample, acidified with dilute hydrochloric acid, barium chloride is added and allowed to stand for thirty minutes. The solution is filtered, if necessary, then 10 ml of 10 per cent sodium nitrite is added and the solution digested on a water-bath until the supernatant liquid is clear. After filtering and washing, the precipitate of barium sulphate is ignited. $BaSO_4 \times 0{\cdot}92606 = C_{12}H_{24}O_6N_2S_2Ca, 2H_2O$.

Sodium cyclamate, $C_6H_{12}O_3NSNa$, Mol. Wt. 201·2. This substance is also assayed in the *N.F.* through its nitrogen content; in compounded preparations, the method given above under calcium cyclamate is applicable. $BaSO_4 \times 0{\cdot}8621 = C_6H_{12}O_3NSNa$.

1. Richmond, H. D., and Hill, C. A., *J. Soc. Chem. Ind.*, 1918, **37,** 246T.
2. Lerrigo, A. F., and Williams, A. L., *Analyst*, 1927, **52,** 377.
3. Jones, N. R., private communication.
4. Parikh, P. M., and Mukherji, S. P., *Analyst*, 1960, **85,** 25.
5. Richmond, H. D., Royce, S., and Hill, C. A., *Analyst*, 1918, **43,** 402.

SALICYLIC ACID

$C_6H_4OH.COOH$ Mol. Wt. 138·1

The extraction and estimation of free salicylic acid presents little difficulty. It is a comparatively strong organic acid and can be titrated directly in aqueous or ethanolic solution with standard alkali to phenolphthalein or phenol red, the former indicator not being so satisfactory in ethanolic solution. The *B.P.* method employs phenol red in weak ethanolic solution. 1 ml 0·5N = 0·06905 g.

In mixtures salicylic acid and salicylates are often best determined by extracting the salicylic acid with ether. Lerrigo[1] concluded that accurate results may be obtained either by allowing the ethereal solution to evaporate spontaneously and drying the salicylic acid at room temperature or by spontaneous evaporation and drying the residue for two hours in an oven at 35°. Hence the acid may be estimated accurately by weighing if care is taken to follow these requirements (salicylic acid × 1·159 = sodium salicylate). Salicylic acid does not volatilise appreciably until temperatures higher than 40° are reached; between 50° and 60° volatilisation becomes comparatively rapid. Another satisfactory method for isolating the acid from its moist ethereal solution is to add about 5 to 10 g of anhydrous sodium sulphate to the ether solution; after shaking, the ether is passed through cotton wool into a weighed flask and the residue washed with more ether in the usual manner. The ether is then evaporated almost to dryness, the flask removed from the source of heat and the residual ether poured out as vapour; the acid sets to a crystalline mass, which is freed from ether by a gentle current of air from bellows and can be weighed immediately it has cooled. A short period in a vacuum desiccator can be used to check the absence of any volatile matter in the residue.

Salicylic acid may also be estimated by its bromine absorption (Kolthoff[2]).

> Mix 0·03 to 0·035 g of salicylic acid with 25 ml of 0·1N potassium bromate solution (containing 15 g of potassium bromide per litre) and 5 ml of concentrated hydrochloric acid and allow to react in the dark for thirty minutes; add excess of potassium iodide and titrate with 0·1N sodium thiosulphate. Repeat the operation omitting the sample. 1 ml 0·1N bromine = 0·002302 g $C_7H_6O_3$.

The salicylic acid with excess of bromine first forms tribromosalicylic acid, which loses carbon dioxide to form tribromophenol, the latter reacting with more bromine to give tribromophenylhypobromite. On treatment with potassium iodide in acid solution tribromophenol is liberated again; hence 1 mol. of salicylic acid is equivalent to 6 atoms of bromine. Salicylic acid should not be extracted with alkali from ether solutions for subsequent bromination as the dissolved ether causes high results; chloroform also can lead to high results, especially if it is heated, when some decomposition of the chloroform to formic acid may occur.

The bromine process is particularly useful in the presence of benzoic acid (*cf.* Compound Ointment of Benzoic Acid) which does not react with bromine. According to Kolthoff[3] the precipitate of tribromophenol may be filtered off and the benzoic acid isolated from the filtrate.

Salicylic acid may be separated from other phenols by its solubility in sodium bicarbonate solution, phenols being extracted by organic solvents from this medium.

The well-known colorimetric method, which depends on matching the violet colour the acid gives with ferric salts against known amounts of pure acid, may be used for determining **small quantities** of salicylic acid. Nicholls[4] observed that, contrary to the usual statements in the literature, the ferric salicylate test was best performed in slightly, but appreciably, acid solution in order to obtain a satisfactory tint. The minimum acidity required to produce a good violet colour was about 0·001N of mineral acid but the intensity of colour diminished with increasing acidity, 0·002N acidity being found suitable for use. For accurate colorimetric work the quantity of salicylic acid present should not exceed 0·8 mg per 100 ml. The *A.O.A.C.*[5] uses a 2 per cent ferric alum solution which has been boiled until a precipitate appears and then filtered. The acidity of the solution is thereby slightly increased but the turbidity caused by its dilution with water, which interferes with the exact matching of the colours, is much less and does not interfere as much as when the unboiled solution is used.

Application of Salicylic Acid and Sulphur, *B.P.C.* Contains 2·08 per cent each of salicylic acid and sublimed sulphur in aqueous cream.

The salicylic acid can be assayed by refluxing about 5 g for fifteen minutes with 20 ml of 5 per cent sodium hydroxide, filtering through a wet filter paper, washing and diluting to 100 ml in a graduated flask; 50 ml of this solution is brominated as above.

The sulphur can be determined directly by the method for Sulphur Ointment (see p. 614) or by flask-combustion.

Collodion of Salicylic Acid, *B.P.C.* Contains 12 per cent of salicylic acid dissolved in flexible collodion. The salicylic acid can be determined by direct titration: 2 ml is washed out from a pipette with a mixture of three parts of ether and one part of ethanol, previously neutralised to phenol red, and titrated directly with 0·1N sodium hydroxide to this indicator. 1 ml = 0·01381 g.

Compound Dusting-powder of Salicylic Acid, *B.P.C.* Consists of 3 per cent salicylic acid and 5 per cent boric acid with talc.

For routine purposes the salicylic acid may be determined directly by bromination as above, and the boric acid by a short ignition to remove salicylic acid and titration of the residue; the loss of boric acid by volatilisation is negligible if the ignition is not protracted.

The *B.P.C.* method of assay dissolves the boric acid and salicylic acid with dilute alkali followed by filtration. The salicylic acid is extracted as usual with ether after acidification and after evaporation of the ether is determined by titration with sodium hydroxide in ethanolic solution. The boric acid is titrated in the aqueous residue after neutralisation to methyl orange.

Dusting-powder of Zinc and Salicylic Acid, *B.P.C.* Zinc oxide, 20 per cent and salicylic acid, 5 per cent, with starch.

Some combination between zinc oxide and salicylic acid may occur in the presence of moisture and low results are obtained if the salicylic acid is titrated directly. Mitchell[6] recommends extraction of the salicylic acid with ether after acidification and titration after evaporation of the solvent; this is the method employed by the *B.P.C.* The zinc oxide may be determined by titration of the aqueous solutions with standard acid in the presence of ammonium chloride or by EDTA (see p. 696).

Lotion of Salicylic Acid and Mercuric Chloride, *B.P.C.* Mercuric chloride 0·114 per cent, salicylic acid 2·29 per cent with castor oil, acetone and alcohol.

Assay for salicylic acid: To 20 ml, diluted with 30 ml of water, add 20 per cent sodium hydroxide solution until just alkaline to litmus paper and extract with two 20-ml quantities of ether, washing each extract with the same 5 ml of water. Discard the ether extracts, add the aqueous washing to the alkaline layer, make acid to litmus paper with concentrated sulphuric acid and determine the salicylic acid as usual, by titration with alkali after extraction with ether and evaporation of the solvent.

For mercury, see p. 416.

Ointment of Salicylic Acid, *B.P.* 2 per cent salicylic acid in ointment of wool alcohols.

A somewhat empirical, but reasonably accurate, estimation of the salicylic acid can be obtained by direct titration of about 10 g of ointment in ether and ethanol with 0·1N alkali to phenol red. Deduct 0·10 per cent from the percentage obtained to allow for the acidity of the wool alcohols present in the ointment which titrate to phenol red.

A more accurate determination is by boiling a weighed quantity of ointment with portions of dilute alkali solution until the acid is completely extracted, and then determining the salicylic acid in the aqueous liquid by bromination as above.

Ointment of Salicylic Acid and Sulphur, *B.P.C.* Salicylic acid 3 per cent and sublimed sulphur 3 per cent in oily cream.

Assay for salicylic acid: Dissolve in light petroleum (b.p. 40° to 60°), extract with 0·5 per cent sodium carbonate solution, make just acid to phenolphthalein by the cautious addition of concentrated hydrochloric acid and then just alkaline with 0·5N sodium hydroxide and complete by Kolthoff's method above.

For sulphur, determine as for Sulphur Ointment, p. 614, or by flask-combustion.

Salicylic Acid Self-adhesive Plaster, *B.P.C.* Suitable cloth spread evenly with a self-adhesive plaster mass containing 20 per cent of salicylic acid.

The salicylic acid is leached out with boiling water. Since it is appreciably volatile in steam the *B.P.C.* method should be modified by using a reflux condenser.

To 3 g, accurately weighed and cut into strips, in a round-bottomed flask fitted with a reflux condenser, add 200 ml of water and boil for twenty minutes. Filter through glass wool, return the residue on the filter to the flask, boil with a further 100 ml of water for ten minutes and filter. Continue the process with further quantities, each of 50 ml, of water, boiling for ten minutes each time, until the salicylic acid is completely extracted, combine the filtrates and titrate with 0·1N sodium hydroxide using phenolphthalein as indicator. 1 ml 0·1N = 0·0138 g.

SALICYLATES

The *B.P.* method for the estimation of **sodium salicylate,** $C_7H_5O_3Na$, Mol. Wt. 160·1, is the same as for sodium benzoate (p. 125) and is a modification of Henville's method,[7] using bromophenol blue instead of methyl orange. 1 ml 0·5N = 0·08005 g.

The estimation of sodium salicylate by the determination of the alkalinity of its ash was shown by Harrison and Carter[8] to be inaccurate when the ash was titrated directly. They suggested the following modification as being preferable:

Ash about 1·5 g, without fusion, to a carbonaceous residue; extract with boiling water and filter. Repeat the extraction and filtering. Ash the filter paper and carbon at dull red heat, dissolve the white ash obtained in water and add it to the other filtrates. Add excess of standard acid, heat to boiling, filter again and titrate back to methyl orange. 1 ml 0·5N = 0·08005 g.

Mixture of Colchicum and Sodium Salicylate, *B.P.C.* Contains 6·86 per cent each of sodium salicylate and potassium bicarbonate, with tincture of colchicum and extract of liquorice in chloroform water.

Assay for sodium salicylate: To 5 ml add 10 ml of dilute hydrochloric acid and extract with six 25-ml quantities of chloroform. Combine the extracts, wash with successive small quantities of water until the washings are free from chloride and then evaporate the chloroform at as low a temperature as possible, under a jet of air. Dissolve the residue in 10 ml of neutral 95 per cent ethanol and titrate with 0·1N sodium hydroxide using phenolphthalein as indicator. 1 ml 0·1N = 0·01601 g.

For potassium bicarbonate: Boil 10 ml for ten minutes under a reflux condenser with 150 ml of water and 25 ml of 0·5N hydrochloric acid, cool and titrate the excess acid with 0·5N sodium hydroxide to phenolphthalein. 1 ml 0·5N = 0·05005 g $KHCO_3$.

Mixture of Sodium Salicylate, *B.P.C.* Contains 4·57 per cent of sodium salicylate and 3·43 per cent of sodium bicarbonate, with sodium metabisulphite, concentrated orange peel infusion and chloroform water.

The assays for sodium salicylate and sodium bicarbonate are the same as given for Mixture of Colchicum and Sodium Salicylate, using 10 ml of the preparation.

Tablets of Sodium Salicylate, *B.P.C.* Usually contain 5 grains.

Dissolve an amount of powdered tablets equivalent to 0·3 g of sodium salicylate as completely as possible, in 25 ml of water, add 2 ml of concentrated hydrochloric acid and extract with successive 20-ml quantities of ether until complete extraction is effected, washing each extract with the same 5 ml of water. Combine the extracts, evaporate the ether (observing the precautions given on p. 557), dissolve the residue in 3 ml of neutral 95 per cent ethanol, add 15 ml of water and titrate with 0·1N sodium hydroxide to phenol red. 1 ml 0·1N = 0·01601 g.

AMINOSALICYLIC ACID, $C_7H_7O_3N$, Mol. Wt. 153·1

Aminosalicylic acid and its salts may be determined either by bromination or by titration with nitrite. The acid itself, official in the *U.S.P.*, is determined by titration with nitrite, the end-point being detected externally with starch-iodide paste. A more satisfactory method is to determine the end-point electrometrically by the 'dead-stop' technique (see p. 867). A suitable method is as follows:

> Dissolve 0·5 g in 75 ml of water in a beaker and add 10 ml of concentrated hydrochloric acid. Then add 1 g of potassium bromide and stir mechanically until dissolved. Titrate slowly with 0·1M sodium nitrite, running the solution in below the surface of the liquid in the beaker and stirring continuously; determine the end-point electrometrically ('dead-stop' technique). 1 ml 0·1M = 0·01531 g $C_7H_7O_3N$.

Sodium aminosalicylate, $C_7H_6O_3NNa,2H_2O$, Mol. Wt. 211·2, is determined in the *B.P.* by titration with bromine as follows:

> Dissolve 0·3 g in 80 ml of a mixture of equal volumes of water and glacial acetic acid, warm to 40°, add 10 ml of concentrated hydrochloric acid and titrate with 0·5N bromine until the mixture, after being allowed to stand for one minute, immediately gives a distinct blue ring when a drop is placed on starch-iodide paper. 1 ml 0·5N = 0·01459 g $C_7H_6O_3NNa$.

The nitrite titration described above is equally applicable (1 ml 0·1M = 0·01751 g $C_7H_6O_3NNa$) and for formulated products, such as sugar-coated tablets, it is preferable since it is less susceptible to error caused by tablet excipients and coating.

Tablets of Sodium Aminosalicylate, *B.P.* Usually contain 0·5 g. They may be determined by the following method, although some workers claim that a more satisfactory end-point is obtained if potassium bromide is included, as in the method given above and in the method of the *U.S.P.*

> Shake a weight of powdered tablets equivalent to about 0·6 g of sodium aminosalicylate with 75 ml of water until the sodium aminosalicylate is completely dissolved and dilute to 100 ml. Filter if necessary, rejecting the first 20 ml of the filtrate and to 50 ml of the solution add 150 ml of water, 25 g of crushed ice and 10 ml of concentrated hydrochloric acid and titrate slowly with 0·1M sodium nitrite, stirring vigorously and continuing the titration until the mixture, after being allowed to stand for two minutes, immediately gives a blue colour when a drop is drawn across the surface of a film of starch-iodide paste. 1 ml 0·1M $NaNO_2$ = 0·02112 g $C_7H_6O_3NNa$, $2H_2O$.

Calcium aminosalicylate, $C_{14}H_{12}O_6N_2Ca,\frac{1}{2}H_2O$, Mol. Wt. 353·4, or $C_{14}H_{12}O_6N_2Ca$, $3H_2O$, Mol. Wt. 398·4, may be determined by the method given for the sodium salt. Calcium can be assayed either by permanganate titration after precipitation as oxalate, or by EDTA.

p-HYDROXYBENZOIC ACID, $C_6H_4(OH)COOH$, Mol. Wt. 138·1

The methyl and propyl esters of this acid and the sodium derivatives of these esters are all widely used in pharmaceutical preparations. Direct bromimetric assay as under Salicylic Acid leads to high results for the esters because of the immediate hydrolysis of a small portion of the ester in the presence of alkali necessary for solution. It is preferable to hydrolyse the material completely before bromination.

Boil about 0·1 g with 50 ml of N sodium hydroxide for thirty minutes under reflux. Cool, add 50 ml of 0·1N bromine and 10 ml of concentrated hydrochloric acid. Allow to stand for half an hour, shaking repeatedly during the first fifteen minutes, add 2 g of potassium iodide and titrate the liberated iodine with 0·1N sodium thiosulphate. 1 ml of 0·1N bromine = 0·002536 g methyl hydroxybenzoate, $C_8H_8O_3$; 0·002902 g sodium salt of the methyl ester; 0·003003 g propyl hydroxybenzoate, $C_{10}H_{12}O_3$, and 0·003370 g sodium salt of the propyl ester.

The hydrolysis can be used quantitatively although the neutralisation point is difficult to assess. The *U.S.P.* uses the following method:

Weigh 2 g into a flask and add 40 ml of N sodium hydroxide, rinsing the sides of the flask with water. Cover with a watch-glass, boil gently for one hour and then cool. Add 5 drops of bromothymol blue indicator and titrate the excess alkali with N sulphuric acid, titrating to pH 6·5 by matching the colour with that of phosphate buffer solution, pH 6·5 containing the same proportion of indicator. 1 ml N sodium hydroxide = 0·1522 g $C_8H_8O_3$ or 0·1802 g $C_{10}H_{12}O_3$.

The *para* acid is not volatile in steam and can thus be separated from benzoic acid. After hydrolysis the acid is extracted from the acidified solution with ether. It can be determined colorimetrically in the extract with Millon's reagent by the method of Edwards, Nanji and Hassan.[9]

Extract the hydrolysed material in acid solution with three portions of ether, and re-extract the bulked ethereal extracts with 10-ml portions of dilute ammonia solution. Remove the excess of ammonia by boiling until neutral. Cool the neutral solution and dilute to 100 ml. To 20 ml of the neutral solution, containing not more than 2 mg of *para* acid, add 2 ml of Millon's reagent. Prepare a series of standards containing from 1 to 10 ml of an aqueous solution of *para* acid (1 ml = 0·1 mg) each diluted to 20 ml with water and add 2 ml of Millon's reagent to each. Heat the test solution and standards in a water-bath for exactly two minutes, dilute immediately to 50 ml and compare the rose-red colour produced. Salicylic acid interferes with this determination.

Although the esters of *p*-hydroxybenzoic acid are not directly determinable by the 4-aminophenazone method (see p. 514) they can easily be converted to the acid by a preliminary hydrolysis and the general method can then be applied. Johnson and Savidge[10] have found the following procedure to be satisfactory for the determination of methyl and propyl *p*-hydroxybenzoates in a number of preparations.

Transfer 10 ml of sample containing 0·2 per cent of methyl *p*-hydroxybenzoate to a flask, washing in with 10 ml of water. Add 25 ml of N sodium hydroxide and reflux gently for two hours. Wash down the condenser with water, cool and transfer to a 1-litre graduated flask containing 5 ml of 25 per cent ammonium chloride solution, washing the original flask with water and adding the washings to the graduated flask. Dilute to volume with water, mix and filter, rejecting the first few millilitres of filtrate. Pipette 10 ml of the filtrate into a 150-ml separator and proceed as described in the general method (chloroform extraction procedure)—

see under Phenol (p. 514)—beginning with the words 'add 1 ml of 4-aminophenazone solution . . .'.

1. Lerrigo, A. F., *Analyst*, 1926, **51,** 79.
2. Kolthoff, I. M., *Pharm. Weekblad.*, 1921, **58,** 699.
3. Kolthoff, I. M., *Pharm. Weekblad.*, 1932, **69,** 1159.
4. Nicholls, J. R., *Analyst*, 1928, **53,** 19.
5. *A.O.A.C.*, 1960, p. 399.
6. Mitchell, J. V., *Pharm. J.*, 1954, **172,** 102.
7. Henville, D., *Analyst*, 1927, **52,** 149.
8. Harrison, J. B. P., and Carter, F. E., *Pharm. J.*, 1919, **103,** 230.
9. Edwards, F. W., Nanji, H. R., and Hassan, M. K., *Analyst*, 1937, **62,** 178.
10. Johnson, C. A., and Savidge, R. A., *J. Pharm. Pharmacol.*, 1958, **10,** 171T.

SANTONICA

Santonica (wormseed) consists of the dried, unexpanded flower-heads of *Artemisia cina* Berg, and is almost exclusively used as a source of the lactone **santonin,** $C_{15}H_{18}O_3$, Mol. Wt. 246·3, of which it contains 2 to 3·5 per cent. Methods of assay are designed for the determination of this substance.

Various processes have been devised, of which the method of Fromme (Engelhardt and O'Brian[1]) is probably the most widely applied. The barium salt of santonin is filtered from inert matter and the liberated santonin is extracted and recrystallised:

Shake 13 g of the drug, well-bruised in a mortar, with 130 g of chloroform in a conical flask occasionally for an hour. Filter, keeping the funnel covered, and take 102·5 g of the solution (= 10 g of drug) in a tared 200-ml conical flask. Distil off the chloroform until the residue weighs 7 to 8 g. Add 100 g of 5 per cent barium hydroxide solution, mix and drive off the residue of chloroform by means of a water-bath. Filter, wash the filter with a little boiling water and acidify with 5 g of hydrochloric acid (25 per cent w/w HCl). Heat on a water-bath for two minutes to convert the lactone into acid and, while lukewarm, transfer to a separator. Rinse the flask with 20 ml of chloroform and run this into the separator. Shake briskly for two minutes, draw off the chloroform into a 100-ml flask and extract the aqueous liquid twice more with chloroform, using 20 ml each time. Evaporate the chloroform and take up the residue in 7·5 g of ethanol with the aid of heat, then mix with 42·5 g of hot water. Filter the milky solution immediately into a tared 100-ml flask, rinse the flask and filter with two 10-ml portions of a mixture of ethanol 3 g and hot water 17 g and allow to stand for twenty-four hours. Collect the santonin on a tared filter, wash the flask and filter with two portions each of 10 ml of a mixture of ethanol 3 g and water 17 g; dry the flask and filter to constant weight. To the weight of santonin thus found add 0·04 g, the amount of santonin remaining dissolved in the ethanolic solution.

The crystals of santonin are large and the washing with dilute ethanol is not believed to dissolve any appreciable amount. The crystals generally contain resin; this can be titrated in ethanolic solution to phenolphthalein and subtracted from the total weight of santonin crystals.

Although reasonably accurate results can be obtained by this method it is not completely satisfactory, since the correction for the santonin left in solution is equivalent to 20 per cent of the santonin actually recovered in the assay and this correction figure must vary with temperature.

By a modification of the quantity of liquid from which the crystallisation was made, Corfield[2] found it possible to reduce the correction and obtain very accurate results.

To avoid processes for which solubility corrections have to be applied Coutts[3] devised a gravimetric method of assay which he claims is applicable to the examination of all classes of crude drugs containing santonin. In this process, similar in principle to that of Fromme, crystallisation is induced from aqueous solution, no correction for solubility being necessary:

> Extract 14 g of dried, coarsely powdered drug, by shaking frequently during six hours with 140 ml of crystallisable benzene; filter off 101 ml of the liquid and shake briskly for five minutes in a separator with 35 ml of 8 per cent sodium carbonate solution. Allow separation to take place (thirty minutes), and decant 80·5 ml of the benzene solution, corresponding to 8 g of the drug, into a flask and evaporate to dryness on a water-bath. Extract the residue by heating for ten minutes with 60 ml of saturated barium hydroxide solution at 95°, and immediately filter the solution into a flask. Wash the flask and filter paper with two 10-ml portions of saturated barium hydroxide solution at 95° and unite the filtrates. Plug the flask with cotton wool and allow the solution to cool, make slightly acid by the addition of 5 ml of 25 per cent hydrochloric acid and set aside for twenty-four hours to crystallise, gently agitating the mixture occasionally. Collect the crystals in a tared Gooch crucible, washing any crystals remaining in the flask into the crucible with small portions of the filtrate. Finally wash the crucible and crystals with 10 ml of cold water and dry to constant weight at 100°. Cool in a desiccator. The weight of santonin is that present in 8 g of the crude drug.

The accuracy of the method appears to be controversial, Corfield[4] asserting that it gives results 30 per cent too low. Conversely other analysts have at least obtained comparable results (Coutts,[5] Janot and Estève[6]).

A further gravimetric method, which has given satisfactory results with plant material, has been published by Qazilbash[7] and the method, with later modifications,[8] is the following:

> Shake 15 g of finely powdered santonica thoroughly with 1·5 g of powdered anhydrous sodium carbonate. Shake the mixture in a 500-ml separator with 15 ml of 15 per cent ammonia solution for a few minutes, add 150 ml of benzene and shake thoroughly at frequent intervals during three hours. After allowing to stand overnight shake thoroughly for fifteen minutes and allow to settle for half an hour, then carefully filter

through cotton wool, previously moistened with benzene, into a 100-ml measuring cylinder. During filtration cover the stem of the cylinder to avoid the loss of benzene by evaporation. Transfer 100 ml of the filtrate to a distilling flask; this represents 10 g of the drug. Rinse the measuring cylinder with a little benzene and add the washing to the distilling flask. Concentrate the benzene extract to about 15 ml and transfer to a beaker, rinsing the distilling flask two or three times with 5 ml of benzene. Evaporate the combined benzene extract completely to dryness. Heat the residue for about twenty minutes on a water-bath with 110 ml of 5 per cent w/v barium hydroxide solution, freshly prepared and filtered, stirring the contents of the beaker carefully with a glass rod during this time. A yellowish-green or dark green resinous solid separates. Filter the hot solution of the barium salt through a double filter paper, previously moistened with water, wash the filter and beaker twice with 10 ml of hot water and acidify the filtrate with dilute hydrochloric acid. Add a slight excess of acid and leave the mixture in a water-bath for about twenty minutes, stirring gently at short intervals. After fifteen minutes test the solution with congo red paper, and if the acid reaction is not well marked, add 1 or 2 ml of acid. Allow the acidified solution to cool and transfer to a separator when lukewarm. Rinse the beaker with 25 ml of chloroform, add the washing to the separator and shake the contents for five minutes. After separation pass the chloroform layer through a pledget of cotton wool, moistened with chloroform, into an Erlenmeyer flask. Repeat the process with three successive quantities of 20, 15 and 10 ml of chloroform. Evaporate the combined chloroform solutions to dryness and blow air through the residue to free from traces of chloroform. Boil the residue with 50 ml of 15 per cent w/w ethanol under a reflux condenser for 15 minutes and filter hot. Wash the flask and filter three times with 5 ml of warm 15 per cent ethanol. Heat the filtrate with 100 mg of a mixture of equal parts of animal charcoal and kieselguhr under a reflux condenser for about ten minutes to remove resinous and colloidal impurities, then filter hot into an Erlenmeyer flask. Rinse the residue and filter three times with 5 ml of 15 per cent ethanol. Allow the filtrate to crystallise, scratching the sides of the dish gently with a glass rod to hasten crystallisation. Keep the dish in the dark at 15° to 17° for twenty-four hours. Collect the crystals of santonin carefully on a weighed filter paper, and measure the volume of the filtrate. Wash the crystals twice with 5 ml of 15 per cent ethanol, dry to constant weight at 100° to 105° and place in a desiccator over concentrated sulphuric acid for twenty-four hours. Determine the weight of santonin and add 6·4 mg per 100 ml of filtrate as a solubility correction. The total weight multiplied by 10 gives the percentage of santonin.

The *A.O.A.C.*[9] use 2,4-dinitrophenylhydrazine as precipitant but Janot and Mouton[10] criticise this method for, although santonin can be recovered from dilute ethanolic solution as the dinitrophenylhydrazone to an accuracy of 3 per cent, too high results are obtained in the evaluation of wormseed. Other ketonic compounds are present, the chief of which is artemisin, which will also be precipitated.

A colorimetric method for the determination of santonin in *Artemisia* has recently been published by Khan and Mohiuddin;[11] the colour development has been found applicable to the determination of santonin isolated from formulated products.

Extraction of santonin: Grind 2 g of finely powdered sample in a mortar with 0·5 g of calcium oxide and then triturate with 5 ml of hot water. Transfer the mixture to a 400-ml beaker with 120 ml of hot water, heat to boiling-point and boil gently for ten minutes. Filter while hot, wash the residue with 120 ml of boiling water and acidify the filtrate with 10 ml of concentrated hydrochloric acid. Allow to stand on a water-bath for five minutes, cool and transfer to a separator. Extract with four successive quantities of 30, 20, 20 and 10 ml of chloroform, shaking vigorously each time and combining the extracts in a second separator. Shake the contents of the second separator with two 15-ml quantities of 4 per cent sodium hydroxide solution and then wash with 10 ml of water to remove the alkali. Filter through a cotton-wool plug into a 250-ml flask, add 0·1 g of animal charcoal and reflux gently on a water-bath for ten minutes. Filter rapidly through a double filter paper (Whatman No. 41) into a second 250-ml flask and wash the first flask and the filter with two 5-ml quantities of chloroform, adding the washings to the filtrate. Evaporate the chloroform and gently dry the residue. Add 2 ml of 95 per cent ethanol and again evaporate to dryness to ensure complete removal of chloroform. Then add 20 ml of 18 per cent v/v ethanol and 0·1 g of animal charcoal and reflux gently on a water-bath for ten minutes. Filter rapidly while hot through a double filter paper into a 50-ml graduated flask, wash the flask and filter with two 5-ml quantities of hot 18 per cent v/v ethanol and dilute to volume with 95 per cent v/v ethanol.

Colour development: Pipette 3 ml of the prepared solution into a second 50-ml graduated flask and add 2 ml of a freshly prepared 7·5 per cent solution of hydroxylamine hydrochloride in N sodium hydroxide followed by 5 ml of N sodium hydroxide. Allow to stand for five minutes, add 3 drops of a 0·1 per cent solution of 2,4-dinitrophenol in 90 per cent ethanol and titrate with N hydrochloric acid to a colourless end-point. Dilute to volume with water. Transfer a 5-ml aliquot to a dry test-tube, add 1 ml of 2·0 per cent aqueous ferric chloride solution and shake thoroughly to mix. Within three minutes, measure the extinction at the maximum at about 500 mμ, using 1-cm cells with water in the comparison cell and taking care that the solution is free from air bubbles. Correct for a reagent blank determined using 2 ml of 50 per cent v/v ethanol instead of the sample solution and read the per cent santonin from a standard curve.

Prepare the standard curve using suitable volumes, covering the range 1 to 5 mg, of a standard solution of santonin, *B.P.*, in 50 per cent v/v ethanol, containing 1 mg of santonin per ml.

Tablets of Santonin, *B.P.C.* Usually contain 1 grain of santonin and are prepared in a chocolate basis. These tablets need a preliminary extraction of the fat with light petroleum saturated with santonin before extraction of the santonin with chloroform.

François[12] suggests the following method for the analysis of santonin chocolate tablets:

Add 10 g of slaked lime to 10 tablets, finely ground in a glass mortar, and triturate well to give a homogeneous mixture. Transfer to a 125-ml conical flask and heat with 50 ml of 95 per cent ethanol to just below the boiling-point under reflux for an hour. Filter and repeat the digestion of the residue twice. Add 100 ml of water and distil off the ethanol. Cool, filter off the fat, add 10 drops of concentrated hydrochloric acid to the aqueous residue and extract with chloroform, wash the chloroform, evaporate, dry and weigh the santonin.

If the base of the tablets consists only of sugar and gums, the santonin may be extracted from a known weight in solution, slightly acidified with hydrochloric acid, by chloroform and weighed.

1. ENGELHARDT, H., and O'BRIAN, L. E., *Drugg. Circ.*, 1913, **57**, 443.
2. CORFIELD, C. E., *Quart. J. Pharm.*, 1932, **5**, 553.
3. COUTTS, J., *Quart. J. Pharm.*, 1932, **5**, 369.
4. CORFIELD, C. E., *Quart. J. Pharm.*, 1934, **7**, 594.
5. COUTTS, J., *Quart. J. Pharm.*, 1934, **7**, 595.
6. JANOT, M. M., and ESTÈVE, C., *Bull. Sci. Pharmacol.*, 1933, **40**, 280.
7. QAZILBASH, N. A., *J. Pharm. Pharmacol.*, 1951, **3**, 105.
8. QAZILBASH, N. A., *J. Pharm. Pharmacol.*, 1956, **8**, 27.
9. *A.O.A.C.*, 1960, p. 545.
10. JANOT, M. M., and MOUTON, M., *Bull. Sci. Pharmacol.*, 1936, **43**, 708.
11. KHAN, R. A., and MOHIUDDIN, H., *J. Pharm. Pharmacol.*, 1960, **12**, 544.
12. FRANÇOIS, M., *J. Pharm. Chim.*, 1922, **26**, 339.

SILVER

Ag At. Wt. 107·87

Silver nitrate, $AgNO_3$, Mol. Wt. 169·9, has limited use in pharmacy. In the *B.P.* it is assayed by the classical method of precipitation as silver chloride.

Dissolve 0·5 g in water, add 3 ml of concentrated nitric acid and dilute with water to 300 ml. Protect the solution from light. Heat to about 70° and add 0·2N hydrochloric acid, dropwise, until precipitation is complete and 2 or 3 drops of the acid are present in excess. Stir until the precipitate has completely coagulated, keeping the solution hot, and then allow to cool and stand for several hours protected from light. Filter through a tared No. 4 sintered-glass filter, transferring the precipitate to the filter with the aid of 0·01N hydrochloric acid, wash several times with 0·01N hydrochloric acid and then twice with water and finally dry to constant weight at 160°. $AgCl \times 1{\cdot}185 = AgNO_3$.

The *U.S.P.* however use a volumetric assay which is also used by the *B.P.* and *B.P.C.* for other silver preparations.

Weigh 0·7 g of sample, previously powdered, and dried in the dark for four hours over silica gel, and dissolve in 50 ml of water. Add 2 ml of concentrated nitric acid and titrate with 0·1N ammonium thiocyanate, using ferric alum as indicator. 1 ml 0·1N = 0·01699 g $AgNO_3$.

Toughened Silver Nitrate, *B.P.* Contains 95 parts of silver nitrate and 5 parts of potassium nitrate, fused together and poured into suitable moulds.

It is assayed by dissolving 0·5 g in 50 ml of water, adding 5 ml of concentrated nitric acid and titrating with 0·1N ammonium thiocyanate to ferric alum, shaking vigorously when nearing the end-point. 1 ml 0·1N = 0·01699 g $AgNO_3$.

Mitigated Silver Nitrate, *B.P.C.* Contains 20 parts of $AgNO_3$ and 40 parts of KNO_3, fused together and poured into suitable moulds.

Assayed as Toughened Silver Nitrate using 1·5 g.

The organic compounds **silver protein** and **mild silver protein** may be assayed for silver by the following methods. Each in its turn has been adversely criticised but they all give reasonably accurate results:

(i) To 1 g in a Kjeldahl flask add 10 ml of concentrated sulphuric acid and 5 ml of concentrated nitric acid. Heat until colourless, adding more nitric acid if necessary. Cool, add 20 ml of water and boil off the oxides of nitrogen. Finally, add 100 ml of water and 5 ml of concentrated nitric acid and titrate with 0·1N ammonium thiocyanate, adding a small crystal of iron alum as indicator. 1 ml 0·1N = 0·01079 g Ag.

(ii) Destroy organic matter by incinerating about 2 g in a porcelain crucible, add 10 ml of concentrated nitric acid, heat until no more coloured fumes are evolved, dilute with water and titrate as in (i).

A rapid method of estimation by Kogan[1] gives good results:

(iii) To 1 g in a conical flask, add 15 ml of 1 : 1 nitric acid and boil for a few minutes until a pale yellow solution is obtained. Cool and dilute with 30 to 40 ml of water. Add potassium permanganate until a pink colour persists for one minute and finally titrate the solution as above. The end-point of this method is not always quite sharp.

Eye-drops of Silver Protein, *B.P.C.* (containing 5 per cent), and **Eye-drops of Mild Silver Protein,** *B.P.C.* (containing 20 per cent), are assayed by method (ii) above after evaporating to dryness.

1. Kogan, G., *Pharm. Zentralhalle,* 1928, **69**, 228.

SOAPS

The estimation of soaps in pharmaceutical preparations is generally made by acidifying an aqueous solution with hydrochloric acid, extracting the liberated fatty acids with ether or light petroleum, washing the solvent free from mineral acid, and evaporating the solvent. If ether is used the residual fatty acids contain moisture; the latter is eliminated by re-evaporating after adding ethanol or acetone. Slight esterification is probable by this procedure when ethanol is used. The fatty acids should be examined by the methods given under Oils and Fats.

SOAPS

The quantitative analysis of soap requires the determination of moisture, insoluble matter, total and free alkali, uncombined fat, total and free fatty acids, resin acids and fillers. Fillers are unusual in pharmaceutical soaps.

Moisture. The moisture determined by drying at 110° is usually sufficiently accurate so long as only a thin layer of soap is used; the portion of soap for analysis should be taken from the centre of the cake. Alternatively the soap may be dissolved in ethanol and evaporated on sand to constant weight at 110°.

Another method is to determine the moisture by distillation with toluene or xylene in a Dean and Stark apparatus (p. 803), adding 10 g of lump resin, stearic acid, or anhydrous barium chloride to prevent frothing.

Alcohol-insoluble matter (carbonate, chloride, silica, fillers, etc.). This is determined as the residue obtained after refluxing 5 to 10 g of dried soap with neutral 95 per cent ethanol (or preferably dehydrated ethanol), filtering hot through a tared Gooch crucible, washing with hot 95 per cent ethanol, drying and weighing. This is sufficiently accurate for sodium soaps, but the solubility of potassium carbonate in ethanol is large enough to introduce serious errors (see Determination of Free Carbonate Alkali).

Silica is determined by washing the weighed residue with hot water until free from soluble matter; the Gooch is again dried and weighed.

Carbonate and chloride dissolve in the aqueous washings, and after neutralisation the chloride can be titrated with 0·1N silver nitrate.

The results are calculated to sodium salts for hard soaps and potassium salts for soft soaps. The titration solution should be tested for borate and silicate, since if these were present they would be included in any determination of alkalinity and methods would have to be modified accordingly.

Total Alkali. The total alkali is measured by dissolving a known weight of the soap in hot water and titrating with 0·5N acid to methyl orange, 1 ml 0·5N = 0·02355 g K_2O or 0·0155 g Na_2O; also the soap may be ashed first and then titrated.

Total Free Alkali. The Analytical Methods Committee of the *S.A.C.*[1] has exhaustively studied the methods for the determination of free alkali, and its conclusions (which counter some previously accepted methods, particularly that for determination of free alkali in potash soaps) are given below. The recommendations have been adopted by the *B.P.*

Boil 100 ml of re-distilled industrial methylated spirit (95 per cent) in a 400-ml flask, add 0·5 ml of a 0·5 per cent phenolphthalein solution, allow to cool to 70° and neutralise at that temperature with 0·1N ethanolic potassium hydroxide. Add 10 g of the soap in thin shavings and dissolve it as quickly as possible by heating. Immediately after complete solution of the soap add 3 ml of N sulphuric acid and boil on a water-bath for at least ten minutes to ensure complete removal of carbon dioxide. If the solution is colourless, cool to 70° and titrate back with N sodium hydroxide until the pink colour reappears. If, after the boiling with acid, the pink colour returns, a further quantity of N sulphuric acid must be added and the boiling repeated, the titration being completed as described above. The excess of N sulphuric acid titrated should be not less than 1 ml. From the amount of standard acid absorbed calculate the total free alkali in terms of Na_2O (or of K_2O in the case of a potash soap).

Free Caustic Alkali. As potassium carbonate was found to be appreciably soluble even in dehydrated ethanol, direct titration methods for potash soaps are impracticable, but for sodium soaps only slightly high results are obtained.

(*a*) For sodium soaps (in the absence of much carbonate and in the absence of more than about 0·4 per cent total free alkali, calculated as Na_2O):

> Boil 100 ml of industrial methylated spirit (95 per cent) to remove carbon dioxide. Add 0·5 ml of 0·5 per cent phenolphthalein solution and neutralise at 70° with 0·1N acid or alkali. Add 10 g of the soap in shavings or powder and heat until dissolved. Cool to 70° and titrate at that temperature with 0·1N sulphuric acid.

When more than 0·4 per cent of total free alkali is present it is necessary to remove this with barium chloride. As addition of barium chloride to an ethanolic solution of a soap, neutral to phenolphthalein, causes the reaction to become slightly acid (probably owing to the precipitation of a basic barium compound), the results obtained for free caustic alkali by this method tend to be low. The error due to this cause may be reduced by increasing the weight of soap taken and by keeping the quantity of barium chloride as low as possible.

(*b*) For soaps containing potassium or more than 0·4 per cent of total free alkali:

> Dissolve 10 g of the soap in 100 ml of neutral industrial methylated spirit (95 per cent) containing 0·5 ml of 0·5 per cent phenolphthalein solution. Add 5 ml of hot neutral 10 per cent aqueous solution of barium chloride in a thin stream, mix thoroughly and titrate with 0·1N hydrochloric acid at 70° until the pink colour disappears.

Free Carbonate Alkali. This may be determined by difference from total free alkali and free caustic alkali and, except for direct determination of carbon dioxide by any of the recognised methods, this is the only way for potassium soaps. The carbonate in sodium soaps can be determined by the usual 'alcohol-insoluble' method.

> Boil 100 ml of neutral industrial methylated spirit (95 per cent) in a 400-ml conical flask, add 10 g of the soap in thin shavings and dissolve it as quickly as possible by heating. Filter rapidly while hot and wash the residue on the paper with hot ethanol until it is free from soap. Extract the residue with hot water until the washings are no longer alkaline. Titrate the combined aqueous washings with 0·1N hydrochloric acid, using methyl orange as indicator. Calculate the result as Na_2O per cent.

Total and Free Fatty Acids. The total fatty acids are determined by extraction as given above for the method of determination of soap in pharmaceutical preparations. For an oleic acid soap, the fatty acids × 0·968 (to correct for the water formed by combination) plus the combined alkali will give the percentage of anhydrous soap. For an olive oil soap, the error involved by calculating the fatty acids as oleic acid would be negligible.

Free fatty acids cannot be present if the ethanolic filtrate from the determination of insoluble matter is alkaline in reaction. If free fatty acids are present, the ethanolic filtrate is titrated with 0·1N potassium hydroxide to phenolphthalein. 1 ml 0·1N = 0·0282 g oleic acid.

Titre. The titre is the highest temperature reached when the liberated water-insoluble fatty acids are crystallised under arbitrarily controlled conditions and is generally taken to represent the solidification point of the fatty acids, although they actually solidify over a range of temperature. Duplicate determinations should be carried out.

Apparatus: This consists of a glass tube, provided at the top with a lip or flange; the tube is 9 cm long by 2·75 cm diameter with sides 0·30 cm thick and is inserted in an ebonite or wooden cover so that it may be held centrally in an outer glass vessel, 13 cm deep by 10 cm diameter (for samples with a titre of less than 35° a wide-mouthed bottle is suitable) and a thermometer suspended centrally in the inner tube; thermometers complying with B.S. 593, Schedules A.40C and A.70C are suitable.

Determination: Dissolve 40 to 50 g of the soap in 400 ml of hot water in a 600-ml beaker and then add, gradually with stirring, an excess of dilute sulphuric or hydrochloric acid. Heat the mixture, with stirring, until the liberated fatty acids form a clear layer on the top and then syphon or draw off the aqueous layer as completely as possible. Wash the fatty acids with two 500-ml quantities of boiling water, drawing off each washing as completely as possible. Filter the fatty acids through dry filter paper until free from moisture and then allow to solidify.

If the titre of soaps containing carbolic acid or mineral oil is required the carbolic acid and mineral oil must be removed; the former can be removed by heating the soap at 100° to 105° and the latter by extracting the soap with ether.

Assemble the apparatus and immerse the outer vessel (if a wide-mouthed bottle is used, to within 1 cm of the shoulder) in a water-bath maintained at 10° to 15° below the expected titre temperature. Melt the fatty acids and introduce to the inner tube sufficient to immerse the thermometer bulb to a depth of not less than ½ in. When crystals of acid first begin to appear, stir the mass vigorously with the thermometer, alternately, three times, first clockwise and then anticlockwise, until the bulb is no longer visible when hanging freely. Allow to stand, without further stirring, and note the temperature; this should at first rise several tenths of a degree and then remain stationary before falling. The maximum temperature reached is the approximate titre. Remelt the fatty acids in the tube by warming on a water-bath, stirring with the thermometer and heating to about 3° above the approximate titre. Replace the tube in the outer vessel, stir the mass slowly until the temperature has fallen to the approximate titre and then stir vigorously, as described above, until the temperature ceases to fall. Allow to stand without further stirring and note the maximum temperature reached; this is the accepted titre.

Unsaponified Fat. The Analytical Methods Committee of the *S.A.C.*[2] recommends three determinations to obtain a correct indication of the total free fat or unsaponified saponifiable matter in soaps, (*i*) free fatty acids by direct titration as above, (*ii*) unsaponified neutral fat and unsaponifiable matter by the method described below, (*iii*) unsaponifiable matter by saponification and extraction of (*ii*). Hence the unsaponified neutral fat is (*ii*) — (*iii*), and the total free fat or unsaponified saponifiable matter is (*ii*) — (*iii*) + (*i*).

As strict adherence to the prescribed details is essential for accurate results the method recommended is given in full:

Weigh 5 g of the soap in thin shavings and dissolve it in about 80 ml of a mixture of 50 ml of redistilled industrial methylated spirit (95 per cent) and 100 ml of water without heating more than is necessary; transfer to a 500-ml separator, washing the beaker with the remaining 70 ml of the dilute spirit. Extract with 100 ml of ether while still slightly warm, run off the ethanolic soap layer into a second separator and repeat the extraction with 50 ml of ether. Extract the lower layer again with a further 50 ml of ether, and pour the three ether extracts into a separator containing 20 ml of water. Rotate the separator gently without violent shaking and, after allowing to separate, run off the wash water. Repeat the washing with water in this way until the water run off is not more than faintly turbid on acidification. Wash the ethereal solution twice more by shaking vigorously with 20 ml of 0·5N aqueous potassium hydroxide solution, each washing with alkali being immediately followed by washing with 20 ml of water, shaking vigorously each time. Acidify the last washing with alkali after separating it, and, if the liquid becomes turbid, repeat the washings with alkali and water until the final washing with potassium hydroxide remains clear on acidification. Finally, wash with successive quantities of 20 ml of water until the water no longer gives a pink colour with phenolphthalein. Transfer the ethereal solution to a weighed flask and distil off the ether. When nearly all the ether is evaporated, add 2 to 3 ml of acetone. By the aid of a gentle current of air remove the solvent completely from the flask, which is preferably almost entirely immersed, held obliquely and rotated in a water-bath. Repeat this operation until the weight is constant. The residue obtained consists of unsaponified neutral fat and unsaponifiable matter (*ii* above).

After weighing, dissolve the contents of the flask in 10 ml of freshly boiled and neutralised industrial methylated spirit, and titrate with 0·1N ethanolic potassium hydroxide solution to phenolphthalein; not more than 0·1 ml should be required for neutralisation. If more is required, the test has not been effectively carried out and must be repeated.

Evaporate the solution remaining from the above titration until the bulk of the ethanol is removed. Add 25 ml of 0·5N ethanolic potassium hydroxide and boil under a reflux condenser for half an hour. Transfer the ethanolic soap solution to a separator with 50 ml of water, and repeat the process of ether extraction, washing, etc., described above. Weigh the final residue of unsaponifiable matter (*iii* above). Subtraction of this weight from the weight obtained above gives unsaponified neutral fat.

Resin Acids. These are often present in household soaps and are determined by the method given under Colophony (p. 196).

Silicated Soaps. The determination of free alkali and silica in silicated soaps is embodied in a report of the Analytical Methods Committee of the *S.A.C.*[3] to which reference should be made if required.

Phenolic Soaps. The Analytical Methods Committee of the *S.A.C.*[4] studied the conditions for the accurate determination of phenol and cresol and for these it recommended a bromination method after separation by steam distillation which is applicable to the majority of commercial soaps.

Transfer 5 g of the soap to a 400-ml round-bottomed flask. Dissolve the soap in about 250 ml of water and add 20 ml of N sodium hydroxide. Steam distil until the distillate is free from turbidity. Discard the distillate, allow the contents of the distilling flask to cool and acidify with 25 ml of 6N sulphuric acid. Steam distil and collect the distillate in a 500-ml graduated flask until approximately 450 ml has been collected or until the distillate no longer gives a precipitate with bromine water. Make the distillate alkaline with 25 ml of 0·5N sodium hydroxide, add a few ml of 0·5M calcium chloride and dilute with water to 500 ml or to a definite volume in excess of this. Filter through paper. Shake 50 ml of the filtrate in a stoppered cylinder with an excess of bromine water to ascertain whether the soap contains phenol or higher homologues. If the precipitate formed by the bromine water is crystalline and silky, phenol only is present; if the solution becomes and remains milky, cresols or high-boiling tar acids are present.

Introduce into three ground-glass stoppered flasks:

Into flask I: 25 ml of water.

Into flask II: 25 ml of standard cresol or phenol solution prepared as described below.

Into flask III: $\frac{1}{20}$th of the filtered distillate from the soap.

Add to each of the three flasks 25 ml of bromide-bromate solution (prepared by dissolving 19·8 g of potassium bromide and 5·6 g of potassium bromate in water and diluting the solution to 1 litre) followed by 5 ml of concentrated hydrochloric acid. Shake each flask well and allow to stand for sixty minutes, then add 30 ml of approximately 0·5N potassium iodide to each flask, rinsing the stoppers with the same solution, mix the contents well, allow to stand five minutes and titrate with 0·1N sodium thiosulphate, using starch solution as indicator.

If W be the weight in grams of soap taken and
a ml of thiosulphate be required for the blank,
b ml of thiosulphate be required for the standard and
c ml of thiosulphate be required for the sample distillate, then

percentage of phenolic substances

$$= \frac{a-c}{a-b} \times \frac{20 \times 100}{40W} = \frac{50}{W} \times \frac{a-c}{a-b}$$

The cresol used in the preparation of the soap, or as agreed between the parties, should be used as a standard for the purposes of the test.

Where either of these is not available, it is recommended that a mixture of 35, 40 and 25 per cent of *o*-, *m*- and *p*-cresols respectively should be used, as this mixture has been found to agree closely with the quality of cresylic acid usually employed in soap manufacture. The standard solution is prepared by dissolving 1·0 g of the cresols in 10 ml of N sodium hydroxide and diluting to 1 litre. When phenol is the ingredient 1 g of phenol is substituted for the 1 g of cresol mentioned above.

When high-boiling tar acids of variable and unknown composition are present the above standard method may give seriously inaccurate results; the following process will give results probably sufficiently accurate for most purposes.

Weigh 50 g of the soap, finely chipped, into a 1-litre graduated flask, add 600 ml of water and 20 ml of 10 per cent sodium hydroxide solution and heat until the soap is dissolved. Cool, add 100 ml of 24 per cent anhydrous calcium nitrate solution (sp. gr. 1·2), mix thoroughly and dilute to volume with water. Filter through a Buchner funnel, measure the volume of the filtrate (V_1), transfer to a separator and acidify with hydrochloric acid. Saturate the solution with sodium chloride and extract successively with 50, 50, 50 and 25 ml of pure benzene. Extract the combined benzene extracts in succession with 25, 25, 10 and 5 ml of 15 per cent sodium hydroxide solution. Combine the alkaline extracts and, after separating from any small residue of benzene, transfer to a 150-ml flask with graduated neck, rinsing out the separator with a further 5 ml of sodium hydroxide solution. Warm the flask and remove traces of benzene by means of a vacuum pump. Saturate the alkaline solution with sodium chloride, acidify with hydrochloric acid and add sufficient saturated brine to bring the phenols into the neck of the flask. Immerse the flask in boiling water until separation appears to be complete. Cool to 37° and keep preferably in an incubator or in a warm place overnight. Again immerse the flask in a water-bath for two hours and then cool and read off the volume (V_2) of the phenols. If the tar acids are of a viscous nature, greater accuracy may be attained by adding a known volume of cresylic acid to assist the separation and subtracting it from the reading obtained.

Calculate the percentage from the formula

$$\text{phenols} = \frac{V_2 \times 2 \times 1{,}000}{V_1} \text{ ml per 100 g.}$$

Soaps from oils and fats most likely to be encountered in pharmaceutical preparations are those of castor oil (iodine value of fatty acids, 87 to 93); coconut oil (iodine value of fatty acids, 8 to 9); palm-kernel oil (iodine value of fatty acids, 12); cottonseed oil (iodine value of fatty acids, 111 to 115); tallow (used for curd soap; iodine value of fatty acids, 35 to 41). Soaps made from the first three oils mentioned are commonly encountered in saponaceous disinfectants. The official soaps (**Curd Soap,** *B.P.C.*, made from sodium hydroxide and purified animal fat; **Hard Soap,** *B.P.C.*, from sodium hydroxide and a suitable vegetable oil; **Soft Soap,** *B.P.*, from potassium or sodium hydroxide and a suitable vegetable oil) should all be free from resin.

Liniment of Soap, *B.P.* A solution of soap prepared by the interaction of 4 per cent w/v of oleic acid with potassium hydroxide and 4 per cent of camphor in diluted alcohol, containing a small proportion of rosemary oil.

The fatty acids are determined as follows:

Add 7 ml of 10 per cent sodium hydroxide solution to 25 ml of liniment in a separator and extract twice with portions of light petroleum. Wash the light petroleum layers with water and add the washings to the main aqueous solution. Acidify with dilute sulphuric acid and extract the fatty acids with light petroleum, evaporate, add 5 ml of acetone, again evaporate, dry the residue at 80° for two hours, and weigh.

The extracted oleic acid should have an acid value of 195 to 202 and an iodine value of 85 to 92.

Spirit of Soap, *B.P.C.* Soft soap, 65 per cent w/v in 90 per cent alcohol. Determine the fatty acids by direct extraction after diluting and acidifying (calculated 28·6 per cent w/v fatty acids).

Ethereal Solution of Soap, *B.P.C.* A potash soap made from oleic acid with alcohol and ether, perfumed with oil of lavender.

The error due to lavender oil in the extracted fatty acids is a maximum of 0·2 per cent; to eliminate this a preliminary extraction by the *B.P.* method for unsaponifiable matter in oils would be necessary, otherwise acid soap would be retained by the solvent. The customary three extractions of the fatty acids is unnecessary; by experiment a third extraction with ether, which was washed with water and evaporated, yielded no weighable residue. The *B.P.C.* assay uses light petroleum for extraction; either solvent can be used.

To 10 ml in a separator add 20 ml of water and 20 ml of N hydrochloric acid; extract with two successive quantities of 20 ml of ether. Mix the ether solutions in a separator and wash with two 10-ml portions of water. Transfer the ether solutions to a weighed flask, remove the solvent, add 5 ml of acetone, evaporate, dry the residue at 80° and weigh to obtain the proportion of oleic acid by weight in volume. Multiply the weight found by 1·121 and calculate the proportion by volume in volume.

Minimum content of oleic acid should be 33 per cent by volume. Free alkali should be absent.

1. *Analyst*, 1937, **62,** 36.
2. *Analyst*, 1935, **60,** 537.
3. *Analyst*, 1937, **62,** 865.
4. *Analyst*, 1946, **71,** 301.

STARCH

A simple, accurate determination of starch is not possible, and it is usually determined by a 'difference' figure; but if it is present as a pure product a close approximation may be obtained by Lintner's[1] method. This is rapid and yields satisfactory results if details are adhered to, but it is only useful for fairly pure material (*e.g.* it can be employed successfully for estimation of starch in Dusting-powders).

Digest about 2·5 g of material with 10 ml of water. Add 20 ml of concentrated hydrochloric acid in small portions at a time; the suspension will clear gradually with stirring. Wash into a 100-ml graduated flask with 12 per cent hydrochloric acid, if proteins are present add 5 ml of 4 per cent phosphotungstic acid solution, then dilute to volume with more 12 per cent hydrochloric acid. Shake the mixture well, filter bright (with Dusting-powders the solution does not need filtration) and determine the optical rotation of the solution in a 2-dm tube.

The following specific rotations are given by Ewers[2] for observations at 20° based on a slightly different hydrolysis procedure. However, when using these figures in pharmaceutical practice, they have been found to give satisfactory results with the Lintner method.

Wheat . . .	+182·7°	Potato	+195·4°
Barley . . .	+181·5°	Rye	+184·0°
Rice . . .	+185·9°	Maize	+184·6°
Oats . . .	+181·3°	Arrowroot. . .	+193·8°

On account of possible hydrolysis, the starch must not be left in contact with the hydrochloric acid longer than is necessary to complete the estimation.

Chinoy, Edwards and Nanji[3] introduced a procedure for estimating starch which depends on the precipitation of starch iodide under standardised conditions and weighing it as such. The original experiments described, using pure natural starches, suggest that the method is of considerable accuracy:

Dissolve 0·5 g of the starch by warming with 100 ml of 0·7 per cent potassium hydroxide solution (in which the hemicelluloses in maize, rice and wheat starches are not appreciably soluble) at 60° to 70° on a water-bath for thirty minutes. After cooling, make up to 100 ml, take 10 ml of the dilution and just neutralise with dilute acetic acid, using phenolphthalein as indicator. Add 1 ml of 0·1N iodine (which must be in excess so that the degree of adsorption of iodine by starch may be constant), *followed* by the coagulating agent; 20 ml of 90 per cent ethanol may be used as coagulant but 2 ml of 10 per cent potassium acetate solution per 10 ml of starch solution is preferable. After allowing the mixture to stand for ten minutes, filter through a tared alundum or sintered-glass crucible (medium variety), Gooch crucibles with asbestos being found not so suitable. Wash with 200 ml of 90 per cent ethanol (the degree of washing has some slight effect and a fixed quantity of ethanol is used), dry at 100° for twelve hours and weigh.

To calculate the percentage of starch present in solution, multiply the weight of starch iodide obtained by the factor 0·8865; this factor was ascertained by determining the weight of starch iodide from a weighed quantity of different pure starches. Allowance for moisture must be made unless the determination has been performed on the dried material.

STARCH

Only with potato starch was gelatinisation with boiling water found to be quite satisfactory; with rice starch, after gelatinisation with 0·7 per cent potassium hydroxide solution, it was found necessary to leave the mixture overnight after coagulation and before filtration. Maize, potato and wheat starches could be filtered a few minutes after coagulation.

To determine starch in the presence of dextrin, Edwards, Nanji and Chanmugam[4] found a modification of the original method necessary:

> Carry out the gelatinisation and neutralisation of the mixture as above. Add 1 ml of 0·1N iodine, followed by 40 ml of a reagent made by adding 4 ml of 10 per cent potassium acetate solution to 100 ml of 50 per cent ethanol. Leave the mixture for ten minutes. Decant the bulk of the liquid into a tared medium alundum crucible, wash the precipitate in the beaker twice with 50 per cent ethanol and twice with 95 per cent ethanol; then transfer the precipitate to the crucible, wash with a little more ethanol, dry and weigh.

Soluble starch is also completely separated from dextrin by the modified method.

A method has been published by Viles and Silverman[5] for the determination of small amounts of starch colorimetrically with anthrone.

> Boil the sample with water, cool and dilute with water to give a solution containing 10 to 200 μg of starch in 2 ml. If the solution contains suspended material, filter through dry paper. Pipette 2 ml of the clear solution into a test-tube and at the same time pipette 2 ml of water into a second test-tube for the blank and prepare one or more 2-ml standards using suitable weights of pure starch (100 μg is suitable) in 2 ml dissolved in water by boiling. To each test-tube add, rapidly from a pipette or burette, 4 ml of a 0·1 per cent solution of anthrone in concentrated sulphuric acid (prepared at least four hours and not more than nine days before use); it is important that the reagent be added in exactly the same way to all the tubes. Mix the contents of each tube, allow to cool in air for ten to fifteen minutes and then cool completely in a bath of cold water.
>
> Measure the extinctions at 625 mμ of the sample and standard solutions against the blank solution and calculate the starch content by comparison.

Beer's law applies over the range 10 to 200 μg and the colour is stable for three hours.

1. LINTNER, *Z. Untersuch. Lebensm.*, 1907, **14,** 205.
2. EWERS, E., *Z. Öffentl. Chem.*, 1908, **14,** 150.
3. CHINOY, J. J., EDWARDS, F. W., and NANJI, H. R., *Analyst*, 1934, **59,** 673.
4. EDWARDS, F. W., NANJI, H. R., and CHANMUGAM, W. R., *Analyst*, 1938, **63,** 697.
5. VILES, F. J., Jnr., and SILVERMAN, L., *Anal. Chem.*, 1949, **21,** 950.

STEROIDS

A large number of steroids, both natural and synthetic, are now used in pharmaceutical practice. For convenience these have been subdivided into four main groups, depending upon their action, although it is appreciated that the assignment of a particular substance to any one group is not always strictly correct.

Since the text refers to the formulæ of the various steroids from time to time, a numbered general formula is reproduced here to assist the reader.

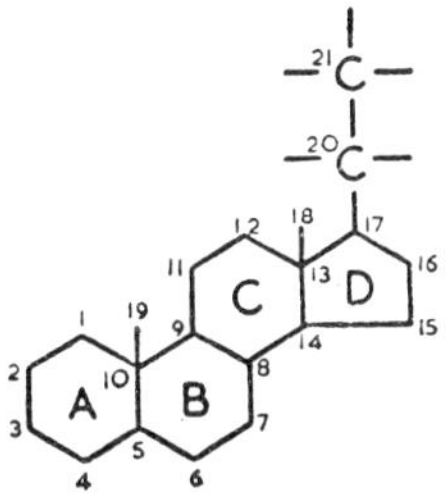

ŒSTROGENIC AGENTS

The œstrogens are characterised by having a phenolic ring A but colour reactions depending on this are not easy to apply and are, of course, entirely non-specific. The œstrogens may be further subdivided into those having an oxo group at position 17 and those having a hydroxyl or esterified hydroxyl group. The only pharmaceutically important member of the first group is **œstrone,** which is official (as Estrone) in the *U.S.P.*, although this is often associated with the less active equilin and equilinin which both show unsaturation in the B ring. No official assay is prescribed for œstrone. It has been determined by reaction of the 17-ketosteroid group with Girard's T reagent[1] but since this steroid is of diminishing pharmaceutical interest the method is not given in detail here.

The non-ketonic œstrogens are more important pharmaceutically; the parent materials are usually not assayed as such, but are controlled by measurement of physical characteristics such as optical rotation or ultra-violet absorption (see Table 29). Where they appear in formulations (frequently as oily injections) the reaction most commonly employed for their determination is that due to Kober[2] in which a magenta colour is formed by reaction of the œstrogen with phenolsulphonic acid and sulphuric acid; the colour produced has an absorption maximum at about 525 mμ, but other œstrogens also react to give a brownish colour with absorption maximum at 420 mμ. The method is further complicated by the fact that the reaction proceeds in two stages, a yellow colour being formed before the magenta. The course of the reaction is influenced by various factors such as temperature, reagent composition and time. A number of procedures have been published for this determination and that given below for the determination of Injection of Œstradiol Benzoate is probably as satisfactory as any; rigid attention to detail is essential.

Œstradiol. Œstradiol exists in two epimeric forms, depending on the configuration of the 17-hydroxyl group. The 17β material is the more potent and it is this form which is official. Since the less potent 17α-epimer* is always in œstradiol obtained from pregnant mares' urine and sometimes in that obtained by the reduction of œstrone a determination of the proportion of the two epimers present is of value. A method has been described by Carol and Molitor[3] based on the fact that in the initial phase of the Kober reaction α-œstradiol reacts with the reagent in the cold while β-œstradiol does not. A limit test for α-œstradiol, based on this fact, is included in the *N.F.* monograph for Estradiol.

Haenni, Carol and Banes[4] have described a simple chromatographic method for the separation of α- and β-œstradiols in complex mixtures of œstrogens, using 0·4N sodium hydroxide as immobile solvent on Celite and benzene as mobile solvent with subsequent determination of the isomers using a sensitive Iron-Kober reagent.

Œstradiol benzoate. This is a monobenzoate, the œstradiol being esterified in the 3-position only. It is frequently administered in the form of an oily injection such as **Injection of Œstradiol Benzoate,** ***B.P.***, which is a sterile solution of the œstrogen in ethyl oleate or a suitable fixed oil. Other suitable esters may be used as solvent, or a mixture of esters and fixed oil. Antoxidants such as gallates or butylated hydroxyanisole may be encountered in preparations of this type and their presence is likely to interfere seriously with the Kober reaction. It is possible that a preliminary chromatographic separation such as that described below under Œstradiol Dipropionate might be used with advantage in such cases. The injection may be assayed by the following method, in which full details of the Kober reaction are given:

> Iron-phenol solution. Dissolve 1·054 g of ferrous ammonium sulphate [$FeSO_4,(NH_4)_2SO_4,6H_2O$] in about 20 ml of water and add 1 ml of concentrated sulphuric acid and 1 ml of strong hydrogen peroxide solution (27 per cent w/w). Mix, heat until effervescence ceases and dilute with water to 50 ml. Transfer 3 ml of this solution to a 100-ml graduated flask and, while cooling, dilute to volume with concentrated sulphuric acid. Redistil phenol, discarding the first 10 per cent and the last 5 per cent of the distillate and taking precautions to exclude moisture and collect the distillate in a tared, dry, glass-stoppered flask of capacity

* Some confusion might arise in that at the time of Carol and Molitor's paper this, the higher-melting epimer, was known as β-œstradiol but later work proved that the lower-melting epimer had the β configuration and the nomenclature given here was adopted.

about twice the volume of the phenol. Cool the flask in ice to solidify the phenol, breaking the top crust with a glass rod to ensure complete crystallisation. Add to the phenol 1·13 times its weight of the iron/sulphuric acid solution, stopper the flask and allow to stand, without cooling but with occasional mixing, until the phenol is liquefied (about thirty minutes or less). Allow to stand in the dark for twenty-four hours and then add to the mixture 23·5 per cent of its weight of a mixture of 10 volumes of concentrated sulphuric acid and 11 volumes of water. Store, protected from light, in dry, glass-stoppered bottles; the reagent should be used within six months.

Determination: Transfer a volume of sample equivalent to about 1 mg of œstradiol benzoate or an equivalent amount of other œstrogen to a separator, dissolve in 30 ml of 2,2,4-trimethylpentane, add 40 ml of 70 per cent ethanol and shake for two minutes. Separate the ethanol layer and wash with 20 ml of 2,2,4-trimethylpentane. Repeat the extraction with five 15-ml quantities of 70 per cent ethanol, washing each extract with the same 20 ml of 2,2,4-trimethylpentane. Combine the extracts, add 5 ml of a 10 per cent solution of anhydrous sodium carbonate and boil gently in a water-bath until the volume is about 15 ml. Cool, add 20 ml of 10 per cent sodium hydroxide solution and transfer to a separator with water. Add 30 ml of 2,2,4-trimethylpentane, shake for two minutes, allow to separate and wash the trimethylpentane layer with two 10-ml quantities of 10 per cent sodium hydroxide solution. Combine the alkaline layers, make acid with 50 per cent v/v sulphuric acid, cool and extract with two 20-ml quantities of benzene, shaking for two minutes each time and washing each benzene extract successively with the same two 5-ml quantities of a 10 per cent solution of anhydrous sodium carbonate, followed by two 5-ml quantities of water. Clarify the benzene layers with anhydrous sodium sulphate, combine in a 50-ml graduated flask and dilute to volume with benzene. Transfer a 2-ml aliquot to a test-tube, evaporate until boiling just ceases and immediately dry the tube and transfer to a vacuum desiccator. Evacuate the desiccator continuously for one hour, remove the tube, add 1 ml of iron-phenol solution, stopper the tube and allow to stand for thirty minutes, shaking at intervals of five minutes. Heat in a water-bath for thirty-five minutes, shaking for a few seconds after the first five minutes. Cool for two minutes in ice, add 4·0 ml of a mixture of 35 volumes of concentrated sulphuric acid and 65 volumes of water, allow to stand for five minutes, mix and measure the extinction at the absorption maximum at about 520 mμ (E_{Sa} 520 mμ) and at 420 mμ (E_{Sa} 420 mμ) with, in the comparison cell, a solution prepared by treating 1 ml of iron-phenol solution as described above, beginning with 'stopper the tube . . .'.

Repeat the procedure using a solution of 1·00 mg of œstradiol benzoate in 5 ml of benzene in place of the sample to obtain E_{St} 520 mμ and E_{St} 420 mμ.

Weight in mg of œstradiol benzoate in volume of sample taken for analysis

$$= \frac{E_{Sa}\ 520\,\text{m}\mu - (E_{Sa}\ 420\,\text{m}\mu/2)}{E_{St}\ 520\,\text{m}\mu - (E_{St}\ 420\,\text{m}\mu/2)}$$

Œstradiol dipropionate. In this case the œstradiol is esterified at both the 3- and 17- positions. Snair and Schwinghammer[5] have described a method for the determination of œstradiol dipropionate in oils in which interfering substances present in the oils are removed by partition chromatography. The dipropionate is then hydrolysed with acid and determined colorimetrically as œstradiol using the Kober reaction. The detailed method is as follows:

Preparation of chromatographic column: Triturate 5 g of Celite 545 with 25 ml of 2,2,4-trimethylpentane and 2 ml of polyethylene glycol 600 until a thick, uniform mixture is obtained. Transfer to a chromatographic tube, 10 mm in diameter, fitted with a fritted disc of coarse porosity at its lower end, and pack down firmly.

Preparation of extract: To an oily solution of œstradiol dipropionate containing about 1·0 mg in 1 to 2 ml add 5 ml of *n*-hexane and transfer to the chromatographic column. Wash into and through the column with small quantities of *n*-hexane until a total of 75 ml has been used. Collect the eluate 25 ml at a time in a 50-ml round-bottomed flask and evaporate the *n*-hexane on a water-bath under a jet of air. To the oily solution remaining add 10 ml of methanol, 0·5 ml of concentrated hydrochloric acid and two glass beads and reflux on a water-bath for fifteen minutes. Remove the condenser and evaporate the acid and methanol on the water-bath under a jet of air. When the oily residue stops bubbling and appears dry transfer it quantitatively to a 125-ml separator with four 15-ml quantities of light petroleum (b.p. 30° to 60°) and extract with five 10-ml quantities of N sodium hydroxide, rinsing the flask with the alkali before adding to the separator. Combine the alkaline extracts and carefully make acid (pH 2 to 3) with 10N sulphuric acid. Allow to stand for one hour and, after checking to ensure that the mixture is still acid, extract with four 15-ml quantities of chloroform, combining the extracts in a beaker. Evaporate the chloroform on a water-bath, dissolve the residue in dehydrated ethanol and dilute to 100 ml with the same solvent in a graduated flask.

Determination of œstradiol: Transfer an aliquot of the prepared solution equivalent to 10 to 20 μg of œstradiol dipropionate to a 10-ml graduated flask and evaporate to dryness on a water-bath. Prepare a blank by evaporating 1 ml of dehydrated ethanol in a second 10-ml graduated flask and treat each flask, respectively, as follows. Add 1·5 ml of dilute iron-phenol solution (prepared by diluting 1 volume of the iron-phenol solution described above with 0·45 volume of water immediately before use), allow to stand for thirty minutes with frequent shaking and then place in a water-bath. After two to three minutes stopper the flasks and after a further five minutes shake well. Leave in the water-bath for a further one hour and then cool, add 6 ml of 35 per cent v/v sulphuric acid and mix. Measure the extinction at 520 mμ of the solution in the first flask against the blank solution and read the œstradiol content from a standard curve prepared by carrying out the colorimetric procedure on suitable volumes, covering the range 5 to 20 μg, of a standard solution of œstradiol in dehydrated ethanol.

The chromatographic separation was found to remove interfering impurities present in solutions of the œstrogen in sesame, cottonseed and arachis oils.

Ethinylœstradiol. This is a synthetic œstrogen which has an ethinyl group in the 17α-position. It may be evaluated by ultra-violet absorption measurements. Unlike the natural œstrogens this substance is administered orally, usually in the form of tablets which contain only a very small dose. The following method may be used to assay the tablets:

Acid-ethanol reagent: Separately cool 20 ml of 95 per cent ethanol and 80 ml of concentrated sulphuric acid to about $-5°$. Carefully add the acid to the ethanol, keeping as cool as possible, and mix gently. The reagent should be stored in a cool place.

Determination: Weigh and powder 30 tablets. Transfer a quantity, accurately weighed, of the powdered material, expected to contain about 200 μg, to a small separator, add 15 ml 0·1N sodium hydroxide and shake mechanically for thirty minutes. Add 15 ml of ether, acidify with a few drops of concentrated hydrochloric acid, shake vigorously and allow to separate. Transfer the aqueous phase together with as much as possible of any insoluble material to a second separator and continue the extraction with five 10-ml quantities of ether, bulking the extracts in the first separator and washing with two 3-ml quantities of water, washing each with the same two 10-ml quantities of ether. Mix the ether extracts and washings, filter through a plug of anhydrous sodium sulphate into a 100-ml graduated flask, washing the sodium sulphate with a little ether, and dilute to volume with ether.

Transfer 10 ml of this ethereal solution (= 20 μg of ethinylœstradiol) to a 25-ml conical flask, evaporate to dryness under vacuum and dissolve

TABLE 29

ŒSTROGENIC AGENTS	FORMULA	MOL. WT.	$[\alpha]_D$* (1 PER CENT IN DIOXAN)	$E^{1\%}_{1cm}$*	SOLVENT
Œstradiol, *B.P.C.*	$C_{18}H_{24}O_2$	272·4	+78°		
Œstradiol Benzoate, *B.P.*	$C_{25}H_{28}O_3$	376·5	+60°		
Œstradiol Dipropionate, *U.S.P.*	$C_{24}H_{32}O_4$	384·5	+38°		
Œstradiol Cyclopentylpropionate, *N.F.*	$C_{26}H_{36}O_3$	396·6	+42°†		
Ethinylœstradiol, *B.P.*	$C_{20}H_{24}O_2$	296·4	0° to + 3°	71 at 281 mμ	Dehydrated ethanol
Œstrone, *U.S.P.*	$C_{18}H_{22}O_2$	270·4	+162°	85 at 280 mμ	Dehydrated ethanol
Piperazine Œstrone Sulphate, *N.F.*	$C_{22}H_{32}O_5N_2S$	436·6			

* Values for $[\alpha]_D$, E(1 per cent, 1 cm) and wavelength of maximum absorption are approximate.

† 2 per cent in dioxan.

the residue in 5 ml of acid-ethanol reagent. Measure the maximum intensity of the colour (after about two and a half minutes) at 532 mμ. In the same way measure the colour produced from an aliquot of a standard solution of ethinylœstradiol and from the readings calculate the content of ethinylœstradiol in each tablet of average weight.

Note: Vessels containing ethinylœstradiol in solution should be protected from light.

One or two other œstrogenic substances are used pharmaceutically, and these are noted in Table 29.

PROGESTATIONAL AGENTS

The pharmaceutically important members of this group are five in number, and they are listed in Table 30. The naturally occurring hormone, progesterone, has a low activity when administered orally and so it is commonly encountered in the form of an oily injection. The other substances, which are synthetic modifications, are usually administered in tablet form. In all these substances except one, ring A possesses an α, β-unsaturated carbonyl grouping, that is a keto group at position 3 and a double bond between C atoms 4 and 5; the exception is norethynodrel, in which the double bond occurs between C atoms 5 and 10. The other analytically significant centre is the oxo group at position 20, which occurs in progesterone only. The basic procedure most commonly employed for the determination of progesterone in formulations depends upon the formation of a bis-2,4-dinitrophenylhydrazone which can be determined either gravimetrically or colorimetrically. The other members of the group could presumably be assayed in a similar way but in these cases a mono-dinitrophenylhydrazone would be formed. Another method, applicable to substances possessing the Δ^4-3 oxo structure (all except norethynodrel), depends upon the formation of a yellow colour on reaction with *iso*nicotinic acid hydrazide (isoniazid). This procedure has yielded excellent results in our hands and is given in detail under Testosterone, p. 589.

Progesterone. The substance itself may be assayed by light absorption measurements of a 0·001 per cent solution in dehydrated ethanol and may also be controlled by physical characteristics such as optical rotation.

Injection of Progesterone, *B.P.* Consists of a sterile solution, usually containing 10 mg of progesterone in 1 ml of a suitable fixed oil, or of ethyl oleate or other suitable ester; it may also consist of a sterile solution of progesterone in ethyl oleate and suitable alcohols.

Cohen and Bates[6] proposed a 'direct' method for the determination of progesterone in oily solution using 2,4-dinitrophenylhydrazine as the precipitant and the *U.S.P.* employs a method which differs little from their procedure. In our hands more reliable results have been obtained by the following modification of the method:

Weigh an amount of sample containing about 20 mg of progesterone into a 25-ml flask and add 20 ml of light petroleum (b.p. 60° to 80°), 75 mg of 2,4-dinitrophenylhydrazine and 30 ml of dehydrated ethanol. Connect the flask to a reflux condenser and heat for thirty minutes. Then add 1 ml of concentrated hydrochloric acid, reflux for fifteen minutes and cool. Filter through a No. 3 sintered-glass crucible and wash the precipitate, first with three 5-ml quantities of cold light petroleum (b.p. 60° to 80°) and then with two 3-ml quantities of a 6 per cent w/v solution of concentrated hydrochloric acid in dehydrated ethanol. Dry at 110° to constant weight. 1 mg residue = 0·4661 mg progesterone. Calculate the percentage w/v from the weight per ml.

A useful check on the purity of the sample can be made by determination of the m.p. of the dinitrophenylhydrazone obtained in the assay; the m.p. of progesterone dinitrophenylhydrazone is about 270°.

The method of the *B.P.* is substantially as above after mixing the sample with light petroleum (b.p. 40° to 60°) and extracting the progesterone with 90 per cent ethanol. The common antoxidants do not interfere with this assay. Owing to the mutual solubility of light petroleum and ethanol only about 5 ml of the light petroleum layer remains after the last extraction and it is preferable to equilibrate the solvents by shaking equal volumes together and separating before use.

Elvidge[7] in pointing out the difficulties of determination in oily solutions where absorption of the base is sufficient to upset the spectrographic determination of œstrogens, proposed a colorimetric determination of progesterone in ethyl oleate by adapting the reaction of ketones with salicylic aldehyde in alkaline solution to quantitative use. It was found necessary to control conditions strictly and prepare a calibration curve for each determination. The best range for determination is 50 to 800 μg of progesterone in 25 ml; correction for the colour of ethyl oleate is slight.

Into four 25-ml graduated flasks introduce volumes of standard progesterone solution (500 μg per ml in dehydrated ethanol) containing respectively, 50, 100, 200 and 400 μg of progesterone and add to each sufficient dehydrated ethanol to give a total volume of 2 ml. Introduce 2 ml of dehydrated ethanol into a fifth 25-ml graduated flask for the standard blank. At the same time, into a sixth 25-ml graduated flask, pipette a volume of sample containing 250 μg of progesterone and, if a sample of the ethyl oleate used in preparing the oily solution is available, 1·25, 0·5 or 0·25 ml of a 10 per cent v/v solution of the ethyl oleate in dehydrated ethanol for samples containing 2, 5 or 10 mg of progesterone per ml, respectively. In a seventh 25-ml graduated flask prepare a sample blank containing the same volume of the 10 per cent ethyl oleate solution as in the sixth graduated flask and dilute the contents of the sixth and seventh flasks to 2 ml with dehydrated ethanol. Treat the contents of each flask, respectively, as follows. Add 1 ml of a 10 per cent solution of salicylic aldehyde in dehydrated ethanol and 10 ml of 7·5N sodium hydroxide. Immerse in a water-bath at 80° ± 2° for ten minutes, cool immediately, dilute to about 22 ml with dehydrated ethanol and then dilute to volume with water.

Measure the extinction of each solution at 550 mμ using 4-cm cells

TABLE 30

PROGESTATIONAL AGENTS	FORMULA	MOL. WT.	$[\alpha]_D$*	SOLVENT	$E^{1\%}_{1cm}$ AT 240 mμ*	SOLVENT
Progesterone, *B.P.*	$C_{21}H_{30}O_2$	314·5	+191°	1% in dehydrated ethanol	540	Dehydrated ethanol
U.S.P.			+179°	2% in dioxan		
Ethisterone, *B.P.*	$C_{21}H_{28}O_2$	312·5	+31°	1% in pyridine	520	Dehydrated ethanol
Dimethisterone	$C_{23}H_{32}O_2,H_2O$	358·5	+17°	2% in chloroform	467 (anhyd. material)	Dehydrated ethanol
Norethisterone	$C_{20}H_{26}O_2$	298·4	−25°	1% in chloroform	571	Dehydrated ethanol
Norethynodrel	$C_{20}H_{26}O_2$	298·4	+120°	1% in dioxan	560 (isomerised substance)	Methanol

* Values for $[\alpha]_D$, E(1 per cent, 1 cm) and wavelength of maximum absorption are approximate.

with the standard blank or sample blank in the comparison cell, as appropriate. Prepare a calibration curve from the extinctions of the standards and read the μg of progesterone in the sample solution from the curve.

A third procedure which may be used is that due to Umberger[8] for the determination of Δ^4-3 oxosteroids using *iso*nicotinic acid hydrazide. Full details of the method are given under Injection of Testosterone Propionate (see p. 589).

Ethisterone, dimethisterone and **norethisterone** may all be determined by measurement of light absorption of a 0·001 per cent solution in dehydrated ethanol. For the assay of tablets of these substances simple extraction is satisfactory, although it is advisable to make a preliminary extraction with a solvent in which the steroid is insoluble. Both ethisterone tablets and norethisterone tablets, for example, can be assayed by extracting first with light petroleum, discarding this solvent and then extracting the active material with chloroform followed by evaporation, drying and weighing. Dimethisterone tablets, where the dosage level is somewhat lower, may be assayed by shaking a quantity of the powdered tablets with spectroscopically pure *n*-hexane, centrifuging, and measuring the light absorption of the clear supernatant liquid at 232 mμ.

Norethynodrel, in which the double bond in the A ring occurs between C atoms 5 and 10 rather than 4 and 5, must first be isomerised before a light absorption assay can be applied. A suitable method is as follows:

Dissolve 0·1 g in sufficient methanol to produce exactly 100 ml and transfer a 10-ml aliquot of this solution to a second 100-ml graduated flask. Add 40 ml of methanol and a mixture of 3 ml of concentrated hydrochloric acid and 2 ml of water, allow to stand for one hour and then dilute to volume with methanol. Dilute a 10-ml aliquot of this solution to exactly 100 ml with methanol and, within three minutes, measure the extinction at the absorption maximum at about 240 mμ, using 1-cm cells with, in the comparison cell, a 0·001 per cent solution of the sample in methanol. For the purposes of the calculation use a value of 560 for E(1 per cent, 1 cm) of norethynodrel when subjected to this treatment.

ANDROGENIC AND ANABOLIC AGENTS

The members of this group listed in Table 31, all have a keto-group in position 3, a double bond between C atoms 4 and 5, and an OH group at the 17 position, although this is esterified in some cases. **Testosterone, methyltestosterone, fluoxymesterone** and **methandienone** are all based on the androstane structure, having methyl groups in both the 10 and 13 positions and **norethandrolone** and **nandrolone** have a methyl group at C 13 only. In addition, methandienone has a second double bond in the

A ring, between C atoms 1 and 2. Fluoxymesterone is further characterised by having a fluorine atom attached at C 9 and an OH group at C 11.

The keto-group in ring A is again the most significant feature for analytical purposes. Reliable assay procedures have been based on semicarbazone formation, 2,4-dinitrophenylhydrazone formation and reaction with *iso*nicotinic acid hydrazide (isoniazid). This latter reaction depends on unsaturation in ring A as well as on the keto-group. For the steroids themselves physical characteristics can be used for control and the two most common are optical rotation and light absorption. Particulars of the more important members of the group are given in Table 31.

The most common formulations are tablets (or implants) and, for the esters, oily injections.

Injection of Testosterone Propionate, *B.P.* Usually contains 10 mg in 1 ml. It is assayed gravimetrically as the semicarbazone by a method based on that described by Madigan, Zenno and Pheasant.[9] The following method is satisfactory although gallates, if present as antoxidants, may cause the result to be about 10 to 15 per cent high:

> Transfer a volume of the sample equivalent to about 50 mg of testosterone propionate to a separator, add 40 ml of light petroleum (b.p. 40° to 60°) saturated with 90 per cent ethanol and mix. Extract with eight 20-ml quantities of 90 per cent ethanol saturated with light petroleum (b.p. 40° to 60°), combine the extracts and evaporate the solvent almost completely on a water-bath. Transfer the residue, with the aid of a little methanol, to a 25- to 50-ml round-bottomed flask and add 3 ml of semicarbazide acetate solution (prepared as follows: triturate 2·5 g of semicarbazide hydrochloride with 3·3 g of sodium acetate trihydrate, mix with 10 ml of methanol, transfer to a flask with 20 ml of methanol, allow to stand at 4° for thirty minutes and dilute to 100 ml with methanol after filtration). Connect the flask to a reflux condenser, heat for two hours and then cool to room temperature. Add 10 ml of 2,2,4-trimethylpentane and pour the resulting mixture into 75 ml of ice-cold water, rinsing the flask first with two 2-ml quantities of 2,2,4-trimethylpentane and then with two 2-ml quantities of methanol. Stir thoroughly, allow to stand at 4° for three hours and then filter the entire mixture (two phases) through a tared, No. 3, sintered-glass crucible. Wash the precipitate with 2,2,4-trimethylpentane, suck dry and wash with water. Finally dry to constant weight at 105°. Semicarbazone × 0·8579 = testosterone propionate.

As a means of identification, the melting-point of the semicarbazide may be determined; it should be about 208°.

Injection of Testosterone Phenylpropionate may also be assayed by the above method, or by dissolving the sample in hexane, shaking with 0·5N sodium hydroxide, washing the alkaline solution with hexane, extracting the original hexane solution and the washings with 90 per cent ethanol saturated with hexane, evaporating the ethanolic solution, dissolving the residue in dehydrated ethanol and measuring the extinction at about 240 mμ.

Umberger[8] has described a colorimetric method for the determination of Δ^4-3-ketosteroids using isoniazid as reagent.

Dissolve the steroid in dehydrated ethanol to give a solution containing about 100 μg per ml. To 2 ml of this solution add 2 ml of isoniazid reagent (prepared by dissolving *iso*nicotinic acid hydrazide to a concentration of 1·0 mg per ml in dehydrated ethanol acidified with 1·25 ml of concentrated hydrochloric acid per litre), mix and allow to stand at room temperature for one hour. Measure the extinction at the absorption maximum at about 380 mμ using 1-cm cells with a reagent-blank solution in the comparison cell, and compare with the extinction given by a standard solution of the steroid (100 μg per ml) in dehydrated ethanol treated similarly.

For oil solutions of testosterone propionate and progesterone containing 10 mg per ml and more:

Prepare a solution of the sample in dehydrated ethanol containing not more than 1 ml of the sample per 100 ml of solution and pipette a volume of the solution containing 50 μg of the steroid into a 25 × 150 mm cylindrical centrifuge tube fitted with a ground-glass joint. Evaporate the ethanol, add to the residue 2 ml of dehydrated ethanol and 2 ml of the isoniazid reagent, stopper the tube and shake to dissolve. Complete as above from allow to stand at room temperature . . .'.

If the solution contains less than 10 mg per ml and a sample of the same oil is not available, the steroid should be separated from the oil on a chromatographic column before colorimetric determination.

Tablets of Methyltestosterone, *B.P.* Usually contain 5 mg. They may be determined by formation of the dinitrophenylhydrazone and measurement of the extinction of a solution in chloroform. The method given below is based on precipitation in a hydrochloric acid solution and measurement of the extinction at 390 mμ:

Weigh an amount of powdered tablets equivalent to about 5 mg of methyltestosterone into a 50-ml graduated flask, dilute to volume with chloroform and shake for twenty minutes. Allow to settle, centrifuge in a stoppered tube and pipette 5 ml of the supernatant liquid into a flask. Evaporate to dryness, dissolve the residue in 2 ml of aldehyde-free, 95 per cent ethanol and add 10 ml of a hot, freshly prepared and filtered 0·25 per cent solution of 2,4-dinitrophenylhydrazine in 2N hydrochloric acid. Mix gently and heat for thirty minutes on a water-bath, taking precautions to avoid loss of liquid by evaporation. Cool, allow to stand overnight and filter through a No. 4 sintered-glass crucible. Wash the precipitate with 50 ml of 2N hydrochloric acid followed by 50 ml of water, dry at 105° for thirty minutes and dissolve in sufficient chloroform to produce 100 ml. Measure the extinction of the solution at 390 mμ against a blank solution prepared by treating 2 ml of aldehyde-free, 95 per cent ethanol exactly as above beginning with 'add 10 ml of a hot . . .'.

Repeat the operation using a suitable quantity of an authentic sample of methyltestosterone and calculate the methyltestosterone content of the tablets by comparison.

A preferable method uses an alkaline medium, when the pale yellow

TABLE 31

ANDROGENIC AND ANABOLIC AGENTS	FORMULA	MOL. WT.	$[\alpha]_D$*	SOLVENT	$E^{1\%}_{1cm}$*	mμ*	SOLVENT
Testosterone, *B.P.*	$C_{19}H_{28}O_2$	288·4	+109°	1% in dehydrated ethanol	560	240	Dehydrated ethanol
Testosterone Propionate, *B.P.*	$C_{22}H_{32}O_3$	344·5	+86°	1% in dioxan	490	240	Dehydrated ethanol
Testosterone Phenylpropionate	$C_{28}H_{36}O_3$	420·6	+88°	1% in dioxan	395	240	Dehydrated ethanol
Testosterone Cyclopentylpropionate, *U.S.P.*	$C_{27}H_{40}O_3$	412·6	+88°	2% in chloroform	420	241	Dehydrated ethanol
Testosterone Enanthate, *U.S.P.*	$C_{26}H_{40}O_3$	400·6	+80°	2% in dioxan			
Methyltestosterone, *B.P.*	$C_{20}H_{30}O_2$	302·5	+82°	1% in 95% ethanol	535	240	Dehydrated ethanol
Methandienone	$C_{20}H_{28}O_2$	300·4	+9°	1% in 95% ethanol	516	245	Dehydrated ethanol
Norethandrolone	$C_{20}H_{30}O_2$	302·5	+22°	2% in methanol	565	241	Methanol
Nandrolone Phenylpropionate	$C_{27}H_{34}O_3$	406·6	+50°	1% in dioxan	430	240	Dehydrated ethanol
Fluoxymesterone	$C_{20}H_{29}O_3F$	336·5	+107°	1% in 95% ethanol	495	240	Dehydrated ethanol

* Values for $[\alpha]_D$, E(1 per cent, 1 cm) and wavelength of maximum absorption are approximate.

colour of the 2,4-dinitrophenylhydrazone is converted to a deep red. Gornall and Macdonald[10] used the following procedure for biological extracts:

Reagents:
Acid/methanol. Mix one volume of concentrated hydrochloric acid with three volumes of analytical-reagent grade methanol. Use within one week.
2,4-Dinitrophenylhydrazine reagent. This is a solution of analytical-reagent grade 2,4-dinitrophenylhydrazine in acid/methanol containing 1 mg per ml and should be freshly prepared or, if stored in a refrigerator, may be used within one week of preparation.
Determination: Transfer to a 20 × 150 mm test-tube a volume of extract containing 1 to 20 μg of the steroid and evaporate to dryness under a stream of nitrogen by gentle warming. Dissolve the residue in 0·5 ml of analytical-reagent grade methanol and to a second, similar test-tube transfer 0·5 ml of the methanol for the blank. Treat the contents of each tube, respectively, as follows. Add 0·5 ml of 2,4-dinitrophenylhydrazine reagent, mix, and allow to stand in a water-bath at 59° ±1° so that 2 cm of tube are immersed in the water and the tube projects well above the sides of the bath. Protect from direct light and leave for ninety minutes. Then remove from the bath, allow to cool slightly and add, with gentle shaking, 0·50 ml of carbonate-free 4N sodium hydroxide. Add exactly 5 ml of analytical-reagent grade methanol, mix and allow to stand at room temperature for twenty to thirty minutes. Measure the extinction at the absorption maximum between 425 and 500 mμ of the solution in the first test-tube against the blank solution and read the steroid content from a standard curve prepared by treating a series of standard solutions of the steroid in analytical-reagent grade methanol, covering the range 0 to 20 μg, exactly as described above.

For Tablets of Methyltestosterone the *U.S.P.* relies upon extraction of the tablets with chloroform, evaporation, solution of the residue in ethanol and measurement of the extinction value at 241 mμ. A similar method may be applied to the determination of other formulations, such as Tablets of Fluoxymesterone.

CORTICOSTEROIDS

The members of this large group of steroids, based on pregnane (which has twenty-one carbon atoms), all have

(*a*) in the A ring, an oxo group at position 3 and a double bond between C 4 and 5 (Δ^4). In addition, some have a double bond between C 1 and 2 (Δ^1).
(*b*) a 21-hydroxy-20-oxo group ($CH_2OH—CO—$) which confers mildly reducing properties on the corticosteroids and provides the basis for useful methods of assay.
(*c*) a hydroxyl group at position 17 and either a hydroxyl or oxo group at position 11 (with the exception of deoxycortone).

Three of the corticosteroids considered below are fluorinated in the 9 position; these are fludrocortisone, triamcinolone and dexamethasone. The principal corticosteroids are as follows:

TABLE 32

	RING A	POSITION 11	OTHER CHARACTERISTICS
Cortisone	Δ^4	=O	
Hydrocortisone	Δ^4	—OH	
Prednisone	Δ^1 and Δ^4	=O	
Prednisolone	Δ^1 and Δ^4	—OH	
Methylprednisolone	Δ^1 and Δ^4	—OH	—CH_3 at position 6
Deoxycortone	Δ^4	—H	No —OH at position 17
Fludrocortisone	Δ^4	—OH	—F at position 9
Dexamethasone	Δ^1 and Δ^4	—OH	—F at position 9 —CH_3 at position 16
Triamcinolone	Δ^1 and Δ^4	—OH	—F at position 9 —OH at position 16

The various official steroids are listed in Table 33, which also shows details of the optical rotation and light absorption characteristics. In the *B.P.* official corticosteroids are assayed by ultra-violet absorption, but such a method is non-specific since any steroid having the Δ^4-3 oxo grouping in ring A is likely to have a maximum light absorption in the region of 240 mμ. For this reason a method based on the reducing activity of the characteristic C 17 side-chain is to be preferred.

For some years tetrazolium salts have been used for the determination of reducing sugars and they were applied to the determination of steroids by Chen and Tewell[11] and by Mader and Buck.[12] The reaction depends upon reduction of the tetrazolium salt to give a highly coloured compound known as a formazan. Under controlled conditions the amount of formazan developed is proportional to the quantity of steroid present. Earlier versions of this method were unsatisfactory, since various factors affecting the reaction had not been recognised. During the period between Mader and Buck's publication (in 1952) and 1960 many papers appeared showing that pH, water concentration, temperature and, particularly, light, all had significant effects on the course of the reaction. The methods given for determination of hydrocortisone in Ointment of Hydrocortisone, *B.P.*, and for determination of prednisolone in Prednisolone Tablets, *U.S.P.*, are examples of procedures incorporating careful control of these factors. When applied to a corticosteroid itself, however, rather than to a formulated product, the method still gave results which lacked precision. In 1960 Johnson, King and Vickers[13] recognised the effect which oxygen can play on the reaction and suggested that the colour development should be carried out under nitrogen. Using the conditions they recommended, collaborative work in a number of laboratories has shown that colour development and measurement can be reproduced with a satisfactory degree of precision. This is important because it enables an extinction value E(1 per cent, 1 cm) to be quoted with confidence and thus permits determinations to be made without use of a reference sample.

Most published methods have made use of either 2,3,5-triphenyltetrazoliumchloride or of tetrazolium blue [3,3′-dianisole-bis-4,4′-(3,5-diphenyl)-tetrazolium chloride]. Johnson, King and Vickers preferred the former reagent because, although more sensitive to oxygen, it gave low and predictable blanks whereas tetrazolium blue gave high and continuously varying blank readings. Calibration graphs constructed by applying the method recommended below give straight lines over the range 100 μg to 500 μg of steroid in the final 25 ml; these do not pass through the origin, however, but cut the x abscissa at a slight positive value. For this reason the extinction value quoted in Table 34 applies only if the recommended weight of steroid has been used for colour development. The use of 350 μg of hydrocortisone rather than the specified 400 μg might result in an error of about 1 per cent.

The recommended method, together with details of its application to a number of types of preparation, is as follows:

Reagents:

I. Dehydrated ethanol, aldehyde-free. Reflux dehydrated ethanol of the *B.P.* Appendix I for four hours with sodium hydroxide pellets and redistil.

II. Triphenyltetrazolium chloride solution. Dissolve 0·1 g of 2,3,5-triphenyltetrazolium chloride in 20 ml of reagent I; the solution should be freshly prepared.

III. Dilute tetramethylammonium hydroxide solution. Dilute 4 ml of an aqueous solution containing 25·0 to 26·0 per cent w/w of tetramethylammonium hydroxide to 100 ml with reagent I; the solution should be freshly prepared.

Determination: Protect the solution from light throughout the determination. Pipette 10 ml of a solution containing the specified weight of steroid (see Table 34) in reagent I into an amber-coloured, 25-ml graduated flask. Add 2·0 ml of reagent II, displace the air from the flask with a stream of oxygen-free nitrogen, immediately add 2·0 ml of reagent III and again displace the air from the flask. Stopper the flask, mix by gentle swirling and allow to stand in a water-bath at 30° for one hour. Cool rapidly to 20° and dilute to volume with reagent I. Mix the contents of the flask by shaking gently and measure the extinction of the resulting solution at the absorption maximum at about 485 mμ using closed 1-cm cells with, in the comparison cell, a solution prepared exactly as above but substituting 10 ml of reagent I for the 10 ml of sample solution. Calculate E(1 per cent, 1 cm) of the sample and, from the given E(1 per cent, 1 cm) of the particular steroid (see Table 34) calculate the steroid content of the sample.

TABLE 33

CORTICOSTEROIDS	FORMULA	MOL. WT.	$[\alpha]_D$*	SOLVENT	$E^{1\%}_{1cm}$ AT 240mμ*	SOLVENT
Cortisone Acetate, *B.P.*	$C_{23}H_{30}O_6$	402·5	+214°	0·2% in dioxan	390	Dehydrated ethanol
Hydrocortisone, *B.P.*	$C_{21}H_{30}O_5$	362·5	+166°	1% in 95% ethanol	435	Dehydrated ethanol
Hydrocortisone Acetate, *B.P.*	$C_{23}H_{32}O_6$	404·5	+162°	1% in dioxan	390	Dehydrated ethanol
Hydrocortisone Hydrogen Succinate, *B.P.*	$C_{25}H_{34}O_8$	462·5	+150°	1% in dehydrated ethanol	341	Dehydrated ethanol
Hydrocortisone Sodium Succinate, *B.P.*	$C_{25}H_{33}O_8Na$	484·5	+140°	1% in 95% ethanol	327	Dehydrated ethanol
Prednisone, *B.P.*	$C_{21}H_{26}O_5$	358·4	+171°	1% in dioxan	430	Dehydrated ethanol
Prednisone Acetate, *B.P.*	$C_{23}H_{28}O_6$	400·5	+186°	0·5% in dioxan	385	Dehydrated ethanol
Prednisolone, *B.P.*	$C_{21}H_{28}O_5$	360·5	+100°	1% in dioxan	415	Dehydrated ethanol
Prednisolone Acetate, *B.P.*	$C_{23}H_{30}O_6$	402·5	+114°	1% in dioxan	370	Dehydrated ethanol

Prednisolone Diethylaminoacetate Hydrochloride	$C_{27}H_{40}O_6NCl$	510·1	+122°	1% in water	296	95% ethanol
Prednisolone Sodium Phosphate	$C_{21}H_{27}O_8PNa_2$	484·4	+97°	1% in water	312‡	Water
Prednisolone Trimethylacetate	$C_{26}H_{36}O_6$	444·6	+108°	1% in dioxan	340	Dehydrated ethanol
Methylprednisolone	$C_{22}H_{30}O_5$	374·5	+82°	1% in dioxan	400	Dehydrated ethanol
Deoxycortone Acetate, *B.P.*	$C_{23}H_{32}O_4$	372·5	+180°	1% in dehydrated ethanol	450	Dehydrated ethanol
Deoxycortone Trimethylacetate	$C_{26}H_{38}O_4$	414·6	+157°	1% in dioxan	395	Dehydrated ethanol
Fludrocortisone Acetate, *B.P.C.*	$C_{23}H_{31}O_6F$	422·5	+132°	0·5% in acetone	400	Methanol
Dexamethasone	$C_{22}H_{29}O_5F$	392·5	+76°	1% in dioxan	395	Methanol
Dexamethasone Acetate	$C_{24}H_{31}O_6F$	434·5	+85°	1% in dioxan	355	Dehydrated ethanol
Triamcinolone	$C_{21}H_{27}O_6F$	394·4	+75°	acetone	380	95% ethanol
Triamcinolone Acetonide	$C_{24}H_{31}O_6F$	434·5	+109°	chloroform	345	95% ethanol
Spironolactone†	$C_{24}H_{32}O_4S$	416·6	−34°	1% in chloroform	470	Methanol

* Values for $[\alpha]_D$, E(1 per cent, 1 cm) and wavelength of maximum absorption are approximate.

† Spironolactone is not a corticosteroid but is included in this ble tafor convenience. It is 7α-acetylthio-17β-hydroxy-3-oxo-17α-pregn-4-ene-21-carboxylic acid γ lactone.

‡ At 247mμ.

Application of the method to preparations (Reagents, as above).

Injections. Pipette a volume containing about 50 mg of steroid into a separator, add 20 ml of water and extract with three 30-ml quantities of chloroform. Filter the extracts through a cotton-wool plug into a dry, 100-ml graduated flask and dilute to volume with chloroform. Transfer a 10-ml aliquot of this solution to a 50-ml graduated flask and dilute to volume with chloroform. Transfer a 4-ml aliquot of the solution so obtained to an amber-coloured, 25-ml graduated flask and evaporate the chloroform under a jet of air. Then add 10 ml of reagent I and continue by the general method from 'Add 2·0 ml of reagent II . . .'.

Applies to **Injection of Cortisone Acetate,** ***B.P.***; **Injection of Hydrocortisone Acetate,** ***B.P.***

TABLE 34

CORTICOSTEROID	WEIGHT OF SAMPLE (IN μg) REQUIRED TO BE PRESENT IN 10 ML OF SAMPLE SOLUTION	$E^{1\%}_{1cm}$ AT THE ABSORPTION MAXIMUM AT ABOUT 485 mμ
Cortisone Acetate	440-460	392
Deoxycortone Acetate	440–460	405
Dexamethasone	390-410	402
Dexamethasone Acetate	440–460	363
Fludrocortisone Acetate	440–460	374
Hydrocortisone	390–410	435
Hydrocortisone Acetate	440–460	390
Methylprednisolone	390–410	421
Prednisolone	390–410	438
Prednisolone Acetate	440–460	392
Prednisone	390–410	440
Prednisone Acetate	440-460	394

Tablets. Weigh an amount of powdered tablets equivalent to about 10 mg of the steroid (3 mg for Fludrocortisone Acetate Tablets) into a separator and extract completely with successive quantities of chloroform. Filter each extract through a cotton-wool plug and filter paper, both moistened with chloroform, into a 250-ml graduated flask and dilute to volume with chloroform. Transfer a 5-ml aliquot of this solution to a flask, just evaporate the chloroform and dissolve the residue in reagent I. Dilute with reagent I to give a solution containing the specified amount of steroid in 10 ml (see Table 34). Pipette 10 ml of the solution into an amber-coloured, 25-ml graduated flask and complete by the general method from 'Add 2·0 ml of reagent II . . .'.

Applies to **Tablets of Cortisone Acetate,** ***B.P.***; **Tablets of Dexamethasone; Tablets of Dexamethasone Acetate; Tablets of Fludrocortisone Acetate; Tablets of Methylprednisolone; Tablets of Prednisolone,** ***B.P.***; **Tablets of Prednisone,** ***B.P.***

Ointments. Weigh an amount of sample equivalent to about 13 mg of the steroid into a beaker, add 20 ml of reagent I and heat on a water-bath until melted, stirring with a glass rod. Cool in ice and decant the ethanolic liquid through a cotton-wool plug into a 100-ml graduated flask. Repeat the extraction and decantation with three further 20-ml quantities of reagent I, using a fresh cotton-wool plug for each filtration and transferring the previous plug to the beaker each time. Dilute the combined extracts to volume with reagent I, mix and filter. Pipette 10 ml of the filtrate into a 50-ml graduated flask and dilute to volume with reagent I. Transfer a 10-ml aliquot of this dilution to the first of three 25-ml, amber-coloured graduated flasks, into the second flask pipette 10 ml of a 0·0026 per cent solution of the steroid in reagent I and into the third flask pipette 10 ml of reagent I. To each flask add, in succession, 2·0 ml of reagent II and displace the air from the flask with a stream of oxygen-free nitrogen. Immediately add 2·0 ml of reagent III and again displace the air from the flask. Stopper the flasks, mix by gentle swirling and allow to stand, protected from light, in a water-bath at 30° for sixty minutes. Cool rapidly to 20° and dilute to volume with reagent I.

Mix the contents of each flask by shaking gently and immediately measure the extinction of the solution in the first flask at 485 mμ, using closed 1-cm cells with the solution from the third flask in the comparison cell and compare with the extinction of the solution in the second flask similarly measured.

Applies to **Ointment of Hydrocortisone,** *B.P.*; **Ointment of Hydrocortisone Acetate,** *B.P.*; **Cream of Hydrocortisone,** *B.P.C.*; **Eye Ointment of Hydrocortisone,** *B.P.C.*

Injection of Deoxycortone Acetate, *B.P.* An oily preparation which may be determined as follows:

Solvent I; Solvent II. Shake together equal volumes of 90 per cent ethanol and 2,2,4-trimethylpentane in a separator for ten to fifteen minutes and allow to separate. Transfer the layers to separate containers; the lower layer is Solvent I and the upper layer is Solvent II.

Determination: Using a pipette calibrated for content, transfer a volume of sample equivalent to about 4·5 mg of deoxycortone acetate to a small separator containing 50 ml of Solvent II, wash out the pipette with about 5 ml of Solvent II, adding the washings to the separator, and mix. Extract with six 20-ml quantities of Solvent I, combine the extracts in a beaker and just evaporate the solvent on a water-bath under a current of air. While still warm add 20 ml of hot aldehyde-free dehydrated ethanol and stir gently with a glass rod for three to five minutes. Pour the solution through a small funnel into a 100-ml graduated flask, rinsing the rod with a few millilitres of hot aldehyde-free dehydrated ethanol and the beaker with four 5-ml quantities of the same solvent and collecting the rinsings in the flask. Cool and dilute to volume with aldehyde-free dehydrated ethanol.

Transfer a 10-ml aliquot of this solution to an amber-coloured 25-ml graduated flask and complete by the general method from 'Add 2·0 ml of reagent II . . .'.

The method is not satisfactory when applied to triamcinolone, for colour development continues to increase gradually and, even after four hours, does not reach a maximum value. This observation applies to any corticosteroid having an —OH group in the 16 position, vicinal to that in the 17 position. The method is also inapplicable to hydrocortisone sodium succinate, possibly due to hindrance of the reaction by the large esterifying group. In this case colour development is slow, and after an hour reaches a value only about one quarter of that to be expected from the amount of hydrocortisone present. A similar slowing of the reaction makes the method inapplicable where the esterifying group is trimethylacetate. Phosphate, as in prednisolone sodium phosphate, also interferes with the reaction. A more detailed review of the use of tetrazolium salts for quantitative colorimetric analysis has been published by Johnson.[14]

For the determination of triamcinolone it is necessary to rely on an ultra-violet absorption assay; the fluorine content may be determined by flask-combustion and determination of fluoride in the absorbing liquid (see p. 300 and Appendix IV). The fluorine contents of dexamethasone and fludrocortisone may be determined in the same way. Such a determination, in conjunction with the tetrazolium assay, gives a satisfactory control of the fluorinated corticosteroids.

For preparations containing hydrocortisone sodium succinate, such as the injection, a method based upon that of Umberger[8] for Δ^4-3 oxo steroids is convenient and accurate.[15]

Dissolve the contents of one sealed container (equivalent to 100 mg of hydrocortisone) in a mixture of equal volumes of chloroform and dry methanol and dilute to volume with the same solvent in a 50-ml graduated flask. Transfer a 5-ml aliquot of this solution to a 200-ml graduated flask and dilute to volume with the chloroform/methanol mixture. Transfer a 5-ml aliquot of this solution to a 25-ml graduated flask and at the same time into a second 25-ml graduated flask pipette 5 ml of a freshly prepared standard solution of hydrocortisone sodium succinate in chloroform/methanol (1 : 1) containing, in 5 ml, 350 μg of hydrocortisone sodium succinate. Pipette 5 ml of the chloroform/methanol mixture into a third 25-ml graduated flask for the blank. Treat the contents of each flask, respectively, as follows. Add, by pipette, 10 ml of isoniazid reagent (prepared by dissolving *iso*nicotinic acid hydrazide to a concentration of 1·0 mg per ml in absolute methanol acidified with 1·25 ml of concentrated hydrochloric acid per litre) and swirl to mix. Allow to stand in a water-bath at $55° \pm 1°$ for twenty-five minutes, cool to room temperature, dilute to volume with the chloroform/methanol mixture and mix. Measure the extinctions of the solutions in the first and second flasks at 383 mμ, using 1-cm cells with the blank solution in the comparison cell in each case, and calculate the hydrocortisone sodium succinate content by a comparison of the extinctions.

Other methods for determining this group of steroids have been examined from time to time. These include colorimetric determination as dinitrophenylhydrazones (Porter and Silber[16]); this has found application in biochemical work but is not suitable for determination of corticosteroids in pharmaceuticals. Clark[17] has described the reaction of corticosteroids with a diphenylamine reagent; a violet colour, having maximum absorption in the region of 530 mμ, is produced with those having an oxo group in the 11 position, and a green colour with maximum absorption at about 650 mμ with those having a hydroxyl group in the 11 position. Attempts have been made[18] to apply this reaction for quantitative use, but without success.

Schulz and Neuss[19] described a method based upon reaction of the steroid with 2,6-di-*tert*-butyl-*p*-cresol in alkaline solution. The butyl-*p*-cresol is added to an ethanolic solution of corticosteroid in a solution made alkaline with sodium hydroxide; after refluxing for thirty minutes the solution is cooled as rapidly as possible and the extinction value measured at the appropriate wavelength. Steroids having an oxo group at position 3 and an —OH or —H at position 11 give a blue colour; those having an oxo group at position 11 give a yellow-brown colour; the presence of a double bond between carbon atoms 1 and 2 prevents the formation of colour. Thus, of the corticosteroids in Table 33, hydrocortisone, deoxycortone and fludrocortisone will give a blue colour having a maximum absorption at about 625 mμ and cortisone will give a yellow-brown colour having a maximum absorption at about 470 mμ. The other steroids, having a double bond between C atoms 1 and 2, give no colour. In our experience, however, the conditions of colour development are so critical that the method could not be put to quantitative use although it might be useful for qualitative separation of steroids into groups. A later paper[20] on this method gives slightly modified conditions for development of colour but in our hands it has still not been found suitable for accurate quantitative use.

In assessing corticosteroids, which are pharmacologically very potent and which might provide quite different actions from each other, it is of considerable importance to limit the presence of any foreign related material. In the *U.S.P.* a paper chromatographic test for Related Foreign Steroids is included in all the corticosteroid monographs. Although good results have been obtained with this procedure it has several drawbacks in that (*a*) it requires six mobile phases, (*b*) the drying time for chromatograms is twelve to eighteen hours and (*c*) the solvent front moves a distance of only about 15 cm and in some cases separation of steroids of similar Rf values is not very good as the spots obtained tend to be diffuse. The following limit test, which makes use of descending paper chromatography, requires only two mobile phases and gives good separation, the solvent front moving about 45 cm. The drying time for chromatograms is much shorter than with the *U.S.P.* method.

Reagents:

Mobile phase A. This is a saturated solution of formamide in chloroform.

Mobile phase B. This is a saturated solution of formamide in a mixture of equal volumes of benzene and chloroform.

Developing solution: Add 1 volume of a 0·1 per cent solution of

2,3,5-triphenyltetrazolium chloride in water to 9 volumes of 2N sodium hydroxide just before use.

Impregnation of paper: Cut strips of chromatographic paper, about 15 cm wide and 55 cm long, saturate with a 40 per cent v/v solution of formamide in methanol and dry without the aid of heat.

Test: Prepare 0·5 per cent solutions, in acetone, of the sample and of an authentic specimen of the substance being tested and pipette 0·005 ml of each solution on to one of the prepared filter-paper strips at points 10 cm from the top. Suspend the paper in a chromatographic tank, at a temperature of 25° to 27°, the atmosphere of which is saturated with the appropriate mobile phase (see below) and allow to stand for one and a half hours. Elute with the specified mobile phase until the solvent approaches the bottom of the paper (about four hours for mobile phase A and about two and a half hours for mobile phase B), remove the paper from the tank and dry, at room temperature, for five minutes and then at 105° for forty minutes. Develop the chromatograms by passage through a shallow layer of the developing solution. The sample and the authentic specimen should each yield, equidistant from the top of the paper, a red spot of approximately the same size and intensity; no secondary spots should appear.

Dry the developed paper at 105° for thirty minutes and examine under ultra-violet light, including light of wavelength 366 mμ. The spots obtained with cortisone, hydrocortisone and fludrocortisone fluoresce; those obtained with dexamethasone, methylprednisolone, prednisolone and prednisone do not fluoresce.

The order of increasing Rf values of a number of important corticosteroids, together with the appropriate mobile phase, is as follows:

	Mobile Phase
Methylprednisolone	B
Prednisolone	A
Dexamethasone	A
Hydrocortisone	B
Prednisone	B
Prednisolone Acetate	B
Hydrocortisone Acetate	B
Fludrocortisone Acetate	B
Prednisone Acetate	B
Cortisone Acetate	B

Triamcinolone, when examined by this method, remains at the point of application.

Triphenyltetrazolium chloride is preferred to tetrazolium blue as the staining reagent since it only stains the corticosteroid spots and does not leave a blue background on the paper. Great care must be taken in staining the chromatograms and the directions must be strictly adhered to, otherwise the paper tends to crumble and becomes difficult to handle.

The following procedure, which avoids staining of the paper, has been found useful. View the chromatogram through a Chance OB4 filter while it is being subjected to short-wave ultra-violet light (a Mazda germicide lamp fitted with a Chance OX7 filter may be used). The steroid zones can be seen as dark blue areas against a lighter blue background. Should a permanent record of the chromatogram be required the light from a suitable ultra-violet source, such as that given above, may be passed through the unstained paper on to a Duostat paper.

If it is necessary to identify any related foreign steroids which may be present, the sample load applied to the paper should be increased to 50 to 75 μg when the subsidiary spots are more clearly visible; loads in excess of 75 μg tend to give diffuse spots.

1. CAROL. J., and ROTONDARO, F. A., *J. Amer. Pharm. Ass., Sci. Edn.*, 1946, **35,** 176.
2. KOBER, S., *Biochem. J.*, 1938, **32,** 357.
3. CAROL, J., and MOLITOR, J. C., *J. Amer. Pharm. Ass., Sci. Edn.*, 1947, **36,** 208.
4. HAENNI, E. D., CAROL, J., and BANES, D., *J. Amer. Pharm. Ass., Sci. Edn.*, 1953, **42,** 162.
5. SNAIR, D. W., and SCHWINGHAMMER, L. A., *J. Pharm. Pharmacol.*, 1961, **13,** 148.
6. COHEN, H., and BATES, R. W., *J. Amer. Pharm. Ass., Sci. Edn.*, 1951, **40,** 35.
7. ELVIDGE, W. F., *Quart. J. Pharm.*, 1946, **19,** 260.
8. UMBERGER, E. J., *Anal. Chem.*, 1955, **27,** 768.
9. MADIGAN, J. J., ZENNO, E. E., and PHEASANT, R., *Anal. Chem.*, 1951, **23,** 1691.
10. GORNALL, A. G., and MACDONALD, M. P., *J. Biol. Chem.*, 1953, **201,** 279.
11. CHEN, C., and TEWELL, H. E., *Federation Proc.*, 1951, **10,** 377.
12. MADER, W. J., and BUCK, R. R., *Anal. Chem.*, 1952, **24,** 666.
13. JOHNSON, C. A., KING, R. E., and VICKERS, C., *Analyst*, 1960, **85,** 714.
14. JOHNSON, C. A., *Proc. Feigl Anniversary Symp.*, 1962, 183.
15. KING, R. E., private communication.
16. PORTER, C. C., and SILBER, R. H., *J. Biol. Chem.*, 1950, **185,** 201.
17. CLARK, I., *Nature*, 1955, **175,** 123.
18. VICKERS, C., private communication.
19. SCHULZ, E. P., and NEUSS, J. D., *Anal. Chem.*, 1957, **29,** 1662.
20. SULTANA ANSARI and RIAZ AHMED KHAN, *J. Pharm. Pharmacol.*, 1960, **12,** 122.

STRAMONIUM

Stramonium leaf contains up to 0·5 per cent of alkaloids, but the *B.P.* requirement of 0·25 per cent is rather high, much of the normal leaf contains somewhat less, 0·20 to 0·22 per cent. It is assayed as for Belladonna Herb (see p. 107).

Dry Extract of Stramonium, *B.P.* Contains 1 per cent of alkaloids, calculated as hyoscyamine.

See Dry Extract of Belladonna for assay.

Liquid Extract of Stramonium, *B.P.* Contains 0·25 per cent of alkaloids, calculated as hyoscyamine.

Assay by transferring 10 ml to a separator, adding 5 ml of water and 1 ml of dilute ammonia solution and continuing as for Tincture of Belladonna by shaking with successive 25-ml portions of chloroform.

Tincture of Stramonium, *B.P.* Contains 0·025 per cent of alkaloids, calculated as hyoscyamine.

Assay as under Tincture of Belladonna, which is essentially the method due to Caines[1] for Tincture of Stramonium.

Tablets of Stramonium, *B.P.C.* Usually contain 1 grain of dry extract of stramonium.

Assay as under Dry Extract of Belladonna using a sample obtained by evaporating to dryness a solution prepared by warming 20 powdered tablets for thirty minutes on a water-bath with 50 ml of 70 per cent ethanol, shaking frequently, and then percolating slowly with warm 70 per cent ethanol until extraction is completed.

1. Caines, C. M., *Quart. J. Pharm.*, 1930, **3,** 342.

SUGARS

Analysis of only the simplest sugar mixtures is generally required for pharmaceutical preparations and the subject will be discussed briefly and yet in sufficient detail for undertaking the estimation of simple sugars or mixtures of sucrose, invert sugar and glucose or lactose.

Polarimetric Estimation. As sugar analysis depends so much upon the polarimeter, various modifications of this instrument have been designed to show the percentage of sugar directly by use of an arbitrary scale when using a definite weight or 'normal weight' of sugar dissolved in 100 ml and determining the polarisation in a 2-dm tube. The simplest formulæ for sugar calculations are those derived for use with these 'saccharimeters.' The following methods are based on the Ventzke scale for which the normal weight is 26·00 g. If an ordinary polarimeter is used, 1 degree of sugar scale is equivalent to 0·3462 angular degree.

(*a*) For a simple sugar the specific rotation, using sodium light, can be calculated from the formula:

$$[\alpha]_D^{20} = \frac{100a}{l \times c} \quad \text{where} \quad [\alpha]_D^{20} = \text{specific rotation at } 20°$$

a = observed rotation in degrees
c = concentration in g/100 ml
l = length of tube in decimetres

$$\therefore c = \frac{100a}{l \times [\alpha]_D^{20}}$$

For some sugars the specific rotation varies slightly with concentration. All readings in polarimetric work are taken at 20° unless otherwise stated. The specific rotations, observed in 25 per cent w/v solution, of a few common sugars are: **dextrose** ($C_6H_{12}O_6$, Mol. Wt. 180·2) +53·5°, **lævulose** ($C_6H_{12}O_6$, Mol. Wt. 180·2) −94·6°, invert sugar −20·6°, **lactose** (anhydrous, $C_{12}H_{22}O_{11}$, Mol. Wt. 342·3) +55·2°, and **sucrose** ($C_{12}H_{22}O_{11}$, Mol. Wt. 342·3) +66·5°. Mutarotation of the solutions of dextrose, lævulose and lactose should be completed by the addition of a few drops of ammonia before being adjusted to volume (see also p. 604).

(*b*) Sucrose in the presence of a reducing sugar (*e.g.* lactose or invert sugar).

By the action of acids or invertase, sucrose is converted to a mixture of equal parts of dextrose and lævulose (inversion); if the optical rotation of any mixture containing sucrose is determined before and after inversion, the change of rotation observed is equivalent to the quantity of sucrose present, and by simple calculation the proportion may be ascertained.

Dissolve the normal weight in 60 ml of water, clarify if necessary (see below) and make up to 100 ml. Observe the rotation (*D*) in a 2-dm tube.

Acid Inversion. Jackson and Gillis[1] critically examined the Herzfeld method of inversion, and the following was recommended as the best procedure:

Pipette 50 ml of the prepared sugar solution into a 100-ml flask and dilute to 70 ml. Add 10 ml of 6·34N hydrochloric acid, immerse the flask in a water-bath at 60°, agitate it continuously for about three minutes and leave in the bath for a total of nine minutes; then quickly cool and make up to volume at 20° for polarisation. The strength of the acid in the final solution is identical with that of the Herzfeld process. Observe the rotation again in a 2-dm tube; multiply the reading by two (*I*).

The temperature at which the reading of the rotation of the inverted solution is taken is important, and it must either be determined exactly at 20° or any variation must be noted.

When the normal weight of sucrose has an $[\alpha]_D$ of 100, invert sugar at 0° has a rotation of −42·5°, which decreases by 0·5° for each 1° of temperature; hence (Clerget formula):

$$\text{Per cent sucrose } (S) = \frac{(D - I) \times 100}{142{\cdot}5 - t/2}$$

or if $t = 20°$, sucrose $= 0{\cdot}754\ (D - I)$ (subtract algebraically).

Invertase Inversion. This process should be used with impure sucrose products, since it has no influence on the optical activity of any other constituents of the solution except raffinose (if present), whereas hydrochloric acid has a destructive effect on lævulose if this sugar is present in considerable quantity. The procedure for invertase hydrolysis is:

To 50 ml of the prepared solution (freed from lead, if this has been used for clarification) in a 100-ml graduated flask, add glacial acetic acid in sufficient quantity to render the solution distinctly acid to methyl red. Then add 10 ml of invertase solution, place the flask in a water-bath at 55° to 60° and allow to stand at that temperature for fifteen minutes with occasional shaking. Cool, add sodium carbonate solution until alkaline to litmus paper, dilute to 100 ml at 20°, mix well and determine the polarisation at 20° in a 2-dm tube.

The inversion factor is slightly different and for invertase inversion with readings at 20° the sucrose is calculated from the formula, $S = 0{\cdot}757 (D - I)$.

For the other sugar in the mixture (*e.g.* invert sugar or lactose):
Let S = percentage of sucrose found by the above method,
V = invert sugar to be found.

$$\text{Then } V = (D - S) \times \frac{[\alpha]_D \text{ sucrose}}{[\alpha]_D \text{ invert sugar}} = (D - S) \times \frac{66{\cdot}5}{-20{\cdot}6}$$

Similarly for lactose (L):

$$L = (D - S) \times \frac{66{\cdot}5}{55{\cdot}2}$$

Clarifying agents may be required for dark or turbid solutions, the general reagents being a slight excess of basic or neutral lead acetate or alumina cream, added before adjusting the volume (but some slight adsorption of reducing sugars is likely). Alumina cream is prepared by adding a slight excess of ammonia to a saturated solution of alum and washing the precipitate by decantation until almost free from sulphates. Special reagents are used for definite processes and should always be employed where directed. Excess of lead may be removed by addition of anhydrous sodium carbonate to the filtered solution, the excess of alkali catalysing **mutarotation,** which may occur if dextrose or other reducing sugars were present in the original sugar in a crystalline form or in solution at high density. Mutarotation may also be completed by boiling the neutral solution of the sugar or by adding a few drops of ammonia and then neutralising with an equivalent of acetic acid before making up to volume.

The above formulæ do not apply when a third optically-active substance is present (*e.g.* glucose in the presence of cane sugar and invert sugar). For such mixtures the copper reducing power must also be determined, as described below.

Determination of Reducing Sugars by Copper Reduction. The gravimetric copper determination of reducing sugars has been almost entirely superseded by volumetric methods. Many modifications have been proposed, each of which claims to give the most accurate results; but if the analyst gains experience in any one method and standardises his titrations against pure sugars, he will be well advised to adhere to that process rather than to experiment with others. The method of Lane and Eynon[2] by reduction of Fehling's solution is the most generally applied volumetric method, the use of methylene blue as an internal indicator increasing the accuracy of the process. If strict attention be given to the details of the procedure and the tables published by the authors are used to calculate the results, a high degree of accuracy can be obtained:

Prepare a solution of the sugar of such concentration that more than 15 ml and less than 50 ml will be required to reduce all the copper in 10 ml or 25 ml of Fehling's solution (0·1 to 0·8 g per 100 ml of dextrose and 0·13 to 1·1 g per 100 ml of lactose). For preliminary titration, measure accurately 10 ml or 25 ml of Fehling's solution into a conical flask of about 300-ml capacity. From a burette add 15 ml of the sugar solution and heat to boiling over an asbestos-covered wire gauze. Continue adding the sugar solution in fairly large portions at fifteen-second intervals, until, from the colour of the mixture, the copper appears to be nearly reduced; then boil for a minute or two, add 3 to 5 drops of 1 per cent methylene blue solution and continue the titration until the blue colour is discharged. Repeat the titration, adding, before heating, almost the full amount of sugar solution required to reduce all the copper. After boiling has commenced maintain a moderate degree of ebullition for two minutes, and, without removing the flame, add 3 to 5 drops of indicator and continue the titration so that it is just complete in a total boiling time of exactly three minutes. The end-point is clearly indicated by the disappearance of the blue colour, the solution becoming orange. The flask must not be removed from the gauze at any stage of the titration.

Fehling's Solution. No. 1 contains 34·64 g of $CuSO_4,5H_2O$ and 0·5 ml of H_2SO_4 in water to 500 ml. No. 2 contains 176 g of sodium potassium tartrate and 77 g of sodium hydroxide in water to 500 ml. Mix equal volumes of No. 1 and No. 2 solutions immediately before use.

The factors given (see Appendix XVIII, p. 888) are only strictly valid for the actual procedure specified by the authors as above, but some latitude in the time of boiling is permissible with the monose sugars when only a small amount of sucrose is present. With large percentages of sucrose a correction is necessary (given in Appendix). The end-point of the titration may be difficult to see in artificial light; Tritton[3] recommends the use of transmitted light for determining the end-point in these circumstances (open wire gauze, white tile and 40-watt opal bulb).

The above method is applicable to a mixture of sucrose and invert sugar, titrations before and after inversion giving free and total invert sugar, from which the sucrose may easily be calculated. Total invert sugar — free invert sugar × 0·95 = sucrose.

If inversion has been obtained by acid, the solution should be neutralised with sodium carbonate before making up to the volume for titration with Fehling's solution.

Mixtures of Cane Sugar with Liquid Glucose. For calculations with mixed sugars, the copper-reducing power, or '*K*' value, is often required, *i.e.* the relative reducing power of carbohydrates and solutions thereof referred to dextrose equal to 100. Thus a syrup which contains 45 per cent of reducing sugars expressed as dextrose, would have a 'K' value of 45.

The commercial variety of glucose, which contains dextrin and maltose, is used to adulterate syrups; as this is not a pure chemical compound, the calculation of the percentage present is based on the approximation for glucose syrup of a mean 'K' value of 36·5 and a rotation of +179° on the Ventzke scale.

The presence of glucose is easily confirmed by the high positive rotation remaining after inversion; if glucose is present, determine the 'K' value before inversion by the volumetric method given above. Then the following equations are necessary:

Calculate 'S' from the Clerget formula given on p. 603.

Then $0{\cdot}365G + 1{\cdot}0\,I = K$

$1{\cdot}79\ G - 0{\cdot}326\,I = D - S$

where G, I and S are percentages of glucose, invert sugar and sucrose respectively.

Another method for determination of glucose depends on the proportional change of rotation of lævulose with temperature compared with dextrose, until at 87° the rotation of invert sugar, which consists of equal parts of dextrose and lævulose, is zero. The following is the *A.O.A.C.*[4] procedure for determining dextrose and lævulose in the presence of cane sugar, as applied to honey:

> From the direct and indirect polarisation at 20° determine the sucrose. Observe the direct polarisation reading at 87° (which is obtained by use of a jacketed metal tube), multiply by 1·0315 to correct for the water expansion at that temperature and subtract the product from the direct polarisation at 20°; divide the difference by 2·3919 (the variation in polarisation of 1 g of lævulose in 100 ml of solution between 20° and 87°), to obtain the grammes of lævulose in a normal weight of the product, and hence calculate the percentage in the original sample. To determine the dextrose, obtain the percentage of total reducing sugars, as dextrose, by Fehling's titration in the direct polarisation solution, multiply the percentage of lævulose found by 0·915 to give its dextrose equivalent in copper-reducing power and subtract from the total to obtain the percentage of dextrose in the sample.

Commercial glucose may be determined approximately by observing the rotation at 87° after inversion. The figure obtained is divided by 1·63 to obtain the percentage of commercial glucose, as it is found that commercial glucose polarising at 175° in the cold, when subjected to inversion and neutralisation, gives a true polarisation at 87°, about 93 per cent of theoretical.

Determination of Aldose Sugars with Chloramine-T. Mention might be made of the titration of aldose sugars with chloramine-T and potassium iodide, devised by Hinton and Macara,[5] in which dextrose or lactose may be determined in the presence of sucrose and lævulose. The method has the advantage of suppressing secondary action on the sugars; the necessary gradual addition of alkali is obtained by its liberation during the reaction:

> Pipette 20 ml or 25 ml of a solution of sugar of suitable strength (dextrose 0·08 g, lactose or invert sugar 0·15 g) into a 250-ml flask and add 20 ml of 10 per cent potassium iodide solution, followed by 50 ml of 0·05N chloramine-T (7·04 g per litre). Close the flask with a rubber bung and keep it at ordinary temperature in the dark for one and a half hours, after which acidify the solution with 10 ml of 2N hydrochloric acid and titrate at once with 0·05N thiosulphate, using starch as indicator. Treat in exactly the same manner a control in which water is used in place of sugar solution. Calculate the difference in titrations to grammes of iodine. The iodine equivalent per gramme of sugar is, dextrose 1·410, lactose 0·705 and invert sugar 0·744.

If the amount of sugar oxidised varies much from the above specified quantities, the factor used differs a little. Sucrose is attacked slightly and allowance must be made in estimating lactose or glucose if this be present (estimating it independently either by chloramine after inversion, or by other means). A table of sucrose corrections, *i.e.* ml of 0·05N thiosulphate to be deducted for grammes of sucrose present in the titration solution, is given in Appendix XIX.

Sucrose may be inverted with hydrochloric acid by the method given above, but, after cooling, the solution must be exactly neutralised with sodium hydroxide, using litmus paper as indicator, before being made up to a definite volume.

Purified Honey. The *B.P.C.* article is commercial honey which has been strained and adjusted to a weight per ml of 1·355 g by the addition of water.

The specific rotation (using a 20 per cent w/v solution containing a few drops of concentrated ammonia to complete mutarotation) should be $+3°$ to $-15°$. If added glucose be suspected it may be determined by the method given above.

Oxymel. A mixture of acetic acid with water and honey. The specific rotation (using a 25 per cent w/v solution) should be $+2{\cdot}4°$ to $-12{\cdot}0°$, which is approximately equivalent to the specific rotation of the official honey, allowing for the proportion in the formula. The acetic acid is determined by titration of 10 ml after dilution, with N sodium hydroxide using phenolphthalein as indicator, 1 ml N = 0·06003 g.

1. JACKSON, R. F., and GILLIS, G. L., *Int. Sugar J.*, 1920, **22,** 509.
2. LANE, J. H., and EYNON, L., *J. Soc. Chem. Ind.*, 1923, **42,** 32T.
3. TRITTON, S. M., *Analyst*, 1943, **68,** 147.
4. *A.O.A.C.*, 1960, p. 436.
5. HINTON, C. L., and MACARA, T., *Analyst*, 1927, **52,** 668.

SULPHONAMIDES

The official sulphonamides are all derivatives of sulphanilamide and the assay for all members of the group by diazotisation follows that of the parent substance either directly or after preliminary hydrolysis or reduction (para-nitrosulphathiazole) except for sulphafurazole and sulphafurazole diethanolamine. Sulphafurazole cannot be diazotised quantitatively since the product consumes more than one equivalent of nitrous acid. Non-aqueous titration can also be applied.

The diazotisation method is now generally used with the following procedure:

> Weigh about 0·5 g into a 250-ml beaker fitted with a magnetic stirrer and dissolve in 75 ml of water and 10 ml of concentrated hydrochloric acid. Titrate electrometrically with 0·1M sodium nitrite using the 'dead-stop' technique (see p. 867).

The sodium nitrite volumetric solution is preferably standardised against a specimen of pure sulphanilamide. In the absence of apparatus for the electrometric end-point, starch-iodide paste may be used as external indicator. It is necessary to titrate slowly and to keep the temperature of the reaction mixture below 15°.

> Weigh about 0·5 g into a beaker, add 20 ml of concentrated hydrochloric acid and 50 ml of water and stir until dissolved. Cool to 15°, add about 25 g of crushed ice and titrate slowly with 0·1M sodium nitrite, with vigorous stirring, until the solution, after being allowed to stand for one minute, immediately gives a blue colour when a drop is drawn across the surface of a film of starch-iodide paste.

The method suffers from the defect that the end-point is not easily seen without suitable experience of the titration. Acriflavine has been used by Frost[1] who found that a very dilute solution could be used as internal indicator, the colour change being from yellow to violet; just before the end-point the colour is purple owing to the presence of unchanged acriflavine.

As previously mentioned, sulphafurazole cannot be determined by the nitrite method but it can be assayed by non-aqueous titration:

> Dissolve about 0·2 g of sulphafurazole in 5 ml of dimethylformamide, maintaining an atmosphere of nitrogen in the flask, add 0·1 ml of a 0·5 per cent solution of thymol blue in dimethylformamide and titrate with 0·1N lithium or sodium methoxide, until the colour changes from yellow to blue. Protect the lithium methoxide from moisture and carbon dioxide. Carry out a blank determination omitting the sample. 1 ml 0·1N = 0·02673 g $C_{11}H_{13}O_3N_3S$.

Non-aqueous titration is applicable to other sulphonamides. Bromimetric assay of sulphonamides has been proposed from time to time but it is not to be recommended. Excess of bromine, temperature of reaction and time of standing all affect the results. Bromination is not applicable to the assay of tablets since many of the excipients themselves react with bromine.

Table 35 on page 610 summarises the official sulphonamides, the factor for 0·1M sodium nitrite assay in all cases is 1×10^{-4} of the molecular weight.

Preparations (tablets and injections) are assayed exactly as the parent substance; tablet excipients do not interfere but it may be desirable to warm the powdered tablets in the acid to aid solution. **Tablets of Sulphafurazole,** *B.Vet.C.*, should be first extracted with dimethylformamide before non-aqueous titration.

Mixture of Succinylsulphathiazole for Infants, *B.P.C.* Contains 13·7 per cent. For assay 5 g should be heated with 10 ml of 20 per cent sodium hydroxide on a water-bath for two hours before neutralising with hydrochloric acid, adding 5 ml of 5N acid in excess and titrating with 0·1M sodium nitrite. **Tablets of Succinylsulphathiazole,** *B.P.*, are best hydrolysed by this method.

Eye Ointment of Sulphacetamide, *B.P.* Usually contains 6·0 per cent of sulphacetamide sodium. It can be assayed as the parent substance after preliminary extraction with dilute hydrochloric acid from a solution of the sample in a mixture of light petroleum and ether.

For the determination of **small amounts** of sulphonamides the colour reaction depending on diazotisation and a subsequent coupling with an amine has advantages over the colour development with *p*-dimethylaminobenzaldehyde since, in the latter reaction, the yellow colour is difficult to match and the sensitivity of the test varies with the pH.

The method of Bratton and Marshall[2] was developed for the estimation of sulphonamides in body fluids; for mixtures in which the concentration of sulphonamides is sufficiently large (this also generally applies to urine) the determination is done as for the filtrate in the method described below. The absence of substances such as local anæsthetics, which would give the same colour reaction as the sulphonamides, must be ascertained. To determine the total drug if conjugated sulphonamides are present a portion of the prepared test solution must be hydrolysed by heating on a water-bath for one hour in 0·2N hydrochloric acid and subsequent adjustment to volume. The following method is that applied to blood:

Measure 2 ml of oxalated blood into a flask, dilute with 30 ml of water and precipitate with 8 ml of 15 per cent trichloroacetic acid solution. Determine the free drug in the filtrate as follows:

To 10 ml of the filtrate add 1 ml of freshly prepared 0·1 per cent sodium nitrite solution, allow to stand for three minutes, add 1 ml of

TABLE 35

SULPHONAMIDE	FORMULA	MOL. WT.	
Acetyl Sulphafurazole, *U.S.P.*	$C_{13}H_{15}O_4N_3S$	309·4	Dissolve in 15 ml glacial acetic acid, add 2 ml concentrated H_2SO_4
Para-nitrosulphathiazole, *N.F.*	$C_9H_7O_4N_3S_2$	285·3	Heat on a water-bath with 30 ml glacial acetic acid, add 15 ml concentrated HCl in 1-ml portions and heat until colourless. Cool, dilute with equal volume of water, filter, add 10 ml of dilute H_2SO_4 and boil for five minutes
Phthalylsulphacetamide, *N.F.*	$C_{16}H_{14}O_6N_2S$	362·4	Reflux for two hours with 40 ml of concentrated HCl
Phthalylsulphathiazole, *B.P.*	$C_{17}H_{13}O_5N_3S_2$	403·4	Reflux for thirty minutes with 50 ml of dilute HCl. Cool and add 50 ml of water
Succinylsulphathiazole, *B.P.*	$C_{13}H_{13}O_5N_3S_2,H_2O$	373·4	Reflux for thirty minutes with 50 ml of dilute HCl. Cool, add 50 ml of water
Sulphacetamide, *B.P.C.*	$C_8H_{10}O_3N_2S$	214·3	
Sulphacetamide Sodium, *B.P.*	$C_8H_9O_3N_2SNa,H_2O$	254·2	
Sulphadiazine, *B.P.*	$C_{10}H_{10}O_2N_4S$	250·3	Warm, if necessary, to dissolve
Sulphadiazine Sodium, *B.P.C.*	$C_{10}H_9O_2N_4SNa$	272·3	
Sulphadimethoxine	$C_{12}H_{14}O_4N_4S$	310·3	
Sulphadimidine, *B.P.*	$C_{12}H_{14}O_2N_4S$	278·3	
Sulphadimidine Sodium, *B.P.*	$C_{12}H_{13}O_2N_4SNa$	300·3	
Sulphafurazole, *B.P.C.*	$C_{11}H_{13}O_3N_3S$	267·3	Non-aqueous titration
Sulphafurazole Diethanolamine, *U.S.P.*	$C_{11}H_{13}O_3N_3S,C_4H_{11}O_2N$	372·5	Non-aqueous titration
Sulphaguanidine, *B.P.*	$C_7H_{10}O_2N_4S,H_2O$	232·3	
Sulphamerazine, *B.P.*	$C_{11}H_{12}O_2N_4S$	264·3	
Sulphamerazine Sodium, *B.P.C.*	$C_{11}H_{11}O_2N_4SNa$	286·3	
Sulphamethizole	$C_9H_{10}O_2N_4S_2$	270·3	
Sulphamethoxypyridazine, *U.S.P.*	$C_{11}H_{12}O_3N_4S$	280·3	Also by non-aqueous titration (*U.S.P.*)
Sulphanilamide, *B.P.C.*	$C_6H_8O_2N_2S$	172·2	
Sulphaphenazole	$C_{15}H_{14}O_2N_4S$	314·4	
Sulphapyridine, *B.P.C.*	$C_{11}H_{11}O_2N_3S$	249·3	
Sulphapyridine Sodium, *B.Vet.C.*	$C_{11}H_{10}O_2N_3SNa$	271·3	
Sulphaquinoxaline, *B.Vet.C.*	$C_{14}H_{12}O_2N_4S$	300·3	Dissolve in 5 ml of N NaOH and 20 ml of water
Sulphasomidine, *B.P.C.*	$C_{12}H_{14}O_2N_4S$	278·3	
Sulphathiazole, *B.P.C.*	$C_9H_9O_2N_3S_2$	255·3	
Sulphathiazole Sodium, *N.F.*	$C_9H_8O_2N_3S_2Na,1\frac{1}{2}H_2O$	304·3	

0·5 per cent ammonium sulphamate solution and, after two minutes, add 1 ml of a 0·1 per cent aqueous solution of *N*-(1-naphthyl)ethylenediamine dihydrochloride. Measure the extinction at the maximum at about 545 mμ (sulphanilamide 540 mμ, sulphapyridine 544 mμ, sulphadiazine 545 mμ, sulphathiazole 548 mμ) and compare with that of the appropriate sulphonamide when similarly treated; the measurement can be made immediately and the colour is stable for at least one hour in subdued light.

The most convenient standards to prepare are 1·0, 0·3 and 0·1 mg of the corresponding sulphonamide per 100 ml. The *N*-(1-naphthyl)-ethylenediamine dihydrochloride solution should be kept in a dark-coloured bottle and stored in a refrigerator; when the solution becomes at all yellow it should be discarded. *p*-Aminosalicylic acid will interfere with this colorimetric assay.

Shepherd[3] proposed a colorimetric method for pyrimidines substituted in the 2-position based on the red colour formed with 2-thiobarbituric acid. Since no colour is produced when the pyrimidine is substituted in either the 4- or the 6-position this reaction may be used for the determination of sulphadiazine in the presence of other sulphonamides, including sulphamerazine and sulphadimidine.

Tablets of Trisulphonamides, *B.P.C.* Although officially only the total sulphonamides are determined, Marzys[4] has proposed a method for the determination of sulphadiazine, sulphamerazine and sulphathiazole in mixtures, using the thiobarbituric acid colorimetric method for sulphadiazine and an ultra-violet absorption method for the other two. The detailed method is as follows:

Reagent: Thiobarbituric acid solution. Dissolve 5 g of 2-thiobarbituric acid in 20 ml of N sodium hydroxide diluted with 500 ml of water. Add 250 ml of citrate buffer solution (prepared by dissolving 37 g of sodium citrate dihydrate in water, adding 32 ml of concentrated hydrochloric acid and diluting to 250 ml with water) and adjust the pH to 2·0. Store in glass-stoppered bottles in a refrigerator.

Preparation of sample solution: To an amount of powdered sample equivalent to about 0·1 g of mixed sulphonamides add 50 ml of N hydrochloric acid and shake intermittently during ten minutes. Filter if necessary and dilute the filtrate and washings to 100 ml with water in a graduated flask. Transfer a 5-ml aliquot to a second 100-ml graduated flask, add 7·5 ml of N hydrochloric acid and dilute to 100 ml with water. (Solution A.)

Preparation of standard solutions: Prepare a standard solution of each of the three sulphonamides in exactly the same way as solution A but using 0·100 g of the sulphonamide in place of the sample.

Method: Dilute a 5-ml aliquot of the standard sulphadiazine solution to 10 ml with 0·1N hydrochloric acid in a graduated flask to give a solution containing 25 μg of sulphadiazine per ml.

Dilute 5-ml aliquots of each of the three standard sulphonamide solutions to 25 ml respectively in graduated flasks to give solutions containing 10 μg of the sulphonamide per ml.

Sulphadiazine: Transfer a 1-ml aliquot of solution A to a 10-ml graduated flask and at the same time transfer a 1-ml aliquot of standard sulphadiazine solution, 25 μg per ml, to a second 10-ml graduated flask and pipette 1 ml of 0·1N hydrochloric acid into a third 10-ml graduated flask for the blank. Dilute the contents of each flask to volume with thiobarbituric acid solution and place the flasks in a water-bath, inserting the stoppers when the solutions have attained the temperature of the bath and allowing to stand for one hour thereafter. Remove the stoppers, allow to cool and add water to volume, if necessary, to compensate for any evaporation.

Measure the extinctions of the sample and standard solutions at the absorption maximum at about 533 mμ, using 1-cm cells with the blank solution in the comparison cell in each case and calculate the sulphadiazine content by comparison.

Sulphamerazine and sulphathiazole: Transfer a 5-ml aliquot of solution A to a 25-ml graduated flask and dilute to volume with 0·1N hydrochloric acid. Measure the extinctions at 243 mμ (E 243 mμ) and 280 mμ (E 280 mμ), using 1-cm cells with 0·1N hydrochloric acid in the comparison cell.

Measure the extinctions at 243 mμ and 280 mμ of each of the standard sulphonamide solutions, 10 μg per ml, using 1-cm cells with 0·1N hydrochloric acid in the comparison cell in each case and calculate the value of E(1 per cent, 1 cm) for each sulphonamide at each wavelength. Let the E(1 per cent, 1 cm) of sulphadiazine be A at 243 mμ and D at 280 mμ. Let the E(1 per cent, 1 cm) of sulphamerazine be B at 243 mμ and E at 280 mμ. Let the E(1 per cent, 1 cm) of sulphathiazole be C at 243 mμ and F at 280 mμ. Then, since the extinction of the mixture is equal to the sum of the extinctions of the constituents,

$$1{,}000 \text{ E } 243 \text{ m}\mu = Ad + Bm + Ct$$
$$1{,}000 \text{ E } 280 \text{ m}\mu = Dd + Em + Ft$$

where d, m and t are the concentrations of sulphadiazine, sulphamerazine and sulphathiazole, respectively, in mg per 100 ml.

Since d is known from the determination of sulphadiazine, if

$$(1{,}000 \text{ E } 243 \text{ m}\mu - Ad) = \text{E}'243 \text{ m}\mu$$
$$(1{,}000 \text{ E } 280 \text{ m}\mu - Dd) = \text{E}'280 \text{ m}\mu$$

then $\text{E}'243 \text{ m}\mu = Bm + Ct$; $\text{E}'280 \text{ m}\mu = Em + Ft$ and m and t can be calculated by substituting the values found for B, C, E and F and solving the equations.

1. Frost, H. F., *Analyst*, 1943, **68**, 51.
2. Bratton, A. C., and Marshall, E. K., *J. Biol. Chem.*, 1939, **128**, 537.
3. Shepherd, R. G., *Anal. Chem.*, 1948, **20**, 1150.
4. Marzys, A. E. O., *Analyst*, 1961, **86**, 460.

SULPHUR

S At. Wt. 32·06

The original determination of elemental sulphur in pharmaceutical preparations, by oxidation to sulphate and determination of the latter by precipitation as barium sulphate, has mainly been superseded by more rapid processes depending on the conversion of the sulphur to thiocyanate or thiosulphate for their volumetric determination.

Conflicting opinions have been expressed on the accuracy of the volumetric methods, since low results have been found with them by some analysts, as compared with an oxidation process (which undoubtedly might give high values); but experience has shown concordant results with volumetric methods. They are advantageous for their simplicity and the results are unaffected by sulphates which may be present.

The estimation of sulphur by methods depending on its degree of solubility in various solvents is quite inaccurate. Henville[1] has drawn attention to the fact that precipitated sulphur is easily soluble in carbon disulphide and slowly soluble in ether and light petroleum, whilst sublimed sulphur is soluble to a great extent in all three solvents. Hence, for example, it is quite useless to try to extract the fat from a sulphur ointment in order to estimate the sulphur in the residue.

The gravimetric determination of elemental sulphur adopted by the *U.S.P.*, depending on oxidation of sulphur to sulphate with hydrogen peroxide, is essentially the following:

> Dry about 1 g over silica gel for four hours and transfer to a flask with 50 ml of 10 per cent ethanolic potassium hydroxide. Boil until the solution is transparent and the sulphur has dissolved, cool and dilute with water to 250 ml in a graduated flask. Oxidise 25 ml by adding hydrogen peroxide solution in excess (50 ml) and heat on a water-bath for one hour. Acidify with hydrochloric acid, dilute to 250 ml and precipitate as barium sulphate in the usual manner (see Sulphuric Acid). A blank is necessary as hydrogen peroxide often contains sulphate. $BaSO_4 \times 0{\cdot}1374 = S$.

A method of oxidation using nitric acid and bromine (Evers and Elsdon[2]), since adopted by the *U.S.P.* for sulphur ointment, has been shown to give high results (Fleck and Ward[3]) unless nitric acid is removed before precipitation of the sulphate with barium chloride; barium nitrate is probably adsorbed and co-precipitated with barium sulphate. Oxidation to sulphate with bromine in sodium hydroxide solution (Allport[4]) avoids the nitric acid contaminant and yields results comparable with volumetric methods:

> Treat a weighed quantity of material, containing about 0·1 g of sulphur, with 10 g of sodium hydroxide dissolved in a small quantity of water. Heat and add slowly, while rotating the flask, an excess of a solution containing 30 per cent each of bromine and potassium bromide until a clear solution is obtained. Dilute with water, acidify with hydrochloric acid, boil to expel bromine and precipitate the sulphate as usual. $BaSO_4 \times 0{\cdot}1374 = S$.

A simple and rapid volumetric assay of elemental sulphur was devised by Fleck and Ward,[5] which gives good results with both **sublimed sulphur** and **precipitated sulphur.** The process depends on the quantitative formation of thiosulphate when free sulphur is refluxed with a solution of sodium sulphite, paraffin being added to accelerate the combination. Excess sulphite is eliminated by formaldehyde and acetic acid and the thiosulphate is titrated with iodine:

> Boil the weighed material, containing preferably about 0·1 g of sulphur, in a conical flask attached to a reflux air condenser, with 2 g of crystalline sodium sulphite and 30 to 40 ml of water, until the sulphur has dissolved completely, adding 1 g of soft paraffin to accelerate the reaction. Cool the solution and, if necessary, pour off from the paraffin. Extract the paraffin twice with small quantities of hot water and cool; pour off the washings and add to the main bulk of liquid. Add 10 ml of 40 per cent formaldehyde solution and 10 ml of 20 per cent acetic acid. Dilute to 150 ml ensuring that the solution is quite cold before titrating without delay with 0·1N iodine. 1 ml 0·1N = 0·003206 g S.

Starch is recommended as indicator, but it is preferable to titrate without it except in the case of Compound Powder of Liquorice, where it is necessary. The rapidity of solution of the sulphur depends upon its state of division and the nature of the material to be analysed, the time required being longest with flowers of sulphur. The simple expedient of using a broad 250-ml conical flask is an advantage to aid rapid solution of the sulphur.

The oxygen-flask combustion method (see Appendix IV) has been applied[6] to a number of sulphur-containing materials of pharmaceutical and horticultural interest. The method is suitable for the determination of sulphur in organic compounds except those containing a high proportion of nitrogen.

Ointment of Sulphur, *B.P.* Contains 10 per cent of sublimed sulphur in simple ointment.

The observation by Fleck and Ward[5] that paraffin greatly accelerated the combination of sulphur in their method, makes the application of the method to the determination of sulphur in the ointment particularly useful. The further addition of paraffin is obviously unnecessary.

The oxygen-flask combustion method can be employed for this preparation using 50 mg. The absorbing liquid is 25 ml of water and 2 ml of 20 volume hydrogen peroxide, neutralised to methyl red with 0·02N sodium hydroxide. After rinsing, a further 100 ml of water is added, shaken for one minute and then boiled until the volume is reduced to about 50 ml. After cooling rapidly it is titrated with 0·02N sodium hydroxide using methyl red as indicator. 1 ml 0·02N = 0·0003206 g S.

Compound Powder of Liquorice, *B.P.C.* Contains 8 per cent of sublimed sulphur.

The determination of sulphur is preferably carried out by the volumetric method of Fleck and Ward given above, since the other ingredients may contain small quantities of sulphate, 0·2 to 0·4 per cent having been found in commercial specimens of this galenical. As stated previously, the end-point is easily visible with starch as indicator in the titration with iodine. A more satisfactory end-point is obtained without the use of paraffin; one and a half hours' boiling with the sodium sulphite is necessary.

SULPHIDES

Commercial **barium sulphide** is a variable article consisting of barium sulphide, barium sulphate and, sometimes, free sulphur.

The percentage of barium sulphide may be determined by reduction of iodine:

> Weigh about 0·2 g into a flask containing 25 ml of 0·1N iodine, stopper the flask, mix and allow to stand for five minutes. Then add 5 ml of dilute hydrochloric acid, mix, allow to stand for one hour and titrate the excess of iodine with 0·1N sodium thiosulphate after diluting with 25 ml of water. 1 ml 0·1N = 0·008471 g BaS.

Another method by titration with standard zinc solution is:

> Make a standard zinc solution by dissolving 7·70 g of zinc in about 75 ml of dilute hydrochloric acid, adding excess of ammonia solution and diluting to 1 litre. Make an alkaline lead solution by dissolving 1 g of lead acetate in about 20 ml of hot 5 per cent potassium hydroxide solution and diluting to 100 ml. Heat to boiling about 1 g of barium sulphide in about 50 ml of water and titrate with the standard zinc solution until no black or brown colour is obtained by adding a drop of the *filtered* barium solution to a drop of the lead indicator, spotted on a porcelain tile. 1 ml zinc solution = 0·0201 g BaS.

The grey commercial powder contains about 50 per cent of barium sulphide and the yellow (containing free sulphur) 70 per cent.

Selenium sulphide, SeS_2, Mol. Wt. 143·1, is determined in the *U.S.P.* as follows:

> Digest 100 mg with 25 ml of fuming nitric acid, over gentle heat, until no further solution occurs. Cool, transfer to a 250-ml graduated flask containing 100 ml of water, again cool, and dilute to volume with water. Transfer a 50-ml aliquot to a small flask, add 25 ml of water and 10 g of urea and heat to boiling-point. Cool, add 10 ml of 10 per cent potassium iodide solution and immediately titrate the liberated iodine with 0·05N sodium thiosulphate using starch, added towards the end of the titration, as indicator. Repeat the operation omitting the sample. 1 ml 0·05N sodium thiosulphate = 0·000987 g Se.

Sulphurated potash (Liver of Sulphur) consists of a mixture of potassium polysulphides, thiosulphate and other salts. It is standardised on its total sulphur content determined by the alkaline bromine oxidation method given above under Sulphur.

ORGANIC SULPHUR COMPOUNDS

Busulphan, $C_6H_{14}O_6S_2$, Mol. Wt. 246·3, can be assayed by hydrolysis with boiling water and titrating with sodium hydroxide to phenolphthalein, 1 ml 0·1N NaOH = 0·01232 g, or from its sulphur content by the flask-combustion method (p. 801).

Tablets of Busulphan, *B.P.*, are sugar-coated and contain only milligram quantities, hence the flask-combustion method is not applicable because of the large amount of organic matter. It is necessary to extract the busulphan with acetone and decompose it in a sealed tube with nitric acid.

Triturate an accurately weighed quantity of powdered tablets equivalent to about 2 mg of busulphan with 10 ml of hot acetone, decant the liquid through a filter into a Carius tube and evaporate to small volume under a jet of warm air. Extract in the same way with two further 10-ml quantities of acetone, decanting and evaporating after each extraction and evaporating to dryness after the third extraction. Add 0·5 ml of fuming nitric acid, seal the tube and heat at 300° for two hours. After opening the Carius tube transfer its contents to a small dish with 15 ml of water, evaporate to dryness, dissolve the residue in water and acidify with concentrated hydrochloric acid. Add an excess of 10 per cent barium chloride solution, heat on a water-bath for three hours, filter through a platinum filtering crucible, ignite at 800° for one hour, cool and weigh. Each mg of residue = 0·5276 mg of $C_6H_{14}O_6S_2$.

Mesulphen, $C_{14}H_{12}S_2$, Mol. Wt. 244·4, is assayed in the *B.P.C.* by heating in a sealed glass tube with fuming nitric acid and precipitating with barium chloride. This is not necessary and it could be assayed satisfactorily by the flask-combustion method (p. 801).

Monosulfiram, $C_{10}H_{20}N_2S_3$, Mol. Wt. 264·5, and **phenothiazine,** $C_{12}H_9NS$, Mol. Wt. 199·3, could also be determined by the flask-combustion method (p. 801) although they are assayed officially from their nitrogen content.

Ichthammol is a mixture of the ammonium salts of the sulphonic acids of an oily substance prepared from a bituminous schist or shale, together with ammonium sulphate and water. It contains not less than 10·5 per cent w/w of organically combined sulphur, calculated with reference to the substance dried to constant weight at 105° and not more than one-quarter of the total sulphur in the form of sulphates.

For organically combined sulphates: Weigh 0·5 g into a porcelain crucible of about 50-ml capacity, add 4 g of anhydrous sodium carbonate and 3 ml of chloroform and mix. Warm the mixture, with stirring, until all the chloroform has evaporated and then add 10 g of coarsely powdered copper nitrate, mix thoroughly and heat very gently over a small flame. When the initial reaction has subsided, heat slightly more strongly until most of the material has blackened and then allow to cool. Transfer the crucible to a large beaker and add 20 ml of concentrated hydrochloric acid. When the reaction has ceased add 100 ml of water and boil until all the copper oxide has dissolved. Filter, dilute with 400 ml of water and precipitate the sulphate with barium chloride as usual. $BaSO_4 \times 0{\cdot}1374 = S$. This gives the total sulphur. Deduct the percentage sulphur in the form of sulphates to obtain the organically combined sulphates.

For sulphur in the form of sulphates: Weigh 2 g into a 200-ml graduated flask, dissolve in 100 ml of water, add a solution of 2 g of cupric chloride in 80 ml of water and dilute to volume with water. Shake thoroughly and filter. Precipitate the sulphur, as usual, using 100 ml of the filtrate (equivalent to one-half the weight of sample taken) and weigh as barium sulphate.

1. Henville, D., *Analyst*, 1930, **55**, 385.
2. Evers, N., and Elsdon, G. D., *Analyst*, 1922, **47**, 197.
3. Fleck, H. R., and Ward, A. M., *Analyst*, 1936, **61**, 28.
4. Allport, N. L., *Quart. J. Pharm.*, 1933, **6**, 431.
5. Fleck, H. R., and Ward, A. M., *Quart. J. Pharm.*, 1934, **7**, 179.
6. Vickers, C., and Wilkinson, J. V., *J. Pharm. Pharmacol.*, 1961, **13**, 72.

SULPHURIC ACID

H_2SO_4 Mol. Wt. 98·08

Sulphuric acid is titrated direct using 1 g (precautions should be taken with concentrated acid during weighing to avoid moisture uptake) with standard alkali to methyl orange or methyl red. 1 ml N = 0·04904 g. The sulphate may be checked by the usual precipitation method with barium chloride. $BaSO_4 \times 0{\cdot}4202 = H_2SO_4$.

SULPHATES

Some observations by Newton Friend and Wheat[1] on the gravimetric estimation of alkali sulphates by precipitation with barium chloride may be of interest. The authors adopt the following precautions to obtain satisfactory results:

(1) The concentration of the alkali sulphate should not exceed about 0·01 g-mol. per litre.

(2) The concentration of hydrochloric acid is best kept near 0·01N.

(3) The solution is heated to boiling and a dilute solution of barium chloride added dropwise, with constant stirring, until about twice the amount of barium chloride theoretically necessary for precipitation has been added.

(4) The solution is kept near the boiling-point for ten minutes and then allowed to stand overnight before filtering, *i.e.* the solution is always filtered cold.

(5) The supernatant liquid is decanted through a filter paper as completely as possible, an approximately equal quantity of water is added to the precipitate and the whole heated for not less than two hours in a water-bath with frequent stirring (this is necessary to remove adsorbed material); after cooling the solution is filtered and the precipitate washed with the minimum of hot water.

(6) The precipitate is ignited with the usual precautions in a porcelain crucible.

> Dissolve about 0·25 g of the substance in 250 ml of water, add 1 ml of concentrated hydrochloric acid and heat to boiling. Add slowly a small excess of 10 per cent barium chloride solution and heat on a water-bath for ten minutes. Cool, allow to stand overnight, filter, wash, ignite and weigh. $BaSO_4 \times 0{\cdot}6085 = Na_2SO_4$.

Conditions (1) and (2) above are observed in the *B.P.* determination of **sodium sulphate,** $Na_2SO_4,10H_2O$, Mol. Wt. 322·2, $BaSO_4 \times 1{\cdot}3802$; **anhydrous sodium sulphate,** Na_2SO_4, Mol. Wt. 142·0, $BaSO_4 \times 0{\cdot}6085$, and **potassium sulphate,** K_2SO_4, Mol. Wt. 174·3, $BaSO_4 \times 0{\cdot}7465$, but no special directions are given for cooling the solution and for washing the precipitate.

Volumetric methods for the estimation of soluble sulphates, and conversely barium, have been devised from time to time but none has reached a high degree of accuracy, and owing to many sources of interference they are limited in their application.

Two methods deserve mention. Köszegi[2] modified Hinman's chromate method:

> Heat an aqueous solution, containing approximately 0·1 g of sulphate, to boiling in a beaker, the solution being slightly acidified if alkaline. Run in 0·1N barium chloride until about 5 ml in excess, *i.e.* use about 30 ml. Boil the solution containing the precipitate for a further five minutes, add 5 or 6 g of crystallised sodium acetate to ensure complete precipitation of barium chromate, and then precipitate the excess of barium with 20 or 25 ml of 0·1N dichromate. Cool; transfer to a 200-ml graduated flask with water and dilute to volume. Filter, pipette 100 ml of the filtrate into a flask, add 1 g of potassium iodide and 10 ml of concentrated hydrochloric acid and titrate the liberated iodine with 0·1N thiosulphate, 1 mol. $K_2Cr_2O_7 = 6I$ but only $= 4BaCl_2$.

The method of Giblin[3] is unusual in the use of the sodium salt of rhodizonic acid as an external indicator. The method is applicable in moderately acid solution.

> Spot drops of a 0·1 per cent solution of the indicator on a filter paper to form yellow stains. Place a known volume of sulphuric acid or sulphate solution in a titration flask, add standard barium chloride from a burette and mix well. Allow the precipitate to settle, remove drops of supernatant liquid and spot on to the filter paper. The appearance of a pink or red colour indicates the completion of the reaction. Reverse the

process using the sulphuric acid in the burette and standard barium chloride in the flask, titrate until drops of supernatant liquid cease to give a red colour on the filter paper. By taking a mean of the two results a final figure of reasonable accuracy can be obtained, not less accurate than other volumetric methods employing external indicators.

The indicator must be freshly prepared since it will not keep longer than one day.[4] The 'spotted' filter papers will keep only for about an hour without fading unless dried in an evacuated desiccator over calcium chloride; thus preserved *in vacuo* they remain effective for several days.

Strebinger and von Zombery[5] employ the indicator internally, but in this case only titration of the barium with acid is possible. Hence in the volumetric estimation of sulphates an excess of standardised barium chloride is added and the excess is titrated by standard sulphate until the red barium salt is converted to yellow sodium salt at the end-point.

Tetrahydroxyquinone is recommended as an internal indicator by Schroeder.[6]

Measure a 25-ml sample, containing from 2 to 20 mg of sulphate, into a 150- or 250-ml conical flask for titration. (If the sample is turbid, filter 50 ml and transfer 25 ml of the filtrate to the flask for titration.) Add a few drops of phenolphthalein indicator. Add 0·02N hydrochloric acid (not stronger than 0·03N) from a burette until just sufficient acid is added to neutralise the sample to the acid side of phenolphthalein. If the sample is originally acid, 0·02N potassium hydroxide should be used for neutralisation so that the sample will have a resulting pH value between 4·0 and 8·3. The temperature of sample should be below 30° and it is advisable to work between 20° and 25°.

To the neutralised sample add 25 ml of *iso*propyl alcohol (ethanol or denatured alcohol can be employed). Introduce 0·2 g of the tetrahydroxyquinone/potassium chloride indicator (prepared by grinding 1 part of the disodium salt of tetrahydroxyquinone with 400 parts of dried potassium chloride) and swirl the flask to dissolve the indicator. Titrate the sample thus prepared with 0·025N barium chloride (standardised gravimetrically). Add the barium chloride at a steady dropping rate, with constant swirling of the flask, until a brown colour begins to form, indicating the approach of the end-point. Then add the titrant 2 or 3 drops at a time, with steady swirling, until a red colour appears throughout the body of the solution and not as spots of colour; this is the end-point. After deducting a blank of 0·1 ml from the volume of titrant required (this is the volume of 0·025N barium chloride required to give a visible precipitate with the indicator when no sulphate is present) 1 ml 0·025N barium chloride = 1·2 mg sulphate.

If more than 0·6 mg of phosphate is present the blank should be increased; for 0·6 to 1·2 mg deduct 0·3 ml; for 1·2 to 1·8 mg deduct 0·6 ml.

When iron or other heavy metals are present in any appreciable concentration, they should be precipitated with potassium carbonate or potassium hydroxide, removed by filtration, and the sample subsequently neutralised before the sulphates are determined.

Various EDTA methods have been suggested for the determination of sulphate. Those based on precipitation of the sulphate with barium, followed by complexometric titration of the excess barium, are not satisfactory because of the low stability constant of the barium-EDTA complex; as would be expected, end-points are sluggish and uncertain. Sporek[7] suggested a method based on precipitation of lead sulphate in 50 per cent *iso*propyl alcohol containing a little nitric acid, followed by titration of the excess lead with EDTA. King,[8] in attempting to apply this method to pharmaceuticals, found consistently high recoveries due to co-precipitation of lead nitrate with the lead sulphate and also a serious interference with chloride. A number of modifications were introduced and some improvement to the method was achieved, but it was still considered to be unsuitable for routine pharmaceutical work.

The most satisfactory volumetric method for determination of sulphate is probably that based on titration with barium perchlorate using Thoron as indicator and a medium of aqueous ethanol.[9] Details of this titration are given under the Appendix on flask-combustion titration of sulphur on page 801.

1. Newton Friend, J., and Wheat, W. N., *Analyst*, 1932, **57,** 559.
2. Köszegi, D., *Z. Anal. Chem.*, 1929, **77,** 203.
3. Giblin, J. C., *Analyst*, 1933, **58,** 752.
4. Godbert, A. L., and Belcher, R., *Analyst*, 1939, **64,** 346.
5. Strebinger, R., and von Zombery, L., *Z. Anal. Chem.*, 1929, **79,** 1.
6. Schroeder, W. C., *Ind. Eng. Chem., Anal. Edn.*, 1933, **5,** 403.
7. Sporek, K., *Anal. Chem.*, 1958, **30,** 1033.
8. King, R. E., private communication.
9. Fritz, J. S., and Yamamura, S. S., *Anal. Chem.*, 1955, **27,** 1461.

SULPHUROUS ACID

H_2SO_3 Mol. Wt. 82·08

The determination of sulphurous acid is best undertaken with standard iodine, but for accurate results it is essential to add the solution to be assayed to an excess of standard iodine and, after a short interval to allow for complete oxidation, to titrate back with thiosulphate. 1 g of approximately 5 per cent acid is used with 25 ml of 0·1N iodine. 1 ml 0·1N = 0·003203 g SO_2.

For determination of sulphur dioxide in **small amounts,** the only reliable method is distillation with the necessary precautions against oxidation in the flask. The distilled sulphur dioxide is oxidised in the receiver and estimated either by precipitation of the resulting sulphate with barium chloride, or by titration of the sulphuric acid formed.

Add about 5 ml of 20 per cent phosphoric acid solution to 20 to 100 g of the sample; distil (adding recently boiled water, if necessary) in a current of carbon dioxide until 150 ml has passed over. Collect the distillate in about 100 ml of saturated bromine water, allowing the end of the condenser to dip below the surface. The method and apparatus may be simplified, without material loss in accuracy, by omitting the current of carbon dioxide, adding 10 ml of the phosphoric acid instead of 5 ml and by dropping into the distillation flask, immediately before attaching the condenser, an amount of sodium bicarbonate weighing not more than 1 g. The carbon dioxide liberated is not sufficient to expel all the air from the apparatus but it will prevent any appreciable amount of oxidation occurring. When the distillation is finished, boil off the excess of bromine, dilute the solution to about 250 ml, add 5 ml of concentrated hydrochloric acid, and precipitate the sulphate with barium chloride as usual (see under Sulphuric Acid, p. 618). Conduct a blank determination on the apparatus and reagents used and correct the result accordingly. $BaSO_4 \times 0{\cdot}2745 = SO_2$.

Titration methods allow an estimation to be made in a much shorter time. Black and Warren[1] showed that distillation into standard iodine and titration of the excess with 0·1N thiosulphate gave satisfactory results with gelatin and glucose syrup; but spices such as nutmeg and mustard, after a short time, yielded iodine-reducing substances even in the absence of sulphur dioxide.

Monier-Williams[2] reviewed the methods of estimation and concluded that titration after oxidation was accurate if volatile organic acids were eliminated, and that gravimetric methods were satisfactory in nearly all cases. Bromine was found to be a satisfactory oxidising agent except when the distillate contained appreciable quantities of volatile sulphur compounds; in such cases oxidation with hydrogen peroxide followed by cold precipitation with barium chloride was necessary to permit of sharp distinction between sulphur dioxide and volatile sulphur compounds, including hydrogen sulphide. He recommended distillation in the presence of carbon dioxide, through an upward sloping condenser, into an absorption tube containing a solution of 3 per cent hydrogen peroxide (free from sulphate and previously neutralised to bromophenol blue; the indicator is unaffected by carbon dioxide and traces of volatile organic acids). The advantage of the use of hydrogen peroxide is that after titration of the distillate with 0·1N alkali to bromophenol blue (1 ml 0·1N = 0·0032 g SO_2) the result may be checked by gravimetric means using cold precipitation as recommended above, and all titrations of less than 0·5 ml 0·1N alkali should be so checked.

The Monier-Williams technique has been adopted in principle by the *B.P.* for the determination of sulphur dioxide.

Sodium sulphite, $Na_2SO_3,7H_2O$, Mol. Wt. 252·2, and **sodium thiosulphate,** $Na_2S_2O_3,5H_2O$, Mol. Wt. 248·2, are both determined by direct titration with 0·1N iodine or after weighing into excess of iodine as given below; no indicator is required. 1 ml 0·1N = 0·01261 g of $Na_2SO_3,7H_2O$ and 0·02482 g $Na_2S_2O_3, 5H_2O$.

Sodium metabisulphite, $Na_2S_2O_5$, Mol. Wt. 190·1, should be weighed into excess of 0·1N iodine, and after complete solution and then acidification, the excess iodine is titrated with 0·1N thiosulphate. 1 ml 0·1N = 0·004753 g.

Injection of Sodium Thiosulphate, *B.P.C.* A 50 per cent w/v solution in water for injection. It is assayed as sodium thiosulphate above, using 2 ml of injection.

1. Black, J. W., and Warren, B. J. W., *Analyst*, 1928, **53**, 130.
2. Monier-Williams, G. W., Report on Public Health and Medical Subjects, No. 43.

SURFACE-ACTIVE AGENTS

Surface-active agents are substances which bring about a lowering of the surface tension of the solvent in which they are dissolved. They may be classified into three groups according to their physical properties as anionic, cationic and non-ionic agents and it is convenient to use these categories in a discussion of analytical methods.

ANIONIC SURFACE-ACTIVE AGENTS

(*a*) *Colorimetric methods.* The most widely used colorimetric methods for anionic surface-active agents are based upon that described by Jones[1] which consists in shaking an aqueous solution of the sample with methylene blue and chloroform, followed by absorptiometric measurement of the blue chloroform extract. Subsequent workers have introduced modifications in an attempt to overcome interferences and of the variations suggested that of Longwell and Maniece[2] is probably the best:

To a volume of sample solution containing 0·02 to 0·15 mg in a 250-ml separator, add 10 ml of alkaline phosphate buffer prepared by dissolving 10 g of reagent-grade anhydrous disodium hydrogen phosphate in water, adjusting to pH 10·0 with dilute sodium hydroxide solution and diluting to 1 litre with water. Then add 5 ml of a 0·035 per cent aqueous solution of methylene blue and 15 ml of chloroform and shake gently and evenly twice a second for one minute. Allow the layers to separate, breaking up any emulsion formed by gentle agitation with a flat-ended glass rod. Run the chloroform layer into a second separator containing 110 ml of water and 5 ml of acid methylene blue solution (prepared by dissolving 0·35 g of methylene blue in 500 ml of water, adding 6·5 g of reagent-grade concentrated sulphuric acid and diluting to 1 litre with water). Rinse the first separator with 2 ml of chloroform, added from a burette, and add to the second separator. Shake the second separator as above, allow the layers to separate and run the chloroform layer into a 50-ml graduated flask, through a small funnel plugged with cotton wool, previously rinsed with chloroform. Rinse with a further 2 ml of chloroform. Repeat the extraction in the second separator with two 10-ml quantities of chloroform, combine the extracts in the graduated flask after filtration and dilute to volume with chloroform. Measure the extinction at 650 mμ against a reagent blank and read the sample content from a standard curve, prepared by carrying out the operation described above using suitable volumes, covering the range 50 to 200 mμ, of a standard solution of Manoxol O.T. (sodium dioctylsulphosuccinate) in water, made to contain 10 p.p.m.

Sulphide interferes and if present should be destroyed by oxidation with 2 ml of 20-volume hydrogen peroxide, after adding the alkaline phosphate buffer.

(*b*) *Anionic-cationic titration.* A method which is applicable generally to anionic surface-active agents is their titration with cationic products. Early techniques were based on the fact that when anionic and cationic agents are present together in aqueous solution they will neutralise the surface activity of each other and the end-point is shown by a sharp rise in surface tension. Better precision became possible when a two-phase titration procedure was introduced. In this method one type of surface-active agent is titrated against the other in the presence of an indicator and a solvent, the transfer of colour from one phase to the other giving the end-point.[3] Barr, Oliver and Stubbings[4] introduced a method, based on Jones' colorimetric extraction procedure, in which the anionic material is titrated with 0·001M cetyl trimethylammonium bromide in the presence of chloroform, bromothymol blue being used as indicator. Another method which has been found satisfactory in our hands is an adaptation of the method due to Carkhuff and Boyd[5] given below under cationic surface-active agents.

(*c*) *p-Toluidine method.* A method by Marron and Schifferli[6] suitable for sulphonated compounds is based on the fact that alkyl-aryl sulphonates react in aqueous solution with an amine salt of a mineral acid, *p*-toluidine hydrochloride, to produce an amine salt which can be extracted with carbon tetrachloride. The carbon tetrachloride extract is mixed with neutral ethanol and titrated with 0·1N sodium hydroxide; simple aryl sulphonates do not interfere.

It is essential that the molecular weight of the alkyl-aryl sulphonate is known. This molecular weight can be ascertained by carrying out determinations on samples of known composition.

Weigh out by difference from a weighing bottle 2 to 3 g of the surface-active agent into a 250-ml separator. Add 100 ml of *p*-toluidine hydrochloride solution (3·4 per cent of the pure recrystallised salt), stopper and shake well. Continue with alternate shaking and settling until all the solid dissolves. Add 50 ml of carbon tetrachloride and shake well. Allow to stand until there is complete separation of the phases. Run off the lower layer into a 500-ml iodine flask. Make further extractions with 25 and 10 ml respectively of carbon tetrachloride. To the combined extracts add 100 ml of neutral industrial methylated spirit and 6 drops of 0·5 per cent *m*-cresol purple indicator. Titrate with 0·1N sodium hydroxide with vigorous shaking between the additions. At the end-point, the grey colour of the emulsion takes on a blue or lavender tint. The two phases will separate if allowed to stand and a reddish-purple colour in the upper layer denotes the end-point.

Carry out a blank determination of the *p*-toluidine hydrochloride solution. Subtract any value found for the blank, which should not exceed 0·3 ml of 0·1N sodium hydroxide, from the value obtained when the sample is present.

The percentage of alkyl-aryl sodium sulphonate contained in the sample is given by:

$$\frac{\text{ml of 0·1N NaOH required for the titration} \times M}{\text{weight of sample taken} \times 100}$$

where M is the molecular weight of the alkyl-aryl sodium sulphonate.

Sodium lauryl sulphate, *B.P.*, is a mixture of sodium normal primary alkyl sulphates and can be assayed by the anionic-cationic titration method. The official method requires weighing of the alcohols liberated on hydrolysis; it is inadvisable to dry the residue at 105° and is preferably dehydrated by rapid evaporation with small quantities of dry acetone.

Dioctyl sodium sulphosuccinate, $C_{20}H_{37}O_7SNa$, Mol. Wt. 444·6. This is assayed by anionic-cationic titration. The sample solution is titrated against tetra-*n*-butylammonium iodide solution to which has been added 50 ml of a solution containing 10 per cent anhydrous sodium sulphate and 1 per cent sodium carbonate, in the presence of chloroform, bromophenol blue being used as indicator.

CATIONIC SURFACE-ACTIVE AGENTS

Cationic surface-active agents are frequently compounds of the quaternary ammonium type.

(*a*) *Colorimetric methods*. These are essentially the same as for anionic agents, except that methylene blue is replaced by reagents such as bromothymol blue and the pH must be controlled. A method using bromothymol blue due to Ballard, Isaacs and Scott[7] is given below; strict attention to detail is essential and the bromothymol blue used should pass the purity test given by Wilson[8] or, if not, should be purified as he describes using a buffer solution of pH 7·5.

To 20 ml of chloroform in a separator add 5·0 ml of a solution of the sample containing not more than two micromols of univalent quaternary ammonium salt, 1·0 ml of bromothymol blue solution (an aqueous solution containing 0·15 per cent of bromothymol blue and 0·15 per cent of anhydrous sodium carbonate) and 20·0 ml of buffer solution, pH 7·5, prepared by diluting 7·5 ml of freshly prepared 0·1M citric acid to 100 ml with 0·2M sodium phosphate (7·16 per cent $Na_2HPO_4,12H_2O$). Shake vigorously for two minutes, allow the layers to separate, slowly invert the separator to mix the chloroform phase and allow to stand for two minutes. Run the chloroform layer into a flask containing 0·4 g of glass wool and repeat the extraction procedure twice more with 20-ml quantities of chloroform, combining the extracts. Stopper the flask, shake for one minute and allow to stand for five minutes. Decant the chloroform through a small glass-wool plug into a 100-ml graduated flask containing 25·0 ml of a solution prepared by dissolving 5·0 g of boric acid in dehydrated ethanol, adding 20·0 ml of water and diluting to 250 ml with dehydrated ethanol. Wash the flask and filter with successive small quantities of ethylene dichloride or ethanol-free chloroform, collecting the washings in the graduated flask and finally diluting to volume with the solvent. Measure the extinction at 420 mμ using 2-cm cells with chloroform in the comparison cell. Read the corresponding amount of quaternary ammonium salt from a calibration curve prepared using samples of known cationic materials.

(*b*) *Anionic-cationic titration.* The same considerations apply as to the determination of anionic surface-active agents above. Sodium lauryl sulphate is a commonly used titrant and is standardised by titration with a standard solution of the compound under examination. Carkhuff and Boyd[5] described a method for the determination of dicyclomine hydrochloride which is of general application to many substances having cationic surface-active properties. For compounds other than dicyclomine hydrochloride the same procedure is used but the sodium lauryl sulphate is standardised appropriately. The quality of the end-point in titrations of this type may be affected by the relative solubility of the quaternary ammonium compound in the two phases of the titration system. For a sharp end-point the compound being titrated should be appreciably more soluble in chloroform than in the aqueous acid. This is the case with dicyclomine hydrochloride and many other substances, but with certain compounds which would be expected to titrate well, *e.g.* benactyzine hydrochloride, the solubility in the two phases is similar and a very sluggish end-point is obtained.

Standard dicyclomine hydrochloride solution. Dissolve exactly 0·1 g of dicyclomine hydrochloride in sufficient water to produce exactly 100 ml.

Determination: Dissolve 1·2 g of sodium lauryl sulphate in sufficient water to produce 1 litre and standardise the solution as follows. Pipette 20 ml of the standard dicyclomine hydrochloride solution into a 100-ml, glass-stoppered, graduated cylinder and add 10 ml of water, 5 ml of dilute sulphuric acid, 1 ml of a 0·01 per cent ethanolic solution of dimethyl yellow (4-dimethylaminoazobenzene) and 20 ml of chloroform. Stopper the cylinder and shake vigorously; the chloroform layer becomes bright yellow. Titrate with the sodium lauryl sulphate solution, shaking after each addition, until the first appearance of an orange-pink colour in the chloroform layer. (The colour of the drop of chloroform that appears on the surface of the aqueous phase may be used as a more precise guide to the end-point but this is not always possible because in some instances the drop does not form.)

Repeat the operation using, in place of the standard dicyclomine hydrochloride solution, an amount of sample containing 10 to 25 mg of dicyclomine hydrochloride.

(*c*) In a method originating in Scandinavia (a form of it being the official procedure for benzalkonium chloride in the Addendum to the 9th edition of the Danish Pharmacopœia) the surface-active agent is reacted with iodide in acid solution, extracted into chloroform and then titrated non-aqueously with perchloric acid in acetic acid.

A version of the method applicable to cetrimide and several other cationic agents, *e.g.* cetylpyridinium chloride, benzalkonium chloride and domiphen bromide, is as follows:

Dissolve about 0·7 g in 20 ml of water in a separator and add 0·8 ml of dilute hydrochloric acid and 8 ml of 10 per cent potassium iodide solution. Mix well and extract with three 30-ml quantities of chloroform, collecting the extracts in a dry beaker. Stir, allow to stand for five minutes and then pour the chloroform solution into a dry conical flask, avoiding transference of aqueous droplets. Rinse the beaker with two 4-ml quantities of chloroform, adding the rinsings to the main chloroform solution, again avoiding the transference of aqueous droplets and then add 12 ml of a 5 per cent solution of mercuric acetate in glacial acetic acid, 0·2 ml of oracet blue B indicator and 0·5 ml of acetic anhydride. Titrate with 0·1N perchloric acid until the colour changes from the initial intense blue to a less intense purple. Repeat the operation omitting the sample. 1 ml 0·1N = 0·03364 g $C_{14}H_{29}(CH_3)_3NBr$ (cetrimide) or 0·03580 g $C_{21}H_{38}NCl,H_2O$ (cetylpyridinium chloride). For benzalkonium chloride take 1·4 g, 1 ml 0·1N = 0·0354 g $C_{22}H_{40}NCl$.

(*d*) *Titration with sodium tetraphenylboron.* This substance reacts with quaternary ammonium compounds and may be used to titrate them, use again being made of the removal of a dyestuff (in the form of its complex with the quaternary) from chloroform to indicate the end-point.[9]

The method, as applied to benzethonium chloride, is as follows:

Dissolve 0·3 g in about 75 ml of water in a separator and add 0·4 ml of bromophenol blue test solution (0·1 g of bromophenol blue dissolved in 3 ml of 0·05N sodium hydroxide and diluted to 200 ml with water), 10 ml of chloroform and 1 ml of N sodium hydroxide. Titrate with 0·02M sodium tetraphenylboron to the disappearance of the blue colour from the chloroform layer, adding the titrant dropwise towards the end of the titration and shaking vigorously after each addition. 1 ml 0·02M = 0·008962 g $C_{27}H_{42}O_2NCl$.

This method can also be applied to benzalkonium chloride and certain other quaternary ammonium compounds.

(*e*) *Gravimetric methods.* Several methods that make use of precipitation reactions with complex anions have been proposed for the determination of quaternary ammonium compounds. These methods have been reviewed by Chinnick and Lincoln[10] who recommend the phosphotungstate method[11] since all previous methods, which include precipitation with ferrocyanide, ferricyanide, dichromate and reineckate, require the molecular weight of the quaternary compound to be known before the amount present in a sample can be determined. In the phosphotungstate method, however, it is possible to calculate the amount of quaternary cation in an unknown sample and also the ionic weight of the quaternary salt by weighing the quaternary phosphotungstate after drying and again after ignition. The detailed method is as follows:

Weigh an amount containing the quaternary ammonium compound equivalent to 0·0002 to 0·0006 gram-molecules into a 400-ml beaker and dilute to about 250 ml with water. Make slightly acid with hydrochloric acid and then add 10 ml of dilute hydrochloric acid followed by about 2 g of sodium chloride. Heat to boiling-point, add 10 ml of a 10 per cent solution of phosphotungstic acid ($P_2O_5,24WO_3,xH_2O$) and continue to boil for two to three minutes, or until the precipitate has coagulated. Test for complete precipitation by the addition of a few drops of phosphotungstic acid, cool to room temperature and filter quantitatively through a tared, No. 3 sintered-porcelain crucible, washing with 100 to 200 ml of water. Dry at 105° to constant weight and then ignite at a dull-red heat and reweigh.

If the molecular weight of the quaternary ammonium compound is known, then

$$\text{per cent quaternary ammonium compound} = \frac{100W_1M}{W(M - X + 959{\cdot}3)}$$

M = molecular weight of quaternary ammonium compound
X = ionic weight of anion
W = weight of sample taken
W_1 = weight of precipitate dried at 105°

If the molecular weight of the quaternary ammonium compound is unknown, then

$$M = \frac{954{\cdot}3(W_1 - W_2)}{W_2} - 5 + X$$

where M, X and W_1 are as above and W_2 = weight of residue left on ignition.

If the molecular weight of the quaternary ammonium compound is unknown, and it is required to calculate the percentage present in the sample without intermediate determination or calculation of the molecular weight, then, combining the above equations,

$$\text{per cent quaternary ammonium compound} = \frac{100}{W}\left[W_1 - W_2\left(1 - \frac{X - 5}{954{\cdot}3}\right)\right]$$

As only a few anions are normally present in quaternary ammonium compounds, the equation may be simplified as follows:

$$\frac{100}{W}(W_1 - KW_2)$$

K = 0·9681 for chlorides
= 0·9215 for bromides
= 0·8722 for iodides

Amines interfere in the above method and so, if present, they should be removed by one of the procedures given by the authors.

The following official cationic surface-active agents are assayed by the ferricyanide method given under Flavines, p. 255, with the minor modifications of using 3 to 3·5 g and keeping the solutions cool during the precipitation and subsequent titration:

Benzalkonium chloride, *U.S.P.*, $[C_6H_5CH_2N(CH_3)_2R]Cl$, in which R represents a mixture of the alkyls from C_8H_{17} to $C_{18}H_{37}$, 1 ml 0·05M = 0·0540 g.

Benzalkonium chloride solution, *B.P.C.*, equivalent to 50 per cent w/v of $C_6H_5,CH_2,N(CH_3)_2,C_{13}H_{27}Cl$, 1 ml 0·1M = 0·1062 g.

Benzalkonium bromide solution, *B.P.C.*, equivalent to 50 per cent w/v of $C_6H_5,CH_2,N(CH_3)_2,C_{13}H_{27}Br$, 1 ml 0·1M = 0·1195 g.

Cetrimide, *B.P.*, chiefly $C_{14}H_{29}(CH_3)_3NBr$, 1 ml 0·1M = 0·1009 g.

Domiphen bromide, *B.P.C.*, chiefly $[C_6H_5O(CH_2)_2N(CH_3)_2(C_{12}H_{25})]Br$, 1 ml 0·1M = 0·1243 g.

Methylbenzethonium chloride, *U.S.P.*, $C_{28}H_{44}O_2NCl,H_2O$, 1 ml 0·05M = 0·06932 g.

All these products can also be assayed by the modified Scandinavian method given on p. 626, and this method is also applicable to **Cetylpyridinium chloride,** *U.S.P.*, $C_{21}H_{38}NCl,H_2O$, Mol. Wt. 358·0.

Dequalinium chloride, *B.P.C.*, $C_{30}H_{40}N_4Cl_2$, Mol. Wt. 527·6, and **Dequalinium acetate,** $C_{34}H_{46}O_4N_4$, Mol. Wt. 574·8, can both be assayed by non-aqueous titration with perchloric acid to crystal violet indicator (see p. 792); addition of mercuric acetate is necessary in the presence of chloride, 1 ml 0·1N = 0·02638 g $C_{30}H_{40}N_4Cl_2$ and 0·02874 g $C_{34}H_{46}O_4N_4$.

Benzethonium chloride, *U.S.P.*, $C_{27}H_{42}O_2NCl$, Mol. Wt. 448·1, is officially assayed by titration with sodium tetraphenylboron, method (*d*) above.

Cetrimide Emulsifying Ointment, *B.P.C.* Contains 30 per cent of cetrimide emulsifying wax. It can be standardised by the anionic-cationic titration method (*b*) described above.

Warm 0·3 g with 25 ml of water and transfer to a stoppered bottle with two 25-ml quantities of water followed by two 25-ml quantities of ethylene dichloride. Add 50 ml of 0·03 per cent sodium lauryl sulphate solution and 0·5 ml of bromothymol blue indicator. Make alkaline with 10 per cent sodium carbonate decahydrate solution, using phenolphthalein as an external indicator, and titrate with 0·001M cetrimide solution, shaking gently after each addition, until there is a rapid separation of the solvent layer. Continue the titration slowly until a permanent blue colour is produced in the ethylene dichloride layer. Repeat the operation omitting the sample. The difference between the two titrations represents the amount of cetrimide in the sample. 1 ml 0·001M cetrimide = 0·0003364 g $C_{14}H_{29}(CH_3)_3NBr$.

Cetrimide Emulsifying Wax, *B.P.C.* Contains 10 per cent of cetrimide in cetostearyl alcohol and can be assayed as the ointment above using about 0·1 g.

Cream of Cetrimide, *B.Vet.C.* Contains 0·5 per cent of cetrimide and can be assayed as the ointment above using about 1·5 g.

NON-IONIC SURFACE-ACTIVE AGENTS

The non-ionic surface-active agents used in pharmaceutical products may be divided into three main groups: (i) long-chain carboxylic acid esters of polyhydric alcohols, of sorbitan and of polyoxyethylene glycols, (ii) ethers of long-chain alcohols and (iii) polyoxyethylene glycols of high molecular weight.

(i) This group includes **Glyceryl monostearate,** *N.F.*, **Self-emulsifying monostearin,** *B.P.C.*, **Polysorbate 80,** *U.S.P.*, and **Polyoxyl 40 stearate,** *U.S.P.*, all of which may be analysed by a determination of saponification value together (for the fatty-acid esters) with a determination of free acids. For self-emulsifying monostearin the *B.P.C.* determines the content of α-monoglyceride as follows:

Warm 0·8 g with 20 ml of chloroform in a separator until dissolved, add a mixture of 2 ml of glacial acetic acid and 25 ml of water and shake for one minute. Allow to separate, run off the chloroform layer and extract with three portions, each of a mixture of 2 ml of glacial acetic acid and 20 ml of water, shaking for one minute each time. Combine the extracts and wash with 5 ml of chloroform. Combine the chloroform solutions in a 100-ml graduated flask and dilute to volume with chloroform. Transfer 25 ml of this solution to an iodine flask, evaporate the chloroform on a water-bath and dissolve the residue in 1 ml of chloroform. Add 10 ml of glacial acetic acid followed by 20 ml of periodic-acetic acid solution (prepared by dissolving 5 g of periodic acid in 200 ml of water and diluting to 1 litre with glacial acetic acid; the solution should be stored in amber-coloured, glass-stoppered bottles). Warm on a water-bath at a temperature not exceeding 45° until the mixture is just molten and then shake for one minute. Rinse the flask walls and stopper with glacial acetic acid and allow to stand for thirty minutes at 20° to 30°. Add 5 ml of freshly prepared, 20 per cent potassium iodide solution and titrate the liberated iodine with 0·1N sodium thiosulphate using starch mucilage as indicator. Repeat the operation omitting the sample. 1 ml 0·1N sodium thiosulphate = 0·01793 g $C_{21}H_{42}O_4$.

(ii) Ethers of long-chain alcohols may be analysed by determining the hydroxyl value, but since they are almost always polyoxyalkylene derivatives they are better determined by specific methods for that grouping (see below). An important example of this type of material is **Cetomacrogol 1000,** *B.P.C.*, which is polyethylene glycol 1000 monocetyl ether (the number refers to the approximate molecular weight of the polyoxyethylene chain) and is assayed in the *B.P.C.* by a determination of hydroxyl value.

(iii) Polyoxyalkylene glycols of high molecular weight included in this group are the macrogols or polyethylene glycols, which are also distinguished by a number in their title indicating the average molecular weight. The analysis of the *B.P.C.* and *U.S.P.* macrogols [**Hard macrogol,** *B.P.C.*, **Polyethylene glycol 4000,** *U.S.P.*, **Liquid macrogol,** *B.P.C.* (polyethylene glycol 300) and **Polyethylene glycol 400,** *U.S.P.*] is based on physical characteristics such as viscosity and pH, together with freezing-point (for hard macrogol) and refractive index (for liquid macrogol) but that of the *N.F* for **Polyethylene glycol 300** and **Polyethylene glycol 1500** includes a determination of average molecular weight. In this determination the sample is heated under pressure with a solution of phthalic anhydride in pyridine and the unchanged phthalic anhydride is hydrolysed and titrated with standard sodium hydroxide.

Most of the methods available for the specific determination of polyoxyethylene derivatives involve precipitation with complex anions. The precipitants generally used are ferrocyanide[12] and in conjunction with barium, molybdophosphate,[13] phosphotungstate[11] and silicotungstate.[14] Since the reactions are not stoichiometric it is necessary to know the nature of the non-ionic agent present in order to determine the empirical factor required for the calculation of results. Barber, Chinnick and Lincoln[15] found that phosphotungstic acid not only gave more accurate results than phosphomolybdic acid but that with the former acid the precipitate could be filtered off after two to three hours standing instead of after standing overnight, as is necessary with phosphomolybdic acid.

> To a solution of the sample in about 200 ml of water, add 10 ml of dilute hydrochloric acid followed by 10 ml of 10 per cent barium chloride solution. Heat to boiling-point, add 10 ml of 10 per cent phosphotungstic acid ($P_2O_5,24WO_3,xH_2O$) solution and continue to boil for two to three minutes. Allow to stand for two to three hours, filter through a No. 3 sintered-glass crucible, wash the precipitate with about 100 ml of water and dry to constant weight at 105°. Repeat using a sample of known type.

Instead of weighing the precipitate, various methods (both volumetric and colorimetric) have been described for determination of the excess precipitant in the filtrate and for the colorimetric determination of the molybdate or molybdate complex in the dissolved precipitate. These include a method due to Stevenson[16] in which the precipitated phosphomolybdate is dissolved in sulphuric acid and the extinction of the solution measured at 520 mμ.

More recently a quite different approach has been adopted to the determination of polyoxyethylene derivatives by Gatewood and Graham.[17] These authors showed that when anhydrous samples of surface-active agents containing polyoxyethylene or polyoxypropylene groups are heated in an acidic solution of carbonyl-free, methanolic, 2,4-dinitrophenylhydrazine and 10 per cent ethanolic potassium hydroxide is added to the reaction product, an intense purple colour with an absorption maximum at 560 mμ results.

MIXTURES OF SURFACE-ACTIVE AGENTS

When anionic and non-ionic agents are present together, the usual procedure is to separate the non-ionic fraction from the anionic either by solvent extraction or, preferably, by passing through an anion-exchange resin when the anionic fraction is retained and the non-ionic eluted. The anionic agent may subsequently be eluted from the column with ethanolic hydrochloric acid.[18] A similar method can be used for the separation of cationic and non-ionic agents except that, of course, a cation exchange column is employed. A suitable procedure has been described by Barber, Chinnick and Lincoln.[15]

Occasionally, in pharmaceutical formulations, the rather unusual combination of a quaternary ammonium compound and sodium lauryl sulphate may occur. Ion-exchange techniques have not been successful in separating these substances, at least on a quantitative basis. A reasonable approximation to the true figures may be obtained by carrying out a cationic-anionic titration on the formulated product (using as titrant either the quaternary ammonium compound in question or sodium lauryl sulphate—depending on which is in excess) and then carrying out another titration after acid hydrolysis of the anionic material. The exact conditions of the hydrolysis must be carefully chosen, according to the particular quaternary present, so that an optimum balance is achieved between destruction of as much sodium lauryl sulphate as possible and avoidance of any degradation of the cationic material.

SOAPLESS DETERGENTS

Many of the methods described above are applicable to the analysis of non-soapy detergent products. A detailed discussion of methods applicable to this class of materials is outside the scope of the present book, but useful methods and reviews on the subject are available.[19,20,21]

1. JONES, J. H., *J.A.O.A.C.*, 1945, **28,** 398.
2. LONGWELL, J., and MANIECE, W. D., *Analyst*, 1955, **80,** 167.
3. EPTON, S. R., *Trans. Faraday Soc.*, 1948, **44,** 226.
4. BARR, T., OLIVER, J., and STUBBINGS, V. W., *J. Soc. Chem. Ind.*, 1948, **67,** 45.
5. CARKHUFF, E. D., and BOYD, W. F., *J. Amer. Pharm. Ass., Sci. Edn.*, 1954, **43,** 240.
6. MARRON, T. V., and SCHIFFERLI, J., *Ind. Eng. Chem., Anal. Edn.*, 1946, **18,** 49.
7. BALLARD, C. W., ISAACS, J., and SCOTT, P. G. W., *J. Pharm. Pharmacol.*, 1954, **6,** 971.
8. WILSON, J. B., *J.A.O.A.C.*, 1951, **34,** 343.
9. PATEL, D. M., and ANDERSON, R. A., *Drug Standards*, 1958, **26,** 189.

10. Chinnick, C. C. T., and Lincoln, P. A., Proceedings, 1st World Congress on Surface-Active Agents, Paris 1954, Chambre Syndicale Tramagras, Paris 1955, Volume 1, p. 209.
11. Lincoln, P. A., and Chinnick, C. C. T., *Analyst,* 1956, **81,** 100.
12. Schonfeldt, N., *J. Amer. Oil Chemists' Soc.*, 1955, **32,** 77.
13. Oliver, J., and Preston, C., *Nature,* 1949, **164,** 242.
14. Schaffer, C. B., and Critchfield, F. H., *Anal. Chem.*, 1947, **19,** 32.
15. Barber, A., Chinnick, C. C. T., and Lincoln, P. A., *Analyst,* 1956, **81,** 18.
16. Stevenson, D. G., *Analyst,* 1954, **79,** 504.
17. Gatewood, L., Jnr., and Graham, H. D., *Anal. Chem.*, 1961, **33,** 1393.
18. Voogt, P., *Rec. Trav. Chim.*, 1959, **78,** 899.
19. Analytical Methods Committee, Examination of Detergent Preparations, *Analyst,* 1951, **76,** 279.
20. Smith, W. B., *Analyst,* 1959, **84,** 77.
21. Longman, G. F., and Hilton, J., Methods for the Analysis of Non-Soapy Detergent (NSD) Products, *S.A.C.* Monograph No. 1.

TARTARIC ACID

$(CHOH.COOH)_2$ Mol. Wt. 150·1

Free tartaric acid may be titrated direct with standard alkali to the dibasic salt using phenolphthalein as indicator. The end-point is very sharp but a considerable volume, say 200 ml, of water should be used or the solution heated to avoid precipitation of the acid tartrate during titration, with subsequent difficulty in redissolving. 1 ml N = 0·07505 g.

The estimation of tartaric acid in mixtures, especially in the presence of citric acid, presents difficulties and there is no very satisfactory rapid method for directly determining the relative quantities of tartaric and citric acids in a mixture of the two. A much criticised but reasonably good method of direct estimation of tartaric acid is to precipitate the acid as potassium hydrogen tartrate by a slight modification of the *A.O.A.C.*[1] technique recommended for the determination of the total tartaric acid in wines.

> To 100 ml of a neutral solution of a suitable weight of the sample to contain 0·3 g tartaric acid, add 2·0 ml of 20 per cent potassium acetate solution, 2 ml of glacial acetic acid and 15 g of potassium chloride. After the potassium chloride has dissolved, add 15 ml of 95 per cent ethanol, stir vigorously until the potassium hydrogen tartrate begins to precipitate and allow to stand at a temperature of 15° to 18° overnight. Filter the precipitate through a Gooch crucible or a small Büchner funnel containing a filter paper, using portions of the cold filtrate to transfer the precipitate to the filter. Wash the precipitate three times with a few ml of a mixture of 15 g of potassium chloride, 20 ml of 95 per cent ethanol and 100 ml of water, using not more than 20 ml of wash solution in all. Transfer the precipitate to the beaker in which the precipitation was

made, wash the crucible with 50 ml of hot water, heat to boiling and titrate the hot solution with 0·1N alkali, using phenolphthalein as indicator. Add 1·5 ml to the titration figure to allow for the solubility of the precipitate. 1 ml 0·1N = 0·015 g tartaric acid.

Steuart,[2] using this method for ciders, found the solubility correction to vary from 0·7 ml 0·1N sodium hydroxide at 15° to 1·15 ml at 20° and 1·6 ml at 25°. If the tartrate present is low, precipitation will be incomplete, and a known quantity of about 0·2 g of pure potassium hydrogen tartrate should be added.

Hartmann and Hillig's modification[3] of the *A.O.A.C.* method was devised for fruit products, the acid being isolated first as a lead salt. It can be adapted for use in the assay of drugs.

To a solution containing about 0·3 g of tartaric acid in 20 ml of water, neutral to phenolphthalein and to which 3 drops excess N potassium hydroxide have been added, slowly add 2 ml of glacial acetic acid with stirring, and 80 ml of 95 per cent ethanol. After allowing the solution to stand in a refrigerator overnight, filter the precipitate through a Gooch crucible and wash with ice-cold 80 per cent ethanol. Remove the precipitate with about 100 ml of hot water, boil and titrate with 0·1N alkali to phenolphthalein. 1 ml 0·1N = 0·015 g tartaric acid.

Citric acid does not interfere. If no potassium salts are present 2 ml of 20 per cent potassium acetate solution should be added. Often inexplicable results have been obtained with this method, a heavy precipitation occurring with the ethanol but no acid salt being formed.

King[4] improved the Kling method for estimation of tartaric acid, which depends upon the insolubility of calcium racemate in dilute acetic and hydrochloric acids. This method is applicable only to *d*-tartaric acid, but as the commercial tartaric acid in this country appears to be exclusively the *d*-acid, the method can be generally used. As applied to pharmaceutical preparations it is:

Take a portion of the sample which contains not more than 0·2 g of tartaric acid and dilute to 150 ml. Run a control experiment at the same time using 0·2 g of tartaric acid in 150 ml of water. Add to each 15 ml of reagent (*a*), 25 ml of reagent (*b*), and 20 ml of reagent (*c*), stir vigorously until calcium racemate begins to precipitate, and allow the mixture to stand overnight at room temperature. Filter through a Gooch crucible, transferring the precipitate entirely with a portion of the filtrate. Wash the contents of the crucible five times with water, filling it about half full each time. Treat the precipitate and mat after removal from the crucible with 20 ml of reagent (*d*), wash the crucible thoroughly and make up to 150 ml with water. Heat 50 ml of reagent (*e*) to boiling-point and add it, through the crucible, to the 150 ml of liquid. Heat the mixture to 80°, cool, stir vigorously and stand for at least four hours, stirring occasionally. Filter and wash as before. Wash the precipitate into a beaker with 150 ml of water, add 50 ml of 10 per cent by volume sulphuric acid and heat to 80°. Add, immediately, an excess of 0·2N permanganate (about 90 ml for 0·2 g tartaric acid), again heat to 80°, add an additional 5 ml of permanganate and allow to stand for one minute. Reheat to 80°, add 10 ml of 0·2N oxalic acid and titrate back with permanganate. (King uses special permanganate and oxalic acid solutions.) From the control experiment calculate the equivalence of 1 ml of permanganate to tartaric acid.

The reagents mentioned above are (*a*) Diammonium citrate. Dissolve 29 g of citric acid in about 200 ml of water, carefully neutralise to methyl red with ammonia, add 14·5 g of citric acid and make up to 1 litre with water. (*b*) Ammonium *l*-tartrate. Dissolve 3·2 g of the salt, entirely free from *d*-tartrate, in water, add 1 ml of formalin as a preservative (or preferably make up as required) and dilute to 200 ml. (*c*) Calcium acetate. Dissolve 16 g of calcium carbonate in a dilution of 120 ml of glacial acetic acid, make up to 1 litre and filter. (*d*) Hydrochloric acid, 34 ml of concentrated acid per litre. (*e*) Calcium and sodium acetate. Dissolve 5 g of calcium carbonate in 20 g of acetic acid and sufficient water, add 100 g of sodium acetate, make up to 1 litre and filter.

Although the method is rather long, excellent results can be obtained with it, and it is recommended for its accuracy.

TARTRATES

Alkali tartrates are determined by the general method for alkali salts of organic acids, *i.e.* heating about 2 g until carbonised, boiling the alkali residue with excess of standard acid, filtering and titrating the filtrate to methyl orange; or preferably by boiling the charred residue with water, filtering, re-igniting the carbonaceous residue to a white ash, adding this to the aqueous filtrate and titrating with standard acid to methyl orange. **Sodium potassium tartrate,** $COONa(CHOH)_2COOK,4H_2O$, Mol. Wt. 282·2. 1 ml 0·5N = 0·07055 g. Normal **potassium tartrate,** $C_8H_8O_{12}K_4$, H_2O, Mol. Wt. 470·5. 1 ml 0·5N = 0·05881 g.

Potassium acid tartrate, $COOH(CHOH)_2COOK$, Mol. Wt. 188·2, is titrated similarly to tartaric acid with 0·2N alkali to phenolphthalein, using about 1·5 g in boiling water. 1 ml 0·2N = 0·03764 g.

Compound Effervescent Powder, *B.P.C.* (*Seidlitz Powder*). The No. 1 powder (blue) consists of 10 g of a mixture of 75 per cent of sodium potassium tartrate with 25 per cent of sodium bicarbonate.

Direct titration of the bicarbonate to methyl orange is not possible owing to buffering. For sodium bicarbonate:

Weigh exactly 2 g, dissolve in 25 ml of water, add 25 ml of 0·5N hydrochloric acid, boil for some minutes to drive off carbon dioxide and titrate back with 0·5N alkali to phenolphthalein. 1 ml 0·5N = 0·04201 g $NaHCO_3$.

For sodium potassium tartrate:

Weigh exactly 2 g, char, digest the residue with water, filter, ignite the filter paper and carbonaceous matter to a white ash and add it to the filtrate. Add excess of 0·5N acid, boil and titrate back with 0·5N alkali to methyl red. From the ml of 0·5N acid required subtract that due to bicarbonate. 1 ml 0·5N = 0·07055 g $NaKC_4H_4O_6,4H_2O$.

The No. 2 powder (white) consists of 2·5 g of *B.P.* tartaric acid.

1. *A.O.A.C.*, 1960, p. 143.
2. STEUART, D. W., *Analyst*, 1934, **59**, 532.
3. *J.A.O.A.C.*, 1930, **13**, 103.
4. KING, J., *Analyst*, 1933, **58**, 135.

THIOURACILS

An assay of these substances (**thiouracil,** $C_4H_4ON_2S$, Mol. Wt. 128·2, **methylthiouracil,** $C_5H_6ON_2S$, Mol. Wt. 142·2, and **propylthiouracil,** $C_7H_{10}ON_2S$, Mol. Wt. 170·2) has been based on the insolubility of their silver salts. As they are insoluble in water they must be dissolved in a slight excess of standard sodium hydroxide before adding a slight excess of silver nitrate; the nitric acid liberated is then titrated. The total alkali used is calculated to the appropriate thiouracil.

Dissolve 0·25 g in 30 ml of 0·1N sodium hydroxide and 20 ml of water, heat to boiling and add 42 ml of 0·1N silver nitrate. Boil gently for five minutes and titrate the hot solution with 0·1N sodium hydroxide to a distinct pale green colour, using solution of bromothymol blue as indicator. 1 ml 0·1N sodium hydroxide (total amount) = 0·00641 g $C_4H_4ON_2S$, 0·007109 g $C_5H_6ON_2S$ and 0·008512 g $C_7H_{10}ON_2S$.

Propylthiouracil is assayed in the *U.S.P.* by this method.

Abbott[1] proposed a method for the determination of thiouracils by direct titration with mercuric acetate, which appears to be more precise and accurate than the argentimetric method. The detailed method is as follows:

Dissolve 0·3 to 0·4 g of thiouracil or methylthiouracil, or 0·35 to 0·45 g of propylthiouracil, in 50 ml of 0·1N sodium hydroxide and 200 ml of water, warming to complete solution. Cool, add 10 g of sodium acetate trihydrate and make acid to litmus paper with 33 per cent w/w acetic acid. Add 1 ml of a freshly prepared 0·5 per cent solution of diphenylcarbazone in ethanol and titrate with 0·05M mercuric acetate to the first appearance of a rose-pink colour persisting for two to three minutes, shaking the mixture well when nearing the end-point. 1 ml 0·05M = 0·01282 g thiouracil, 0·01422 g methylthiouracil and 0·01702 g propylthiouracil.

The addition of sodium acetate is not essential but was found to increase the sharpness of the end-point. This method has been adopted by the *B.P.* for propylthiouracil and methylthiouracil.

Of the more common tablet excipients only lactose was found to interfere, giving a yellow colour on boiling with sodium hydroxide which subsequently interfered with the end-point (for tablets the sodium hydroxide/water/thiouracil mixture was boiled for at least two minutes to ensure that the excipient was fully dispersed and all the thiouracil was dissolved). However, if the following modification of the method is used the interference will be overcome.

Boil the tablet mixture with 200 ml of water for two to three minutes to dissolve the thiouracil compound, cool to 70° before adding the sodium hydroxide and allow to stand for five minutes with occasional shaking. Complete as above beginning with 'add 10 g of sodium acetate . . . ,' cooling to room temperature before titrating. (If no stearic acid is present in addition to the lactose, the addition of the sodium hydroxide solution may be omitted.)

The thiouracils may also be titrated in non-aqueous medium (dimethylformamide) with sodium methoxide to thymol blue (see p. 794).

Tablets of Methylthiouracil, *B.P.* Usually contain 50 mg.

The tablets can be assayed directly by the mercury method given above using a weight of powdered tablets equivalent to about 0·35 g of methylthiouracil. The silver precipitation method may also be used directly on the powdered tablets provided that in the presence of lactose, which causes darkening of the silver precipitate, the precipitate is filtered from hot solution through kieselguhr with suction and washing with a little hot water before continuing the titration.

Tablets of Propylthiouracil, *B.P.* Usually contain 50 mg.

The tablets can be assayed directly by the mercury method given above using a weight of powdered tablets equivalent to about 0·4 g of propylthiouracil. The silver precipitation method, however, is not applicable to the tablets since an interfering red colour completely obscures the end-point.

OTHER ANTITHYROID SUBSTANCES

Carbimazole, $C_7H_{10}O_2N_2S$, Mol. Wt. 186·2, has an absorption maximum at 291 mμ, E(1 per cent, 1 cm) in 0·1N hydrochloric acid = 557.

The substance is, however, almost insoluble in water and the *B.P.* assay using 6 mg per 100 ml for the original solution must lead to the possibility of serious errors.

Methimazole, $C_4H_6N_2S$, Mol. Wt. 114·2.

This substance is assayed in the *U.S.P.* by the silver precipitation method given above. 1 ml 0·1N sodium hydroxide = 0·01142 g.

1. Abbott, C. F., *J. Pharm. Pharmacol.*, 1953, **5**, 53.

THYMOL

$CH_3.C_6H_3OH.C_3H_7$ Mol. Wt. 150·2

Thymol is phenolic and is extracted by solutions of fixed caustic alkalis. For the same reason it can be determined by the general Koppeschaar method (see Phenol, p. 513). The bromination can be directly estimated by titration, using the bleaching of a solution of methyl orange as an indication of the end-point.[1]

To about 2 g of powdered thymol in a 500-ml graduated flask add 25 ml of 25 per cent sodium hydroxide solution, and when the thymol has dissolved, dilute to the mark with water. To 25 ml of the dilution in a 250-ml stoppered flask, add 20 ml of hot 1 : 1 hydrochloric acid and immediately run in 1 to 3 ml less than the theoretical amount of 0·1N potassium bromate-bromide solution (determined by a preliminary titration). Warm to 70° or 80°, add 2 drops of 1 per cent aqueous methyl orange solution, and titrate slowly with the bromine solution, swirling vigorously after each addition. When the colour of the methyl orange is bleached, add alternately two drops of the bromine solution and one drop of methyl orange solution, shaking vigorously for ten seconds between each addition until the red colour disappears after addition of methyl orange. 1 ml 0·1N = 0·003753 g. To the cooled titration liquid resulting from the above determination, add 3 to 5 ml more of bromine solution. Shake, add 1 g of potassium iodide and titrate the liberated iodine with 0·1N sodium thiosulphate. The total bromine added less the thiosulphate required should equal the original bromine titration value.

Thymol gives with 4-aminophenazone[2] a dye soluble in chloroform and may, therefore, be determined by the general method given under Phenol (p. 514); the chloroform solution is of a moderately strong yellow colour, with a wavelength of maximum absorption at about 470 mμ.

Compound Glycerin of Thymol, *B.P.C.* A mixture of sodium bicarbonate, 1 per cent w/v, borax, 2 per cent w/v, sodium benzoate, 0·80 per cent w/v, and sodium salicylate, 0·52 per cent w/v, with glycerin and a number of volatile constituents.

A determination of the salts present can be made as follows:

(*i*) Evaporate 10 ml of sample in a platinum dish on a water-bath until the residue is apparently free from moisture, ash gently and dissolve the residue in hot water. Titrate with 0·1N hydrochloric acid to methyl orange for total alkali = '*a*' ml.

Boil, add mannitol and titrate back with 0·1N alkali to phenolphthalein for boric acid = '*b*' ml.

(*ii*) Acidify 20 ml of sample, extract the organic acids with ether, wash the mixed ethers, dry the solvent and evaporate it cautiously. Titrate the acids in dilute ethanol with 0·1N alkali to phenolphthalein = '*c*' ml. Make the titration solution up to 100 ml. Determine the salicylic acid in 20 ml of the dilution by bromination, as given under Salicylic Acid (p. 558). Calculate the 0·1N alkali equivalent to the salicylic acid present in the 100 ml of dilution (1 ml 0·1N alkali = 0·0138 g salicylic acid) = '*d*' ml.

Then per cent w/v sodium benzoate $= (c-d) \times 0{\cdot}01221 \times 1{\cdot}180 \times 5$
sodium salicylate $= d \times 0{\cdot}0138 \times 1{\cdot}159 \times 5$
borax $= b \times 0{\cdot}009536 \times 10$
sodium bicarbonate $= (a - b/2 - c/2) \times 0{\cdot}0084 \times 10$

1. *A.O.A.C.*, 1960, p. 525.
2. Johnson, C. A., and Savidge, R. A., *J. Pharm. Pharmacol.*, 1958, **10**, 171T.

THYROID

The *B.P.* requires that thyroid be standardised by means of a chemical determination in terms of the content of 'thyroxine-iodine', whereas the *U.S.P.* relies on the determination of total 'iodine in thyroid combination'. Johnson and Smith[1] have shown that both of these determinations may not indicate the biological activity of the drug. For a proper standardisation of thyroid, therefore, recourse to a biological method must be made. Several biological systems have been described for the assay of thyroidal activity, but from our experience the choice of method lies between that based on the reduction of asphyxiation time in mice (Smith *et al.*[2]) and that depending on the anti-thiouracil-goitre test in rats (Reineke *et al.*[3]) but whichever method is used there will be some difficulty in deciding what should be used as a reference standard and by what route the drug should be administered. It has been suggested that thyroxine is not a suitable choice for standard since the dosage response curves of thyroid and thyroxine are not parallel. This was not the experience of Johnson and Smith[1] who chose to use L-thyroxine in order to avoid the difficulty of assigning an arbitrary potency to a sample of thyroid selected to serve as a standard and which in the end might still not be identical with the samples of thyroid to be tested, since the activity of thyroid is due not only to thyroxine, but also to tri-iodothyronine and these are not likely to be present in constant ratios. It is to be expected also that routes of administration will affect the relative activity of dissimilar substances and it is not unknown for the same biological system to yield different results at different times in different hands when mixtures are being examined.

However, although the use of a biological assay may give somewhat inaccurate results and although it is certain that the degree of precision which will have to be accepted is less than that which has hitherto been considered to apply in the chemical standardisation of thyroid, it must be true that a biological method provides a more suitable standardisation than the present chemical methods depending on the determination of total or 'thyroxine-iodine'.

Mouse anoxia method

Mice weighing 16 to 20 g, of one sex and preferably males, are dosed on days 1, 3 and 5 with a standard preparation at more than one dose level with a dose interval of the order 2 : 1. An identical group is similarly treated with the sample under test. On day 7 the mice are placed individually in jars of 1-qt capacity, which can be rendered gas tight. The elapsed time for death to occur through asphyxiation is recorded, and although the potency may be calculated from the relationship of asphyxiation time and log dose, Webb[4] has found that there is advantage in transforming asphyxiation time to logs. The response is affected by temperature, and the whole test, including dosing and reading, should be carried out at a uniform temperature. Smith *et al.*[2] claim that an assay conducted at 23° using 40 mice should give a result within 80 to 124 per cent of the true value in 19 out of 20 tests.

The test has been successfully applied by some workers, but others have experienced little success with it.

Anti-thiouracil-goitre test in rats

The method as described by Reineke *et al.*[3] requires the use of male rats weighing 100 to 200 g. These are apportioned as evenly as possible into groups of 8 to 10 animals and are dosed daily with the standard and preparation under test, during which time all animals receive 0·1 per cent of thiouracil in their feed. After fourteen days the animals are sacrificed, their thyroids dissected out cleanly on moist filter paper and weighed rapidly to avoid evaporation loss. The thyroid weights are inversely proportional to the dose of thyro-active substance administered.

In practice it has been found convenient to dissect the trachea with thyroids attached, to fix overnight in Bouin's fluid, to separate the thyroids, to immerse in 95 per cent ethanol for two hours and to allow to become air dry before weighing.

Despite the fact that a biological method is the only way to obtain a reliable estimate of the potency of thyroid, chemical assessment is still quite frequently required. The *B.P.* method is a determination of so-called 'iodine in combination as thyroxine' and is based on the observations of Harington and Randall[5] that, after hydrolysis of the thyroid with sodium hydroxide, an acid-insoluble fraction can be separated which consists essentially of thyroxine. There have always been mechanical difficulties associated with this assay, especially when an attempt is made to apply it to formulated products such as tablets. Further considerations, however, indicate that it is an unreliable guide to the potency of thyroid. Firstly, the discovery of the highly potent 3,5,3′-tri-iodothyronine (liothyronine) invalidates the assumption that the amount of total iodine in the acid-insoluble fraction is related to the proportion of thyroxine and hence to potency; secondly it has been shown that when lactose is present during the hydrolysis stage a greater proportion of iodine is present in the subsequent acid-precipitated fraction than if the lactose is absent. This observation was first made by Doery[6] and has since been confirmed in a number of laboratories; an additional stage was introduced into the assay by the Addendum 1960 to the *B.P.*, whereby any lactose present (and it is present in most samples of Thyroid *B.P.* since it is the officially permitted diluent for adjustment of dried, defatted material to the appropriate strength) is removed by washing with cold 0·5 per cent w/v sulphuric acid prior to the alkaline hydrolysis. However, it has been shown that, in addition to removing lactose, this treatment may also produce a significant lowering of the content of iodine in the acid-insoluble fraction.[1] The chemical standardisation of thyroid by such a determination is thus open to considerable criticism and it seems certain that the use of methods of this type will be abandoned in the future.

The *U.S.P.* rely upon a determination of total iodine, together with a statement that thyroid is free from iodine in inorganic or any form of combination other than that peculiar to the thyroid gland. It is obvious that such a standardisation can give no accurate index of biological activity but at least it is free from interference due to the diluent present and could very well be used for comparative purposes to assess, say, the quantity of a given batch of thyroid present in tablets made from it. The total iodine determination may be carried out by fusion with sodium carbonate and subsequent treatment as described for the determination of iodine in organic combination on p. 315. Alternatively, the flask-combustion method (see p. 796), which is convenient and much more rapid than the fusion method, may be used. Certain modifications to the general method described in Appendix IV need to be made, since an unusually large amount of organic matter must be burned. The following procedure is suitable:

Apparatus: This is essentially the same as that described in Appendix IV but a 2-litre iodine flask is used and the platinum gauze is 2·5 cm wide and 2 cm long. Since the sample should be suspended about two-thirds of the way from the base of the stopper to the bottom of the flask it is preferable to reduce the length of the platinum wire by fusing a length of glass rod to the stopper and attaching the platinum wire to its lower end.

Method: Weigh about 0·2 g of the sample and transfer to a piece of light-weight tissue about 7 cm wide and 10 cm long. Continue as described in Appendix IV, using a mixture of 50 ml of water and 2 ml of N sodium hydroxide as absorbing liquid and titrating with 0·005N sodium thiosulphate. 1 ml 0·005N = 0·1058 mg iodine in thyroid combination.

In this determination ensure that the flask is filled with oxygen by passing a steady stream of the gas for at least five minutes and take particular care to sweep out all traces of excess bromine from the flask before titration.

Since thyroid contains a number of iodine-containing substances of different degrees of activity, it would seem that the only possible form of chemical standardisation is that the more important constituents be separated and determined individually. From the known potency of each constituent, some assessment of the overall potency of the sample might then be possible. A number of paper chromatographic systems for the separation of thyroxine and related compounds have been suggested from time to time and these have been conveniently reviewed by Wilkinson and Bowden.[7] However, the main difficulties associated with a possible determination of this type rest in the initial quantitative hydrolysis, and in the final elution and determination of the separated substances. The hydrolysis can be accomplished by alkaline or enzymic attack; the use of alkaline hydrolysis is convenient and clean, but it suffers from the disadvantage that the liberated iodo-amino acids may be partially decomposed; enzymic hydrolysis, on the other hand, may be much more carefully controlled but is liable to give rise to considerable amounts of impurities in the hydrolysate. Jende[8] has recommended a hydrolysis with papain activated by hydrocyanic acid in citric acid buffer at pH 4·7 to 4·8 for forty-eight hours at 55° and Devlin and Stephenson[9] one with trypsin and erepsin for ninety-six hours at 37°. After hydrolysis the iodinated thyronines are extracted from the hydrolysate with a solvent such as *n*-butanol and then subjected to paper chromatography. Determination of the minute amounts of separated material on the paper also presents many problems; the type of method which seems most promising is based on the ceric sulphate–arsenious acid catalytic reaction (see p. 295) and this has been applied by Block and his colleagues[10] and by Devlin and Stephenson.[9] It seems certain that more work is required before this type of chemical standardisation can be applied to commercial samples of thyroid.

Tablets of Thyroid, *B.P.* Usually contain ½ grain of thyroid. At present the only standardisation possible is by biological assay unless a sample of the thyroid used is available; in the latter case for control purposes a total iodine content is satisfactory. Weigh and powder twenty tablets, or more if necessary, and carry out the assay described above under Thyroid using a weight of powder, not exceeding 0·4 g, equivalent to about 0·2 g of thyroid.

Thyroxine sodium, $C_{15}H_{10}O_4NI_4Na,5H_2O$, Mol. Wt. 889·0, is the sodium salt of L-thyroxine. It may be assayed by the oxygen-flask combustion method as described in Appendix IV using about 13 mg and titrating with 0·02N sodium thiosulphate. 1 ml 0·02N = 0·0006657 g anhydrous.

Tablets of Thyroxine Sodium, *B.P.* Usually contain 0·05 mg. These tablets contain too much organic matter for application of the flask-combustion method.

Weigh an amount of powdered tablets equivalent to about 1·5 mg of thyroxine sodium into a nickel crucible about 6 mm in diameter and about 6 mm deep and add 3 ml of water followed by 5 g of sodium hydroxide in small pieces. Heat on a water-bath to remove the water, add a further 4 g of sodium hydroxide and heat over a Bunsen flame, at first gently and then sufficiently strongly to maintain the mixture in a molten state, with continuous gentle swirling, until the evolution of gas ceases and the mixture is clear. Allow to cool, dissolve the residue in 350 ml of water and complete the assay described under chiniofon sodium (p. 315) beginning with the words 'Add three drops of 0·04 per cent . . .' and titrating with 0·05N sodium thiosulphate. 1 ml 0·05N = 0·1852 mg of $C_{15}H_{10}O_4NI_4Na,5H_2O$.

Adamson *et al.*[11] recommended a colorimetric method based upon nitrosation for the determination of small amounts of thyroxine. Extraction of thyroxine from tablets for this method presents little difficulty; most of the commonly used excipients are either soluble in the reagents without interfering or can be removed by some simple extraction and filtration technique.

Transfer a quantity of powder, equivalent to 1·5 to 2·0 mg of anhydrous thyroxine sodium, to a 50-ml graduated flask. Add 17·5 ml of 95 per cent ethanol and 25 ml of sodium chloride reagent (prepared by dissolving 170 g of sodium chloride in sufficient N hydrochloric acid to produce 1 litre). Heat the flask in a water-bath until the solution boils, cool and dilute to volume with sodium chloride reagent. Filter and collect 35 ml of filtrate. Transfer 15·0 ml of clear filtrate to a 20-ml graduated flask, add 2·0 ml of freshly prepared 1 per cent sodium nitrite solution, mix and allow to stand in the dark for twenty minutes. Dilute to volume with strong ammonia solution, mix and determine the extinction at 470 mμ using 2-cm cells. Carry out a blank determination with 2·0 ml of water in place of the 2·0 ml of sodium nitrite solution and apply the necessary correction to the extinction. Calculate the thyroxine sodium content of the material by reference to a standard curve prepared with known amounts, covering the range 0 to 0·8 mg, of pure thyroxine sodium.

The method is not suitable for determination of thyroxine in thyroid preparations.

Liothyronine sodium, $C_{15}H_{11}O_4NI_3Na$, Mol. Wt. 673·0, is the sodium salt of L-tri-iodothyronine. It may be assayed by the oxygen-flask combustion method, using about 15 mg and titrating with 0·02N sodium thiosulphate. 1 ml 0·02N = 0·0007478 g.

Tablets of Liothyronine Sodium, *B.P.* May be of any strength between 5 and 50 micrograms. These tablets contain too much organic matter in relation to iodine content for application of the flask-combustion method.

Weigh an amount of powdered tablets not exceeding 0·5 g, equivalent to between 0·5 and 1 mg of liothyronine sodium, and transfer to a nickel crucible about 10 cm in diameter and 10 cm deep. Add 5 ml of water, 5 g of sodium carbonate decahydrate and 25 g of sodium hydroxide and heat in a water-bath for one hour, mixing thoroughly. Then heat over a Bunsen flame, at first gently and then sufficiently strongly to maintain the mixture in a semi-molten state, with continuous gentle swirling, until the evolution of gas ceases and the mixture is free from yellow uncarbonised material. Do not attempt to burn off all the carbon. Allow to cool, dissolve the residue in hot water, filter through a cotton-wool plug and wash the crucible and filter with hot water until the volume of filtrate is about 500 ml. Cool and complete the assay described under chiniofon sodium, p. 315, beginning with the words 'Add three drops of 0·04 per cent . . .' and titrating with 0·05N sodium thiosulphate, immediately after the addition of potassium iodide. 1 ml 0·05N = 0·1870 mg of liothyronine sodium.

1. Johnson, C. A., and Smith, K. L., *J. Pharm. Pharmacol.*, 1961, **13**, 133T.
2. Smith, A. U., Emmens, C. W., and Parkes, A. S., *J. Endocrinology*, 1947, **5**, 186.
3. Reineke, E. P., Mixner, J. P., and Turner, C. W., *Endocrinology*, 1945, **36**, 64.
4. Webb, F. W., *J. Pharm. Pharmacol.*, 1961, **13**, 136T.
5. Harington, C. R., and Randall, S. S., *Quart. J. Pharm.*, 1929, **2**, 501.
6. Doery, H. M., *Quart. J. Pharm.*, 1945, **18**, 384.
7. Wilkinson, J. H., and Bowden, C. H., Chromatographic and Electrophoretic Techniques. Vol. I (Ed. Ivor Smith), 2nd ed., p. 166, (London) Heinemann, 1960.
8. Jende, S., *Pharm. Ztg.*, 1960, **105**, 243.
9. Devlin, W. F., and Stephenson, N. R., *J. Pharm. Pharmacol.*, 1962, **14**, 597.
10. Block, R. J., Werner, S. C., Mandl, R. H., Row, V. V., and Radichevich, T., *Arch. Biochem. Biophys.*, 1960, **88**, 98.
11. Adamson, D. C. M., Domleo, A. P., Jefferies, J. P., and Shaw, W. H. C., *J. Pharm. Pharmacol.*, 1952, **4**, 760.

BALSAM OF TOLU

The *B.P.* estimation of total balsamic acids is due to Cocking.[1] The acids from the saponified balsams are converted into the corresponding magnesium salts and the salts of the balsamic acids are separated from the salts of the resin acids by filtration and from aromatic alcohols by extraction with sodium bicarbonate. The *B.P.* quantities directed to be used must be adhered to and the manipulative details must be closely followed to prevent precipitation of gummy matter and formation of clots.

Reflux 1 to 1·5 g of the sample with 25 ml of 0·5N ethanolic potassium hydroxide for one hour, evaporate the ethanol, add 50 ml of water and warm until the residue is diffused throughout the liquid. Cool, add 80 ml of water and a solution of 1·5 g of magnesium sulphate heptahydrate in 50 ml of water, mix thoroughly and allow to stand for ten minutes. Filter, wash the residue with 20 ml of water and acidify the combined filtrate and washings with concentrated hydrochloric acid. Extract with four 40-ml quantities of ether, discard the aqueous liquid and extract the combined ether extracts with 20, 20, 10, 10 and 10 ml of 5 per cent sodium bicarbonate solution, washing each extract with the same 20 ml of ether. Discard the ether liquids, combine the aqueous extracts, acidify with concentrated hydrochloric acid and extract with 30, 20, 20 and 10 ml of chloroform, filtering each extract through a cotton-wool plug covered with a layer of anhydrous sodium sulphate. Evaporate the chloroform in a current of air and, immediately the last trace of chloroform has been removed, add to the residue 10 ml of 95 per cent ethanol, previously neutralised to phenol red, and warm until dissolved. Cool and titrate with 0·1N sodium hydroxide using phenol red as indicator. 1 ml 0·1N NaOH = 0·01482 g total balsamic acids, calculated as cinnamic acid.

Cocking used ether for extraction of the purified balsamic acids and this solvent is preferable. Further, the *B.P.* directs the mixed benzoic and cinnamic acids to be titrated but they should be weighed after drying *in vacuo* over sulphuric acid as they are present in variable proportions; the amount of cinnamic acid present may be determined by bromination.

Tolu balsam contains 35 per cent to 50 per cent of total balsamic acids, calculated on the dry alcohol-soluble matter.

In the original method Cocking[1] included a determination of free balsamic acids:

Dissolve 2·5 g of balsam of tolu, or the alcoholic extractive from 2·5 g of benzoin, in 15 ml of hot 95 per cent ethanol in a 300-ml flask. Add all at once a mixture of 10 ml of 5 per cent potassium hydroxide solution and 50 ml of water; mix and dilute with 150 ml of water. To the mixture add 2·5 g of magnesium sulphate dissolved in 50 ml of water, and stand the flask on a water-bath for five minutes. Cool, and continue the determination of total balsamic acids as given above.

Omission of the preliminary warming of the magnesium precipitate prevents satisfactory filtration, but the solution should be allowed to become quite cold before filtering.

Syrup of Tolu, *B.P.* Contains an aqueous extract from balsam of tolu (mostly aromatic acids) in syrup.

The percentage of total acids present is small and varies considerably; the cinnamic acid can be determined by bromination.

STORAX

Assayed for total balsamic acids by the method given above for balsam of tolu. Prepared storax should contain at least 30 per cent of total balsamic acids calculated on the substance dried on a water-bath for one hour.

1. Cocking, T. T., *Quart. J. Pharm.*, 1931, **4,** 330.

TRAGACANTH

Tragacanth is imported in different grades of natural flake or ribbon with large variations in colour and amount of extraneous vegetable tissue and is often bought on appearance and assessed from the experience of the dealers. However, the viscosity of the mucilage obtained by treatment of the gum with water is of paramount importance since commercial evaluation largely depends on this property.

The Analytical Methods Committee of the *S.A.C.*[1] investigating this determination considered that since the mucilage formed is a non-Newtonian fluid the expression of its viscosity in absolute units has no validity and that the Redwood viscometer method yielded the most reproducible results when used by different analysts. Further, since in grading of gums it would be desirable to obtain the weight of gums to give similar viscosities, a method was evolved of determining the concentration of dry gum that would be required to produce a mucilage with a standard efflux time for a known volume of mucilage.

Place a quantity of the powdered gum equivalent to the required weight of dry gum (the dried gum must not be used for the preparation of the mucilage) in a dry 500-ml conical flask and add 5 ml of 95 per cent ethanol. Ensure that the gum is completely wetted and dispersed evenly over the inner surface of the flask. Add 195 ml of cold water as quickly as possible and shake. Connect the flask to a reflux condenser and place in a vigorously boiling water-bath, so that the surface of the water is about 1 inch above the surface of the mucilage. Continue the heating for one hour, gently swirling the mucilage at intervals of fifteen minutes without removing the flask from the water-bath. At the end of one hour remove the flask from the water, stopper it and allow to cool naturally to room temperature.

After it has stood for twenty-four hours, determine the efflux time of 50 ml in a Redwood No. 1 viscometer at 20°. Record the mean of six readings. Correct to a water efflux time of 27 seconds by multiplying the result by $27/x$, where x is the efflux time of 50 ml of water at 20° for the same instrument. If the efflux time of the mucilage is not between 75 and 125 seconds repeat the test with a fresh mucilage of suitable concentration. If a mucilage is found to give a higher efflux time than 125 seconds an approximate result may be obtained by diluting with water to bring the efflux time within the required range, but for accurate results it is recommended that a fresh mucilage be prepared.

Calculate the concentration of dry gum (C_Q) required to give an efflux time of 100 seconds from the equation:

$$C_Q = \text{antilog}\,(\log C_E - 0{\cdot}002E + 0{\cdot}2)$$

in which C_E = concentration of dry gum giving an efflux time of E seconds, when E lies between 75 and 125 seconds.

The method has been extended to flake gum.[2]

After sifting out any accompanying powder, grind a representative sample, preferably not less than 50 g, until the whole passes through a No. 30-mesh sieve. The grinding may be effected in a coffee mill or a laboratory disintegrator of the Christy and Norris type or by any other method in which the process of grinding is not prolonged and does not appreciably heat the gum. Determine the moisture in the powder; weigh out a quantity of the powdered gum equivalent to the required weight of dry gum into a dry 500-ml conical flask and add 5 ml of 95 per cent ethanol. Ensure that the gum is completely wetted and dispersed evenly over the inner surface of the flask. Add 195 ml of cold water as quickly as possible and shake. Allow to stand for one hour, swirling frequently. Connect the flask to a reflux condenser and place in a vigorously boiling water-bath, so that the surface of the water is about 1 inch above the surface of the mucilage. Complete the determination by the method as described above.

The determination of volatile acidity is of value in detecting adulteration of tragacanth with Karaya gum (also known as Indian tragacanth) from Sterculia species and with Gum Ghatti (Indian gum) from *Anogeissus latifolia*, and the following method[3] is recommended:

Treat 1 g of the whole or powdered sample in a 700-ml round-bottomed long-necked flask in the cold with 100 ml of water and 5 ml of phosphoric acid (85 per cent by weight) for several hours or until the gum is completely swollen. Boil gently for two hours under reflux; a very small quantity of cellulose substance will remain undissolved. Tragacanth yields a practically colourless solution, Karaya gum gives a pink or rose solution. This reaction may be used as a preliminary test for detection of Karaya gum. Distil the hydrolysed product with steam, using a scrubber to connect the distillation flask with the condenser. Continue the distillation until the distillate amounts to 600 ml and the acid residue to about 20 ml. To avoid scorching of the residue, do not permit concentration of the contents of the distilling flask to less than 20 ml. Titrate the distillate with 0·1N sodium hydroxide, using 10 drops of phenolphthalein indicator. Correct the results by a blank determination and express as 'volatile acidity', the number of ml of 0·1N sodium hydroxide required to neutralise the volatile acid obtained.

Figures obtained using this method on twenty-eight samples of tragacanth gave a range of 2·3 to 4·0 ml with a mean of 3·46 ml of 0·1N sodium hydroxide. One sample of Indian gum (Gum Ghatti) gave 12·75 ml and a sample of Karaya gum 22·2 ml.

1. *Analyst*, 1948, **73**, 368.
2. *Analyst*, 1949, **74**, 2.
3. *A.O.A.C.*, 1960, p. 545.

TRIETHANOLAMINE

Commercial triethanolamine consists mainly of the base tri(2-hydroxyethyl)amine, $(CH_2OH.CH_2)_3N$, together with di(2-hydroxyethyl)amine and smaller amounts of 2-hydroxyethylamine.

It has become an important compound for use in toilet preparations, and in combination with fatty acids it is of value as an emulsifying agent.

The gravimetric determination of triethanolamine was first described by Fleck,[1] in which an addition compound, very insoluble in *iso*propyl alcohol, was formed with hydriodic acid.

> To about 0·5 g in a glass dish add 6 ml dilute hydriodic acid; evaporate to dryness on a water-bath. Stir the residue with 5 ml *iso*propyl alcohol and filter through a tared sintered-glass crucible, washing the dish and residue with three portions each of 5 ml of *iso*propyl alcohol. Dry the residue at 105° and weigh. Add to the weight obtained 1 mg for each ml of *iso*propyl alcohol used. 1 g residue = 0·536 g of pure triethanolamine.

In this and the method to be described below the mono- and di-ethanolamine present do not interfere, and only the triethanolamine is determined; hence the amount of original commercial triethanolamine can only be assessed approximately from the result obtained. The total bases can be determined by titration with standard acid to methyl red. 1 ml N = 0·1492 g $C_6H_{15}O_3N$.

Eastland, Evers and West[2] found Fleck's method unsatisfactory for many preparations, since the base is not easily completely extracted and it is often contaminated with substances not readily removed in the subsequent treatment. The necessary technique for separating the triethanolamine from emulsions, and for its subsequent determination, is:

> Mix about 5 g of the emulsion with 20 ml of water and heat on a water-bath for five minutes. Add sulphuric acid until a blue colour is given with congo red paper (about pH 3) and continue heating on the water-bath for another minute, adding more sulphuric acid if required. Transfer the cooled mixture to a separator and extract the fat with two 25-ml quantities of ether. Shake the ethereal extracts with 20 ml of approximately 0·1N sulphuric acid, and distil off the ether so that the ether-soluble matter is left floating in the acid. Re-extract this with ether and add the aqueous layer to that obtained from the previous extraction. Remove the ether from the acid extract by heating on a water-bath and precipitate the sulphuric acid by adding barium hydroxide solution. Any remaining haziness due to incomplete extraction of the fatty matter is carried down with the precipitate of barium sulphate. Warm the mixture, centrifuge, pour off the liquid from the sediment and wash it with a little water. Precipitate the excess of barium by passing carbon dioxide into the boiling solution. Cool, filter and concentrate under reduced pressure to about 3 ml. Wash into a 50-ml beaker with 15 ml of ethanol, removing any insoluble material by filtering through a Hirsch funnel.

Remove the ethanol by evaporation and add 2 ml of concentrated hydrochloric acid to the residue. Evaporate the solution to dryness, when the hydrochloride forms a hard skin on the bottom of the beaker. Dry in a steam-oven for half an hour and allow to cool in a desiccator. Wash the crystals on to a sintered-glass crucible (IG.3) using four 5-ml quantities of pure *iso*propyl alcohol, and dry at 105° to constant weight. Triethanolamine hydrochloride × 0·8035 = triethanolamine. Add 0·003 g to the weight obtained as a correction for the slight solubility of the hydrochloride in *iso*propyl alcohol.

Glycerin and ethylene glycol do not interfere in the determination, but when the proportion of polyhydric alcohol is relatively great, it is an advantage to leave the hydrochloride residue for two hours in the steam-oven before treating it with the *iso*propyl alcohol.

ETHANOLAMINE, $NH_2.CH_2.CH_2OH$, Mol. Wt. 61·09

Ethanolamine is a strong base and can be titrated directly with acid to methyl red. 1 ml N acid = 0·06109 g.

Injection of Ethanolamine Oleate, *B.P.* Contains ethanolamine oleate equivalent to about 4·1 per cent w/v oleic acid and about 0·89 per cent w/v ethanolamine with benzyl alcohol in water for injection.

Oleic acid: Transfer 10 ml to a separator, add 20 ml of 0·1N sulphuric acid and extract with three 25-ml quantities of chloroform, washing each extract with the same 10 ml of water. Add the washings to the acid layer and retain for the determination of ethanolamine. Combine the chloroform extracts, evaporate the chloroform and dissolve the residue in 95 per cent ethanol, previously neutralised to phenolphthalein. Titrate with 0·1N sodium hydroxide using phenolphthalein as indicator. 1 ml 0·1N = 0·02825 g $C_{17}H_{33}.CO_2H$.

For ethanolamine: Titrate the excess acid in the combined acid layer and washings, retained above, with 0·1N sodium hydroxide using methyl orange as indicator. 1 ml 0·1N = 0·006109 g C_2H_7ON.

1. Fleck, H. R., *Analyst*, 1935, **60,** 77.
2. Eastland, C. J., Evers, N., and West, T. F., *Analyst*, 1937, **62,** 261.

TUBOCURARINE CHLORIDE

$C_{38}H_{44}O_6N_2Cl_2,5H_2O$ Mol. Wt. 785·8

In water tubocurarine chloride has an absorption maximum at about 280 mμ, E(1 per cent, 1 cm) = 105.

Tubocurarine chloride possesses a specific rotation of + 190°, equivalent to $[\alpha]^{20}_D$ + 215° for the anhydrous salt, and it is practically independent of the concentration. It is officially assayed for its chlorine content directly by the Volhard method (see p. 290). 1 ml 0·1N silver nitrate = 0·003546 g Cl.

Injection of Tubocurarine Chloride, *B.P.* Contains 1 per cent in water for injection.

The *B.P.* assay is spectrophotometric after diluting 5 ml to 1 litre.

Colorimetric determination[1] is based on Folin and Ciocalteu's phenol reagent which gives a brilliant blue colour with as little as 0·01 mg of the alkaloid.

Measure 2 ml of the standard solution (prepared by dissolving 10 mg of crystalline tubocurarine chloride in water and making up to 100 ml) or 2 ml of the test solution (prepared by diluting the solution under examination to approximately the same concentration as the standard) into a 25-ml glass-stoppered measuring cylinder. Add 3 ml of Folin and Ciocalteu's phenol reagent (see p. 476) and adjust the volume to 25 ml with water. Add 2 ml of 20 per cent sodium carbonate solution, mix and heat a suitable volume (5 ml) in a test-tube placed in a water-bath for three minutes. Cool the reaction mixture.

Prepare under identical conditions reaction mixtures from the standard and test solutions and compare them in a suitable colorimeter. From the readings obtained calculate the tubocurarine chloride content of the test solution.

If a phenol is present as a bacteriostat it will interfere unless removed by extraction with chloroform in slightly acid solution.

A number of compounds of similar pharmacological action are available. They are all assayed by non-aqueous titration with perchloric acid (see p. 792) although their injections are determined gravimetrically as reineckates (or from the iodide content in the case of gallamine triethiodide injection).

The substances are the following:

Decamethonium iodide, $C_{16}H_{38}N_2I_2$, Mol. Wt. 512·3
Gallamine triethiodide, $C_{30}H_{60}O_3N_3I_3$, Mol. Wt. 891·6
Hexamethonium bromide, $C_{12}H_{30}N_2Br_2$, Mol. Wt. 362·2
Hexamethonium tartrate, $C_{20}H_{40}O_{12}N_2$, Mol. Wt. 500·6
Pentolinium tartrate, $C_{23}H_{42}O_{12}N_2$, Mol. Wt. 538·6
Suxamethonium bromide, $C_{14}H_{30}O_4N_2Br_2,2H_2O$, Mol. Wt. 486·3
Suxamethonium chloride, $C_{14}H_{30}O_4N_2Cl_2,2H_2O$, Mol. Wt. 397·4

Injection of Gallamien Triethiodide, *B.P.* A sterile solution in water for injection containing sodium sulphite.

This preparation is assayed with silver nitrate by Volhard's method (see p. 290) using 5 ml. 1 ml 0·1N = 0·02972 g.

Injection of Suxamethonium Chloride, *B.P.* It usually contains 50 mg in 1 ml of injection.

This preparation can be assayed gravimetrically as reineckate.

To a volume equivalent to about 0·1 g suxamethonium chloride add

10 ml of water, 10 ml of dilute sulphuric acid and 30 ml of a 1 per cent aqueous solution of ammonium reineckate. Allow to stand for thirty minutes, filter and wash the residue with a saturated solution of suxamethonium reineckate until the washings are free from chloride and sulphate. (The suxamethonium reineckate is prepared by mixing equal volumes of a 1 per cent solution of suxamethonium chloride and a 1 per cent solution of ammonium reineckate, acidifying with dilute sulphuric acid, filtering and washing the precipitate of suxamethonium reineckate with water until the washings are free from chloride and sulphate.) Wash the residue with 2 ml of 95 per cent ethanol followed by 50 ml of ether and dry to constant weight at 80°. 1 g residue = 0·4285 g $C_{14}H_{30}O_4N_2Cl_2,2H_2O$.

Injection of Hexamethonium Tartrate, *B.P.* A sterile solution in water for injection, adjusted to pH 7·0.

This preparation can be assayed as reineckate similarly to suxamethonium chloride injection above. The method is modified by heating the solution to boiling before adding the warm reagent, cooling and allowing to stand in ice for one hour before filtering. Hexamethonium reineckate solution for washing the precipitate is prepared similarly using hexamethonium tartrate. 1 g residue = 0·5964 g $C_{20}H_{40}O_{12}N_2$.

Injection of Pentolinium Tartrate, *B.P.* A sterile solution in water for injection, adjusted to pH 6·5 with sodium hydroxide.

This preparation can be assayed as reineckate similarly to hexamethonium tartrate injection above. Pentolinium reineckate solution for washing the precipitate is prepared similarly using pentolinium tartrate. 1 g residue = 0·6140 g $C_{23}H_{42}O_{12}N_2$.

Tablets of Pentolinium Tartrate, *B.P.*

For assay an amount of powdered tablets equivalent to about 0·12 g of pentolinium tartrate should be extracted with warm water, filtered and the insoluble matter washed before evaporating the total filtrate and washings to about 10 ml and then continuing as for the injection.

1. Foster, G. E., *Analyst*, 1947, **72**, 62.

VANILLIN

$CH_3O.C_6H_3(OH).CHO$ Mol. Wt. 152·2

Vanillin is obtained from the vanilla pod, in which it occurs to the extent of from 2 to 3 per cent, or more generally it is prepared synthetically.

Titration of the hydroxyl group in vanillin with 0·1N alkali is not very satisfactory; thymolphthalein has been recommended as an indicator (Schimmel[1]), titration being continued to a distinct blue colour, but the end-point is not sufficiently definite. The determination of the methoxyl group is too long for general practical use, although it is quite accurate.

A volumetric method has been proposed by Sharp[2] dependent on oxidation of the vanillin to aliphatic acids with hydrogen peroxide in alkaline solution. However, the result depends on an arbitrary factor calculated from titrations on pure vanillin, hence it would not be reliable for impure products; for commercially pure vanillin it may be of value since direct titration is not very satisfactory.

Dissolve about 0·4 g of sample in 20 ml of N sodium hydroxide and add 40 to 60 ml of hydrogen peroxide solution (20 vol). Heat on a water-bath until all effervescence has ceased, then cool to room temperature. Titrate the excess of sodium hydroxide with N hydrochloric acid using phenolphthalein as indicator. Repeat the determination omitting the vanillin. 1 ml of N NaOH = 0·2954 g of $C_8H_8O_3$.

The gravimetric estimation of vanillin by means of its aldehyde group offers the best chances of success. Phillips[3] could not obtain good results by use of substituted hydrazines as precipitants but found accurate results with semicarbazide:

Weigh exactly 1 g of sample into a 100-ml beaker and add 13·6 ml of 0·5N sodium hydroxide from a burette; warm on a water-bath and shake to effect solution. Add a filtered solution of 2·4 g of semicarbazide hydrochloride and 3·0 g of anhydrous sodium acetate dissolved in 30 ml of water. Heat the mixture by immersing it in a water-bath for ten minutes and then allow to cool for four hours. Meanwhile dry a filter paper in an oven at 100° for one hour and weigh. Filter the precipitate on to the weighed filter and wash with cold water until the filtrate gives no precipitate with silver nitrate solution, the total volume of filtrates not exceeding 200 ml. Place the filter and funnel containing it in an oven at 100° and, after one hour, transfer the paper to a porcelain basin and dry to constant weight. Weight of semicarbazone × 0·7273 = vanillin.

If an impurity such as **piperonal** is present, the vanillin is separated by dissolving the semicarbazone in ammonium hydroxide solution, since the phenolic group produces a soluble ammonium salt; piperonal semicarbazone is insoluble. After weighing the precipitate, obtained as above, it is removed from the paper into a beaker and warmed to about 50° with a mixture of 40 ml of strong ammonia solution and 60 ml of water. After cooling it is filtered and washed free from the yellow solution of vanillin compound, dried and weighed, and the weight found subtracted from that previously obtained, the remainder being calculated to vanillin.

Rubin and Bloom[4] found the determination of vanillin as 2,4-dinitrophenylhydrazone satisfactory, even in the presence of coumarin or 10 per cent of alcohol, with the following technique.

To a solution of 0·06 g of vanillin in 20 per cent ethanol, diluted with water to about 90 ml, add, slowly and with constant stirring, 40 ml of reagent (prepared by triturating 0·4 g of 2,4-dinitrophenylhydrazine with 21 ml of concentrated hydrochloric acid, diluting with water to 100 ml and filtering before use). Allow to stand for thirty minutes at room temperature, filter through a weighed Gooch crucible, wash the precipitate with 40 ml of 2N hydrochloric acid, then with 10 ml of water, and dry at 105°. 1 g precipitate = 0·4579 g vanillin.

A determination of vanillin in vanilla extracts is by Folin and Denis' colorimetric method[5] on which the details given below are based. The method is applicable in the presence of coumarin, which has often been used as an adulterant.

Pipette, respectively, into five 500-ml graduated flasks, 2·5, 5·0, 7·5, 12·5 and 20·0 ml of a standard vanillin solution (1 mg per ml) prepared by dissolving 0·100 g of vanillin in 3 ml of ethanol and diluting to 100 ml with water in a graduated flask. Into a sixth 500-ml graduated flask pipette 2 ml of the extract. (If the concentration of vanillin is more than 1·0 per cent dilute 50 ml to 100 ml with water and use the dilution.) Dilute the contents of each flask to about 80 ml with water and at the same time transfer 80 ml of water to a seventh 500-ml graduated flask for the blank. Treat the contents of each flask, respectively, as follows. Add, from a graduated pipette, 2·0 ml of a solution of lead acetate (prepared by dissolving 50 g each of neutral and basic lead acetate in hot water, diluting to 1 litre, cooling and filtering) and dilute to volume with water. Mix and filter through a dry, 18·5-cm fluted filter paper (Whatman No. 12 is suitable), discarding any cloudy filtrate. Pipette 10 ml of the clear filtrate into a 100-ml graduated flask, add 5 ml of Folin and Denis reagent (see p. 474) and allow to stand for exactly five minutes after mixing. Then add 10 ml of a solution of 40 g of anhydrous sodium carbonate in 160 ml of water, mix and allow to stand for exactly ten minutes. Dilute to volume with water, mix and filter through a dry, fluted filter paper (Whatman No. 12 is suitable), discarding any cloudy filtrate.

Immediately measure the extinctions of the sample and standard solutions at 610 mμ, against the blank solution. Plot the extinctions against the concentration for the standards (the curve may not obey Beer's law) and read the concentration of vanillin in the sample from the curve.

Coumarin (applicable to vanilla, vanilla containing added vanillin and/or coumarin, and imitation vanilla).

Diazonium reagent: Dissolve 0·7 g of *p*-nitroaniline in 9 ml of concentrated hydrochloric acid and dilute to 100 ml with water. Dissolve 5 g of sodium nitrite in sufficient water to produce 100 ml. Cool both solutions and a 100-ml graduated flask to about 3° and pipette 5 ml of each solution into the flask. Mix and allow to stand for five minutes at about 3°. Add a further 10 ml of the sodium nitrite solution, allow to stand for five minutes at about 3° and dilute to volume with ice-cold water. Allow to stand for fifteen minutes and discard after twenty-four hours.

Determination: Pipette, respectively, into five 200-ml graduated flasks 1·0, 2·0, 3·0, 4·0 and 5·0 ml of standard coumarin solution (2 mg per ml), prepared by dissolving 0·200 g of coumarin in 3 ml of ethanol and diluting to 100 ml with water in a graduated flask. Into a sixth 200-ml graduated flask pipette 5 ml of the sample and dilute the contents of each flask to about 80 ml with water. To each flask add 5 ml of lead acetate solution, prepared as described in the method for vanillin, above, and at the same time add 5 ml of the lead acetate solution to 80 ml of water in a seventh 200-ml graduated flask for the blank. Treat the contents of each flask, respectively, as follows. Dilute to volume with water, mix and filter through an 18·5-cm fluted filter paper (Whatman No. 12 is suitable), discarding any cloudy filtrate. Add 0·2 g of anhydrous sodium oxalate to the clear filtrate, swirl to dissolve and again filter through an 18·5-cm fluted filter paper, discarding any cloudy filtrate. Pipette 5 ml of the clear filtrate into a 100-ml graduated flask, add 15 ml of water and 10 ml of 1 per cent sodium carbonate solution and heat in a water-bath for five minutes. Allow to cool gradually to room temperature, then add 10 ml of the diazonium reagent, dilute to volume with water and mix. Allow to stand for one and a half hours and filter through an 18·5-cm fluted filter paper.

Measure the extinctions of the sample and standard solutions at 490 mμ, against the blank solution. Plot the extinctions against the concentration for the standards and read the concentration of coumarin in the sample from the standard curve.

Since several related compounds give the same colour reactions as vanillin and coumarin the above methods are not specific and a method has been developed[6] in which coumarin, vanillin and ethyl vanillin are separated from each other by partition chromatography and subsequently determined spectrophotometrically.

1. SCHIMMEL & CO., *Annual Reports*, 1929, p. 123.
2. SHARP, L. K., *Analyst*, 1951, **76**, 215.
3. PHILLIPS, S. B., *Analyst*, 1923, **48**, 367.
4. RUBIN, N., and BLOOM, A., *Amer. J. Pharm.*, 1936, **108**, 387.
5. FOLIN, O., and DENIS, W., *J. Ind. Eng. Chem.*, 1912, **4**, 670.
6. ENSMINGER, L. G., *J.A.O.A.C.*, 1955, **38**, 730; 1956, **39**, 715.

VITAMIN A

$C_{20}H_{29}OH$ Mol. Wt. 286·5

Several methods now exist for the quantitative estimation of vitamin A alcohol and acetate in solutions which are comparatively free from interfering substances. These include the Carr-Price (antimony trichloride colorimetric) method, the ultra-violet spectrophotometric absorption method, the dichlorhydrin and the Budowski Bondi anhydro methods. When these methods are applied to simple extracts of natural products and complex mixtures analytical accuracy is affected by contaminants carried through from the parent material. In the ultra-violet spectrophotometric method an attempt is made to correct for irrelevant absorption by a geometric (Morton and Stubbs[1]) technique. The alumina chromatographic technique[2] aims at removing as much contaminant as possible but loss and degradation of vitamin A may occur during attempts at purification. When vitamin A solution is exposed to even small amounts of actinic light, isomerisation first occurs, resulting in increased absorption, followed by rupture of the molecule giving non-linear absorption at a reduced level. The analytical purification process may thus be accompanied by chemical breakdown and distortion of the spectral curve.

ULTRA-VIOLET SPECTROPHOTOMETRIC ASSAY AND GEOMETRIC CORRECTION

The spectral curve of vitamin A alcohol and acetate in various solvents has a maximum at 325–328 mμ, with the steeper slope at wavelengths greater than 325 mμ and a pronounced shoulder at about 312 mμ. If extraneous material in vitamin A solution absorbs linearly within the wavelength region of this curve a simple geometrical correction can be applied. This correction holds if the irrelevant absorption is constant or increases and decreases uniformly. However, gross errors are introduced if the formula is used in cases of non-linear irrelevant absorption. The formula usually ascribed to Morton and Stubbs takes the form—

$$E_{Corr.} = \frac{1}{1-f}[E_{\lambda_{max.}} - K\,E_{\lambda_1} - (1-K)\,E_{\lambda_2}]$$

In order to take advantage of the shoulder at 312 mμ and also to limit the mathematical uncertainty of an equation of this type Morton and Stubbs chose points on the curve such that

$$\frac{E_{\lambda_1}}{E_{\lambda_{max.}}} = \frac{E_{\lambda_2}}{E_{\lambda_{max.}}} = f = 6/7$$

and

$$K = \frac{\lambda_2 - \lambda_{max.}}{\lambda_2 - \lambda_1}$$

Under these conditions, using light petroleum as solvent, the above formula reduces approximately to—

$$E_{Corr._1} = 7(E_{325} - 0{\cdot}39E_{310} - 0{\cdot}61E_{334.5})$$

The precise formula will vary slightly with the instrument and the accuracy of wavelength calibration; it is also different for each solvent.

The wavelength scale of the ultra-violet spectrophotometer should be calibrated by reference to the hydrogen lines at 486·1 mμ and 656·3 mμ. Where instrument design permits easy replacement of a mercury lamp for the hydrogen lamp the calibration should also be checked at 253·6 mμ, 365·5 mμ and 546·1 mμ.

It is not certain that vitamin A alcohol and acetate can be purchased in the pure all-trans form and slight variations may be found between supplies. It is therefore advantageous to derive a single formula to satisfy local conditions. In using the above formula the difference figures are multiplied by 7 and therefore absorption at each wavelength must be read accurately to the third place of decimals.

The formula presupposes linear irrelevant absorption between 310 and 335 mμ. The truth of this assumption can be checked by choosing points on the curve such that $E_{\lambda_1}/E_{\lambda max.}$ is a value greater than 6/7. In selecting a second ratio it should be borne in mind that the denominator of the ratio is the multiplicand of the geometric equation. Thus, if the ratio is chosen as 13/14 (at median points with respect to those of the 6/7 ratio) the error is now multiplied by 14. The irrelevant absorption is normally greatest between 310 and 325 mμ. The greatest deviation between non-linearity of irrelevant absorption commensurate with mathematical inaccuracy would be exposed by using a $E_{\lambda_1}/E_{\lambda max.}$ ratio of 9/10 when—

$$E_{Corr._2} = 10(E_{325} - 0{\cdot}41E_{315} - 0{\cdot}59E_{332})$$

The two corrected values for absorption should agree to ± 3 per cent and certainly should not lie outside ± 5 per cent.

Many of the impurities present in naturally occurring foods are not removed during the analytical process and absorb in the region 310 to 335 mμ. This irrelevant absorption is generally more linear in the case of fish oils than with synthetic vitamin A additions to starch-protein-mineral based materials. In the latter case the irrelevant absorption is greatest on the shorter wavelength side of the maximum. If the base material containing no vitamin A is available, this should be run through the selected analytical process as a blank. In the case of minerals, and particularly when the chromatographic step is omitted, the blank consists of a small non-linear irrelevant absorption, the amount varying slightly according to conditions of saponification. The observed absorption of the vitamin A solution should be corrected for the blank at each wavelength before the geometric correction is applied.

Choice and use of solvents: If solutions of vitamin A alcohol are exposed to even diffuse sunlight, distortion of the spectral curve occurs. At first the absorption at peak wavelength increases and than falls rapidly; at the same time the ratios on either side of the peak increase rapidly, with the greater increase at lower wavelengths. Exposure to light therefore increases the magnitude of the geometrical correction and the analytical process itself creates the need for correction against irrelevant absorption.

Table 36 shows the extinction of pure vitamin A alcohol and acetate in various solvents.

The selection of solvent is frequently a matter of individual choice but may be dictated by the following considerations.

TABLE 36

	VITAMIN A ACETATE			VITAMIN A ALCOHOL		
	max. mμ	$E^{1\%}_{1cm}$	Factor†	max. mμ	$E^{1\%}_{1cm}$	Factor†
Light petroleum (b.p. 40° to 60°)	325	1600	1830	325	1820	1830
*cyclo*Hexane	327·5	1530	1900	326·5	1755	1900
*iso*Propyl alcohol	325	1600	1830	325	1820	1830

† To convert $E^{1\%}_{1cm}$ to units per g (see later).

Transfer from one solvent to another should be avoided because exposure of vitamin A in a thin film on walls of flasks renders it susceptible to actinic breakdown.

*cyclo*Hexane has been preferred because the spectral differences in the 310 to 335 mμ region between *neo-* and *all-trans* vitamin A are less pronounced in this solvent than in *iso*propyl alcohol and light petroleum.

Light petroleum is volatile and losses of solvent occur by evaporation during measurements of optical density in spectrophotometric cells. This loss can be reduced if stoppered cells are used. Soapy emulsions are more easily broken down with light petroleum than with ether. No change of solvent is required if light petroleum can be used throughout the analytical process.

Processing losses: The Brunius vitamin A Commission[3] reported losses of 2·4 per cent during saponification due to isomerisation and 1·5 per cent during column chromatography. During normal analysis it is not unreasonable to expect total losses as high as 5 per cent. In certain methods losses or distortion (and consequent corrective loss) occur when solutions are dried by repeated evaporation even though this operation is carried out in an atmosphere of nitrogen. These losses are particularly pronounced if the vitamin has been extracted from mineral base. It is, therefore, apparent that a correction factor must be evaluated for given laboratory conditions.

Vitamin A may be estimated using ultra-violet spectrophotometric techniques after simple extraction with solvent, saponification followed by extraction, or saponification and extraction followed by chromatography. The resulting extinction may need correction by the geometric technique.

It may be that a greater processing error is incurred by taking the extra purification step than if the analysis were simplified. The need for refinement in technique must be assessed independently for each type of material and under typical laboratory conditions.

No geometric correction holds for the Carr-Price colorimetric assay of vitamin A. The reagent does however react with degraded vitamin A and therefore the saponification and chromatographic purification steps may form part of the analytical process.

Methods of analysis: Various methods of analysis are detailed below. Many follow the pattern of saponification followed by chromatography with different means of assaying the purified vitamin present in the final solution. The alumina-column method is given in full because it is incorporated in a statutory order for foodstuffs, is recommended by the Brunius Committee, the *A.O.A.C.*[4] and also the Analytical Methods Committee of the *S.A.C.*[5] Some form of chromatography is recommended under given conditions by the *B.P.* These methods differ only in the criterion dictating acceptance of the purity of the spectral curve:

(*a*) The statutory order mentioned above accepts ratios in light petroleum of

$$\frac{E_{(\lambda-15)}}{E_{\lambda}} \quad \text{and} \quad \frac{E_{(\lambda+10)}}{E_{\lambda}} \quad \text{not greater than } 0{\cdot}88$$

where E_{λ} = wavelength of maximum absorption

(*b*) The *S.A.C.* method accepts similar ratios not greater than 0·90.

(*c*) The Brunius Committee applies a geometric correction after chromatography.

(*d*) The *B.P.* prescribes in detail when chromatography shall be carried out dependent on the wavelength of maximum absorption and also ratios on either side of the peak. In addition conditions are given under which saponification, chromatography and/or geometric correction may be omitted.

Concentrated vitamin preparations are available commercially in which the vitamin A is protected from oxidation with a protective coating of wax or protein, such as gelatin. These products need special treatment to liberate the vitamin A before extraction.

EXTRACTION AND PURIFICATION OF VITAMIN A FOR INSTRUMENTAL ESTIMATION

A. Simple Extraction

Applicable to concentrates of vitamin A in simple admixture or solution. Potency levels greater than 100 units per g and ester or alcohol form known to be present.

(*a*) For high potency or synthetic vitamin A: Dissolve and dilute the sample in *cyclo*hexane to give a concentration of 10 units per ml.

(*b*) For wax protected vitamin A: Transfer the sample, accurately weighed, to a dry stoppered cylinder, add a measured quantity of ether and shake for up to two hours. Allow to settle and pipette an aliquot of the supernatant liquid into a flask. Remove the solvent in a stream of nitrogen and dissolve the residue in *cyclo*hexane to give a concentration of about 10 units per ml.

(*c*) For gelatin protected vitamin A: Transfer the sample, accurately weighed, to a mortar. Grind thoroughly with 3 to 5 ml of water and decant into a 100-ml cylinder. Grind and decant in turn with 15 ml of ethanol, 25 ml of ether, 45 ml of light petroleum and 10 ml of water. Shake well and allow to separate. Note the volume of the light petroleum layer. Pipette an aliquot into a flask. Remove the solvent in a stream of nitrogen and dissolve the residue in *cyclo*hexane to give a concentration of about 10 units per ml.

(*d*) For vitamin A in liquid or pellet formulations: Weigh the sample accurately into a 200-ml stoppered cylinder. Add 1 ml of water and thoroughly disperse the sample. Add 20 ml of ethanol followed by 75 ml of *cyclo*hexane. Replace the air in the cylinder with nitrogen and shake for up to twenty minutes. Add 20 ml of water and again replace the air with nitrogen and shake for a further ten minutes. Allow to settle and note the volume of the *cyclo*hexane layer. Filter a portion of the *cyclo*hexane layer to remove turbidity and dilute if necessary to produce a final vitamin A concentration of about 10 units per ml.

(*e*) For vitamin A concentrate in liquid formulations: Transfer the sample, accurately weighed, to a beaker or small mortar containing 2 to 3 g of anhydrous sodium sulphate. Grind the mixture until it is homogeneous. Add 10 ml of 20 per cent acetone in light petroleum and slurry for ten minutes. Decant the solution into a flask and repeat the extraction with a further four 10-ml quantities of the solvent. Remove the solvent under a stream of nitrogen. Dissolve the residue in *cyclo*hexane to give a final vitamin A concentration of about 10 units per ml.

If the vitamin A is present in ester form in *cyclo*hexane the following limitation must be accepted.

If the wavelength of maximum absorption lies between 326·5 and 328·5 mμ and the observed relative extinctions are within 0·02 of those in Table 37 the potency of the sample in units per g is calculated from the expression:

$$E(1 \text{ per cent, } 1 \text{ cm})\ 327{\cdot}5\ \text{m}\mu \times 1{,}900$$

If the wavelength of maximum absorption lies between 326 and 329 mμ but the relative extinctions are not within 0·02 of those in Table 37 calculate a corrected extinction at 327·5 mμ by applying the observed values to the equation:

$$E_{327\cdot5}\ (\text{Corr.}) = 7(E_{327\cdot5} - 0{\cdot}405\ E_{312\cdot5} - 0{\cdot}595\ E_{337\cdot5})$$

When the extinction ratio $E_{327\cdot5}$ (Corr.)/$E_{327\cdot5}$ lies between 0·85 and 1·00 the potency of the sample in units per g is calculated from the expression:

$$E(1 \text{ per cent, } 1 \text{ cm})\ 327{\cdot}5\ \text{m}\mu\ (\text{Corr.}) \times 1{,}900$$

TABLE 37

WAVELENGTH (mμ)	RELATIVE EXTINCTION
300	0·555
312·5	0·857
327·5	1·000
337·5	0·857
345	0·695
360	0·299

Note: (i) Where the corrected absorption differs from the gross absorption by more than ± 3 per cent, the applicability of the above equation can be shown by a second equation with $E_{\lambda}/E_{max.} = f = 9/10$ and corresponding values of K. The value of the two corrected absorptions should not differ by more than 3 per cent.

(ii) Absorbance ratios of vitamin A alcohol in light petroleum at $(\lambda_{max.} - 15)$ and $(\lambda_{max.} + 10)$ to $\lambda_{max.}$ should each be not greater than 0·88. (Statutory order.)

(iii) Absorbance ratios of vitamin A alcohol in light petroleum at $(\lambda_{max.} - 15)$ and $(\lambda_{max.} + 10)$ to $\lambda_{max.}$ should each be not greater than 0·90. (*S.A.C.*)

If the Morton and Stubbs' correction is in excess of +3 per cent or −15 per cent or if the absorbance ratio requirements are not met proceed as below.

Certain heavily waxed or gelatin protected synthetic vitamin A must be saponified before extraction and measurement.

B. Saponification and Extraction

Applicable to certain wax or gelatin protected synthetic vitamin A mixtures (*e.g.* vitaminised feed-stuffs); oil-based natural vitamin A materials.

Single-stage saponification: Weigh a quantity of sample equivalent to not less than 100 units and preferably about 2,000 units into a 250-ml flat-bottomed amber-coloured flask. Add 50 ml of dehydrated ethanol, 0·2 g of quinol and 15 ml of freshly prepared 50 per cent aqueous potash (prepared by dissolving 160 g of potassium hydroxide in 100 ml of water). Boil under reflux on a water-bath for thirty minutes with occasional swirling. Remove from the water-bath and cool prior to transferring to a separator.

Double-stage saponification: Simple saponification is sometimes not entirely successful in freeing vitamin A from heavily waxed or gelatinised protective coatings particularly where formaldehyde has been used to 'harden' the protection. In these cases saponification is first carried out for twenty minutes, the bulk of the soluble material removed and the residue re-saponified for one hour. The soluble fractions are pooled and processed as below. This system avoids degradation of the bulk of vitamin A caused by prolonged heating.

In the absence of solid material transfer the contents of the saponification flask to a separator (250 or 500 ml) with 10 ml of ethanol and 60 ml of water. Rinse the flask with 50 ml of light petroleum followed by three 25-ml quantities and add the washings to the contents of the separator, shake and allow the phases to separate.

Use only gentle shaking to avoid the formation of emulsions.

In the presence of solid material use three 500-ml separators for the extraction (A), (B), (C). Filter the contents of the saponification flask through a Büchner funnel (7 cm), using a No. 54 Whatman filter paper, into separator (B). Use an adaptor fitted with a side arm to permit the application of gentle suction to draw the solution through the filter paper. Allow the solution to filter at first without suction and then apply gentle suction until most of the solution has passed through the paper. Wash the flask and insoluble material with two portions, each of 5 ml, of 50 per cent ethanol. Wash the flask and insoluble material with 50 ml of light petroleum. Wash further with three 25-ml quantities of light petroleum. Remove the Büchner funnel. Add 50 ml of water and shake the contents of the separator.

Allow the phases to separate completely (about five minutes) and run off the lower aqueous/ethanolic layer into separator (C). Swirl the light petroleum solution in (B), allow to settle for about thirty seconds and run off any further aqueous/ethanolic solution into (C). Introduce a few millilitres of water into (A) to act as a seal and transfer the light petroleum solution from (B) to (A) through the neck of (B). Rinse the neck of (B) inside and outside with a little light petroleum. Rinse (B) thoroughly with three portions of light petroleum and transfer each portion in turn to (C) via the top of (B). Close the top and return (B) to its stand. Insert the stopper into (C), shake vigorously and allow the phases to separate for five minutes. Transfer the lower layer to (B) and the upper to (A) in the manner described above and repeat the operations until four extractions have been completed and all the light petroleum extracts are combined in (A).

Wash the light petroleum extract in (A) as follows. By means of a wash-bottle (preferably plastic) direct a jet of water at 35° to 40° into (A) so that at first the water flows down the inside of the separator and then through the light petroleum. Swirl the separator gently and allow it to stand until the phases have separated. Run off the aqueous layer, swirl the contents of the separator and run off any further water. Repeat the washing twice more with water at 30° to 35° and swirl more vigorously or shake gently. Test the last wash with phenolphthalein and, if alkaline, give further washes. If emulsions occur at any stage, add 2 to 3 ml of ethanol.

Filter the solution through a cotton-wool plug into a suitable flask, If the concentration of vitamin A is sufficiently high, make up to a suitable volume in a graduated flask to give a final concentration of about 10 units per ml. For lower concentrations of vitamin A, evaporate the extract to about 5 ml in a stream of nitrogen and remove the last 5 ml without the application of heat. Dissolve the residue in *iso*propyl alcohol to give a final vitamin A concentration of about 10 units per ml.

Applicable to solutions in light petroleum and *iso*propyl alcohol:

If the wavelength of maximum absorption lies between 323 and 327 mμ and the absorption at 300 mμ relative to that at 325 mμ does not exceed 0·73, a corrected absorbance is derived from the equation:

$$E_{325}(\text{Corr.}) = 6{\cdot}815\ (E_{325} - 0{\cdot}375\ E_{310} - 0{\cdot}625\ E_{334})$$

The potency of the sample in units per g is calculated from the expression:

$$E(1 \text{ per cent, } 1 \text{ cm})\ 325\ m\mu \times 1{,}830$$

except that when the corrected absorption lies within ±3 per cent of the uncorrected absorption, the corrected absorption is ignored and the potency estimated from the uncorrected absorption.

Note: (i) See A, Notes (i), (ii) and (iii), above.

(ii) If the wavelength of maximum absorption lies outside the range 323 to 327 mμ, if the Morton and Stubbs' correction exceeds +3 to −15 per cent, if the absorbance ratio requirements are not met, or if the relative absorption at 300 mμ to that at the wavelength of maximum absorption exceeds 0·73, the unsaponifiable fraction of the sample must be chromatographed.

C. **Chromatographic Purification**

Simple chromatographic purification on alumina.

Apparatus: A glass chromatographic tube, 6 to 7 mm internal diameter and fitted with a stopcock. To facilitate the application of pressure (nitrogen) the column is fitted with a B24 joint.

Preparation of alumina: De-activate alumina (aluminium oxide for chromatographic absorption analysis) by adding 3·0 per cent of water. Mix well until no lumps are observed. Allow to stand in a stoppered bottle for at least forty-eight hours before use.

Preparation of chromatographic column: Pour sufficient alumina to produce a 4-cm length column into a chromatographic tube containing light petroleum (b.p. 40° to 60°) and a glass-wool plug. The column should run, under slight nitrogen pressure, at a rate of about 2 ml per minute. Allow the level of light petroleum to fall to within 1 cm of the top of the alumina (the column must not be allowed to dry) and the column is ready for use.

Take a large aliquot of the light petroleum solution obtained at the extraction stage and dry over anhydrous sodium sulphate. Centrifuge and pipette an aliquot equivalent to 100 to 200 units of vitamin A on to the column previously prepared. Wash the column with 5 ml of light petroleum, five 10-ml portions of 2 per cent acetone (analytical-reagent grade dried over anhydrous sodium sulphate) in light petroleum and elute the vitamin A with five portions each of 10 ml of 10 per cent acetone in light petroleum.

Evaporate the solvents in a stream of nitrogen, removing the last 5 ml without the application of heat to avoid degradation of the vitamin A. Dissolve the residue in a suitable solvent to give a final concentration of about 10 units per ml.

Double chromatographic purification on alumina. This procedure is normally applied to low-potency materials of less than 100 units per g.

Preparation of alumina: Prepare the alumina for the chromatography from aluminium trihydrate.*

Type 1: Activate the fraction which passes through a B.S.S. 150 mesh by heating at 800° for seven hours. Cool, add 2 g of water for each 98 g activated alumina, mix well and store in a stoppered bottle.

Type 2: Alkaline alumina. Weigh 20 g of Type 1 into a 100-ml round-bottomed flask fitted with a B19 neck, add 20 ml of 10 per cent sodium hydroxide solution, and attach an adaptor through which passes a glass tube drawn to a coarse capillary, extending to about one-quarter

* Suitable quality can be obtained from the British Aluminium Company, Norfolk House, St. James's Square, London, S.W.1.

of an inch from the bottom of the flask. Connect the incoming tube to a cylinder of hydrogen or nitrogen and a vacuum lead to a water pump, apply suction and pass a slow stream of gas from the cylinder; leave for one hour (Fig. 12). Immerse the flask in an oil-bath and raise the temperature gradually during one hour to 135° ± 2°; maintain the flask at 135° ± 2° for a further hour. Discontinue the gas stream, remove the

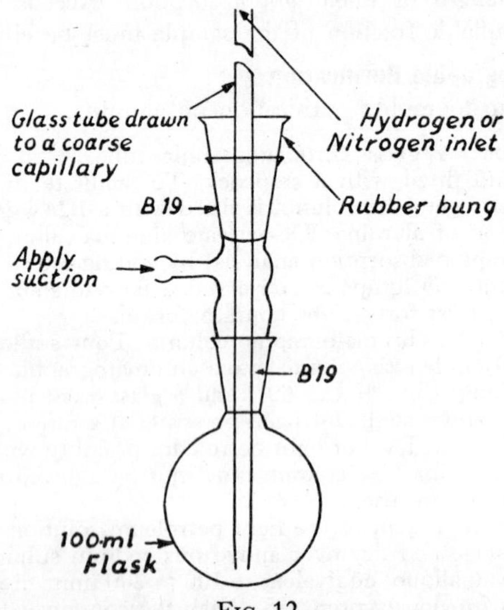

FIG. 12

Apparatus for preparation of alkaline alumina (Type 2)

flask from the oil-bath and allow to cool under vacuum (preferably overnight). Release the vacuum with hydrogen or nitrogen and determine the moisture content of the product (loss on heating at 500° for two hours).

Adjust the moisture to 12·5 per cent ± 1 per cent. Store the product in small glass tubes sealed with wax. Each tube to contain the amount of alumina (about 1 g) required for the lower column.

Note: A preliminary run should be carried out to ensure that vitamin A comes off the column at the 24 per cent solvent stage (see below).

Dry the light petroleum extract from the extraction with anhydrous sodium sulphate, transfer to a flat-bottomed flask with a little light petroleum and evaporate to dryness under the inert gas; repeat this twice and finally dissolve in 3 to 5 ml of light petroleum and chromatograph using the apparatus shown in Fig. 13.

Place a small wad of cotton wool in the lower tip of the upper column, pour in sufficient light petroleum to fill the middle of the 10-mm diameter tube and add alumina (Type 1) to fill the 5-mm diameter tube. Apply the inert gas pressure to the top of the column, and when the excess of light petroleum has been forced through the column, release the pressure and transfer the light petroleum extract to the column.

Develop under pressure first with 5 ml of light petroleum and then

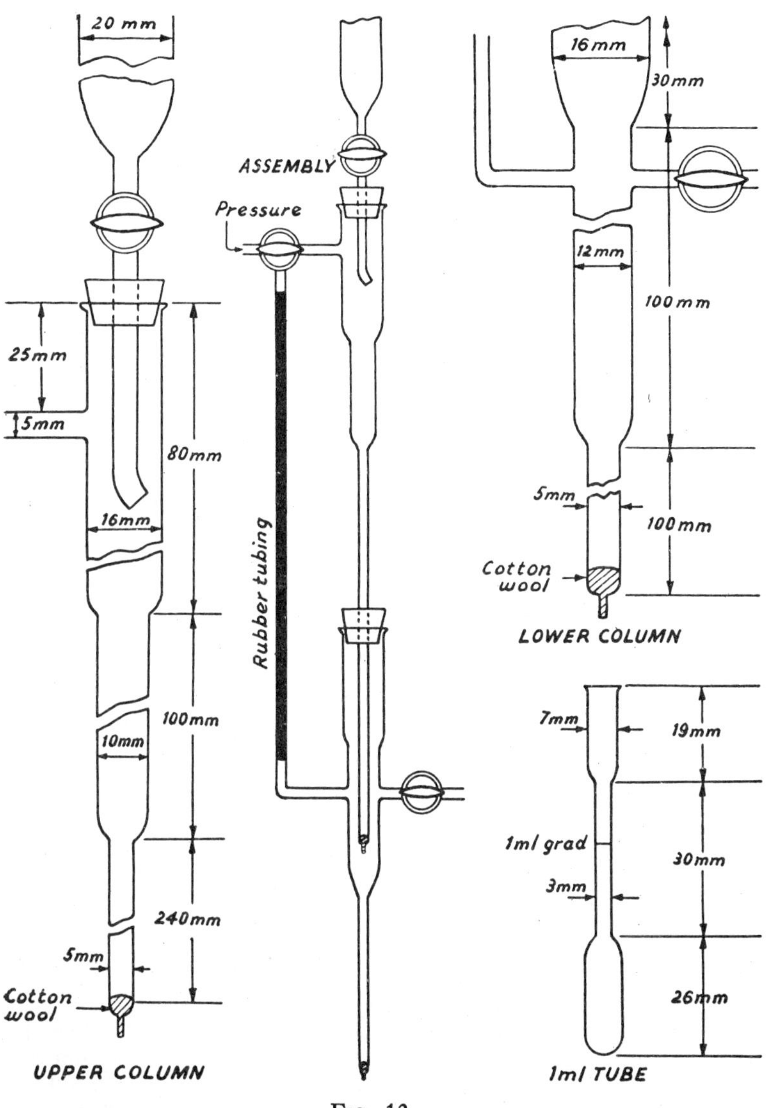

FIG. 13

with 5-ml quantities of light petroleum containing, respectively, 4, 8, 12, 16, 20, 24 and 36 per cent of anæsthetic ether (peroxide-free). Immediately prior to adding the 16 per cent ether developing solvent, attach the lower column containing about 1 g of alkaline alumina, type 2, to the bottom of the upper column. Then continue developing with 20,

24 and 36 per cent ether solvents until all the vitamin A has been eluted. Collect the eluate—starting when the lower column is in position—in calibrated 1-ml tubes and mix the solution in each tube by blowing through the liquid a few air bubbles with a 0·5-ml pipette with the tip drawn to a capillary. Withdraw from each tube approximately 0·3 ml of solution and test for vitamin A with antimony trichloride solution (see below).

Pipette 0·5-ml aliquots from the fractions that give a positive test with the antimony trichloride reagent and make up to a suitable volume in a graduated flask with light petroleum.

Note: If the spectral purity requirements listed previously are not met with, the whole determination must be repeated.

INSTRUMENTAL DETERMINATION OF VITAMIN A AFTER EXTRACTION

A. Ultra-violet Spectrophotometric Determination

Take a suitable aliquot from the extraction process and adjust the volume to contain 8 to 10 units per ml in light petroleum or *iso*propyl alcohol. Measure the extinction of the solutions at about 300, 310, 325, 335 mμ with the solvent in the reference cell. The exact wavelengths are determined by the applicability requirements and local conditions previously described.

Calculate the corrected extinction at the maxima and the potency of the sample from the expression:

$$E(1 \text{ per cent, } 1 \text{ cm}) \text{ max. corrected} \times \text{FACTOR}$$

B. Colorimetric Determination with Antimony Trichloride Reagent

The blue colour produced by the reaction of vitamin A and antimony trichloride fades rapidly. Mixing and measurement must take place within ten seconds. The satisfactory use of null-point instruments is precluded by the time required to make adjustments.

Antimony trichloride reagent: Wash *B.P.* chloroform two or three times with its own volume of water and dry over anhydrous potassium carbonate. Pour off and distil, rejecting the first 10 per cent of the distillate. To 200 g of antimony trichloride, add sufficient chloroform to make 1 litre. Warm and shake to dissolve. Cool and add 30 ml of acetic anhydride. If the solution is not clear, allow the residue to settle and decant off. Store in brown stoppered bottles.

Method: Evaporate an aliquot of the solution from the extraction process (equivalent to about 40 μg of vitamin A) under vacuum on a water-bath at 60°. Dissolve the residue in 1 ml of alcohol-free chloroform.

Place 0·5 ml of alcohol-free chloroform in a 1-cm path-length cell, preferably with external rectangular dimensions 3 cm × 4 cm. Arrange the cell in the instrument together with a small funnel of large stem bore, the end of which is flattened to act as a mixing device. Fit the funnel into a clamp in a manner which allows vertical motion of the stem within the cell but away from the light path. Quickly measure, by pipette, 4·5 ml of antimony trichloride reagent into a beaker and pour it rapidly into the funnel. At the same time lift the funnel up and down three or four times. Set the instrument to read 100 per cent transmission. Dry the cell and funnel and replace in the instrument. Add 0·5 ml of the vitamin A solution, followed by 4·5 ml of reagent, and record the maximum deflection.

Repeat with aliquots of vitamin A in chloroform of known potency and prepare a calibration graph.

C. Determination of Absorbance after Sulphuric Acid Treatment

The destruction of the vitamin A alcohol with sulphuric acid has been applied by Tardif[6] to the determination of the potency of cod-liver oil samples. The procedure involves the extraction of the non-saponifiable fraction of the oil into purified hexane and the measurement of the absorption at 325 mμ before and after destruction of the vitamin A with 60 per cent sulphuric acid. The author claims the results by this method are more accurate than those given by the three-point correction procedure, with standard deviations of about 1/10 of those from the three-point correction procedure.

Take an aliquot from the extraction process so that the final solution contains 8 to 10 units of vitamin A per ml. Use purified *n*-hexane (acid-washed and dried) as the extracting solvent of the unsaponifiable material.

Transfer 50 ml of hexane extract to a 150-ml separator and also 50 ml of purified hexane to a second separator to act as the reagent blank. To each, add 10 ml of 60 per cent sulphuric acid and shake one hundred and fifty times. Discard the sulphuric acid and repeat with further 10-ml portions of acid until this layer is colourless; wash it acid-free with water and filter through a cotton-wool plug. Measure the extinction at 325 mμ with the similarly treated reagent blank in the comparison cell.

$$A_1 \text{ corr.} = \frac{\text{Destroyed absorbancy at 325 m}\mu}{\text{Tan } \alpha + (\tan \beta - \tan \alpha)\dfrac{(1 + \tan^2 \beta)}{(1 + \tan^2 \alpha)}}$$

$$\text{Tan } \beta = \frac{\text{Extinction of sample destroyed at 325 m}\mu}{\text{Extinction of sample at 325 m}\mu}$$

$$\text{Tan } \alpha = \frac{\text{Extinction of standard destroyed at 325 m}\mu}{\text{Extinction of standard at 325 m}\mu}$$

Potency may then be calculated from the following expression:

$$E(1 \text{ per cent, 1 cm}) \times \text{factor } (1940)$$

where $$E(1 \text{ per cent, 1 cm}) = \frac{A_1}{\text{per cent concentration}}$$

D. Determination by Conversion to Anhydro-Vitamin A

In the method of Budowski and Bondi[7] vitamin A alcohol is converted to anhydro-vitamin A in benzene solution at room temperature with toluene-*p*-sulphonic acid as a catalyst. The increase in absorption at 399 mμ which results from the dehydration is directly proportional to the amount of vitamin A present. The reaction has to be stopped by the addition of alkali.

VITAMIN A

The method is given in full because the 'anhydro' method is a good screening test for vitamin A in feeding-stuffs, although the method has not found general application.

Preparation of benzene: Add a small quantity of toluene-*p*-sulphonic acid to a quantity of benzene (analytical-reagent grade) in a 2-litre flask. Heat the liquid to boiling on a heating mantle under a reflux condenser fitted with a calcium chloride guard. Allow to stand overnight. Distil off the benzene and discard the first fraction (10 per cent) which contains any water present in the original solution. Store the benzene in clean, dry, stoppered containers.

Preparation of catalyst reagent: Take 15 g of toluene-*p*-sulphonic acid monohydrate which has been stored in an open dish over phosphorus pentoxide in a desiccator and add to 100 ml of benzene in a clean, dry flask. Heat under reflux with a calcium chloride-guarded condenser until all the solid has dissolved. Distil off about 10 ml of benzene to remove any moisture, allow to cool and re-adjust the volume to 100 ml with dry benzene.

Prepare the reagent each day as required and store in a stoppered flask over calcium chloride in a desiccator if not required for immediate testing.

Take the light petroleum solution obtained as directed in Method B above for final spectrophotometric determination and dry over anhydrous sodium sulphate (previously dried at 105° for three hours and cooled over calcium chloride). Dry any glass apparatus required for the estimation in an oven and cool in a desiccator over calcium chloride.

Evaporate the light petroleum to a volume of 50 ml and adjust the volume to 50 ml with light petroleum (or adjust the concentration to about 40 units per ml of vitamin A). Take two 100-ml conical flasks and pipette 10-ml aliquots into each flask and evaporate to dryness under vacuum at 40°. To one of the dried extracts add 5 ml of dry benzene (Solution B). To the other add 1 ml of benzene and 4 ml of the catalyst solution (Solution A). Mix by shaking and allow to stand for one minute. Add 1 g of anhydrous sodium carbonate, shake and allow to stand for at least one minute. Pour off the supernatant layer into two separate centrifuge tubes. Spin to obtain a clear solution.

Measure the extinction at 399 mμ of the solution (A) using the solution (B) in the reference cell.

The potency of the vitamin A is given by the expression:

$$\text{Units per aliquot} = \frac{\text{E(difference)}}{0{\cdot}0122}$$

Note: The absorption of 0·0122 is the increase corresponding to 1 unit of vitamin A (*U.S.P.* standard) being put through the method described.

The following vitamin A-containing materials are prepared for determination by one of the above methods as detailed:

Cod-liver Oil

Weigh 1 g of oil into a saponification flask and proceed as described in method B above, dissolving the final residue in 100 ml of *cyclo*hexane.

Emulsion of Cod-liver Oil, *B.P.C.* (a minimum of 285 units per g). Extract 2 g as described under Malt Extract with Cod-liver Oil and dissolve the final residue in 100 ml of *cyclo*hexane for spectrophotometric assay.

Extract of Malt with Cod-liver Oil, *B.P.* (a minimum of 60 units per g).

For assay the oil is extracted by a modified Rose-Gottlieb method (see p. 401) followed by hydrolysis as follows:

> Transfer about 2 g to a separator with the aid of 25 ml of warm water, add 10 ml of 95 per cent ethanol, 10 ml 0·5N ethanolic potassium hydroxide and 25 ml anæsthetic ether. Shake vigorously, add 15 ml of light petroleum (b.p. 40° to 60°), shake and allow to separate. Extract the aqueous layer with two further quantities, each of 25 ml of anæsthetic ether and 15 ml of light petroleum (b.p. 40° to 60°). Wash the combined extracts with three 10-ml quantities of water and filter. Evaporate the filtrate to dryness under oxygen-free nitrogen and boil the residue with 15 ml 95 per cent ethanol and 1·5 ml 50 per cent w/w potassium hydroxide under a reflux condenser in a stream of oxygen-free nitrogen for fifteen minutes. Cool rapidly, add 20 ml of water and continue as under method B above (single saponification). Dissolve the final residue in 20 ml of *cyclo*hexane or *iso*propyl alcohol for spectrophotometric assay. Apply the appropriate factor for the solvent used.

Halibut-liver Oil

Weigh out 0·5 g of oil, dissolve in *cyclo*hexane and make up to 100 ml. Dilute 5 ml to 100 ml in *cyclo*hexane and determine the vitamin A as described in method A above.

Capsules of Halibut-liver Oil, *B.P.* (4,500 units per capsule).

Express as much oil as possible from ten capsules. Weigh out 0·5 g and determine the vitamin A as described under Halibut-liver Oil above.

Extract of Malt with Halibut-liver Oil, *B.P.C.* (a minimum of 60 units per g).

Extract 2 g as described above under Extract of Malt with Cod-liver Oil.

Capsules of Vitamins, *B.P.C.* (2,500 units per capsule).

Express as much as possible of the contents of ten capsules. Weigh out 0·25 g into a saponification flask and proceed as described in method B above, dissolving the final residue in 50 ml of *cyclo*hexane and diluting a further 10 ml to 100 ml in *cyclo*hexane.

Capsules of Vitamins A and D, *B.P.C.* (4,500 units per capsule).

Express as much oil as possible from ten capsules. Weigh out 0·5 g, dissolve in *cyclo*hexane and make up to 100 ml. Dilute 5 ml to 100 ml in *cyclo*hexane. Determine the vitamin A as described in method A above.

1. Morton, R. A., and Stubbs, A. L., *Analyst*, 1946, **71**, 348.
2. Food Standards (Margarine) Order S.I. 1954, No. 613.
3. Brunius, E., *J.A.O.A.C.*, 1959, **42**, 657.
4. *A.O.A.C.*, 1960, p. 649.
5. *Analyst*, 1963, **88**, in the press.
6. Tardif, R., *J. Amer. Pharm. Ass., Sci. Edn.*, 1960, **49**, 741.
7. Budowski, P., and Bondi, A., *Analyst*, 1957, **82**, 751.

VITAMIN B_6

Naturally-occurring vitamin B_6 consists of a mixture of pyridoxine, pyridoxal and pyridoxamine in varying proportions according to the source. This makes accurate assessment difficult, since various biological and microbiological methods show different responses to the three forms and physical and chemical methods do not differentiate. The latter are only satisfactory for almost pure pyridoxine and its preparations.

In the ultra-violet the three forms of vitamin B_6 show no common light absorption maxima, but close estimates of the total may be made from readings at 325 mμ taken on solutions buffered to pH 6·75, provided there is no irrelevant light-absorbing material. This wavelength is one of maximum absorption for both pyridoxine and pyridoxamine, while the curve for pyridoxal (which shows maximum absorption at 316 mμ) almost coincides with the two maxima at 325 mμ. The E(1 per cent, 1 cm) value for all three forms at this wavelength, expressed in terms of the free bases, is about 440.[1] The absorption curve of pyridoxine itself changes markedly with change in pH; in 0·1N hydrochloric acid there is a single absorption maximum at 291 mμ, but in neutral and alkaline solutions there are two peaks:

TABLE 38

SOLVENT	WAVELENGTH OF MAX. ABSORPTION (mμ)	E(1 PER CENT, 1 CM)
0·1N hydrochloric acid	291	430
Phosphate buffer, pH 7	254	180
	324	350
0·1N sodium hydroxide	244	326
	309	338

The blue colour produced when a phenol is coupled with 2,6-dichloro-*p*-benzoquinone-4-chloroimine is the basis of a method for pyridoxine first suggested by Scudi.[2] A subsequent version of this method[3] has been found to be fairly satisfactory for the determination of pyridoxine hydrochloride in pharmaceutical preparations. However, when the preparation contains less than 0·1 mg per unit of product, a level that falls within the lower sensitivity of the method, decomposition occurs before maximum colour development is obtained. Sweeney and Hall[4] modified the method so as to give greater sensitivity and stability and their method, applicable to capsules or to tablets, is given below. The boric acid which is added to the blank tube (as originally suggested by Scudi, Bastedo and Webb[5]) increases the specificity of the method since one molecule of it reacts with two of pyridoxine to give a compound that no longer reacts with the chloroimine. Other phenolic substances likely to be present, and in particular pyridoxamine and pyridoxal, are not inactivated in this way since the reaction with boric acid is due to the $-CH_2OH$ group of pyridoxine being adjacent to the phenolic $-OH$. Ascorbic acid, if present, interferes with the reaction of pyridoxine with 2,6-dichloro-*p*-benzoquinone-4-chloroimine and this is overcome by oxidation, shaking the alkaline extract with manganese dioxide.

Weigh an amount of sample equivalent to between 100 and 500 μg of pyridoxine into a 25-ml graduated cylinder and add 15 ml of 0·5N sodium hydroxide. Heat in a water-bath for a few minutes, break up the material with a glass rod and continue to heat, with occasional stirring, for fifteen minutes. Cool, dilute to 20 ml with water, add 200 mg of manganese dioxide and shake for five minutes. Pipette a volume of the suspension containing between 10 and 50 μg of pyridoxine into a centrifuge tube containing sufficient *iso*propyl alcohol to make a total volume of 25 ml, centrifuge, filter and pipette 5 ml of the filtrate into each of three test-tubes. To each tube add 1 ml of ammonia buffer solution (prepared by mixing 40 g of ammonium chloride with 40 ml of strong ammonia solution and diluting to 170 ml with water) followed by 1 ml of a 20 per cent solution of sodium acetate trihydrate. Then, to the first tube (the blank) add 1 ml of 5 per cent boric acid solution to inhibit the colorimetric reaction, to the second tube (the sample tube) add 1 ml of water and to the third tube (the internal standard) add 1 ml of a standard solution of pyridoxine hydrochloride (4 μg per ml), prepared by diluting 1 ml of a 0·01 per cent solution of pyridoxine hydrochloride in 0·1N hydrochloric acid to 25 ml with water. To the blank add 1 ml of chloroimine reagent (prepared by dissolving 0·1 g of 2,6-dichloro-*p*-benzoquinone-4-chloroimine in 250 ml of *iso*propyl alcohol) and set a spectrophotometer to read 100 per cent transmittance at 650 mμ exactly one minute after the addition of the reagent. Add 1 ml of the chloroimine reagent to the sample and internal standard tubes in turn and without altering the setting of the spectrophotometer measure the extinction at 650 mμ exactly one minute after adding the reagent.

A = extinction of the sample solution
B = extinction of the internal standard solution

μg per ml pyridoxine hydrochloride in sample

$$= \frac{A}{B - A} \times (\mu\text{g per ml in standard})$$

When the Hochberg method[3] is used for some elixirs a turbidity develops when the highly concentrated buffer is added to the sample solution but this difficulty was eliminated by Sweeney and Hall by the following preliminary treatment:

Pipette a suitable volume of sample into a graduated flask and dilute with 95 per cent ethanol to the required volume to make the alcohol concentration at least 70 per cent. Filter and use aliquots of the filtrate for colour development, as described above.

Sweeney and Hall[4] have also shown that when solutions, in *iso*propyl alcohol, of the three forms of the vitamin, buffered with sodium acetate alone, are reacted with the chloroimine reagent, relative intensities at 650 mμ may vary widely. Since the total amount of the three forms can be determined by measurement of the extinction of a pH 6·75 solution at 325 mμ (see above) a separate determination of pyridoxine, pyridoxal and pyridoxamine is possible. The pyridoxamine is absorbed on a cation-exchange resin, while the pyridoxal and pyridoxine pass through the column. The pyridoxamine is eluted with 0·5N hydrochloric acid and determined independently by a version of the chloroimine reaction. If slight differences in molecular weight of the three forms of the vitamin are ignored, the amount of pyridoxine and pyridoxal present can be calculated by subtracting the pyridoxamine content from the total vitamin B_6. Subsequently the solution from which the pyridoxamine has been removed is suitably diluted and the colour developed with chloroimine and measured at 650 mμ. The ratio of the two forms can then be derived by interpolation from a standard curve prepared by carrying out the colour reaction on known mixtures of the two forms. Extinction readings are taken at the time of maximum colour (about ten minutes after the addition of the reagent).

Pyridoxine is frequently determined microbiologically (see p. 813) but the method is not suitable for very low concentrations such as found in animal feeding-stuffs.

Pyridoxine hydrochloride, $C_{18}H_{11}O_3N,HCl$, Mol. Wt. 205·6. The pure substance may be determined by non-aqueous titration (see p. 792). 1 ml 0·1N perchloric acid = 0·02056 g.

Strong Compound Tablets of Aneurine, *B.P.C.* These tablets contain 2 mg of pyridoxine hydrochloride together with nicotinamide (20 mg), aneurine hydrochloride (5 mg) and riboflavine (2 mg). The *B.P.C.* prescribes a microbiological test for determination of the aneurine and pyridoxine, but the alginic acid separation method of Foster and Murfin is also applicable (see p. 461).

1. Melnick, D., Hochberg, M., Himes, H. W., and Oser, B. L., *J. Biol. Chem.*, 1945, **160**, '.
2. Scudi, J. V., *J. Biol. Chem.*, 1941, **139**, 707.
3. Hochberg, M., Melnick, D., and Oser, B. L., *J. Biol. Chem.*, 1944, **155**, 119.
4. Sweeney, J. P., and Hall, W. L., *J.A.O.A.C.*, 1955, **38**, 697.
5. Scudi, J. V., Bastedo, W. A., and Webb, T. J., *J. Biol. Chem.*, 1940, **136**, 399.

VITAMIN D

The term vitamin D embraces two different substances: **calciferol,** $C_{28}H_{43}OH$, Mol. Wt. 396·7 (vitamin D_2 or activated ergosterol), and **7-dehydrocholesterol** (vitamin D_3). Both forms have similar chemical and ultra-violet spectrophotometric properties and their separation has proved extremely difficult; the difficulty is emphasised by the low content of most natural materials. The major problem of analysis is separation from vitamin A which is usually present at a comparatively high level. It is, therefore, not surprising that the method of choice for analysis of vitamin D has been biological assay.

Vitamin D can be assayed using either rachitic rats or chicks. Vitamin D_2 and vitamin D_3 are equipotent on rats but vitamin D_2 has little antirachitic effect in chicks. It could be assumed therefore that vitamin D preparations intended for chick use should be assayed on chicks but if the source of the vitamin is known the rat result is of course quite acceptable.

Rats from parents allowed a diet in which the vitamin D is minimal up to the isolation of the doe and absent until the young are weaned are fed on a Vitamin D-free diet in which the calcium-phosphorus ratio has been increased. One diet which has been found convenient has the composition:

Ground yellow maize	76 per cent
Wheat gluten	20 ,, ,,
Calcium carbonate	3 ,, ,,
Sodium chloride	1 ,, ,,

After about three weeks the rats develop a rachitic condition which may be demonstrated by X-ray photographs of the proximal end of the tibia. Rats showing a uniform degree of rickets are distributed over four groups to be dosed, respectively, with the standard preparation and the sample under test at two levels. When litters of eight or of four are available two or one rat from each litter are assigned to each group. An economical usage of other litter sizes is to distribute them on a basis suggested by the twin cross-over test so that pairs of litter mates are distributed to the groups which will receive the high dose of standard and the low dose of test or to the groups receiving the low dose of standard and the high dose of test.

The rats are at best dosed daily for ten to fourteen days although other dosing schedules may be used. Fourteen days after the initial dose the rats are killed and the extent to which the rickets have been cured is estimated by means of X-ray photographs or by examination of the bones after staining in either instance by reference to a standard scale. To stain the bones the distal ends of the ulnæ and radii may be removed, immersed in 4 per cent w/v solution of formaldehyde, cut by longitudinal section, immersed in a 1·5 per cent solution of silver nitrate and exposed to light for a few minutes and then transferred to water.

Suitable daily doses for the higher level of standard are of the order of 0·25 unit with a lower dose of half this amount.

The method given above is based on a curative effect but the test may be satisfactorily conducted as a prophylactic test, the dosing being commenced as soon as the rats are weaned and placed on the rachitogenic diet. The daily dose required is then reduced to about 50 per cent of that required by the curative test. If X-ray photography is used the progress of the test may be followed and the test continued until a suitable differentiation between the two levels of dosing is achieved. Under these conditions the test is most likely to be completed in a shorter time than is required when the curative effect is being used.

Several physico-chemical methods are available for determination of vitamin D, the measure of individual success depending on the potency of the material and the nature and amount of interfering contaminants.

In the assay of pharmaceutical preparations containing calciferol in the absence of vitamin A interference may be due to decomposition products of calciferol or the vehicle used in the preparation. The subject has been investigated by Brealey and Stross.[1] A spectrophotometric procedure has been shown to be free from interference from decomposition products of calciferol since they no longer show its selective absorption and their minor effect can be corrected for by application of a geometric three-point correction. However, the absorption peak of calciferol is rather flat and the correction is of limited value unless the composition of the preparations is known and blank readings are available, but the method is of particular value for control purposes.

Decomposition products of calciferol appear to give practically no colour with antimony trichloride–acetyl chloride reagent, and the colorimetric method applied direct to a chloroformic extract of a decomposed sample of calciferol, or of ground tablet material, gives the same result before and after chromatography. In the case of the comparatively low-potency oily solutions of calciferol where the phytosterols present in the oil give colours which interfere, chromatography is necessary.

The presence of antoxidants such as gallate esters or butylated hydroxyanisole do not interfere with the determination.

The solvent recommended by Brealey and Stross was *n*-hexane but light petroleum has been shown to be equally suitable. Amber-coloured glassware must be used throughout.

Tablets of Calciferol, *B.P.* Contain 1·25 mg, equivalent to 50,000 units of vitamin D.

Finely powder about 20 tablets and weigh out accurately an amount equivalent to about 250,000 units of calciferol into a stoppered cylinder. Add by pipette 20 ml of light petroleum (b.p. 40° to 60°) and shake for one hour. Allow the insoluble material to settle and pipette 2 ml of the clear supernatant liquid into a 150-ml flask. Evaporate to dryness under nitrogen and dissolve the residue in 20 ml ethanol-free chloroform.

Proceed as described under 'Solution of Calciferol' beginning 'Mix 1 ml of this solution with 9 ml of antimony trichloride reagent . . .'.

Tablets of Calcium with Vitamin D, *B.P.C.* Contain the equivalent of 500 units of vitamin D.

Finely powder 5 tablets in a beaker with about 10 ml of ethanol and transfer to a 250-ml saponification flask, rinsing the beaker with two portions, each of 20 ml, of ethanol.

Add 14 ml of glycerol and 20 ml of 50 per cent (w/v) aqueous potassium hydroxide and boil under a reflux condenser for thirty minutes with occasional swirling. Add 110 ml water and allow to stand for ten minutes with occasional swirling. Cool and transfer the contents of the flask to a 250-ml graduated flask, rinsing in and making up to volume with ethanol. Mix and allow the insoluble material to settle.

Pipette 50 ml of the supernatant liquid into a 250-ml separator and extract with three portions, each of 30 ml, of light petroleum (b.p. 40° to 60°). Combine the extracts and wash with successive portions, each of 50 ml, of water until the washings are no longer alkaline to phenolphthalein solution. Evaporate the extract to dryness under nitrogen.

Dissolve the residue in exactly 1 ml of ethanol-free chloroform and add 9 ml antimony trichloride reagent. Determine the units of vitamin D per tablet as described under Solution of Calciferol.

Solution of Calciferol, *B.P.* A solution in a suitable vegetable oil to contain 3,000 units of vitamin D per ml.

Weigh out accurately about 1·5 g sample and 0·1 g hydroquinone into a 150-ml flask, add 25 ml of 0·5N ethanolic potassium hydroxide and boil under a reflux condenser for twenty minutes. Cool, add 50 ml water and transfer to a 250-ml separator. Extract with three successive portions, each of 30 ml, of anæsthetic ether. Combine the ether extracts, wash with 20 ml water, then with 20 ml 0·5N aqueous potassium hydroxide, and finally with successive portions, each of 20 ml, of water until the washings are no longer alkalinc to phenolphthalein solution.

Filter the ether solution through a cotton-wool plug, wash with two portions, each of 10 ml, of anæsthetic ether and evaporate the combined extracts and washings to dryness under nitrogen on a water-bath.

Dissolve the residue in about 20 ml of a mixture of 10 per cent anæsthetic ether in light petroleum (b.p. 40° to 60°) and transfer to the top of an alumina column 20 cm long and 1 cm in diameter, prepared as in C, p. 661, by slurrying alumina in light petroleum. Wash the column with two portions, each of 25 ml, of 10 per cent anæsthetic ether in light petroleum, and then with two portions, each of 25 ml, of 20 per cent anæsthetic ether in light petroleum. Elute the vitamin D with four portions, each of 25 ml, of 10 per cent ethanol in a mixture of equal volumes of anæsthetic ether and light petroleum. Evaporate the eluate to dryness under nitrogen on a water-bath at 50°. Dissolve the residue in exactly 5 ml chloroform (ethanol-free).

Mix 1 ml of this solution with 9 ml of antimony trichloride reagent (prepared by dissolving 22 g antimony trichloride in ethanol-free chloroform, making up to 100 ml, adding 2·5 ml acetyl chloride and allowing to stand for thirty minutes). Measure the extinctions at 500 mμ and 550 mμ in a 1-cm cell one and a half to two minutes after adding the reagent.

Carry out the colorimetric procedure on a 1-ml aliquot of a standard solution containing 0·003 per cent of calciferol in ethanol-free chloroform.

Let the extinctions of the sample at 500 mμ and 550 mμ be E_1 and E_2 respectively, and the extinctions of the standard at 500 mμ and 550 mμ be S_1 and S_2 respectively.

$$\text{Units of vitamin D per g} = \frac{E_1 - E_2}{S_1 - S_2} \times \frac{0{\cdot}003}{100} \times \frac{5 \times 40 \times 10^6}{\text{wt. of sample taken}}$$

In the presence of vitamin A the vitamin may be extracted with organic solvent either directly or after saponification with ethanolic potassium hydroxide. Both vitamins D_2 and D_3 have identical spectra with broad bands having maxima at 265 mμ in hexane but the extinction coefficients in this solvent are comparatively low, being 459 for D_2 and 474 for D_3, and the more intense absorption of vitamin A, with its peak at 328 mμ, may completely overshadow the absorption of vitamin D. The spectrophotometric method therefore requires separation of vitamin D from vitamin A and other absorbing materials and can only be applied to comparatively high-potency materials.

For the separation of vitamin D from related sterols and from vitamin A the first step in most methods is removal of saponifiable matter after treatment with hot ethanolic potassium hydroxide. In many instances sterols are then removed by precipitation with digitonin. The vitamins D are then separated by either column or paper chromatography.

Antimony trichloride reacts with vitamin D producing an orange colour with a maximum at 500 mμ. The reagent also reacts with vitamin A (transient blue colour with a maximum at 620 mμ), sterols and allied compounds. The colour produced with a vitamin D is not stable, its intensity increasing with time at a rate dependent on the nature and quantity of residual impurities. Purification of solvents and use of different grades of solid have not perceptibly improved this condition. The addition of acetyl chloride and use of ethylene dichloride as solvent have given some improvement.

The method detailed below has been applied, with some success, in the authors' laboratory to simple multivitamin preparations. It has not proved successful with oil-based materials such as halibut-liver and cod-liver oils where bioassay is necessary. Amber glassware must be used throughout.

Antimony trichloride reagent:

Solution *A*. Dissolve approximately 100 g of the crystalline solid in about 350 ml of redistilled ethylene dichloride as quickly as possible. Add 2 or 3 g of anhydrous alumina, mix thoroughly, and filter the solution through filter paper into a reagent bottle, then make up to a previously marked 440 ml volume with ethylene dichloride.

Solution *B*. Mix 100 ml acetyl chloride and 400 ml ethylene dichloride and store in a reagent bottle.

For the colour reagent mix 45 ml of *A* and 5 ml of *B*. Prepare fresh daily.

Standard solution of vitamin D: Vitamin D_2 standard solution in ethylene dichloride containing 10 μg (400 units) of crystalline vitamin D_2 per ml. Store in a refrigerator.

Equilibrate 200 ml of *iso*-octane with excess of polyethylene glycol 600. Take 100 ml of the clear supernatant liquid, add 25 g of Celite 545 and shake vigorously until a thin slurry is formed. Add, dropwise,

10 ml of polyethylene glycol 600 with vigorous stirring and shake for two minutes to ensure uniformity. Plug a chromatographic tube (28 cm long by 22 mm internal diameter) with a pledget of glass wool and with the aid of a disc plunger consolidate aliquots of the slurry to a height of 15 cm.

Determine the volume in which the vitamin D is recovered as follows: Add 2 ml of a 0·03 per cent solution of vitamin D_2 in *iso*-octane to the column and rinse into the latter with small portions of *iso*-octane. Up to 5 ml can be used without altering the recovery volume of the vitamin. Maintain a 2 to 3 ml flow rate and elute the vitamin D with *iso*-octane, collecting 5-ml fractions of eluate, and measure their extinctions at 263 mμ.

Vitamin D is recovered in a volume slightly less than 25 ml, usually between the 35th and 75th ml of eluate. This volume and the interval of recovery remain constant for each column and are used in subsequent analyses. (Recoveries of vitamin D have consistently been between 97 and 99 per cent.)

Weigh the sample into a 150-ml flat-bottomed flask. Add 15 ml 50 per cent potassium hydroxide and 50 ml ethanol. Reflux on a water-bath for thirty minutes. Cool and transfer to a 500-ml separator with 50 ml water in several portions. Add 75 ml ether, shake vigorously and allow to separate for a few minutes. Run the aqueous layer into a second 500-ml separator and extract with three quantities, each of 30 ml, of ether. Add each ether layer in turn to the original ether extract. Pour 100 ml of water through the combined ether extracts, allow for complete separation and run the aqueous layer into another separator. Extract this with two quantities, each of 50 ml, of ether, shaking vigorously, and add each to the original ether extract.

Pour two quantities, each of 100 ml, of water through the ether extract without shaking, allow to separate and discard these aqueous fractions. Add successive 10-ml portions of water to the ether extract with gentle agitation, removing each until the rinse water is alkali-free when tested with phenolphthalein.

Run the ether into a 500-ml beaker containing anhydrous sodium sulphate and stir for about two minutes. Transfer the ether quantitatively to a suitable flask and evaporate to about 5 ml by heating on a water-bath.

Remove the remaining solvent in a stream of nitrogen without the application of heat and dissolve the residue in 5 ml of *iso*-octane.

Transfer the *iso*-octane solution to the Celite column using a further 5 ml of solvent. Add 5-ml portions of *iso*-octane and collect the fraction previously found to contain vitamin D.

Prepare a 5-g column of Florex XXS in *iso*-octane in a chromatographic tube of 6 mm internal diameter, 20 cm long, plugged with glass wool. Transfer the vitamin D fraction from the Celite to this column, rinsing with 10 ml of *iso*-octane, and discard the washings.

Elute the vitamin D with 50 ml of redistilled benzene. Evaporate to about 5 ml by heating on a water-bath, removing the remaining solvent in a stream of nitrogen without the application of heat. Dissolve the residue in 4 ml of ethylene dichloride.

Measure the extinctions at about 500 mμ of the following three solutions in 1-cm stoppered cells exactly one minute after adding the antimony trichloride reagent, using a blank of ethylene dichloride.

E_1, 1 ml of sample solution + 1 ml ethylene dichloride + 10 ml antimony trichloride reagent

E_2, 1 ml of sample solution + 1 ml acetic anhydride/ethylene dichloride (1 : 1) + 10 ml antimony trichloride reagent

E_3, 1 ml of sample solution + 1 ml standard vitamin D solution + 10 ml antimony trichloride reagent

Units of vitamin D/ml of sample solution

$$= \frac{E_1 - E_2}{E_3 - E_1} \times \text{units of vitamin D/ml of standard solution}$$

Thus, units of vitamin D/g of sample

$$= \frac{\text{units of vitamin D per ml of sample solution}}{\text{wt. of sample (g) per ml of sample solution}}$$

Recent work has shown that Haloport F (a perfluorocarbon polymer) offers some advantages over polyethylene glycol 600 and Florex columns in the separation of vitamin A from vitamin D.

The irregular variation of colour intensity with time has proved an obstacle to precise measurement of extinction particularly in the comparison of samples with standards. This difficulty has partly been overcome by using a recording spectrophotometer; the instrument is equipped with a voltage-controlled photomultiplier detector. The amplified signal from the photomultiplier is fed into a 10-millivolt recorder having a chart speed of 1 inch per minute. With this system, narrow slit widths can be employed and the sensitivity adjusted so that 2 μg per ml of vitamin D solution gives 25 per cent full-scale traverse of the recorder pen. A large cross-section 1-cm cell is mounted in the cell holder so that the light path is offset. A small funnel and stirrer projects into the other half of the cell, through the light-tight cell holder cover and to one side of the light path. With the phototube slide closed the recorder pen is adjusted to zero. With 0·5 ml of standard or sample solution in the cell the recorder is adjusted to read 100 per cent transmission. In quick succession, 0·5 ml of ethylene dichloride and 5 ml antimony trichloride are poured into the funnel and the stirrer operated for a few seconds. The recorder traces a curve showing colour development with time. With simple vitamin D solutions the curve reaches a maximum in approximately one minute. With materials such as fish oils, after chromatographic separation of the vitamin D, the recorder trace shows increasing absorption even after several minutes. An approximate analysis of impure vitamin D extracts can be inferred by examination of the recorder curves.

Vitamin D_2 is known to undergo thermal cyclisation at temperatures above 200° yielding pyrocalciferol and *iso*pyrocalciferol. Quantitative separation of vitamin D_2 from other sterols by gas chromatography has been achieved[2] (using 0·75 per cent *neo*pentyl glycol succinate on 100 to 140-mesh Chromosorb P with 6 feet by 4 mm columns at 220° and β-ionisation detection). Two peaks are recorded but their areas are relatively constant under steady operating conditions. With this system it is possible to estimate 0·2 μg of vitamin D and to separate vitamin D_2 from vitamin D_3. Preliminary separation of major impurities is still necessary.

1. BREALEY, L., and STROSS, P. S., *J. Pharm. Pharmacol.*, 1955, **7**, 739.
2. ZIFFER, H., VANDEN-HEUVEL, W. J. A., HAAHTI, E. O. A., and HORNING, E. C., *J. Amer. Chem. Soc.*, 1960, **82**, 6411.

VITAMIN E

Although the determination of tocopherols (vitamin E) is required for materials from natural sources, pure **tocopheryl acetate,** $C_{31}H_{52}O_3$, Mol. Wt. 472·8, is available commercially and is stable; the free tocopherol is rapidly oxidised on exposure to air and light.

Chemical assay of the official compound is by use of its reducing action on ceric sulphate after acid hydrolysis of the ester, since tocopherols are unstable in alkaline solutions.

Heat about 0·025 g, accurately weighed, under a reflux condenser with 7 ml of dehydrated ethanol until solution is complete; add 5 ml of a 12 per cent v/v solution of sulphuric acid in dehydrated ethanol, and boil for three hours. Cool, transfer to a 25-ml graduated flask and add dehydrated ethanol to volume; to 10 ml of this solution add 2 drops of a 1 per cent solution of diphenylamine in nitrogen-free concentrated sulphuric acid and titrate with 0·01N ceric ammonium sulphate, using a microburette, until the colour changes to bluish-violet. 1 ml 0·01N = 0·002364 g of $C_{31}H_{52}O_3$.

***d*-Alpha tocopheryl acid succinate,** $C_{33}H_{54}O_5$, Mol. Wt. 530·8, is official in the *N.F.* with the following assay:

Heat about 0·25 g with 50 ml of dehydrated ethanol under a reflux condenser until dissolved and for at least one minute longer. While the solution is boiling, add, through the condenser, 1 g of potassium hydroxide pellets, one at a time to avoid over-heating. Continue to reflux for twenty minutes and then add, dropwise, without cooling, 2 ml of concentrated hydrochloric acid through the condenser. Cool to room temperature and transfer to a 500-ml, amber-coloured separator, rinsing the flask with 100 ml of water and 100 ml of ether and adding to the separator. Shake vigorously, separate and extract the aqueous layer with two 50-ml quantities of ether. Combine the ether extracts and wash them with four 100-ml quantities of water. Transfer the ether solution to a flask and evaporate the ether, on a water-bath in a current of nitrogen or under reduced pressure, until the volume is reduced to about 7 or 8 ml. Remove the flask from the water-bath and evaporate the solution to dryness without heating. Immediately dissolve the residue in 0·5N ethanolic sulphuric acid and transfer quantitatively to a 200-ml graduated flask and dilute to volume with 0·5N ethanolic sulphuric acid. Transfer a 50-ml aliquot of this solution to a 250-ml flask, add 50 ml of 0·5N ethanolic sulphuric acid and 2 drops of a 1 per cent solution of diphenylamine in concentrated sulphuric acid and titrate with 0·01N ceric sulphate at a rate of approximately 25 drops per ten seconds, with constant swirling, until a blue colour persists for ten seconds. Carry out a blank titration using 100 ml of 0·5N ethanolic sulphuric acid, 20 ml of water and 2 drops of the diphenylamine solution. 1 ml 0·01N ceric sulphate = 0·002654 g $C_{33}H_{54}O_5$.

The reducing property of the tocopherols forms the basis of the colorimetric assay of vitamin E and the most useful methods are modifications of the original technique of Emmerie and Engel[1] in which the ferrous salt formed in the reduction of ferric chloride is determined colorimetrically with 2,2′-dipyridyl. The reaction is not specific, fats cause a marked depressing effect on the colour, and substances such as cholesterol, vitamin A and carotenoids interfere with the colour reaction; these effects are reduced by suitable purification, although many recommended modifications have subsequently been shown to cause loss of tocopherols. It is now known that seven tocopherols exist in naturally occurring materials and a method has been developed by the Analytical Methods Committee of the *S.A.C.*[2] which enables them to be determined individually in whatever amounts and proportions they might be present, whether in a single raw material or a complex mixture. The analysis may involve all or most of the seven stages enumerated below with their purposes.

(*a*) Solvent extraction of a representative sample with a lipid solvent, for quantitative separation of all tocopherols present along with other fatty material.

(*b*) Saponification of the lipoid extract and separation from it of the unsaponifiable matter.

(*c*) Separation of most of the steroid material by freezing from solution in methanol.

(*d*) Column chromatography on floridin earth to remove carotenoids and residual steroids.

(*e*) Two-dimensional paper chromatography, to separate the tocopherols into five zones, and individual elution.

(*f*) Treatment of the eluates with the Emmerie-Engel reagent and reading of the extinctions at 520 mμ.

(*g*) Calculation of tocopherol equivalents from extinctions by using the established factor for each tocopherol.

The seven stages enumerated above may not all be necessary. The obvious omission is of stage (*a*) when the sample to be examined is a clean oil or fat. Stage (*c*) is only necessary for materials of low potency. Stage (*d*) can be omitted during the analysis of samples containing more than 5 to 10 mg of tocopherols per g of oil, and possibly in certain other circumstances not easy to define or forecast.

The recommended method, given below, is primarily for vegetable oils but the Committee states that it should be applicable to the fat-soluble extracts of other biological materials and that, in their opinion, the tocopherols are sufficiently stable to involve no special hazards or difficulties when one of the several normal methods of fat extraction is used.

Reagents:

Ether. Analytical-reagent grade or anæsthetic ether, *B.P.* If the material contains peroxides they should be removed by shaking 500 ml of the reagent, for six minutes, with a mixture of 4 g of silver nitrate in 30 ml of water and 2 g of sodium hydroxide in 50 ml of water; the reagent is then decanted, after separation, and used without distillation.

Dehydrated ethanol. Purify by distillation in an all-glass apparatus over potassium permanganate and potassium hydroxide (1 and 2 g, respectively, per litre of ethanol).

Diluted ethanol. Add 75 volumes of the dehydrated ethanol to 25 volumes of water.

Floridin earth. Specially selected material should be used; it is available as 'Floridin earth XS for the determination of Vitamin E' from the British Drug Houses Limited.

Ferric chloride solution. This is a 0·2 per cent solution of analytical-reagent grade ferric chloride hexahydrate in dehydrated ethanol; since the solution is extremely liable to photochemical reduction it must be prepared directly in the amber bottle in which it is to be stored and the bottle, which must not be exposed even to moderate daylight, is best masked by a covering of black paper or black paint.

Dipyridyl solution. This is a 0·5 per cent solution of analytical-reagent grade 2,2′-dipyridyl in ethanol.

The following reagents should be of analytical-reagent grade: stannous chloride, concentrated hydrochloric acid, methanol, benzene, *cyclo*hexane, zinc oxide, strong ammonia solution and ammonium carbonate.

Determination:

1. *Saponification of the oil:* Weigh accurately about 1 g of the oil into a round-bottomed flask (50 to 150 ml is a suitable size). Add 4 ml of a freshly prepared 5 per cent solution of pyrogallol in dehydrated ethanol and heat in a water-bath, using a cold-finger condenser or a small reflux condenser fitted with a ground-glass joint. When the mixture boils, remove the condenser, and add 1 ml of a solution of 160 g of analytical-reagent grade potassium hydroxide in 100 ml of water. Replace the condenser, immerse the flask in the water-bath, and heat under vigorous reflux for three minutes, with occasional shaking.

Remove the flask from the water-bath, cool the contents, and add 20 ml of water. Extract the unsaponifiable matter, as rapidly as possible, with three 25-ml quantities of ether. If the phases fail to separate quickly and sharply, add 1 or 2 ml of ethanol. Sometimes emulsions are formed; they can usually be dispersed by adding a few millilitres of ethanol. If they persist, it may be because the directions have not been followed closely enough; the proportions of reagents are somewhat critical, and too much ethanol may even encourage the formation of emulsions. Vigorous shaking at any stage is unnecessary and should be avoided, especially as some biological materials are naturally rich in emulsifying agents. Wash the combined ether extracts with 20-ml quantities of water until neutral to phenolphthalein, avoiding vigorous shaking at first. Three or four washes are usually necessary. Transfer the ether solution to a round-bottomed flask, and remove the ether by evaporation in a current of nitrogen, or under reduced pressure while warming the solution on the water-bath. Dry the residue, if necessary, by adding a little dehydrated ethanol and benzene and re-evaporating. Do not dry the solution with magnesium sulphate or sodium sulphate, because these chemicals may contain traces of iron. Dissolve the dry residue either in 5 ml of benzene for step 3 or in methanol for step 2.

2. *Removal of sterols.* It is rarely necessary to remove sterols before chromatography. However, with extracts of certain materials, poor separation on paper may be due to the presence of sterols. These may be removed as follows. Dissolve the unsaponifiable residue in boiling methanol and transfer the solution to a 15-ml centrifuge tube using, in all, 12 ml of solvent. Cool to about $-10°$ in a suitable bath, centrifuge in a previously cooled centrifuge cup and pour the supernatant liquid into a flask. Redissolve the sterol precipitate in 5 ml of hot methanol and repeat the process twice. Evaporate the combined methanol solutions to dryness under reduced pressure and dissolve the residue in 5 ml of benzene.

3. *Floridin earth separation:* Preparation of chromatographic column. Mount a glass chromatographic tube, not less than 1·2 to 1·4 cm in internal diameter and not less than 16 to 20 cm long, in a vertical position. Mix 5 g of Floridin earth and 0·5 g of stannous chloride with 20 ml of concentrated hydrochloric acid, and bring to boiling-point. With rapid stirring, pour the slurry into the chromatographic tube in one continuous operation, so that the earth settles with an even gradation. After the liquid has passed through, wash the column successively, with five 5-ml quantities of dehydrated ethanol, and then with five 5-ml quantities of benzene.

Column chromatography. Pass the benzene solution from step 1 (or step 2) through the prepared Floridin earth column. Elute the column with seven 5-ml quantities of benzene, the complete elution taking not less than forty-five minutes. Nitrogen under pressure or gentle suction may be used to hasten both the preparation of the columns and the chromatography, provided the latter process takes not less than forty-five minutes. If total reducing substances are to be determined, an aliquot may be taken at this stage. It is safe to store the benzene solution overnight in a refrigerator.

4. *Paper chromatography:* (*a*) Preparation of zinc-ammine solution. Dissolve 16 g of zinc oxide and 25 g of ammonium carbonate in a mixture of 150 ml of strong ammonium hydroxide and 600 ml of water. Add 5 ml of a 0·1 per cent aqueous solution of sodium fluorescein. This zinc-ammine solution is indefinitely stable in a stoppered bottle.

(*b*) Preparation of zinc carbonate impregnated paper: Use Whatman papers No. 1 grade 'for chromatography' in sheets 51·2 cm × 46·4 cm. Some batches of chromatographic paper have contained reducing material that raised the blank value. This may be removed by continuous extraction of the paper with hot methanol in a Soxhlet apparatus or by extraction and decantation in a measuring cylinder. Because solvents move faster along the machine direction of filter paper than across it, all the papers should be similarly orientated. The procedure described below ensures the most evenly coated papers with the minimum handling of the working portion; the position of the written date gives a clue to the machine direction of the paper. Cut the large sheets of paper into four equal parts, as indicated in Fig. 14. Pour the zinc-ammine solution into a large dish. Immerse each sheet separately in the solution to within about 5 cm of one short edge, and hang all the sheets to drain at room temperature for about an hour. The dry margin allows the use of clips for supporting the papers. Dry the papers, hanging vertically, at 95° to 100° for three hours in an oven with or without forced air circulation. Remove the dried papers, cut a 20-cm square from the coated portion

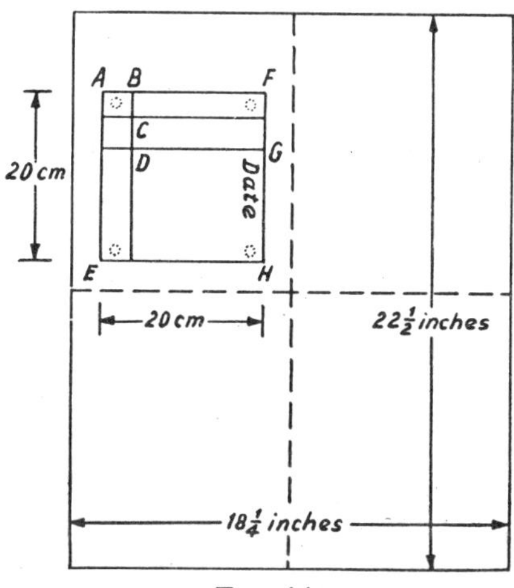

FIG. 14

Dimensions of zinc carbonate impregnated paper. Care should be taken to preserve the machine direction of the paper (as indicated on the package). AB = BC = 2 cm. CD = 3 cm. The letters need not be copied; they are inserted here only for explanatory purposes

of each sheet, and write the date close to the edge GH. The prepared papers may be stored for a few weeks in a thoroughly dry place, but they are soon spoiled by humidity.

Rule each paper lightly in pencil, as shown by the thin lines in Fig. 14. Punch holes in the corners, if necessary, for use on a frame.

(*c*) Apparatus: Chromatography in both dimensions is done by the ascending-solvent method, and should be carried out in a glass tank large enough to hold the 20-cm × 20-cm papers in a vertical position. It is advisable to use a separate tank for each dimension. Alternatively, both runs may be carried out in the same tank; the necessary change of solvent must then be made before running the second dimension. The inside walls of each tank must be lined with a sheet of filter paper, saturated with the mobile phase. The tanks must have gas-tight lids, and they should be shielded from strong light.

When less than four papers are run together, and provided that the chromatograms are to be examined later under ultra-violet light (method (i) of section (*f*) below), they may be supported in each tank by glass rods, arranged so that the papers hang evenly, with their edges dipping into the solvent. It is, however, more convenient to use some sort of two-dimensional chromatographic frame for carrying the papers, and this is recommended. If spot location is to be by spraying (method (ii) of section (*f*) below), or, if four or more papers are to be run together, such a frame is essential. Its use enables the papers to be manipulated easily and simultaneously during the various stages of the chromatographic separation, and ensures that the chromatograms are uniform and reproducible.

(*d*) First-dimension chromatography: Evaporate the solution from step 3 to dryness under reduced pressure or in nitrogen. Dissolve the residue in 0·5 to 3 ml of benzene in a stoppered flask, to give a solution containing 0·5 to 2·0 mg of tocopherol per ml, if possible. (Polar solvents must not be used for preparing this solution.) Set the tocopherol solution, by means of discrete additions of 10 to 20 μl, as a narrow band across the starting line CD (Fig. 14), so that, in all, 5 to 30 μg of each tocopherol are present. The total solution set should not contain more than 100 μg of total tocopherols. Use three replicate papers for each test sample and a fourth paper as a blank. The additions should be made from a fine-tipped glass capillary, calibrated by weight, from a 10-μl blood pipette, from a Trenner pipette with a curved tip or from an Agla micrometer syringe. It is important to apply the solution as a regular band.

Into the first chromatographic tank pour enough 30 per cent v/v benzene in *cyclo*hexane to produce a depth of about 0·5 to 1 cm. Support test and blank papers with the dates at the top and their edges AE just immersed in the solvent. Leave the papers in the tank until the solvent front has migrated about 15 cm. This usually takes about one hour.

(*e*) Second-dimension chromatography: If no frame is being used, remove the papers individually from the first tank and dip each one in a 3 per cent w/v solution of liquid paraffin *B.P.* in light petroleum (b.p. 60° to 80°), with edge EH at the bottom, to within 0·5 cm of the line DG. If a frame is used, remove it with the papers from the first tank, and, with edges EH at the bottom, immerse the assembly in a bath of the liquid paraffin solution to within 0·5 cm of the line DG. Remove the papers from the paraffin solution, drain, and allow the light petroleum to evaporate in the air. Then place the papers in the second tank with edge AF just immersed in the diluted ethanol as the mobile phase. Run the papers for two to three hours or until the front has migrated to within 4 or 5 cm from the top of the papers.

Remove the papers from the tank, and dry them by means of a current of nitrogen or air.

(*f*) Removal of spots from chromatograms: Remove the papers from the frame, if one is used. Use either of two methods for spot location and removal for analysis. Method (i) is much to be preferred, but method (ii) can be used when no ultra-violet lamp is available. Even when method (i) is used, it is still desirable to spray one of the papers as in the first part of method (ii) in order to confirm the position of reducing spots.

(i) Examine the dry papers in a dark room under ultra-violet light; the lamp should not be nearer to the paper than 10 cm. Tocopherol spots are visible as dark patches on a fluorescing background, less than 1 μg being easily detected. (See Fig. 15.) Mark the spots by ringing with a hard pencil as quickly as possible, with a slight margin round each spot. Remove the paper, and cut out the marked spots with sharp scissors, cutting within the pencilled lines. With the minimum of handling, roll the cut-out pieces of paper into cylinders and drop each one separately into a numbered

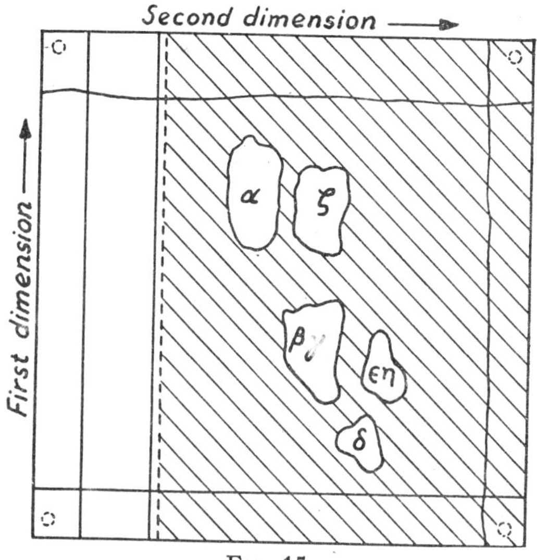

FIG. 15

Reproduction, one-third full size, from a paper, marked to show the positions of tocopherol zones after two-dimensional chromatography. The shaded area shows the part of the paper impregnated with paraffin after running in the first dimension. The wavy lines show approximate levels reached by the solvent fronts

test-tube (measuring about 10 cm × 1·5 cm and fitted with a B14 ground-glass stopper) containing 3 ml of ethanol and 0·5 ml of the dipyridyl solution (when large numbers of tubes are to be filled, it is convenient to use 3·5 ml of 0·07 per cent 2,2′-dipyridyl solution instead of 0·5 ml of 0·5 per cent dipyridyl solution plus 3 ml of dehydrated ethanol. This solution is conveniently dispensed from a 3·5-ml automatic pipette). Mark the blank chromatogram correspondingly, and cut out the blank areas similarly.

(ii) Spray one of the test papers heavily from a fine glass atomiser with the mixed reagent (equal parts of the ferric chloride solution and the dipyridyl solution). Tocopherols appear as red spots, which should be ringed with a hard pencil. If no ultra-violet lamp is available use these spots to locate tocopherols on the assay papers. Remove the sprayed spots and a generous margin by cutting outside the pencilled rings, and use the resulting series of holes as a template for marking another test paper, and a blank paper. Alternatively, trace the sprayed paper on to a clean sheet of thin paper, and use the latter as a template. Having marked the tocopherol positions, cut out the areas from both test and blank papers, and drop them into tubes containing dipyridyl solution, as in (i) above.

5. *Positions of the spots on the chromatogram:* The seven tocopherols separate as shown in Fig. 15. Depending on the material being analysed, one spot or several spots may be visible. Although by this method, β- and γ-tocopherol are inseparable, as are ε- and η-tocopherol, instructions for their distinction are given below. Other spots appearing on the papers are normally distinguished from the tocopherols by their positions. It must be emphasised that, depending on the degree of purification of the sample and the relative proportions of the different tocopherols present, some distortion of the movements of the spots may occur. Absolute R and R_F values may be disregarded, however; provided separation occurs according to the general pattern shown in Fig. 15, the next stage may be carried out.

6. *Colorimetric determination:* Gently swirl the stoppered test-tubes, each containing 3·5 ml of ethanolic dipyridyl solution and the slip of paper, for a few seconds. Transfer to a darkened room, and carry out the rest of the determination under dim *artificial* light. To one of the solutions add 0·5 ml of the ferric chloride solution from a fast-delivery pipette, shake the stoppered tube for a moment, and then transfer the contents to a glass spectrophotometer cell 1 cm in path length. Exactly two minutes after adding the ferric chloride, measure the extinction at 520 mμ against a similar cell containing ethanol. Repeat this procedure with each tube. Subtract the reading of each 'blank' tube from the reading obtained from the corresponding 'test' tube. This gives the 'net extinction' reading. Multiplication of the net extinction reading by the spectrophotometric factor for the tocopherol being measured gives directly the number of micrograms of tocopherol in the cut-out spot.

7. *Blanks:* The tocopherol-containing solution has been indirectly measured against a corresponding blank solution. The highest accuracy can only be obtained, therefore, if it can be safely assumed that the blank reaction of the mixed reagents is identical in both 'blank' and 'test' tubes. The 'blank' has two components, namely (*a*) that derived from the residual reducing material in the paper, and (*b*) the reaction between the dipyridyl and traces of ferrous iron in the ferric chloride. Component (*a*) amounts to an extinction of about 0·010; component (*b*) can be reduced to about 0·050 by suitable precautions, such as preparing and keeping the ferric chloride solution in the dark and the observance of scrupulous cleanliness in the use of the pipettes for ferric chloride. Ferric chloride is converted to the ferrous state photochemically; hence the solution should not be exposed to daylight in transparent glass. The total blank value can be reduced to about 0·060 to 0·080. Blanks that give extinctions of over 0·100 are likely to be unstable and should be suspect. If high blank values continue, and other forms of contamination have

been eliminated, it is best to prepare a new ferric chloride solution in a dark bottle previously cleaned with chromic acid solution.

8. *Calculations:*

Where G = grams of oil taken,
V = volume of benzene in millilitres to prepare solution for paper chromatography,
v = volume in microlitres spotted on paper,
D = net extinction, and
F = spectrophotometric factor for 4 ml,
then each tocopherol, in micrograms per gram, is given by—

$$\frac{D \times F \times V \times 1{,}000}{v \times G}$$

The recommended factors, F, are: α-tocopherol, 98; β-tocopherol, 96; γ-tocopherol, 90; δ-tocopherol, 75; ε-tocopherol, 96; ζ-tocopherol, 94; η-tocopherol, 88.

The β- and ε-tocopherol are determinable when spots in their respective positions give no colour on spraying with the dianisidine reagent (see below). However, if the dianisidine reaction shows the presence of γ- or η-tocopherol the analyst may either assume that β- and ε-tocopherol are absent or attempt a differential analysis of the four substances by chromatographic separation of nitroso-derivatives, such as has recently been described by Marcinkiewicz and Green.[3] Factors for γ- and η-tocopherol should be used even though β- or ε-tocopherol, or both, may be present but masked.

Detection of γ-, η- and δ-tocopherol by diazotised *o*-dianisidine.

Reagent: Diazotised *o*-dianisidine. Dissolve 0·5 g of *o*-dianisidine dihydrochloride in 60 ml of water. Add 6 ml of concentrated hydrochloric acid and then 12 ml of 5 per cent aqueous sodium nitrite. Mix thoroughly. After five minutes add 12 ml of 5 per cent aqueous urea solution.

Test: Spray one of the test papers (it is advisable to run an extra paper if the presence of γ-, η- or δ-tocopherol is suspected) heavily with 5 per cent sodium carbonate solution and then with the diazotised *o*-dianisidine from a fine glass atomiser. The tocopherols may be identified by the resultant colours: γ-, blue-green changing to indigo; η-, brownish purple changing to purple; δ-, reddish brown changing to purple. The colours may be stabilised by washing the papers in water after spraying.

The presence of colour in either the γ- or the η-position does not exclude the presence of β- or ε-tocopherol, respectively.

Estimation of α-tocopheryl acetate by a simplified procedure is sometimes possible where (i) the vitamin is present in sufficient quantity to yield organic solvent extracts which have measurable ultra-violet absorption, (ii) interference from such material as steroids and vitamin A is small and constant in magnitude and (iii) simple chromatography removes sufficient of the interfering material to apply baseline correction techniques to ultra-violet spectra recorded continuously in the region 220 mμ to 350 mμ.

VITAMIN E

The following method has been found suitable for a tonic containing 0·025 per cent of α-tocopheryl acetate with other vitamins and minerals:

Pipette 30 ml of the tonic into a 250-ml stoppered cylinder; add 20 ml of water, 20 ml of ethanol and 75 ml of *cyclo*hexane. Replace the air above the solution with nitrogen, stopper the cylinder immediately and shake for twenty minutes. Add a further 30 ml of water, again replace the air with nitrogen, stopper and shake for a further ten minutes. Allow the solution to separate and measure the volume of the *cyclo*hexane layer (V ml). Pipette 50 ml of the *cyclo*hexane layer into a 150-ml round-bottomed flask, evaporate to dryness under nitrogen, dissolve the residue in 20 ml of ethanol, add 3 ml of 60 per cent potassium hydroxide solution and 3 ml of a 5 per cent solution of pyrogallol in ethanol. Reflux for twenty minutes, cool and transfer to a 500-ml separator, washing in with 50 ml of water and 50 ml of solvent ether. Shake and allow to separate. Run off the aqueous layer into a second separator and extract with four 20-ml quantities of solvent ether. Combine the ether extracts and wash with 50 ml followed by four 30-ml quantities of water. Transfer the ether extract to a 250-ml flask and evaporate to dryness under nitrogen. Remove any traces of water in the residue by re-evaporation with acetone. Dissolve the final residue in 5 ml of toluene.

Place a pledget of glass wool just above the tap of a 50 cm × 1 cm chromatographic column. Add to it a previously-boiled slurry of 5 g of Florex XXS (retained by No. 72 B.S.S.), 0·5 g of stannous chloride and 20 ml of concentrated hydrochloric acid. Run off the acid and wash the column with five quantities of 10 ml of ethanol and then five quantities of 10 ml of toluene without letting the column run dry.

Transfer the 5 ml of toluene solution of the sample onto the column, wash in with about 5 ml of toluene and collect the eluate. Wash the column five times with 10-ml quantities of toluene and evaporate the combined toluene washings to dryness under nitrogen. Re-evaporate with three 10-ml quantities of acetone to remove any residual toluene and dissolve the residue in exactly 50 ml of light petroleum (b.p. 40° to 60°). Record the spectrum of this solution with a recording spectrophotometer from 220 mμ to 350 mμ, using light petroleum in the reference cell.

Draw a baseline between the minimum absorption at about 255 mμ and the inflection at about 315 mμ. Measure the difference between the maximum absorption at 298 mμ and the baseline at this wavelength. Let this value be E corr.

$$\frac{\text{mg of } \alpha\text{-tocopheryl acetate}}{\text{in 30 ml of the sample}} = \frac{E \text{ corr.}}{E \text{ std.}} \times \frac{(V)}{100} \times 1000$$

where E std. is the corrected E(1 per cent, 1 cm) at 298 mμ for pure α-tocopheryl acetate (*i.e.* 72·2) which has been saponified and extracted as above.

1. EMMERIE, A., and ENGEL, C., *Rec. Trav. Chim.*, 1938, **57**, 1351.
2. *Analyst*, 1959, **84**, 356.
3. MARCINKIEWICZ, S., and GREEN, J., *Analyst*, 1959, **84**, 304.

ZINC

Zn At. Wt. 65·37

The determination of zinc in pharmaceutical preparations may be carried out in a number of ways. In general, the use of EDTA (see below) is superseding most other methods but there may be occasions when alternative methods are useful and these are given in detail.

(i) When present as the oxide, which is basic, zinc may be titrated with acid; the sample is dissolved in excess of N hydrochloric or sulphuric acid and back-titrated to methyl red or to methyl orange. With the latter indicator the addition of 2·5 g of sodium chloride or ammonium chloride before titration sharpens the end-point considerably. 1 ml N acid = 0·04069 g ZnO.

(ii) The determination of zinc oxide in many pharmaceutical preparations can be carried out by simple ignition. Although such a procedure is often criticised because of the possibility of volatilisation of zinc metal produced by reduction during the carbonisation of organic matter, no appreciable loss occurs when the ignition is carried out at the temperature of the ordinary Bunsen flame.

Gently ignite a suitable weight of the sample until the basis is completely volatilised or charred, taking precautions against loss by decrepitation, increase the heat until the carbon is removed and ignite the residue of zinc oxide to constant weight. 1 g of residue = 0·8034 g Zn.

The residue so obtained may be titrated acidimetrically (see (i), above) or with EDTA (see (viii), below), but this is only necessary when other inorganic matter remains in the residue as, for example, in the case of Cream of Zinc and Ichthammol.

(iii) By precipitation from a hot solution with a minimum excess of sodium carbonate.

Heat an approximately neutral solution, containing between 0·2 and 1·0 g of zinc in about 100 ml of water, to about 90° and add, dropwise, just sufficient of a 10 per cent solution of sodium carbonate decahydrate to precipitate all the zinc (a large excess of carbonate should be avoided). Boil for about five minutes, allow to stand until the precipitate has settled and filter quantitatively through a tared Gooch crucible. Wash the precipitate with water until free from alkali and then dry the residue and ignite to constant weight as zinc oxide. ZnO × 1·675 = $ZnCl_2$; × 1·984 = $ZnSO_4$; × 3·534 = $ZnSO_4,7H_2O$; × 5·059 = $C_{12}H_{10}O_8S_2Zn$ (zinc phenolsulphonate).

(iv) By titration as ferrocyanide. The only metals which interfere with the ferrocyanide titration and are likely to be met with in pharmaceutical practice are lead, copper and iron; the latter has no effect if only present in very small amount. Titration may be carried out directly on the ammoniacal filtrate after precipitation of iron; if much iron is present, reprecipitation is necessary, the filtrates from the reprecipitation being added to the main bulk of liquid. Formerly the end-point of this reaction was determined with an external indicator such as uranyl acetate which gives a light-brown colour when excess of ferrocyanide is present; indeed, some workers still prefer to use such an external indicator. More commonly nowadays, however, an internal oxidation-reduction indicator such as diphenylbenzidine, sodium diphenylamine sulphonate or 3,3′-dimethylnaphthidine is used. These rely upon the ratio of ferrocyanide to ferricyanide in the solution; the titrant used is an approximately 0·05M ferrocyanide solution which is also about 0·001M with respect to ferricyanide. While an excess of zinc is present in solution all the ferrocyanide is used and the ratio of ferricyanide to ferrocyanide is high. As soon as the end-point is reached, however, this position is reversed and there is a sudden decrease in the oxidation potential. If such an end-point indication as this is to be used, of course, it is essential that both reducing and oxidising agents should be absent.

The following details are based on those given by Richardson and Bryson.[1]

> Prepare the 0·05M potassium ferrocyanide by dissolving 21·12 g of potassium ferrocyanide trihydrate and 0·3 g of potassium ferricyanide in water free from carbon dioxide and making up to 1 litre. Take a volume of sample solution such that the concentration of zinc at the end-point will be at least 0·4 mg per ml and add sufficient sulphuric acid to give an acidity of 1·7 to 2·1N at the end-point, sufficient ammonium sulphate to give a concentration of 1 to 2 g per 100 ml at the end-point and 2 to 4 drops of a 1 per cent solution of diphenylbenzidine in concentrated sulphuric acid per 100 ml. Titrate at room temperature with the 0·05M potassium ferrocyanide solution until the colour change from purple to yellowish green is permanent. With amounts of zinc below 30 mg the titration should be carried out slowly; the purple colour of the indicator will, as the reaction proceeds, be replaced by a blue which persists until shortly before the true end-point and then fades (the false end-point) but if subsequent titration is carried out dropwise the original purple colour will re-appear and sharply change to yellow-green at the final end-point. With amounts of zinc greater than 30 mg the rate of titration has no effect and it is not necessary to wait for the false end-point to come to completion. Standardise the ferrocyanide solution by repeating the operation described above using, instead of the sample solution, a suitable volume of 0·05M zinc solution prepared by dissolving 14·34 g of analytical-reagent grade zinc sulphate heptahydrate in water and making up to 1 litre.

Nitrates at low concentration have no effect on the above titration, but even small amounts of nitrites give unsatisfactory end-points.

(v) By precipitation as zinc mercuric thiocyanate. Zinc forms with mercury thiocyanate an insoluble precipitate, $ZnHg(SCN)_4$, which can either be weighed after filtering through a sintered-glass crucible, washing and drying at 105°, or titrated by Jamieson's method with potassium iodate.

For the titration method. To 100 ml of a solution containing a maximum of 0·1 g of zinc and not more than 5 per cent of free acid, add 25 ml of a precipitating reagent consisting of 30 g of ammonium thiocyanate and 27 g of mercuric chloride in 1 litre of water. Allow to stand for five minutes, stir briskly and then allow to stand for one hour. Filter through a sintered-glass crucible (porosity No. 3) and wash four or five times with a solution containing 2 per cent of the precipitating reagent. Transfer the washed precipitate to a stoppered bottle or flask of about 300-ml capacity, add a cooled mixture of 35 ml of concentrated hydrochloric acid and 10 ml of water, and titrate at once with standard potassium iodate, using chloroform as indicator, to the disappearance of the violet colour from the chloroform layer. 1 ml 0·2M = 0·002179 g Zn; 0·002713 g ZnO.

For the gravimetric method. Precipitate as above, but allow the reaction mixture to stand for three hours before filtering through a tared sintered-glass crucible and washing as above. Dry the precipitate to constant weight at 105°. Weight of precipitate × 0·1633 = ZnO; × 0·2735 = $ZnCl_2$; × 0·5770 = $ZnSO_4,7H_2O$.

(vi) By precipitation with 8-hydroxyquinoline. This method still finds occasional use although it has now been largely superseded by complexometric titration methods.

To 50 ml of a neutral solution containing 20 to 50 mg of zinc, add 8 ml of dilute acetic acid. Heat to 70° to 90° and, while maintaining at this temperature and stirring continuously, add 10 ml of a solution prepared by dissolving 5 g of oxine (8-hydroxyquinoline) in 12 ml of glacial acetic acid, diluting to 100 ml with water and filtering. Add 15 per cent ammonium acetate solution until a permanent precipitate forms and then add 20 ml of the solution in excess. (If a permanent precipitate is already present after the addition of oxine, add only 20 ml of the ammonium acetate solution.) Heat at just below the boiling-point for five minutes, stirring gently, allow to stand for one hour and filter through a tared sintered-glass crucible (porosity No. 4). Wash the precipitate with water and dry to constant weight at 130°. Weight of precipitate × 0·2303 = ZnO.

Under the conditions given above, zinc may be separated from aluminium and magnesium which form oxinates soluble in glacial acetic acid. The drying temperature of 130° is necessary to volatilise co-precipitated reagent.

(vii) By precipitation as zinc ammonium phosphate. The classic version of this method finishes with an ignition of the residue to pyrophosphate, but satisfactory results may be obtained by weighing as the ammonium phosphate provided that strict attention is paid to detail. The method still finds occasional use in pharmaceutical analysis although it is of limited application because of the many elements which form sparingly soluble phosphates.

To 140 ml of a neutral solution containing about 0·08 g of Zn or 0·1 g of ZnO, add 10 ml of 2M sodium acetate and 5 g of ammonium chloride and heat on a water-bath. Then add, dropwise and with continuous stirring, 10 ml of a 10 per cent ammonium phosphate solution and continue to heat on a water-bath for two hours. Filter through a tared sintered-glass crucible (porosity No. 4), wash the precipitate first with 150 ml of water and then with 5 ml of 95 per cent ethanol and dry to constant weight at 105°. Weight of precipitate × 0·4561 = ZnO.

(viii) By titration with EDTA. Zinc forms a strong complex with EDTA and may be titrated under both slightly acid (acetate buffer or at pH 5 to 6 in the presence of hexamine) and alkaline (ammonia buffer) conditions. Either method of titration is very satisfactory and in many cases both are equally applicable; in some cases, however, a particular system may be chosen to avoid interference from another metal. For example, zinc may be titrated at pH 5 in the presence of magnesium which does not form a complex under these conditions; on the other hand at pH 10, and in the presence of triethanolamine, zinc may be titrated without interference from aluminium. Many versions of these methods are available, using different buffer conditions and indicators, but the following have proved themselves reliable, rapid and accurate when applied to a wide range of pharmaceutical products.

(*a*) To an approximately neutral solution containing about 0·08 g of zinc add 10 ml of ammonia buffer solution (see Appendix II) and 0·5 ml of solochrome black indicator and titrate with 0·05M EDTA to the full blue colour of the indicator.

(*b*) To a solution containing about 0·08 g of zinc at a pH of approximately 6·0 add 3 g of hexamine followed by 4 drops of xylenol orange indicator and titrate with 0·05M EDTA to the bright yellow colour.

1 ml 0·05M = 0·004069 g ZnO; 0·006815 g $ZnCl_2$; 0·01438 g $ZnSO_4,7H_2O$.

(ix) Zinc is conveniently determined by atomic absorption techniques. The resonance line is at 2139A and according to David[2] the concentration range over which measurements can usefully be made is 0·1 to 100 p.p.m., depending on the length of flame through which the light from the hollow cathode source passes (see p. 873). The method is convenient and rapid and no serious interferences have been reported to date.

Although for the assay of zinc salts and preparations below alternative methods are given, in almost every case an EDTA titration may be used with advantage because of its speed, accuracy and convenience.

Sylvester and Hughes[3] published a comparatively rapid method for the determination of **small amounts** of zinc. Diphenylthiocarbazone in chloroform will extract zinc, copper, mercury, silver, bismuth and cadmium from a solution buffered with ammonium acetate at about pH 4·5. From this extract zinc, bismuth and cadmium are removed with dilute hydrochloric acid (silver is precipitated as chloride). The extracted zinc can be titrated by a micro-method based on Lang's process,[4] in which zinc, in the presence of potassium ferricyanide, liberates an equivalent amount of iodine from potassium iodide. The method is specific for zinc and is not affected by any other of the metals which are extracted with it; it is recommended for amounts up to 0·3 mg. Ashing the sample at 500° to 550° causes no loss of zinc and saves considerable time as compared with wet combustion (see Appendix XI). This method has proved reliable and is comparatively easily manipulated.

If organic matter is present, ash the material, containing preferably between 0·1 and 1·0 mg of zinc, in a silica dish in a muffle-furnace at 500° to 550°, until a carbon-free ash is obtained. Treat the ash with 5 ml of 5N hydrochloric acid, heat to boiling, dilute with 10 ml of water and boil again; ensure complete solution of the ash. Wash the solution into a separator with 20 ml of water and add 10 ml of 5N ammonium acetate. Shake vigorously with 5 ml of 0·15 per cent diphenylthiocarbazone in chloroform and allow to separate. Wash the extract with a mixture of 6 ml of 5N ammonium acetate, 3 ml of 5N hydrochloric acid and 10 ml of water, and then with 20 ml of water. Repeat the extraction of the original solution with 5-ml portions of diphenylthiocarbazone solution until the liquid is completely extracted, as indicated by the colour of the reagent appearing unchanged after shaking. Wash the chloroform layers with the same wash liquors as the first extraction and bulk the chloroform in a fourth separator. Shake the combined extracts with 10 ml of 0·5N hydrochloric acid, run off the chloroform layer and transfer the acid solution to a small Pyrex beaker. Wash the separator with about 10 ml of water, adding the washings to the contents of the beaker. Repeat the extraction of the chloroform layer and the washing of the separator as before, adding the acid extract and the washings to the liquid in the beaker. Evaporate the aqueous liquid to dryness. Add five drops of perchloric acid and five drops of 30 per cent hydrogen peroxide solution and take to dryness on a hot-plate. Repeat this treatment until all organic matter is destroyed and a white residue is obtained. Wash down the sides of the beaker, if necessary take an aliquot part, and again evaporate to dryness.

To an amount containing less than 0·3 mg of zinc, add 0·1 ml of glacial acetic acid and about 0·01 g of ammonium hydrogen fluoride, followed by 2 ml of 5 per cent potassium iodide solution and 2 drops of 1 per cent starch solution. If a blue colour appears after the addition of the starch, add 0·002N sodium thiosulphate until the colour is just discharged. Add about 0·5 ml of freshly prepared 1 per cent potassium ferricyanide solution, and, stirring with a glass rod, titrate with freshly prepared 0·002N sodium thiosulphate. The blue starch-iodide colour may be adsorbed on the precipitated zinc ferrocyanide, and in this case the precipitate serves as an indicator (0·51 ml of 0·002N thiosulphate = 0·10 mg of zinc).

The titration is preferably carried out by artificial light; the blue starch-iodide colour returns after a few minutes, but this should be ignored.

ZINC

Colorimetric methods depending on the use of diphenylthiocarbazone have been developed for the determination of traces of zinc and the following method, recommended by the Analytical Methods Committee of the *S.A.C.*,[5] is of sufficient accuracy for most purposes although a reference method[6] has also been published. After the destruction of organic matter zinc is determined volumetrically by titration with standard dithizone solution at pH 4·2. With feeding-stuffs sufficient accuracy may be obtained by this method which aims at eliminating the troublesome blank and avoids the purification of reagents. Reagents tend to pick up metallic contamination from bottles on storage.

Destroy the organic matter by dry ashing, method A (see Appendix XI). When all the organic matter has been destroyed, cool the basin and contents, add 10 ml of hydrochloric acid (1 + 1 v/v) and evaporate to dryness on a water-bath. Extract the soluble salts with two 10-ml quantities of boiling hydrochloric acid (1 + 5 v/v), decanting the solution each time through the same Whatman No. 541 filter paper into a 50-ml graduated flask. Then add 5 ml of hydrochloric acid (1 + 1 v/v) and about 5 ml of nitric acid (1 + 2 v/v) to the residue in the basin and evaporate to dryness on a hot-plate at low heat to remove all the nitric acid. Finally extract the residue with a further 10 ml of boiling hydrochloric acid (1 + 5 v/v) and filter the solution through the same filter paper into the graduated flask. Dilute the combined extracts to volume with water, washing the filter paper in the process. This final solution should be approximately normal with respect to hydrochloric acid.

Transfer a suitable volume of the acid solution (containing not more than 100 μg of zinc) to a 150-ml separator (A). Into a second separator (B) pipette 2 ml of 50 per cent citric acid solution, neutralise to litmus paper with strong ammonia solution (usually about 1 ml) and add 3 drops of the ammonia in excess. Extract with 5 ml of dithizone solution (approximately 0·01 per cent of diphenylthiocarbazone in carbon tetrachloride; 100 μg of zinc should require about 20 to 25 ml for titration as described below) and reject the carbon tetrachloride layer. Add the aqueous layer to separator (A) and test for alkalinity. Rinse separator (B) with water, add to separator (A) and then add about 10 ml of the dithizone solution and shake vigorously. Allow to separate and run the lower layer into separator (B). Continue to extract the aqueous solution in separator (A) with 5-ml quantities of the dithizone solution until the lower layer remains green, adding the lower layer each time to separator (B). To this extract add 5 ml of 0·02N hydrochloric acid and shake for one minute. If the dithizone layer is not green add 2-ml quantities of the acid until the dithizone layer remains green after shaking. Run the carbon tetrachloride layer into a third separator and re-extract with 3 ml of 0·02N hydrochloric acid. Add the acid layer to the acid solution in separator (B) and wash with 2 ml of carbon tetrachloride. Discard the lower layer.

In a clean separator mix 5 ml of acetate buffer (prepared by dissolving 27·2 g of sodium acetate trihydrate in water, adding 12 ml of glacial acetic acid and diluting to 200 ml with water) with 1 ml of 25 per cent sodium thiosulphate solution and extract with about 3 ml of dithizone solution. Run off the lower layer and wash the aqueous layer with 3 ml of carbon tetrachloride, discarding the washing. Add the aqueous layer to the contents of separator (B). (The pH should be between 4·0 and 4·5; if it is not make the necessary adjustment.) Titrate with the dithizone solution by adding decreasing amounts, shaking for one minute and running off the lower layer each time, until the dithizone layer remains green. The amount of dithizone solution to add for each successive extraction depends on the speed with which the previous extraction turns red. (With 100 μg of zinc convenient portions might be 15 ml, then 5 ml and then 1 ml.) Note the total volume used ('*a*' ml) and then make a final extraction with 3 ml of dithizone solution, which should remain green. Run off the lower layer and discard.

Wash the aqueous layer with 3 ml of carbon tetrachloride, discard the washing and add exactly 10 ml of standard zinc solution (prepared by dissolving 0·044 g of zinc sulphate heptahydrate in 50 ml of 0·01N sulphuric acid and diluting to 1 litre with water; this solution contains 10 μg of Zn per ml). Repeat the titration with the dithizone solution as described above. Let the ml of dithizone solution required be '*b*.'

Then the μg of zinc in the weight of sample taken is $\frac{100\,a}{b}$.

'*a*' should not differ from '*b*' by more than 20 per cent.

Alternatively, for amounts of zinc up to 10 p.p.m., the following method, with a spectrophotometric finish, may be used.

In this method the dithizone solution must be purified immediately before use as follows: Extract 10 ml of a stock solution (0·1 per cent of diphenylthiocarbazone in redistilled carbon tetrachloride) with two 50-ml portions of a solution prepared by diluting 4 ml of 10M ammonium hydroxide to 100 ml with water. Reject the lower layer and, if necessary, filter the combined ammoniacal extracts. Acidify the combined extracts with 1 per cent hydrochloric acid and extract the precipitated dithizone with 100 ml of carbon tetrachloride. Wash the extract with two 10-ml quantities of water and filter the carbon tetrachloride solution through a dry filter paper.

Method: Proceed as described in the above method to the end of the titration of the test solution with dithizone, retaining the lower layers run off after each addition of dithizone solution in the titration. To the combined dithizone extracts add 10 ml of 0·04 per cent sodium sulphide solution and shake for ten seconds to remove excess dithizone. Allow the layers to separate and run the lower layer into a clean separator (C). Wash the aqueous layer in separator (B) with 1 ml of carbon tetrachloride and add this washing to the main solution in separator (C). Extract the carbon tetrachloride solution with further 10-ml quantities of 0·04 per cent sodium sulphide solution until the aqueous layer is no longer yellow. Shake the carbon tetrachloride layer with 1 g of anhydrous sodium sulphate and filter through a dry 9-cm Whatman No. 41 filter paper into a 25-ml graduated flask. Wash the separator and filter paper with a few millilitres of carbon tetrachloride, adding the washings to the solution in the flask, and dilute to volume with carbon tetrachloride. Dilute the solution further with carbon tetrachloride to give a solution with an extinction within the normal range for measurement.

Repeat the entire operation omitting the sample to obtain a blank solution.

Measure the extinctions of the sample and blank solutions at 532 mμ, using 1-cm cells with carbon tetrachloride in the comparison cell in each case. Read the number of microgrammes of zinc equivalent to the observed extinctions of the sample and blank solutions from a standard curve and so obtain the net amount of zinc in the sample.

Preparation of standard curve: Measure suitable amounts of standard zinc solution 10 μg per ml (for preparation, see above method), covering the range 0 to 100 μg of zinc, into a series of separators (B). Extract the zinc in each as described for the test solution, beginning with 'In a clean separator mix 5 ml of acetate buffer . . .', taking care that the treatment with sodium sulphide is exactly the same as in the test, *i.e.* duration of shaking, etc. Measure the extinctions using 1-cm cells and prepare a curve relating extinctions to the number of microgrammes of zinc.

ZINC SALTS

The following zinc salts are of pharmaceutical interest:

TABLE 39

	FORMULA	MOL. WT.	OFFICIAL ASSAY	ALTERNATIVE METHODS
Zinc chloride, *B.P.C.*	$ZnCl_2$	136·3	(v), 0·2 g	(viii)(*a*), 2 g, 5 ml dil. HCl to 100 ml, take 10 ml; (iii), 1 g
Zinc oxide, *B.P.*	ZnO	81·38	(i)	(viii) (*a*), after soln. in HCl
Zinc phenol-sulphonate, *N.F.*	$C_{12}H_{10}O_8S_2Zn,8H_2O$	555·9	(iii), 2 g	
Zinc sulphate, *B.P. U.S.P.*	$ZnSO_4,7H_2O$	287·6	(v), 0·5 g (iii), 1 g	(viii)(*b*), 0·5 g

Zinc stearate, *B.P.*, a zinc soap, and **zinc undecenoate,** *B.P.*, $C_{22}H_{38}O_4Zn$, Mol. Wt. 431·9, can both be assayed by boiling 1 g with an excess of 0·1N hydrochloric acid for ten minutes, filtering and washing, the excess of acid being titrated in the total filtrate and washings with 0·1N sodium hydroxide to methyl red. 1 ml 0·1N acid = 0·004069 g ZnO. Alternatively the combined filtrate and washings can be neutralised with dilute ammonia solution, 3 ml of dilute hydrochloric acid added and the zinc determined by method (viii) (*b*) above. 1 ml 0·05M = 0·004069 g ZnO and 0·02160 g $C_{22}H_{38}O_4Zn$.

Calamine was originally a native basic zinc carbonate containing iron and siliceous matter, but it is now almost entirely manufactured from precipitated zinc carbonate and zinc oxide. For a complete analysis, the loss at 105°, residue on ignition, carbon dioxide, hydrochloric acid-insoluble matter, iron, and total zinc by ferrocyanide titration should be determined. Calcium carbonate is a common adulterant, magnesium carbonate and oxide have also been found in place of the zinc.

The following preparations can all be assayed for zinc oxide by direct ignition (method (ii) above).

TABLE 40

	ZnO %	WEIGHT OF SAMPLE TAKEN
Compound Application of Calamine, *B.P.C.*	11·8	0·5 g
Cream of Calamine*	5·8	4 g
Cream of Zinc, *B.P.**	32	0·5 g
Oily Lotion of Calamine	3·55	2 g
†Compound Ointment of Benzocaine	6·75	4 g
Ointment of Calamine*	11·8	1 g
Compound Ointment of Calamine*	21·4	1 g
Ointment of Zinc, *B.P.**	15	0·5 g
Ointment of Zinc and Castor Oil, *B.P.**	7·5	0·5 g
‡Paste of Coal Tar, *B.P.C.*	23·2	1 g
Paste of Resorcinol and Sulphur, *B.P.C.*	37·5	0·5 g
Compound Paste of Zinc, *B.P.**	25·0	1 g
‡Paste of Zinc and Coal Tar, *B.P.C.*	6·25	4 g
Paste of Zinc and Salicylic Acid, *B.P.**	24·0	1 g

* Alternatively the zinc may be determined directly as follows:

To a quantity equivalent to about 0·1 g of zinc oxide add 20 ml of ether, 2 ml of industrial methylated spirit and 2 ml of dilute hydrochloric acid. Warm to dissolve the fatty basis, shake well for about five minutes and dilute to about 200 ml with water. Complete by method (viii) (*a*). 1 ml 0·05M EDTA ≡ 0·004069 g ZnO.

† For benzocaine, see p. 189.

‡ Paste of Coal Tar and Paste of Zinc and Coal Tar cannot be assayed by direct titration with EDTA. In preparations containing coal tar the sample must be ignited until all the carbon is destroyed; the residue is then dissolved in dilute hydrochloric acid and the solution neutralised before titrating with EDTA as in method (viii) (*a*).

Cream of Zinc and Ichthammol, *B.P.C.* Contains 26·2 per cent of zinc oxide.

The ichthammol interferes with a direct ignition because it yields an inorganic residue.

In the *B.P.C.* the zinc oxide is assayed by gently igniting about 0·7 g, dissolving the cooled residue in dilute sulphuric acid, adding 40 ml of water and (after filtering if necessary and washing the filter with water) making just alkaline to litmus paper with dilute ammonia solution and then just acid with dilute sulphuric acid. After diluting to 100 ml with water the assay is completed by method (v) from the addition of the mercuric ammonium thiocyanate.

Another method is to dry and gently ignite about 0·4 g, dissolve the cooled residue in about 10 ml of dilute sulphuric acid, add 40 ml of water and adjust to pH 10 with dilute ammonia solution, completing by method (viii) (*a*).

Dusting-powder of Alum and Zinc for Infants, *B.P.C.* Zinc oxide 40 per cent and potash alum 20 per cent with talc.

Alum interferes with the direct titration of zinc with EDTA. Triethanolamine has been used to mask aluminium in the determination of magnesium by complexometric titration[7] and a similar method is used in the *B.P.C.* for the determination of zinc oxide in this preparation.

> To a weight of sample equivalent to about 0·1 g of zinc oxide, add 10 ml of water and 10 ml of N sulphuric acid and shake until dissolution is as complete as possible. Add 0·5 g of ammonium chloride and a slight excess of dilute ammonia solution and then add sufficient triethanolamine so that the precipitate which first forms redissolves and add a further 3 ml. Dilute to about 200 ml with water and complete by method (viii) (*a*) above from the addition of the ammonia buffer solution. 1 ml 0·05M EDTA = 0·004069 g ZnO.

Potash alum may be determined as sulphate after dissolving in dilute hydrochloric acid and filtering from the talc. $BaSO_4 \times 0{\cdot}553 = KAl(SO_4)_2$. But see also under Aluminium (p. 35).

Compound Dusting-powder of Zinc, *B.P.C.* Zinc oxide 25 per cent and boric acid 5 per cent with starch and talc.

The zinc oxide may be determined by extracting the zinc by boiling about 1·5 g with dilute hydrochloric acid, filtering, washing and completing by method (iii) on the filtrate and washings, or better by EDTA titration:

> Boil 4 g for two minutes with 50 ml of water and 20 ml of 5N nitric acid, cool and filter quantitatively through a Whatman No. 41 filter paper into a 200-ml graduated flask, washing the filter with water. Dilute the combined filtrate and washings to volume with water. Dilute a 20-ml aliquot of this solution to about 100 ml with water and complete by method (viii) (*b*). 1 ml 0·05M EDTA = 0·004069 g ZnO.

For boric acid, see p. 135.

Dusting-powder of Zinc and Salicylic Acid, *B.P.C.* Zinc oxide, 20 per cent, and salicylic acid, 5 per cent, with starch.

Some combination between zinc oxide and salicylic acid may occur in the presence of moisture and low results are obtained if the salicylic acid is titrated directly. Mitchell[8] recommends extraction of the salicylic acid with ether after acidification and titrating after evaporation of the solvent. The zinc oxide may be determined by direct ignition on the aqueous solution remaining after extraction of salicyclic acid, by method (i) above or complexometrically by the method given for Dusting-powder of Alum and Zinc for Infants, omitting the addition of triethanolamine.

Dusting-powder of Zinc, Starch and Talc, *B.P.C.* 25 per cent of zinc oxide with starch and talc.

This preparation may be assayed by the methods given under Compound Dusting-powder of Zinc.

Dusting-powder of Zinc Undecenoate, *B.P.C.* Contains 10 per cent of zinc undecenoate with undecenoic acid, pine oil, starch and kaolin.

Although the official method is to extract the zinc undecenoate with hot chloroform, which is evaporated and the residue ignited to zinc oxide, quantitative recoveries could not be obtained either by this method or by complexometric titration.

The *B.P.C.* eye-drops and eye lotions are simple solutions of zinc sulphate with one or more of the following substances: sodium chloride, adrenaline solution, chlorbutol and boric acid. None of these substances interferes with the assay of zinc sulphate by EDTA titration, method (viii) (*a*), 1 ml 0·02M EDTA = 0·00575 g $ZnSO_4,7H_2O$; adrenaline solution tends to mask the end-point but the amount present in these preparations is not sufficient to prevent the end-point being readily detected. For titration take 30 ml of **Eye-drops of Zinc Sulphate,** *B.P.C.* (0·25 per cent), 30 ml of **Eye-drops of Zinc Sulphate and Adrenaline,** *B.P.C.* (0·25 per cent), and 50 ml of **Compound Eye Lotion of Zinc Sulphate,** *B.P.C.* (0·34 per cent with 2·29 per cent of boric acid); if boric acid is to be determined in the last-mentioned preparation, the zinc must first be precipitated with sodium carbonate (see p. 134).

Gelatin of Zinc, *B.P.* (Unna's Paste). Zinc oxide and gelatin, 15 per cent each, with glycerin, 35 per cent w/w and water.

Zinc oxide may be determined using 4 g by method (i) above after warming with 25 ml of water until the base is dissolved and cooling. Methyl orange-xylene cyanol FF indicator is an improvement on methyl orange.

The zinc can also be determined by method (viii) (*a*) using 0·5 g after dissolving in 20 ml of warm water and 2 ml of dilute hydrochloric acid and diluting to about 200 ml with water.

Gelatin can be estimated approximately from a nitrogen figure by the Kjeldahl method (× 6·25 = gelatin), using 1·5 g of paste. For glycerol:

Dissolve about 20 g in a small quantity of hot water in a beaker, precipitate by adding a considerable bulk of ethanol, the gelatin and zinc oxide coagulating on the sides of the beaker. Pour off the ethanol, repeat the solution and precipitation of the gelatin, bulk the ethanol, allow to stand and then filter through cotton wool. Evaporate the ethanol after adding water and make up to 25 ml. Filter if necessary, take the specific gravity of the solution and calculate the percentage of glycerol from the table given in Appendix XX.

Gelatin of Zinc and Ichthammol, *B.P.C.* Contains 15 per cent of zinc oxide.

The zinc can be assayed by the method given above under Cream of Zinc and Ichthammol or by complexometric titration as given under Gelatin of Zinc.

Lotion of Zinc Sulphate, *B.P.C.* Contains 1 per cent of zinc sulphate.

For determination of zinc, either dilute 25 ml with 100 ml of water, add 1 ml of 0·1N sulphuric acid and complete by method (v), weighing the residue, wt. × 0·5770 = $ZnSO_4,7H_2O$, or assay by method (viii) (*a*) using 30 ml; since the lotion contains amaranth the colour change at the end-point is from red to purple.

Mouth-wash of Zinc Sulphate and Zinc Chloride, *B.P.C.* Contains 2·29 per cent of zinc sulphate and 1·14 per cent of zinc chloride.

The official method of assay is to dilute 5 ml with 100 ml of water, acidified with 0·1 ml of dilute sulphuric acid, and complete by method (v), titrating with 0·2M KIO_3 and calculating the percentage as Zn. 1 ml 0·2M = 0·002179 g Zn. It can also be assayed by method (viii) (*a*) using 10 ml; since the preparation contains tartrazine the colour change at the end-point is from red to green.

Compound Ointment of Resorcinol, *B.P.C.* Contains 4 per cent of zinc oxide.

The zinc in this ointment is best determined by complexometric titration after removal of the bismuth, as follows:

> Gently ignite about 6 g in a silica dish to destroy the fat, and then ignite more strongly, but at a temperature not exceeding 500°, until all the carbon is destroyed. Dissolve the residue in a mixture of 5 ml of concentrated nitric acid and 10 ml of water and dilute to 50 ml with water in a graduated flask. To a 10-ml aliquot of this solution add 2 ml of dilute hydrochloric acid and 150 ml of water and then make just alkaline to litmus with dilute ammonia solution. Boil for two minutes, cool to 15°, filter, wash the residue with water and dilute the combined filtrate and washings to 250 ml with water in a graduated flask. Determine the zinc by method (viii) (*a*) using a 50-ml aliquot of this solution diluted to about 100 ml with water. 1 ml 0·05M EDTA = 0·004069 g ZnO.
>
> The bismuth can be determined by complexometric titration on a further 20 ml of the acid solution prepared above (see p. 127).

Ointment of Zinc Undecenoate, *B.P.* Contains 20 per cent of zinc undecenoate.

The zinc can be determined by method (i) after dissolving the fatty base in 20 ml of chloroform. 1 ml N sulphuric acid = 0·2160 g $C_{22}H_{38}O_4Zn$. A better method is:

> Reflux 2 g with 20 ml of dilute hydrochloric acid for at least twenty minutes or until the fatty layer is clear, filter, and wash the residue with hot water. Cool the combined filtrate and washings, neutralise to litmus paper with dilute ammonia, add 3 ml of dilute hydrochloric acid, 5 g of hexamine and 0·4 ml of xylenol orange indicator and titrate with 0·05M EDTA to the bright yellow colour of the indicator. 1 ml 0·05M = 0·02160 g $C_{22}H_{38}O_4Zn$.

Compound Paste of Aluminium, *B.P.C.* Contains 40 per cent of zinc oxide and 20 per cent of powdered aluminium in a paraffin base.

Both the zinc and aluminium may be determined by EDTA titration as follows:

Stir 1 g with 20 ml of chloroform in a 150-ml beaker and decant the chloroform through a filter paper. Repeat this operation four or five times, discard the chloroform washings and transfer the filter paper to the beaker. Dissolve the solid residue in hydrochloric acid (1 + 1), warming on a water-bath to assist solution. Filter into a 100-ml graduated flask, wash the beaker and filter paper with water and dilute the combined filtrate and washings to volume with water.

Transfer a 20-ml aliquot of this solution to a flask, add 1 g of ammonium chloride and sufficient triethanolamine to dissolve the precipitate that first forms (usually 25 to 40 ml) and then add 200 ml of water, 5 ml of ammonia buffer solution and sufficient solochrome black to give a full red colour. Titrate immediately with 0·05M EDTA to a full blue colour. 1 ml 0·05M = 0·004069 g ZnO.

The aluminium is determined on a 10-ml aliquot of the acid solution prepared above as follows: Neutralise to congo red paper with 20 per cent sodium hydroxide, add 40 ml of 0·05M EDTA and warm on a water-bath for thirty minutes. Cool, add about 3 g of hexamine and titrate with 0·1N zinc solution to the purple-red end-point of xylenol orange indicator. From the ml 0·05M EDTA absorbed subtract half the ml required in the zinc determination. 1 ml 0·05M EDTA (remainder) = 0·001349 g Al.

The zinc oxide may also be determined by method (i) above after shaking with 30 ml of chloroform to dissolve the fatty material.

Paste of Resorcinol and Sulphur, *B.P.C.* Contains 37·5 per cent of zinc oxide.

For zinc oxide: Warm about 2 g with 10 ml of chloroform until the fatty basis has dissolved, cool, add 25 ml of N sulphuric acid and shake until the residue has dissolved. Titrate the excess acid with N sodium hydroxide to methyl orange after the addition of 1 g of ammonium chloride. 1 ml N acid = 0·04069 g ZnO.

For resorcinol and sulphur, see p. 551.

1. Richardson, M. R., and Bryson, A., *Analyst*, 1953, **78,** 291.
2. David, D. J., *Analyst*, 1960, **85,** 779.
3. Sylvester, N. D., and Hughes, E. B., *Analyst*, 1936, **61,** 734.
4. Lang, R., *Z. Anal. Chem.*, 1929, **79,** 161.
5. Determination of Trace Elements, *S.A.C.*, p. 34.
6. *Analyst*, 1948, **73,** 304.
7. Brookes, H. E., and Johnson, C. A., *J. Pharm. Pharmacol.*, 1955, **7,** 836.
8. Mitchell, J. V., *Pharm. J.*, 1954, **118,** 102.

SYNTHETIC ORGANIC COMPOUNDS

Of recent years there has been a steady decline in the use of drugs from natural sources and a rapid growth in the number of synthetic organic materials. This change in the practice of pharmacy is reflected in the new problems which face the pharmaceutical analyst; it might be thought that the control of 'pure' organic substances of synthetic origin would present few difficulties compared with the examination of natural products where much interfering material might be present. In fact, however, the 'pure' organic substance is likely to be contaminated with small amounts of other materials such as intermediates or products of side-reactions. These other materials will probably be of closely related structure to the main compounds but may have very different, and sometimes undesirable, pharmacological actions. There is little evidence, from an examination of various pharmacopœias, that this problem is, as yet, being dealt with effectively. All too often highly potent substances are controlled by little more than a determination of melting-point together with some non-specific assay such as a non-aqueous titration or a Kjeldahl nitrogen. Such tests as these are possibly of value but only when they are augmented by additional requirements designed to limit the presence of undesirable impurities. In some cases this is being done; it is now, for example, common practice to examine synthetic steroids for the presence of foreign related materials by a paper chromatographic test (see p. 599). Much more remains to be done, however, before the analyst can feel that he has effective control.[1]

In the meantime a variety of methods, mostly of a fairly non-specific nature, are in use for the determination of organic compounds. These methods will be briefly reviewed and an indication given as to some of the compounds to which they can be applied. Where they fall into recognisable groups many organic substances have been dealt with in other sections; the present discussion is largely concerned with the heterogeneous group of compounds which it has not been convenient to classify. In conclusion, methods which might be of increasing importance for the more critical examination of synthetic organic compounds will be considered.

(i) *Non-aqueous titration.* This is perhaps the most frequently used method for determination of organic compounds and is dealt with in detail in Appendix III (p. 792). Basic substances and salts are titrated with perchloric acid in glacial acetic acid and acidic substances with sodium or lithium methoxide or, increasingly, with tetrabutylammonium hydroxide

Table 41

Basic Substances

	FORMULA	MOL. WT.	WEIGHT TO TAKE (G)	EQUIVALENT (G) FOR 1 ML 0·1N
Acepromazine Maleate	$C_{23}H_{26}O_5N_2S$	442·5	0·5	0·04425
Benactyzine Hydrochloride, *B.P.C.*	$C_{20}H_{25}O_3N,HCl$	363·9	0·7	0·03639
Benzhexol Hydrochloride, *B.P.*	$C_{20}H_{31}ON,HCl$	337·9	0·7	0·03379
Benztropine Methanesulphonate,* *N.F.*	$C_{22}H_{29}O_4NS$	403·5	0·06	0·004035 (0·01N)
Bephenium Embonate, *B.Vet.C.*	$C_{57}H_{58}O_8N_2,H_2O$	917·1	1	0·04585
Bephenium Hydroxynaphthoate	$C_{28}H_{29}O_4N$	443·5	1	0·04435
Bisacodyl	$C_{22}H_{19}O_4N$	361·4	0·5	0·03614
Caramiphen Hydrochloride	$C_{18}H_{27}O_2N,HCl$	325·9	0·7	0·03259
Carbachol, *B.P.*	$C_6H_{15}O_2N_2Cl$	182·7	0·4	0·01827
Chlorhexidine Gluconate Solution, *B.P.*	—	—	5 g evaporated to low vol.	0·02245 $C_{22}H_{30}N_{10}Cl_2, 2C_6H_{12}O_7$
Chlorhexidine Hydrochloride, *B.P.*	$C_{22}H_{30}N_{10}Cl_2,2HCl$	578·4	0·4	0·01446
Chlorpromazine Hydrochloride, *B.P.*	$C_{17}H_{19}N_2SCl,HCl$	355·3	0·7	0·03553
Choline Theophyllinate, *B.P.C.*	$C_{12}H_{21}O_3N_5$	283·3	0·8	0·02833
Dequalinium Chloride, *B.P.C.*	$C_{30}H_{40}N_4Cl_2$	527·6	0·7	0·02638
Dicyclomine Hydrochloride, *B.P.C.*	$C_{19}H_{35}O_2N,HCl$	346·0	0·6	0·03460
Diethazine Hydrochloride	$C_{18}H_{22}N_2S,HCl$	334·9	0·7	0·03349
Diethylthiambutene Hydrochloride, *B.Vet.C.*	$C_{16}H_{21}NS_2,HCl$	327·9	0·7	0·03279
Dipipanone Hydrochloride, *B.P.C.*	$C_{24}H_{31}ON,HCl,H_2O$	404·0	0·4	0·03860 $C_{24}H_{32}ONCl$
Edrophonium Chloride	$C_{10}H_{16}ONCl$	201·7	0·6	0·02017
Ethopropazine Hydrochloride, *B.P.*	$C_{19}H_{24}N_2S,HCl$	348·9	0·7	0·03489
Isothipendyl Hydrochloride	$C_{16}H_{19}N_3S,HCl$	321·9	0·3	0·03219
Mepyrium	$C_{14}H_{20}N_4Cl_2$	315·3	0·3	0·03153
Metronidazole	$C_6H_9O_3N_3$	171·2	0·45	0·01712
Orphenadrine Citrate	$C_{18}H_{23}ON,C_6H_8O_7$	461·5	1	0·04615
Orphenadrine Hydrochloride	$C_{18}H_{23}ON,HCl$	305·9	1	0·03059
Pempidine Tartrate	$C_{10}H_{21}N,C_4H_6O_6$	305·4	0·8	0·03054
Perphenazine	$C_{21}H_{26}ON_3ClS$	404·0	0·5	0·02020
Phenazocine Hydrobromide	$C_{22}H_{27}ON,HBr,\frac{1}{2}H_2O$	411·4	0·75	0·04024 $C_{22}H_{27}ON,HBr$
Phenglutarimide Hydrochloride	$C_{17}H_{24}O_2N_2,HCl$	324·9	0·5	0·03249
Phenmetrazine Hydrochloride, *B.P.C.*	$C_{11}H_{15}ON,HCl$	213·7	0·3	0·02137
Pipamazine	$C_{21}H_{24}ON_3ClS$	402·0	0·6	0·04020
Pipradrol Hydrochloride, *B.P.C.*	$C_{18}H_{21}ON,HCl$	303·8	0·5	0·03038
Potassium Gluconate	$C_6H_{11}O_7K$	234·3	0·5	0·02343
Prochlorperazine Ethanedisulphonate,* *U.S.P.*	$C_{20}H_{24}N_3ClS,C_2H_6O_6S_2$	564·2	0·75	0·02821
Prochlorperazine Maleate, *U.S.P.*	$C_{20}H_{24}N_3ClS,2C_4H_4O_4$	606·1	0·6	0·03030
Propantheline Bromide, *B.P.*	$C_{23}H_{30}O_3NBr$	448·4	0·5	0·04484
Propoxyphene Hydrochloride, *U.S.P.*	$C_{22}H_{29}O_2N,HCl$	375·9	0·6	0·03759
Pyridostigmine Bromide, *B.P.*	$C_9H_{13}O_2N_2Br$	261·1	0·85	0·02611
Thiambutosine	$C_{19}H_{25}ON_3S$	343·5	0·7	0·03435
Thiopropazate Hydrochloride	$C_{23}H_{28}O_2N_3ClS,2HCl$	519·0	0·5	0·02595
Trimeprazine Tartrate	$(C_{18}H_{22}N_2S)_2,C_4H_6O_6$	747·0	1	0·03735

* On extracted base.

Non-aqueous Titrations

TABLE 42

ACIDIC SUBSTANCES

	FORMULA	MOL. WT.	WEIGHT TO TAKE (G)	EQUIVALENT (G) FOR 1 ML 0·1N
Bendrofluazide	$C_{15}H_{14}O_4N_3S_2F_3$	421·4	0·4	0·02107
Chlorothiazide, *B.P.*	$C_7H_6O_4N_3ClS_2$	295·7	0·6	0·02957
Diloxanide Furoate	$C_{14}H_{11}O_4NCl_2$	328·2	0·3	0·03282
Diphenylhydantoin, *U.S.P.* (Phenytoin)	$C_{15}H_{12}O_2N_2$	252·3	0·5	0·02523
Disulphamide	$C_7H_9O_4N_2S_2Cl$	284·8	0·2	0·01424
Hydrochlorothiazide, *U.S.P.*	$C_7H_8O_4N_3ClS_2$	297·7	0·3	0·01489
Hydroflumethiazide	$C_8H_8O_4N_3F_3S_2$	331·3	0·3	0·01657

in benzene. Tables 41 and 42 list a number of substances which may be conveniently determined in this way.

(ii) *Kjeldahl nitrogen.* This method, although it is hardly less specific than the non-aqueous titration, is not now used so frequently as formerly. A full consideration of the method has been given on p. 447 and a number of substances to which it is applicable are given in Table 43.

(iii) *Light absorption.* Because of the somewhat imprecise nature of ultra-violet absorption spectrophotometry, due largely to instrumental variation, this method has not been successfully applied to the determination of pure compounds as widely as might be expected. The effect of instrumental variation can be greatly minimised by the use of reference substances which are purified samples of the material under examination and which are treated in the same way so that a comparative, rather than an absolute, response is measured. The *U.S.P.* has a large collection of such reference materials[11] but as yet none has been prepared in the United Kingdom; when official reference substances are freely available the use of light absorption measurements as a criterion of purity may be considerably extended. A list of some substances which may be examined by this technique is given in Table 44 although this could obviously be augmented.

In certain cases, use is made of light absorption measurements at two wavelengths to give a measure of a principal ingredient in the presence of a subsidiary one. Thus, Anthralin, *U.S.P.* (dithranol), is determined by measuring the E(0·001 per cent, 1 cm) at 354 mμ and at 432 mμ and comparing with measurements made on anthralin and dihydroxyanthraquinone reference standards at the same wavelengths.

Nitrogen Assays

TABLE 43

	FORMULA	MOL. WT.	WEIGHT TO TAKE (G)	EQUIVALENT (G) FOR 1 ML 0·1N ACID
Acinitrazole,* *B.Vet.C.*	$C_5H_5O_3N_3S$	187·2	0·23	0·00624
Aminometradine, *B.P.C.*	$C_9H_{13}O_2N_3$	195·2	0·2	0·006508
Aminonitrothiazole,* *B.Vet.C.*	$C_3H_3O_2N_3S$	145·1	0·18	0·004838
Amiphenazole Hydrochloride, *B.P.C.*	$C_9H_{10}N_3SCl$	227·7	0·15	0·007591
Bemegride, *B.P.*	$C_8H_{13}O_2N$	155·2	0·3	0·01552
Bemegride Sodium, *B.Vet.C.*	$C_8H_{12}O_2NNa$	177·2	0·3	0·01772
Chlorpropamide	$C_{10}H_{13}O_3N_2ClS$	276·8	0·3	0·01384
Chlorthalidone	$C_{14}H_{11}O_4N_2ClS$	338·8	0·25	0·01694
Crotamiton, *B.P.C.*	$C_{13}H_{17}ON$	203·3	0·5	0·02033
Dichlorphenamide	$C_6H_6O_4N_2Cl_2S_2$	305·2	0·5	0·01526
Dimidium Bromide, *B.Vet.C.*	$C_{20}H_{18}N_3Br$	380·3	0·3	0·01268
Dinazine Aceturate	$C_{22}H_{29}O_6N_9,4H_2O$	587·6	0·3	0·007365† $C_{22}H_{29}O_6N_9$
Disulfiram, *B.P.C.*	$C_{10}H_{20}N_2S_4$	296·6	0·4	0·01483
Ethotoin	$C_{11}H_{12}O_2N_2$	204·2	0·5	0·01021
Homidium Bromide, *B.Vet.C.*	$C_{21}H_{20}N_3Br$	394·3	0·3	0·01314
Imipramine Hydrochloride	$C_{19}H_{24}N_2,HCl$	316·9	0·25	0·01584
Lucanthone Hydrochloride, *B.P.*	$C_{20}H_{24}ON_2S,HCl$	377·0	0·5	0·01885
Mebhydrolin Naphthalene-disulphonate	$C_{48}H_{48}O_6N_4S_2$	841·1	0·5	0·02103
Meprobamate, *B.P.C.*	$C_9H_{18}O_4N_2$	218·3	0·3	0·01091
Mercaptopurine, *B.P.*	$C_5H_4N_4S,H_2O$	170·2	0·15	0·003805 $C_5H_4N_4S$
Methoin, *B.P.*	$C_{12}H_{14}O_2N_2$	218·3	0·27	0·01091
Monosulfiram, *B.Vet.C.*	$C_{10}H_{20}N_2S_3$	264·5	0·35	0·01322
Paracetamol, *B.P.*	$C_8H_9O_2N$	151·2	0·3	0·01512
Pentamidine Isethionate, *B.P.*	$C_{23}H_{36}O_{10}N_4S_2$	592·7	0·4	0·01482
Phenamidine Isethionate, *B.Vet.C.*	$C_{18}H_{26}O_9N_4S_2$	506·6	0·3	0·01266
Phenothiazine, *B.Vet.C.*	$C_{12}H_9NS$	199·3	0·5	0·01993
Pholedrine Sulphate, *B.Vet.C.*	$C_{20}H_{32}O_6N_2S$	428·5	0·5	0·02143
Primidone, *B.P.*	$C_{12}H_{14}O_2N_2$	218·3	0·2	0·01091
Prochlorperazine Methane-sulphonate	$C_{20}H_{24}N_3SCl,2CH_4O_3S$	566·2	0·6	0·01887
Quinapyramine Chloride, *B.Vet.C.*	$C_{17}H_{22}N_6Cl_2,2H_2O$	417·3	0·2	0·006355 $C_{17}H_{22}N_6Cl_2$
Quinapyramine Sulphate, *B.Vet.C.*	$C_{17}H_{22}N_6,2CH_3SO_4$	532·6	0·25	0·008877
Quinuronium Sulphate, *B.Vet.C.*	$C_{23}H_{26}O_9N_4S_2$	566·6	0·35	0·01417
Urethane, *B.P.*	$C_3H_7O_2N$	89·10	0·2	0·008910

Most of the compounds listed above can be determined by Method A (see p. 449); in some cases (*e.g.* dimidium bromide) it is essential to use potassium rather than sodium sulphate for quantitative decomposition; where the substance is a salt of a halogen acid it should be heated for fifteen minutes with the nitrogen-free concentrated sulphuric acid before addition of the mercury.

* By Dickinson's method (see p. 451).

† Only 7 nitrogen atoms are converted to ammonia on decomposition.

Light Absorption

TABLE 44

	FORMULA	MOL. WT.	SOLVENT	mμ	$E^{1\%}_{1cm}$
Acetazolamide, *B.P.*	$C_4H_6O_3N_4S_2$	222·3	0·1N HCl	265	474
Acetazolamide Sodium, *U.S.P.*	$C_4H_5O_3N_4S_2Na$	244·2	0·1N HCl	265	
Benoxinate Hydrochloride, *U.S.P.*	$C_{17}H_{28}O_3N_2,HCl$	344·9	Water	308	430
Benzthiazide	$C_{15}H_{14}O_4N_3S_3Cl$	432·0	0·01N ethanolic HCl	283	284
Carbimazole, *B.P.*	$C_7H_{10}O_2N_2S$	186·2	0·1N HCl	291	557
Cyclocoumarol, *B.P.C.*	$C_{20}H_{18}O_4$	322·4	Dehydrated ethanol	282	396
Cyclomethycaine Sulphate	$C_{22}H_{33}O_3N,H_2SO_4$	457·6	0·01N HCl	261	400
Dithiazanine Iodide	$C_{23}H_{23}N_2IS_2$	518·5	0·2% v/v dimethylformamide in methanol	652	4,800
Furazolidone, *B.Vet.C.*	$C_8H_7O_5N_3$	225·2	2% v/v glac. acet. acid and 1% v/v pyridine in water	367	746
Hydroxystilbamidine Isethionate, *U.S.P.*	$C_{20}H_{28}O_9N_4S_2$	532·6	0·01N HCl	344	530
Nicarbazin, *B.Vet.C.*	$C_{19}H_{18}O_6N_6$	426·4	5% v/v dimethylformamide in 95% ethanol	345	885
Nitrofurantoin	$C_8H_6O_5N_4$	238·2	1% v/v dimethylformamide in sod. acetate/acetic acid buffer*	367	765
Nitrofurazone, *B.P.C.*	$C_6H_6O_4N_4$	198·1	0·5% 95% ethanol in water	375	810
Phenoxybenzamine Hydrochloride	$C_{18}H_{22}ONCl,HCl$	340·3	$CHCl_3$	272	56·3
Piperonyl Butoxide	$C_{19}H_{30}O_5$	338·4	Dehydrated ethanol	290	130
Sodium Anoxynaphthonate	$C_{26}H_{16}O_{10}N_3S_3Na_3$	695·6	Buffer solution, pH 7·4†	570	555
Warfarin Sodium	$C_{19}H_{15}O_4Na$	330·3	0·01N NaOH	308	430

* Sod. acetate/acetic acid buffer. Dissolve 18 g hydrated sod. acetate and 1·4 ml glac. acet. acid in sufficient water to produce 1 litre (pH of solution should be 5·6).

† Buffer solution pH 7·4. Dissolve 7·6 g sod. phosphate and 1·81 g pot. dihydrogen phosphate in sufficient water to produce 1 litre.

Quantitative application of infra-red measurements is similarly limited by the lack of suitable reference standards. Diethyltoluamide is examined for content of meta isomer by making E(10 per cent, 0·1 mm) measurements in carbon disulphide at 14·1μ and 14·5μ and comparing with *U.S.P.* Reference Standard material.

(iv) *Base extraction.* The principle of the extraction of a base liberated from its salt into an organic solvent is used considerably in pharmaceutical analytical work. Exact details of the method such as choice of solvent and alkali, number and volume of extractions, etc., may vary considerably. Sometimes this variation is justifiable on scientific grounds; in other cases it may be due to lack of correlation between laboratories and indicates the fairly wide deviation from conditions laid down which is often tolerable in this type of method.

Some considerations that might guide the choice of organic solvent for an extraction method of this type are:

(*a*) The nature of the base being extracted and in particular its partition coefficient between the aqueous layer and the organic solvent.

(*b*) The nature of possible impurities and other substances which might be present; obviously it is desirable to choose a solvent which will minimise their extraction.

(*c*) The physical requirements of the method; in some cases it may be more desirable to have the liberated base extracted into the upper layer, rather than the lower.

(*d*) The boiling-point of the solvent; this may be of importance if the liberated base is heat-labile.

In general, chloroform is the most efficient solvent for organic bases (with notable exceptions as, for example, in the case of morphine). Naturally, however, it shows little selectivity. Two disadvantages of chloroform are its readiness to form emulsions (more often encountered when examining natural products rather than synthetics) (see p. 887) and its possible decomposition to yield hydrochloric acid.

Ether is not such a good solvent as chloroform but it is often more selective and its low boiling-point makes it useful in dealing with heat-labile materials. However, the tendency of peroxides to form in ether constitutes a hazard because of the danger of explosion on distillation; in commercial solvent ether substances may be added as stabilisers to prevent peroxide formation and the presence of these may cause interference with assay procedures. Further disadvantages are its fairly high solubility in water (although it is possible to reduce this by saturating the aqueous layer with sodium chloride) and the fact that it forms the top layer during an extraction procedure; this latter property can, however, sometimes be turned to advantage.

Light petroleum, which is not a good solvent for many organic bases, is useful in limited cases since, when it can be used, it often has a high degree of selectivity.

Many other solvents and mixtures of solvents are used in base-extraction assays but it is difficult to generalise since the choice of a particular system may be due to personal preference or experience.

The choice of alkali for liberation of the base is simpler. Whenever it is possible to use it, ammonia is the most satisfactory; it is sufficiently basic to liberate most organic bases without danger of causing decomposition and has the considerable advantage of being volatile and thus readily removable by evaporation. In some cases the use of a mild alkali such as sodium bicarbonate has advantages; in particular for the determination of phenolic bases which would be fixed in a solution of a stronger base. The use of sodium hydroxide is rarely justifiable, especially when dealing with synthetic materials, although it is necessary in certain cases, particularly for alkaloids present as tannates in naturally occurring materials.

When the base has been extracted it may be determined in a number of ways, the most common being back-titration with standard alkali after addition of an excess of standard acid. A number of substances to which base extraction methods are applicable are listed in Table 45.

(v) *Miscellaneous titrimetric methods.* Depending on the type of compound, it is often possible to apply a titration procedure to the material itself. Substances which are sufficiently acidic or basic can be titrated directly, or by back-titration, with standard sodium hydroxide or standard

Base Extractions

TABLE 45

	FORMULA	MOL. WT.	EQUIVALENT (G) FOR 1 ML 0·1N ACID
Cyclopentolate Hydrochloride, *U.S.P.*	$C_{17}H_{25}O_3N,HCl$	327·9	0·03279
Diethylcarbamazine Citrate, *B.P.*	$C_{16}H_{29}O_8N_3$	391·4	0·03914
Eucatropine Hydrochloride, *U.S.P.*	$C_{17}H_{25}O_3N,HCl$	327·9	0·03279
Guanethidine Sulphate	$(C_{10}H_{22}N_4)_2,H_2SO_4$	494·7	0·02474
Procyclidine Hydrochloride, *B.P.*	$C_{19}H_{29}ON,HCl$	323·9	0·03239
Promazine Hydrochloride	$C_{17}H_{20}N_2S,HCl$	320·9	0·03209
Thioridazine Hydrochloride	$C_{21}H_{26}N_2S_2,HCl$	407·1	0·04071
Tolazoline Hydrochloride, *B.P.*	$C_{10}H_{12}N_2,HCl$	196·7	0·01967

TABLE 46

	FORMULA	MOL. WT.	WEIGHT TO TAKE (G)	TITRANT	INDICATOR	EQUIVALENT (G) FOR 1 ML OF TITRANT
Titrations with Acid or Alkali						
Bialamicol Hydrochloride	$C_{28}H_{42}O_2N_2Cl_2$	509·6	0·5	0·1N NaOH	Phenolphthalein	0·02548
Dehydrocholic Acid, *U.S.P.*	$C_{24}H_{34}O_5$	402·5	0·5	0·1N NaOH	Phenolphthalein	0·04025
Ethyl Biscoumacetate, *B.P.*	$C_{22}H_{16}O_8$	408·4	0·4	0·1N NaOH	Bromophenol blue	0·04084
Ethylenediamine Hydrate, *B.P.*	$C_2H_4(NH_2)_2,H_2O$	78·12	1·5	N HCl	Bromophenol blue	0·03906
Maleic Acid, *B.P.*	$CH(CO_2H):CH(CO_2H)$	116·1	2	N NaOH	Phenolphthalein	0·05804
Mandelic Acid, *B.P.C.*	$C_6H_5.CH(OH).CO_2H$	152·2	0·3	0·1N NaOH	Phenolphthalein	0·01522
Phenylbutazone, *B.P.C.*	$C_{19}H_{20}O_2N_2$	308·4	1	0·1N NaOH	Phenolphthalein	0·03084
Probenecid, *U.S.P.*	$C_{13}H_{19}O_4NS$	285·4	1	0·1N NaOH	Phenolphthalein	0·02854
Sulphinpyrazone	$C_{23}H_{20}O_3N_2S$	404·5	0·6	0·1N NaOH	Phenolphthalein	0·04045
Undecenoic Acid, *B.P.*	$CH_2:CH.(CH_2)_8.CO_2H$	184·3	3	0·5N NaOH	Phenolphthalein	0·09214
Back Titrations						
Propylhexedrine,* *B.P.C.*	$C_{10}H_{21}N$	155·3	0·3	0·1N NaOH	Methyl red	0·01553
Glutethimide,† *B.P.C.*	$C_{13}H_{15}O_2N$	217·3	0·5	0·2N HCl	Phenolphthalein	0·04346
Amine Distillation						
Neostigmine Bromide, *B.P.*	$C_{12}H_{19}O_2N_2Br$	303·2	0·15	0·02N H_2SO_4	Methyl red	0·006064
Neostigmine Methyl-sulphate, *B.P.*	$C_{13}H_{22}O_6N_2S$	334·4	0·15	0·02N H_2SO_4	Methyl red	0·006688
Paramethadione, *B.P.*	$C_7H_{11}O_3N$	157·2	0·3	0·1N HCl	Methyl red	0·01572
Troxidone, *B.P.*	$C_6H_9O_3N$	143·1	0·3	0·1N HCl	Methyl red	0·01431
Triple Bonds						
Ethchlorvynol,‡ *N.F.*	C_7H_9OCl	144·6	0·11	0·05N NaOH	Methyl red/ methylene blue	0·007230
Ethinamate,‡ *N.F.*	$C_9H_{13}O_2N$	167·2	0·2	0·05N NaOH	Methyl red/ methylene blue	0·008361
Methylpentynol,‡ *B.P.C.*	$C_6H_{10}O$	98·15	0·3	0·1N NaOH	Bromothymol blue	0·009815
—SH Groups						
Methimazole,‡ *U.S.P.*	$C_4H_6N_2S$	114·2	0·25	0·1N NaOH	Bromothymol blue	0·01142

* After dissolving in excess 0·1N H_2SO_4 † After refluxing with excess 0·25N ethanolic KOH ‡ Titrated after reaction with $AgNO_3$

acid; naturally a non-aqueous method would also be applicable but there is no advantage in using such a system when aqueous titration is adequate. If possible, the sample should be dissolved in recently boiled and cooled water or, failing that, in ethanol or in a mixture of acetone and water, in each case neutralised to the indicator to be used in the titration (Table 46).

Certain substances yield volatile amines on distillation with sodium hydroxide and this fact may be utilised for assay purposes. For example, troxidone and paramethadione yield methylamine which may be distilled into standard acid and titrated; the neostigmine salts (bromide and methylsulphate) give dimethylamine (Table 46).

Table 46 also lists a number of compounds which contain triple bonds (*e.g.* methylpentynol) and one which contains an —SH group (methimazole). These may be conveniently determined by reacting with silver nitrate; an equivalent of nitric acid is liberated and this is titrated with standard sodium hydroxide.

Table 47 lists some substances that are determined by other titrimetric methods.

(vi) *Acetylation.* Substances having a hydroxyl group may be determined by an acetylation method; the following version is applicable in the majority of cases:

> Reflux the specified weight of substance with 10 ml of a freshly prepared mixture of 1 volume of acetic anhydride and 3 volumes of pyridine for one hour. Cool, add 20 ml of water, swirl to mix and allow to stand for two minutes; titrate with 0·5N sodium hydroxide using phenolphthalein as indicator. Repeat the operation omitting the sample; the difference between the two titrations corresponds to the amount of acetic anhydride required by the sample.

In certain cases it may be found necessary to reflux for a longer period. An alternative procedure is to filter off the acetylated product, wash with water until no odour of pyridine remains and then to dry to constant weight in a vacuum desiccator. Some compounds to which the acetylation method is applicable are given in Table 48.

(vii) *Miscellaneous gravimetric methods.* A number of fairly general precipitants are available for the determination of basic organic compounds; these include picric acid, nitranilic acid, phosphotungstic acid, ammonium reineckate, sodium tetraphenylboron and trichloracetic acid. The use of gravimetric methods is declining, however, and wherever possible, alternative procedures are used. Some examples of their use are given in Table 49. In certain cases the use of a precipitation reaction can be combined with a subsequent titration procedure to give a convenient and useful method of determination of basic substances; for example, excess tetraphenylboron may be determined, after precipitation of the organic substance, by titration with cetylpyridinium chloride (see p. 116) and excess

Titrations with Other Titrants

TABLE 47

	FORMULA	MOL. WT.	WEIGHT TO TAKE (G)	TITRANT	INDICATOR	EQUIVALENT (G) FOR 1 ML TITRANT
Carbachol, *B.P.*	$C_6H_{15}O_2N_2Cl$	182·7	0·5	0·1N $AgNO_3$	Phenosafranine	0·01827
Cyanacetohydrazide[A]	$C_3H_5ON_3$	99·1	0·15	0·05M KIO_3	Chloroform	0·00495
Dimercaprol,[B] *B.P.*	$CH_2(SH).CH(SH).CH_2OH$	124·2	0·1	0·1N iodine	—	0·006211
Ditophal[C]	$C_{12}H_{14}O_2S_2$	254·4	0·075	0·1N bromine	—	0·002120
Hydrallazine Hydrochloride,[D] *N.F.*	$C_8H_8N_4,HCl$	196·6	0·15	0·05M KIO_3	Amaranth	0·009831
Lachesine Chloride, *B.P.C.*	$C_{20}H_{26}O_3NCl$	363·9	0·8	0·1N $AgNO_3$	Potassium chromate	0·03639
Mannomustine Hydrochloride[E]	$C_{10}H_{24}O_4N_2Cl_4$	378·1	0·03	0·1N iodine to titrate excess periodic acid	Starch	0·03781
Phanquone[F]	$C_{12}H_6O_2N_2$	210·2	0·2	0·1N ceric ammonium sulphate	*o*-Phenanthroline ferrous complex	0·01051
Phenelzine Sulphate	$C_8H_{12}N_2,H_2SO_4$	234·3	0·25	0·1N sodium thiosulphate to titrate excess iodine	Starch	0·00585
Phenindione,[G] *B.P.*	$C_{15}H_{10}O_2$	222·2	0·3	0·1N sodium thiosulphate	Starch	0·01111
Suramin,[H] *B.P.*	$C_{51}H_{34}O_{23}N_6S_6Na_6$	1429·2	1	0·1M sodium nitrite	'Dead stop' end-point	0·02382
Volhard (see p. 290)						
Bethanechol Chloride, *U.S.P.*	$C_7H_{17}O_2N_2Cl$	196·7	0·4	0·1N NH_4CNS to titrate excess $AgNO_3$	Ferric alum	0·003546 g Cl
Chlorambucil[I]	$C_{14}H_{19}O_2NCl_2$	304·2	0·5	0·1N NH_4CNS to titrate excess $AgNO_3$	Ferric alum	0·01521
Mustine Hydrochloride,[I] *B.P.*	$CH_3.N(C_2H_4Cl)_2,HCl$	192·5	0·2	0·1N NH_4CNS to titrate excess $AgNO_3$	Ferric alum	0·006418
Piperoxan Hydrochloride, *B.P.C.*	$C_{14}H_{20}O_2NCl$	269·8	0·4	0·1N NH_4CNS to titrate excess $AgNO_3$	Ferric alum	0·02698

A. After refluxing with conc. HCl.
B. After addition of 20 ml 0·1N HCl.
C. Dissolve in 40 ml glacial acetic acid, add 25 ml conc. HCl, 10 ml water and 2 g KBr, heat to 60° and titrate to the first pale yellow (denoting free bromine); maintain solution at 60° throughout titration.
D. Andrews' method, see p. 292.
E. Dissolve in 10 ml water, add 10 ml 0·1M periodic acid, shake, add 2 g $NaHCO_3$, 25 ml 0·1N sod. arsenite and 0·5 g KI. Stand for 20 min. and titrate with 0·1N iodine. Repeat without sample.
F. Dissolve in 40 ml dil. HCl, gradually add 5 g $Na_2SO_3,7H_2O$, boil 5 min. and add 40 ml dil. HCl. Maintain temp. between 40° and 50° during titration.
G. Warm with 50 ml 95% ethanol until dissolved. Cool, add 10 ml 10% v/v soln. of bromine in 95% ethanol and stand 10 min. with occasional shaking. Add 1 g 2-naphthol and shake until colour of bromine discharged. Remove any bromine vapour in flask with current of air, add 50 ml water and 10 ml 10% KI soln. and titrate liberated iodine.
H. Reflux for 1 hr with 20 ml 50% v/v H_2SO_4.
I. After refluxing with ethanolic KOH.

Acetylation

TABLE 48

	FORMULA	MOL. WT.	WEIGHT TO TAKE (G)	EQUIVALENT (G) FOR 1 ML 0·5N
Chlorphenesin*	$C_9H_{11}O_3Cl$	202·6	1·3	0·05066
Ethohexadiol, *U.S.P.*	$C_8H_{18}O_2$	146·2	1	0·03656
Monobenzone, *N.F.*	$C_{13}H_{12}O_2$	200·2	0·4	1 g acetate = 0·8265 g $C_{13}H_{12}O_2$
Phenoxyethanol, *B.P.C.*	$C_8H_{10}O_2$	138·2	2	0·06908

* Reflux for two hours.

Gravimetric Methods

TABLE 49

	FORMULA	MOL. WT.	PRECIPITANT	EQUIVALENT FOR 1 G PRECIPITATE
Betazole Hydrochloride, *U.S.P.*	$C_5H_9N_3,2HCl$	184·1	Phospho-tungstic acid	0·09058
Bretylium Tosylate	$C_{18}H_{24}O_3NSBr$	414·4	Ammonium reineckate	0·7378
Histamine Acid Phosphate, *B.P.*	$C_5H_9N_3,2H_3PO_4$	307·1	Nitranilic acid	0·9001
Phentolamine Hydrochloride, *B.P.C.*	$C_{17}H_{19}ON_3,HCl$	317·8	Trichloro-acetic acid	0·7146
Phentolamine Methane-sulphonate, *B.P.C.*	$C_{17}H_{19}ON_3,CH_3SO_3H$	377·5	Trichloro-acetic acid	0·8487
Trimetaphan Camphor-sulphonate, *B.P.C.*	$C_{32}H_{40}O_5N_2S_2$	596·8	Picric acid	1·005

of a metal salt, after a similar precipitation, by titration with EDTA (see p. 790).

Of the techniques which might become of increasing importance in the critical study of synthetic organic substances, methods for separation of closely related compounds are probably the most important but certain other procedures also suggest themselves. A number of these are briefly reviewed below.

(i) *Column chromatography*. Methods based on partition chromatography have been used for the determination of impurities in such substances as 2,4-dichlorophenoxyacetic and chloromethylphenoxypropionic acids; although these materials are not of pharmaceutical interest, it is obvious that the technique is of potential application. Where the amount of impurity is small (of the order of 1 per cent) difficulties might be encountered because of the necessity to overload the column in order to obtain sufficient of the separated impurity for quantitative determination; this consideration applies equally to other forms of chromatography.

(ii) *Paper chromatography.* This is likely to be the most extensively used technique for the separation of impurities and is already being applied routinely for the determination of foreign related steroids in such substances as prednisolone and for detection of noradrenaline in adrenaline and other alkaloids in ergometrine maleate.

(iii) *Gas chromatography.* The application of this technique for the determination of impurities in organic solvents has been established practice for some years. Its use for less volatile substances is being developed rapidly, however. In the pharmaceutical field successful applications to the qualitative separation of barbiturates and steroids have been made.

(iv) *Thin-layer chromatography.* In this more recently developed method a thin, even layer (about 250 μ thick) of an adsorbant (usually silicic acid but sometimes alumina, kieselguhr or other material) is coated onto a glass plate with the aid of some binding material such as starch or plaster of Paris. The size of the glass plate will vary according to the nature of the separation, but 4 inches by 10 inches is convenient for many purposes. After drying in an oven, the plates are stored in an air-tight container with a desiccant until required for use. Spots are applied to the plates and development is carried out in a chromatographic chamber by techniques similar to those used in paper chromatographic work.

The advantages of this type of chromatographic separation are speed (most systems require less than one hour development time), sharpness of separation (there is frequently less 'tailing' of spots than on paper), the fact that results can often be applied to column separation on a preparative scale, the small size of chromatographic chambers used which makes for more rapid equilibration and uses less bench space and, in particular, the possibility of using corrosive spray reagents such as strong sulphuric and phosphoric acids.

This technique has been applied to the separation of ergot alkaloids,[2,3] synthetic analgesics[4,5] and steroids,[6,7,8] to mention only a few of the many recently published applications. It would appear to have a considerable potential use for the examination of synthetic organic materials for closely related compounds.

(v) *Electrophoresis.* Although it is used widely in clinical work for the determination of drugs in body tissues and fluids there has been little application of this technique to the examination of the purity of compounds.

It would not seem that, in the majority of cases in this context, the method would offer any advantage over other separation techniques.

(vi) *Countercurrent distribution.* This method is based on the carrying out of many individual extractions rapidly and in sequence. Fractionation is accomplished by distribution, transfer and recombination of various fractions. The technique has been applied to a number of problems in pharmaceutical work where complex mixtures of closely related compounds have to be separated. A full discussion of countercurrent methods is outside the scope of this book but a comprehensive review has been given by Weisiger.[9] There are several considerations which make this method of potential value; the solute is not exposed to abnormal conditions of temperature or pH, no assumptions of solubility, volatility or even of distribution coefficient are necessary and it is frequently possible to completely separate the components of a mixture and recover them in a suitable form, and in sufficient quantity, for use as reference materials.

(vii) *Phase solubility analysis.* In this method precise solubility measurements are used for determination of the purity of a substance. The technique consists of mixing, in separate containers, increasing quantities of the sample with the same amounts of solvent; the mixtures in the containers are then allowed to reach a state of equilibrium under identical conditions of temperature and pressure. Any solid phase remaining is then separated from the solutions and the concentration of material dissolved in each solution is determined by a suitable means. A plot is then made of the weight of material dissolved per unit of solvent (on the y axis) against the weight of material added per unit of solvent (on the x axis).

If a pure substance is being examined, the total amount of material dissolved per unit of solvent is equal to the weight added per unit of solvent until the solubility limit of the sample is reached; after this the weight dissolved remains constant. When plotted, the results give a diagram similar to that shown in Fig. 16*a*.

If an impurity is present a similar line is obtained until the solubility limit of the principal material is reached; this is then followed by a less steep line, the slope of which gives a measure of the concentration of the impurity. (See Fig. 16*b*.)

For successful application of this method strict attention to detail must be observed and the amount of impurity present should be at least 0·1 per cent. In some cases the technique is sufficiently sensitive to distinguish between optical isomers. It has been used widely in the examination of amino acids and is specified in the *U.S.P.* for determining mecamylamine hydrochloride in the presence of isomeric material as follows:

> Into seven tared, numbered, scrupulously-cleaned glass ampoules, introduce respectively, about 50, 100, 140, 175, 200, 225 and 250 mg of the sample and reweigh. Treat each ampoule, respectively, as follows. Add by pipette, 5 ml of freshly distilled *iso*propyl alcohol, cool in a mix-

ture of 'dry ice' and acetone and flame seal, retaining any separated glass. Weigh, together with the separated glass, and then rotate end over end in a water-bath maintained at 25° until equilibrium is attained (seven to fourteen days), if necessary shaking by hand occasionally to break up the solid when caking of the solute occurs. Support vertically in the water-bath with the neck of the ampoule above the level of the water and

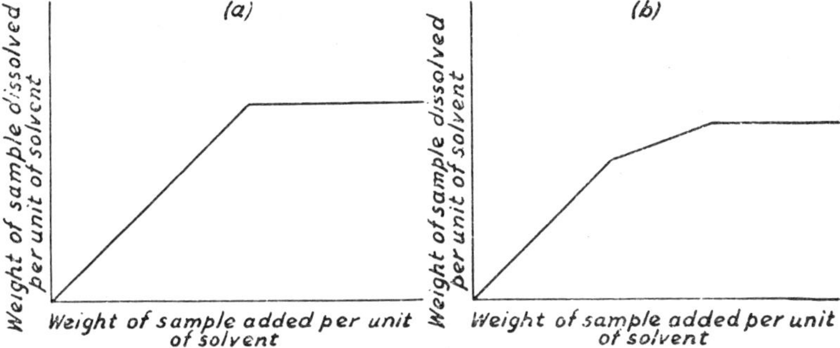

FIG. 16

allow the solid phase to settle completely. Open the ampoule and, taking precautions to avoid transference of solid particles, transfer 2 ml of the clear supernatant liquid to a tared solubility flask fitted with a ground-glass capillary stopper of inside diameter about 2 mm. Immediately weigh the flask to determine the weight of solution transferred, cool in a mixture of dry ice and acetone and transfer to a vacuum oven. Evaporate the solvent at a pressure not exceeding 5 mm of mercury and then increase the temperature of the oven to 100° and dry the flask and contents to constant weight.

Prepare a graph plotting the weight of residue obtained per g of solvent for each ampoule as ordinate and the corresponding weight of sample added per g of solvent as abscissa. The first point (for the solution prepared from 50 mg of sample and 5 ml of solvent) represents an unsaturated solution and should fall on a line of slope 1 passing through the origin. The points corresponding to saturated solutions should fall on another straight line whose slope represents the fraction of impurity in the sample. (If the points do not fall on a straight line, equilibrium has not been attained.) Calculate the percentage of $C_{11}H_{21}N,HCl$ in the sample by the formula, $100 - 100S - C$, where S is the slope of the line representing the fraction of impurity and C is the percentage loss on drying for one hour at 105° at a pressure not exceeding 5 mm of mercury.

Another application of this type of analysis to the determination of the purity of compounds has been made by Tarpley and Yudis[10] who used the technique for various steroids. They found that best results were obtained when the sample had a solubility of between 0·1 and 1 per cent and the boiling-point of the solvent was between 65° and 100°. Thus, for cortisone acetate, they chose benzene as solvent and used six ampoules, the first containing just sufficient sample to complete solution at the equilibration temperature, the second to allow of 5 to 10 per cent of solid phase out of solution and the subsequent ones to allow from 20 to 50 per cent. Solubilities were determined after equilibration for two weeks at a temperature of 25° ± 0·02° (although a bath temperature controlled to ±0·1° is satisfactory). By this means three samples of cortisone acetate, representing successive stages in a purification procedure, were shown to contain 14 per cent, 4·5 per cent and 0·8 per cent of impurity respectively.

It will be realised from the details of the above method that a serious shortcoming of the technique (from the point of view of routine analysis) is the long time necessary to ensure that a state of equilibrium has been reached in all containers. Unless this can be assured the method is valueless.

(viii) *Non-aqueous titration.* In an earlier part of this discussion non-aqueous titration has been dismissed as a non-specific method. However, if a form of recorded titration is used in which the titrant is added automatically and at a controlled rate and in which the e.m.f. change of the titration liquid is followed with a sensitive meter coupled with a chart recorder it is often possible to observe small 'steps' in the titration curve which correspond with the titration of impurities.

(ix) *Polarography*. Polarographic methods have been introduced in the first supplement to the *U.S.P.* XVI to provide more specific methods of analysis for certain organic substances, particularly when potentially interfering substances such as excipients are present. Thus polarographic methods are employed for determination of acetazolamide sodium in tablets, for chlorothiazide in tablets and for nitrofurantoin in both suspension and tablets. When organic compounds are being determined polarographically the reduction is almost invariably irreversible. The pharmaceutically interesting groups which are susceptible to polarographic reduction are (*a*) conjugated double bonds, (*b*) aldehydes, (*c*) ketones, (*d*) nitro and nitroso compounds, (*e*) quaternary ammonium groups, (*f*) most halogens. A typical application of a polarographic method is to the determination of acetazolamide in acetazolamide sodium, *U.S.P.* The use of a reference standard is again necessary:

> Weigh accurately an amount of sample equivalent to about 0·25 g of acetazolamide into a 500-ml graduated flask, dissolve in water, dilute to volume with water and mix. Pipette 3 ml of this solution into a 25-ml graduated flask, add 2·0 ml of M hydrochloric acid, dilute to volume with water and mix. Transfer a quantity of this solution to a polarographic cell that is immersed in a water-bath maintained at 25° ± 0·5° and bubble oxygen-free nitrogen through the solution for ten minutes. Insert the dropping-mercury electrode of a suitable polarograph and record the polarogram from −0·20 volt to −0·75 volt, using a saturated calomel electrode as the reference electrode. Measure the height of the diffusion current at −0·70 volt. Prepare a solution of *U.S.P.* Acetazolamide Reference Standard in water to contain about 60 μg per ml, record the polarogram under the conditions described above and calculate the per-

centage acetazolamide in the sample by comparing the diffusion currents at −0·70 volt of the two solutions.

1. GARRATT, D. C., *J. Pharm. Pharmacol.*, 1961, **13,** 9T.
2. ROCHELMEYER, H., *Pharm. Ztg.*, 1958, **103,** 1269.
3. NÜRNBERG, E., *Arch. Pharm.*, 1959, **292,** 610.
4. GÄNSHIRT, H., and MALZACHER, A., *Arch. Pharm.*, 1960, **293,** 925.
5. LIEBICH, M., *Dtsch. Apoth.-Ztg.*, 1959, **99,** 1246.
6. DAM, M. J. D. VAN, KLEUVER, G. J. DE, and HEUS, J. G. DE, *J. Chromatog.*, 1960, **4,** 26.
7. BARBIER, M., JÄGER, H., TOBIAS, H., and WYSS, E., *Helv. Chim. Acta*, 1959, **42,** 2440.
8. STRUCK, H., *Mikrochim. Acta*, 1961, 634.
9. WEISIGER, J. R., Organic Analysis, Vol. II. Interscience Publishers, Inc., New York 1954, p. 277.
10. TARPLEY, W., and YUDIS, M., *Anal. Chem.*, 1953, **25,** 121.
11. HAYDEN, A. L., SAMMUL, O. R., SELZER, G. B., and CAROL, J., *J.A.O.A.C.*, 1962, **45,** 797.

ESSENTIAL OILS

The assessment of the purity of essential oils requires a long and specialised experience to interpret the results of analysis. The expert relies considerably on odour, but to the casual investigator this is of little value except when comparison is made with an oil of known authenticity.

Owing to the latitude that must be allowed for variation in the characteristics of individual oils, mainly due to seasonal conditions and methods of distillation, the range of constants for normal oils is so wide that it may permit sophistication to a considerable extent, and owing to the complex nature and similarity of many of the oils, the detection of adulteration is difficult.

As many oils, other than those included in the official publications, are met with in pharmaceutical practice, the most useful chemical methods of analysis are given briefly below. The Analytical Methods Committee of the *S.A.C.* (referred to below as the *S.A.C.*) has carried out a considerable amount of useful work on standardisation of methods for the analysis of essential oils, and many of its recommendations have been embodied in the official monographs.

ALCOHOLS. The determination of alcohols depends upon their esterification with acetic anhydride and estimation of the proportion of the resulting acetates by hydrolysis with ethanolic potassium hydroxide.

As even slight variations in the technique used to determine the acetylisable constituents of essential oils are responsible for serious differences in the results obtained, the *S.A.C.*[1] recommended method should be followed in detail.

> Mix 10 ml of the oil, 20 ml of acetic anhydride (95 to 100 per cent), and 2 g of freshly fused anhydrous sodium acetate in a long-necked, round-bottomed, 200-ml Kjeldahl flask; add a fragment of broken glass and boil the contents gently under an air reflux condenser for two hours. Support the flask on a sheet of asbestos board, in which has been cut a hole about 1½ inches in diameter, and heat by a small naked flame, placed about 1 inch below, and not impinging on the bottom of the flask.
>
> At the expiration of two hours, remove the flame and allow the flask to cool; add 50 ml of water and heat the flask and contents on a water-bath for fifteen minutes, with frequent and thorough shaking. After cooling, transfer the contents of the flask to a separator and reject the lower aqueous layer. Then wash the acetylated oil successively with (i) 50 ml of brine; (ii) 50 ml of brine containing 1 g of sodium carbonate in solution; (iii) 50 ml of brine; (iv) 20 ml of water. Mixtures (i), (ii) and (iii) should be shaken vigorously, but the final washing with water must be conducted with gentle shaking only.

If the washing operations have been properly conducted, the aqueous layer from the second washing should be alkaline to phenolphthalein (ethanolic phenolphthalein must not be added to the mixture in the separator).

When the washing is complete, remove the aqueous layer as completely as possible, pour the oil out and mix it with about 3 g of powdered anhydrous sodium sulphate. Stir for fifteen minutes or until 1 drop of the oil produces no cloudiness when added to 10 drops of carbon disulphide in a dry test-tube. Then filter the oil through a dry filter paper in a covered funnel.

Method of hydrolysis: Accurately weigh about 2 g or other suitable quantity, so that the volume of 0·5N ethanolic potassium hydroxide to be added is at least twice that theoretically required, of the dried and filtered oil into a hard glass flask, add 2 ml of water, and titrate the free acidity with 0·1N aqueous potassium hydroxide, using 1 ml of 1 per cent solution of phenolphthalein in 60 per cent ethanol as indicator. Then add 40 ml of 0·5N ethanolic potassium hydroxide and boil the mixture under a reflux condenser on a water-bath for one hour; cool the flask rapidly, add 20 ml of water, and titrate the excess of alkali with 0·5N sulphuric acid.

Carry out a blank determination of the ethanolic potassium hydroxide simultaneously with the hydrolysis of the acetylated oil, and under conditions conforming as nearly as possible with those employed therein.

The percentage of total alcohols in the oil is obtained from the formula:

$$\text{Percentage of total alcohols} = \frac{M \times x}{20(w - 0{\cdot}021x)} \times [1 - (E \times 0{\cdot}0021)]$$

M = molecular weight of the alcohol
x = ml of 0·5N potassium hydroxide absorbed
w = wt. of acetylated oil taken
E = percentage of esters calculated as acetate (see p. 727).

The percentage of free alcohols may be calculated from the same data:

$$\text{Percentage of free alcohols} = \frac{(b - a)M}{0{\cdot}42 \times (1{,}335 - b)}$$

a = ester value of original oil
b = ester value after acetylation (see p. 718).

Molecular weights of borneol, citronellal, geraniol and linalol are 154·3; menthol and citronellol, 156·3; santalol, 220·4.

The use of 0·5N hydrochloric acid for titration has the advantage of not precipitating insoluble sodium sulphate in the reaction mixture.

Linalol and terpineol cannot be determined accurately by acetylation, owing to partial decomposition. Other methods have been devised, such as by estimation of the alcohols with cold acetoformic anhydride (Glichitch[2]); this method gave good results in collaborative trials (Analytical Methods Committee of the *S.A.C.* report[3]) but the work of Holness[4] using gas-liquid chromatography has shown them to be a fortuitous balancing of errors and the method less reliable than that of Fiore published by the Essential Oil Association of the U.S.A. and now recommended by the

S.A.C.[5] The method is more rapid and suitable for determination of linalol in oils such as bois-de-rose and in the isolate. Although higher results can be obtained with modifications, such increases do not necessarily indicate the true content. Details of the *S.A.C.* modification are the following:

Dry the sample with anhydrous sodium sulphate, take 10 ml in a 125-ml conical flask and cool in ice-water. Add 20 ml of analytical-reagent grade dimethylaniline free from monomethylaniline, mix thoroughly and then add 8 ml of acetyl chloride and 5 ml of acetic anhydride (both of analytical-reagent grade). Cool for a few minutes, allow to stand at room temperature for thirty minutes, then immerse in a water-bath at 40° (±1°) for three hours.

Wash the acetylated oil as follows, shaking for thirty seconds each time and allowing to separate: with two 75-ml quantities of a 10 per cent solution of anhydrous sodium sulphate, with 50-ml quantities of a 2·5 per cent solution of concentrated sulphuric acid in the sodium sulphate solution until the washings are free from dimethylaniline (usually five washings are necessary), with two 25-ml quantities of a 5 per cent solution of sodium bicarbonate in the sodium sulphate solution and finally with two 25-ml quantities of the 10 per cent sodium sulphate solution.

Dry the oil with anhydrous sodium sulphate and determine the ester value of the acetylated oil as described below (p. 727) and calculate the total linalol from the formula:

$$\text{Percentage of linalol} = \frac{A \times 154{\cdot}2}{561 - 0{\cdot}42A}$$

A = ester value of the acetylated oil.

The dried acetylated oil should be almost neutral and, in the determination of ester value, not more than one drop of 0·1N potassium hydroxide should be required to give a pink colour; the first pink colour is taken as the neutral point since linalyl acetate is readily hydrolysed.

Unless the reagents have been freshly prepared it may be necessary to extend the acetylation time to ensure complete reaction. In such cases the reaction mixture may have to stand at 40° for at least sixteen hours. The optimum time for acetylation can be established by trial for individual conditions.

A new method for determination of hydroxyl groups in primary alcohols and secondary alcohols, but not tertiary alcohols, has been described by Sully[46] in which stearic anhydride is used instead of acetic anhydride. Among the compounds successfully assayed were citronellol, geraniol, benzyl alcohol, phenylethyl alcohol and menthol. The procedure has also been used for determining phenols including eugenol.

Stearic anhydride. Mix 1000 g of stearic acid (a commercial grade of stearic acid is suitable, provided that it has a good heat stability, an iodine value below 4 and crystallises well) and 550 g of acetic anhydride and boil under a reflux condenser for eight hours. Remove the excess of acetic anhydride and the acetic acid formed during the reaction, under vacuum, taking care that the temperature does not rise above 135°.

Purify the stearic anhydride by crystallisation from 1500 g of light petroleum (b.p. 60° to 80°) and then grind the crystals to a powder to ensure homogeneity. Determine the purity by boiling for fifteen minutes with an excess of methanol, which produces one molecular equivalent of methyl stearate and one of stearic acid from each molecular equivalent of stearic anhydride, and titrate while still hot with N sodium hydroxide using phenolphthalein as indicator. Boil a further portion of the reagent for fifteen minutes with pyridine containing 10 per cent v/v of water and titrate while hot with N sodium hydroxide using phenolphthalein as indicator. Calculate the per cent free stearic acid in the stearic anhydride from the two titres; the reagent may contain up to 10 per cent of stearic acid but this is unimportant.

Determination. Weigh a suitable amount of sample (see Note below) into a 250-ml, round-bottomed flask with 12 to 13 g of stearic anhydride, also accurately weighed. Add 10 ml of analytical-reagent grade xylene (the volume is important because an excess will hinder the decomposition of the unreacted stearic anhydride in the final stage of the determination) and reflux for thirty minutes (or longer, if necessary) using a water-cooled condenser with a ground-glass joint. Decompose the unreacted stearic anhydride by procedure A or B, below.

Procedure A. (To be used for alcohols of unknown chemical constitution or under conditions in which the alcohol is accompanied by unstable compounds.) Cool the xylene solution, add 40 ml of pyridine containing 4 ml of water and boil for fifteen minutes.

Procedure B. Cool the xylene solution, add 4 ml of water and 0·6 g of sodium stearate and reflux for fifteen to thirty minutes. Dilute the mixture with 40 ml of neutral, industrial methylated spirit.

Titrate the mixture resulting from Procedure A or B, while still hot, with N sodium hydroxide using phenolphthalein as indicator; the phenolphthalein indicator must not be added before the stearic anhydride is completely decomposed, since it is normally made up in spirit solution. If unchanged stearic anhydride is present the phenolphthalein will bleach during the titration with alkali and, if this is the case, the determination must be abandoned.

Carry out a blank determination by repeating the entire operation omitting the sample.

Note: The weight of sample taken should be such that the titre is approximately two-thirds of that equivalent to the stearic anhydride used—found from the blank determination—which corresponds to a 50 per cent excess over the theoretical.

$$\text{Percentage of alcohol or phenol} = \frac{(x - y) \times M}{w}$$

x = ml of N sodium hydroxide equivalent to the weight of stearic anhydride used with the sample, calculated from the blank determination

y = ml of N sodium hydroxide required to neutralise the excess of stearic anhydride used in the assay

M = molecular weight of the alcohol or phenol

w = wt. of sample taken.

ALDEHYDES AND KETONES. Formerly aldehydes and ketones were usually determined by absorption with neutral sodium sulphite or sodium bisulphite solutions, but from the investigation by Bennett and Salamon[6] of the hydroxylamine method (see below), the latter has been adopted, with modification, by the *S.A.C.* for the estimation of all aldehydes and ketones except pulegone.

As oils are still commonly sold in the trade on the figure obtained by neutral sulphite or bisulphite absorption, these methods are briefly described below. They act as a useful check on the hydroxylamine method and the neutral sulphite method is especially suitable for caraway and dill oils, separation being particularly clean and the results less likely to be complicated by adulterants than in the case of other oils.

The original bisulphite method:

> Heat 5 ml of the oil in a 150-ml Hirschsohn flask with 100 ml of a clear 35 per cent solution of sodium bisulphite in a water-bath for an hour (or longer if necessary) with frequent agitation, allowing it to remain in the water-bath until the solid compound formed is completely dissolved. Drive the uncombined oil into the neck of the flask by the addition of more bisulphite solution and measure the residual oil after some hours.

In the case of cassia oils containing much resin three or four hours' heating is sometimes necessary, and citronellal bisulphite compound takes much longer than the citral compound to form a clear solution. The method is still commonly employed for cassia and lemon grass oils.

The neutral sulphite modification was generally used for aldehydes in cinnamon and lemon grass oils and it can be used for most aldehydes and ketones. Pulegone can be determined, but in this case four hours' absorption is necessary (see Pennyroyal Oil).

> Place 5 ml of oil in a Hirschsohn flask and add about 50 ml of 20 per cent sodium sulphite solution and a few drops of phenolphthalein solution. Heat the flask on a water-bath with continuous shaking, keeping the reaction mixture neutral by the continuous addition of 10 per cent acetic acid solution from a burette, until no further alkali is liberated. The process usually occupies from one-half to one hour. Drive the uncombined oil into the neck of the flask by the addition of more sulphite solution and measure the volume of non-aldehydic residue after some hours.

The hydroxylamine method in which the mineral acid, liberated from hydroxylamine salts by oxime formation with the aldehyde, is titrated direct, requires to be modified according to the particular aldehyde or ketone being determined (Bennett and Cocking[7]). The advantages of the hydroxylamine process over the absorption methods given above are recognised as (*a*) the hydroxylamine method is a definite determination of aldehydic or ketonic substances, whereas the absorption methods include impurities such as water-soluble organic acids and adulterants such as alcohol; (*b*) a small quantity only of the oil is required and the determination can be completed in a much shorter time. Yet it must be pointed out that except for cinnamon oil, which may contain free acid, and cassia oil, where alcohol is often present and where emulsions are likely in the case of the absorption methods owing to the presence of resin, the impurities mentioned are not of frequent occurrence. The hydroxylamine method has the disadvantage that the end-point is frequently quite difficult to determine with certainty, but in spite of this the method is a great improvement. The *S.A.C.* methods are summarised below.

Aldehydes other than citronellal may be determined by a general method.[8]

Weigh out exactly, into a glass-stoppered tube, approximately 150 mm long by 25 mm in diameter, a suitable quantity of the oil; add 5 ml of benzene and 15 ml of 0·5N hydroxylamine hydrochloride. This reagent is prepared by dissolving 3·475 g of pure hydroxylamine hydrochloride in 95 ml of 60 per cent v/v ethanol, adding 0·5 ml of 0·2 per cent solution of methyl orange, adjusting to the full yellow colour of the indicator with 0·5N ethanolic potassium hydroxide and making up to 100 ml with 60 per cent ethanol. Shake vigorously and titrate with 0·5N potassium hydroxide in 60 per cent ethanol until the red colour changes to yellow. Continue the shaking and titrating until the full yellow colour of the indicator is permanent in the lower layer after shaking vigorously for two minutes and then allowing to stand for the liquids to separate. The reaction is slow towards the end, but should be complete in about fifteen minutes. It is preferable to confirm the result by a second determination, using the first reaction mixture slightly over-titrated as a colour-standard for the end-point. Obtain the percentage *by weight* of aldehydes by multiplying the number of ml of 0·5N ethanolic potassium hydroxide used, corrected by the factor 1·008 (necessary owing to the fact that the end-point of the titration occurs at a pH different from that of neutral hydroxylamine hydrochloride), by the factor for the appropriate aldehyde, and by 100, and dividing by the weight of oil taken.

Use about 0·6 g of oil of bitter almond, 0·7 g of oil of cassia, 1·0 g of oil of cinnamon, 1·5 g of oil of cumin, 1·0 g of oil of lemon grass, 1·2 g of sesquiterpeneless oil of lemon, and 1·5 g of terpeneless oil of lemon, terpeneless and sesquiterpeneless oil of orange.

Particular attention must be paid to the adjustment of the reagent and the end-point of the reaction. Standardise the 0·5N ethanolic potassium hydroxide by running it into a known volume of 0·5N acid until the full yellow colour of the indicator (a 0·2 per cent solution of methyl orange in 60 per cent ethanol) is obtained, *i.e.* that colour not changed by further addition of alkali. The necessity for the correction factor in this method is questionable in view of the limited degree of accuracy obtainable with the somewhat difficult assessment of the end-point.

The original indicator, bromophenol blue, proposed by Bennett and Salamon,[6] is preferred by many workers.

Citronellal has been found to be quickly destroyed by free hydrochloric acid, and as its reaction with hydroxylamine hydrochloride proceeds rapidly only in slightly acid solution, certain precautions are necessary in its determination. The *S.A.C.*[9] recommendation is the following modification; differences to be noted in the reagents are the strength of ethanol in the ethanolic potassium hydroxide used, and the difference in strength and indicator for the hydroxylamine solution.

> Into a stoppered tube approximately 150 mm long by 25 mm diameter, weigh accurately such a quantity of the oil as contains about 0·8 g of citronellal and cool to a temperature of 0°, or lower. Add 10 ml of the N hydroxylamine hydrochloride previously cooled to 0°. (The reagent is prepared by dissolving 6·95 g of pure substance in 95 ml of 90 per cent v/v ethanol, adding 0·4 ml of 0·2 per cent dimethyl yellow solution, adjusting to the full yellow of the indicator with 0·5N ethanolic potassium hydroxide and making up to 100 ml with 90 per cent ethanol.) Titrate the liberated acid immediately with 0·5N potassium hydroxide in 90 per cent ethanol, adding the alkali very cautiously and taking great care to avoid going beyond the orange colour of the indicator. Continue the titration as long as the red colour develops, then allow the mixture to stand at laboratory temperature for one hour and complete the titration to the full yellow colour of the indicator. Calculate the percentage by weight of citronellal in a manner similar to that for the general method for aldehydes, above.
>
> Record the results as total aldehydes by the hydroxylamine method, calculated as citronellal.

Rowaan and Koolhaus[10] claim that bromophenol blue gives a sharper end-point with citronellal.

The *S.A.C.* method[11] recommended for the determination of **citral in lemon oil** is a great advance over the previously used method of Bennett. The method is similar in procedure to that for aldehydes other than citronellal, with a difference in the relative proportions of the reacting substances; to ensure a reasonably sharp end-point being obtained these proportions must be adhered to. About 10 g of lemon oil is used, without the addition of benzene, and 7 ml of hydroxylamine reagent (containing an extra drop of indicator) is added; the determination is carried out as directed above. The volume of hydroxylamine reagent should be 1 or 2 ml in excess over the ethanolic potassium hydroxide required in all cases and so must be varied according to the citral content of the oil; high-grade Sicilian oils may contain up to 5·8 per cent of citral. The method is also used for oils of sweet and bitter orange, mandarin, grapefruit and lime.

Bennett and Cocking[7] observed that the hydroxylamine method for aldehydes was unsuitable for ketones as the oxime formation proceeded too slowly for completion within a reasonable time. By varying conditions, especially temperature, better results were obtainable. On their findings, the *S.A.C.*[12] recommended the following modification for the ketones **carvone** and **menthone.** The procedure is similar to the method for aldehydes, using the same hydroxylamine reagent and dimethyl yellow indicator, as in the case of citronellal (above). The modified method is as follows:

Weigh a suitable quantity of the oil (1·5 g) into a glass-stoppered tube, approximately 25 mm in diameter and 150 mm in length, and add 10 ml of hydroxylamine hydrochloride reagent in 90 per cent ethanol. (The reagent is prepared by dissolving 7 g of hydroxylamine hydrochloride in 90 ml of 90 per cent ethanol, adding 0·4 ml of a 0·2 per cent solution of dimethyl yellow in 90 per cent ethanol, adjusting to the full yellow of the indicator with N ethanolic potassium hydroxide and diluting to 100 ml with 90 per cent ethanol; the reagent should comply with the following test: to 10 ml add one drop of N ethanolic potassium hydroxide; no change in colour is produced. To a further 10 ml add one drop of N hydrochloric acid; the colour changes slightly to orange.) Titrate with N ethanolic potassium hydroxide (in 90 per cent ethanol) until the red colour changes to yellow. Place the tube in a water-bath at 75° to 80° and neutralise the liberated acid at five-minute intervals; at the end of forty minutes complete the titration to the full yellow colour of the indicator. Confirm the result by a second determination and calculate the percentage by weight of ketone in a manner similar to that for the general method for aldehydes, above.

It is essential to allow the reaction to proceed for a definite time only, as experiments appear to indicate that a secondary reaction takes place very slowly and continues for some hours.

The following factors, which have been corrected for the pH end-point, should be used for aldehydes, titrating with 0·5N ethanolic potassium hydroxide:

Benzaldehyde	0·05348
Cinnamic aldehyde	0·06661
Citral	0·07672
Citronellal	0·0777
Cuminaldehyde	0·0747
Decylic aldehyde	0·0787

and for ketones, titrating with N ethanolic potassium hydroxide:

Carvone	0·1514
Menthone	0·1555

ASCARIDOLE. The *B.P.C.* method for the determination of ascaridole is that of Cocking and Hymas[13] based upon the oxidising action of the peroxide radical present in the molecule on a strongly acidified solution of potassium iodide and titration of the iodine liberated, under specified conditions. It was found necessary to resort to an empirical method based on the titration of pure ascaridole (standardised by titanous chloride—a method inapplicable to general determination as it has to be carried out in an inert atmosphere) as the reaction which takes place is complex and not yet fully understood. The conditions adopted result in the maximum liberation by a normal peroxide. Obviously, to obtain accurate and concordant results, it is essential to adhere strictly to the conditions laid down.

The original method has been recommended for adoption without alteration by the *S.A.C.*[14]

Dissolve about 2·5 g, accurately weighed, in sufficient 90 per cent acetic acid to produce 50 ml and place the solution in a narrow burette with 0·05-ml graduations and which delivers 5 ml in not more than five seconds. Place 3 ml of an 83 per cent w/v solution of potassium iodide in water, 5 ml of concentrated hydrochloric acid and 10 ml of glacial acetic acid in a stoppered tube, about 150 mm long and 25 mm in diameter, cool to $-3°$, run in about 5 ml of the solution from the burette, mixing as quickly as possible, and allow to stand for two minutes before taking the burette reading. Allow to stand for five minutes, maintaining the temperature below 10°, and without prior dilution, titrate the liberated iodine with 0·1N sodium thiosulphate. Repeat the operation omitting the sample, adding 20 ml of water before the final titration. The difference between the two titrations represents the amount of iodine liberated by the sample. 1 ml 0·1N sodium thiosulphate = 0·00665 g $C_{10}H_{16}O_2$.

The end-point must be sharp, and the final solution white, if the determination has been carried out correctly. Starch must not be used in the titration.

Since in the official method it is necessary to adhere rigidly to the conditions laid down and the factor is an empirical one, based on the titration of a specimen of ascaridole, Beckett and Jolliffe[15] consider the use of the same factor questionable for oil of chenopodium, because of the change in the ratio of ascaridole to the acidified potassium iodide solution. This was confirmed experimentally under conditions which were constant except for the weight of sample used and consequently the use of a constant factor for oil of different ascaridole content must yield incorrect results. Based on polarographic determinations a suitable quadratic expression was derived for the conversion of the titration figures obtained by the *B.P.C.* procedure into correct figures of ascaridole percentages. However, since this depends on the use by the authors of a sample of ascaridole which had not been proved 100 per cent pure, it must still be considered empirical. The *B.P.C.* method is satisfactory as a comparative method.

CINEOLE. The *ortho*-cresol process of Cocking[16] has entirely superseded the older methods of determining cineole (based on the formation of additive compounds with phosphoric or arsenic acids). The accuracy of the *ortho*-cresol process has been fully substantiated by the *S.A.C.*[17] for eucalyptus, cajuput and camphor oils, but it has been shown that, with oils containing alcohols, esters, aldehydes and ketones in quantity, the method indicates a higher result than the actual content as these substances raise the freezing-point of the *ortho*-cresol. No means has been found for carrying out accurate determinations in these circumstances, but the *S.A.C.* recommends that, as the apparent cineole content thus obtained for oils of rosemary, spike lavender and sage (which are frequently adulterated with fractions of eucalpytus oil) would be of value, the determination of the 'apparent cineole content by *ortho*-cresol' should be made with these oils.

The method of determination of cineole in eucalyptus and cajuput oils by the *ortho*-cresol method depends on the lowering of the freezing-point of a mixture of cineole and *ortho*-cresol by the other constituents of the oil. A mixture is made of approximately molecular proportions for cineole and *ortho*-cresol, and the freezing-point is taken.

Into a stout-walled test-tube, about 15 mm in diameter and 80 mm in length, place 2·1 g, accurately weighed, of melted *o*-cresol together with 3 g, accurately weighed, of the oil previously dried by shaking with anhydrous calcium chloride. Insert a thermometer graduated in fifths of a degree and stir the mixture well with a loop of glass or wire to induce crystallisation; note the highest reading of the thermometer. Warm the tube gently until the contents are completely melted, insert the tube through a bored cork into a wide-mouthed bottle which is to act as an air jacket and allow to cool slowly until crystallisation commences, or until the temperature falls to the point previously noted. Stir the contents of the tube vigorously with the loop, rubbing the latter on the side of the tube with an up and down motion to induce rapid crystallisation; continue the stirring and rubbing as long as the temperature rises. Take the highest point as the freezing-point.

Remelt the mixture and repeat the determination of the freezing-point until two consecutive concordant results are obtained, because the first temperature noted is always lower than the true freezing-point.

Find the percentage w/w of cineole corresponding to the freezing-point from the following Table, obtaining intermediate values by interpolation:

TABLE 50

FREEZING-POINT	PER CENT W/W OF CINEOLE	FREEZING-POINT	PER CENT W/W OF CINEOLE
24°	45·6	41°	68·6
25°	46·9	42°	70·5
26°	48·2	43°	72·3
27°	49·5	44°	74·2
28°	50·8	45°	76·1
29°	52·1	46°	78·0
30°	53·4	47°	80·0
31°	54·7	48°	82·1
32°	56·0	49°	84·2
33°	57·3	50°	86·3
34°	58·6	51°	88·8
35°	59·9	52°	91·3
36°	61·2	53°	93·8
37°	62·5	54°	96·3
38°	63·8	55°	99·3
39°	65·2	55·2°	100·0
40°	66·8		

The method gives an accurate determination of cineole if the following points are noted: (*a*) the oil must be dry; (*b*) the weights of oil and *ortho*-cresol must not vary from the required weights by more than 0·02 g; (*c*) the *ortho*-cresol must be pure and dry, with a minimum freezing-point of 30°. Berry and Swanson[18] obtained a freezing-point of 56·3° for the pure cineole-cresol mixture instead of 55·2° given in the *B.P.*

This method is satisfactory for oils containing 50 per cent and upwards of cineole. Those, such as camphor oil, containing less than 50 per cent may be mixed with an equal weight of pure cineole or a high-content oil before carrying out the test. The *S.A.C.* suggests that a better way is to perform the test in the usual manner first, and then, if the mixed liquids do not crystallise, add an equal weight (5·1 g) of pure recrystallised cresol-cineole compound (obtained from a high-percentage oil by draining and pressing the magma and recrystallising from a small quantity of light petroleum), warm until liquefied, determine the freezing-point as before, and make the necessary corrections. This method gives a rather unmanageable bulk of material in a tube of the size recommended for the test. In the case of light camphor oil, *i.e.* one distilling below 200°, the modified test is carried out directly on the oil. When a camphor oil contains high-boiling constituents, such as camphor and safrole, it is necessary to distil the oil through a fractionating column and carry out the test on the fraction boiling below 200°. The cineole content of the original oil is then obtained by calculation.

CITRONELLOL. Several methods have been proposed from time to time for the determination of citronellol in the presence of geraniol, none of which is entirely satisfactory. As the amount of citronellol in geranium oils is often required by dealers, and the determination of its proportion in otto of rose is of value in the detection of adulteration, a method giving useful comparative results only and not an accurate means of determination is given below. It depends on the conversion of geraniol to terpenes by anhydrous formic acid, whilst citronellol is esterified to citronellyl formate. Actually, geraniol is incompletely decomposed and citronellol is incompletely esterified but gives high results owing to decomposition.

Heat 10 ml of the oil with 20 ml of 90 per cent formic acid for one hour on a water-bath. Then dilute the mixture with water and transfer to a separator. Wash the formylated oil with water until free from acid, dry with anhydrous sodium sulphate and filter. Saponify a weighed portion of the oil in the same manner as for acetylated oil. From the amount of potassium hydroxide absorbed, calculate the percentage of citronellol.

$$\text{Citronellol per cent} = \frac{15{\cdot}6 \times x}{\text{wt. of formylated oil taken} - (0{\cdot}028x)}$$

x = ml N potassium hydroxide absorbed.

A number of hot formylation methods have been studied by Holness for the *S.A.C.*[19] and from gas-liquid chromatography evidence the general conclusions confirm that such methods are not satisfactory.

ESTERS. These are determined by hydrolysis with ethanolic potassium hydroxide, and it is pointed out by the *S.A.C.*[20] that unless the conditions of the tests are standardised somewhat closely, variations in results are likely to occur. The following method is given:

Weigh into the saponification flask, 2 g of the oil, or other suitable quantity so that the amount of alkali added is at least double that required for saponification. Add 5 ml of freshly well-boiled and neutralised ethanol and titrate the free acid with 0·1N ethanolic potassium hydroxide, using 0·2 ml of phenolphthalein solution (1 per cent in 95 per cent ethanol) as indicator. Calculate the result to acid value.

To the neutralised solution add 20 ml of approximately 0·5N ethanolic potassium hydroxide in 95 per cent ethanol and boil under a reflux condenser for one hour, at the end of which time add 20 ml of water and titrate the excess of alkali immediately with 0·5N hydrochloric acid, using an additional 0·2 ml of phenolphthalein solution as indicator.

Carry out at the same time a blank determination by boiling for one hour under reflux 5 ml of ethanol, 20 ml of the approximately 0·5N ethanolic potassium hydroxide and 0·2 ml of phenolphthalein indicator and then titrating immediately with 0·5N hydrochloric acid after the addition of 20 ml of water and a further 0·2 ml of phenolphthalein solution. Calculate the difference between the two titrations to the percentage of esters from the following formula:

$$\text{Percentage of esters} = \frac{x \times M}{w \times 20}$$

x = ml of 0·5N potassium hydroxide absorbed
M = molecular weight of the ester
w = wt. of oil taken.

Molecular weights of common esters are: bornyl acetate, geranyl acetate, linalyl acetate, 196·3; menthyl acetate, 198·3; menthyl valerianate, 240·3; geranyl tiglate, 236·4; santalyl acetate, 262·4; methyl salicylate, 152·2.

Special consideration with regard to oils of wintergreen, sweet birch and bergamot will be found under the notes on the individual oils. A number of esters, particularly terpinyl acetate and menthyl valerianate, are not readily saponified in one hour by 0·5N ethanolic potassium hydroxide, but Perry and West[21] observed that saponification was complete in thirty minutes with a solution of potassium hydroxide in ethylene glycol monoethyl ether. After neutralising 1·5 g of the sample dissolved in 5 ml of ethylene glycol monoethyl ether with 0·1N sodium hydroxide to phenolphthalein, 40 ml of 0·5N potassium hydroxide in the solvent is added and the mixture refluxed for thirty minutes before titrating with acid.

PHENOLS. The usual method of determination of phenols is by alkali absorption of the phenol, and the *S.A.C.* method[22] is the following. It has been found that, in order to obtain uniform results, standard conditions must be strictly observed.

Place 80 ml of 5 per cent aqueous potassium hydroxide solution (sodium hydroxide does not give good separations) in a 150-ml Hirschsohn flask, followed by 10 ml of the clear oil. Shake the mixture thoroughly at five-minute intervals during thirty minutes, at room temperature. Raise the unabsorbed portion of the oil into the neck of the flask by the gradual addition of more of the alkaline solution, rotating the flask between the hands and gently tapping to facilitate separation of the oily layer. Allow to stand for twenty-four hours and read the volume of unabsorbed oil, taking the bottom line of the meniscus. If a maximum of 0·4 ml of emulsion is formed between the liquids, take a mean reading of this. If an emulsion is formed which will not separate, repeat the experiment after the addition of 2 ml of xylene (b.p. 137° to 142°). The proportion of oil absorbed, multiplied by 10, will give the percentage by volume of the phenolic content of the oil under examination.

Some points are to be noted, especially (*a*) the flask should be previously cleaned with concentrated sulphuric acid; (*b*) the potassium hydroxide solution should be prepared from pure sticks and not differ by more than 0·1 per cent from 5 per cent; (*c*) small variations in the size of the flasks used make no appreciable differences in the results obtained; (*d*) in some cases treatment with hot potassium hydroxide, although giving a more rapid separation, gives higher results which are incorrect.

ARTIFICIAL ESTERS. The number of artificial esters available for adding to oils to increase their apparent natural ester content might appear to be very large, but sophisticators are limited in their choice to those of slight odour, comparatively high ester value and commercial accessibility.

Glyceryl acetate can be detected and estimated in bergamot and lavender oils by its solubility in 5 per cent ethanol.

Shake 10 ml of oil with 20 ml of 5 per cent ethanol, separate and filter the ethanolic layer. Saponify 10 ml of filtrate after neutralising to phenolphthalein. Under these conditions 1 per cent of glyceryl acetate absorbs approximately 0·6 ml of 0·5N ethanolic potassium hydroxide. The oil, after a further two or three washings with 5 per cent ethanol, may be dried and the ester value taken again, a large difference confirming a soluble ester.

Terpinyl acetate is detected by its rate of hydrolysis. Natural esters are saponified within thirty minutes; terpinyl acetate requires one and a half to two hours. In this difference of time of saponification, 5 per cent of terpinyl acetate will show a difference of at least three units in ester value, whilst pure oils will not differ by more than 0·5 unit.

The volatility of the acids occurring in natural esters was utilised in a method by Schimmel[23] for the detection of **esters of fixed acids.** Bennett and Garratt[24] proved the method unreliable and proposed a simple test for the detection of esters of fixed acids dependent on the insolubility of their potassium salts in dehydrated ethanol.

Place 1 ml of the oil with 3 ml of an approximately 10 per cent solution of potassium hydroxide in dehydrated ethanol in a test-tube, immerse in a water-bath for a few minutes and then allow to cool. If no precipitate forms within, at the most, one hour, the oil may be considered unadulterated with the esters of citric, tartaric, succinic, benzoic, phthalic and cinnamic acids. All these esters show a crystalline precipitate if present to the extent of 2·5 per cent in the oil.

The test is especially delicate for the detection of **phthalic esters** and can be made roughly quantitative by filtering the precipitate, washing it with dehydrated ethanol and weighing after drying. These esters have been found commercially in geranium and bergamot oils. Phthalic esters are also detected by heating the less volatile fractions of an oil with concentrated sulphuric acid and resorcinol, adding alkali hydroxide and pouring into water, when fluorescein is formed in the presence of phthalate and a strong green fluorescence is obtained.

SOLUBILITIES OF ESSENTIAL OILS. In the determination of the solubility of an essential oil it is necessary that the alcohol used should be of exactly the required spirit strength, slight deviations causing a considerable difference in solubility in many cases. The limits of specific gravity for the alcohol used are:

Alcohol 90 per cent,	specific gravity (20°/20°)	0·8289 to 0·8319
,, 80 ,, ,,	,, ,, ,,	0·8599 to 0·8621
,, 70 ,, ,,	,, ,, ,,	0·8860 to 0·8883
,, 60 ,, ,,	,, ,, ,,	0·9103 to 0·9114

Prepared by diluting alcohol (95 per cent by volume) with water to 1 litre, the final adjustment of volume being made at the same temperature, about 20°, as that at which the alcohol was measured.

For 90 per cent dilute	947 ml
,, 80 ,, ,, ,,	842 ,,
,, 70 ,, ,, ,,	737 ,,
,, 60 ,, ,, ,,	632 ,,

If the solution of essential oil under test is not clear, the appearance is described as 'with opalescence'.

Table 51

ESSENTIAL OIL	WT./ML AT 20°	OPT. ROTATION	REF. INDEX AT 20°	SOLUBILITY‡	OTHER DATA
Ajowan	0·910–0·930†	0/+2	1·485–1·510	4/90	Phenols not less than 40%
Almond	1·055–1·065†	—	1·534–1·542	—	Benzaldehyde 85%, HCN 2–4%
Almond purified	1·042–1·046	—	1·542–1·546	2/70	Benzaldehyde 95% min.
Anise	0·978–0·992	−2/+1	1·553–1·560	3/90	F.p. min. 15°. M.p. min. 19°
Bay	0·940–0·985	0/−4	1·500–1·520	1/95§	Phenols 45% min. § Freshly dist.
Bergamot	0·876–0·881	+8/+24	1·464–1·467	—	Esters 36–43% (L.A.)
Cade	0·970–1·010	—	1·510–1·530	—	
Cajuput	0·910–0·923	+1/−4	1·464–1·472	2/80	Cineole 50–65%
Camphor (rect.)	0·870–0·918	+2/+20	1·462–1·470	3/90	Cineole 30% min.
Camphor (heavy)	1·00–1·08	0/+12	1·500–1·510	3/90	
Cananga	0·905–0·940	−15/−55	1·493–1·505	1–2/95	
Caraway	0·902–0·912	+74/+80	1·485–1·492	7/80	Carvone 53–63%
Cardamom	0·917–0·940	+20/+44	1·461–1·467	6/70	Ester value 90–156
Cassia (rect.)	1·052–1·063	−1/+1	1·600–1·606	2/80	Aldehyde 80% min. (C.A.)
Cedar Wood	0·936–0·970	−25/−60	1·495–1·510	10–20/90	
Chamomile	0·897–0·910	—	1·442–1·450	6/70	Sap. value 260–296. Acid v. 1·5–14
Chenopodium	0·955–0·975	−4/−8	1·474–1·480	10/70	Ascaridole min. 65·0%
Cinnamon bark	1·000–1·035	0/−2	1·573–1·595	3/70	Aldehyde 60–75% (C.A.)
Cinnamon leaf	1·045–1·065†	−1/+1	1·530–1·540	3/70	Eugenol 75–90%
Citronella (Ceylon)	0·895–0·905	−9/−18	1·480–1·485	4–10/80	Total alcohols 59% min. G.
Citronella (Java)	0·880–0·895	−5/+2	1·468–1·473	4–10/80	Total alcohols 85% min. G.
Clove	1·041–1·054	0/−1·5	1·528–1·537	2/70	Eugenol 85–90%
Copaiba	0·895–0·908†	−7/−35	1·495–1·500	—	
Coriander	0·863–0·877	+8/+12	1·462–1·472	3/70	
Cubebs	0·905–0·925	−20/−43	1·480–1·502	18/90	B.p. 60% distils between 250–280°
Cummin	0·900–0·935†	+3/+8	1·495–1·509	10/80	Aldehyde min. 30% (CuA)
Dill	0·895–0·910	+70/+80	1·481–1·492	10/80	Carvone 43–63%
Eucalyptus	0·904–0·924	−5/+10	1·458–1·470	5/70	Cineole min. 70%
Fennel	0·953–0·983	+4/+24	1·525–1·545	5/90	F.p. min. +3°
Fir (Siberian)	0·900–0·920	−32/−45	1·466–1·476	1/90	Esters 33–45% (B.A.)
Geranium (Afr.)	0·889–0·900	−7/−12	1·466–1·473	3/70	Esters min. 20% (G.T.)
Geranium (Bbn.)	0·883–0·892	−8/−14	1·462–1·468	3/70	Esters min. 25% (G.T.)
Geranium (Fr.)	0·889–0·900	−7/−12	1·466–1·473	3/70	Esters min. 20% (G.T.)
Ginger	0·877–0·888†	−28/−45	1·488–1·494	—	
Grapefruit (expressed)	0·854–0·860†	+91/+96	1·475–1·478	—	
Juniper	0·859–0·890	+1/−15	1·476–1·484	4/95	
Lavender (English)	0·875–0·895	−5/−13	1·460–1·474	3/80	Esters 7–15% (L.A.). E.v. acetyl 165–200
Lavender (foreign)	0·878–0·892	−5/−12	1·457–1·464	4/70	Esters 35–50% (L.A.). E.v. acetyl 220–280
Lavender, spike	0·894–0·915	−4/+6	1·462–1·469	4/65	Free alcohols 35% min. (L.)

Lemon	0·850–0·856	+57/+65	1·474–1·476	12/90	Citral min. 3·5%. Non-vol. 2–3%
Lemon, terpeneless	0·890–0·900	−4/+1	1·478–1·485	1/80	Citral 40–50%. Ester value 40–75
Lemongrass (E. Ind.)	0·893–0·906	−3/+1	1·483–1·489	3/70	Citral min. 70%
Lemongrass (W. Ind.)	0·870–0·895	−3/+1	1·483–1·489	1/70	Citral min. 70%
Limes (expressed)	0·872–0·885†	+35/+40	1·476–1·485	—	Citral 6–10%
Mustard, volatile	1·005–1·020	—	1·525–1·530	10/70	Allyl *iso*thiocyanate min. 92%
Neroli	0·865–0·880	0/+8	1·468–1·477	2/80	Sap. value max. 70
Nutmeg, (E. Ind.)	0·880–0·915	+10/+25	1·475–1·488	3/90	Non-vol. max. 3%
Nutmeg, (W. Ind.)	0·860–0·880	+25/+45	1·472–1·477	4/90	Non-vol. max. 3%
Nutmeg, terpeneless	—	+1/+14	1·500–1·533	3/80	
Orange, bitter	0·845–0·851	+92/+97	1·472–1·475	7/90	Ald. 0·3–1·0 (D). Residue on evap. 2–4%
Orange, sweet	0·842–0·848	+94/+99	1·472–1·476	7/90	Ald. 1·0–3·0 (D). Residue on evap. 1–5%
Origanum	0·915–0·970†	−1/−13	1·500–1·510	3/70	Carvacrol 25–85%
Palmarosa	0·885–0·895†	−2/+2	1·474–1·485	3/70	Geraniol 75–95%
Parsley	1·040–1·100†	−5/−11	1·510–1·519	8/80	
Patchouli	0·950–0·960†	−40/−68	1·505–1·520	10/90	
Pennyroyal	0·930–0·960†	+14/+28	1·475–1·490	3/70	Pulegone min. 85%
Peppermint	0·897–0·910	−16/−30	1·460–1·470	4/70	Free menthol min. 45%. Esters 4–9% (M.A.
Peppermint (Jap. Dem.)	0·895–0·905†	−25/−35	1·460–1·465	4/70	Total menthol 46–60%. Esters 5–12% (M.A.)
Petitgrain (French)	0·885–0·900†	−5/+3	1·462–1·465	3/70	Esters 50–80% (L.A.)
Petitgrain (S. Amer.)	0·884–0·895†	−2/+8	1·462–1·465	2/80	Esters 35–60% (L.A.)
Pimento	1·030–1·045	0/−5	1·500–1·536	3/70	Eugenol min. 60%
Pine (aromatic)	0·927–0·942	+7/+15	1·479–1·487	2/70	
Pine (pumilio)	0·858–0·870	−4/−15	1·470–1·480	10/95	Esters 4–10% (B.A.)
Rose	0·852–0·862§	−2/−4	1·458–1·465	—	§ At 30°. F.p. 18–22°. M.p. 19–23°
Rosemary	0·893–0·910	−5/+10	1·466–1·474	1/90	E.v. 5·5 min.; E.v. acetyl 37–65
Rue	0·832–0·845†	0/+3	1·430–1·440	3/70	F.p. 8–10°
Sandalwood (E.I.)	0·968–0·983	−15/−20	1·505–1·510	5/70	Esters 2% min. (S.A.). Free alcohol 90% (S.)
Sandalwood (W. Aus.)	0·964–0·974	−3/−10	1·498–1·508	3–6/70	Free alcohol 90% (S.)
Sassafras (Amer.)	1·064–1·078	+1/+5	1·523–1·532	3/90	Safrole 80–90%. Congealing p. min. 5°
Sassafras (Brazil)	1·080–1·094	0/−3	1·532–1·536	4/90	Safrole 85–95%. Congealing p. min. 8°
Savin	0·905–0·930†	+43/+66	1·470–1·478	2/90	Sap. value 101–169
Spearmint	0·917–0·934	−45/−60	1·484–1·491	1/80	Carvone 55% min.
Succini	0·845–0·900	−12/+12	1·465–1·500	8/95	
Tea-tree	0·890–0·900	+6/+10	1·476–1·481	3/90	Ester value 2–7, after acet. 80–90. Cineole max. 10%
Thyme	0·900–0·955	—	1·483–1·510	2/80	Phenols min. 40%
Turpentine (rect.)	0·855–0·868	—	1·467–1·477	7/90	Non-vol. max. 0·5%
Wintergreen	1·176–1·186	−0·5/+0·5	1·534–1·538	6/70§	§ At 25°. Esters min. 98% (M.S.)
Ylang-Ylang	0·930–0·960†	−38/−56	1·494–1·505	1–2/95	Sap. value 95–138

† Sp. gr. at 15·5°/15·5°.
Alcohols: G, calculated as geraniol, L as linalol, S as santalol, B as borneol.
Aldehydes: CA, calculated as cinnamic aldehyde, CuA as cumminic aldehyde, D as decanal.
Esters: BA, calculated as bornyl acetate, GT as geranyl tiglate, LA as linalyl acetate, MA as menthyl acetate, MS as methyl salicylate, SA as santalyl acetate.

‡ Solubility: 4/90 = soluble in 4 volumes of 90% alcohol.

Table 52

Constants: Synthetics and Isolated Products

	Specific Gravity	Solubility* or Melting-Point	Ref. Index at 20°	Boiling-Point	
Acetophenone	1·0295	M.p. 19·6–19·7	1·534–1·536	202·5	
Amyl acetate	0·870–0·875	S. 21/45	1·399–1·402	138–142	
Amyl benzoate	0·994–1·003	S. 4/80	1·4945	261	
Amyl butyrate	0·863–0·869	—	—	169–181	
Amyl cinnamate	1·001	S. 7/80	1·534–1·535	—	
Amyl salicylate	1·054–1·056	S. 3/90	1·505–1·507	277·5	
Anethole	0·985–0·987	M.p. 21–22	1·558–1·561	234–235	
Anisic aldehyde	1·126–1·239	S. 2/60	1·572–1·574	248·5	
Benzaldehyde	1·051–1·055	S. 1/70	1·545–1·546	178	
Benzyl acetate	1·060–1·062	S. 1·5/70	1·502–1·503	215·5	
Benzyl alcohol, *B.P.*	1·043–1·060†	S. misc./95	1·538–1·541	200–208	Min. 97·0% by acetylation
Benzyl benzoate, *B.P.*	1·115–1·119†	F.p. min. 17·0	1·568–1·570	About 323	Min. 99·0% (2 hours boiling)
Bornyl acetate (*iso*)	0·990–0·991	M.p. 29	1·465–1·466	98§	§ At 10 mm
Bromstyrol	1·41–1·43	S. 13/80	—	219	M.p. −2·5/−2·0°
Cinnamic aldehyde	1·054–1·058	S. 3·5/70	1·615–1·619	252	
Citral	0·893–0·897	S. 7/60	1·486–1·488	228–229	
Citronellal	0·855–0·860	S. 5/70	1·446–1·450	205–208	
Citronellol	0·861–0·870	—	1·456–1·458	225–226	Opt. Rot. −1/+4°
Coumarin	0·9348	S. 9/70	—	300–301	M.p. 69–70°
Dibutyl phthalate, *B.P.*	1·042–1·049†	S. misc./95	1·492–1·495	About 330	Min. 99·0%
Dimethyl phthalate, *B.P.*	1·186–1·192†	S. misc./95	1·515–1·517	About 280	Min. 99·0%
Diphenyl oxide	Solid	S. 15/80	—	259	M.p. 26–27°
Ethyl acetate	0·905–0·906	—	1·373	77	
Ethyl butyrate	0·885–0·886	S. 1·5/45	1·388	115–140	
Ethyl benzoate	1·051–1·053	S. 7/60	1·505–1·506	212	
Ethyl cinnamate	1·053–1·055	S. 6/70	1·559–1·561	271	
Ethyl formate	0·9295	S. 9/aq.	1·362	53–57	

Ethyl phthalate, *B.P.C.*	1·111–1·126	S. misc./90	1·4805–1·5060	295	Min. 98%
Ethyl salicylate	1·135–1·137	S. 4/80	1·523–1·524	234	
Eucalyptol (cineole) *B.P.*	0·922–0·924	S. 2/70	1·456–1·460	176–177	Opt. Rot. −1/+1°. F.p. 0·3–1·2 ≡ 98–100% (min. 0°)
Eugenol, *B.P.C.*	1·064–1·068	S. 2/70	1·540–1·542	254	
Geraniol	0·880–0·885	S. 3/60	1·471–1·478	229–230	
Geranyl acetate	0·910–0·917	S. 2/80	1·460–1·464	245	
Heliotropin	Solid	S. 10/70	—	263	M.p. 37°
Hydroxycitronellal	0·955–0·956	S. 3/70	1·449–1·456	115–135§	§ At 10 mm
Ionone alpha	0·9338	S. 4/50	1·499	123–124§	§ At 10 mm
Ionone beta	0·9488	S. 2–3/70	1·5198	132§	§ At 10 mm
Isoeugenol	1·085–1·090	S. 4/50	1·570–1·576	266·5	
Linalol	0·87	S. 1–3/70	1·463	197–220	
Linalyl acetate	0·905–0·913	S. 5/70	1·453–1·456	220	
Menthol (lævo), *B.P.*	Solid	M.p. 42–44	—	211–222	Opt. Rot. −49/−50°
Menthol (racemic), *B.P.*	Solid	M.p. 32·5–34	—	211–222	F.p. 27–28° (30–32°)
Methyl anthranilate	1·168	S. 3·5/70	—	255	M.p. 24–25°
Methyl ionone	0·910–0·920	S. 12/70	1·515	—	
Methyl salicylate, *B.P.*	1·180–1·184†	S. misc./90	1·536–1·538	—	Min. 99·0%
Musk ambrette	Solid	S. 60/95	—	—	M.p. 84–86°
Musk ketone	Solid	S. 100/95	—	—	M.p. 131–136°
Musk xylol	Solid	S. 200/95	—	—	M.p. 110–113°
Phenylacetic acid	1·077	S. 1·5/45	—	265·5	M.p. 76–77°
Phenylacetic aldehyde	1·560	S. 3/70	1·52–1·53	206	
Phenylethyl acetate	1·037–1·038	S. 1/70	1·498–1·499	232	
Phenylethyl alcohol	1·023–1·024	S. 2/50	1·531–1·533	222	
Safrol	1·096–1·100†	S. 3/90	1·536–1·539	About 233	M.p. min. 11. F.p. min. 10°
Salicylic aldehyde	1·169–1·173	S. 2/90	1·571–1·572	197	
Terpineol, *B.P.C.*	0·931–0·935†	S. 2/70	1·4825–1·4855	214–224	
Terpinyl acetate	0·962–0·965	S. 4–6/70	1·465	220	
Thymol, *B.P.*	Solid	S. 1/90	—	—	F.p. min. 49·3°
Vanillin, *B.P.*	Solid	M.p. 81–83	—	—	

* Solubility: 40/80 = soluble in 4 volumes of 80 per cent alcohol.
† For sp. gr. read wt./ml at 20°.

NOTES ON INDIVIDUAL ESSENTIAL OILS

The analysis of essential oils consists of determining the physical constants of weight per ml, optical rotation, refractive index and solubility, with sometimes boiling-range, melting-point and non-volatile matter, and the percentage of the chemically reactive constituents present by the methods outlined above. Any adulteration is detected mainly by the interpretation of the results obtained for these constants and very little further quantitative work is possible. However, a few notes are given below on some of the individual oils, but standard works on the subject should be consulted for more detailed information which cannot be included in a small monograph such as this.

Almond Oil. Benzaldehyde may be determined by the general method for aldehydes, using 0·6 g. In the determination of oils containing benzaldehyde allowance should be made for the amount of acid titratable to methyl orange.

The oil used in pharmacy has been freed from prussic acid, but where the crude oil is used it is adjusted to contain from 2 to 4 per cent. The free prussic acid may be determined as follows:

> Dissolve about 1 g in 25 ml of 90 per cent ethanol, add 1 ml of 10 per cent potassium iodide solution and 1 ml of dilute ammonia solution. Titrate with 0·1N silver nitrate to a permanent opalescence. 1 ml 0·1N = 0·0054 g HCN.

Another method is:

> Dissolve 0·75 g of magnesium sulphate in 50 ml of water, add 5 ml of 0·5N alkali and 2 drops of potassium chromate solution. Titrate with 0·1N silver nitrate to the production of a permanent reddish tint. Pour this mixture into a flask containing a weighed portion of about 1 g of almond oil; titrate again to a red tint. Conduct this titration as rapidly as possible. 1 ml 0·1N = 0·0027 g HCN.

Almond oil is frequently adulterated with synthetic benzaldehyde and methods of detection of the latter depend upon the presence of traces of chlorine compounds in the adulterant. But benzaldehyde free from chlorinated bodies is now a commercial article, and hence the absence of chlorine is not an infallible indication of the genuineness of the almond oil. Salamon's method[25] is somewhat objectionable in technique and has many disadvantages, particularly the difficulty of controlling the violent reaction.

> In a stoppered retort, the beak of which dips beneath the surface of 10 ml of 0·1N silver nitrate, place 40 ml of concentrated sulphuric acid, add 1 g of almond oil, mix and add 10 ml of concentrated nitric acid. Distil for thirty minutes, using caution at first, until frothing subsides. To the distillate add 1 ml of concentrated nitric acid, boil until colourless and weigh the precipitate.

Daubney[26] modified Schimmel's method of burning the oil and estimating the chloride formed. He obtained total recovery of known amounts of chlorine added to almond oil in the form of organic chlorine compounds. The advantage of the method is that the determination can proceed as long as is necessary to give weighable amounts of silver chloride. The process requires the special Richardson lamp used by the Institute of Petroleum Technologists[27] for determination of sulphur in petroleum products, and the technique given by Daubney should be followed, for details of which the original paper must be consulted. Bitter almond oil was shown to contain about 0·001 per cent of chlorine, whilst commercial benzaldehydes examined contained between 0·005 and 0·03 per cent.

Bay Oil. In the determination of phenols in this oil a secondary liquid layer frequently occurs at the bottom of the separated non-phenols; this should be included in the unabsorbed portion.

Garratt[28] suggested the use of the furfural test as used for peppermint oil (p. 738) to detect clove oil in bay oil. The ten-minute red value of a bay oil under the conditions of test was about 1·4, whereas that for clove oil was as high as 23.

Bergamot Oil. In the determination of esters, the first disappearance of the colour of the indicator should be taken as the end-point and any re-appearance of the pink colour on standing should be ignored.[29] This oil is very frequently adulterated, especially with artificial esters. A modification of the method given above, to detect terpinyl acetate, consists of determining the saponification value by allowing to stand in the cold for twenty-four hours, and comparing the result with that obtained by hot saponification.

The non-volatile residue obtained by evaporating 2 g of the oil rapidly in a flat-bottomed dish, 9 cm in diameter and 1·5 cm in depth, on a water-bath for four hours should be between 4 and 6 per cent.

Cajuput Oil. The cineole is best estimated by the modification used for light camphor oil, in which the mixture is enriched with cineole before determination.

Camphor Oil. Note the modification recommended in the general method described on p. 725 for the determination of cineole in this oil. Heavy fractions of camphor oil contain safrole and are known as Brown Oil of Camphor.

Cananga Oil. Simmons[30] has suggested that adulteration with light fractions of petroleum oil might be indicated by the flash-point. The pure oil flashes at 93°, but some obviously adulterated samples flashed at 82° and 83°. The refractive index probably gives the most definite conclusion as to purity, increasing considerably with this type of adulteration.

Caraway Oil. Use 1·5 g for the determination of ketones.

Cassia Oil. Use 0·8 g for the determination of aldehydes by the hydroxylamine method. It is very common in the trade still to buy and sell this oil on the bisulphite absorption method, the standard adopted by this method being 80 to 85 per cent cinnamic aldehyde; an oil of this quality gives only 75 to 78 per cent by the hydroxylamine method. Schimmel[31] has shown that the flash-point of the oil is lowered by alcohol. A rectified cassia oil had a flash-point of 117°, but the addition of 1 per cent of alcohol lowered it to 70° and 3 per cent of alcohol to 45°. In their opinion cassia oil should not flash below 75°.

Artificial esters, such as ethyl phthalate, may be present in adulterated oils, and may be detected in the unabsorbed portion from a bisulphite absorption test.

The acidity of the oil increases with age if stored under poor conditions; the acid value should not exceed 10.

Chenopodium Oil. Schimmel[32] criticised the *B.P.C.* ascaridole evaluation as being based on a method of assay not sufficiently tested as to its reliability.

Cinnamon Bark Oil. Use 1 g for the determination of aldehydes. By experiment, the usually accepted ferric chloride test for absence of leaf oil was found to admit from 30 to 40 per cent adulteration. A determination of phenols should be made, not more than 10 per cent being present in bark oils.

Cinnamon Leaf Oil. As much as 10 per cent of aldehyde does not appreciably affect the phenol determination by the usual method.

Citronella Oil. As citronellal, which is present in the oil, is converted by acetic anhydride into *iso*pulegyl acetate, the 'total acetylisable constituents' are determined and calculated as geraniol. The determination is made by the method for Alcohols given above, the percentage of 'total acetylisable' being calculated from the formula:

$$\text{Percentage of total acetylisable constituents} = \frac{7{\cdot}707x}{\text{wt. of acetylated oil} - 0{\cdot}021x}$$

x = ml 0·5N ethanolic potassium hydroxide absorbed by saponification of the acetylated oil.

The citronellal may be determined by the method on p. 722 and the geraniol obtained by difference. Java oil contains 30 to 40 per cent, and Ceylon oil 7 to 15 per cent of citronellal.

Clove Oil. Eugenol and aceteugenol are both absorbed in the determination of phenols.

Cummin Oil. Use 1·0 g for the determination of aldehydes.

Dill Oil. Use 1·5 g for the determination of ketones. The neutral sulphite absorption method (p. 720) is also suitable for this oil.

Eucalyptus Oil. The limit for aldehydes imposed by the *B.P.* is equivalent to 1·5 per cent of cuminal. Hendry and Berry[33] have suggested that the range of specific gravity should not be too stringent, especially as oils containing less than the standard limit of aldehydes are generally lower in specific gravity; the lower limit should be reduced to 0·905, equivalent to a weight per ml of 0·900. The *N.F.* minimum congealing-point for the oil, −15·4°, is equal to 70 per cent of cineole.

E. Citriodora Oil. The figures in the literature for citronellal content (85 to 95 per cent), using bisulphite absorption, are high. The hydroxylamine method gives more accurate figures.

Lavender Oil. Many good French oils have an ester content below the *B.P.C.* minimum of 35·0 per cent. Linalyl acetate increases the 'apparent cineole content' which is really low; adulteration with spike lavender oil also increases this 'apparent cineole content.'

Lemon Oil. The *B.P.C.* minimum citral content of 3·5 per cent admits inferior oils, good oils containing 4·4 to 4·8 per cent. Lemon terpenes are generally used as the adulterant. Romeo and Giuffre[34] claim that the percentage of volatile esters present is an index of adulteration, 1·25 to 1·75 per cent as linalyl acetate being present in the original oil and only 0·30 to 0·60 per cent in terpene residues, but sophisticators could easily circumvent this test. The residue obtained by rapidly evaporating 5 g in a dish, as described under Bergamot Oil, should be from 2 to 3 per cent.

Terpeneless Lemon Oil. Use 1·0 g for the determination of aldehydes. Dalton[35] found the aldehyde: ester ratio for genuine terpeneless oil to be 5 : 2, any considerable deviation from this pointing to adulteration. The genuine oil should not be soluble in 75 per cent alcohol.

Lemon Grass Oil. Use 1 g for the determination of aldehydes by the hydroxylamine method. Of the absorption methods, neutral sulphite gives somewhat higher results (up to 2 per cent) than bisulphite, the latter method being generally used.

Mustard Oil. The assay for allyl *iso*thiocyanate is the following:

> Dissolve about 4 g in sufficient 95 per cent ethanol to produce 100 ml. To 5 ml of this solution add 50 ml of 0·1N silver nitrate and 5 ml of strong ammonia solution; heat under a reflux condenser on a water-bath for thirty minutes, cool, dilute to exactly 100 ml with water and filter. To 50 ml of the filtrate add 5 ml of concentrated nitric acid, and titrate the excess of silver nitrate with 0·1N ammonium thiocyanate, using iron alum as indicator. 1 ml 0·1N = 0·004958 g C_3H_5NCS.

Nutmeg Oil. The size of the dish and time of evaporation are important factors in the *B.P.C.* test for non-volatile matter and have been standardised to the details given under Bergamot Oil (limit, 2 per cent).

Orange Oil. Washed citrus oils are detected by the low percentage of non-volatile matter, which should not be less than 2·0 per cent in pure oils. When distilled, the first 10 per cent of distillate should have an optical rotation differing by not more than 2° from that of the original oil. Use 5 to 10 g for the determination of aldehydes; the oil contains 1·0 to 3·0 per cent as decanal, $C_{10}H_{20}O$.

Terpeneless Orange Oil. Use 0·6 g for the determination of aldehydes; the oil contains 20 to 30 per cent.

Pennyroyal Oil. The estimation of pulegone (and other ketones, menthone also being present) presents some difficulties, the ketone reacting much more slowly than others. Since the *S.A.C.* hydroxylamine method is inapplicable, the neutral sulphite method must be employed, and the absorption and neutralisation continued for at least four hours. A 40 per cent sodium sulphite solution assists the absorption and should be used in place of the usual 20 per cent solution.

Peppermint Oil. The esters are often above the *B.P.* maximum of 9·0 per cent and the *U.S.P.* gives no upper limit. Use 3 g for the determination of menthone. Parry and Ferguson[36] have published figures for a large number of English and American oils, the menthone varying from 24 to 42 per cent in English oils and from 17 to 30 per cent in American oils. Hence this constituent varies too much in its proportion to be used as a limiting characteristic.

Garratt[37] used the variable proportion of furfuraldehyde present in different types of oil as a means of detecting Japanese mint oil in peppermint oil. As the quantity of furfuraldehyde was found to be approximately the same for all oils of the same type, a roughly quantitative method was developed.

Mix 0·1 ml of the oil, measured from a 1-ml pipette (graduated in 1/100th of a ml), in a test-tube with 5·0 ml of a 2 per cent solution of freshly redistilled aniline in glacial acetic acid, added from a burette. Examine the reaction mixture in a 1-cm cell of the Lovibond tintometer after an interval of ten minutes.

The reaction mixture must be protected from bright light. For American oils the red value obtained was from 0·5 to 0·7 unit, for European oils 0·1 to 0·3 and English oils 0·4 to 1·2; but with dementholised Japanese oils the red value rose to from 4·5 to 7·4 units, and the following table was constructed for a roughly quantitative application of the test.

TABLE 53

	Ten-minute Red Values	
	American	French and Italian
Containing 10 per cent Japanese oil	1·1–1·4	0·6–0·9
,, 20 ,, ,, ,,	1·4–1·8	0·9–1·3
,, 30 ,, ,, ,,	1·8–2·4	1·3–1·9
,, 40 ,, ,, ,,	2·4–2·8	1·9–2·3
,, 50 ,, ,, ,,	above 2·8	above 2·3

For English oils the figures may be taken as similar to those for American oils, with the caution that, in view of the wider range shown for the pure oils, too much stress must not be laid on any results which slightly exceed these limits. As it would not be difficult to fractionate a Japanese mint oil to eliminate furfural and circumvent the test, only a positive result would be of value.

Although the original method was developed using a Lovibond tintometer for colour measurement, a more precise instrumental method could be employed. The colour absorbs at a maximum at 525 mμ and a 1-cm layer of a 0·008 per cent furfural solution under the given conditions has an extinction of 0·70.

Pimento Oil. Garratt[28] suggested the use of the furfural test described under Peppermint Oil to detect admixture of clove oil with pimento oil, the latter having a red value of about 1·0 unit under the conditions of the test, whereas that of clove oil, without dilution, was 23; admixture of 10 per cent was easily detected.

Rose Oil. Geraniol and citronellol constitute about 70 to 75 per cent of the oil, the latter being one-third to a half of the total alcohols. An approximate estimation of the citronellol present may be obtained by the method given above (p. 726). The amount of **stearoptene** (a mixture of hydrocarbons which occurs in variable proportions in oils from different sources) may be a useful criterion for assaying the quality of commercial rose oil. It may be determined by dissolving a weighed quantity of the oil in 70 per cent ethanol, in which the stearoptene is insoluble, filtering through a weighed filter paper and drying *in vacuo* to constant weight. The melting-point of the stearoptene from rose oil varies between 32° and 37°; paraffin wax, spermaceti and stearin may be used as adulterants.

Any appreciable difference in refractive index of the washed oil will show adulteration with alcohol.

It has been stated that citronellol raises the specific gravity of rose oil, but Parry[38] has pointed out that, as the specific gravity of this adulterant is 0·850 at 30°, it will lower the figure.

Rosemary Oil. The 'apparent cineole content' (*cf.* Cineole determination) helps detection of adulteration with light camphor oil fractions; the freezing-point of the *o*-cresol mixture after the addition of an equal quantity of pure cineole-cresol complex should not be above 39·8°.

Sandalwood Oil. Benzyl alcohol is a common adulterant, one part being equivalent to two parts of santalol; it can be detected by heating the oil with potassium dichromate and dilute sulphuric acid in a test-tube immersed in a water-bath, the odour of benzaldehyde being easily recognised.

Sassafras Oil. The freezing-point of sassafras oil gives a method of determination of the safrole content which is present to the extent of about 80 to 90 per cent.

Determine the congealing-point of the sassafras oil in the apparatus used for cineole (see p. 725). Construct a graph correlating freezing-point and percentage safrole from Table 54 (Shukis and Wachs[39]).

TABLE 54

SAFROLE per cent by wt.	FREEZING-POINT ° C.	SAFROLE per cent by wt.	FREEZING-POINT ° C.
69·1	2·4	90	8·3
73·3	3·7	91	8·6
76	4·4	92	8·8
79	5·2	93	9·2
82	6·1	94	9·4
85	6·9	95	9·7
86	7·2	96	10·0
87	7·5	97	10·3
88	7·8	98	10·6
89	8·0	99·5	11·0

Spearmint Oil. Use 1·5 g for the determination of ketones. The *N.F.* requires the oil to contain not less than 55 per cent by volume of carvone when determined by the neutral sulphite method, using saturated sodium sulphite solution and keeping neutrality to phenolphthalein with 30 per cent sodium bisulphite solution.

Thyme Oil. To estimate the components of the mixture of thymol and carvacrol present in the oil, the melting-point of the dried mixed phenols obtained by light petroleum extraction was taken by Sage and Dalton[40] and the percentage read from a curve prepared from known mixtures.

Turpentine Oil. Petroleum products are frequently used for the adulteration of turpentine and are to be suspected if a low weight per ml and refractive index are found. The original method of polymerisation and sulphonation proposed by Armstrong[41] for the direct determination and separation of petroleum spirit has been recommended by Coste[42] for confirmation of these suspicions, and in his opinion was in every way preferable to the various drastic processes suggested by other workers. As small a quantity as 100 ml of turpentine should, with care, give reliable results by this method.

Treat 500 ml of the oil with about 150 ml of sulphuric acid (two volumes of acid to one of water), cautiously agitating the mixture and cooling in running water. When no more heat is developed, transfer to a separator, run off the acid and wash the oil layer; transfer this to a flask and steam-distil. Treat the distillate similarly with half its bulk of 4 : 1 acid and again steam-distil. The residue from this second operation, consisting of cymene and a small quantity of paraffin hydrocarbons, should not be more than 4 to 5 per cent of the original oil. If it is more it is advisable to repeat the treatment with the 4 : 1 acid. The proportion of petroleum, which is not affected by this treatment, may be estimated by subtracting 5 per cent from the percentage volume of residue.

Armstrong effected a further purification by treating the residue with concentrated sulphuric acid heated to 50° to 60°, separating and again steam-distilling; genuine oil will not give more than 0·5 to 1 per cent of residue.

A similar method has been included in the *N.F.* for paraffin hydrocarbons in turpentine. The method has also been used for detection of paraffin in Ceylon citronella oil when in known mixtures recovery of added kerosene was only about 85 per cent. Both pure turpentine and citronella oils give negligible residues by this method.

Place 20 ml of fuming sulphuric acid, containing 15 per cent free sulphur trioxide, in a graduated narrow-necked Babcock bottle of 50-ml capacity, cool in an ice-bath for ten minutes; keep the bottle in the bath and add 5 ml of oil of turpentine dropwise at such a rate that the bottle remains cold. Incline the bottle and rotate continuously during the addition which should require about five minutes. When no further action is apparent remove from the ice-bath, bringing slowly to room temperature with frequent cautious shaking. Wash down the neck with 3 or 4 ml of fuming sulphuric acid.

When no further action is apparent on cautious shaking, shake vigorously for thirty seconds. Place the bottle in a water-bath and heat slowly to 60° with frequent agitation. (Caution is required, as escaping gas may force some of the solution from the bottle.) Heat at 60° to 65° for fifteen minutes, shaking the contents carefully but vigorously eight to ten times during the period. Remove from the bath and, without cooling, carefully add concentrated sulphuric acid until the bottle is about three-quarters full. Shake well (no material should adhere to stem and sides at this point), cool to room temperature, add sulphuric acid until the liquid is about two-thirds up in the neck of the flask. Allow to stand overnight and read. Pure oil of turpentine should show not more than 1 per cent of readable separation.

Liniment of Turpentine, *B.P.* Contains 65 per cent by volume of oil of turpentine and 5 per cent by weight of camphor emulsified with soft soap.

The total oils can be determined by steam distillation after acidification with dilute sulphuric acid, preferably in the apparatus used for the determination of volatile oils in drugs.

Wintergreen and **Sweet Birch Oils.** In the determination of esters in these oils, the *S.A.C.*[43] recommend that the free acid be determined in a separate experiment by shaking 5 g of the oil with 25 ml of water and titrating with 0·1N aqueous potassium hydroxide, using 1 ml of phenol red (0·04 per cent in 20 per cent ethanol) as indicator. The saponification should be carried out without the preliminary neutralisation of the free acid, the boiling should be continued for an hour and a half, and from the volume of alkali required the equivalent of that used in the separate determination of the free acid should be deducted.

Ylang-Ylang Oil. The saponification value should be 95 to 138. In adulterated oils it is much less.

ALCOHOLIC SOLUTIONS AND FLAVOURING EXTRACTS

Determination of Essential Oils

Randall[44] proposed a method for determining small percentages of oil, using Babcock milk-test bottles.

For extracts containing 3 to 5 per cent of oil, pipette 10 ml into a clean Babcock bottle, fill to the shoulder with a clear solution of calcium chloride, sp. gr. 1·30, containing 4 per cent, by volume, of concentrated hydrochloric acid, and shake. Run in exactly 1 ml of light petroleum (b.p. 40° to 60°), stopper with a soft cork, shake violently for one or two minutes and centrifuge for two minutes. Then remove the cork and quickly add enough of the calcium chloride solution to bring the whole of the petroleum layer within the graduated part of the neck and centrifuge again. Read the volume of the petroleum column, taking the mean graduation between the upper and lower meniscus. The lower meniscus should be flat and sharp, any whitish collar indicating insufficient hydrochloric acid in the calcium chloride solution. Conduct a control estimation using 10 ml of alcohol in place of the extract and calculate the volume of light petroleum introduced in terms of the bottle graduation; deduct this volume from that of the petroleum and oil solution, and multiply the remainder by two to give the percentage of oil in the extract. The factor may vary with the composition of the light petroleum which should be tested by an estimation of the oil in a standard 5 per cent orange extract.

This method is official in the *U.S.P.*, only differing in detail (particularly in the use of kerosene in place of light petroleum) for compound spirit of orange and spirit of peppermint.

In practice the use of light petroleum has not been found satisfactory, owing to its volatility. A modification of the method can be used, employing round Gerber milk-tubes, which has given quite good results with the concentrated waters and spirits of the *B.P.* and *B.P.C.*

The reagent is a saturated solution of sodium chloride to which 2 per cent by volume of concentrated hydrochloric acid is added, and the solution filtered. If the strength of the oil in the alcoholic solution be between 7 and 15 per cent, take 2 ml (but for lower strengths use 5 ml) and introduce it into a Gerber milk-tube containing 20 ml (17 ml if 5 ml of alcoholic solution is used) of the reagent. Then add exactly 0·5 ml of kerosene delivered from a 1-ml pipette. Close the tube immediately with a rubber cork, shake, centrifuge for three minutes and measure the paraffin layer at room temperature exactly as for milk fat. A control experiment must be made, using 0·5 ml of the kerosene and a quantity of ethanol approximately equivalent to the amount present in the test solution.

The blank varies considerably under different conditions, *e.g.* for a particular sample of kerosene, with 5 ml and 2 ml of ethanol the readings were 3·76 and 3·90 respectively; in the former case the percentage of oil present for 2 ml of sample would be

$$\frac{(\text{scale reading} \times 1{\cdot}33) - 5{\cdot}0}{0{\cdot}2}$$

If *iso*propyl alcohol has been used as the solvent for the oil, the strength of the sodium chloride solution must be lowered considerably to avoid 'salting out' of the alcohol, and a fresh blank determined.

Another modification has been worked out by Valaer[45] using saturated magnesium sulphate solution containing a little hydrochloric acid, and equal parts of mineral oil and kerosene as solvent. For cinnamon, cassia and clove essences most of the ethanol is removed by an air current after introducing the sample into the Babcock bottle.

The following summary gives a list of the oil contents of the usual pharmaceutical spirits and concentrated waters made by the solution of essential oils in aqueous alcohol. The alcohol may be determined by the method described in Appendix I (p. 778) and the figures are recorded therein.

Concentrated Waters. Anise, caraway, cinnamon (*B.P.*), **dill** (*B.P.*), **peppermint** (*B.P.*), and **spearmint** all contain 2 per cent, by volume, of oil.

Spirit of Peppermint, *B.P.*, contains 10 per cent, by volume, of oil; **Compound Spirit of Orange,** *B.P.C.*, approximately 8·9 per cent, by volume, of oils. If sufficient sample is available a simpler method of determination of volatile oil in spirits is illustrated by the method given below:

> Place 90 ml of 10 per cent solution of sodium chloride containing 1 per cent of concentrated hydrochloric acid in a Hirschsohn flask which has previously been cleaned with sulphuric acid. Add 25 ml of the compound spirit of orange and 5 ml of xylene and shake thoroughly. Raise the undissolved oil into the graduated part of the neck of the flask with more sodium chloride solution. Allow to stand overnight and read the volume of oil.
>
> $$\text{Percentage oil v/v} = (\text{ml oil layer} - 5) \times 4$$

The oil content of most of these preparations may be somewhat lower than the formula requires as, if necessary, they are filtered through talc; this generally applies to concentrated waters.

1. *Analyst*, 1928, **53,** 214.
2. Glichitch, M. L., *Bull. Soc. Chim. France*, 1923, **33,** 1284.
3. *Analyst*, 1957, **82,** 974.
4. Holness, D., *Analyst*, 1959, **84,** 3.
5. *Analyst*, 1960, **85,** 165.
6. Bennett, C. T., and Salamon, M. S., *Analyst*, 1927, **52,** 693.
7. Bennett, C. T., and Cocking, T. T., *Analyst*, 1931, **56,** 79.

8. *Analyst*, 1934, **59**, 105.
9. *Analyst*, 1932, **57**, 773.
10. Rowaan, P. A., and Koolhaus, D. R., *Chem. Weekblad*, 1935, **32**, 405.
11. *Analyst*, 1930, **55**, 109.
12. *Analyst*, 1932, **57**, 378.
13. Cocking, T. T., and Hymas, F. C., *Analyst*, 1930, **55**, 180.
14. *Analyst*, 1936, **61**, 179.
15. Beckett, A. H., and Jolliffe, G. O., *J. Pharm. Pharmacol.*, 1953, **5**, 869.
16. Cocking, T. T., *Y.B. Pharm.*, 1920, 395.
17. *Analyst*, 1927, **52**, 276; 1931, **56**, 738.
18. Berry, P. A., and Swanson, T. B., *P.E.O.R.*, 1933, **24**, 224.
19. *Analyst*, 1959, **84**, 690; 1961, **86**, 231.
20. *Analyst*, 1937, **62**, 541; 1951, **76**, 387.
21. Perry, H. M., and West, T. F., *Analyst*, 1942, **67**, 159.
22. *Analyst*, 1928, **53**, 215.
23. Schimmel, H., *Semi-Annual Reports*, 1910.
24. Bennett, C. T., and Garratt, D. C., *P.E.O.R.*, 1923, **14**, 359.
25. Salamon, M. S., *P.E.O.R.*, 1917, **8**, 41.
26. Daubney, C. G., *Analyst*, 1935, **60**, 29.
27. 'Standard Methods of Testing Petroleum and Its Products', London, 1929. Method G. 4a, p. 16.
28. Garratt, D. C., *Analyst*, 1935, **60**, 595.
29. *Analyst*, 1937, **62**, 451.
30. Simmons, W. H., *P.E.O.R.*, 1934, **25**, 167.
31. Schimmel, H., & Co., *P.E.O.R.*, 1928, **19**, 353.
32. Schimmel, H., & Co., Reports Abs. *C. & D.*, 1935, **122**, 422.
33. Hendry, J., and Berry, P. A., *P.E.O.R.*, 1935, **26**, 117.
34. Romeo, D., and Giuffre, U., *Atti. Congr. Naz. Chim. Pura ed Appl.*, 1923, 322.
35. Dalton, W. G., *P.E.O.R.*, 1928, **19**, 7.
36. Parry, E. J., and Ferguson, G., *C. & D.*, 1936, **124**, 37.
37. Garratt, D. C., *Analyst*, 1935, **60**, 369.
38. Parry, E. J., *C. & D.*, 1935, **122**, 338.
39. Shukis, A. J., and Wachs, H., *Anal. Chem.*, 1948, **20**, 248.
40. Sage, C. E., and Dalton, W. G., *P.E.O.R.*, 1924, **15**, 345.
41. Armstrong, H. E., *J. Soc. Chem. Ind.*, 1882, **1**, 480.
42. Coste, J. H., *Analyst*, 1908, **33**, 219.
43. *Analyst*, 1937, **62**, 541.
44. Randall, W. W., *J.A.O.A.C.*, 1924, **7**, 425.
45. Valaer, D., *Spice Mill*, 1932, **55**, 1410.
46. Sully, B. D., *Analyst*, 1962, **87**, 940.

DRUGS CONTAINING ESSENTIAL OILS

Estimation of Essential Oils in Drugs and Spices

Numerous methods have been devised for the determination of oils in drugs and spices.

The chief difficulties which have to be overcome in the direct methods, in which the distilled oil is weighed or measured, are adherence of oil drops to the sides of vessels, solubility of the oil in the aqueous distillate and volatilisation of the oil when the solvent containing it is evaporated. Methods in which the solvent has to be evaporated should, as far as possible, be avoided.

In order to reduce the volume of aqueous distillate, apparatus has been designed to return the aqueous portion automatically to the distillation flask. Of these the apparatus of Cocking and Middleton[1] claims to measure the oil directly to an accuracy within about 2 per cent and is shown to scale in Fig. 17, the proportions adopted are the final result of a number of trials. It consists of a 1-litre round-bottomed flask A, the neck of which has been cut down in order to reduce the total height of the apparatus (this is convenient but not essential). The neck of the flask carries, by means of a rubber bung, the vertical tube B, the upper portion of which is reduced in diameter in order to decrease the area of cooling surface. This tube is bent round to join the top of the vertical condenser C, which is designed to permit good drainage of the condensed liquid. Below the condenser is a length of graduated tubing of such an internal diameter that 1 ml corresponds to 40 to 45 mm in length. The lower end of this tube is bent up and joined to B to form the return tube F. Between the bottom of the condenser and the graduated tube is a vent D carrying at its upper end a ground stopper with a long seating. A tap G is added for convenience in removing the contents of the receiver for examination, but it is not essential. The flask is supported on an asbestos-gauze and clamped so as to allow the flask to be raised and swirled without difficulty.

In order to avoid adherence of oil drops to the sides of the measuring tube the necessity for cleanliness of the inner surface of the glass is emphasised. Before use the apparatus is rinsed out with ethanol, ether and then with water. The stopper is inserted at D (which, with the tap, must never be greased), the apparatus is filled with sulphuric acid and dichromate mixture, allowed to stand overnight and then rinsed out with water. It is not necessary to use the chromic acid mixture for cleaning before each determination.

The estimation is carried out on quantities of from 4 to 20 g of the drug.

Bring about 300 ml of water nearly to boiling in the flask, add a weighed quantity of the drug and connect the flask to the apparatus. Fill the return tube F with water through the vent D, place a slip of paper on the ground portion of the seating to provide a vent for the air displaced by the steam when the stopper is inserted, and hold the stopper in position by a rubber band. Heat the flask by a Bunsen burner or electric heating-mantle, swirling round at frequent intervals until the contents commence to boil, when, if this is too vigorous, the flask may be lifted from the gauze for a moment. When ebullition has become steady, moderate the heating so that the condensed liquid in the tube E remains cold. When distillation is complete (two to five hours) read the volume of the separated oil, after allowing five to ten minutes for drainage.

For heavy oils and those which do not separate well or which crystallise, 1 ml of oil of turpentine is first added to the apparatus and distilled with water, the volume of distilled oil being determined before and after introduction of the drug.

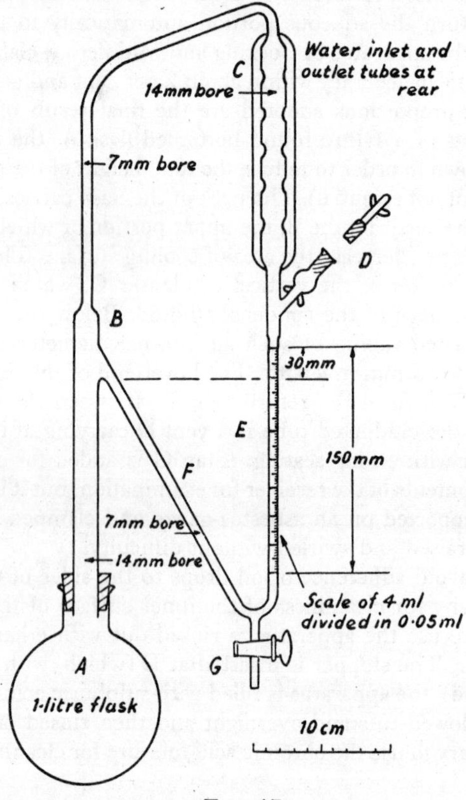

FIG. 17

The figures obtained by an apparatus of this kind do not usually agree closely with yields from large-scale factory distillation, partly owing to the difficulty of correctly representing a bulk with such a small quantity of drug as that used in the assay, and partly owing to decomposition. The method must be looked upon as an estimation of the amount of oil that can be distilled from a drug rather than the amount present.

A further complication has been observed by Kofler and Krämer,[2] who showed that the state of division of the sample had a bearing on the yield. With drugs belonging to the families of *Labiatæ* and *Compositæ* (rosemary herb being an exception) in which the oil is present in external glandular hairs, a greater amount was obtained from the whole drug than when powdered. As would be expected, in other cases where the oil is present in internal cells, the powdered drug gave considerably higher yields.

Meek and Salvin[3] critically discussed the various types of apparatus used and described one they found most convenient. This is shown in Fig. 18.

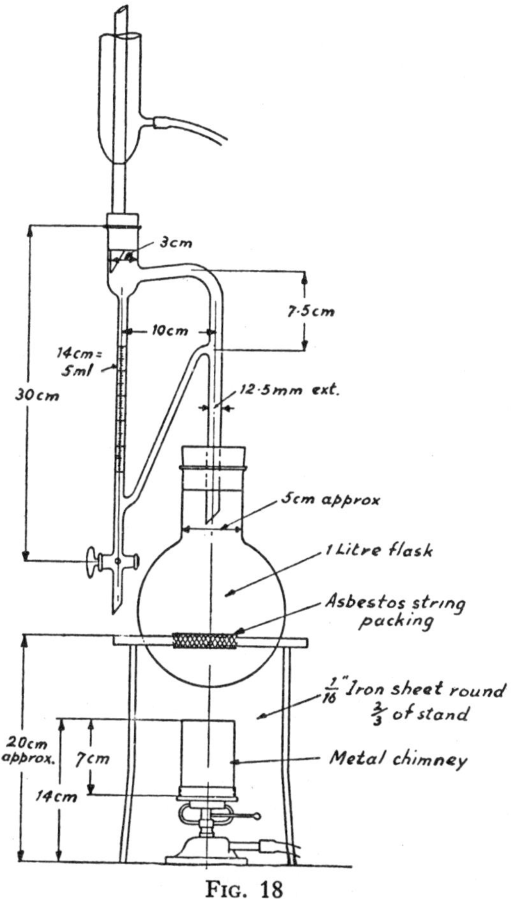

FIG. 18

Place about 350 ml of water (to which, as a matter of routine, a little powdered pipe-clay is added) and the weighed quantity of material in a bolt-head globular flask of resistance glass. Fit to this the receiver which is filled with water, and connect with the condenser, decentred as shown in Fig. 18. By means of a controlled source of heat, supplied by use of the luminous flame of an Argand burner, adjust the rate of distillation so that about 60 drops per minute fall from the end of the condenser; this can be increased, if thought necessary, after the first hour. If it is necessary to remove material which appears to be adhering to the upper part of the flask, ease the condenser clamp and lift the whole apparatus about 2 inches, so that the flask can be rotated. The time needed to complete the distillation will obviously depend on the nature and condition of the material and the quantity taken, but it is not often that more than four hours are required. Allow the oil to cool to laboratory temperature before taking the final reading, the cooling being assisted by very gradually pouring through the top of the condenser a few ml of cold water.

In cleaning the apparatus it is most important to concentrate on the graduated part of the receiver, which is washed with ethanol and water, followed by warm chromic and sulphuric acid mixture. To assist this a glass rod is inserted into the tube and the sides gently rubbed. For oils that do not readily separate from water, various devices have been suggested. Cocking and Middleton used a known volume of turpentine in the flask and Wasicky used pinene. Kuhn put xylene on to water in the graduated tube, and Sage and Fleck used toluene.

The apparatus designed by Cocking and Middleton has been adopted by the *B.P.* but the drug is mixed with cold water. The improvement suggested by Meek and Salvin of using xylene in place of turpentine has also been substituted where this is necessary.

A useful correction if xylene has been used is the addition of 0·01 ml for every hour during which distillation has continued.

TABLE 55

CONDITIONS FOR THE DETERMINATION OF ESSENTIAL OILS IN DRUGS

DRUG	WEIGHT TO BE TAKEN G	CONDITION WHEN DISTILLED	METHOD	APPROXIMATE TIME OF DISTILLATION (HOURS)
Bitter-Orange Peel, Dried, *B.P.*	20	In small pieces	I	3
Buchu, *B.P.C.*	25	Whole	*	4
Caraway, *B.P.C.*	20	Whole	I	4
Cardamom Fruit, *B.P.*	20	Seeds only, whole	I	5
Cinnamon, *B.P.*	40	No. 10 powder	*	5
Clove, *B.P.C.*	4	Coarsely crushed	*	4
Coriander, *B.P.* .	40	No. 10 powder	I	3
Fennel, *B.P.C.*	25	Whole	*	4
Lemon Peel, Dried, *B.P.*	20	In small pieces	I	3
Nutmeg, *B.P.C.*	15	No. 20 powder	I	3

* Method II. *i.e.* with xylene added.

CRUDE FIBRE. In the determination of crude fibre the method employed has an influence on the result, and to obtain comparable figures the same process must be used and strictly adhered to in every detail. In this country the usual method followed is that contained in the Fertilisers and Feeding Stuffs Regulations, 1960, p. 58, in which the details of the procedure are clearly stated. They are:

> Extract 2·7 to 3·0 g (weighed to the nearest mg) with light petroleum (b.p. 40° to 60°) in an extraction apparatus, dry the residue in air and transfer to a 1-litre, conical flask. Add 200 ml of 0·255N sulphuric acid, measured at ordinary temperature and brought to boiling-point, the first 30 or 40 ml being used to disperse the sample. Heat the flask so that the contents come to boiling within one minute (adding an appropriate amount of anti-foaming agent if necessary) and boil gently and continuously for exactly thirty minutes, the original volume being maintained. Rotate the flask every few minutes in order to mix the contents and remove particles from the sides. At the end of thirty minutes allow to stand for one minute and then pour the contents of the flask at once into a shallow layer of hot water remaining in a funnel fitted with a pump-plate or, alternatively, into a similar layer remaining in a Büchner funnel. To prepare the funnel, cut a piece of cotton cloth or filter paper to cover the holes, so as to serve as a support for a disc of ordinary filter paper; pour boiling water into the funnel and allow it to remain until the funnel is hot, and then apply suction. Discard the experiment if the time of filtration of the bulk of the 200 ml exceeds ten minutes. Wash the residue with boiling water until free from acid. Wash the residue from the filter paper back into the flask with 200 ml of 0·313N sodium hydroxide, measured at ordinary temperature and brought to boiling-point. Boil the contents of the flask for exactly thirty minutes, observing the precautions given for the treatment with acid. Allow to stand for one minute then filter the contents immediately through an ordinary filter paper. Transfer the whole of the insoluble material to the filter paper by means of boiling water and wash the precipitate first with boiling water, then with 1 per cent hydrochloric acid and finally with boiling water until free from acid. Then wash twice with 95 per cent ethanol and three times with ether. Transfer the insoluble matter to a dried weighed ashless filter paper; dry at 100° to constant weight. Determine the ash of the paper and contents by incineration at a dull red heat and subtract the weight of ash obtained from the increase of weight found on the paper. Report the difference as fibre.

1. Cocking, T. T., and Middleton, G., *Quart. J. Pharm.*, 1935, **8**, 435.
2. Kofler, L., and Krämer, F., *Arch. Pharm.*, 1931, **269**, 416.
3. Meek, H. O., and Salvin, F. G., *Quart. J. Pharm.*, 1937, **10**, 471.

OILS, FATS AND WAXES

The analysis of oils, fats and waxes is too extensive a subject for comprehensive consideration in a book of this character, and hence this section has been restricted to those oils which are of pharmaceutical interest. Comments of interest made on the determination of the commoner chemical constants applicable to oil and fat analysis and useful data on individual oils have been included.

The examination of mixtures, such as ointments, containing oils or fats is mostly for the estimation of the proportions of known constituents to ensure that the preparation has been made to the prescribed formula. If the usual constants are determined and average values for normal individual oils used in calculation, a reasonably accurate result can be obtained well within the limits of probable error in the compounding of the article.

DETERMINATION OF FATTY OILS. The following method should prove satisfactory in all cases:

> Extract a weighed quantity of the sample, placed in an extraction thimble, with light petroleum (b.p. 40° to 60°) in a Soxhlet apparatus for three to four hours. Remove and dry the thimble, grind the contents finely in a mortar, return the substance to the thimble and continue the extraction for another hour. After evaporation of the solvent, dry the oil at 100° and weigh.

The determination of fatty oils in emulsions presents some difficulties. Four general methods are available, each being suitable for particular emulsions:

(*a*) Werner-Schmidt method:

> Heat 5 to 10 g of emulsion, accurately weighed, with 20 ml of a mixture of equal parts of concentrated hydrochloric acid and water, on a water-bath until the emulsion is destroyed. Cool, transfer to a separator and extract three times with large quantities of ether. Wash the mixed ethers, evaporate, dry and weigh. After weighing the flask and contents, wash out the oil with light petroleum, dry and weigh the flask and any residue which may have been extracted from non-fatty material by the ether. The difference in weight obtained represents the oil present in the quantity taken.

(*b*) Röse-Gotlieb method:

> Transfer about 2·5 g of emulsion or extract to a stoppered 100-ml measure by means of about 7·5 ml of water (or weigh in this amount by difference and add water) to obtain about 10 ml of aqueous liquid. Add 1 ml of strong ammonia solution and 5 ml of ethanol. Add 25 ml of ether, using part to rinse in any oil remaining in the original weighing

vessel. Stopper and shake vigorously for five minutes. Add 25 ml of light petroleum (b.p. 40° to 60°) and shake again. Allow the mixture to stand half an hour to separate; then either take off an aliquot part of the ether layer or, preferably, siphon off the total ethers, shaking with a further two portions of mixed ethers. Evaporate, dry and weigh the oil.

If free fatty acids are present ammonia should not be added. Emulsions can be cleared by further small additions of ethanol.

(*c*) Sodium sulphate desiccation and extraction:

Weigh 0·5 to 1·0 g of emulsion, add anhydrous sodium sulphate in considerable excess, sufficient so that on massing the product is quite dry, powdery and free from clots. Transfer the whole to a Soxhlet thimble and extract with light petroleum (b.p. 40° to 60°) for two hours. Evaporate the solvent, dry and weigh the oil.

This method is also useful for obtaining a quantity of fat rapidly from an emulsion, but often lengthy extraction is necessary to obtain quantitative results.

(*d*) Ethanol precipitation:

To about 2·5 g in a beaker add 0·5 g of kaolin and mix. Add 5 ml of 70 per cent ethanol, stir thoroughly, then add a further 45 ml of ethanol and stir again. Filter through a pleated open-texture filter paper, transferring the precipitate to the filter with further portions of the ethanol. Place the filter paper and precipitate in an extraction thimble, transfer to a continuous extraction apparatus and exhaust with ether, continuing the extraction for about two hours. Transfer the ethereal extract to a separator, and wash with two 15-ml portions of water. Transfer the solution to a weighed flask, remove the solvent, add 5 ml of acetone and evaporate. Repeat the addition and evaporation of acetone until the residue is free from water. Dry at 100° for fifteen minutes and weigh the oil.

Free fatty acids are soluble in aqueous ethanol and would not be included in the figure for oil obtained by this method.

ACETYL VALUE. This test gives a measure of the hydroxylated acids in an oil or fat and of the free alcohols present in a wax. For most oils and fats the acetyl value is insignificant although, as sterols are present, all oils and fats give a small value. The method is important for determining castor oil, which has a very high acetyl value (150) compared with other common fatty oils (maximum values under 20).

The acetyl value is defined as the number of milligrammes of potassium hydroxide required to neutralise the acetic acid obtained when 1 g of an acetylated oil, fat or wax is saponified. The following procedure is that devised by Lewkowitsch.[1]

Boil 10 g or any convenient quantity of the material with twice its weight of acetic anhydride for two hours under a reflux condenser. Pour the solution into a large beaker, mix with 500 to 600 ml of boiling water and boil for thirty minutes, passing a fine stream of carbon dioxide through the liquid to prevent bumping. Allow the mixture to separate, siphon off the water and repeat the heating with water three times until all trace of acetic acid is removed. Filter the acetylated fat through a dry filter paper until free from water, or preferably mix the wet fat with anhydrous sodium sulphate and when clear, filter.

Saponify about 2·5 g of this acetylated fat in an exactly similar manner to that employed in carrying out the saponification value. The ethanolic potassium hydroxide used must be accurately measured. After saponification, remove the ethanol and dissolve the soap in water. To the solution add 0·5N sulphuric acid exactly equivalent to the ethanolic potassium hydroxide used plus 0·5 ml in excess, in order to cause the fatty acids to separate easily. Warm gently until these separate completely as an oily layer. Filter the acids through a wet filter paper, wash with boiling water until the washings are no longer acid and titrate the total filtrate with 0·1N potassium hydroxide to phenolphthalein. From the result obtained subtract 2·5 ml, being allowance for the excess of 0·5N sulphuric acid added.

$$\text{Acetyl value} = \frac{\text{ml } 0{\cdot}1\text{N alkali} \times 5{\cdot}61}{\text{wt. of acetylated oil taken}}$$

Although this is the generally accepted method, in view of the possibility of slight hydrolysis by continued washing with boiling water, it is preferable to wash the acetylated oil free from acid by repeated shaking with warm water in a separator. Any small amount of free acidity not removed after three or four washings may be titrated before saponification of a weighed quantity of the acetylated product.

A simpler method of determination of acetyl value, which is superseding the original Lewkowitsch method, is by double saponification:

Acetylate 15 to 20 g of oil with twice its volume of acetic anhydride as usual. Wash the acetylated oil free from acid by repeated extraction with warm brine then with water in a separator, and dry. Determine the saponification value of the acetylated oil, using 2·5 g and 50 ml of 0·5N ethanolic potassium hydroxide (S_1). Determine the saponification value of the original oil (S). Then:

$$\text{Acetyl value} = \frac{(S_1 - S)}{1 - 0{\cdot}00075S}$$

In the case of fats containing volatile acids the figure obtained will include these acids. In such cases, therefore, the amount of alkali required when the same weight of unacetylated fat is treated in an exactly similar manner is subtracted from the apparent acetyl value to give the true acetyl value.

ACID VALUE. This is a measure of the free fatty acids and indicates the condition of the oil, since rancidity is accompanied by formation of free fatty acids.

Weigh about 10 g of the substance, add 50 ml of hot 95 per cent ethanol, previously boiled and neutralised to phenolphthalein, and titrate with 0·1N alkali, shaking constantly.

$$\text{Acid value} = \frac{\text{ml of } 0{\cdot}1\text{N alkali} \times 0{\cdot}00561 \times 1000}{\text{wt. of substance taken}}.$$

The *B.P.* method of determination uses a mixture of equal parts of ethanol and ether to dissolve the fat; the ethanol-ether mixture must be neutralised to phenolphthalein before dissolving the fat in it. This method is satisfactory as long as the volume of alkali required is not large.

The acidity may be required in terms of percentage of oleic acid; this may be calculated from the acid value by the factor 0·5027, or 1 ml 0·1N = 0·0282 g oleic acid.

Rancidity. Although the presence of free fatty acids is generally concurrent with a state of rancidity it is not necessarily so, especially in refined oils.

The presence of peroxide oxygen resulting from autoxidation is an indication of incipient rancidity and can be measured by the method of Lea:[2]

> Weigh 1 g of the oil or fat into a pyrex test-tube (15 cm × 17 mm), add approximately 1 g of powdered potassium iodide and 20 ml of glacial acetic acid-carbon tetrachloride (or chloroform) mixture (2 : 1 by volume). Heat the liquid to boiling-point over a small flame impinging on the bottom of the tube. Continue boiling for half a minute, the heavy vapour of the liquid minimising the diffusion of oxygen back into the tube. Then cool the tube under the tap, pour the contents into 30 ml of water and titrate with 0·002N sodium thiosulphate. Carry out a blank on the reagents and deduct from the test figure.

The peroxide figure is the number of ml of 0·002N thiosulphate required to titrate the liberated iodine from 1 g of oil or fat. The peroxide value at which rancidity is just perceptible is between 10 and 20.

IODINE VALUE. As this is a constant of considerable importance in the analysis of oils and fats, numerous methods and modifications have been devised for its determination. As variations in the iodine value are obtained by different methods, the one used should always be stated and the conditions laid down by the particular method should be strictly adhered to.

Hübl's method is now little used owing to the time required for the absorption and the irregular results obtained, although De Conno *et al.*[3] have claimed uniform results, using a Hübl solution containing 3 per cent of hydriodic acid.

The well-known Wijs' method[4] is considerably shorter and is used by the *B.P.* Briefly it is:

> To a quantity of the oil in 10 ml of solvent, add 20 ml of iodine monochloride solution. Allow the mixture to stand in the dark at

between 15° and 25° for the appropriate time, then add an excess of potassium iodide and water. Titrate the excess of iodine with 0·1N thiosulphate. Conduct a control experiment.

$$\text{Iodine value} = \frac{\text{ml } 0{\cdot}1\text{N iodine absorbed} \times 0{\cdot}01269 \times 100}{\text{wt. of substance taken}}$$

The iodine monochloride reagent is best prepared by dissolving 8 g of iodine trichloride in about 200 ml of glacial acetic acid and 9 g of iodine in 300 ml of carbon tetrachloride before mixing the two solutions and diluting to 1 litre with glacial acetic acid. It should be stored in a cool place in a stoppered bottle protected from light.

The points to be particularly noted in using the method are: (*a*) the iodine absorbed should only be about one-third of the total employed; to obtain the approximate amount of substance to be taken, use the weight in grammes obtained by dividing the highest probable iodine value into 20; (*b*) as the coefficient of expansion of glacial acetic acid is comparatively high a control determination must be made at the same time, using identical conditions; (*c*) to avoid substitution reactions the mixture must be kept in the dark for the appropriate time; generally one hour is sufficient for absorption with two to three hours for drying oils and marine oils. However, the *B.P.* has stipulated a half-hour period for all oils and fats, hence the figures obtained by the *B.P.* method will be somewhat arbitrary values in cases of highly unsaturated oils; (*d*) to dissolve the oil before contact with the iodine solution either carbon tetrachloride or chloroform is used, but this must be of analytical-reagent quality.

Hanus' method, used by the *U.S.P.*, is equivalent to the Wijs method and the same process is followed, thirty minutes being allowed for absorption of all oils and fats except castor, cod-liver and linseed oils, which are allowed to stand for one hour. The Hanus iodobromide solution is made by dissolving 13·2 g of iodine in 1 litre of glacial acetic acid and then, to the cold solution, a quantity of bromine is added equivalent to that of the iodine present; the iodine present is determined by titration.

A method of halogen absorption using pyridine sulphate bromide, introduced by Rosenmund and Kuhnhenn,[5] has the advantage of great rapidity. With this reagent a small excess is sufficient, though a large one is not deleterious. It is claimed that the reagent forms additive compounds with oils without any substitution or oxidation. The reagent is prepared by dissolving 8 g of pyridine and 10 g of concentrated sulphuric acid in 20 ml of glacial acetic acid, adding 8 g of bromine dissolved in another 20 ml of glacial acetic acid and diluting the mixture to 1 litre with glacial acetic acid; this gives a reagent of approximately 0·1N strength. The procedure follows the lines of the Wijs method except that ten minutes' absorption is sufficient. The method is certainly of advantage with fats or residues containing a high proportion of sterols. Copping[6] showed that results were reliable with all sterols except ergosterol, whilst Garratt[7] obtained theoretical figures for cholesterol but probably abnormal results with lanosterol. Hence figures by this method on wool fat, although concordant, would not be of theoretical value. It must be particularly stressed that iodine values thus obtained are not strictly comparable with those obtained by the Wijs or Hanus method.

Another method worthy of mention is the absorption of bromine vapour by thin films of oils and fats, devised by Toms.[8] To obtain quantitative results comparable with the Wijs method only a very thin layer of oil must be used, sufficiently thin to prevent the formation of a pellicle on the surface. The method is extremely simple.

Spread a single drop of oil (0·02 to 0·03 g) in a thin film, about 0·2 mm thick, on a weighed microscope slide and place it in a wide tube closed at each end with a waxed cork and containing a boat in which are placed a few drops of bromine. After twenty to thirty minutes take out the slide and remove the excess of bromine, either by heating to 50° to 60°, or by a current of warm air. From the increase in weight of the slide the bromine value can be calculated.

For the less unsaturated oils larger amounts are needed, and then it is advisable to use a larger plate, with a similar one for a counterpoise. The iodine value is obtained by the factor 1·588 and was shown to agree closely with the iodine value obtained by Wijs' method, except for notable differences unassociated with oils of pharmaceutical use, other than castor oil, which gave a lower bromine absorption, probably owing to the presence of ricinoleic acid. The appearance of the film after absorption is in many cases characteristic of the particular oil.

SAPONIFICATION VALUE. This is a measure of the glycerides present in an oil and is determined as follows:

To about 2 g of substance, add 25 ml of approximately 0·5N ethanolic potassium hydroxide and reflux on a water-bath for thirty minutes. Add phenolphthalein as indicator and, while still hot, titrate the excess of alkali with 0·5N acid. Repeat the experiment omitting the oil.

$$\text{Saponification value} = \frac{\text{ml } 0{\cdot}5\text{N alkali absorbed} \times 0{\cdot}02805 \times 1{,}000}{\text{wt. of substance taken}}$$

The following points should be noted:

(*a*) The control experiment in this determination is essential, since even a good quality 0·5N ethanolic potassium hydroxide diminishes each week by about 0·1 ml titration value per 20 ml of solution.

(*b*) A small piece of pumice added before heating the mixture produces even boiling.

(*c*) The titration of excess alkali after saponification should be made as soon as possible, since carbon dioxide is quickly absorbed by the alkali and affects the phenolphthalein end-point.

(*d*) Titration of the alkali with standard hydrochloric acid is preferable to sulphuric acid, as the former gives a more soluble potassium salt.

(*e*) A more accurate method of determining the end-point of the titration is to add a small excess of 0·5N acid and titrate back with 0·1N alkali.

UNSAPONIFIABLE MATTER. A report of the Analytical Methods Committee of the *S.A.C.* on the 'Determination of Unsaponifiable Matter in Oils and Fats and of Unsaponified Fat in Soaps'[9] defines unsaponifiable matter thus: 'Unsaponifiable matter consists of that material present in oils and fats which, after saponification of the oil or fat by caustic alkali and extraction by the solvent specified (under the conditions detailed in the description of the method given later in this report), remains non-volatile on drying at 80°.' A footnote adds that unsaponifiable matter as defined includes, among other things, hydrocarbons and higher alcohols, such as cholesterol and phytosterol.

Smith[10] pointed out that the choice of a suitable solvent is very important, the partition coefficients for unsaponifiable matter between organic solvents and soap solution being surprisingly low in many cases. Although light petroleum dissolves less soap and water than ether, and unsaponifiable matter is completely soluble in light petroleum, yet the unsaponifiable matter is not necessarily completely extracted by that solvent as the partition coefficient is too high in favour of the soap solution. He affirms that 'although the degree of hydrolysis of even dilute soap solutions is fairly small, the presence of the ethereal layer causes a wide displacement of the position of equilibrium, since the fatty acid produced by hydrolysis is withdrawn from the aqueous phase owing to its much greater solubility in ether. In the case of dilute soap solutions in contact with ether the degree of hydrolysis may exceed 50 per cent, and increases with dilution. Thus attempts to extract soap from an ethereal solution result in removal of rapidly decreasing portions of the soap in the first two or three washings, after which further washing is entirely ineffective to remove the fatty acid resulting from hydrolysis of the remainder.' Although washing the ether with fairly strong alkali results in converting fatty acids to soap, which is partly removed by subsequent extraction with water or dilute ethanol, it seems impossible to remove the last traces of fatty acids by any means, hence residual fatty acids must be determined by titration.

These observations are of interest in comparison with the following details, which form a summary of the Committee's report[9] of the method recommended for general determination of unsaponifiable matter.

Saponify 2·0 to 2·5 g of oil or fat by boiling for one hour under a reflux condenser with 25 ml of approximately, but not less than, 0·5N ethanolic potassium hydroxide. After saponification, wash the solution into a separator with a total of 50 ml of water. Extract the soap solution, while still just warm, with three portions of 50 ml of ether. Transfer the ethereal solutions to a second separator containing 20 ml of water, filtering any solid suspended matter and washing the filter paper subsequently with ether. Rotate the total extracts gently, without violent shaking, with the 20 ml of water and reject the wash-water. Then wash the ethereal solution twice with 20 ml of water, shaking vigorously on each occasion. Shake the ethereal solution three times with 20 ml of 0·5N aqueous potassium hydroxide, washing between each alkali treatment with 20 ml of water. Wash with water until the aqueous layer gives no alkaline reaction to phenolphthalein. Transfer the ethereal extract to a weighed flask, distil off the ether and dry the residue to constant weight, preferably with the aid of 2 or 3 ml of acetone, not allowing the temperature to exceed 80°. After attaining constant weight, dissolve the contents of the flask in 10 ml of freshly boiled and neutralised 95 per cent ethanol and titrate with 0·1N ethanolic potassium hydroxide, phenolphthalein being used as indicator. If the amount of 0·1N alkali does not exceed 0·1 ml take the unsaponifiable matter as the amount weighed; if this quantity is exceeded, repeat the determination from the start, as this limit may correspond with 0·11 per cent of free fatty acid or much larger quantities of acid soap.

The only oils of pharmaceutical interest requiring special consideration were found to be those containing a high proportion of wax esters such as wool fat and sperm oil, in the case of which, in the opinion of the Committee, complete saponification is difficult or impossible to secure in one operation; it is necessary to use only 0·5 g and to resort to re-saponification of the unsaponifiable material as first obtained.

A shortened method was also recommended by the Committee, for it is known that with many oils and fats the method described above may be shortened by reducing the number of washing treatments. For this modification:

After the three preliminary water washes, wash the ethereal solution twice with 20 ml of 0·5N aqueous potassium hydroxide by shaking vigorously on each occasion and then with two or more successive quantities of 20 ml of water until the wash water no longer reacts alkaline to phenolphthalein. Continue then as under the directions described in the full method.

To ensure uniformity, emphasis is laid upon the necessity for attention to detail at every stage.

The Committee maintains that it is almost impossible to obtain complete extraction with light petroleum in the case of some of the marine animal oils, and also that, although titration of the unsaponifiable matter gives an index of the free fatty acids present, to apply a correction involves the use of an arbitrary equivalent of such acidic material which, if acid soap is present, may be far from the correct figure.

In the analysis of mixtures of oils, fats and waxes the determination of the unsaponifiable matter is of considerable value; but where only a small quantity of wax is present with the oils, the unsaponifiable matter of the oils must be taken into account in the calculation, the amount present being sufficient to affect the result seriously.

Phytosterol Acetate Test. The sterols contained in the unsaponifiable fraction of oils offer a means of detecting vegetable oils and fats in animal fats, but the test is only resorted to if simpler methods have been inconclusive. The method depends on the difference of melting-points and solubilities of the acetates of cholesterol (obtained from animal fats only) melting at 114°, and phytosterols (obtained from plant products) with acetates melting between 127° and 133°. Steuart[11] has shown that the method is useless for the detection of animal fats in vegetable oils and fats, as the sterol acetates from some vegetable oils contain fractions of lower melting-point.

The test is somewhat cumbersome and can be found in all standard works on the examination of oils and fats, but the modification by Hawley[12] of the method of Fritzsche, using digitonin, for routine examination of butter fats with border-line Reichert-Meissl values, considerably shortens the time and reduces the amount of material required and the manipulations involved. The method appears to be based on sound principles and sufficient practical detail is given in the original paper to ensure that it can be followed with ease. The procedure is:

> 25 g of butter-fat (the original Fritzsche method was evolved for oils and fats other than butter-fat) with 10 ml of chloroform and 15 ml of a 1 per cent solution of digitonin in 95 per cent ethanol are shaken by hand in a small flask for about ten minutes in a bath of water at 65° to 70°. The mixture is then filtered hot through a Jena filter (No. 11aG4). This has a disc of 40 mm diameter, is 90 mm high above the disc and holds about 100 ml. For this filtration it is essential that the No. 4 (fine grade) be used. The filter is jacketed with water at about 60° to 70°. A jacket is easily arranged by fixing the filter through a bung in the neck of an inverted wide shallow bell jar which is filled with hot water. The filtrate is turbid, and gives the impression that some of the digitonide has passed through the filter. This will be found not to be the case. The turbidity is due to separation of the fat-chloroform-ethanol mixture on cooling. On adding more chloroform, or warming, the filtrate becomes clear. The digitonide on the filter is washed five or six times with chloroform, each addition being made just before the precipitate is dry, otherwise channels form, and thorough washing (which is essential) becomes difficult. Air is now drawn through the filter until the precipitate appears to be dry. The filter is then placed in a vacuum desiccator at 2 or 3 mm pressure for half an hour or longer. It will be found that the digitonide has assumed a paper-like texture. The bulk of it is easily removed with a mounted needle.
>
> The pure digitonide is transferred to a long-form Stokes tube, in which it is boiled with 5 ml of acetic anhydride over a very small flame, the neck of the tube acting as an air condenser. Heating is continued for a minute or so after the precipitate has dissolved (about five minutes in all). The tube is then rinsed out with 20 ml of 50 per cent ethanol into a small beaker, where the liquid is allowed to crystallise. The crystals

are filtered off on a Jena filter; No. 3 (medium grade) is sufficient, and size 3G3 (capacity 30 ml) is convenient. The crystals are washed thoroughly with 50 per cent ethanol and dissolved off the filter with ether, the solution being received in a 10-ml stoppered, tube-form, weighing bottle. Ether is removed by warming and blowing in air. The dry sterol acetate is then dissolved by warming in 5 ml of 90 per cent (by vol.) ethanol and allowed to crystallise. Dehydrated ethanol is unsatisfactory with such small quantities of material. The crystals are filtered off through a Jena micro-filter (No. 12G3, capacity 2 ml) and washed four times with 1 ml of cooled 90 per cent ethanol from a pipette. In India ice is used to assist this crystallisation; in temperate climates this might be unnecessary. The filter is then dried overnight in a vacuum desiccator, and the melting-point determined. In the absence of vegetable fat the melting-point is invariably between 114° and 115°. By repeated crystallisation it is possible to raise it to about 115·2°. In the presence of as little as 10 per cent of vegetable oil, the melting-point is over 117°, and can be raised usually to over 120° by another crystallisation. Melting-points are determined in the apparatus described by Junge,[13] supplied by Albert Dargatz, Hamburg.

HYDROGENATED OILS AND FATS. The detection of hydrogenated oils depends on the presence of esters of *iso*-oleic acid. This is an unsaturated acid but is distinguished by forming a lead salt which is insoluble in solvents whereas those of other unsaturated acids are soluble. Of the methods employed for the determination of *iso*-oleic acid that due to Twitchell[14] is to be recommended. The method has objections, particularly the difficulty of filtration and incomplete separation of liquid and salt, but is preferred by many workers:

Dissolve 2 g of fatty acids of solid fat or 10 g of oil in hot ethanol and add a boiling solution of 1·5 g of lead acetate in ethanol to give a total volume of 100 ml. Cool slowly to 15° for eighteen hours. Filter through a Büchner funnel and wash thoroughly with 95 per cent ethanol until the filtrate remains clear when diluted with water. Transfer the precipitate to a beaker, boil with 100 ml of ethanol and 0·5 ml of acetic acid, cool as before, filter and wash. Wash the precipitate into a beaker with ether, add nitric acid to decompose the lead salts, transfer to a separator and draw off the acid solution. Wash the ethereal solution with water until free from acid, evaporate, dry and weigh the residue of fatty acids.

The method has been criticised by Cocks, Christian and Harding[15] as giving low figures for solid unsaturated acids which are partially soluble in the ethanol, since *iso*-acids other than the preponderating elaidic acid are present. It can be improved by increasing the amount of lead acetate for precipitation but the authors modify the method after precipitation in ethanol by washing with a different solvent (light petroleum). Briefly, the method is the following:

Dissolve 3·5 g of fatty acids in 50 ml of 95 per cent ethanol and, for mixtures with over 25 per cent solid acids, use 3·45 g of lead acetate, otherwise add 1 g of lead acetate dissolved in 50 ml ethanol. Heat both solutions to boiling-point and pour in the lead solution. Cool slowly and allow to stand overnight at 15° to 20°. Filter on a Büchner funnel, change the flask and wash with 100 ml of light petroleum. Remove the solvent from the washings and boil the residue under reflux with 20 ml of ethanol containing 1 drop of glacial acetic acid. Crystallise for three hours, filter and wash with 20 ml of ethanol. Work up the total solid acids as in the Twitchell method and weigh.

Determine the iodine value allowing a value of 90 for unsaturated acids. Figures for natural oils (except rape) were about 2 to 3 per cent but partially hydrogenated oils gave values of 20 to 50 per cent.

TABLE 56

CONSTANTS: SYNTHETICS AND ISOLATED PRODUCTS

	FORMULA	MOL. WT.	MELTING POINT	ACID VALUE MAX.	IODINE VALUE MAX.	
Ethyl oleate, *B.P.*	$C_{20}H_{38}O_2$	310·5	—	0·5	75–84	Esters 98·0–103·0% Wt./ml at 20° 0·869–0·874
Glyceryl monostearate, *N.F.*	—	—	min. 55°	18	6·0	Sap. value 164–170
Isopropyl myristate	$C_{17}H_{34}O_2$	270·5	—	0·5	1·0	Esters min. 99% R.I. at 20° 1·434/6 Wt./ml at 20° 0·850–0·855
Stearic acid, *B.P.C.*	$C_{18}H_{36}O_2$	284·5	min. 54°	200–210	4	Pure acid m.p. 69·3°
Stearyl alcohol, *U.S.P.*	$C_{18}H_{38}O$	270·5	56° to 60°	2	2	Hydroxyl value 200–220

NOTES ON INDIVIDUAL OILS, FATS AND WAXES

The assessment of adulteration in oils and fats is mainly made by the interpretation of the constants, or detection of the specific adulterant by some qualitative test and judging the extent of the adulteration from the usual constants. Hence in order that these notes should be of greater value the information has not been strictly confined to quantitative measurements.

Almond Oil (Valencia sweet-almond oil). The saponification value is sometimes as high as 198 to 200. Almond oil is often adulterated with other kernel oils, and although peach-kernel oil is practically unknown on the market, apricot-kernel oil is comparatively common; the iodine value of this latter oil is distinctly higher than almond oil but insufficiently so to give a definite indication of admixture.

Bieber's test for kernel oils, given in the *B.P.*, is not very satisfactory, Lewkowitsch being unable to detect less than 25 per cent of apricot-kernel

Table 57

Constants: Fixed Oils, Fats and Waxes

Oil, fat or wax	Wt./ml at 20°	Ref. index at 20°	Maximum acid value	Saponification value	Iodine value	Other data
Almond	0·910–0·915	1·470/3	2·0	188–196	95–102	
Apricot kernel	0·917–0·921†	1·4715/25	8·0	189–193	100–110	
Arachis	0·911–0·915	1·468/72	2·0	188–196	85–100	
Beeswax (white)	0·958–0·970†	1·438/42§	18–24	Ester V. 70–80	8–11	Unsap. 52–55%. § At 80°; m.p. 62/64°; Ratio No. 3·3/4·2
Carnauba wax	0·990–0·999†	—	4–7	79–95	10–14	M.p. 83/86°; unsap. 55%
Castor	0·953–0·964	1·477/81	2·0	177–187	82–90	Opt. Rotn. min. +3·5°; acetyl v. min. 140
Chaulmoogra	0·935–0·960	—	13	196–213	93–104	M.p. 25°, $[\alpha]_D$ +48/60°. M.p. acids 44/45°
Coconut	0·912–0·940†	1·456/8	6	250–264	7·0–10·5	S.p. 21·5/23°
Cod-liver	0·917–0·924	1·478/82	1·2	180–190	155–180	Unsap. max. 1·5%. Vit. A, 600u; vit. D, 85u
Cottonseed	0·915–0·920	1·472/4	0·5	190–198	103–117	
Croton	0·940–0·950	1·478/81	—	205–220	105–118	Sol. pet. ether; acetyl v. 20–40
Halibut-liver	0·915–0·925	1·478/91	2·0	Max. 180	Min. 112*	Unsap. min. 7·0%. * Pyridine bromide. Vit. A 30,000u; i.v. glycerides 112–150
Hydnocarpus	0·946–0·956‡	1·480/4	6·0	198–204	97–103	‡ At 25°; m.p. 20/25°, $[\alpha]_D$ min. +53°
Japan wax	0·975–0·993†	1·450/2§	7	218–222	12–14	§ At 40°; m.p. 50/60°; unsap. 1·1–1·6%
Lard	0·859–0·864*	1·452/5§	1·0	192–198	50–66	§ At 60°; m.p. 33/41°; unsap. max. 0·5%. * At 100°/15°
Linseed	0·925–0·930	1·480/4	4·0	188–195	175–200	Unsap. max. 1·5%
Maize	0·915–0·923	1·472/5	1·0	188–195	110–128	Unsap. max. 2·0%
Neatsfoot	0·913–0·917†	1·468/70	—	192–203	65–78	
Olive	0·910–0·913	1·468/71	2·0	190–195	79–88	
Palm	0·921–0·924†	1·458/67	24–200	197–202	49–57	
Palm-kernel	0·918–0·922†	1·449/52§	6	245–255	14–22	§ At 40°; s.p. 20/26°; m.p. 21/24°
Poppy seed	0·924–0·926†	1·476/7	—	192–196	130–138	Unsap. 0·5%
Rape (Colza)	0·907–0·912	1·471/5	4	170–178	97–107	Unsap. max. 1·5%
Sesame	0·916–0·919	1·472/6	2·0	188–195	103–116	
Sperm	0·878–0·884†	1·462/5	—	120–137	81–90	
Spermaceti (Cetaceum)	0·950–0·960†	—	1·0	120–136	3·0–4·4	Cryst. p. max. 18°; unsap. min. 48%
Soya	0·924–0·927†	1·475/6	5·0	190–194	130–137	Unsap. 0·7–1·5%
Teaseed	0·915–0·920†	1·460/4	0·6	188–196	80–90	
Theobroma	0·950–0·976†	1·456/8§	4·0	188–195	35–40	§ At 40°; unsap. 1·2%; m.p. 31/35°
Tung	0·939–0·943†	1·517/20	5·0	190–195	155–167	
Whale	0·917–0·924†	1·473/6	5·0	184–194	116–128	
Wheat-germ	0·920–0·940	—	10	180–195	128–145	Unsap. 5·5–7·5%
Wool fat	0·932–0·945†	1·478/82§	1·0	90–106*	18–32‡	§ At 40°; * 2 hours; ‡ 1 g; m.p. 36/42°

† Sp. gr. at 15·5°/15·5°

oil and Mohler and Benz[16] less than 20 per cent. The latter workers suggest a modification claimed to detect as little as 5 per cent of apricot-kernel oil.

Many other foreign oils are differentiated by the *N.F.* solubility test on the fatty acids. One volume of the fatty acids obtained from the oil by saponification and acidification in the usual manner should yield a clear solution when mixed with one volume of ethanol (95 per cent by volume) and this solution does not deposit any fatty acid at 15° or become turbid upon the further addition of one volume of ethanol.

See also under Arachis Oil.

Arachis Oil. This may be adulterated with cottonseed, sesame, poppy seed or rape oils.

For detection and determination of arachis oil, Evers[17] re-investigated Mansfeld's modification of Bellier's test as applied to olive and almond oils, and found that the constancy of the turbidity temperature depended on the pH of the solution. He devised the following modified test for olive oil which has been adopted by the *B.P.*:

> Saponify 1 ml of the oil by heating with 5 ml of 1·5N ethanolic potash on a water-bath for five minutes, avoiding loss of ethanol. Add 50 ml of 70 per cent ethanol (saponification with 15 ml of 0·5N ethanolic potassium hydroxide can be followed by the addition of 25 ml of dehydrated ethanol and 15 ml of water), followed by 0·8 ml of concentrated hydrochloric acid. After heating to dissolve any precipitate which may be formed, cool the solution in water, stirring continuously with a thermometer, so that the temperature falls at the rate of about 1° per minute. If a turbidity appears before the temperature reaches 9°, the usual confirmatory test for arachis oil must be applied; if the liquid remains clear at this temperature, arachis oil may be regarded as absent.

It was also shown that in the absence of oils other than olive and arachis oils the turbidity temperature is a reliable quantitative measure of the arachis oil present. The turbidity temperature of arachis oil itself is remarkably constant at 39·0° to 40·0°; the test thus forms an excellent guide to the purity of arachis oil.

The modified test is not suitable for the detection of arachis in other oils, except almond and maize oils. The turbidity temperature of almond oil was found to be lower than that of olive oil, at about 1·0°. In the presence of 5 per cent of arachis oil the clouding temperature was 4·5° to 5·5°; hence it is necessary to cool to 4° with almond or apricot-kernel oils to detect such a small addition. With 10 per cent or more of arachis oil present, the curve follows that of olive/arachis oil mixtures. The turbidity temperature of maize oil in this test is 11°.

If a positive qualitative reaction has been obtained, the confirmatory test must be applied. The *B.P.* confirmatory test is a qualitative modification of Evers' quantitative method,[18] in which the arachidic acid is determined; the percentage found can be calculated back to the oil, since the arachidic and lignoceric acids are present in fairly constant proportions.

Boil 5 g of the oil in a 200-ml conical flask with 25 ml of 1·5N ethanolic potassium hydroxide under a reflux condenser for five minutes to saponify. To the hot soap solution add 7·5 ml of 33 per cent acetic acid

TABLE 58

CORRECTION PER 100 ML OF 90 PER CENT ETHANOL USED FOR CRYSTALLISATION AND WASHING

WEIGHTS OF FATTY ACIDS	GRAMMES AT		
	15°	17·5°	20°
0·1 g or less	0·033	0·039	0·046
0·2 g ,,	0·048	0·056	0·064
0·3 g ,,	0·055	0·064	0·074
0·4 g ,,	0·061	0·070	0·080
0·5 g ,,	0·064	0·075	0·085
0·6 g ,,	0·067	0·077	0·088
0·7 g ,,	0·069	0·079	0·090
0·8 g ,,	0·070	0·080	0·091
0·9 g and upwards	0·071	0·081	0·091

CORRECTION PER 100 ML OF 70 PER CENT ETHANOL USED FOR WASHING

WEIGHT OF ACIDS (CORRECTED FOR 90 PER CENT ETHANOL)	CORRECTION PER 100 ML 70 PER CENT ETHANOL		
	M.P. 71°	M.P. 72°	M.P. 73°
Above 0·10 g	0·013 g	0·008 g	0·006 g
0·08 to 0·10 g	0·011 g	0·007 g	0·006 g
0·05 to 0·08 g	0·009 g	0·007 g	0·005 g
0·02 to 0·05 g	0·007 g	0·006 g	0·005 g
Less than 0·02 g	0·006 g	0·005 g	0·004 g
Factor for conversion of percentage of fatty acids to arachis oil	17	20	22

and 100 ml of 70 per cent ethanol containing 1 per cent v/v of concentrated hydrochloric acid, and cool to 12° to 14° for an hour. Filter and wash with 70 per cent ethanol containing 1 per cent of concentrated hydrochloric acid, at 17° to 19°, the precipitate being broken up occasionally by means of a platinum wire bent into a loop. The washing is continued until the filtrate gives no turbidity with water, the washings being measured. Dissolve the precipitate, according to its bulk, in 25 to 70 ml of hot 90 per cent ethanol, and cool to a fixed temperature between 15° and 20°. If crystals appear in any quantity, allow to stand at this temperature for one to three hours, filter, wash with a measured volume of 90 per cent ethanol (about half the volume used for crystallisation), and finally with 50 ml of 70 per cent ethanol. Wash the crystals into a weighed flask with warm ether, distil off the ether, dry at 105°, and weigh.

If the melting-point is lower than 71° recrystallise from 90 per cent ethanol. Add the correction for the solubility in 90 per cent ethanol from Table 58 (above), and also for the total volume of 70 per cent ethanol used in precipitating and washing (including the 100 ml added in the first instance) from the same table. If there are no crystals from 90 per cent ethanol, or if they are only in very small amount, add a sufficient quantity of water to reduce the strength of the ethanol to 70 per cent (31 ml of water to 100 ml 90 per cent ethanol). Crystallise at 17° to 19° for an hour, filter, wash with 70 per cent ethanol, and weigh as before, adding the correction for the 70 per cent ethanol from Table 58. If the melting-point is below 71° recrystallise from a small quantity of 90 per cent ethanol, or again from 70 per cent ethanol. From the amount of arachidic acid present the corresponding amount of arachis oil is found by multiplying by the factor given in the table appropriate to the melting-point of the acid.

Beeswax. Other waxes (such as carnauba, Japan, and tallow), paraffin and resin are all likely adulterants. The ratio value (*i.e.* ratio of ester value to acid value) being constant between 3·6 and 3·8 for normal beeswax, will exclude a large number of adulterants.

Ceresin and paraffin wax may be detected in beeswax by Salamon and Seaber's method,[19] depending on the solubility of the unsaponifiable matter of beeswax in ethanol. The conditions of test must be closely observed.

Boil about 1 g for one hour under reflux with 10 ml of 0·5N ethanolic potassium hydroxide and 10 ml of ethanol. Detach the flask, insert a thermometer and allow to cool, stirring constantly. The liquid does not become cloudy above 61° but becomes cloudy between 61° and 59° and the precipitation of large flocks occurs at not more than 2° below the point at which the liquid becomes cloudy.

The temperature of 'clouding' is notably raised by even small additions of paraffin wax and flocculation does not occur until a lower temperature is reached.

Japan wax and resin are also excluded by a *B.P.* test, these being partially saponified by aqueous sodium hydroxide, beeswax being unaffected.

The *U.S.P.* includes a test to detect carnauba wax.

Place 0·1 g of beeswax in a test-tube and add 20 ml of *n*-butanol. Place the test-tube in boiling water and shake the mixture gently until solution is complete. Immerse the test-tube in a beaker of water at 60° and allow it to cool to room temperature during a period of two hours.

A loose mass of fine, needle-like crystals separates from a clear mother liquor. Under the microscope the crystals are loose needles or stellate clusters, without the presence of amorphous masses.

Castor Oil. The outstanding characteristics are the acetyl value and the wt. per ml, which are the highest of any commonly occurring natural fatty oil. These constants, together with the solubility in ethanol test, will detect the presence of most adulterants although this oil is not commonly sophisticated.

Medicinal oil is practically colourless and usually described as 'cold pressed,' having been obtained by pressure below about 40°.

Theobroma Oil (Cocoa Butter). The *A.O.A.C.*[20] gives the following method to detect the presence of coconut or palm-kernel oil, depending on the property of these oils of not being easily 'salted out' from solution after saponification.

Saponify 5 g of the sample with 15 ml of 12·5 per cent ethanolic potassium hydroxide solution and evaporate the ethanol. Add 5 ml of water and again evaporate to remove the last trace of ethanol. Dissolve the soap in 100 ml of water, cool to room temperature and add, while stirring, 100 ml of saturated salt solution. Allow to stand for fifteen minutes and then filter through a Büchner funnel. To 100 ml of filtrate add 100 ml of saturated salt solution and again filter after fifteen minutes. To the filtrate add a drop of phenolphthalein indicator, neutralise with 1 + 3 hydrochloric acid and then add 0·5 ml in excess. If coconut or palm-kernel oil is present, the solution will become milky or turbid.

These adulterants may also be detected by the Polenské value.[21] Paraffin, beef stearin and tallow may be detected by Björklund's test.

Dissolve 1 g in 3 ml of ether at 17° in a test-tube and place in water at 0°, the solution does not show any deposit in less than three minutes; after it has congealed expose it to a temperature of 15·5°, the solution is not more than slightly turbid.

This test is not applicable in the case of Borneo tallow. The latter, which resembles cocoa butter very closely, is difficult to detect. Bywaters *et al.*[22] observed a characteristic difference in behaviour of these two fats when allowed to cool without stirring. The temperature at which separation occurs is a constant for each fat and the proportions present in mixtures can be ascertained by determination of the turbidity temperature. Ashmore[23] devised a simple but ingenious apparatus whereby this temperature can be determined accurately on as little as about 2 g of fat.

Coconut Oil. This is not often sophisticated except by extraction of stearin. The unusually high saponification value and low iodine value are to be noted. Coconut oil is used as an adulterant of butter, but the abnormal Reichert-Polenské[21] values would indicate its presence.

Cod-liver Oil. The only common adulterants are inferior fish oils. The unsaponifiable matter and iodine value are important constants for indicating purity. The oil is affected by light.

Emulsion of Cod-liver Oil, *B.P.C.* Contains 50 per cent v/v of cod-liver oil with gums and flavouring material, in water.

No difficulty should be experienced in the determination of the oil content, since only small quantities of sample are required and the emulsion is easily broken, but care is necessary to obtain an oil fit for vitamin A determination. The Bond and Druce method given under Extract of Malt with Cod-liver Oil (p. 401) is recommended for determination of the oil in this preparation since the extracted oil is suitable for both determination of the acid value of stored samples and for vitamin A assay (see p. 667).

The vitamin A content does not deteriorate much in well-stored preparations. The iodine value of the oil obtained is a good indication of its freedom from oxidation.

Cottonseed Oil. The *B.P.* modification of Halphen's test, in which the oil (2·5 g) and reagent (2·5 ml of equal volumes of amyl alcohol and 1 per cent precipitated sulphur in carbon disulphide) are heated under slight pressure, will detect less than 5 per cent of cottonseed oil and may be made roughly quantitative up to 20 per cent by the use of comparison mixtures. Kapok oil also gives this reaction, and fats from animals fed on cottonseed cake may show a slight positive test. The reaction is not given by oils which have been previously heated to above 200°. The amyl alcohol may be replaced by a drop of pyridine which is said to make the test more sensitive (Gastaldi[24]).

Halibut-liver Oil. Fish-liver oils have been thoroughly examined by Evers and Smith[25] with particular attention to the unsaponifiable matter extracted by ether (see p. 756) and it is shown that the composition of this varies according to the zoological classification of the fish. The iodine value (Rosenmund and Kuhnhenn) of the unsaponifiable matter, combined with the light petroleum soluble and insoluble acid-phthalic ester value (determined by a method described in the paper), should be found useful in determining the type of fish from which an unknown oil has been obtained. For further details the original paper must be consulted.

The iodine value of the glycerides is a good indication of the purity of the oil. It is determined by obtaining the unsaponifiable matter quantitatively, taking precautions against oxidation by evaporating solvents under nitrogen and doing the iodine value (pyridine bromide method) on the residue without delay. The iodine value of the glycerides is given by the formula $(100x - Sy)/(100 - S)$, where $x =$ iodine value of oil, $S =$ percentage unsaponifiable matter and $y =$ iodine value of unsaponifiable matter.

Hydnocarpus and **Chaulmoogra Oils.** Chaulmoogra oil (*Taraktogenos kurzii* King) has now been mainly replaced by the more easily obtainable hydnocarpus oil (*Hydnocarpus wightiana* Blume) and the latter is now official in the *B.P.C.*, although certain amounts of the former are still demanded. The main differences which may be used to distinguish them are the odour, specific rotation and acid values. The odour of chaulmoogra oil may be described as resembling rancid palm, that of hydnocarpus as artichoke or sunflower.

Lard. Lard is adulterated extensively with beef stearin, cottonseed, sesame and arachis oils. Evers' method for determination of arachis oil is not conclusive with lard.

Sutton, Barraclough, Mallinder and Hitchin[26] indicate that a greater range of iodine value may be shown by genuine commercial lards, most specimens falling between the values 57 to 73, whereas the refractive index tends to be concentrated between 1·4593 and 1·4606 at 40°.

BÖMER VALUE. Although the *B.P.C.* test for detection of beef fat, by determination of melting-point of the glycerides which separate from an ethereal solution, is a good deductive test, it has been improved by the use of acetone at 30° for crystallisation.

Using the acetone technique, the lowest figure for the melting-point of the separated glycerides from genuine lard found by Sutton *et al.*[26] was 64·5°. The authors extended their observations to the melting-point of the constituent fatty acids of these glycerides (Bömer[27]) and used the factor Mg + 2d, which is the melting-point of the glycerides plus twice the difference. This factor is employed in the tentative *A.O.A.C.* method for determination of beef-fat in lard;[28] this is claimed to detect 10 per cent of beef fat with certainty. The method is not applicable to hydrogenated pork fats.

Treat 20 g of filtered sample with acetone at 30° until a total volume of 100 ml is obtained. Shake and leave at 30° ± 2° for eighteen hours; centrifuge or siphon off the supernatant liquid. Add another 20 ml of acetone at 30° and remove as before. Repeat with 20 ml of acetone but transfer the mixture to a filter paper. Wash the crystals with five small portions of acetone at 30°; dry thoroughly at a temperature below the melting-point of the glycerides. Determine the m.p. in a sealed capillary tube.

Saponify the remainder of the glycerides, liberate and extract the fatty acids and dry for a few minutes at 100°. Dip a capillary tube into the melted acids so that the sample stands about 1 cm high in the tube. Seal the open end in a gas flame and leave the tube for half an hour in ice-water or overnight in a refrigerator. Determine the m.p. simultaneously with that of the glycerides. The m.p. is the point at which the samples become clear and liquid.

If the m.p. of the glycerides, plus twice the difference between the m.p. of the glycerides and that of the fatty acids, is less than 73° the lard is regarded as adulterated.

Since a difference of only 0·1° in each of the two melting-points may result in a difference of 0·5° in the value Mg + 2d the standardised procedure must be followed exactly.

Williams[29] has amplified the details of the test to obtain satisfactory results. If after obtaining a clear solution at 30° as directed no crystals are formed in eighteen hours, the assumption that hard fat is absent and the sample is pure may be incorrect. The difficulty originates in the abnormal stability of some supercooled lard solutions, and may be simply overcome by making a clear solution of the lard as directed, cooling it until crystallisation has started and then placing it in the constant-temperature bath at 30° for eighteen hours. Variations in the speed with which the initial crystallisation is allowed to take place do not affect the melting-point of the glycerides or fatty acids, and it makes no difference whether cooling is allowed to proceed until a heavy deposit has formed or is checked while the deposit is still small. It is also pointed out that the 4° temperature variation should not be allowed since crystals may often be obtained at the lowest permitted temperature but not at the highest; if such crystals are of low melting-point, as may happen, conflicting deductions can be drawn from the results. Such conflict would be avoided if temperature variations permissible were reduced to a fraction of a degree.

The following table obtained by Sutton *et al.*[26] illustrates the gradations in the figures obtained for lard and mixtures with beef fat.

TABLE 59

	MELTING-POINTS (° C) GLYCERIDES	MELTING-POINTS (° C) FATTY ACIDS	DIFFERENCE (° C)	Mg+2d
Lard	65·0	59·7	5·3	75·6
Lard + 2 per cent of beef fat	64·4	58·8	5·6	75·6
5 " " " " "	64·0	59·3	4·7	73·4
10 " " " " "	63·9	60·3	3·6	71·1
20 " " " " "	63·3	60·5	2·8	68·9
40 " " " " "	62·6	61·1	1·5	65·6
60 " " " " "	61·8	61·2	0·6	63·0
80 " " " " "	61·4	61·0	0·4	62·2
Beef fat	61·6	60·9	0·7	63·0

If a low figure is obtained in the Bömer test a search for *iso*-oleic acid must be made and the melting-point of the sterol acetates determined. If these tests preclude the presence of hydrogenated oils and fats, the adulterant is beef fat (or mutton or horse fat), and an approximate measure of the proportion of beef fat can be obtained by comparison with known mixtures. For detection of hydrogenated oils and fats in lard, Sutton *et al.* prefer the method of Twitchell (see p. 759) since in their opinion it effects more complete separation of the liquid unsaturated acids, also with genuine lards the iodine values of the 'solid' acids thus separated are so uniformly low (about 1·0) that the test may be used to obtain confirmatory evidence of the presence of substantial amounts of beef fat (iodine value of solid acids 4·4 to 7·6).

Linseed Oil. The very high iodine value should be noted. Mixtures of oils or fatty acids containing linseed oil must be protected from oxidation during analysis. Usual adulterants are fish oils, resin oil and rape oil.

A figure of value for the detection of fish oils in linseed oil is the determination of **ETHER-INSOLUBLE BROMIDES.** The test depends upon the separation of the linolenic and clupanodonic acids as insoluble bromides, and the presence of the bromide of clupanodonic acid (derived from fish oils) is detected by its melting-point. The insoluble bromides of vegetable oils melt between 170° and 180°, but those from fish oils do not melt under 200°, although they darken above 180°. The following quantitative test is briefly that due to Gemmell:[30]

> Saponify 5 g of the oil with ethanolic potassium hydroxide, evaporate the ethanol, make up to 100 ml and liberate the fatty acids. Cool, extract twice with ether and make the ether extracts up to 100 ml. Pipette 20 ml into a 50-ml flask, add 2 ml of glacial acetic acid and cool in melted ice. Add bromine, drop by drop, from a burette until a permanent brownish-red colour results. Stopper the flask and leave at 0° for at least four hours. Decant the liquid, wash the precipitate three times in the flask with 5 ml of cooled ether, transfer the crystals to a weighed filter, using two more portions of 5 ml of cooled ether for transferring and washing. Dry to constant weight at 100° and determine the melting-point.

The quantitative test has been the subject of much controversy and is generally adversely criticised because of the lack of uniformity of the results obtained.

Olive Oil. The quality of the oil is mainly judged on flavour, and for edible purposes the acid value should be less than 2. A low iodine value (within the usual limits) is a good indication of purity, most oils used as adulterants having higher values. The usual adulterants, arachis, cottonseed, sesame and teaseed oils, do not cause much alteration in the constants of the oil and must be tested for separately by the methods given under the individual oils. Some genuine oils, especially Algerian and Tunisian, give a positive reaction for sesame oil by Baudouin's test, but in these cases, if shaken with ammonia and ethanol and dried before the test, a negative reaction is obtained. Also, Parry[31] observed that certain pure olive oils, especially those from Tunis, give a slight but definite arachidic acid reaction (but see Arachis Oil). The *U.S.P.* has included the *A.O.A.C.*[32]

modification of Renard's method for the detection of arachis oil; this is much more tedious than Evers' method but is quite reliable.

For the detection of solvent-extracted oils (in which carbon disulphide is used) the Olive Oil Committee of the American Oil Chemists' Society[33] recommends the silver benzoate test.

Mix silver nitrate and sodium benzoate in hot aqueous solution; cool and collect, wash and dry the precipitated silver benzoate. Add 0·02 g of the dry benzoate to 5 ml of the oil and heat the mixture to 150° in an oil-bath. A definite brown coloration is obtained, which may, even with a sample containing only 1 per cent of extracted oil, easily be distinguished from that produced by pure olive oil.

Sesame Oil. Baudouin's test (in which 2 ml of the oil is shaken with 1 ml of concentrated hydrochloric acid containing 1 per cent of sucrose, a pink colour developing in the presence of sesame oil) will detect very small amounts of the oil in other oils. Repetition of the test without sucrose will confirm if the colour developed is due to sesame oil or other causes. The test was modified by Villavechia and Fabris, using a few drops of 2 per cent ethanolic solution of furfural in place of the sucrose, and although some olive oils, especially of African or Spanish origin, give pink or crimson colours with Baudouin's test, if the furfural reagent gives a reaction in the absence of sesame oil the colour will disappear after the addition of an equal volume of water. As with cottonseed cake, the reaction may be given by the fat of animals fed on sesame cake. The oil is not often adulterated, but cottonseed and rape oils are those most likely to be used. The oil is optically active (+1° to +3° in a 2-dm tube).

Teaseed Oil. Although this oil is used for edible purposes, its main interest in analytical practice is as an adulterant of olive oil, which it resembles so closely that it is extremely difficult to detect its presence. As a substitute, or if present in large proportion, the oil may be indicated by the titre, which is 23° in the case of olive oil and 13·5° in the case of teaseed oil. The various colour reactions which have been suggested depend on the presence of impurities, which are removed by refining; only one is of value and that is the method introduced by Fitelson.[34]

Measure into a test-tube 0·8 ml of acetic anhydride, 1·5 ml of chloroform and 0·2 ml of concentrated sulphuric acid; mix, cool to room temperature and add 7 drops of the oil to be tested (weighing approximately 0·23 g) by means of a tube of 4 mm external and 2 mm internal diameter. If the mixture is cloudy after mixing, add acetic anhydride drop by drop, with shaking, until a clear solution is suddenly formed. Note the colour after five minutes at room temperature. Teaseed oil gives a colour deep green by reflected and brown by transmitted light, and olive oil a green colour by reflected and transmitted light, with occasional faint fluorescence. Then add 10 ml of anhydrous ether and mix the contents of the tube by one inversion. Teaseed oil shows a brown colour, changing, after a minute or so, to intense red, which reaches a maximum and fades within a few minutes, whilst olive oil gives an initial green colour, slowly fading to brownish-grey, occasionally passing through a faint pink stage.

Mixtures show the characteristic teaseed colour in an intensity proportional to the amount present. For approximately quantitative estimations the procedure is as described, but after the oil and reagent have been mixed and left for five minutes, the test-tube is placed in ice-water for one minute, the previously-cooled 10 ml of ether added and the mixture left in the ice-water for five minutes. The colour is compared with standard mixtures treated simultaneously.

Tunisian olive oil will give a pronounced colour reaction with this test equivalent to approximately 10 per cent of teaseed oil. It is for this reason that a transient pink colour should be allowed without significance, and a positive Fitelson reaction is completely reliable only when more than 15 per cent of teaseed oil is indicated.

Wool Fat (Wool Wax or Anhydrous Lanolin). The analysis of mixtures containing wool fat is difficult as its constants vary considerably according to the conditions of experiment, and mixtures containing it are not easy to separate owing to its emulsifying power with water.

Some difference of opinion exists on the saponification of wool fat. Abraham and Cockton[36] were of the opinion that heating in a stoppered flask with N ethanolic potash on a water-bath (*i.e.* under pressure) for two and a half hours gave the most accurate and concordant results. These findings are not in accordance with the results obtained by Richardson and Bracewell,[35] who tried various methods of saponification, including the ethoxide method, and found no advantage over the use of N ethanolic potash. Garratt[37] also showed that N ethanolic potassium hydroxide saponified wool fat as completely as ethoxide and the values obtained were of the same order as with 0·5N ethanolic potassium hydroxide used in the *B.P.* method. Two hours' boiling is undoubtedly necessary.

That the figure for the iodine value depends on the method of determination employed, and that exact conditions of experiment are necessary in the case of this material, has been conclusively proved. Abraham and Cockton[36] showed the necessity for specifying the exact quantity to be taken in the official iodine monochloride method; using 1·0 g and 25 ml of approximately 0·2N Wijs' solution, the iodine value increased from 27·3 in one hour to 29·9 in five hours, whereas using 0·2 g and the same quantity of iodine solution the results were of the order of 49. The *B.P.* method uses 1 g with an iodine value range of 18 to 32, whilst the *U.S.P.* limits are 18 to 36 with 0·78 to 0·82 g of wool fat. The length of time of exposure to the iodine does not appear to affect the result appreciably.

The determination of the amount of unsaponifiable matter (which includes insoluble alcohols) is a useful figure for calculations on ointments containing wool fat. The most suitable method is that employing light petroleum extraction from 50 per cent aqueous ethanol (but compare 'Determination of Unsaponifiable Matter'), the extraction being made in hot solution.

After adjustment of the saponified mixture with water to contain 50 per cent of ethanol, heat the mixture nearly to boiling, transfer to a separator, wash in with hot 50 per cent ethanol and extract immediately with light petroleum. After separation, which is almost instantaneous, run off the aqueous layer and repeat the extractions two or three times. If the solution cools meanwhile it must be reheated. Wash the mixed light petroleum first with 50 per cent ethanol and finally with water, avoiding much agitation. Filter off any flocculent precipitate, which consists of soap soluble with difficulty in ethanol and water, evaporate the petroleum and weigh the insoluble matter.

Pharmaceutical wool fat contains 48 to 52 per cent of this 'total unsaponifiable matter' consisting mainly of cholesterol, lanosterol and other alcohols of high molecular weight.

Hydrous Wool Fat (Lanolin). This is wool fat with 30 per cent of water. The moisture may be determined by direct drying of a thin layer in an oven at 100°, or preferably, by distillation with an immiscible solvent (p. 803).

Wool Alcohols. Consists of the free alcohols obtained by saponification of wool fat and contains cholesterol, lanosterol and higher fatty alcohols. It is required by the *B.P.* to contain not less than 28·0 per cent of cholesterol by digitonin precipitation; this is a general method of determination of true sterols.

Dissolve about 0·1 g in 12 ml of 95 per cent ethanol and allow to stand overnight for precipitation of some of the fatty alcohols which would otherwise precipitate with the digitonide. Filter and wash with a minimum of ethanol. To the filtrate and washings add 40 ml of hot 0·5 per cent solution of digitonin in 95 per cent ethanol. Collect the precipitate in a Gooch crucible, wash with ethanol and dry at 105°. 1 g digitonide = 0·239 g cholesterol.

ANTIOXIDANTS

Antioxidants are used to prevent rancidity in oils and fats. Hence in pharmaceutical work they may be present in preparations, such as oily injections, made from vegetable oils. The most commonly used antioxidants (indeed, the only ones permitted by The Antioxidant in Food Regulations[38]) are normal propyl, octyl or dodecyl gallates (or any mixture of them) and butylated hydroxyanisole (BHA) or butylated hydroxytoluene (BHT), either separately or together. When such substances are present they may seriously interfere in the assay of the therapeutic material (see, for example, pages 580 and 588).

Propyl gallate, $C_{10}H_{12}O_5$, Mol. Wt. 212·2. This is assayed gravimetrically by precipitation with bismuth; the conditions given below give a readily filterable precipitate, but the precision of the method is not good. An obvious modification, which has been used successfully by some workers, is to add a definite volume of a standard bismuth solution and to determine the remainder complexometrically.

To a boiling solution of 0·2 g in 100 ml of water add 50 ml of a solution prepared by refluxing 5 g of bismuth nitrate with 250 ml of water and 7·5 ml of concentrated nitric acid until dissolved, cooling and filtering. Continue to boil for a few minutes, cool, filter, wash the residue with a mixture of one volume of dilute nitric acid and thirty volumes of water and dry to constant weight at 110°. Weight of residue × 0·4863 = propyl gallate.

A similar method is applicable to the other gallates.

Total gallates in olive oil, up to 200 p.p.m., may be determined by the method of Cassidy and Fisher.[39] These workers state that Beer's Law is obeyed over the range 0 to 0·8 mg of gallate and they obtained recoveries of about 95 per cent.

Weigh 10 g of warm liquid sample into an extraction vessel (a boiling-tube which has had a bulb of capacity 10 to 12 ml blown in its side at the bottom, so permitting separation of an upper layer by tilting the tube) or, if the sample is a solid, weigh 5 g into the extraction vessel and add 5 ml of liquid paraffin, *B.P.* Add 25 ml of 95 per cent methanol, shake vigorously for one minute and then place in a water-bath at 40° to 50° and allow to separate for about fifteen minutes (separation into clear layers is unlikely and unnecessary). Pour the upper layer into a 50-ml graduated flask, repeat the extraction with a further 20 ml of 95 per cent methanol, again pour the upper layer into the graduated flask and dilute to volume with 95 per cent methanol. Add 1 g (or a sufficient quantity) of calcium carbonate to the combined extracts, shake for thirty seconds, filter through a Whatman No. 1 filter paper and reject the first few millilitres of filtrate; the calcium carbonate will neutralise any extracted acidity and assist in the clarification of the solution by coagulating some of the extraneous matter and should be added in sufficient quantity to provide a clear filtrate at this stage. Pipette 10 ml of the filtrate into a glass-stoppered test-tube and add exactly 1 ml of acetone that has been shaken with calcium carbonate for one minute and filtered. Then add about 10 mg of powdered ferrous ammonium sulphate, stopper the tube and shake for one minute. Allow to stand for thirty minutes to allow the blue colour to develop fully and then measure the extinction at the absorption maximum at about 580 mμ using 1-cm cells, or larger cells for very dilute solutions. The amount of gallate present in the 11 ml of final solution is given by the relationship:

Gallate present (mg) = EK where E is the extinction of a 1-cm layer of solution and K has the value 0·622, 0·785 or 0·952 for *n*-propyl, *n*-octyl or *n*-dodecyl gallate respectively. (It is recommended that these factors be determined for each batch of reagents.)

Butylated hydroxyanisole and **butylated hydroxytoluene** may be determined by light absorption methods. For example, BHT in ethanolic solution has an E(1 per cent, 1 cm) of about 87 at 277·5 mμ. Commonly, however, isomeric material might be present and this is not taken into account in simple light absorption measurements. BHA, which is 3-*t*-butyl-4-hydroxy anisole, usually contains a proportion of the 2-*t*-butyl isomer; in such a case an infra-red method is often of value. Measurements made on a 10 per cent solution in carbon disulphide at 11·42 μ give a measure of total BHA, but to obtain a valid answer correction must be made for the amount of 2-*t*-butyl compound present, since this absorbs less strongly at the wavelength in question. The ratio of 3-*t*-butyl to 2-*t*-butyl compound present is determined by making measurements at 10·75 μ and at 10·95 μ, and referring to a calibration line constructed by using known amounts of the two isomers.

For the determination of these antioxidants, either separately or together, in food products and oils, Sloman, Romagnoli and Cavagnol[40] have developed a chemical method, suitable for application to amounts down to less than 10 p.p.m. The sample is steam-distilled, the vapours being passed through a scrubber containing magnesium oxide suspension to remove phenolic and acidic substances before condensing and then, after two simple concentration steps, each antioxidant is determined colorimetrically.

Apparatus: A 1-litre, 3-necked round-bottomed flask A (with all necks parallel), provided with an inlet tube, reaching nearly to the bottom of the flask, connected to a 2-litre steam generator, the outlet tube of which is bent through an angle of about 75°. The outlet tube of flask A is connected to a glass tube that reaches nearly to the bottom of a 100-ml Kjeldahl flask. The Kjeldahl flask is fitted with a ground-glass joint and an outlet tube. This is connected, by means of an adaptor bent through an angle of about 95°, to the side arm of a vessel B, in the shape of a large test-tube, which tapers at its lower end into a narrow open tube from which the distillate is collected through a funnel fitted with a stopcock. B contains a 'cold finger' condenser about 15 cm long attached to the top of the tube by means of a ground-glass joint.

Method: Weigh an amount of sample containing 20 to 100 μg of BHT and/or 20 to 100 μg of BHA into flask A, add 50 ml of *iso*propyl alcohol, 200 ml of water and 1 drop of G.E. silicone Antifoam 60 and mix thoroughly. Introduce 1,500 ml of water into the steam generator and 50 ml of a 2 per cent suspension of magnesium oxide in water into the Kjeldahl flask. Connect the apparatus, ensuring that all joints are tight, heat the water in the steam generator so that vapours entering vessel B will be completely condensed, heat flask A so that its contents boil gently and heat the Kjeldahl flask with a small heating mantle or a micro-Bunsen burner; guard against too vigorous boiling in the steam generator or flask A as this will cause losses of BHA and the blank will be high. The rate of heating should be such that the first 100 ml of distillate is collected in about fifteen minutes and the second 180 ml in a further fifteen to twenty minutes.

Collect the first distillate (Fraction I) in a 100-ml graduated flask and, when exactly 100 ml has been collected, close the stopcock in the funnel and replace the flask with a 250-ml glass-stoppered cylinder. Open the stopcock and continue the distillation until 180 ml of distillate (Fraction II) has collected in the cylinder. Add 50 g of sodium chloride and 50 ml of *iso*butyl alcohol to the contents of the cylinder, stopper, and shake for two minutes. Then allow to stand until the two layers separate and the top layer is clear.

Determination of BHT:

Dimethoxybenzidine reagent. Mix 0·5 g of 3,3′-dimethoxybenzidine and 0·5 g of activated charcoal (50- to 200-mesh) with 100 ml of *iso*propyl alcohol, shake well and filter. Pipette 40 ml of the filtrate into a 100-ml graduated flask, dilute to volume with N hydrochloric acid and mix. This reagent should be freshly prepared on the day it is to be used.

Pipette a 50-ml aliquot of Fraction I into an amber-coloured 125-ml separator, add 10 ml of dimethoxybenzidine reagent and 5 ml of a freshly prepared 0·2 per cent sodium nitrite solution and mix. After exactly ten minutes add 20 ml of chloroform, shake for about thirty seconds, allow to settle for about one minute and run the chloroform layer into a 50-ml flask. Add 7 to 8 g of anhydrous sodium sulphate powder, mix by inverting the flask three times and immediately measure the extinction at the absorption maximum at about 520 mμ using a 4-cm cell, after setting the spectrophotometer to read 100 per cent transmission with a 4-cm layer of a reagent blank prepared as for the sample solution using 50 ml of 50 per cent v/v *iso*propyl alcohol in place of the 50 ml of Fraction I. At the same time prepare a standard curve by repeating the colour development and chloroform extraction using a series of standard solutions covering the range 10 to 100 μg of BHT in a total volume of 50 ml of 50 per cent v/v *iso*propyl alcohol (using suitable volumes of a solution prepared by diluting 1 ml of a 0·1 per cent solution of BHT in *iso*propyl alcohol to 100 ml with 50 per cent v/v *iso*propyl alcohol, giving a solution containing 10 μg BHT per ml), measuring the extinctions and plotting extinction against μg BHT. Determine the μg BHT in the sample by reference to this curve.

Determination of BHA:

Mix a 10-ml aliquot of Fraction I with a 5-ml aliquot of the *iso*butyl alcohol extract from Fraction II in a 25-ml graduated flask and add 5 ml of *iso*butyl alcohol, 1 ml of a 1 per cent solution of borax in water and 0·5 ml of a 0·05 per cent solution of 2,6-dichloro-*p*-benzoquinone-4-chloroimine in *iso*propyl alcohol prepared not more than one week before use and stored in an amber-coloured flask. Stopper the 25-ml flask and shake vigorously. Exactly fifteen minutes after the addition of the reagents measure the extinction at the absorption maximum at about 620 mμ using a 4-cm cell, after setting the spectrophotometer to read 100 per cent transmission with a 4-cm layer of 50 per cent *iso*propyl alcohol. Measure also the extinction at 620 mμ of a reagent blank prepared by mixing 10 ml of *iso*butyl alcohol, 1 ml of 1 per cent borax solution and 0·5 ml of the 2,6-dichloro-*p*-benzoquinone-4-chloroimine solution in a 25-ml graduated flask and diluting to volume with 50 per cent *iso*propyl alcohol. Prepare a standard curve by pipetting suitable volumes of a standard BHA solution (containing 10 μg per ml in *iso*butyl alcohol), covering the range 10 to 50 μg, into a series of 25-ml graduated flasks, adding to each sufficient *iso*butyl alcohol to give a total of 10 ml of *iso*butyl alcohol in each flask, developing and measuring the colour as described above from the addition of the borax solution and plotting extinction against μg BHA. By reference to this curve, calculate the μg BHA in the sample using the extinction of the sample solution corrected for the extinction of the reagent blank.

The amount of *iso*propyl alcohol used in the distillation is critical because it provides the correct concentration of alcohol in the distillate for the reaction of BHT with dimethoxybenzidine and variations in this concentration will cause erratic results and also because this volume of the alcohol will ensure constant volume extraction of the coloured compound with chloroform.

When only BHT is present in the sample omit the second distillation. When only BHA is present, omit the addition of *iso*propyl alcohol to flask A, collect the first 180 ml of distillate and treat this as for Fraction II, above; in addition, since the heating of the magnesium oxide trap is to prevent losses of BHT due to its adsorption by cold magnesium oxide suspension and such adsorption does not occur with BHA, it is not necessary to heat the Kjeldahl flask.

Buttery and Stuckey[41] have described a method for the determination of BHA and BHT using gas-liquid chromatography. In their method the sample is extracted with light petroleum (b.p. 40° to 60°), the extract is concentrated and then a suitable volume (30 μl) of the concentrate is injected on to a 5-ft column packed with 40- to 60-mesh diatomaceous earth firebrick coated with 20 per cent of Apiezon L high vacuum grease (the column should be aged for one week at 220° under the operating conditions given below). The working temperature of the column is 220°, nitrogen being used as carrier gas and a chromatogram is obtained using a flame ionisation detector and a suitable chart recorder. For comparison 30 μl of a standard solution containing 0·10 μg per ml each of BHA and BHT in light petroleum (b.p. 40° to 60°) is treated in a similar way to the concentrated extract from the sample. The authors found an average error of less than 11 per cent from the true concentration for both antioxidants within the range 0·5 to 10 p.p.m. in samples of dehydrated potato granules.

1. Lewkowitsch, J., *J. Soc. Chem. Ind.*, 1897, **16**, 503.
2. Lea, C. H., *Food Investigation Spec. Report*, No. 46 (1938, p. 108).
3. De Conno, E., Finelli, L., and Farsitano, L. *Ann. Chim. Appl. Roma*, 1931, **9**, 436.
4. Wijs, J. J. A., *Ber.*, 1898, **31**, 750.
5. Rosenmund, K. W., and Kuhnhenn, W., *Z. Untersuch. Lebensm.*, 1923, **46**, 154.
6. Copping, A. M., *Biochem. J.*, 1928, **22**, 1142.
7. Garratt, D. C., *J. Soc. Chem. Ind.*, 1933, **52**, 355T.
8. Toms, H., *Analyst*, 1928, **53**, 71.
9. *Analyst*, 1933, **58**, 203.
10. Smith, E. L., *Analyst*, 1928, **53**, 632.
11. Steuart, D. W., *Analyst*, 1923, **48**, 155.
12. Hawley, H., *Analyst*, 1933, **58**, 529.
13. Junge, C., *Chemiker Ztg.*, 1929, **53**, 996.
14. Twitchell, E. J., *Ind. Eng. Chem.*, 1921, 806.
15. Cocks, L. V., Christian, B. C., and Harding, G., *Analyst*, 1931, **56**, 368.

16. Mohler, H., and Benz, H., *Z. Anal. Chem.*, 1933, **94,** 184.
17. Evers, N., *Analyst*, 1937, **62,** 96.
18. Evers, N., *Analyst*, 1912, **37,** 487.
19. Salamon, M. S., and Seaber, W. M., *J. Soc. Chem. Ind.*, 191 5, **34,** 461.
20. *A.O.A.C.*, 1960, p. 153.
21. *Analyst*, 1936, **61,** 404.
22. Bywaters, H. W., and Pool, C. J., *Analyst*, 1927, **52,** 324.
23. Ashmore, S. A., *Analyst*, 1934, **59,** 515.
24. Gastaldi, E., *Giorn. Farm. Chim.*, 1912, **61,** 289.
25. Evers, N., and Smith, W., *Quart. J. Pharm.*, 1932, **5,** 331; 1933, **6,** 329; 1934, **7,** 476.
26. Sutton, R. W., Barraclough, A., Mallinder, R., and Hitchin, O., *Analyst*, 1940, **65,** 623.
27. Bömer, A., Limprich, R., Kronig, R., and Kuhlmann, J., *Z. Untersuch. Lebensm.* 1913, **26,** 559.
28. *A.O.A.C.*, 1960, p. 376.
29. Williams, K. A., *Analyst*, 1940, **65,** 596.
30. Gemmell, A., *Analyst*, 1914, **39,** 297.
31. Parry, E. J., *C. & D.*, 1932, 227.
32. *A.O.A.C.*, 1960, p. 374.
33. *Olive Oil Committee of the American Oil Chemists Society, Oil and Fat Ind.*, 1928, **5,** 206.
34. Fitelson, J., *J.A.O.A.C.*, 1936, **19,** 493.
35. Richardson, F. W., and Bracewell, G. A., *J. Soc. Chem. Ind.*, 1916, **35,** 160.
36. Abraham, E. E. U., and Cockton, W. H., *C. & D.*, 1931, 420.
37. Garratt, D. C., *J. Soc. Chem. Ind.*, 1933, **52,** 141T.
38. The Antioxidant in Food Regulations, 1958 (S. I. 1958 No. 1454).
39. Cassidy, W., and Fisher, A. J., *Analyst*, 1960, **85,** 295.
40. Sloman, K. G., Romagnoli, R. J., and Cavagnol, J. C., *J.A.O.A.C.*, 1962, **45,** 76.
41. Buttery, R. G., and Stuckey, B. N., *J. Agric. Food Chem.*, 1961, **9,** 283.

APPENDIX I

Determination of Alcohol Content

It must be emphasised that the accurate determination of spirit strength requires considerable care and practice. The following method for its assay in drugs is somewhat more in detail and varies a little from the technique described in the *B.P.* (Appendix XII, H).

A. Normal Procedure. Note the temperature of the sample. Pipette 25 ml of sample, when containing over 50 per cent of alcohol, or 50 ml otherwise, into the distillation flask of a Government still containing 100 to 125 ml of tap water. Distil at such a rate as to obtain about 90 ml of distillate in twenty to thirty minutes.

Allow the distillate to stand corked for a short time, and then make up to 100 ml at the temperature of the sample as previously determined. Invert twenty to thirty times for thorough mixing, avoiding violent agitation, and allow to stand for at least two hours. The usual procedure is to take the specific gravity in the afternoon in the case of spirits distilled in the morning, and for afternoon distillations to take the specific gravity the next morning.

Determine the specific gravity of the distillate as described below.

B. Special Procedure where Volatile Compounds are Present. Observe the temperature of the sample as above. Take 25 ml of the sample whatever the strength may be, pipette into a separator containing approximately 100 ml of saturated brine, add 30 to 50 ml of light petroleum (b.p. 40° to 60°), shake well, and then allow to stand for two hours. Separate the aqueous layer into a distillation flask, washing in two or three times without disturbing the light petroleum layer by movement of the separator. Extract the light petroleum with 10 to 20 ml of brine by rotation (avoid agitation) and add to the bulk. Add 50 ml of water and distil as above in *A*, then proceed with the distillate in the usual manner.

C. Procedure for Products which would cause Emulsification with Light Petroleum. Proceed exactly as in *A*, but without making the distillate up to volume. After distilling about 90 ml, transfer the distillate to a separator, wash in with water, add salt sufficient to saturate the liquid, and light petroleum. Shake well, allow to stand for two hours, and proceed as in *B*.

D. Procedure Involving Special Technique

(*a*) It is advisable, although not usually necessary, to make all distillations alkaline with sodium hydroxide solution, using aqueous phenolphthalein as indicator. This must be done where volatile acids are present.

(*b*) For samples containing free iodine, addition of an excess of zinc dust will allow direct distillation as in *A*.

(*c*) Where volatile compounds and ammonia are present, proceed as in *B*, but before distilling make acid to litmus with a slight excess of dilute sulphuric acid, keeping the acid in excess during distillation.

(*d*) Where volatile compounds and soaps are present proceed as in *B*, but separate soaps as fatty acids by adding a slight excess of dilute sulphuric acid before shaking with light petroleum. Make alkaline with sodium hydroxide after separating, and before distilling.

(*e*) Where the spirit strength is very low, or if the liquid is very viscous, a graduated flask is preferable for measuring the original sample, which may be washed into the distillation flask with the 100 ml of tap water. The temperature may be neglected.

(*f*) Spirit of Nitrous Ether. Proceed as in *B*, but place the light petroleum in the separator, then add the 25 ml of sample, rotate and finally add the brine and an excess of salt before reshaking (this clears the aqueous layer of nitrous oxide).

(*g*) Ammoniated Solution of Quinine. Distil direct as in *A*, after acidifying with dilute sulphuric acid, keeping the liquid acid throughout the distillation.

E. Elimination of Frothing. All the following methods have been used to stop frothing. No general rule can be laid down as to suitability, individual samples responding to different treatment.

(*a*) A small piece of paraffin wax or preferably a few drops of liquid paraffin, sometimes with dilute sulphuric acid. (Most mild cases of frothing are stopped by this.)

(*b*) Powdered soap 0·1 to 0·2 g. (Suitable for very obstinate frothing.)

(*c*) Rolled or pleated filter-paper in neck of distilling flask and the flame to one side.

(*d*) Salt.

(*e*) Powdered resin.

(*f*) Capryl alcohol.

(*g*) Silicones.

Capryl alcohol and silicones are required only in very small amounts and are very efficient.

F. Specific Gravity and Calculation of Spirit Strength. Note: the thermometer should be standardised, and not used for other purposes.

For accurate determinations of specific gravity or where only small quantities of alcoholic distillate are available use some form of pycnometer with ground glass stopper.

For more rapid routine work where a number of determinations have to be made in a short time a specific gravity bottle may be used. The specific gravity bottle is of 50 g capacity and standardised with distilled water at 20°. Adjust the temperature of the standardising water in a separate container before quickly transferring it to the bottle.

Wash out the specific gravity bottle twice with the distillate. Bring the temperature of the distillate exactly to 20°, with the thermometer reading steady at this figure, and quickly transfer to the specific gravity bottle. Insert the stopper sharply to avoid air bubbles in the neck, wipe the top at once and do not touch it again; wipe the bottle thoroughly and weigh as quickly as possible. Repeat the whole operation until two successive weighings are within 2 mg (with practice this can be done in two weighings).

When the weight has been obtained to within 2 mg, take the higher figure and calculate the specific gravity to the nearest fourth place of decimals.

From the specific gravity found obtain the percentage of alcohol direct from published tables (issued by the Commissioners of H.M. Customs and Excise, 1954, price 4*s.* 0*d.*, published by H.M. Stationery Office), or from the following condensed table for quadruple bulk.

TABLE 60

ETHYL ALCOHOL (QUADRUPLE BULK) TABLE

SPECIFIC GRAVITY AT 20°/20° OF THE DISTILLATE OBTAINED BY DISTILLATION TO QUADRUPLE BULK	PERCENTAGE V/V OF ETHYL ALCOHOL IN THE ORIGINAL PREPARATION AT 20°	PROPORTIONAL DIFFERENCE	REFRACTIVE INDEX AT 20° OF THE DISTILLATE OBTAINED BY DISTILLATION TO QUADRUPLE BULK
0·9710	95·93		1·34661
0·9720	92·32	3·61	1·34605
0·9730	88·66	3·66	1·34549
0·9740	84·96	3·70	1·34493
0·9750	81·26	3·70	1·34437
0·9760	77·53	3·73	1·34380
0·9770	73·82	3·71	1·34324
0·9780	70·10	3·72	1·34267
0·9790	66·38	3·72	1·34211
0·9800	62·72	3·66	1·34154
0·9810	59·09	3·63	1·34098
0·9820	55·48	3·61	1·34044
0·9830	51·94	3·54	1·33991
0·9840	48·45	3·49	1·33942
0·9850	45·02	3·43	1·33892
0·9860	41·62	3·40	1·33842
0·9870	38·28	3·34	1·33796
0·9880	34·99	3·29	1·33751
0·9890	31·76	3·23	1·33705
0·9900	28·62	3·14	1·33663
0·9910	25·53	3·09	1·33620
0·9920	22·49	3·04	1·33578
0·9930	19·50	2·99	1·33540
0·9940	16·59	2·91	1·33501
0·9950	13·71	2·88	1·33466
0·9960	10·89	2·82	1·33432
0·9970	8·10	2·79	1·33397
0·9980	5·38	2·72	1·33362
0·9990	2·68	2·70	1·33331
1·0000	0·00	2·68	1·33300

The *B.P.* requires the final distillate to comply with purity tests for freedom from methanol and *iso*propyl alcohol. The refractive index of the distillate, when determined with an immersion refractometer, should not differ by more than 0·00007 (equivalent to 0·2 on the immersion refractometer scale) from that corresponding to the specific gravity of the distillate (see table). If it differs by more than 0·00007 the process *B* must be used on an aliquot part. If the refractive index still does not correspond with the specific gravity, the distillate contains some impurity and the specific gravity does not indicate the true proportion of ethyl alcohol. (See also Ethyl Alcohol.)

Table 61 gives the majority of the *B.P.* and *B.P.C.* alcoholic preparations and the procedure for the determination of spirit strength (including any special treatment necessary in the individual cases).

Weights per ml, alcoholic strengths and some figures for total solids are included, but of these latter figures, those marked † have only been inserted as a guide and are *not intended as standards* since in some cases they represent only a few samples.

TABLE 61

	PROCEDURE	SPECIAL TECHNIQUE	ALCOHOL PERCENTAGE BY VOLUME	WT./ML	TOTAL SOLIDS PER CENT W/V
Concentrated Infusions					
Gentian (Compound), *B.P.*	C	—	20–24	—	min. 8·0
Orange Peel	C	—	21–25	1·00–1·03	10–15
Quassia	A	—	21–24	0·97–0·98	0·3†
Rhubarb	A	—	18–21	1·00–1·05	17·0†
Senega	A	E	20–24	1·00–1·03	9·5–13·0
Senna	C	—	20–24	1·00–1·07	20·0†
Valerian	A	—	20–23	0·98–1·00	4–6
Concentrated Waters					
Anise	B	—	51–55	0·917–0·925	—
Caraway	B	—	51–55	0·917–0·925	—
Chloroform	B	—	51–55	0·953–0·969	—
Cinnamon	B	—	52–56	0·914–0·922	—
Dill	B	—	52–56	0·914–0·922	—
Peppermint, *B.P.*	B	—	52–56	0·912–0·920	—
Spearmint	B	—	52–56	0·912–0·920	—
Elixirs					
Diamorphine and Terpin	C	—	20–23	1·17–1·18	—
Ephedrine	C	—	14–16	1·19–1·22	—
Nux Vomica	A	—	10–12	1·14–1·16	—
Phenobarbitone	C	—	37–41	1·03–1·05	—
Flexible Collodion, *B.P.*	C	—	20–23	—	6·6–7·4†
Injection					
Mephenesin, *B.P.*	A	—	21–25	—	—
Inhalations					
Benzoin	B	—	80–84	0·84–0·87	11–14; balsamic acids min. 3·4% w/v
Menthol and Benzoin	B	—	78–82	0·84–0·87	11–14; balsamic acids min. 3·3% w/v

Linctus					
Squill, Opiate	C	Da	17–20	1·16–1·19	—
Liniments					
Aconite	C	—	75–85	0·86–0·89	6–7†
Belladonna	C	—	50–60	0·937–0·995	—
Camphor (Ammoniated), *B.P.*	B	Dc	54–58	0·85–0·88	—
Soap, *B.P.*	B	Dd	60–65	0·880–0·900	—
Liquid Extracts					
Belladonna	A	—	48–66	0·95–1·01	—
Cascara, *B.P.*	A	—	21–24	—	20–26
Cocillana	A	—	52–57	0·92–0·96	2·5–6
Colchicum, *B.P.*	A	—	60–70	—	—
Hamamelis, *B.P.*	A	—	32–40	1·015–1·035	18–25
Hyoscyamus, *B.P.*	A	—	50–60	—	—
Ipecacuanha, *B.P.*	A	—	63–69	—	—
Liquorice, *B.P.*	A	E	16–20	1·125–1·140	40–45
Nux Vomica, *B.P.*	A	—	36–42	—	—
Quillaia	A	Eb	28–34	1·02–1·06	20–30
Senega	A	E	38–42	1·03–1·05	26–34
Senna	A	—	21–24	1·02–1·09	17–25
Squill	A	—	34–50	1·00–1·14	40–55
Stramonium, *B.P.*	A	—	28–44	—	—
Valerian	C	—	43–47	0·98–1·04	15–25
Mixture					
Senna (Compound)	A	De	7·5–9·5	1·10–1·12	22–25†: mag. sulph. 25% w/v
Solutions					
Ammonia (Aromatic)	B	Dc	2·6–3·5	0·980–1·005	—
Chloroxylenol, *B.P.*	B	Dc	16–20	—	—
Coal Tar, *B.P.*	C	—	75–85	—	4†
Hydrocortisone, Alcoholic, *B.P.*	A	—	47–53	—	—
Iodine (Simple)	A	Db	92–94	0·873–0·900	—
Iodine (Strong), *B.P.*	A	Db	74–79	—	—
Iodine (Weak), *B.P.*	A	Db	83–88	—	—

TABLE 61 (*continued*)

	PROCEDURE	SPECIAL TECHNIQUE	ALCOHOL PERCENTAGE BY VOLUME	WT./ML	TOTAL SOLIDS PER CENT W/V
Solutions (cont.)					
Morphine Hydrochloride, *B.P.*	A	—	21–24	—	—
Quinine (Ammoniated)	A	Dg	52–54	0·919–0·927	—
Soap (Ethereal)	B	Dd	13–15	0·860–0·900	Fatty acids min. 33% v/v
Strychnine Hydrochloride, *B.P.*	A	—	21–24	—	—
Tolu	A	Da	23–25	1·140–1·175	—
Spirits					
Ammonia (Aromatic)	B	Dc	64–70	0·880–0·893	—
Camphor	B	—	79–82	0·835–0·843	—
Chloroform, *B.P.*	B	—	83–87	0·856–0·862	—
Ether	B	—	59–65	0·796–0·800	—
Lemon	B	—	84–87	0·814–0·823	3·9–5·1% w/w citral
Nitrous Ether	B	Df	84–87	0·827–0·836	—
Orange (Compound)	B	—	80–83	0·825–0·835	Oils 8·1–9·1% v/v
Peppermint, *B.P.*	B	—	79–82	0·832–0·836	—
Soap	B	Dd	28–32	0·950–0·970	Fatty acids min. 27%
Syrups					
Figs (Compound)	C	—	4·5–5·5	1·25–1·29	80†
Ginger, *B.P.*	C	De	—	1·290–1·310	—
Lemon, *B.P.*	C	De	—	1·29–1·32	Citric acid 2·5% w/w
Orange, *B.P.*	C	De	8–10	1·29–1·31	—
Senna	A	De	4·5–6·0	1·25–1·28	—
Tinctures					
Belladonna, *B.P.*	A	—	64–69	—	—
Benzoin (Simple)	C	—	82–85	0·850–0·865	6·3–6·8†
Benzoin (Compound), *B.P.*	C	Da	70–77	0·875–0·900	16–20
Capsicum	A	Da	57–60	—	1·2†
Cardamom (Aromatic)	B	—	84–88	0·830–0·845	0·5–0·8†

Cardamom (Compound), *B.P.*	A	—	52–57	0·925–0·937	11†
Catechu	A	—	37–40	0·990–1·010	12–17
Chloroform and Morphine	C	De	12–15	1·22–1·26	—
Colchicum, *B.P.*	A	—	67–70	—	—
Digitalis	A	—	65–70	0·895–0·910	3†
Gelsemium	A	—	56–59	0·910–0·925	1·3–1·4†
Gentian (Compound), *B.P.*	A	—	40–45	0·955–0·970	6†
Ginger (Strong), *B.P.*	B	Da	80–88	0·832–0·846	2·0–3·0
Ginger (Weak), *B.P.*	B	Da	86–90	0·825–0·835	min. 0·40
Hyoscyamus, *B.P.*	A	—	66–71	—	—
Ipecacuanha, *B.P.*	A	Da	24–28	—	—
Lemon, *B.P.*	B	—	41–51	0·940–0·965	2·5–3·5
Lobelia (Ethereal)	B	—	55–63	0·800–0·825	1·8–2·0†
Myrrh	C	—	81–87	0·840–0·860	4·5–6·5
Nux Vomica, *B.P.*	A	—	43–46	—	—
Opium, *B.P.*	A	—	41–46	—	—
Opium (Camphorated), *B.P.*	B	Da	56–60	—	0·2–0·3†
Opium (Camphorated, Conc.)	B	Da	54–59	0·910–0·930	—
Orange, *B.P.*	B	—	62–72	0·895–0·920	3·5–4·5
Quillaia	A	Eg	43–45	0·940–0·955	1·0–1·5
Rhubarb (Compound), *B.P.*	A	—	48–53	0·958–0·977	17†
*Senega	A	Ea, c	54–58	0·930–0·940	4·9–7·0
Squill	A	—	52–57	0·925–0·945	4·5–6·5
Stramonium, *B.P.*	A	—	40–45	—	—
Tolu	C	Da	80–84	0·850–0·870	8†
Valerian (Ammoniated)	C	Dc	48–54	0·925–0·940	3–6; NH_3 0·70–1·05% w/v

* A preliminary distillation without addition of acid, followed by acidification and re-distillation of the distillate is necessary for senega preparations to avoid hydrolysis of methyl compounds present in the material (SARGEANT, G. A., *J. Pharm. Pharmacol.*, 1950, **2,** 434).

APPENDIX II

Complexometric Titrations

One of the most significant advances in chemical analysis as applied to pharmaceuticals during the last decade is undoubtedly the introduction and development of the complexometric titration. The ability of certain amino-polycarboxylic acids to react stoichiometrically and instantaneously with certain metal ions was first recognised and described by Schwarzenbach in 1945. Later, the same author, together with co-workers, described the first metal indicator, murexide,[1] and then, perhaps the most important of all,[2] Eriochrome Black T (usually referred to in this country as solochrome black). This was followed quite shortly by the first description of the now classic use of the complexometric titration for the determination of temporary and permanent hardness in water.[3] It was some time, however, before metal indicators capable of functioning at an acid pH were developed; with the availability of such indicators a rapid increase in the application of complexometric titrations took place and there are now few metal ions that are not capable of determination by this means. In the present book reference will be found to the use of complexometric methods for determination of aluminium, bismuth, calcium, copper, iron, lead, magnesium, manganese, mercury and zinc. In addition, indirect methods are described for the determination of certain anions such as fluoride, phosphate and sulphate.

The most widely used titrant for such determinations is diamino-ethane-tetra-acetic acid (ethylenediamine tetra-acetic acid) which is conveniently employed as the disodium salt, referred to throughout this book as EDTA. (The titrant is referred to in the *B.P.* and *B.P.C.* as sodium edetate, but this synonym has not gained universal acceptance.) Many other amino-polycarboxylic acids have been used and in certain special applications they may have some advantage; for routine pharmaceutical work, however, it has not been found necessary to use any titrant other than EDTA. This substance reacts stoichiometrically with most metals to form a 1 : 1 complex and, usually, the reaction is instantaneous (but see Aluminium, p. 32). pH has a marked effect on the stability of the complexes formed; the alkaline earth metals form complexes that are stable in alkaline solution but decompose in neutral and acid solution; aluminium, copper, lead and mercury all complex under mildly acid conditions while bismuth and ferric iron form stable complexes in a solution as acid as pH 1. The monovalent ions of sodium, potassium and silver form complexes that are too weak to be used for titration purposes whilst mercurous mercury forms no complex, being reduced to the metallic form. Those complexes that form in acid conditions are, in general, stable in alkaline solution although in certain cases the stability constant of the corresponding metal hydroxide is sufficiently strong to decompose the complex and cause precipitation in strongly ammoniacal solution (aluminium and ferric iron, for example). The approximate stability constant of some ions of importance in pharmaceutical analysis are listed in Table 62. In general, for a successful titration, the value of log K should be at least 8.

TABLE 62

CATION	LOG K*	CATION	LOG K*
Na^+	1·7	Al^{3+}	15·5
Ag^+	7·2	Zn^{2+}	16·1
Ba^{2+}	7·8	Pb^{2+}	18·0
Mg^{2+}	8·7	Cu^{2+}	18·8
Ca^{2+}	10·7	Hg^{2+}	21·8
Mn^{2+}	13·5	Fe^{3+}	25·1
Fe^{2+}	14·3		

* At 20°, for an ionic strength of 0·1.

It will be seen that the stability of the barium complex is just below the required value and this, in part, explains the unsatisfactory nature of methods for determination of sulphate that depend on precipitation with barium and complexometric titration of the excess.

The complexes of colourless ions are themselves colourless but those of coloured ions are usually more intensely coloured than the ion itself. Since these colours tend to obscure visual indicators, and because convenient alternative titrimetric methods exist, it is seldom of advantage to apply complexometric methods to the determination of copper and of ferric iron.

There are now many metallochromic indicators which may be used in complexometric titrations. For successful end-point indication the pK value of the metal-dye complex should be at least 4 units less than that of the metal-EDTA complex which is formed during the titration; if the difference is less than 4 units the titrant is unable to compete satisfactorily with the indicator dye and a sluggish end-point results. The indicators which are most widely used in the methods described in this book are solochrome black (for titrations carried out in ammoniacal solution), xylenol orange (for titrations carried out between pH 4 and 7) and catechol violet (for titration in mineral acid solution at pH 1 to 2). Table 63 lists the various indicators called for in methods in the monographs. Discussion of the merits of different indicators for specific purposes will be found in various parts of the book.

For titration in alkaline solution an ammoniacal buffer which gives a solution of about pH 10 is used:

APPENDIX II

TABLE 63

INDICATOR	FORM IN WHICH USED
*Acid Alizarin Black SN (Diadem Chrome Black 10 B)	0·1 per cent solution in 95 per cent ethanol
Alizarin S	0·1 per cent solution in water
Calcon	0·4 per cent solution in methanol
Catechol Violet	0·1 per cent solution in water
Murexide	0·2 per cent triturate in sodium chloride with 0·5 per cent Naphthol Green (Colour Index No. 10020)
Methylthymol Blue	1 per cent triturate in potassium nitrate
PAN [1-(2-Pyridyl-azo)-2-naphthol]	0·1 per cent solution in 95 per cent ethanol
Patton and Reeder's Indicator (containing ascorbic acid)	1 per cent triturate of 2-hydroxy-1-(2-hydroxy-4-sulpho-1-naphthylazo)-3-naphthoic acid in anhydrous sodium sulphate containing 5 per cent of ascorbic acid
*Solochrome Black (Eriochrome Black T; Mordant Black 11)	0·5 per cent solution in 95 per cent ethanol
†Xylenol Orange	0·1 per cent solution in 50 per cent ethanol

* Freshly prepared.
† Stable for at least a month.

Ammonia buffer solution. Dissolve 13·5 g of ammonium chloride in 130 ml of strong ammonia solution and dilute to 200 ml with water.

For buffering to a pH suitable for titration with xylenol orange it is convenient to use solid hexamine.

The standard solutions employed in the complexometric methods given in this book are prepared and standardised as described below. Pure zinc, washed with acid and dried before use, has proved a satisfactory material for standardisation of EDTA solutions. An alternative substance, convenient and reliable for use in the routine laboratory, is lead nitrate. Calcium carbonate is favoured by some workers as a primary standard and many pure metals have been investigated. It has been suggested that the disodium salt of diamino-ethane-tetra-acetic acid may be obtained sufficiently pure for use as a primary standard but this is not recommended. If strengths other than those given are required they may be prepared by suitable adjustment of the weights and volumes given.

0·05M EDTA. Dissolve 18·61 g of disodium diamino-ethane-tetra-acetate, $C_{10}H_{14}O_8N_2Na_2,2H_2O$, in 1 litre of water.

Standardise this solution as follows:

Standard: Acid-washed zinc. This is zinc of at least 99·9 per cent purity that has been treated as follows before use: Cover with dilute hydrochloric acid and swirl. Decant the acid and wash the zinc with water, by decantation, until the last washing is not acid to litmus paper. Wash with acetone and ether and allow to dry in air.

Dissolve about 0·7 g of the acid-washed zinc in the minimum quantity of dilute hydrochloric acid and dilute to exactly 250 ml with water. Transfer a 25-ml aliquot to a flask, add 125 ml of water and 10 ml of ammonia buffer solution and titrate with the EDTA solution using solochrome black as indicator. 1 ml 0·05M EDTA = 0·003269 g zinc.

0·05M Calcium chloride. Dissolve 5·478 g of calcium chloride, $CaCl_2,6H_2O$, in sufficient water to produce exactly 1 litre and mix.

Standardise this solution as follows:

Pipette 50 ml into a 250-ml graduated flask and dilute to volume with water. Transfer a 25-ml aliquot of this solution to a flask, add 75 ml of water, heat nearly to boiling-point and add an excess of hot 2·5 per cent ammonium oxalate solution followed by a slight excess of dilute ammonia solution, stirring during the additions. Allow to stand on a water-bath for one hour, allow to cool and transfer, quantitatively, to a No. 4 sintered-glass crucible with a 0·1 per cent solution of ammonium oxalate. Wash the precipitate with water until the washings are free from chloride and then dissolve the precipitate by passing 100 ml of hot dilute sulphuric acid through the filter, in small quantities at a time. Heat the filtrate to about 70° and titrate with 0·1N potassium permanganate, maintaining the solution at 70° throughout the titration. 1 ml 0·1N potassium permanganate = 0·01095 g $CaCl_2,6H_2O$.

0·05M Lead nitrate. Dissolve 16·56 g of lead nitrate in 1 litre of water.

Standardise this solution as follows:

Pipette 30 ml of 0·05M EDTA into a flask, add 1 g of hexamine and 100 ml of water and titrate with the lead nitrate solution using xylenol orange as indicator.

0·05M Thorium nitrate. Dissolve 29·40 g of thorium nitrate, $Th(NO_3)_4,6H_2O$, in 1 litre of water.

Standardise this solution as follows:

Pipette 25 ml of 0·05M EDTA into a flask, add 100 ml of water and neutralise to congo red paper with 10 per cent sodium hydroxide solution. Add 10 ml of 1M sodium acetate, 5 ml of 2M monochloracetic acid and 1·5 ml alizarin S indicator and titrate with the thorium nitrate solution to the bluish-red end-point.

0·05M Zinc. Dissolve about 3·269 g, accurately weighed, of acid-washed zinc (see above under the standardisation of 0·05M EDTA) in the minimum of concentrated hydrochloric acid and dilute to exactly 1 litre with water. Calculate the molarity.

It is often possible to determine two or more metals in the same solution. This may be done either by selection of a pH at which one metal will complex and the other will not (for example, the titration of bismuth in the presence of most other metals at pH 1 to 2, see p. 127, and the titration of aluminium in the presence of alkaline earth metals at pH 6, see p. 32), or by using a suitable masking agent. A masking agent is a substance that will complex more strongly with the metal under the conditions of the titration than does the titrant. Examples of masking agents used in methods given in this book are triethanolamine (for inactivating aluminium and so allowing the selective titration of magnesium at pH 10, see p. 396) and thioglycerol (for masking copper and so allowing the titration of zinc at pH 6, see p. 201) and potassium cyanide can also be used for preventing interference from heavy metals during the titration of alkaline earth metals.

For the selective determination of mercuric mercury in the presence of other metals, potassium iodide is used as a masking agent in the sense that, when it is added to the solution, which has first been titrated to the equivalence point with EDTA, the complexing agent that has reacted with the mercury is quantitatively released due to the preferential formation of a mercuric potassium iodide complex; this liberated EDTA may then be titrated with a standard zinc solution (see p. 408). Ammonium fluoride is also an effective masking agent and can be used to prevent reaction of EDTA with calcium, magnesium and aluminium while zinc is being titrated.[4] Occasionally the use of a demasking agent is of value; for example the metal ions in a solution of lead and zinc can be masked by addition of potassium cyanide and the zinc can then be released for titration with EDTA by addition of formaldehyde or chloral hydrate.

The indirect determination of certain organic substances can be made by complexometric titration methods. Such methods depend on the formation of an insoluble product between the organic material and a metal; then, either the excess metal in solution is determined by a suitable titration with EDTA, or the metal-containing precipitate is decomposed and the liberated metal ions titrated. Thus, for example, narcotine, papaverine, codeine, strychnine and brucine have been determined by formation of iodobismuthate complexes,[5] chlorpromazine[6] and quinine[7] as cadmium iodide complexes, purines and nicotinic acid derivatives by precipitation with mercury[8] and barbiturates by precipitation with zinc.[9]

For a theoretical discussion of complexometric analysis the reader is recommended to Schwarzenbach's book;[10] a useful short account of the subject has been given by Pribil[11] and for a recent account of practical considerations reference should be made to the monograph of West and Sykes.[12]

1. Schwarzenbach, G., Biedermann, W., and Bangerter, F., *Helv. Chim. Acta.*, 1946, **29**, 811.
2. Schwarzenbach, G., and Biedermann, W., *Helv. Chim. Acta.*, 1948, **31**, 678.
3. Biedermann, W., and Schwarzenbach, G., *Chimia (Switz.)*, 1948, **2**, 1.
4. Pribil, R., *Chem. Listy*, 1954, **48**, 51.
5. Buděšínský, B., *Českosl. Farm.*, 1956, **5**, 579.
6. Przyborowski, L., and Krowczanski, L., *Chem. Anal. (Warsaw)*, 1959, **4**, 59.
7. Yuen-Yau Chou and Ju-Cheng Hsu., *Acta Pharm. Sinica*, 1958, **6**, 7.
8. Helmstaedter G., *Mitt. Dtsch. Pharm. Ges.*, 1959, **29**, 91 (publ. in *Arch. Pharm.*, 1959, **292**).
9. Roushdi, I. M., Abdine, H., and Ayad, A., *J. Pharm. Pharmacol.*, 1961, **13**, 153T.

10. SCHWARZENBACH, G., 'Complexometric Titrations,' Methuen & Co. Ltd., London, 1957.
11. PRIBIL, R., *Analyst*, 1958, **83**, 188.
12. WEST, T. S., and SYKES, A. S., 'Analytical Applications of Diamino-ethane-tetra-acetic Acid.' 2nd Edition. The British Drug Houses Ltd., Poole, 1960.

APPENDIX III

Non-aqueous Titrations

The non-aqueous titration has now become an established technique in pharmaceutical analysis and is widely employed in official standardisations. Its use permits the determination of substances, both basic and acidic, that are too weak to be titrated in aqueous solution. A simple introduction to the theory of the non-aqueous titration is given in a monograph by Beckett and Tinley.[1]

Because of the rapid growth in interest in this technique, a multiplicity of solvents, titrants and indicators has been recommended. These variations are seldom justifiable, except on grounds of personal preference, and the purpose of this appendix is to suggest methods that are of fairly general application.

For the determination of basic substances a solution of perchloric acid in anhydrous acetic acid is the most commonly used titrant. Perchloric acid in dioxan is favoured by some workers since the presence of dioxan in the titration liquid results in a sharper end-point in certain cases; for the uses of non-aqueous titration described in this book, however, a dioxan solution of perchloric acid is not necessary. Where dioxan is desirable to obtain an improved end-point it may be added to the solvent system in which the titration is carried out.

Many indicators have been suggested for non-aqueous titrations and it is often a matter of personal choice which one is used; whichever is used, however, the colour change corresponding to the end-point as found potentiometrically should always be determined whenever a substance which has not been titrated before is being examined. Because of the high coefficient of expansion of glacial acetic acid it is necessary to correct for differences in temperature which may occur between the time of standardisation and that at which the titrant is used. The general method given below is suitable for application to many basic substances; crystal violet is still the most widely used indicator, but oracet blue is also very suitable while alpha-naphtholbenzein and quinaldine red find favour with some workers.

Preparation of Standard Solutions

0·1N Perchloric acid. To 900 ml of glacial acetic acid (acid containing not less than 99·6 per cent w/w of $C_2H_4O_2$ should be used throughout) at a temperature not above 25° add 8·2 ml of 72 per cent w/w perchloric acid and mix thoroughly. Then add 30 ml of acetic anhydride, mix again, cool to room temperature and dilute to 1 litre with glacial acetic acid.

Standardise this solution as follows: Weigh about 0·5 g of potassium hydrogen phthalate (of purity 99·9 to 100·1 per cent), previously dried at 120° for two hours, into a dry flask, add 50 ml of glacial acetic acid, previously neutralised to crystal violet with 0·1N perchloric acid, and warm until dissolved. Cool and titrate with the 0·1N perchloric acid to the full blue colour of the indicator. Record the temperature (t_1) at which the standardisation is carried out. 1 ml 0·1N perchloric acid = 0·02042 g of potassium hydrogen phthalate.

0·05N Perchloric acid. Prepare as for the 0·1N acid using 4·1 ml of 72 per cent w/w perchloric acid and 20 ml of acetic anhydride and standardise using about 0·25 g of the potassium hydrogen phthalate.

0·02N Perchloric acid. Prepare as for the 0·1N acid using 1·65 ml of 72 per cent w/w perchloric acid and 13·9 ml of acetic anhydride and standardise using about 0·1 g of potassium hydrogen phthalate.

For work of the highest accuracy, determine the water content of the titrant and adjust to lie between 0·01 and 0·2 per cent by the addition of water or acetic anhydride, as appropriate. This ensures that the end-point will not be impaired by the presence of water, and at the same time prevents an excess of acetic anhydride which can cause erroneous results due to acetylation of titratable groups.

Indicator Solutions

Crystal violet	0·5 per cent in glacial acetic acid
2-Naphtholbenzein	0·2 per cent in glacial acetic acid
Oracet blue B	0·5 per cent in glacial acetic acid
Quinaldine red	0·1 per cent in methanol

Method: Neutralise a suitable volume (about 50 to 80 ml) of glacial acetic acid with 0·1N perchloric acid using the indicator of choice. Add and dissolve the specified weight of sample, warming and cooling if necessary, and, when the sample is a halide, add 10 ml of a 5 per cent solution of mercuric acetate in glacial acetic acid that has been neutralised, if necessary, to the chosen indicator with 0·1N perchloric acid Titrate with standard perchloric acid to the colour of the indicator that corresponds to the maximum value of dE/dV (where E is the electromotive force and V the volume of titrant) in a potentiometric titration of the substance being examined.

When the temperature (t_2) at which the titration is carried out differs from the temperature (t_1) at which the titrant was standardised, multiply the volume of titrant required by $1 + 0{\cdot}001(t_1 - t_2)$ and calculate the result of the assay from the corrected volume.

Potentiometric titration may be carried out using a general-purpose glass electrode as indicator electrode and a saturated calomel half-cell as reference electrode.

For the determination of acidic substances a standard solution of lithium methoxide in benzene containing just enough methanol to maintain a clear solution is frequently used as titrant. Lithium is preferable to sodium since it has much less tendency to produce gelatinous precipitates during the titration. Dimethylformamide (the vapours of which are quite toxic) is a commonly used titration medium and suitable indicators are 0·1 per cent quinaldine red in methanol, 0·3 per cent thymol blue in methanol or 0·2 per cent azo violet, 4-(*p*-nitrophenyl-azo)-resorcinol, in benzene. Tetrabutylammonium hydroxide in a benzene-methanol mixture is a more versatile titrant than lithium methoxide since it will titrate weaker acids. In this case the sample is dissolved in pyridine and, for universal application, the end-point should be determined potentiometrically. The pyridine used should be of analytical-reagent grade, or should be purified either by standing over sodium hydroxide pellets for four hours and then distilling, or by shaking with chromatographic grade basic aluminium oxide for about five minutes and then filtering.[2] Because of the toxicity of benzene and dimethylformamide vapours both titrants described below should be used with caution.

I. *Titration with tetrabutylammonium hydroxide*

Standard Solution:

0·1N Tetrabutylammonium hydroxide in benzene/methanol. Dissolve 80 g of tetrabutylammonium iodide in 180 ml of analytical-reagent grade dehydrated methanol in a flask. Place in an ice-bath, add 40 g of finely ground silver oxide, stopper the flask and agitate intermittently for one hour. Filter through a dry sintered-glass crucible (No. 4), wash the flask and residue with three 50-ml quantities of cold, dry benzene and dilute the combined filtrate and washings to 2 litres with dry benzene.

Alternatively, an equivalent quantity of tetrabutylammonium bromide may be substituted for the tetrabutylammonium iodide in the above preparation and, in this case, the agitation time may be reduced to fifteen minutes.

Standardise this solution as follows:

Apparatus: This consists of a general-purpose glass electrode and a sleeve-type calomel electrode that has been modified by replacing the saturated aqueous solution of potassium chloride, in the outer jacket, by a saturated solution of potassium chloride in dry methanol. The electrodes are connected to a direct-reading pH-meter having an additional scale graduated in millivolts. The electrodes, together with the jet of a 10-ml microburette, are fitted through holes in a cork that will fit into the top of a titration flask (so that the liquid to be titrated is protected from the atmosphere). The top of the burette is also fitted with a guard-tube to protect its contents from carbon dioxide and moisture in the atmosphere. A slight air space is left round the jet of the burette to give an air leak. The titration flask should also contain a stirrer (a stirrer of the magnetic type has been found most convenient).

Method: Weigh into the titration flask about 0·1 g of benzoic acid (of purity at least 99·8 per cent) that has been dried at 100° for thirty minutes before use and dissolve in 50 ml of analytical-reagent grade pyridine. Insert the electrodes in the solution, set the stirrer in motion and adjust the instrument so that the millivolt-scale reading is zero with the electrodes in circuit. Titrate potentiometrically with the tetrabutylammonium hydroxide solution, at the same time preparing a graph by plotting readings on the millivolt-scale against the volume of titrant added. In the region of the equivalence-point take readings every 0·1 ml. Read the volume of titrant added at the point of inflection of the curve.
1 ml 0·1N tetrabutylammonium hydroxide = 0·01221 g benzoic acid.

Apparatus: This is the same as that described above for the standardisation.

Determination: Weigh the specified amount of the sample into the titration flask of the apparatus and dissolve in 50 ml of analytical-reagent grade pyridine. Continue as described above for the standardisation beginning with 'Insert the electrodes . . .' and ending with '. . . at the point of inflection of the curve.'

II. *Titration with lithium methoxide*

Standard Solution:

0·1N Lithium methoxide. Dissolve 0·7 g of lithium in 150 ml of dry methanol, cool in ice-water and dilute to 1 litre with dry benzene.

Standardise this solution as follows. Weigh about 50 mg of benzoic acid (of purity at least 99·8 per cent) that has been dried at 100° for thirty minutes before use, into a dry titration flask and dissolve in 25 ml of dimethylformamide. Titrate with the lithium methoxide solution using a 0·1 per cent solution of quinaldine red in methanol as indicator and protecting the solution from carbon dioxide of the atmosphere. Repeat the titration omitting the benzoic acid. 1 ml 0·1N lithium methoxide = 0·01221 g benzoic acid.

Determination: Dissolve the specified weight of sample in 40 ml of dimethylformamide and titrate with 0·1N lithium methoxide as described in the standardisation. Repeat the titration omitting the sample.

1. BECKETT, A. H., and TINLEY, E. H., 'Titration in Non-aqueous Solvents,' 3rd Edition, The British Drug Houses Ltd., Poole, Dorset, 1961.

2. BANICK, W. M., Jnr., *Anal. Chem.*, 1962, **34,** 296.

APPENDIX IV

The Oxygen-Flask Combustion Technique

The oxygen-flask combustion technique has proved of considerable value in pharmaceutical work since the principle was revived by Schöniger in 1955.[1,2] The method is rapid, elegant and applicable to the determination of several elements in organic samples. In many cases it may be applied directly to the determination of elements in formulated products such as tablets, lozenges, oily solutions and ointments. In pharmaceutical analysis the method has been applied to the determination of halogens (including fluorine), sulphur and mercury although there is no doubt that this list will be extended.

For the determination a suitable size of sample (usually about 10 to 25 mg of compound for semi-micro work) is wrapped in filter paper which is then clamped in a sample holder made of platinum gauze. The gauze is attached by means of stout platinum wire to the stopper of a 500-ml iodine flask. A suitable absorbing liquid (depending on the element being determined) is introduced into the flask which is then filled with oxygen. The paper containing the sample is ignited and is then introduced into the flask by inserting the stopper. When combustion is complete the flask is shaken to absorb liberated gases in the liquid. Finally the flask is opened and, after washing down, the required ions are determined in the absorbing liquid by some suitable method. If the final determination is a simple titration the whole procedure takes about twenty minutes to complete. In considering the application of the oxygen-flask technique to the determination of, say, iodine in an organic compound, it will be seen that the time required compares very favourably with that needed to complete the classical sodium carbonate fusion method.

The general method, to be applied in all cases unless otherwise stated, is as follows:

Apparatus. The apparatus consists of a stout-walled 500-ml iodine flask of resistant glass. Into the stopper is fused one end of a length of platinum wire 1 mm in diameter. To the free end is attached a piece of 36-mesh platinum gauze measuring 1·5 × 2 cm (Fig. 19). This may readily be attached by bending back the wire round the fold in the gauze.

Method. Accurately weigh a suitable quantity of the sample by difference and transfer to a strip of filter paper (Whatman No. 1 is suitable) which has been folded into three along its length. A convenient size has been found to be 3 × 5 cm but this is not critical, provided that both sample and paper burn satisfactorily during the subsequent combustion stage. Enclose the sample in the filter paper by folding in the outer thirds and rolling up the strip. Grip the small packet so obtained in the platinum gauze and insert a narrow strip of filter paper into the roll to act as a fuse.

Moisten the ground-glass joint of the flask with water and fill the flask with oxygen after adding a suitable absorbing liquid, applicable to the element being determined (see below). Ignite the fuse and immediately insert the stopper into the flask. Since a small positive pressure is formed during combustion, hold the stopper firmly in place. Once the sample is burning vigorously turn the flask on its side so as to prevent incompletely-burned material from falling out of the gauze into the liquid. As soon as the combustion is complete shake the flask vigorously for about five minutes; then place a few ml of water in the collar of the flask and withdraw the stopper, when the slight negative pressure will suck the water in to wash down the neck. Rinse the stopper, platinum wire, gauze and walls of the flask with water. Continue by a method applicable to the particular element being determined (see below).

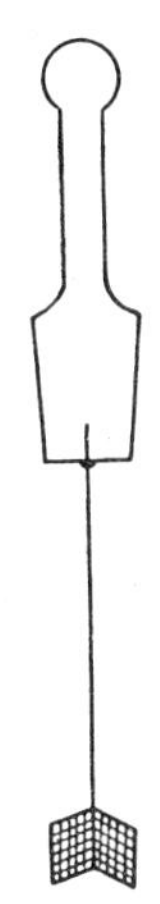

FIG. 19

Stopper with platinum wire and gauze attached as used in the flask combustion method

With ointments, the sample is weighed on to a small square of greaseproof paper which is folded so as to completely enclose the material and is then itself folded in filter paper as usual. In some instances a small amount of carbon may deposit on the wall of the flask during combustion but this does not appear to affect the result.

A liquid sample may be determined by enclosing it in a capsule of gelatin or methylcellulose containing about 20 mg of ashless filter-paper floc to serve as an adsorbent. Methylcellulose capsules are preferable since they burn more gently than gelatin capsules, they give rise to lower blank values and, particularly, because they do not give rise to acidic products on combustion.

Repeated routine use of the oxygen-flask technique has shown it to be rapid, reliable and safe. When a new material is being examined, however, especially if its constitution is not fully known, adequate precautions should be taken against a possible accident. Safety spectacles or, better, a perspex safety screen should be used to protect the operator; alternatively some form of electrical ignition by remote control, such as that described by Haslam, Hamilton and Squirrell,[3] may be used.

With a little experience the oxygen-flask combustion technique is capable of a very satisfactory degree of precision. The reproducibility available will, of course, depend upon the determination used to complete the method. As an example to indicate the precision which is obtainable the case of pheniodol may be quoted. In 24 determinations made at intervals over a period of two to three weeks, results ranging from 98·7 to 99·2 per cent with a standard deviation of 0·161 were obtained.

APPENDIX IV

The size of flask given in the method (500 ml) is suitable for the semi-micro determination of most organic compounds but in some cases, particularly where low content formulations are being determined, a 1-litre or even a 2-litre flask may be used. See Thyroid (p. 640). In general, a sample weighing up to 50 mg may be burnt in a 500-ml flask without the formation of carbon. Samples of certain materials weighing up to 0·6 to 0·7 g have been burnt in a 2-litre flask.

METHODS FOR INDIVIDUAL ELEMENTS

For chlorine-containing substances. Use 20 ml of water and 1 ml of hydrogen peroxide (100 volumes) as the absorbing liquid.

For the titration a number of satisfactory methods are available. (i) A potentiometric titration with silver nitrate, (ii) a comparative titration using mercuric oxycyanide, (iii) a titration with mercuric nitrate using diphenylcarbazone as indicator in an ethanolic titration medium, or an application of the Volhard procedure (see p. 290), have all proved satisfactory. The simplest and most reliable methods are the potentiometric and mercuric nitrate titrations.

(i) *Potentiometric titration with silver nitrate.* After removing the stopper from the combustion flask wash down the wire and gauze with water, collecting the washings in a 250-ml beaker. Rinse down the walls of the combustion flask and to the liquid add a drop of a 0·1 per cent solution of methyl red in 95 per cent ethanol. Neutralise by addition of N sodium hydroxide and then add 0·5 ml in excess. Boil gently for five to ten minutes (using a small air condenser if necessary to avoid mechanical loss) to destroy peroxide. Cool the flask and quantitatively transfer the contents to the 250-ml beaker. Add 1 drop of the methyl red indicator and then N nitric acid until the indicator just changes to red, followed by 2 ml of acetate buffer (50 ml of glacial acetic acid and 50 ml of sodium acetate per litre). Stand the beaker in an ice-bath to cool the contents to about 8° to 10° and titrate potentiometrically with 0·02N silver nitrate using calomel/potassium nitrate or silver/silver chloride electrodes.

(ii) *Comparative mercuric oxycyanide titration.* Rinse down the stopper, wire and gauze with a little water and boil the solution gently for a few minutes to destroy hydrogen peroxide. Cool and neutralise with 0·02N sodium hydroxide to match the colour of an equal volume of previously boiled and cooled water containing the same amount of screened methyl red indicator solution in a similar flask. Add 20 ml of mercuric oxycyanide solution to the test flask and titrate the alkali liberated using 0·02N sulphuric acid until the colour in the control flask is again matched. To the control flask now add the same volumes of mercuric oxycyanide solution and 0·02N sulphuric acid as used above and titrate with 0·02N sodium chloride to match the colour of the test solution. The volume of chloride solution required is used to calculate the chlorine content of the sample.

Reagents:

Screened methyl red indicator solution: Dissolve 0·125 g of methyl red in 50 ml of ethanol (95 per cent); dissolve 0·083 g of methylene blue in 50 ml of ethanol (95 per cent). Store the solutions separately and mix equal volumes when required for use.

Mercuric oxycyanide solution: Dissolve, without the aid of heat, 20 g of mercuric oxycyanide in 1 litre of previously boiled and cooled water. Store in a brown-glass bottle.

The oxycyanide reaction on which the above method is based is not stoichiometric so an excess of reagent must be used. The 20 ml specified is sufficient for the titration of up to 12 mg of chloride but it should be increased to 30 ml if this quantity is exceeded. It should be noted that, at the end-point of the titration with sodium chloride solution, the volumes and temperatures of both the test and comparison solutions should be the same. For many practical purposes it may be sufficiently accurate to calculate the chlorine content of the sample from the volume of 0·02N sulphuric acid used, thus dispensing with the second titration.

(iii) *Mercuric nitrate titration.*[4] In this case the absorbing liquid should also contain about 3 ml of 0·1N sodium hydroxide. After rinsing down the stopper, wire and gauze with 5 ml of water, add 2 drops of a 0·1 per cent solution of bromophenol blue in ethanol and then add 0·1N nitric acid to the yellow-green colour of the indicator followed by a further 0·5 ml of the acid. (If the compound contains sulphur, add a slight excess of 0·1N barium nitrate at this stage.) Add 100 ml of 95 per cent ethanol, using some of it to further rinse the stopper, wire and gauze, and then add 15 drops of a 0·1 per cent solution of diphenylcarbazone in ethanol and titrate with 0·02N mercuric nitrate, added from a 5-ml micro-burette, to the first trace of a pink colour. Carry out a blank determination by repeating the entire operation omitting the sample. 1 ml 0·02N mercuric nitrate = 0·0007092 g Cl.

0·02N mercuric nitrate. Dissolve 6·86 g of mercuric nitrate in 75 ml of 0·1N nitric acid and dilute to about 1,500 ml with water. Add 200 ml of 95 per cent ethanol, dilute to 2 litres with water and filter. (The ethanol is added to reduce the surface tension of the solution as this aids the filling of the micro-burette.) Standardise this solution, not more than one week before use, as follows: Into a 250-ml flask pipette 5 ml of 0·02N sodium chloride (prepared by weighing 1·1690 g of analytical-reagent grade sodium chloride, previously dried at 250° for two hours, and dissolving in sufficient water to produce exactly 1 litre), and add 15 ml of water, 2 drops of the 0·1 per cent solution of bromophenol blue in ethanol and 0·1N nitric acid to the yellow-green colour of the indicator. Add a further 0·5 ml of the acid and then add 100 ml of 95 per cent ethanol and 15 drops of the 0·1 per cent solution of diphenylcarbazone in ethanol and titrate with the mercuric nitrate solution, added from a 5-ml micro-burette, to the first trace of a pink colour. Determine the indicator blank using 20 ml of water, subtract this from the previous titre and calculate the normality of the mercuric nitrate solution.

For bromine-containing substances. Use 20 ml of a 30 per cent solution of analytical-reagent grade sodium chloride, 10 ml of sodium hypochlorite solution and 5 ml of buffer solution (a 20 per cent solution of sodium dihydrogen phosphate in water) as absorbing liquid.

After combustion heat the solution to boiling, add 5 ml of 50 per cent sodium formate solution and again boil for a short time. Draw air through the flask to remove chlorine vapours, cool and dilute to about 100 ml with water. Add 1 g of potassium iodide, 25 ml of 6N sulphuric acid and 1 drop of 0·5N ammonium molybdate and titrate immediately with 0·02N sodium thiosulphate. Carry out a blank determination under the same conditions.

Sodium hypochlorite solution: Pass sufficient chlorine into a 1·1N solution of sodium hydroxide to make the solution about normal in chlorine.

Bromine may also be determined by the mercuric nitrate titration procedure given under chlorine-containing substances. In this case the absorbing liquid should be 20 ml of water, 1 ml of hydrogen peroxide (100 volumes) and 3 ml of 0·1N sodium hydroxide. 1 ml 0·02N = 1·5984 mg Br.

For iodine-containing substances.[5] Use 10 ml of water and 2 ml of N sodium hydroxide as absorbing liquid.

After combustion add an excess (5 to 10 ml) of acetic-bromine solution and allow to stand for two minutes. Remove the excess bromine by addition of formic acid (about 0·5 to 1·0 ml), wash down the sides of the flask with water and sweep out any bromine vapours above the liquid with a current of air. Add 1 g of potassium iodide and titrate with 0·02N sodium thiosulphate, using starch mucilage as indicator.

Acetic-bromine solution: Dissolve 100 g of potassium acetate in glacial acetic acid, add 4 ml of bromine and dilute to 1 litre with glacial acetic acid.

For fluorine-containing substances. For the determination of substances containing fluorine it has been shown[6] that low results are obtained if the combustion is carried out in a flask constructed of borosilicate glass. Acceptable results are obtainable if a soda-glass flask, essentially free from boron, is used, but for the best results a flask constructed of silica should be used. Use 20 ml of water as absorbing liquid.

After combustion transfer the liquid to a 250-ml graduated flask, dilute to the mark and treat an aliquot expected to contain about 25 μg of fluoride by the procedure described below under 'Preparation of Calibration Graph.' At the same time, prepare a standard colour from 5 ml of standard fluoride solution (prepared by dissolving 22 mg of dried analytical-reagent grade sodium fluoride in 2 litres of water) to serve as a check on the calibration graph. For solutions derived from the combustion of sulphur-containing compounds, boil gently for about ten seconds with 1 ml of 100-volume hydrogen peroxide, neutralise to phenolphthalein with N sodium hydroxide and then add 1 ml in excess; boil to destroy excess of peroxide, cool, and adjust the pH to about 4 with N hydrochloric acid. Transfer to a 250-ml graduated flask, dilute to the mark and continue as above.

Preparation of Calibration Graph. In each of a series of 100-ml graduated flasks place 50 ml of water, an aliquot portion of standard fluorine solution (22·1 mg of dried sodium fluoride in 2 litres of water; 1 ml

= 5 μg of fluorine; store in a polythene container) containing from 10 to 40 μg of fluorine, 10 ml of alizarin complexan solution, and 3 ml of acetate buffer solution. Mix each solution, add 10 ml 0·0005M cerous nitrate to each, dilute to the mark with water and set aside, protected from direct light, for one hour. At the same time prepare a blank solution in similar fashion by omitting the standard fluoride solution. Measure the extinction values of the test solutions against the blank in 4-cm cells at 610 mμ, and plot a graph of extinction against amount of fluorine present.

Reagents:

Alizarin complexan solution, 0·0005M: Transfer 0·385 g of alizarin complexan to a 2-litre graduated flask by means of 20 ml of recently prepared 0·5N sodium hydroxide. Dilute to about 1,500 ml with water, add 0·2 g of hydrated sodium acetate, and adjust the pH to about 5 by careful addition of N hydrochloric acid. Dilute to the mark and transfer to a brown-glass bottle, filtering if necessary. This solution is stable for at least four months.

Cerous nitrate, 0·0005M: Standardise an approximately 0·02M cerous nitrate solution by titration with EDTA at pH 6 using xylenol orange as indicator (see p. 300). To a suitable volume of this solution (about 50 ml) add 0·2 ml of concentrated nitric acid, 0·1 g of hydroxylamine hydrochloride and sufficient water to dilute to 2 litres.

Acetate buffer solution, pH 4·6: Dissolve 150 g of hydrated sodium acetate in about 600 ml of water, add 75 ml of glacial acetic acid, dilute to 1 litre with water and filter.

For sulphur-containing substances.[7] Use 15 ml of water and 1 ml of hydrogen peroxide (20 volumes) as the absorbing liquid. For titration of the solution resulting from combustion two methods are applicable:

(i) For substances which do not yield acidic or basic substances, other than sulphuric acid, on combustion.

Boil the solution for about ten minutes to destroy excess peroxide, cool, and titrate with standard sodium hydroxide solution (0·05N or 0·02N according to the material being assayed) using screened methyl red as indicator.

(ii) For all other sulphur-containing substances.

After combustion wash down the stopper, platinum wire, gauze and walls of the flask not with water as specified in the general method, but with 60 ml of industrial methylated spirit. Add 2 drops of a 0·2 per cent solution of Thoron * in water and 2 drops of a 0·0125 per cent solution of methylene blue in water and titrate with 0·02M or 0·01M barium perchlorate until the yellow colour changes to pale pink. The titration should be carried out in a good natural light and the solution should be kept stirred vigorously by means of a magnetic stirrer.

For mercury-containing substances.[8] Use 20 ml of water and 5 ml of saturated bromine water as the absorbing liquid. This should be added to

* The sodium salt of 1-(*o*-arsono-phenyl-azo)-2-naphthol-3,6-disulphonic acid.

the flask *after* it has been filled with oxygen, otherwise loss of bromine will occur.

Wash down the stopper, wire, gauze and walls of the flask with water. Remove the excess bromine from the solution by drawing a stream of air through it until colourless and then for a further five minutes. Rinse the aspiration tube with a little water and to the solution in the flask add 30 ml of 0·005M EDTA (this need not be accurately standardised), 5 ml of ammonia buffer solution and 0·3 ml of PAN indicator solution. Titrate with 0·01M zinc to the first pink colour using a magnetic stirring device; add 2 g of potassium iodide, stir for two minutes, and continue the titration, again to the pink colour; the mercury content of the sample is calculated from the volume of zinc solution required after addition of the potassium iodide.

The above EDTA method for mercury is specific and is discussed on p. 408.

The oxygen-flask combustion technique is also applicable to other elements than those mentioned above. Methods for phosphorus, arsenic and boron have been described and these are discussed in a general review of the topic published by Macdonald.[9]

1. SCHÖNIGER, W., *Mikrochim. Acta*, 1955, 122.
2. SCHÖNIGER, W., *Mikrochim. Acta*, 1956, 869.
3. HASLAM, J., HAMILTON, J. B., and SQUIRRELL, D. C. M., *Analyst*, 1960, **85**, 556.
4. WHITE, D. C., *Mikrochim. Acta*, 1961, 449.
5. JOHNSON, C. A., and VICKERS, C., *J. Pharm. Pharmacol.*, 1959, **11**, 218T.
6. JOHNSON, C. A., and LEONARD, M. A., *Analyst*, 1961, **86**, 101.
7. VICKERS, C., and WILKINSON, J. V., *J. Pharm. Pharmacol.*, 1961, **13**, 72.
8. VICKERS, C., and WILKINSON, J. V., *J. Pharm. Pharmacol.*, 1961, **13**, 156T.
9. MACDONALD, A. M. G., *Analyst*, 1961, **86**, 3.

APPENDIX V

Determination of Water

The direct measurement of moisture by distillation with an immiscible solvent is of wide application and is of considerable use in pharmaceutical analysis, particularly when gravimetric determination is interfered with by the presence of other volatile matter or by decomposition of the substance. The method is rapid and has been shown to be capable of considerable accuracy. Water of hydration is removed by this method.

For most purposes the following method using the apparatus originally due to Dean and Stark,[1] and later modified by Bidwell and Sterling,[2] is satisfactory:

Apparatus: This is as illustrated in the diagram. A 500-ml flask A is connected by means of trap B to a reflux condenser C (of the Liebig type) by ground-glass joints. The trap leads into a graduated receiver E. The source of heat is an electric heating mantle. For most efficient working the upper portion of the flask and the connecting tube D may be insulated with asbestos. A small tube containing a drying agent such as anhydrous calcium chloride may be fitted to the top of the condenser to prevent atmospheric moisture condensing inside the apparatus.

When any evidence of greasiness appears, *e.g.* if there is difficulty in the separation of the water and the entraining liquid, the condenser and receiver should be cleaned with chromic acid cleaning mixture, thoroughly rinsed with water and dried in an oven.

Entraining liquid: This may vary but in most cases xylene or toluene is satisfactory. Tate and Warren[3] preferred to use heptane as, since this boils at about 100°, the results obtained are most nearly comparable with oven-drying tests at that temperature. Glycerol was found to distil slowly when boiled with heptane, with consequent inaccurate results, and therefore this solvent cannot be used as entraining liquid when glycerol is present.

For usual purposes the entraining liquid should be free from water (but see Note). If the apparatus is in continuous use, the use of the liquid already in the flask from a previous determination (providing the liquid and apparatus are not too contaminated) sufficiently fulfils this requirement. If the liquid is not known to be anhydrous it can be made so by distilling in the apparatus before use and using the liquid remaining in the flask.

Determination: Weigh into the flask, which should be half-filled with the entraining liquid, sufficient sample to yield 2 to 4 ml of water and, if necessary, add a little porous pot or a few glass beads to prevent bumping. Connect the apparatus and fill the receiver (if not already filled) with the entraining liquid, poured through the top of the condenser. Heat the flask gently until the liquid begins to boil and then more vigorously until there is no further increase in the volume of water in the receiver (usually about half to one hour). Rinse the inside of the condenser with a further quantity (20 to 30 ml is usually sufficient) of the entraining liquid, which in this case should always be free from water, and continue the distillation for a further ten minutes. Allow the receiver to cool to room temperature and if any drops of water adhere to the sides of the receiver dislodge them with a piece of wire. When the

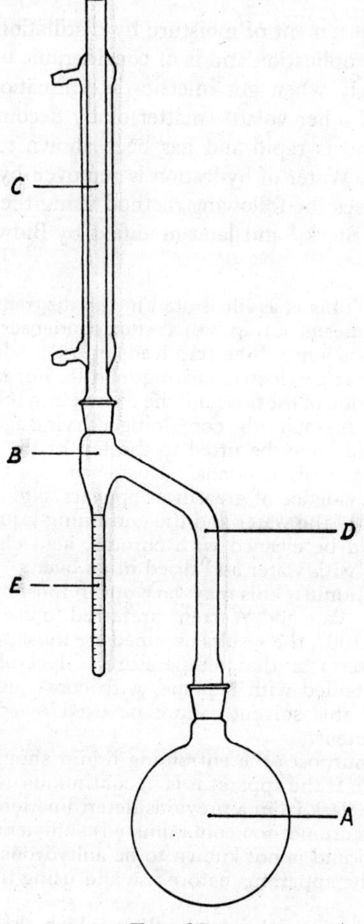

FIG. 20

water and entraining liquid have separated completely, read the volume of water and from it calculate the percentage present in the sample.

Note. The results obtained will be slightly low due to some water being dissolved in the entraining liquid above the water in the receiver. In the case of xylene and toluene the amount is negligible for the normal design of apparatus, providing the receiver used is not much too large for the volume of water collected. If an entraining liquid is used in which the solubility of water is appreciable the liquid should be saturated with water and distilled in the apparatus before the sample is added. The volume of water in the sample is then read by difference.

Jones and McLachlan[4] proposed to release small drops of water from the condenser by the use of a long thin copper spiral which is fitted inside the condenser and, periodically during distillation, is moved up and down, but it does not effect complete removal.

Calderwood and Piechowski[5] working with the Dean and Stark method, using xylene as the immiscible liquid, found the addition of a very small quantity (2 drops) of 95 per cent ethanol through the condenser removed water adhering to the inner wall of the condenser tube. The ethanol should be added only after dehydration of the sample is complete and boiling must not be interrupted for the addition but should be continued for a further five minutes after the violent ebullition and refluxing caused by the addition have ceased. Undoubtedly the best method for eliminating this source of error is by prior treatment of the inner surface of the condenser and the Dean and Stark receiving tube with a silicone; various commercial forms are available. A solution in carbon tetrachloride is placed in the apparatus for an hour; after its removal the surface resists wetting for a considerable time and the apparatus can be used repeatedly without re-treatment with the silicone.

The method given above is particularly useful for the determination of moisture in emulsions and ointments, but high results are obtained in the presence of glycerol.

Small quantities of water may be determined by the Karl Fischer technique.[6] The method is not universally applicable but the limitations of the direct determination can be overcome by some preliminary technique.

The method depends upon the reaction of the water to be determined with iodine and sulphur dioxide in pyridine-methanol solution. The pyridine prevents loss of sulphur dioxide from the reagent by forming an additive compound and also assists completion of the reaction with water by combining with the products of the reaction. The reaction between water and the reagent is complex and the stoichiometrical relationships are uncertain hence it is necessary to standardise the reagent empirically against weighed amounts of water.

Since the reagent is extremely sensitive to water it is necessary to take special precautions in its preparation, storage and use. It should be standardised at frequent intervals under the conditions in which it will be used, by titration against a standard solution of water in methanol or against weighed amounts of a hydrated salt, the most favoured salts being hydrated sodium acetate, which is soluble in methanol, and sodium tartrate dihydrate.

A visual end-point titration is possible for colourless substances, using a control end-point solution of 0·005N iodine in a similar cylinder to that in which the titration is carried out; this is suitable for colourless substances dissolved in dry methanol or for colourless liquids which must be diluted with about 20 per cent by volume of methanol. In this and all cases of direct titration where a solvent is used, the solvent should be titrated to the end-point before the addition of the sample. The usual titration technique uses an electrometric end-point; the principle of the method is that a low e.m.f. (10 to 15 mV) is put across the electrodes of the cell in which the titration is carried out and the polarisation e.m.f. is able to balance it; under these conditions a dead-stop end-point occurs in the titration of all systems in which a sharp transition from the polarisation of at least one electrode to the complete depolarisation of both coincides with the end of the reaction. Two methods of titration are available. In the first, the Karl Fischer reagent is added to the solution of the sample under examination. In these circumstances, the cathode is polarised until there is a slight excess of iodine which, by its oxidising action, depolarises this electrode causing a current to flow; the end-point is taken when the first steady current is recorded. In the second and preferable method an excess of reagent is added and the excess back titrated with a standard solution of water in methanol to a zero reading.

Apparatus: Various forms of apparatus for use in indirect titration are available commercially. Essentially the apparatus is as follows: The Karl Fischer reagent and the standard solution of water in methanol are contained separately in two bottles and from these are pumped into the respective burettes by means of hand bellows; access of moisture is prevented by a suitable arrangement of drying tubes. The burettes, of 10-ml capacity, are graduated in 0·02 ml and are closed by drying tubes while the titration vessel, of about 60-ml capacity, is fitted with an air-tight rubber closure through which pass the two electrodes, the jets of the burettes and a vent tube filled with a desiccant. Stirring is preferably accomplished magnetically.

Reagents:

Karl Fischer reagent. Dissolve 63 g of analytical-reagent grade iodine in 110 ml of dehydrated pyridine in a dry gas wash-bottle (of which the delivery tube is fitted with a screw-clip and the exit tube connected to an efficient drying tube) and weigh the bottle and its contents. Cool in ice-water and pass dry sulphur dioxide into the cold solution, stirring continuously, until the increase in weight is 32 g. Allow the mixture to stand for about thirty minutes and then dilute to 500 ml with dry methanol. When freshly prepared the solution will have a water equivalent of about 5 mg per ml but slowly decomposes. It should be allowed to stand for twenty-four hours before standardisation.

Standard solution of water in methanol. Add 6 ml of water to about 2,500 ml of methanol and mix well. Standardise this solution, if it is necessary to detach the titration vessel for any purpose during a series of determinations and in any case every week, as follows:

Dry about 1 g of sodium tartrate dihydrate at 130° to constant weight (overnight is usually a sufficient length of time); the water content of the dried material is 15·65 per cent w/w.

Introduce an accurately measured volume of Karl Fischer reagent (C ml) into the titration vessel, which must be clean and dry (the volume of reagent added should be sufficient to cover the electrodes), and titrate electrometrically with the solution of water in methanol. Repeat until two successive titrations are in agreement. Let the final volume be A ml.

Weigh about 0·2 g of the dried sodium tartrate dihydrate into the titration vessel, add C ml of Karl Fischer reagent and again titrate with the solution of water in methanol. Repeat this procedure until two successive titrations are in agreement. Let the final volume required be B ml.

If F is the mg of water in 1 ml of the solution of water in methanol and W is the weight (in g) of sodium tartrate dihydrate taken then

$$F = \frac{15{\cdot}65 \times 1{,}000 \times W}{(A-B) \times 100}$$

Determination: Introduce a suitable volume (D ml) of Karl Fischer reagent (sufficient to cover the electrodes) into the titration vessel and titrate electrometrically with the standard solution of water in methanol. Repeat this procedure until two successive titrations are in agreement. Let the final volume required be a ml. Introduce an accurately weighed or accurately measured quantity of the sample into the titration vessel, add D ml of Karl Fischer reagent and again titrate with the standard solution of water in methanol. Let the volume required be b ml.

$$\text{Per cent water in sample} = \frac{(a - b) \times F \times 100}{1{,}000 \times \text{wt. (or vol.) of sample taken}}$$

For more precise work a stream of dry nitrogen should be passed through the apparatus for fifteen minutes before, and during, the titration.

The water in some compounds that react with the Fischer reagent may be extracted with methanol of known water content. For non-volatile compounds that react and from which the water cannot be extracted in this way an azeotropic distillation method using either benzene or pyridine has been described by Roberts and Levin.[7] Types of compounds likely to give rise to difficulties include those containing a reactive carbonyl group, phenolic and highly unsaturated substances, and reactive aromatic amino-compounds.

Water has been determined in a number of pharmaceutical preparations such as creams and ointments by Elvidge and Proctor[8] using a gas chromatographic method. The equipment had a special injection system to prevent non-volatile materials in the sample from reaching the column (see p. 877) and a thermal conductivity detector was used. The method is as follows.

Make up standard solutions containing up to 2·0 per cent of water in dry acetone and add 2·0 per cent of n-pentanol. Shake the sample vigorously with dry acetone and dilute as necessary to bring the water content between 0·50 and 2·0 per cent. Add 2·0 per cent of n-pentanol. Chromatograph the sample and standards under the following conditions: column length—5 feet, column diameter—4 to 5 mm, column temperature—

117°, stationary phase—20 per cent of Carbowax 1,500 on 36- to 85-mesh Chromosorb, carrier gas—hydrogen-nitrogen mixture (4 + 1 by volume) at 100 ml per minute, flash heater temperature—150°, sample size about 30 μl.

Under these conditions the retention volume for water is 225 ml and for *n*-pentanol 525 ml. The water gives a reasonably symmetrical peak and the peak height method can be used for the calculation by reference to the standards (see p. 879).

It has been found in routine practice that the calibration curve relating the ratio of the peak heights of water and *n*-pentanol to water concentration is linear and reasonably reproducible from day to day and so the standards need be examined only occasionally as a check on the calibration.

1. Dean, E. W., and Stark, D. D., *J. Ind. Eng. Chem.*, 1920, **12**, 486.
2. Bidwell, G. L., and Sterling, W. F., *J.A.O.A.C.*, 1925, **8**, 295.
3. Tate, F. G. H., and Warren, L. A., *Analyst*, 1936, **61**, 367.
4. Jones, J. M., and McLachlan, T., *Analyst*, 1927, **52**, 383.
5. Calderwood, H. N., and Piechowski, R. J., *Ind. Eng. Chem., Anal. Edn.*, 1937, **9**, 520.
6. Fischer, K., *Z. Angew. Chem.*, 1935, **48**, 394.
7. Roberts, F. M., and Levin, H., *Anal. Chem.*, 1949, **21**, 1553.
8. Elvidge, D. A., and Proctor, K. A., *Analyst*, 1959, **84**, 461.

APPENDIX VI

MICROSCOPIC ANALYTICAL TESTS FOR PRESENCE OF EXTRANEOUS MATTER IN FOOD AND DRUGS

Although the examination of materials for the presence of extraneous animal matter and insects has mainly been limited to food, an extension to drugs should be considered; however, the stringent standards adopted for food should not be necessary. The micro-analytical test applied is commonly known as the 'Filth Test'; the technique used varies with the nature of the material.

There can be many types of extraneous matter but in general the micro-analytical test is mainly directed to the determination of rodent hairs, and of insect, mould and other fragments. If rodent hairs are found there is likely to be contamination with excreta since rodent fæces always contain a mass of rodent hair. There is a limit to the implications of the test, but while there is no direct evidence of harm to health from the presence of fæcal matter, such contamination is most undesirable.

The technique of the micro-analytical procedure is dealt with at length in the U.S. Food and Drug Technical Bulletin No. 1[1] and the *A.O.A.C.*,[2] but a method suitable for cereals and adaptable to other farinaceous products has been fully described by Kent-Jones, Amos, Elias, Bradshaw and Thackray.[3] This procedure retains rodent hair, insect fragments and even mould fragments without losing their distinctive microscopic features. For the extraction and collection of extraneous matter the following procedure is recommended:

Weigh 25 g of the material, de-fat if necessary, and transfer to a 400-ml beaker. Boil 100 ml of 0·5N hydrochloric acid in a separate beaker, add the boiling acid quickly to the material and stir into a paste thoroughly for thirty seconds before placing the 400-ml beaker over a small flame. Avoid the presence of unwetted material on the bottom of the beaker; any suitable procedure to effect this will suffice. If the paste seems too thick, dilute somewhat with hot water. Boil the mixture for ten minutes, cool and dilute with about 100 ml of water. Add about 9·5 ml of 5N sodium hydroxide, stirring to avoid local concentration; add 2·5 ml of saturated trisodium phosphate solution and adjust the pH to 7·0 by adding a few drops of acid or alkali as necessary using phenol red (0·2 per cent aqueous solution) as external indicator. When the temperature falls below 40°, add 1 g of pancreatin, which should be free from any contamination, suspended in 20 ml of water. Dilute to about 350 ml, mix thoroughly and incubate at about 37° overnight.

Pour the digest into a special separator of about 600-ml capacity prepared by cutting off the tap and replacing it by a wide rubber tube with screw clip. Add 25 ml of petrol; shake gently to distribute the petrol throughout the solution. Allow to separate for twenty to thirty minutes. Run off the bulk of the digest into the original beaker, but leave sufficient to form a small layer under the interface. Keep the removed digest for a second separation. Add to the layers in the separator about 400 ml of distilled water, mix gently by swirling and allow to separate. Draw off and reject the washings and add a further quantity of water. Mix, allow to separate, and draw off most of this second washing. Run the liquids remaining in the separator through ruled filter paper on a Büchner funnel; the paper should rest upon a light layer of kieselguhr to avoid the debris congregating over the holes and the paper should be large enough to extend some distance up the sides of the funnel. Replace the original digest in the separator and extract again with petrol as before. Remove the bulk of the digest and then wash the petrol and the small volume of digest underlying the interfacial layer twice with water as previously described. Reject the washings and collect as before. Wash down thoroughly the inner surface of the separator and of the rubber outlet tube with ethanol from a wash bottle and finally with water. In view of the firmness with which hairs tend to adhere to the glass, the addition of a few drops of a wetting agent, such as Teepol, to this final water wash is advised. Collect any extraneous matter in these washes; serious errors can arise through not properly washing out the glassware.

The rubber exit tube should be renewed fairly frequently, as otherwise minute cracks may develop on the inner surface and retain hairs.

The general methods of procedure of preparation for cereals are not satisfactory for spices. A suitable procedure is described in the *A.O.A.C.*[4]

Weigh 10 g of sample into a 250-ml beaker. Add 150 ml of light petroleum and boil gently for fifteen minutes on a hot-plate, adding light petroleum occasionally to keep the volume constant. Decant the light petroleum on to a smooth 7-cm filter paper on a Büchner funnel. Add 150 ml of chloroform to the beaker and allow to stand with occasional stirring for thirty minutes. Decant the spice and chloroform on to the funnel, leaving the heavy residue of sand and soil, if any, in the beaker. If appreciable spice tissue remains in the bottom of the beaker, add successive portions of chloroform mixed with carbon tetrachloride to give increasingly higher specific gravity until practically all spice tissue is floated off.

Transfer the residue from the beaker to an ashless filter and examine for filth. If there is appreciable quantity of residue, place filter paper in a tared crucible, ignite, and determine sand and soil. Dry the spice in the Büchner funnel thoroughly, scrape the fine material from the paper and transfer to a 1-litre Wildman trap flask. Add about 150 ml of water, heat to boiling and simmer for fifteen minutes with stirring; wash down the inside of the flask with water and cool to below 20°. Add 25 ml of petrol, mix thoroughly and allow to stand for five minutes, then fill the flask with water and allow to stand for thirty minutes. Stir every five minutes, trap off and filter. Add to the flask about 15 ml of petrol and mix well; trap off and filter again after fifteen minutes. If the second extraction yields an appreciable quantity of filth decant most of the liquid from the flask, add 15 ml of petrol and make a third extraction.

The collected extraneous matter can be examined microscopically in the following ways and the appearance of the dirt is influenced by the means employed.

(1) Viewed by reflected light from the filter paper. This procedure is sound, but the counting is often tedious, examination of each filter paper often taking two or three hours.

(2) Viewed by transmitted light either through the filter paper oiled with castor oil, for example, to make it translucent, or through a ruled glass surface direct. The filter paper is allowed to dry naturally and then treated with just as much oil as it will absorb. Castor oil diluted with 25 per cent of ethanol is a convenient medium, but paraffin is also satisfactory. The paper is placed between two glass plates, pressed and examined by transmitted light.

(3) As in (2) but throwing the magnified image on a suitable screen.

The separated and collected extraneous matter is examined microscopically and counted, normally at a magnification of 35 to 70. It is convenient to work at a magnification of about 50 (although 35 would suffice) and a field of view of about 3 mm. With an ordinary microscope this is obtained with a 1-inch objective and a $\times$ 8 eyepiece; some sort of mechanical stage is also desirable. Since the most important factor is the number of rodent hairs reported, only typical rodent hairs should be reported as such; photographs are given by Kent-Jones *et al.*[3]

Flotation methods are not very satisfactory for complete separation of insect fragments from drugs.

Melville[5] proposed a method for the isolation of beetle fragments from powdered vegetable drugs, dependent on solution of the vegetable matter; in this procedure rodent hairs would be destroyed.

> Boil about 5 g of the powdered drug in a flask with 100 ml of dilute nitric acid in water for about one minute with frequent shaking. Filter through a No. 3 sintered-glass filter using suction, and wash the residue with hot water. Return the residue to the flask and boil for about one minute with 100 ml of 2·5 per cent sodium hydroxide solution, filter through the original filter and wash the residue with hot water. Remove the excess of water by suction and the last traces by passing a few ml of glacial acetic acid through the filter. Transfer the residue as completely as possible to a flask of about 50-ml capacity, and wash the remaining fragments into it with 10 ml of acetic anhydride. Add a mixture of 10 ml of acetic anhydride and 2 ml of concentrated sulphuric acid, mix well and heat on a water-bath until the crude fibre has dissolved. Solution is usually complete after about ten to fifteen minutes, during which time the liquid becomes dark reddish-brown. Separate the residue by centrifugation, pour off the supernatant liquid, replace with glacial acetic acid and re-centrifuge.

After pouring off the glacial acetic acid, the residue of insect fragments may be mounted in any desired mountant for microscopical examination. Where infestation is heavy and the finest fragments are not required, the contents of the flask may be passed through the sintered-glass filter and the residue washed with glacial acetic acid followed by water. The larger fragments can then be removed by adding a few drops of water or mounting fluid to the filter and gently brushing with a small stiff brush. Passage of air the reverse way through the filter by connecting the side-arm of the receiving flask to a water tap facilitates the removal. If the drug contains much oil or fat it is preferable to remove most of it by maceration for a short time with one or two changes of light petroleum or similar solvent before preparing the crude fibre.

Identification of insect fragments is aided by the description and sketches in the paper by Melville[5] of the diagnostic microscopical characters of some of the more common beetle pests found in drugs.

The identification of fragments as being of insect origin is not sufficient evidence that the material was infested. Certain drugs, particularly herbs such as hyoscyamus, not infrequently contain small insects which were associated with the growing plant and were not removed during the preparation for the market. Large insects such as the cockroach may also occasionally find their way into drugs, and unless their identity was realised, the powdered material might be reported as highly infested.

1. *Food and Drug Technical Bulletin No.* 1.
2. *A.O.A.C.*, 1960, p. 619.
3. Kent-Jones, D. W., Amos, A. J., Elias, P. S., Bradshaw, R. C. A., and Thackray, G. B., *Analyst*, 1948, **73**, 128.
4. *A.O.A.C.*, 1960, p. 632.
5. Melville, C., *J. Pharm. Pharmacol.*, 1949, **1**, 649.

APPENDIX VII

MICROBIOLOGICAL ASSAYS OF ANTIBIOTICS (ANTIBACTERIAL AGENTS) AND OF VITAMINS (BACTERIAL GROWTH FACTORS)

Microbiological assays can be applied to any substance or preparation which will influence the growth of micro-organisms in a regular manner such that the effect can be measured. In this category fall the antibiotics and other antibacterial agents (especially those used as preservatives at only low concentrations), all of which inhibit the growth of bacteria, and the water-soluble vitamins of the B group together with a wide range of amino acids, each of which is an essential growth factor to different bacteria or fungi, particularly those of the *Lactobacillus* genus.

The method of assessing the effect of these agents is *either* by the plate-diffusion technique, in which measured amounts of the agent, introduced into cups cut into agar plates inoculated with a test organism, diffuse into the agar to produce zones of inhibition or stimulation of growth, *or* by the tube-dilution method in which graded dilutions of the agent introduced into suitable nutrient media suppress or stimulate in a quantitative manner the growth of a test organism which can be measured turbidimetrically, gravimetrically or acidimetrically. Both of these assays are essential comparative ones in which the potency of the sample is assessed in terms of a standard of known potency. Standards for the antibiotics each with a given potency expressed in microgrammes or units per milligramme are obtainable from the National Institute for Medical Research, Mill Hill, London. These standards, being of either British or International designation, are only available in small quantities and so for regular use a laboratory working standard based on the primary standard should be set up. These standards must be carefully preserved and the working standards should be checked at intervals with the official standards to ensure that they maintain their potencies. For the vitamins similar reference standards are available in the United States but not, apart from riboflavine, in Great Britain; here, therefore, a standard of known and agreed chemical purity must be used.

In practice, both the plate-diffusion and the turbidimetric tube-dilution methods are used for antibiotic assays but for vitamin assays the tube-dilution method is preferred. The recommended methods for the antibiotics and vitamins, together with the suggested media, organisms, etc., are given in Tables 64 to 66.

Experience is essential before reliable results can be expected from any of the methods described.

APPENDIX VII

Maintenance of test organisms. The organisms used in microbiological assays, with few exceptions, are best stored in the freeze-dried state. For current use they are kept on nutrient agar slopes or, with the lactobacilli, as stab cultures, starting from a fresh freeze-dried tube occasionally. Keep such cultures at 4° and subculture them at weekly intervals. For use in the assay, prepare the inoculum as given in Tables 64 and 65.

Plate-diffusion method. Rectangular trays with a usable area of about 10 in. by 10 in. and fitted with light-weight lids, or 3½-in. petri-dishes, are suitable; they must be flat-bottomed inside, and washed thoroughly, sterilised and dried between each assay. Large trays are preferred because they are more economical, three samples being simultaneously assayed with only one set of dilutions of standard. Immediately before use, warm each tray (to avoid too rapid setting of the agar medium) and level it on a tripod device; alternatively, assemble the petri-dishes on a levelled surface. Pour into each an amount of the appropriate agar assay medium previously melted in flowing steam, cooled to 45° to 50° and inoculated with a suspension of the chosen assay organism (see Table 64) such that the depth of the medium is about 0·1 in. (this requires about 200 ml of medium in the large trays and 12·5 ml in each petri-dish). Allow the plates to stand for about half an hour before placing the lids in position and then transfer them to the refrigerator. When required for use, cut out cups in the agar by means of a sterile No. 5 cork borer (thus giving cups about 7 mm diameter) and remove each disc of agar with a 'spear' so that the surrounding agar is not lifted. For the large trays 8 rows of 8 cups or 12 rows of 12 cups are required, and for the petri-dishes 4 cups per plate.

Weigh accurately about 20 mg of the standard antibiotic (or other antibacterial) preparation and dissolve in a measured amount of solvent (see Table 64). Dilute further with the appropriate buffer solution to the required concentration per ml to give the desired 'high' and 'low' standard dilutions. Prepare a solution of the sample to be assayed and dilute this also with the same buffer solution to give approximately the same final concentration of the 'high' and 'low' test dilutions as of the standard. In all cases, the differences between the 'high' and 'low' dilutions of the standard and of the test material must be the same, the 'high' dilution being normally 4 or 5 times that of the 'low' one.

By means of a constant-delivery dropping-pipette fill a constant amount (between 0·05 and 0·1 ml) of each dilution of the standard and test samples into each of 8 cups cut in a large plate, using a predetermined Latin square design, or into one cup in each of 16 petri-dishes, and allow to stand at laboratory temperature for about one hour. Incubate for sixteen to twenty hours at a specified temperature (usually 32° to 37°) and then read the zones of inhibition as accurately as possible by means of a projection magnification optical device or with vernier calipers.

Sum the diameters of the zones for each dilution on each large plate or group of 16 petri-dishes and from this check the parallelism of the slope of the standard responses with that of the test sample responses. Then calculate the result either graphically or by formula:

(*a*) *By graph.* Plot a graph of zone diameters against log potency using the sums of the observations for the 'high' and 'low' dilutions of standard and test sample. By interpolation on the standard slope read the potency of the test material.

(*b*) *By formula.* The calculation is:

$$P = \text{antilog}\,(D/B \times I) \times F \times H$$

P = potency of sample
$D = (T_1 + T_2) - (S_1 + S_2)$
$B = (T_1 - T_2) + (S_1 - S_2)$
(T_1 and T_2 = sum of 'high' and 'low' responses with test sample
S_1 and S_2 = sum of 'high' and 'low' responses with standard)
I = log ratio of dilutions used
F = dilution factor of 'high' test sample
H = potency of 'high' standard

Tube-dilution method (*for antibiotics*). All of the manipulations up to the incubation stage must be carried out aseptically using sterilised apparatus, buffer solutions, etc.

Rimless test-tubes ¾ in. in diameter and about 6 in. long are used. They must be cleaned thoroughly each time they are used to remove trace residues which might interfere in subsequent assays. All detergents are not suitable and either one of the non-ionic preparations or a chromic acid-sulphuric acid mixture should be used. After cleaning, rinse the tubes in at least two changes of distilled water, then cover with metal caps or plug with cotton wool and sterilise in the autoclave at 115° (10 lb per sq. in. steam pressure) for twenty minutes.

Weigh accurately about 20 mg of the standard antibiotic and dissolve aseptically in a measured amount of solvent (see Table 64). Dilute further with sterile buffer solution and from this prepare *seven* graded dilutions to cover the required range of potency. Add 1 ml of each dilution to each of 4 sterile tubes. From a solution of the test sample (see monograph under each antibiotic as required) prepare *three* similar graded dilutions also within the required range of potency and add 1 ml to each of 4 sterile tubes. Then add to each tube 9 ml of the assay broth previously inoculated with the appropriate test organism. The appropriate amount of culture to be added to the assay medium is given in Table 64 but this must be checked to ensure that it gives a satisfactory dose-response slope. Incubate all of the tubes together at 37° for two to four hours in a water-bath fitted with a stirrer to minimise any variation in temperature.

Remove the tubes from the water-bath and measure the relative light transmittance of each tube nephelometrically in a photoelectric absorptiometer and calculate the mean reading for each dilution level of standard and test solution. Prepare a standard curve by plotting log concentration of standard against mean galvanometer reading and from this read off the concentration (or amount) of active material at the various levels of the test sample by interpolation on the standard curve; do *not* extrapolate. From the mean of the three amounts so found, calculate the potency of the test sample. (*Note.* The responses from the dilutions of the test sample should run parallel to those of the standard. If they show any significant 'drift' towards higher or lower values as the dilution increases, the assay is invalid.)

Tube dilution method (*for vitamins*). Rimless test-tubes ¾ in. in diameter and about 6 in. long are used. They must be cleaned thoroughly each time they are used to remove residual traces of vitamins, etc., which might interfere in subsequent assays. All detergents are not suitable and

APPENDIX VII

TABLE

DETAILS OF ORGANISMS USED AND OTHER CONDITIONS

ANTIBIOTIC	TEST ORGANISM[1]	MEDIUM[2] AND pH FOR STOCK CULTURE	MEDIUM[2] AND TYPE OF INOCULUM
Bacitracin	*Micrococcus flavus* (NCIB 8166)	B 6·5	B: suspension from 24 hr slope
Benzathine penicillin	see Benzylpenicillin		
Benzylpenicillin	*Bacillus subtilis* (NCTC 8236)	B 6·5	C: spore suspension
Chloramphenicol	*Sarcina lutea* (NCIB 8553)	B 6·5	B: suspension from 24 hr slope
Chlortetracycline	*Bacillus cereus* (NCIB 9231)	G 6·5	G: spore suspension
Demethylchlortetracycline	*Bacillus cereus* (NCIB 9231)	G 6·5	G: spore suspension
Dihydrostreptomycin	*Bacillus subtilis* (NCTC 8236)	B 6·5	C: spore suspension
Erythromycin	*Bacillus pumilus* (NCTC 8241)	B 6·5	C: spore suspension
Neomycin	*Bacillus pumilus* (NCTC 8241)	B 6·5	C: spore suspension
	Staphylococcus aureus (ATCC 6538P)	B 6·5	B: suspension from 24 hr slope
	Klebsiella pneumoniæ (ATCC 10031)	A 6·5	A: suspension from 6 hr slope
Novobiocin	*Sarcina lutea* (NCIB 8553)	B 6·5	B: suspension from 24 hr slope
	Bacillus subtilis (NCIB 8993)	B 6·5	C: spore suspension
	Staphylococcus albus (ATCC 12228)	B 6·5	B: suspension from 24 hr slope
Nystatin	*Saccharomyces cerevisiæ* (NCYC 87)	H 5·8	H: 24 hr broth culture
Oxytetracycline	*Bacillus cereus* (NCIB 9231)	G 6·5	G: spore suspension
Phenoxymethylpenicillin	*Bacillus subtilis* (NCTC 8236)	B 6·5	C: spore suspension
Polymyxin	*Brucella bronchiseptica* (NCTC 8344)	E 7·3	E: suspension from 24 hr slope
Streptomycin	*Bacillus subtilis* (NCTC 8236)	B 6·5	C: spore suspension
Tetracycline	*Bacillus cereus* (NCIB 9231)	G 6·5	G: spore suspension
Tyrothrycin	*Streptococcus fæcalis* (NCIB 8025)	B 7·0	F: 24 hr broth culture
Vancomycin	*Bacillus subtilis* (NCTC 8236)	B 6·5	C: spore suspension
Viomycin	*Bacillus subtilis* (NCTC 8236)	B 7·0	C: spore suspension

[1] NCIB = National Collection of Industrial Bacteria, Torry Research Station, Aberdeen, Scotland.
NCTC = National Collection of Type Cultures, Central Public Health Laboratory, Colindale Avenue, London, N.W.9.
ATCC = American Type Culture Collection, 2112 M-Street N.W., Washington D.C.7, U.S.A.
NCYC = National Collection of Yeast Cultures, Brewing Industry Research Foundation, Nutfield, Surrey.

64

FOR THE MICROBIOLOGICAL ASSAY OF ANTIBIOTICS

APPROX. VOLUME AND OPACITY (BROWN'S TUBE NO.) OF INOCULUM PER 100 ML ASSAY MEDIUM	ASSAY[2] MEDIUM AND pH	METHOD[3] OF ASSAY	BUFFER[4] SOLUTION AND pH	SOLVENT FOR PURE SOLID	POTENCY RANGE OF ASSAY	INCUBATION TEMPERATURE
1 ml No. 9	B 6·5	Plate	I 6·5	Buffer pH 6·5	0·5–0·1 unit/ml	32–35°
1 ml No. 5	A 7·0	Plate	I 7·0	Buffer pH 7·0	5·0–1·0 units/ml	35–37°
1 ml No. 9	B 6·5	Plate	II 6·0	Ethanol 1% of final volume at 1,000 µg/ml in buffer pH 6	80–20 µg/ml	30°
1 ml No. 2	D 6·5	Plate	IV 4·5	Buffer pH 4·5	0·5–0·1 µg/ml	30°
1 ml No. 2	D 6·5	Plate	II 6·0	Buffer pH 6·0	2·5–0·25 units/ml	30°
1 ml No. 5	A 8·0	Plate	II 8·0	Buffer pH 8·0	20–4 units/ml	35–37°
1 ml No. 2	A 8·0	Plate	II 8·0	Methyl alcohol approx. 1% of final volume at 100 µg/ml in buffer pH 8	10–2 µg/ml	35–37°
1 ml No. 4	A 8·0	Plate	II 8·0	Buffer pH 8·0	10–2 µg/ml	35–37°
1 ml No. 8	A 8·0	Plate	II 8·0	Buffer pH 8·0	10–2 µg/ml	35–37°
1 ml No. 4	F 7·0	Tube	II 8·0	Buffer pH 8·0	9–3 µg/tube	35–37°
1 ml No. 9	B 6·5	Plate	II 6·0	Absolute ethanol 25% of final volume at 1,000 µg/ml in buffer pH 6	10–2 µg/ml	30°
1 ml No. 4	A 6·5	Plate	II 6·0		10–2 µg/ml	35–37°
1 ml No. 9	A 6·5	Plate	II 6·0		5–1 µg/ml	35–37°
1 ml No. 8	J 5·0	Plate	I 6·0	Dimethyl formamide 10% of final volume at 800 units/ml in buffer pH 6·0	40–10 units/ml	35–37°
1 ml No. 2	D 6·5	Plate	III 4·5	Buffer pH 4·5	2·5–0·5 µg/ml	30°
1 ml No. 5	A 7·0	Plate	I 7·0	Buffer pH 7·0	2·5–0·5 µg/ml	35–37°
1 ml No. 5	E 7·3	Plate	I 6·0	Buffer pH 6·0	200–20 units/ml	35–37°
1 ml No. 5	A 8·0	Plate	II 8·0	Buffer pH 8·0	20–4 units/ml	35–37°
1 ml No. 2	D 6·5	Plate	IV 4·5	Buffer pH 4·5	2·5–0·5 µg/ml	30°
1 ml No. 3	F 7·0	Tube	I 7·0	Absolute ethanol 1·0 µg/ml	0·05–0·01 µg/tube	35–37°
1 ml No. 5	A 8·0	Plate	II 8·0	Buffer pH 8·0	200–20 µg/ml	35–37°
1 ml No. 5	A 8·0	Plate	II 8·0	Buffer pH 8·0	200–50 µg/ml	35–37°

[2] For types of media, A, B, C, etc., see page 818.
[3] Plate = plate-diffusion.
Tube = tube dilution.
[4] For types of buffer, I, II, III, IV, see page 819.

either one of the non-ionic preparations or a chromic acid-sulphuric acid mixture should be used. After cleaning, rinse in at least two changes of distilled water.

Dilute the stock solution of the vitamin with water to an appropriate level (see Table 65) and from this add to each of 4 tubes *seven* graded amounts to cover the range specified in the Table. From a prepared solution of the test sample (see under each vitamin as required) add *four* graded amounts also within the same range to each of 4 tubes. Make the volume in each tube up to 5 ml with water, add 5 ml of the appropriate assay medium, cover each tube with a metal cap and sterilise as specified.

After growing the test organism as specified, centrifuge and wash the culture three times with sterile saline and finally suspend in sufficient saline to give a faint turbidity. Add one drop of this suspension to each of the tubes above and incubate them together at the appropriate temperature for the required time and measure the response either nephelometrically or titrimetrically.

(*a*) *Nephelometrically.* After incubating the tubes for seventeen to twenty-four hours measure the relative light transmittance of each tube in a photoelectric absorptiometer and calculate the mean reading from each dilution level of standard and test solution. Prepare a standard curve by plotting log concentration of standard against mean galvanometer reading and from this read off the concentration (or amount) of active material at the various levels of the test sample by interpolation on the standard curve; do *not* extrapolate. From the mean of the amounts so found calculate the vitamin content of the test sample. (*Note.* The responses from the dilutions of the test sample should run parallel to those of the standard. If they show any significant 'drift' towards higher or lower values as the dilution increases, the assay is invalid.)

(*b*) *Titrimetrically.* After incubating the tubes for seventy-two hours add to each 0·4 ml of a 0·04 per cent solution of bromothymol blue and titrate the acid produced with 0·1N NaOH which also contains an equivalent amount of bromothymol blue. Calculate the mean of the volume of NaOH solution required for each dilution of standard and test sample. Prepare a standard curve by plotting log concentration of standard vitamin against log volume of alkali used and from this determine the vitamin content of the test sample by the method described in (*a*) above.

Culture Media and Buffer Solutions for Antibiotic Assays

A.	Peptone	0·5 g
	Lab Lemco	0·3 g
	Agar (New Zealand)	1·5 g
	Water to	100 ml
B.	Peptone	0·6 g
	Pancreatic digest of casein	0·4 g
	Yeast extract	0·3 g
	Beef extract	0·15 g
	Dextrose	0·1 g
	Agar (New Zealand)	1·5 g
	Water to	100 ml

C. As B with the addition of 0·0001 per cent $MnSO_4$

D. Yeast extract	0·1 g
Ammonium nitrate	0·5 g
Sodium acid phosphate	0·5 g
Glucose	0·5 g
Agar (New Zealand)	1·5 g
Water to	100 ml

E. Pancreatic digest of casein	1·7 g
Papain digest of soya bean	0·3 g
Sodium chloride	0·5 g
Dipotassium hydrogen phosphate	0·25 g
Dextrose	0·25 g
Polysorbitanmono-oleate	1·0 g
Agar (New Zealand)	1·5 g
Water to	100 ml

F. Peptone	0·5 g
Yeast extract	0·15 g
Beef extract	0·15 g
Sodium chloride	0·35 g
Glucose	0·1 g
Dipotassium hydrogen phosphate	0·368 g
Potassium dihydrogen phosphate	0·132 g
Water to	100 ml

G. Difco Protone	0·5 g
Manganese sulphate	0·0001 g
Agar (New Zealand)	1·5 g
Water to	100 ml

H. (Broth and Agar)	
Tryptone	0·5 g
Malt extract	0·3 g
Yeast extract	0·3 g
Dextrose	1·0 g
(Agar, New Zealand)	(1·5 g)
Water to	100 ml

J. Beef extract	0·25 g
Yeast extract	0·5 g
Peptone	1·0 g
Dextrose	1·0 g
Sodium chloride	1·0 g
Agar (New Zealand)	2·0 g
Water to	100 ml

I 0·05M Phosphate Buffer Solution adjusted to required pH value with 2N NaOH

II 0·1M Phosphate Buffer Solution adjusted to required pH value with 2N. NaOH

III Potassium dihydrogen phosphate	13·6 g
Water to	1,000 ml

Table 65

Details of Organisms Used and Other Conditions for the Microbiological Assay of Vitamins

		Aneurine	Riboflavine	Pyridoxine	Nicotinic Acid	Pantothenic Acid	Vitamin B_{12}	Vitamin B_{12}
Culture	Type and number	*Lactobacillus fermentum* 36 (NCIB 6991) (ATCC 9833)	*Lactobacillus casei* (NCIB 8010) (ATCC 7469)	*Saccharomyces carlsbergensis* (NCYC 74) (ATCC 9080)	*Lactobacillus arabinosus* 17/5 (NCIB 8014) (ATCC 8014)	*Lactobacillus arabinosus* 17/5 (NCIB 8014) (ATCC 8014)	*Lactobacillus leichmannii* (NCIB 7854) (ATCC 4797)	*Ochromonas malhamensis* (Pringsheim strain)
	Stock culture maintained on	Liver tryptone agar stab	Liver tryptone agar stab	Malt agar slope	Liver tryptone agar stab	Yeast agar stab	Stab culture: Single strength basal medium +1·5% agar and 2mμg Vit. B_{12} per ml	Single strength basal medium +1·0 mμg Vit. B_{12} per 10 ml broth
	Inoculum grown in	Single strength basal medium +1·0 μg Aneurine per 10 ml broth	Single strength basal medium +1·0 μg Riboflavine per 10 ml broth	Malt agar slope	Single strength basal medium 1·0 μg Nicotinic Acid per 10 ml broth	Single strength basal medium +0·5 μg Pantothenic Acid per 10 ml broth	Single strength basal medium +2mμg Vit. B_{12} per 10 ml broth	Single strength basal medium +1·0 mμg Vit. B_{12} per 10 ml broth
	Temperature of incubation	37°	37°	28–30°	37°	30°	37°	27–30° (1 ft below a 60 watt tungsten bulb)
	Age of inoculum (hours) (subcultured from stock culture)	15–17	18–24	18–24	18–24	18–24 (subcultured from 1st generation 24 hour broth culture)	18–24	4–5 days

Assay conditions	pH of medium	6·5	6·8	5·0–5·2	6·8	6·8	5·5	5·5
	Concentration of standard (μg/ml) for making final dilutions	0·02	0·1	0·02	0·1	0·02	0·2 (mμg)	0·2 (mμg)
	Range of levels of response (μg/tube)	0·005–0·1	0·05–2·5	0·005–0·1	0·05–2·5	0·005–0·1	0·05–1·0 (mμg)	0·1–1·0 (mμg)
	Conditions of sterilisation	Autoclave 115°/10 min.	Autoclave 115°/10 min.	100°/30 min. in flowing steam	Autoclave 115°/10 min.	Autoclave 115°/10 min.	Autoclave 115°/10 min.	Autoclave 115°/10 min.
	Temperature of incubation	37°	37°	28–30° on shaker	37°	30°	37°	27–30° on shaker
	Light sensitivity		Yes	Yes			Yes	Yes
	Measurement of response *	N only	(a) N (b) T	N only	(a) N (b) T	(a) N (b) T	(a) N (b) T	N only
	Time of incubation (hours)	17–18	(a) 18–24 (b) 72	18–24	(a) 18–24 (b) 72	(a) 18–24 (b) 72	(a) 18–24 (b) 72	72–96
Reference		'The Microbiological Assay of the Vitamin B Complex and Amino Acids' (E. C. Barton-Wright: Pitman, London: 1952)	*Analyst*, 1946, **71,** 397	*Ind.Eng.Chem., Anal. Edn.*, 1943, **15,** 141	*Analyst*, 1946, **71,** 460	*J. Biol. Chem.*, 1944, **156,** 21	*J. Biol. Chem.*, 1950, **184,** 211	*Analyst*, 1956, **81,** 132

* N = nephelometrically
T = titrimetrically

Table 66

Culture Media for the Microbiological Assay of Vitamins

	Aneurine	Riboflavine	Pyridoxine	Nicotinic Acid	Pantothenic Acid	Vitamin B_{12} (*L. leichmannii*)	Vitamin B_{12} (*Ochromonas*)
Acid-hydrolysed casein (vitamin free) (g)	5		10	20	4	10	5
Enzyme-hydrolysed casein (ml)		400					
Alkali-treated peptone solution (ml)	400				200		
Glucose (g)	40	40		40	40	40	10
Xylose (g)				2	2		
Sodium acetate (trihydrate) (g)	20	66		66	44	20	
Sodium chloride (g)	10	10		10	10		
Ammonium sulphate (g)				6	6		
Di-ammonium hydrogen citrate (g)							0·8
Potassium dihydrogen phosphate (g)							0·3
Magnesium sulphate (g)							0·2
Calcium chloride (anhydrous) (g)							0·15
**l*-Cystine (mg)	200	200		400	400	200	100
**dl*-Tryptophane (mg)				200	200	200	100
*Adenine (mg)	20	20		20	20	10	
*Guanine (mg)	20	20		20	20	10	
*Uracil (mg)	20	20		20	20	10	
*Xanthine (mg)				20	20	10	
*Calcium *d*-pantothenate (μg)	200	1,000	5,000	200		2,000	
*Nicotinic acid (μg)	200	1,000	15,000		800	2,000	
*Pyridoxine hydrochloride (μg)	200	2,000		200	200	4,000	
*Pyridoxal (μg)						4,000	

*p-Aminobenzoic acid (μg)	200	200		200	200	1,000	1,000
*Folic acid (μg)	0·5	0·4				1,000	
*Aneurine hydrochloride (μg)		1,000	125	200	200	2,000	2,000
*Biotin (μg)	0·8	0·8	20	3·2	0·8	10	10
**l*-Glutamic acid (μg)		4					
*Asparagine (μg)		4					
Inositol (mg)			50				10
*Riboflavine (μg)	200			400	400	2,000	
dl-Methionine (mg)				50			200
l-Leucine (mg)				20			
Choline hydrochloride (mg)							2
*'Salts A' solution (ml)	10	50		10	10	10	
*'Salts B' solution (ml)	10	10		10	10	10	
*Sugar salts solution (ml)			250				
*Potassium citrate buffer solution (ml)			50				
*'Metals' solution (ml)							10
Thiomalic acid (recrystallised) (g)							
Sodium cyanide solution (ml)							0·2
Tween 80 (TB culture grade) (ml)						1	1
Sodium molybdate (g)							0·05
*Vitamins solution (ml)							2
pH	6·5	6·8	5·0–5·2	6·8	6·8	5·5	5·5
Water to (ml)	1,000	1,000	1,000	1,000	1,000	1,000	200

* Stock solutions (see text below).
The amounts given are for double strength media, except with Vitamin B_{12} (*Ochromonas*) which is five times the final strength.

APPENDIX VII

Media for Maintenance of Stock Cultures for Vitamin Assays

Malt agar

Malt extract	4 g
Yeast extract	1 g
Glucose	0·5 g
Peptone	1 g
Agar (New Zealand)	1 g
Water to	100 ml
Final pH about	5·4

Liver tryptone agar

Tryptone	1 g
Glucose	1 g
Liver extract	1 g
l-Cystine	40 mg
Dipotassium hydrogen phosphate	0·2 g
Calcium chloride	0·3 g
Salts A solution	0·5 ml
Salts B solution	0·5 ml
Agar (New Zealand)	1 g
Water to	100 ml
Final pH about	6·8

Yeast agar

Yeast extract	1 g
Glucose	1 g
Salts A solution	0·5 ml
Salts B solution	0·5 ml
Agar (New Zealand)	1 g
Water to	100 ml
Final pH about	6·8

Dissolve with the aid of flowing steam and adjust so that after distributing in 5 or 6 × ½-in. tubes (about 15 ml per tube) and sterilising at 121° (15 lb per sq. in. steam pressure) for ten minutes the pH value is that stated.

Stock Solutions of Ingredients for Vitamin Assays

Enzyme-hydrolysed casein. Suspend 120 g of casein in 2 litres of a 0·8 per cent sodium bicarbonate solution, previously adjusted to pH 8·0. Add a suspension of 1·0 g of pancreatin and shake. Add a few drops of toluene and incubate for about fifty-six hours at 37°. Heat in flowing steam for thirty minutes, cool, adjust to pH 6·0 with glacial acetic acid (about 28 ml is usually required) and filter. A filter aid, such as supercel, may be used. Add 60 g of activated charcoal, stir for thirty minutes and filter. Adjust to pH 3·8 with hydrochloric acid, add 24 g of activated charcoal, stir for thirty minutes, and filter. Finally, adjust the volume to 2·4 litres with water.

Alkali-treated peptone. Dissolve 40 g of peptone in 250 ml of water and 20 g of sodium hydroxide in a further 250 ml of water, mix the two solutions and autoclave at 121° (15 lb steam pressure) for fifteen minutes. Allow to stand at room temperature for twenty-four hours, neutralise with glacial acetic acid (about 28 ml), add 11·6 g of sodium acetate and make up to a final volume of 800 ml.

'Salts A' solution. Potassium dihydrogen phosphate 10 per cent and dipotassium hydrogen phosphate 10 per cent in water.

'Salts B' solution. Magnesium sulphate 4 per cent, sodium chloride 0·2 per cent, ferrous sulphate 0·2 per cent and manganese sulphate 0·2 per cent in water.

Sugar salt solution. Potassium dihydrogen phosphate 0·4 per cent, potassium chloride 0·34 per cent, calcium chloride 0·1 per cent, magnesium sulphate 0·002 per cent, and glucose 40 per cent in water.

Metals solution. Manganese sulphate 0·6 per cent, zinc sulphate 1·1 per cent, ferrous sulphate 0·1 per cent, cobalt sulphate 0·03 per cent, copper sulphate 0·004 per cent, boric acid 0·006 per cent, potassium iodide 0·0001 per cent and EDTA 0·5 per cent. Prepare the solution by first dissolving the EDTA in hot water and then adding the remaining constituents.

Sodium cyanide solution. 1 per cent solution of sodium cyanide in water.

Potassium citrate buffer. Potassium citrate 20 per cent and citric acid 4 per cent in water. Dissolve with the aid of heat.

l-Cystine solution. Transfer 8 g of *l*-cystine to a beaker containing a small amount of boiling water, and add concentrated hydrochloric acid until the cystine is dissolved. Make up the volume to 500 ml with water so that the final solution contains 16 mg of *l*-cystine per ml.

dl-Tryptophane solution. Transfer 16 g of *dl*-tryptophane to a beaker containing a small amount of boiling water and add concentrated hydrochloric acid until the tryptophane is dissolved. Make up the volume to 500 ml with water so that the solution contains 32 mg of the racemate per ml.

Adenine, guanine and uracil solution. Transfer 0·2 g of adenine, 0·2 g of guanine and 0·2 g of uracil to a beaker containing a small amount of boiling water and add concentrated hydrochloric acid until they are dissolved. Make up the volume to 100 ml with water so that the solution contains 2 mg each of adenine, guanine and uracil per ml.

Xanthine solution. Transfer 0·2 g of xanthine to a beaker containing a small amount of water, and add sodium hydroxide (20 per cent solution) until the xanthine is dissolved. Make up the volume to 100 ml with water so that the solution contains 2 mg of xanthine per ml.

Calcium d-pantothenate solution. A solution in water containing 1,000 μg pantothenic acid per ml (108·7 μg calcium *d*-pantothenate ≡ 100 μg pantothenic acid).

Nicotinic acid. A solution in water containing 1,000 μg nicotinic acid per ml.

Riboflavine hydrochloride solution. A solution in 0·1 per cent glacial acetic acid solution containing 50 μg riboflavine per ml.

Pyridoxine hydrochloride solution. A solution in water containing 1,000 μg pyridoxine per ml (122 μg hydrochloride ≡ 100 μg free base).

Pyridoxal hydrochloride solution. A solution in water containing 1,000 μg pyridoxal hydrochloride per ml.

p-Aminobenzoic acid solution. A solution in water containing 1,000 μg of the acid per ml.

Folic acid solution. Dissolve 10 mg of folic acid in about 250 ml of water and make up to volume with 90 per cent ethanol so that the solution contains 20 μg of folic acid per ml.

Aneurine hydrochloride solution. A solution in water containing 1,000 μg aneurine hydrochloride per ml.

Biotin solution. Dissolve 2 mg of biotin in about 50 ml of water. Make up to volume with 90 per cent ethanol so that the solution contains 20 μg of biotin per ml.

Vitamins solution. Inositol 0·5 per cent, choline chloride 0·1 per cent, *p*-aminobenzoic acid 0·05 per cent, aneurine hydrochloride 0·1 per cent and biotin 0·0005 per cent in 20 per cent ethanol.

APPENDIX VIII

Tests for Sterility

Preparations of drugs administered by injection or applied under some surgical conditions must of necessity be free from contaminating micro-organisms. Therefore, besides the chemical and physical assays on such preparations, tests for sterility are also applied. These tests involve the examination of every lot or batch processed for the presence of aerobic and anaerobic bacteria, and often moulds.

To ensure the complete absence of contamination it would be necessary to culture the whole of a batch of material to destruction, but since this is impossible limited samples only, chosen at random, are examined. The various pharmacopœial and other authorities differ in their requirements concerning the numbers of samples to be examined and the amounts to be tested from each sample. On statistical grounds, a reasonable number of containers to examine is twenty from each batch, regardless, within limits, of the size of the batch; on this basis it is calculated[1,2] that there is a 90 per cent chance of passing a batch of material if one per cent of the containers are contaminated, a 60 per cent chance if five per cent are contaminated, and so on. If the number of samples examined is less than twenty then the stringency of the test falls away markedly; contrariwise, if the number is increased the sensitivity is not greatly enhanced. Because of this hazard in detecting contaminations, it is desirable to ensure that the conditions of treatment and handling of any product are such that they are likely to yield a sterile preparation rather than to rely too heavily on the sterility test result.

GENERAL METHOD

It is essential that all tests for sterility should be carried out under the most strictly aseptic conditions, in order to eliminate contamination from sources other than the actual material being tested. Otherwise, it is quite possible that a batch of material that is, in fact, satisfactory might be rejected because of the accidental introduction of a contaminating organism from the air, or from an operator, while the test is being made.

If possible, tests should be made in a small laboratory that contains a minimum of equipment and that can easily be cleaned down and disinfected. The amount of preparation, cleaning and disinfection necessary will depend to a large extent on the laboratory facilities available—whether there is a supply of sterile air, etc.—but whatever the conditions, operators must 'scrub up' and must disinfect their hands and forearms with a suitable antiseptic solution (one of the chloroxylenol preparations is recommended) before carrying out any tests: pre-sterilised rubber gloves must be worn. If, however, the hermetically sealed screen described by Royce and Sykes (p. 831) is used, many of the foregoing precautions can be dispensed with, but the use of this apparatus depends on a supply of ethylene oxide being available.

In order to check the reliability of the method employed, control tests with materials treated in such a way that they must be sterile should be made at frequent intervals, under the exact conditions of an actual sterility test.

Culture media. The basis of all sterility test media is a nutrient broth containing 1·0 per cent w/v peptone, 0·2 per cent meat extract (Lab-Lemco or other suitable brand), 0·2 per cent yeast extract (Yeastrel or other suitable brand), 0·25 per cent sodium chloride and 0·1 per cent glucose. Alternatively, a medium made from either the papaic or the tryptic digestion of lean meat (ox heart is preferred) may be used.

The usual aerobic medium is plain nutrient broth, adjusted so that it has a final pH value after sterilisation of 7·2–7·8. The anaerobic medium is the same nutrient broth with the addition of 0·5 per cent cystine, 0·05–0·07 per cent agar,* 0·05 per cent glucose, 0·05 per cent sodium thioglycollate and 0·1 per cent of a 1 in 1,000 aqueous solution of resazurin, and adjusted so that the final pH value after sterilisation is between 7·2 and 7·8. Both media may be filled in about 50-ml or 250-ml amounts into tubes plugged with cotton wool or into screw-capped bottles: if bottles are used, they should be of such a size that they are not more than two-thirds filled with the aerobic medium, but for the anaerobic medium they should be filled to the neck to minimise the access of oxygen. If the anaerobic medium shows a pink colour extending to more than about one inch below the surface it should be heated in flowing steam for twenty to thirty minutes, and subsequently cooled immediately prior to use.

The medium for testing for moulds is a plain nutrient broth containing 2 per cent of glucose, and adjusted so that the final pH value after sterilisation is 6·0–6·5. It is filled and treated as for the aerobic medium.

For subculturing aerobic bacteria a plain nutrient agar with a pH value of 7·2–7·8 is used, filled into 'slopes' in 5- or 6-in. tubes plugged with cotton wool: for anaerobic bacteria it is the same nutrient agar, but containing 1 per cent of glucose, and filled into 'stabs,' each 5 or 6 in. × ½-in. tube containing about 15 ml of the medium. The medium for subculturing moulds is the same as that for subculturing anaerobic bacteria, but adjusted to pH 6·0–6·5, and again filled into 'slopes.'

All these media should be sterilised in the autoclave at 115° (10 lb per sq. in. steam pressure) for thirty minutes. Each batch should be checked to see that it will support the growth of a *small* inoculum (less than a hundred viable cells) of suitable test organisms.

Sampling. For all filled products, samples must be taken at random after the whole batch has been filled. The following sampling is recommended:

* New Zealand agar—if agar of another source is used, a different concentration may be required.

No. of containers in batch	*No. of containers examined*
less than 200	4
200/1,000	2 per cent
1,000/20,000	20
20,000/40,000	40
more than 40,000	10 from each day's filling

In each case, if the volume in each container is less than 2 ml, additional samples are required for the test for moulds.

The interpretation of what constitutes a batch may differ, but it should be derived from one bulk batch and should comprise that number of containers which are filled without any substantial break in time or conditions. For preparations sterilised in their final containers, a batch should normally be derived from a single sterilisation treatment.

Amounts of sample tested. When the material is a liquid and the volume in each container is 3 ml or more, inoculate 1-ml portions from each container successively into 50 ml of the aerobic, anaerobic and mould media. Alternatively, aggregated samples of 5 ml comprising 1 ml from each of five containers (or, if more convenient, 4 ml from four containers, etc.) may be inoculated into 250-ml amounts of the three media.

When the volume in each container is less than 3 ml but not less than 2 ml, inoculate one-third portions of the contents from each container successively into 50 ml of the aerobic, anaerobic and mould media. In this case also, aggregated samples from four or five containers may be used as above, except that the amounts inoculated into the 250-ml quantities of the various media will necessarily be less—possibly considerably less—than the normal 5 ml.

When the volume in each container is less than 2 ml, inoculate half the volume in each container into 50 ml of the aerobic medium and the other half into 50 ml of the anaerobic medium (alternatively, aggregated samples, as above, may be used). Additional samples are required for the mould tests, for which 1 ml from each container is inoculated into respective 50-ml quantities of the mould medium.

It should be noted, throughout the above, that 1 ml or less is always inoculated into 50 ml of the aerobic, anaerobic or mould medium and more than 1 ml is always inoculated into 250 ml of the medium.

When the material is a solid, half the contents of each container is inoculated into 50 ml of the aerobic medium and the other half into 50 ml of the anaerobic medium, except that, if the amount of material in each container is more than 2 g, the amount taken for each type of test need not exceed 1 g. No test for moulds is made.

Solids are best handled by suspending or dissolving them in about 5 ml of aerobic medium (transferred by means of a syringe), then withdrawing the suspension or solution back into the syringe and inoculating an appropriate volume into the final test media.

Incubation. Incubate the tests for aerobic and anaerobic bacteria at 37° ± 0·5° for five days,* but this period may be extended to six or seven

* Because of the increasing evidence that surviving organisms appear to recover better in sub-optimal conditions there is a tendency nowadays to incubate at a lower temperature, *i.e.* 30° to 32°, for a longer time, *i.e.* seven days.

days if it is inconvenient to examine them on the fifth day: incubate the tests for moulds at 25° to 28° for seven days. The tests must be examined at regular intervals during this period. If at any time during the incubation period there is any suspicion of growth, the particular culture tube or bottle must be subcultured—for bacteria on to a nutrient agar slope or in a glucose-agar 'shake' tube and for moulds on to a glucose-agar slope—and incubated as required at 37° or at 25° to 28° for forty-eight hours. Should the growth be confirmed, the subculture, and the growth in the nutrient broth, must be retained for identification (see 'Identification of organisms,' below).

Some products react with the culture medium to give an opalescence or precipitate. In such cases growth cannot be observed with certainty and *all* culture tubes must be subcultured, as above, at the end of the normal incubation period.

Identification of organisms. Classification of organisms need not be too rigorous. For the purpose of interpretation of results (see below), bacteria are considered to be 'the same' if they are alike in all of the following particulars: (*a*) morphology, (*b*) colony appearance on nutrient agar, (*c*) cultural appearance in nutrient broth, (*d*) biochemical reaction with glucose, gelatin, starch and litmus milk. Moulds are considered to be 'the same' if they present a similar morphological appearance.

Interpretation of results. The material passes the test for sterility if there is no growth in any of the culture tubes or bottles at the end of the incubation period.

If growth occurs in any tube or bottle, the entire test with all media is repeated. If a growth is obtained the second time, and if this growth is found on examination to be 'the same' organism as in the first test (by the criteria laid down under 'Identification of organisms'), the material does not pass the test for sterility.

If no growth is obtained the second time, the material passes the test for sterility.

If a growth is obtained the second time but this is *not* the same organism as in the first test, then the whole test may be repeated a third time. If a growth is obtained the third time, whatever the organism, bacterium or mould, the material does not pass the test for sterility.

If no growth is obtained the third time, the material passes the test for sterility.

USE OF MEMBRANE FILTERS

Membrane filters,* of a suitable porosity to retain all bacteria, are now established tools for assessing small numbers of micro-organisms and as such they are particularly useful in sterility testing.[3,4] Their virtues are that they virtually eliminate any carry-over of bacteriostatic or other interfering substances which may delay the growth of organisms in the final test medium, and in this context they are of special value in testing streptomycin, neomycin and other antibiotic preparations; they also allow larger samples to be examined when desired without the necessity of using proportionally larger volumes of culture media. They can be used with all solutions, including oily ones, but obviously are unsuitable for suspen-

* Different makes are available in Great Britain, the United States and on the Continent.

sions. A high degree of asepsis is needed to avoid accidental contaminations, and for this reason the membrane filter technique is best carried out in the sealed screen (see below), but it can be handled satisfactorily with the usual sterile room procedure.

Membranes 5 cm in diameter are a convenient size for use in sterility testing. Assemble the membrane in a suitable holder (various types made on the Seitz filter principle are available) with a glass or metal cover-lid and sterilise either with steam in the autoclave or with ethylene oxide. Connect to a convenient receiver and filter the test sample through the membrane, solid samples having previously been dissolved in sterile water or saline. Filtration is rapid if a vacuum is applied. Wash the membrane through several times with water or saline and then remove it aseptically from its holder, cut it in two with the aid of sterile forceps and scissors and culture one part aerobically and the other anaerobically in the appropriate media.

If the membrane is pre-wetted with water or saline it prevents the subsequent seepage of the test solution to the edge of the membrane, which is difficult to wash, and so reduces further the carry-over of highly bacteriostatic substances such as the antibiotics.

THE SEALED-SCREEN METHOD

With every aseptic manipulation carried out under normal 'sterile' conditions there is always the inherent hazard of introducing extraneous contaminants from the atmosphere or from the operator and this can be largely eliminated by the use of the sealed screen with ethylene oxide as described by Royce and Sykes.[5] The screen consists basically of a sheet-metal box, sealed with a removable hatch and fitted with long-sleeved rubber gauntlets. The size is limited by the reach of the arms within the screen, with or without the aid of tongs, etc., and convenient dimensions are 2 ft 6 in. long by 2 ft deep by 1 ft 6 in. high. The screen is provided with two perspex windows, one in the top to admit light and one in the sloping front to enable the operator to see inside, and all joints must be gas-tight. At diagonally opposite corners of each end are fixed short metal tubes joined by rubber tubing to air filters (non-absorbent cotton wool packed into metal tubes about 1 ft long and 1½ in. diameter), the pair of tubes at one end being connected to one air filter and those at the other end to a second filter. The removable hatch is built in the back of the screen and is fixed in position by means of wing nuts and sealed with a sponge rubber gasket: a small tube with a tap is also sealed into the hatch to provide a vacuum lead.

Operation. Because the sterilising agent is a gas, it obviously must not gain access to the samples being tested or to any liquids in which it may dissolve and react; therefore, all samples and culture media must be in sealed containers—the latter in screw-capped bottles. All outer surfaces must also be clean and grease-free otherwise organisms might be protected from the action of the ethylene oxide.

To use the screen for sterility testing, load into it the necessary samples, culture media, syringes, measuring or weighing devices and all other essential equipment, together with a chilled, screw-capped bottle containing an amount of liquid ethylene oxide calculated to give a gaseous concentration in the screen of 12·5 per cent. Seal the hatch in position and immediately pour the liquid ethylene oxide over the floor of the screen, from which it will evaporate within a minute or two. Having allowed the slight excess of air pressure in the screen to escape through the filters, seal them off and allow the sterilisation process to continue for at least sixteen hours at normal temperature (an elevated temperature will accelerate the process). In the morning, flush the screen via the filters with air for about half an hour so that it removes virtually all of the ethylene oxide gas. The operator can then insert his hands and arms into the gauntlets and carry out the necessary transfers of samples to test media, etc., in a fixed, sterile atmosphere without any danger of contamination during the manipulation from the air or from his own hands and arms, unless he should happen to puncture the gloves.

Two points should be borne in mind: (i) because of the explosive nature of ethylene oxide in air, it should only be handled in a flame-free area, and the screens should be flushed with nitrogen or carbon dioxide before introducing the ethylene oxide and at the first stages of its subsequent removal; (ii) rubber absorbs a certain amount of ethylene oxide and this can cause reactions in sensitive skins. This can be obviated by hanging the gauntlets in free air for an hour after flushing the screen.[6]

1. KNUDSEN, L. F., *J. Amer. Pharm. Ass., Sci. Edn.*, 1949, **38,** 332.
2. DAVIES, O. L., and FISHBURN, A. G., *Pharm. J.*, 1948, **160,** 184.
3. HOLDOWSKY, S., *Antibiotics & Chemotherapy*, 1957, **7,** 49.
4. SYKES, G., and HOOPER, Margaret C., *J. Pharm. Pharmacol.*, 1959, **11,** 235T.
5. ROYCE, A., and SYKES, G., *J. Pharm. Pharmacol.*, 1955, **7,** 1046.
6. ROYCE, A., and MOORE, W. K. S., *Brit. J. Ind. Med.*, 1955, **12,** 167.

APPENDIX IX

Pyrogen Testing

Materials intended for intravenous use should be free from undue amounts of pyrogenic substances and this condition may be established by making intravenous injection of prescribed quantities into rabbits and noting the effect on the rectal temperature compared with a control level established for each animal.

Test procedures are described both in the *B.P.* and in the *U.S.P.* The conduct of these differs only in detail although there is some difference in the interpretations of the results obtained. The *B.P.* method will be described and any difference between this and that of the *U.S.P.* noted in parenthesis.

Healthy (mature) rabbits of either sex each weighing not less than 1,500 g with rectal temperatures not exceeding 39·8° (and those on one test within 1° of each other) are used for the test. They should not have been used in similar tests during the previous seventy-two hours (forty-eight hours) nor in the previous three weeks unless the material passed the test. No rabbit should be used if it has appeared in a test where the mean response exceeded 1·2° (two weeks following their having been given a test sample adjudged pyrogenic). One to three days before the test, if it has not been used during the preceding two weeks the rabbit should be submitted to the test procedure using 10 ml per kg body weight of a 0·9 per cent solution of pyrogen-free sodium chloride in water for injection, and animals which show an undue rise or fall in temperature should be excluded from pyrogen tests until they show no such abnormal response in a similar test (conduct a sham test omitting the injection).

The test is conducted in a quiet room which has a temperature within 3° of that of the rabbits' living quarters or in which the rabbits have been kept for eighteen hours prior to the test. (House individually in areas of uniform temperature ±3°.) Food is withheld from the rabbits overnight and water withheld for the duration of the test. (On day of test withhold all food during test but access to water may be allowed.)

The rectal temperatures are measured by means of a tested clinical thermometer or other suitable instrument of equal precision inserting to a depth uniform for each rabbit of 6 to 9 cm (7·5 cm). If the instrument is left in position for the duration of the test the rabbit may be restrained only with loosely fitting neck stocks so designed to allow the rabbit to sit normally. Temperatures are recorded at regular intervals at not more than thirty minutes commencing at least ninety minutes before the injection and continuing for three hours after the injection. The 'mean initial' temperature, the mean of the temperatures recorded in the forty minutes prior to injection, is determined for each rabbit and the difference between this and the maximum temperature reached is taken to be its response. (Take a control temperature within thirty minutes prior to the injection. Record temperatures at one, two and three hours.)

The material to be tested is injected intravenously. The quantity to be used is that stated in the monographs. The solution may be made isotonic with pyrogen-free sodium chloride. If the total volume exceeds 10 ml, it is warmed to 30° to 40° before injection.

Interpretation of Results

The *B.P.* interpretation relies on a sequential sampling plan using sums of responses and permits repetition until 12 rabbits have been used. The *B.P.* records the critical sums as from groups of 3 but in practice the appropriate values for intermediate numbers apply equally well. The *U.S.P.* prescribes that 3 rabbits be used and interprets the results by considering the number of individual rises in excess of 0·6° together with their sum. A repeat test of 5 rabbits is permitted and the whole assessed.

A comparison of the two interpretations is shown in the table.

TABLE 67

	B.P.		*U.S.P.*	
No. of Rabbits	Pass if sum of responses is less than	Fail if sum of responses exceeds	Pass	Fail
3	1·15	2·65	If no response exceeds 0·6 and sum is less than 1·4	If all responses exceed 0·6
6	2·80	4·30		
8	3·9	5·4	If no more than 3 responses exceed 0·6 and sum does not exceed 3·7	If 4 or more responses exceed 0·6 or sum exceeds 3·7
9	4·45	5·95		
12	6·60	6·60		

Discrimination of Two Tests

The *B.P.* test is based on a sequential plan which permits a 10 per cent chance of accepting material which would cause a rise of 0·78°.

Dare[1] examined the discrimination of the *U.S.P.* test using rabbits which had not been previously exposed to pyrogens and considered that such a test allowed only a 4·5 per cent chance of accepting material which would cause a rise of 0·74°.

For all practical purposes the tests of the *U.S.P.* and *B.P.* may be considered interchangeable.

1. DARE, J. G., *J. Pharm. Pharmacol.*, 1953, **5**, 898.

APPENDIX X

Interpretation of Analytical Results

The principles involved in interpretation of analytical data whether these be obtained from biological or chemical methods are essentially the same and differ only in the degree to which certain factors can be established on theoretical grounds. Thus the biological response resulting from a certain dose of drug will vary from laboratory to laboratory, or even from time to time in the same laboratory. It is necessary therefore that in biological assays the response obtained using a test preparation be compared with that obtained using a standard preparation. The change in response which is brought about by a change in dose is most likely to be unique to each laboratory and to vary with time and so must also be established by administering the standard or the test preparation or preferably both at the same time and at more than one dose level. The greater variability of biological responses also makes it necessary to employ statistical treatments of them so that the reliability of the results may be assessed. These treatments can and have been applied similarly to chemical results. To what extent such application is necessary is a matter of opinion but the analyst, even though he is dealing solely with chemical methods, should at least be conversant with the statistical treatment of results, if only to assess for himself the extent to which they are necessary.

The information may be required to indicate, on the basis of previous experience, within what range a single determination could be expected to fall or to indicate the reliability to be attached to a mean of several estimates, to the sum of two estimates, to the difference between them or to their ratio.

All such examinations call for the calculation of the variance (s^2) of a single observation, which is identical with the value described as the 'residual variance' or 'error variance.'

In its simplest concept the error variance may be derived from the repeated observations on a similar quantity of the same substance. Thus if the observed responses (or estimated potencies, etc.) are:

$$y_1 y_2 y_3 \ldots y_n \text{ with mean } \bar{y} = \Sigma y/n$$

then

$$\text{the error variance} = s^2 = \Sigma(y - \bar{y})^2/n - 1$$

which may, perhaps, be more easily calculated as

$$(\Sigma y^2 - (\Sigma y)^2/n)/n - 1$$

and is referred to as being established with $n - 1$ degrees of freedom (d.f.).

The normal methods of interpreting the results of biological assays assume that the estimate of s^2 from the difference dosage groups are homogeneous and methods exist to test this (Bartlett[1]). Homogeneous variances may be combined to give a weighted mean as:

$$\Sigma(\Sigma y - \bar{y})^2/\Sigma(n - 1)$$

The square root of the error variance is termed the standard deviation (s) and the results to be expected from a single determination should then fall in the range:

$$\bar{y} \pm ts$$

the value for t being taken from tables and depending on the d.f. with which s^2 was established and on the risk one wishes to take of being wrong. Thus if one does not wish to be wrong more often than 1 in 20 ($P = 0{\cdot}95$) t has the approximate value of 2.

The distribution of results to be obtained is characterised by the values $\bar{y}$ and s. In certain cases the variation experienced depends on the size of the measurement and for this reason it has been found convenient to record the standard deviation as a percentage of the mean, this expression being termed the coefficient of variation. The results of analytical procedures do not necessarily lend themselves to this treatment for it is not true that the measurement of twice the amount is accompanied by an error twice as large.

Since all the essential characteristics are defined by recording $\bar{y}$ and s the use of these symbols is to be preferred to that of the coefficient of variation which masks some of the information.

Some workers may find the coefficient of variation a convenient expression; here only its use in establishing the limits of error of a ratio will be considered (see variance of a ratio).

Experimental designs exist in which extraneous variables may be eliminated from the responses (such as the use of litter mates, cross-over designs, etc.). The error variance is derived from such designs by an analysis of variance which will be illustrated by reference to data obtained in the assay of heparin, in which, over the dosage range used, the logarithm of the coagulation time is linearly related to the log concentration of heparin.

The variance ratios in the last column are compared with those found by entering the variance ratio tables (Fisher and Yates[2]) with the appropriate d.f. and indicate that the doses have had a highly significant effect, but that there is little variation due to runs.

It will be seen that the error variance for such an assay removing only the effect due to doses is given by:

$$(\Sigma y^2 - \Sigma Y^2 \div \text{number of runs}) \div n - \text{number of runs}$$

which is identical with the simple concept given above for calculating a

TABLE 68

LOG COAGULATION TIME

	STD. 2 UNITS	STD. 1.6 UNITS	TEST 2 UNITS	TEST 1.6 UNITS	SUM = R
	1·03	0·81	1·16	0·81	3·81
	0·99	0·76	1·09	0·90	3·74
	0·93	0·76	1·12	0·91	3·72
	0·96	0·71	1·04	0·88	3·59
Sum = Y	3·91	3·04	4·41	3·50	14·86
Sum of Sq.	3·8275	2·3154	4·8697	3·0686	14·0812

Sum of Squares for doses
$= (3{\cdot}91^2 + \ldots 3{\cdot}50^2) \div 4(=$ number of runs$) = 14{\cdot}0569$
Sum of Squares for runs
$= (3{\cdot}81^2 + \ldots 3{\cdot}59^2) \div 4(=$ number of doses$) = 13{\cdot}8075$
Correction Term
$= (\Sigma y)^2 \div n(=$ number of observations$) = (14{\cdot}86)^2 \div 16 = 13{\cdot}8012$

TABLE 69

ANALYSIS OF VARIANCE

SOURCE	SUM OF SQUARES	CORRECTION TERM	REDUCED SUM OF SQUARES	D.F.	s^2	VARIANCE RATIO
Total	14·0812	13·8012	0·2800	15		
Doses	14·0569	13·8012	0·2557	3	0·0852	42·6
Runs	13·8075	13·8012	0·0063	3	0·0021	1·05
Residual = Total − (Doses + Runs)			0·0180	9	0·0020	

mean error variance. Although in this instance there is no significant effect due to runs the data can be used to illustrate how the calculation is made. The error variance obtained by removing variation due to both runs and doses is then:

$$s^2 = \left\{\left[\Sigma y^2 + \frac{(\Sigma y)^2}{n}\right] - (\Sigma Y^2 \div \text{number of runs} + \Sigma R^2 \div \text{number of doses})\right\} \div n + 1 - (\text{number of runs} + \text{number of doses})$$

Error variance from a twin cross-over test

The error variance from a twin cross-over test may be obtained by considering the difference in response to standard and test preparation for each animal as y and calculating for each cell the value

$$\Sigma(y - \bar{y})^2 \div n - 1 \text{ then } s^2 = \tfrac{1}{2}\Sigma(\Sigma y - \bar{y})^2 \div \Sigma(n - 1)$$

The use of more extensive designs is possible, together with the application of co-variance analysis by which the error variance may be still further reduced by considering the regression of the response upon a pre-treatment observation.

The consideration of such designs is beyond the scope of this book.

Use of range methods

The analysis of variance was developed in the course of experimentation, where the labour of calculation was small compared with the labour of the experiment, and it was desirous to obtain the maximum amount of information. When the demand for such analysis is great there will be some advantage to be gained by estimating the variance from the range of the observations. Methods covering the designs used in biological assay have been described (David, Hartley[3,4]); it is our experience that these methods are perfectly satisfactory for routine assays.

The variance of a mean

The variance of a mean of n determinations is calculated as:

$$\frac{s^2}{n}$$

and the range within which such a mean would be expected to fall on repetition is calculated as:

$$\bar{y} \pm t.\frac{s}{\sqrt{n}}$$

t being the appropriate value for $n - 1$ d.f.

The variance of a sum or difference

The variance of a sum or of a difference of two values is the sum of their individual variances:

$$s^2_{a+b} = s^2_a + s^2_b$$

Thus the range within which the difference of means $\bar{y}_1$ and $\bar{y}_2$ depending on n_1 and n_2 observations respectively would be expected is

$$(\bar{y}_1 - \bar{y}_2) \pm t\sqrt{\left(\frac{s_1{}^2}{n_1} + \frac{s_2{}^2}{n_2}\right)}$$

if this range does not include zero it would be concluded that at the probability level chosen the means differ significantly.

APPENDIX X

By calculating:

$$t = (y_1 - y_2) \Big/ \sqrt{\left(\frac{s_1^2}{n_1} + \frac{s_2^2}{n_2}\right)}$$

and entering the appropriate tables with $n_1 + n_2 - 2$ d.f. one may assess the probability level at which the two values differ.

The variance of a ratio

The variance (V) of a ratio $\left(\frac{a}{b} = R\right)$ of two estimates (a and b) is calculated by considering the individual coefficients of variation ($C.V.$).

$$(C.V. \text{ of } R)^2 = (C.V. \text{ of } a)^2 + (C.V. \text{ of } b)^2$$

i.e.
$$\frac{(V)R}{R^2} = \frac{(V)a}{a^2} + \frac{(V)b}{b^2}$$

which may be transformed to

$$(V)R = \frac{1}{b^2}[(V)a + R^2(V)b]$$

The use of this estimate of variance to assign fiducial limits of error to a ratio will overestimate the precision of an assay unless the coefficient of variation of b is small. Fieller[5] showed that the true fiducial limits are the roots of the quadratic.

$$m^2[b^2 - t^2V(b)] - 2m(ab - t^2 \text{ Cov. } ab) + [a^2 - t^2(V)a] = 0$$

Consideration of this formula allows the fiducial limits to be calculated from that using coefficients of variation as:

$$\frac{R}{1-g} \pm \frac{t}{b(1-g)}\sqrt{\left\{(V)a(1-g) + R^2(V)b\right\}}$$

where $g = t^2(V)b/b^2$

which is the expression used in the *B.P.*

Fieller[5] preferred to calculate

$$C = b^2/b^2 - t^2(V)b \quad i.e.\ C = \frac{1}{1-g}$$

and calculate the fiducial limits as

$$CR \pm \frac{t}{b}\sqrt{C(V)a + C^2R^2(V)b}$$

When the estimates of a and b are independent of one another the roots of the quadratic are

$$CR \pm \sqrt{(C-1)\left(CR^2 + \frac{(V)a}{(V)b}\right)}$$

which is the general form of the formula used in the *U.S.P.* to establish confidence limits of ratios.

Estimation of relative potency and the fiducial limits of error

All estimates of relative potency whether obtained from chemical or biological methods of assay are derived by equating those quantities which produce an equivalent effect and will depend on the calculation of a ratio or a difference. The assay of digitalis in which the individual lethal doses of standard or test preparation are equated provides a practical example of the use of both these treatments. In the *U.S.P.* pigeon assay the actual lethal doses are used to calculate the relative potency as a ratio. In the *B.P.* guinea pig assay their logarithms are used. The application of both these treatments to results obtained in the conduct of a *B.P.* assay will be illustrated.

TABLE 70

	STANDARD		TEST PREPARATION	
	Individual lethal dose ml/kg	log	Individual lethal dose ml/kg	log
	20·43	1·3102	22·43	1·3508
	21·30	1·3284	21·98	1·3420
	25·00	1·3979	20·54	1·3126
	23·51	1·3713	24·34	1·3863
	22·08	1·3439	19·95	1·3000
Total	112·32	6·7517	109·24	6·6917
Mean = $\bar{y}$	22·46	1·3503	21·85	1·3383
Sum of Sq.	2536·3214	9·121926	2398·5550	8·960371
Correction Term	2523·1565	9·117091	2386·6755	8·955770
Reduced Sum of Sq.	13·1649	0·004835	11·8795	0·004601

Using lethal doses

$$R = \bar{y}_{st}/\bar{y}_t = 22{\cdot}46/21{\cdot}85 = 1{\cdot}028$$

$$s^2 = \frac{13{\cdot}1649 + 11{\cdot}8795}{(5-1)+(5-1)} = \frac{25{\cdot}0444}{8} = 3{\cdot}1305$$

$$s^2_{\bar{y}_{st}} = s^2_{\bar{y}_t} = \frac{3{\cdot}1305}{5} = 0{\cdot}6261$$

$$t^2(P = 0{\cdot}95,\ 8\text{ d.f.}) = 5{\cdot}32.\quad t^2 s^2_{\bar{y}_t} = 3{\cdot}3309$$

$$C = \bar{y}_t^2/(\bar{y}_t^2 - t^2 s^2_{\bar{y}_t}) = 477{\cdot}4225/474{\cdot}0916 = 1{\cdot}007$$

$$CR = 1{\cdot}0352 \qquad CR^2 = 1{\cdot}0642$$

the fiducial limits of R are given by the formula

$$CR \pm \sqrt{(C-1)\left(CR^2 + \frac{n_t}{n_{st}}\right)}$$

where n_t and n_{st} are the number of responses on test and standard respectively and in this instance $n_t/n_{st} = 1$.

The fiducial limits (P = 0·95) are then

$$1{\cdot}0352 \pm \sqrt{(0{\cdot}007)(2{\cdot}0642)} = 1{\cdot}0352 \pm 0{\cdot}12 = 1{\cdot}16 \text{ and } 0{\cdot}92$$

Using logs

$$M = \text{log activity ratio} = 1{\cdot}3503 - 1{\cdot}3383 = 0{\cdot}012$$

$$R = \text{Activity ratio} = 1{\cdot}028$$

$$s^2 = \frac{(0{\cdot}004835)}{4} + \frac{(0{\cdot}004601)}{4} = \frac{0{\cdot}009436}{8} = 0{\cdot}001180$$

$$s_M^2 = 0{\cdot}001180(\tfrac{1}{5} + \tfrac{1}{5}) = 0{\cdot}0004720$$

$$s_M = 0{\cdot}02173$$

$$t(\text{P} = 0{\cdot}95;\ 8 \text{ d.f.}) = 2{\cdot}306$$

$$\text{log fiducial limits of error} = 0{\cdot}0120 \pm (2{\cdot}306)(0{\cdot}02173) = 0{\cdot}062 \text{ and } -0{\cdot}038$$

$$\text{Fiducial limits of error (P} = 0{\cdot}95) = 1{\cdot}153 \text{ and } 0{\cdot}916$$

In most biological assays a linear relationship is established between the response or a function of it (= y) and the logarithm of the dose administered (= x). Lines are fitted for standard and test by the method of least squares, and if these lines are parallel within the limits of experimental error, a mean slope is calculated. The log activity ratio is equal to:

$$M = \bar{x}_{st} - \bar{x}_t - \frac{\bar{y}_{st} - \bar{y}_t}{b}$$

where $\bar{x}_{st}$ and $\bar{x}_t$ are the mean log doses of standard and test administered, $\bar{y}_{st}$ and $\bar{y}_t$ the respective mean response and b the combined slope of the log dose response line (l.d.r.l.).

The assays fall into two main groups: (*a*) those in which an 'all or none' effect is noted, such as the occurrence of convulsion, death, purgative effect, etc., and which are called quantal response assays and (*b*) those in which each response is graded in itself such as the measured fall in blood sugar level, or the coagulation time in blood systems, such assays being called continuous response assays.

The assays fall into two main groups: (*a*) those in which an 'all or none' l.d.r.l. and for this purpose the standard, or the test preparation, or preferably both, must be injected at more than one dose level.

When the linearity of the l.d.r.l. can be assumed two dose levels will suffice. The treatments are best given on the assumption that the doses of standard and test are equipotent, for then the data are interpreted so that the potency of the test preparation is expressed as a ratio of the standard, and hence of the potency assumed for the test preparation.

The arithmetical treatment of data from both quantal and continuous response assays are essentially the same, the difference lying in that whereas in continuous response assays the variance of a single response is established from the data itself (current or from previous experience), in quantal response assays the variance is established with infinite precision, and in some treatments (probit transformation) varies according to the level of the response. The arithmetic will be greatly reduced if the numbers in each dosage group are equal and the logarithmic interval between the dose levels the same for standard and test.

Treatment of Quantal Response Assays

For the purpose of example the treatment of a quantal response assay by probit transformation using two doses of standard and two of the test preparation will be considered. The data used are taken from the assay for insulin in which the number of mice displaying hypoglycæmic convulsions is taken as the response.

The calculations can be simply made by following a set pattern such as that shown in Table 71, the values for probit $= y$ and the weighting coefficient $= B \left(\frac{1}{nB} = \text{variance of the response}\right)$ being taken from the appropriate tables (Fisher and Yates[2]). Since the log interval is the same for

TABLE 71

	STANDARD			TEST		
	High Dose	Low Dose	Sum	High Dose	Low Dose	Sum
Response	19/24	4/24		15/24	6/24	
Probit $= y$	5·812	4·033		5·319	4·326	
Weighting coefficient $= B$	0·50	0·45		0·61	0·54	
n	24	24		24	24	
$nB = N$	12·00	10·80	22·8	14·64	12·96	27·60
$x =$ log dose	1	0		1	0	
$N x$	12·0	0	12·0	14·64	0	14·64
$N x^2$	12·0	0	12·0	14·64	0	14·64
$N y$	69·7440	43·5564	113·3004	77·8702	56·0650	133·9352
$N x y$	69·7440	0	69·7440	77·8702	0	77·8702

Ratio of high to low dose = 100/60 = 1·667 log 1·667 = d.

The values accumulated in this table are used to derive those in Table 72 which allows the estimated potency and the limits of error to be calculated.

APPENDIX X

TABLE 72

	$1/\Sigma N$	$\Sigma Nxy - \bar{x}\Sigma Ny = q$	$\Sigma Nx^2 - \bar{x}\Sigma Nx = p$	q^2/p	$\Sigma Ny \div \Sigma N = \bar{y}$	$\Sigma Nx \div \Sigma N = \bar{x}$
Standard	0·0439	10·1140	5·6844	17·9954	4·9693	0·5263
Test	0·0362	6·8310	6·8749	6·7874	4·8527	0·5304
Sum	0·0801	16·9450 = Q	12·5593 = P	24·7828		
Difference					0·1166	−0·0041
Q^2/P				22·8622		
Difference = χ^2 for parallelism with 1 d.f.				1·9206		

both standard and test, the logs for the high and low doses may be scored 1 and 0 respectively, suitable correction being made later for conversion to common logarithms. The simplification this introduces is obvious.

$$M = \text{log activity ratio} = d\left(\bar{x}_{st} - \bar{x}_t - \frac{\bar{y}_{st} - \bar{y}_t}{Q/P}\right)$$

$$= 0{\cdot}2218[-0{\cdot}0041 - (0{\cdot}1166/1{\cdot}349)] = -0{\cdot}0201 = \log 0{\cdot}9548$$

The variance of M is obtained as:

$$s_M^2 = \frac{d^2P^2}{Q^2}\left(\Sigma\frac{1}{N} + \frac{P(\bar{y}_{st} - \bar{y}_t^2)}{Q^2}\right) = 0{\cdot}0022$$

and the limits of error P = 0·95 are $M \pm 1{\cdot}96\, s_M$ $= -0{\cdot}0201 \pm 0{\cdot}0919 = +0{\cdot}0718$ and $-0{\cdot}1120 = \log 1{\cdot}18$ and log 0·7727.

The true fiducial limits are given by the formula:

$$CM \pm t\sqrt{\frac{Cd^2P^2}{Q^2}\left(\Sigma\frac{1}{\Sigma N} + CP\frac{(\bar{y}_{st} - \bar{y}_t)^2}{Q^2}\right)}$$

where $$C = Q^2/Q^2 - t^2P$$

Since the number of mice have been kept constant at each dose the calculation could have been carried out using $n = 1$, suitable correction being made at the end of the calculations.

The scheme shown can be used for all quantal response assays if probit transformations are to be used. When three doses of standard or test are used and the doses are equally spaced on the logarithmic scale, scores 1, 0 and −1 can be used for x, and the linearity of the line checked by comparing $\Sigma N(y-\bar{y})^2$ which may be calculated as $\Sigma Ny^2 - \bar{y}\,\Sigma Ny$ with χ^2 for 1 d.f. If the doses are not equally spaced logarithmically the common logarithm of the dose must be used for x and the value of d then becomes unity. If the assay is to be interpreted using angular transformations the same steps could be followed, but a further simplification is possible since although still established theoretically the error variance is constant at all response levels ($\sigma^2 = 820{\cdot}7$). If the number of responses per group is kept constant the calculation may be made using the angular transformation by itself and suitable correction made later for both number of animals and the variance, but in this instance there would be some convenience in scoring 1 and -1 for the logarithms of the doses. The value to be used for d is then half the log of the extreme dose ratio.

The maximum tabulation which is needed if the number in each group is constant is shown in Table 73 where the appropriate angular transformations for the data in Table 71 are recorded.

TABLE 73

	STANDARD		TEST		Sum	Difference
	High Dose	Low Dose	High Dose	Low Dose		
Responses	19/24	4/24	15/24	6/24		
Angular Transformations	62·8	24·1	52·2	30·0		
Sum	86·9		82·2			$4{\cdot}7 = T$
Difference	$38{\cdot}7 = q_{st}$		$22{\cdot}2 = q_t$		$60{\cdot}9 = Q$	16·5

Ratio high to low dose $= 1{\cdot}667$; $2d = \log 1{\cdot}667 = 0{\cdot}2218$

n = number in each group $= 24$; $\sigma^2 = 820{\cdot}7$

Then $M = -2dT/Q = -(0{\cdot}2218 \times 4{\cdot}7) \div 60{\cdot}9$

$= -0{\cdot}0171 = \log 0{\cdot}9614.$

The values for Q and $T (= \bar{y}_{st} - \bar{y}_t)$ are relevant to the use of $+1$ and -1 for x (= log dose) and under these conditions P has the value 4.

χ^2 slope (1 d.f.) may be calculated as $n\,(q_{st} - q_t)^2 \div P\sigma^2$

$$= 24 \times 16{\cdot}5^2 \div 4 \times 820{\cdot}7 = 1{\cdot}99$$

$$\text{Then } s_M^2 = \frac{P^2d^2\sigma^2}{nQ^2}\left(1 + \left(\frac{M}{2d}\right)^2\right)$$

$$= \frac{4^2 \times 0{\cdot}1109^2 \times 820{\cdot}7}{24 \times 60{\cdot}9^2}\left(1 + \left(\frac{0{\cdot}0171}{0{\cdot}2218}\right)^2\right)$$

$$= 0{\cdot}001825 = 0{\cdot}0427^2$$

The limits of error P $= 0{\cdot}95$ are then $-0{\cdot}0171 \pm 1{\cdot}96 \times 0{\cdot}0427$ $= 0{\cdot}0171 \pm 0{\cdot}0837 = 0{\cdot}0666$ and $-0{\cdot}1008 = \log 1{\cdot}166$ and $0{\cdot}7929$

The true fiducial limits are equal to

$$CM \pm \sqrt{(C-1)[CM^2 + (2d)^2]}$$

where $$C = Q^2/Q^2 - Pt^2\sigma^2$$

APPENDIX X

Reference has been made to the essential similarity in the treatment of continuous and quantal response assays. When the response groups are equal in size the treatment as described for the use of angular transformations may be applied using the mean response for the group. In such assays an estimate of variance is established from the data presented and t has the value appropriate to the degrees of freedom with which it is established. When the groups are not equal in size the more extended method used for probit transformations may be used. Each response could be weighted as $\frac{n}{s^2}$ and the formulæ used for the probit method then applies exactly. Alternatively, the response could be weighted for n and suitable modification made in the subsequent formulæ for s^2.

A twin cross-over test may also be interpreted by suitable entry into the treatments described. It may also be interpreted by considering the difference obtained by subtracting the response to test preparation from that obtained using the standard preparation for each animal $= y$ and calculating for each cell the value, $\bar{y}_1, \bar{y}_2, \bar{y}_3, \bar{y}_4$.

Then $$M = \frac{\bar{y}_1 + \bar{y}_2 + \bar{y}_3 + \bar{y}_4}{\bar{y}_1 - \bar{y}_2 - \bar{y}_3 + \bar{y}_4} \times d$$

where $$d = \text{log dose ratio}$$

$(\bar{y}_1 - \bar{y}_2 - \bar{y}_3 + \bar{y}_4) \div 4d$ is an estimate of b and if the numbers of animals yielding responses to standard and test is n

$$s_M^2 \text{ may be calculated as } \frac{2s^2}{nb^2}\left(1 + \frac{M^2}{d^2}\right)$$

Slope Ratio Assays

There still remains a small group of biological assays in which the response or a function of it is linear to the dose itself, a relationship which is satisfied by the data to be obtained from chemical or physio-chemical methods of assay. The relative activity of the two preparations is, in these assays, the ratio of the slopes of the two regression lines providing the lines converge, within the limits of experimental error, at zero dosage.

The simplest design is that in which the preparations are examined at one level and a blank is also carried out. If the blank gives zero response the ratio of the slopes is the ratio of the two readings themselves or, if the blank has a value, the ratio of the two readings each diminished by the blank value, an operation which is regularly applied in chemical assays.

The simplest design which allows some test of validity to be made is that using two concentrations of each preparation without a blank, and in this case the test for validity is that which ensures that the lines converge at zero dosage. If a blank is introduced a check may be made to ensure that this convergence is at the blank level.

The general formulæ necessary for the interpretation of slope ratio assays is given by Finney.[6] Finney also shows how the arithmetic may be simplified if certain restrictions are imposed, such as keeping the number of responses per group, the number of dosage groups equal for standard and test, and maintaining the same arithmetic interval between the doses for standard and test assuming that the corresponding doses of standard and test are equal.

Combination of results

When a number of estimates of M are available to each of which a variance has been attached, a weighted mean may be calculated by weighting each estimate inversely as its variance, *i.e.*

$$W = \frac{1}{s_M^2} \quad \text{and} \quad \bar{M} = \Sigma WM/\Sigma W$$

the variance of $\bar{M}$ is then $\dfrac{1}{\Sigma W}$.

The combination is valid only if the group of n results are shown to be homogeneous by computing

$$\chi^2 = \Sigma W(M - \bar{M})^2$$

and entering the appropriate tables with $n - 1$ d.f.

The *B.P.* implies that this procedure is only acceptable when the individual values for g at P = 0·95 are less than 0·1. When this approximate method of combination was compared with the more exact method using a series of six tests in which all of the values of g exceeded 0·15 and one was as high as 0·64, the mean estimate by the approximate method was 93·94 per cent (P = 0·95, limits of error 82·35–103·4) and by the more exact method it was 94·19 per cent (P = 0·95, limits of error 85·8–103·4).

We consider, therefore, that the restriction suggested by the *B.P.* is too severe and that the approximate method may be used with confidence when aggregate weights of the order 2,000 are being attained.

Sequential Analysis

The methods generally employed for the estimation of error assume that the calculations are carried out when the experimental work is complete. In practice, when the calculations indicate border-line acceptability, further observations may be made and added to the existing information.

The proper analysis of such data is provided by the method of Sequential Analysis (Wald[7]) which also has the advantage that when the information can or must be collected sequentially its application allows decisions to be made with fewer observations when particularly good or particularly bad samples are being examined.

Suitable models exist for each of the general methods of assay. In those assays where the variance of a single observation may be calculated the critical sum of m observations which will allow a decision to be made to accept or reject, is given by appropriate entry into the formulæ.

$$A_m = \frac{\sigma^2}{\theta_0 - \theta_1} 2{\cdot}3 \log \frac{\beta}{1-\alpha} + m\frac{\theta_0 + \theta_1}{2}$$

$$R_m = \frac{\sigma^2}{\theta_0 - \theta_1} 2{\cdot}3 \log \frac{1-\beta}{\alpha} + m\frac{\theta_0 + \theta_1}{2}$$

θ_1 = acceptable mean level
θ_0 = unacceptable mean level
α = probability of its rejection
β = probability of its acceptance
σ^2 = the variance of a single observation

Application to Pyrogen Testing

The pyrogen test of the *B.P.* fits a sequential plan having the characteristics:

$$\theta_1 = 0{\cdot}32^\circ$$
$$\theta_0 = 0{\cdot}78^\circ$$
$$\alpha = 0{\cdot}009$$
$$\beta = 0{\cdot}10$$
$$\sigma^2 = 0{\cdot}1$$

from which
$$A_m = 0{\cdot}55m - 0{\cdot}50$$
$$R_m = 0{\cdot}55m + 1{\cdot}0$$

The critical values given in the *B.P.* are recorded in terms of responses from successive groups of three rabbits. The test may be applied with equal efficiency by considering the responses singly.

Application to Digitalis Assay

A sequential plan may be established for the assay of digitalis by considering sequentially the difference in the log lethal dose of successive pairs of guinea pigs (each difference representing a single estimate of the log activity ratio). Experience shows that a reasonable estimate of the variance of such a difference is 0·004. The *B.P.* specification implies that there should only be a 5 per cent probability of accepting material with a potency of less than 80 per cent or more than 125 per cent and it would not be unreasonable to allow a 5 per cent probability of rejecting material with a potency greater than 95 per cent or less than 105 per cent.

Transforming these values into the notation used we have

θ_1 = acceptable log activity ratio = $\pm\, 0{\cdot}0223$
θ_0 = unacceptable log activity ratio = $\pm\, 0{\cdot}0969$
$\alpha = 0{\cdot}05$
$\beta = 0{\cdot}05$
$\sigma^2 = 0{\cdot}004$

from which
$$A_m = 0{\cdot}0596m - 0{\cdot}1579$$
$$R_m = 0{\cdot}0596m + 0{\cdot}1579$$

which are shown graphically in Fig. 21.

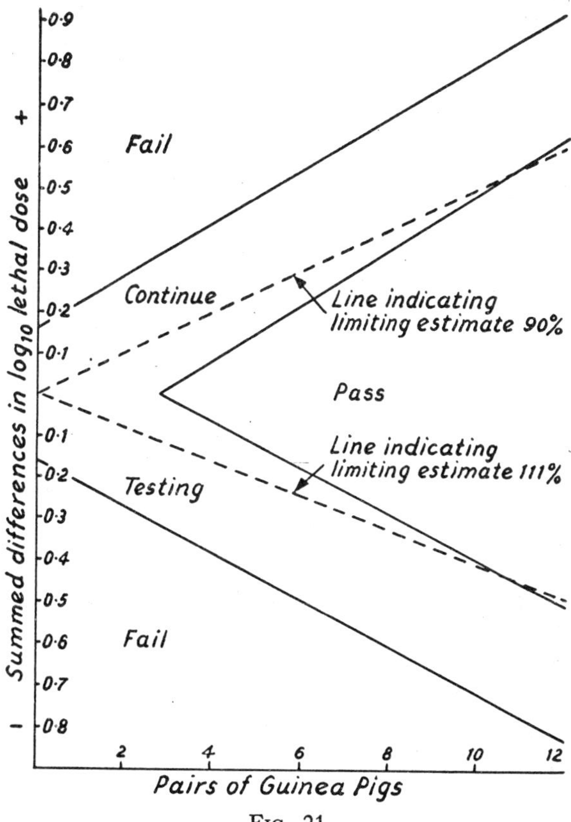

FIG. 21

The *B.P.* also requires that the mean potency estimate shall be between 90 and 111 per cent and the lines indicating this restriction are also drawn. It will be seen that the plan controls the quality until twelve pairs of guinea pigs have been used, but beyond that number the quality is controlled by the estimated potency alone.

Application to Repeated Assays

When more than one assay is carried out a weighted mean of M (= log activity ratio) is calculated weighting each estimate according to the reciprocal of its variance.

A sequential plan may be derived in which these weights are considered sequentially when by definition the variance of a single unit of weight is itself unity.

The interpretation of the *B.P.* criterion for insulin is identical with that for digitalis and the appropriate conditions for acceptance and rejection may be established by entering the formulæ with $\sigma^2 = 1$. In this instance the sequential plan itself controls the quality up to summed weights of 2,500, but beyond that the quality is controlled by the permitted limits of the estimated potency.

1. Bartlett, M. S., *Proc. Roy. Soc. (London)*, **A,** 1937, **160,** 268.
2. Fisher, R. A., and Yates, F., Statistical Tables for Biological, Agricultural and Medical Research, Oliver and Boyd, Edinburgh, 5th Ed., 1957.
3. David, H. A., *Biometrika*, 1951, **38**, 393.
4. Hartley, H. O., *Biometrika*, 1950, **37**, 271.
5. Fieller, E. C., *J. Roy. Statist. Soc., Suppl.*, 1940, **7**, 63.
6. Finney, D. J., Statistical Method in Biological Assay, Chas. Griffin and Co. Ltd. (London), 1952.
7. Wald, A., Sequential Analysis, Wiley (London), 1947.

APPENDIX XI

Methods for the Destruction of Organic Matter

The Analytical Methods Committee of the *S.A.C.*[1] has recommended various methods of combustion, both wet and dry, that may be used when organic matter is to be destroyed as a preliminary to the determination of metallic traces. The choice of method will depend (*a*) on the nature of the organic material and of any inorganic constituent and (*b*) on the metal that is subsequently to be determined and the method to be used for its determination. For application to pharmaceutical materials details of the methods recommended are essentially as follows.

WET DECOMPOSITION

In these methods it is essential to use reagents and distilled water of suitably low metal content, taking into consideration that the concentrated mineral acids are generally used in amounts several times that of the sample. Even when these reagents are used, reagent blank determinations will be necessary; these follow the lines of the determination proper with obvious modifications, but since they must be prepared with the same quantities of reagents as are used in the tests, the measurement and recording of these quantities must not be overlooked.

The Kjeldahl flasks used should be made of borosilicate glass or silica (100- to 250-ml nominal capacity) fitted with an extension to the neck by means of a standard ground joint. The extension serves to condense fumes into an acid-fume condenser and carries a tap funnel through which the reagents are introduced. A suitable apparatus is shown in Fig. 22.

The weight of sample taken will depend (*a*) on the level of the metal content of the material and (*b*) on the methods subsequently to be used for the determination of the metal. For amounts of metal of the order of 10 to 100 p.p.m., 5 g is a convenient quantity, but if ultra-sensitive methods are available 2 g is often enough, with consequent saving of time taken to wet oxidise the material and use of less acid.

For biological samples, 10 to 15 g of blood or tissue or 50 ml of urine or plasma are generally sufficient for all determinations; they should be boiled down to small bulk with nitric acid before sulphuric acid is added.

For other liquids, take 20 to 50 g of the sample, containing not more than 5 g of solids, and boil down to small bulk with nitric acid before adding sulphuric acid. Continue then as for solid samples.

APPENDIX XI

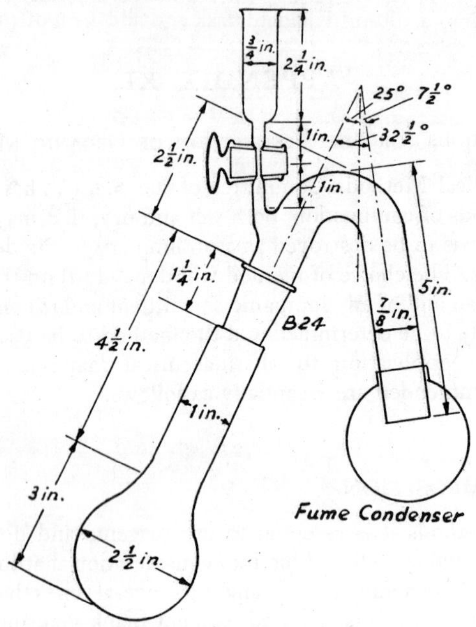

FIG. 22

Dimensions are for a flask of 150-ml capacity

I. Destruction with Nitric and Sulphuric Acids, With or Without the Aid of Perchloric Acid or Hydrogen Peroxide

Method (I) A. Weigh 5 g (or a suitable amount) of the well-mixed sample into a 100-ml Kjeldahl flask and add 10 ml of a mixture of 1 volume of concentrated nitric acid and 2 volumes of water. As soon as any initial reaction subsides, heat gently until further reaction ceases, and then cool the mixture. (When much carbohydrate is present, the initial reaction may be violent and heating should be delayed, if necessary, even overnight. Further nitric acid may then be added as necessary. With some extremely reactive organic compounds it is necessary to carry out the preliminary treatment with dilute nitric acid in a 500-ml beaker, heating the beaker slowly on a water-bath until the initial reaction is completed. If excessive frothing is experienced in the earlier stages, a drop or two of *sec.*-octyl alcohol may be added or the preliminary treatment may be carried out in a 500-ml borosilicate-glass beaker with the addition of glass beads to prevent bumping.) Add, gradually, up to 10 ml of concentrated sulphuric acid, at such a rate as not to cause excessive frothing or heating (five to ten minutes are usually required), and then heat until the liquid darkens appreciably in colour.

Continue as given below in 'Continuation for Methods (I) A to (I) D'.

Method (*I*) *B*. Weigh 5 g (or a suitable amount) of the well-mixed sample into a 100-ml Kjeldahl flask and add 5 ml of concentrated nitric acid. As soon as any vigorous initial reaction subsides, heat gently until further vigorous reaction ceases, and then cool the mixture. Add, gradually, 8 ml of concentrated sulphuric acid, at such a rate as not to cause excessive frothing or heating (five to ten minutes are usually required), and then heat until the liquid darkens appreciably in colour.

Continue as given below in 'Continuation for Methods (I) A to (I) D'.

Method (*I*) *C*. Weigh 5 g (or a suitable amount) of the well-mixed sample into a 100-ml Kjeldahl flask and add a mixture of 8 ml of concentrated sulphuric acid and 10 ml of concentrated nitric acid. Warm cautiously until the reaction subsides, and then boil rapidly until the solution begins to darken owing to incipient charring.

Continue as given below in 'Continuation for Methods (I) A to (I) D'.

Method (*I*) *D*. Treat 5 g (or a suitable amount) of the material in a 100-ml Kjeldahl flask with 20 ml of a mixture of 1 volume of concentrated nitric acid and 2 volumes of water, and warm until the initial vigorous reaction is over. At this point a spongy, tarry cake is formed. Cool the mixture, pour off the acid into a beaker, and wash the tarry residue with a small amount of water (three or four 1-ml portions), adding the washings to the acid liquor in the beaker. Add 8 ml of concentrated sulphuric acid to the tarry residue, agitate to disperse the cake, and introduce concentrated nitric acid, drop by drop, with warming if necessary, until vigorous oxidation ceases. Return the original acid liquor to the flask, and boil until the solution just begins to darken.

Continue as given in 'Continuation for Methods (I) A to (I) D'.

Continuation for Methods (*I*) *A to* (*I*) *D*

(*a*) *Without addition of perchloric acid or hydrogen peroxide*

Add concentrated nitric acid slowly in small portions (1 to 2 ml), heating after each addition, until darkening again takes place. Do not heat so strongly that charring is excessive, or loss of arsenic may occur; a small, but not excessive, amount of free nitric acid must be present throughout. Continue this treatment until the solution fails to darken on prolonged heating to fuming (five to ten minutes). The criterion of completion of oxidation is that the final solution is fuming when hot and colourless when colder, but if much iron is present the solution will be pale yellow in colour, frequently with a granular precipitate soluble on dilution. Allow to cool somewhat, dilute the solution with 10 ml of water (this should give a colourless solution, or a faintly yellow one if iron is present), and boil gently to fuming. Allow the solution to cool again, add a further 5 ml of water, and boil gently to fuming. Finally, cool, and dilute the solution with 5 ml of water.

(*b*) *With the addition of perchloric acid or hydrogen peroxide*

1. With addition of perchloric acid—Add concentrated nitric acid, slowly in small portions, heating after each addition, until darkening takes place. Do not heat so strongly that charring is excessive, or loss of arsenic may occur; a small, but not excessive, amount of free nitric acid must be present throughout. Continue this treatment until the solution fails to darken in colour on prolonged heating (five to ten minutes)

and is only pale yellow in colour. Run into the flask 0·5 ml of 60 per cent w/w perchloric acid, and a little more nitric acid, and heat for about fifteen minutes, then add a further 0·5 ml of perchloric acid, and heat for a few minutes longer. Allow to cool somewhat, and dilute the mixture with 10 ml of water. The solution should be quite colourless, except when much iron is present, when it may be faintly yellow. Boil gently, taking care to avoid bumping, until white fumes appear; allow the solution to cool, add a further 5 ml of water, and again boil gently to fuming. Finally, cool, and dilute the solution with 5 ml of water.

2. With addition of hydrogen peroxide—Proceed as given in section (*b*) 1, above, to the point of addition of perchloric acid. In place of this add analytical-reagent grade 100-volume hydrogen peroxide, in small quantities (1 or 2 ml), with a few drops of concentrated nitric acid. Heat to fuming after each addition of hydrogen peroxide until the residue is colourless or no further reduction of the pale yellow colour can be obtained; cool the solution, dilute it with 10 ml of water, and evaporate to fuming; again dilute the solution with 5 ml of water, and evaporate to fuming. Finally, dilute the solution with 5 ml of water.

Method (I) E: Destruction with Nitric, Perchloric and Sulphuric Acids

(i) Weigh 2 g of the sample into a 500-ml conical flask having a B24 neck, and fit a B24 cone to act as a short air condenser. (For dry, finely divided powders and for materials that might react vigorously with nitric acid it is advisable to moisten the sample with a few millilitres of water at this stage.) Add 15 ml of concentrated nitric acid and shake to wet the sample completely. Allow any reaction to subside and then add 10 ml of 60 per cent w/w perchloric acid and 5 ml of concentrated sulphuric acid, swirling the contents of the flask during additions. Place the flask on a cold hot-plate, and switch to medium heat. (Starting with a cold hot-plate prevents the too rapid evaporation of nitric acid before all the readily reactive material has been oxidised.) As the temperature rises, the material dissolves with the evolution of brown fumes, which clear to leave a quietly boiling solution with some refluxing taking place in the short air condenser. When most of the nitric acid has been driven off, with some materials there may be signs of a more vigorous reaction with further evolution of brown fumes. If this occurs, add a few millilitres of nitric acid, and continue heating. Finally, heat the solution until white fumes are evolved; cool, dilute the solution with 5 ml of water, and again heat until white fumes are evolved.

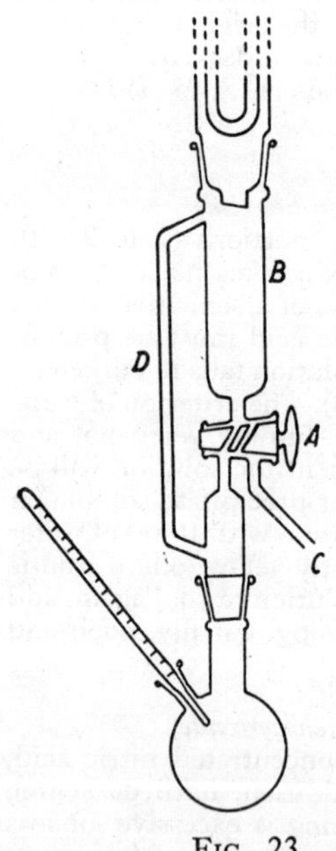

FIG. 23

(ii) Alternative method. Weigh 2 g of the sample into the flask of the apparatus, shown in Fig. 23.

Add 15 ml of concentrated nitric acid, allow any reaction to subside, and then add 10 ml of 60 per cent w/w perchloric acid and 5 ml of concentrated sulphuric acid, by way of the condenser, mixing well during the additions. Set the flask aside for half an hour, then heat gradually to full reflux, and maintain for one hour. Maintaining full heat, turn the tap A through 90° so that liquid distils into the reservoir B. When the temperature has reached 140°, turn the tap through a further 90° so that the distillate runs out through C into a suitable receptacle; then complete the turn through the full 360°, re-establishing the conditions shown in the figure. Allow to reflux for a further hour, then raise the temperature similarly to 180° for an hour, then to 200° for half an hour. Cool, and dilute the residue as required.

II. Destruction with Nitric and Perchloric Acids

Method (II) A. Introduce into a 200-ml Kjeldahl flask an amount of sample containing not more than 2 g of dry matter. Add 25 ml of concentrated nitric acid and boil slowly for thirty minutes. Cool the mixture and add 15 ml of 60 per cent w/w perchloric acid. Boil very gently until the solution is colourless or nearly so and dense white fumes appear in the flask. This latter boiling should take nearly one hour. Dangerous conditions may arise if the flask is allowed to boil dry at any time.

Method (II) B. Introduce into a 100-ml conical borosilicate-glass flask an amount of sample containing not more than 2 g of dry matter. Add 1 ml of water, 3 ml of concentrated nitric acid and 2 ml of 60 per cent w/w perchloric acid and heat the flask on an electric hot-plate, starting the plate from cold. Use a layer of asbestos paper, if necessary, to moderate the heat. When the liquid begins to turn brown, add further nitric acid, drop by drop, to avoid further darkening. (*Note:* The darkening of digestion mixtures containing perchloric acid is regarded by some workers as indicating the onset of dangerous conditions. The real significance of this darkening probably depends upon the nature of the sample, but in any case, the condition should not be allowed to persist longer than can be avoided.) A colourless solution and white fumes of perchloric acid indicate completion of oxidation.

Method (II) C. In a large test-tube ($1\frac{1}{2}$ in. × 9 in.) digest a volume of sample containing about 0·25 g of total solids with 2·0 ml of 60 per cent w/w perchloric acid and 2 ml of concentrated nitric acid. It is advisable to use several fragments of acid-washed porcelain to prevent bumping. Add nitric acid, drop by drop, if the solution does not clear quickly after charring. Evaporate the solution to fumes of perchloric acid.

III. Destruction with Nitric Acid and Ammonium Nitrate

Transfer 1 g of the dried and powdered sample to a 250-ml Kjeldahl flask, and add 10 ml of concentrated nitric acid. Gently warm the flask until solution is complete, add 10 ml of oxidising reagent (a solution of 50 g of ammonium nitrate and 25 g of concentrated nitric acid, made up to 100 ml with water), and heat gently to expel water, so that oxidation (indicated by effervescence) proceeds in a melt of ammonium nitrate. From time to time add more reagent, if necessary, and continue until no browning of the solution is observed and a clear melt has been obtained. In the presence of much fat, oxidation is slower and more reagent may be required, and there may be excessive initial frothing if much carbohydrate is present. When oxidation is complete, heat the clear melt more strongly to volatilise the excess of ammonium nitrate (avoid overheating), holding the flask over a free flame to expel salt subliming on the side. Then dissolve the residue in 2 ml of concentrated hydrochloric acid, evaporate to dryness, fuse the residue in the flask, so as to remove all nitric acid, dissolve it in about 10 ml of N hydrochloric acid, and evaporate the solution to a small bulk to ensure conversion of any metaphosphate to orthophosphate. Evaporate to dryness in a stream of warm air, dissolve the residue in a few millilitres of warm water, add a few drops of N hydrochloric acid, and dilute to 10 ml with water.

In all the above methods employing perchloric acid special precautions should be taken. Full advice on these is given in a Report by the Analytical Methods Committee of the *S.A.C.*[2]

DRY DECOMPOSITION

Method A. No Ashing Aid.

Weigh accurately a suitable quantity of the well-mixed sample in a tared silica or platinum basin. Heat first by means of a soft flame, such as that of an Argand burner, to volatilise as much as possible of the organic matter, then transfer the basin to a temperature-controlled muffle furnace, at a temperature preferably not exceeding 420°.

If it is suspected that all the carbon has not been removed, cool the ash, add a slight excess of dilute hydrochloric acid or a mixture of one volume of concentrated nitric acid and two volumes of water, warm on a water-bath, and note whether any colour is extracted or whether organic matter is still present. If so, evaporate the mixture to dryness on the water-bath, and gently char the residue over a small flame until all the organic matter has been destroyed, or better, repeat the ignition at a higher temperature or for a longer period.

Method B. Ashing Aid, Light Magnesium Oxide.

Weigh a suitable amount of the material into a tared silica or platinum basin containing light magnesium oxide (up to 2 per cent of the weight of the sample) distributed over the base and partly up the sides of the basin. Support the basin in a hole cut in asbestos board so that at least two-thirds of the basin projects below the asbestos. Heat first by means of a soft flame, such as that of an Argand burner, to volatilise as much as possible of the organic matter, then transfer the basin to a temperature-controlled muffle furnace at a temperature preferably not exceeding 420°, and heat until no carbon remains.

Method C. Ashing Aid, Magnesium Nitrate Solution.

Magnesium Nitrate Solution. Adjust the pH of a 50 per cent w/v solution of magnesium nitrate to 9·5 with ammonium hydroxide, using thymol blue as indicator, and extract with successive portions of dithizone solution in chloroform until the dithizone layer remains green.

Weigh a quantity of the sample equivalent to not more than 5 g of solids, into a tared silica or platinum basin. Heat first by means of a soft flame, such as that of an Argand burner, to drive off any moisture and to volatilise as much as possible of the organic matter; continue with increasing heating until white fuming ceases and a dry char is obtained. Break down the char with a clean glass rod, and moisten it with a little magnesium nitrate solution. Transfer the basin to a temperature-controlled muffle furnace, bring the temperature to about 420°, and maintain the furnace at this temperature until no carbon remains.

Method D. Ashing Aid, Sodium Carbonate.

Mix intimately a suitable quantity of the well-mixed sample with anhydrous sodium carbonate (20 per cent of the weight of the sample) in a tared silica or platinum basin. Heat first by means of a soft flame, such as that of an Argand burner, until all volatile carbonaceous matter is driven off. Transfer the basin to a temperature-controlled muffle furnace at a temperature as low as possible, and in any case not exceeding 420°, and heat until a grey powdery ash is obtained. Care must be taken not to fuse the ash, having regard to the fact that its melting-point will possibly be much lower than that of pure sodium carbonate.

The methods employing wet decomposition are of almost universal application although unfamiliar materials must always undergo preliminary treatment on a small scale before the method to be used is selected. This particularly applies to Method (I) E, the most vigorous method of wet decomposition.

Given suitable selection, Methods (I) are applicable to the destruction of most organic materials, including such materials as dyestuffs, intermediates and medicinals, before the determination of most of the common trace metals, but they are not recommended in the presence of appreciable amounts of alkaline-earth metals, since the insoluble sulphates formed absorb a considerable proportion of trace metals, particularly lead. In such instances, Methods (II) should be used. Method (I) B is suitable for less reactive substances than those that Method (I) A is suitable for and Method (I) C, a more rapid method than A or B, is appropriate for substances that decompose quietly. For substances that are liable to deflagrate violently during charring, with risk of incurring appreciable losses of arsenic, Method (I) D must be used.

The choice of continuation method for Methods (I) A to (I) D may be left to the individual operator. The use of perchloric acid or hydrogen peroxide speeds digestion and hence reduces the amount of nitric acid required and shortens the time taken to complete the removal of all the organic matter but, of course, perchloric acid must not be used if the presence of chloride is detrimental in the procedure for determination of the metals.

Method (I) E is suitable for many organic and biological materials and the alternative method (ii) is particularly flexible, since the increases in temperature and the lengths of the periods of refluxing can be altered to suit the type of sample being decomposed. Further, except for the periods during which the temperature is being raised, it needs no supervision.

Method (II) A is capable of dealing with a wide variety of materials of biological origin. It may be used for some chemicals and synthetic materials but these often give very vigorous reactions and care must be taken that the reacting mixtures never boil dry. The disadvantage of this method is that, since conditions are less severe than some other procedures, some types of organic material, notably those containing heterocyclic nitrogen, escape complete destruction. For such materials dry ashing is indicated.

Method (II) B is suitable for sugar products when lead is to be determined and (II) C for small volumes of liquid samples.

Method (III) was originally devised for the determination of calcium, magnesium, sodium, potassium and sulphur all on one sample, since sodium and potassium, which have volatile compounds, cannot be determined after dry ashing and methods involving the use of sulphuric acid as an oxidising agent, which leave unchanged acid in the residue, preclude the determination of sulphur. The method can also be applied when iron, copper and similar elements are to be determined in samples in which the amount of organic matter is small and is easily decomposed.

Dry ashing is applicable to the determination of most of the common metals, usually with the exception of mercury and arsenic, in organic matter. It has been reported that losses occur in certain metals (*e.g.* zinc, tin or antimony) when dry ashing is carried out in the presence of halides; such losses can be minimised by ensuring that an alkaline ash remains. The method is particularly applicable when the use of sulphuric acid is objectionable; for instance, for the determination of lead in materials containing an appreciable quantity of the alkaline earths, whose sulphates occlude lead sulphate. Method A is suitable for the determination of most of the common metals, excluding mercury and arsenic, in organic materials that leave a bulky ash, Method B for those with a low ash content and Method C for sugars, sugar syrups and biological materials, but this last method is unsuitable when magnesium phosphate may interfere with the subsequent procedure. Method D is appropriate for the determination of trace metals (excluding mercury) whose salts may be volatile, in dyestuffs, intermediates and medicinals.

More specific information about the influence of the metal and its method of determination on the choice of decomposition procedure is given in the monograph on the particular metal involved.

A method using hydrogen peroxide with sulphuric acid for wet decomposition of organic matter, which should find increasing use in the future, has been described in a paper by Whalley.[3] The main advantages of the method are that the oxidation is generally smooth and clean, no unpleasant acid fumes are evolved except those from sulphuric acid and only water is formed when the reagent decomposes. In addition, the reagent has extremely low blanks for heavy metals.

1. *Analyst*, 1960, **85**, 643.
2. *Analyst*, 1959, **84**, 214.
3. WHALLEY, C., *Proc. Feigl Anniversary Symp.*, 1962, 397.

APPENDIX XII

THE EXTRACTION OF NON-VOLATILE ORGANIC CHEMICALS FROM VISCERA, VOMITS, ETC.

Although the quantitative determination of individual organic chemicals is considered under the monographs in the text, a systematic procedure for their isolation from complex biological material may usefully be outlined here. It is important that the chemical substances should be separated in as pure a form as possible although the amounts usually obtainable in toxicological work are insufficient for application of any methods other than colorimetric or spectrophotometric; full quantitative recovery cannot be expected and the drug may have been modified during metabolism.

The classical Stas-Otto process which was originally devised to separate alkaloids can be extended to other classes of substances, provided caution is used in the judgement of quantitative results. The method is generally considered too cumbersome and liable to cause losses by adsorption on the precipitated extraneous matter but it is the basis of many later published methods and the procedure given below can be adapted for most materials as a preliminary treatment to eliminate the greater part of the proteins, resinous substances, fat and colouring matter before examination.

> Thoroughly mix a portion of the prepared material, evaporated almost to dryness at a low temperature if a liquid, with dehydrated ethanol (industrial spirit must be distilled over tartaric acid before use) and add sufficient 10 per cent tartaric acid solution to give a very slightly acid reaction after shaking, avoiding a large excess. Heat under a reflux condenser on a water-bath for fifteen minutes. After cooling, filter through a Büchner funnel to remove fat and other insoluble matter as completely as possible, wash the residue with ethanol, replace the solid matter in the flask and reflux with more ethanol. Repeat until the residues are exhausted. Evaporate the acid filtrate and mix the residue thoroughly with cold water, allow to stand for some hours, preferably at low temperature, filter and again evaporate the filtrate to dryness or to a syrup. Mix this residue with a large volume of dehydrated ethanol; a light-coloured viscous residue usually remains undissolved and if it is allowed to stand for a short time frequently becomes granular. Filter, again evaporate the ethanolic filtrate on a water-bath and dissolve the residue in a small volume of water. Filter into a separator after confirming that the solution has remained acid.

Considerable patience must be used in preparing this solution and the possibility of the decomposition of certain substances by too drastic treatment must be remembered. Aconitine and atropine are particularly liable to hydrolysis at high temperatures. Hence, if they are suspected, all distillations and evaporations should be carried out under reduced pressure or at low temperature. The solution should then be ready for extraction.

(*a*) Extract the acid solution three or four times with ether or preferably with ether-chloroform. The residue after evaporation of the solvent may contain acidic, neutral or feebly basic substances, such as barbitones, organic acids, phenacetin, glucosides, caffeine (not soluble in ether) or ergot alkaloids. Papaverine and narcotine are only partly extracted.

(*b*) Make the residual solution alkaline with potassium hydroxide and again extract a number of times with ether. Basic substances, including most of the alkaloids, will be extracted from this solution.

(*c*) To the residual aqueous solution add an excess of ammonium sulphate in order to make it ammoniacal and extract with ether. Phenolic alkaloids are liberated in ammonia solution and will be extracted (except morphine).

(*d*) To the aqueous residues from (*c*) add an equal volume of ethanol and an equal volume of chloroform. Extract, repeat the extraction twice with the addition of half the volume of ethanol and one volume of chloroform. Morphine, and any substance in (*a*) or (*b*) only slightly soluble in ether, will be obtained.

The products from each extraction should be dissolved in 0·1N acid or alkali and made up to a definite volume. After identification in a portion of this solution, they may be determined in an aliquot part by a suitable method as given in the general text of the book.

In the opinion of Daubney and Nickolls[1] the quantitative determination of comparatively large amounts of alkaloids is relatively easy by the classical methods, since in cases where a large dose of poison has been consumed, death usually follows rapidly and the bulk of the poison is in the stomach contents, but difficulty arises in the extraction of relatively small amounts of alkaloids from tissues. A technique was evolved from experiments with a range of alkaloids, sufficiently wide for the method to be assumed of general applicability. Morphine was shown to be unique in being extracted from tissue by saturated ammonium sulphate solution and required special treatment. The general method finally adopted was as follows:

Freeze the tissue overnight in a refrigerator and while still frozen mince 400 g or other suitable quantity, into a tared casserole. Add 50 ml of water and 10 ml of glacial acetic acid and warm, with stirring, to about 50°. Add sufficient ammonium sulphate (200 to 300 g) to leave a small amount undissolved and warm, with stirring, to about 65°; the protein will then have coagulated and the thick gruel will have become quite fluid. Filter on a large Büchner funnel and wash with about 100 ml of warm water. Return the residue to the casserole, macerate at about 65° to 70° with approximately 200 ml of water containing 1 per cent of acetic acid until the mixture has been stirred into a thin gruel free from lumps, and filter. Repeat the maceration of the residue with hot acidulated water until approximately 1·5 litre of total filtrate has been obtained. Any turbidity caused by mixing the ammonium sulphate extract with the water extracts must not be filtered. The filtrate is sufficiently free from protein for the alkaloid to be directly extracted from it in a relatively clean condition.

Transfer the filtrate to a 2-litre separator and make alkaline with ammonia. Extract five times with 100-ml portions of chloroform and filter the chloroform extracts. Combine the filtered solutions and extract successively with 25-, 15- and 10-ml portions of 3N sulphuric acid, followed by 25 ml of water, filtering the aqueous extracts in turn through a small filter. Make the combined aqueous liquors alkaline with ammonia, extract with five 20-ml portions of chloroform, and filter into a small carbon dioxide flask, evaporate and weigh. Dissolve the residue in a little dilute acid and filter the solution through a small paper; wash well with dilute acid. Return any small amount of insoluble matter on the filter to the flask by dissolving it in acetone and then in chloroform. Dry and reweigh the flask, the difference from the previous weight representing the weight of pure alkaloid.

For morphine, add 200 ml of ethanol to the bulked extracts transferred to the separator and repeat the extraction with chloroform and ethanol, or preferably, if morphine only is sought, use the following modification. After coagulation of protein from the original tissue and filtration on a Büchner funnel, as described above in the first paragraph, continue extraction of the residue with successive portions of hot saturated ammonium sulphate solution containing 1 per cent of acetic acid. Remove fat from the combined extracts with light petroleum (b.p. 40° to 60°) and extract in ammoniacal solution, to which ethanol has been added, with a mixture of equal parts of ethanol and chloroform. Evaporate the solvent, extract the morphine from the residue with hot ethyl acetate and again evaporate to dryness.

The adsorption of alkaloids from tissue extracts by suitable adsorbents had been considered by Daubney and Nickolls, but they found that quantitative results were not obtained in the presence of strong ammonium sulphate solutions, the use of which is a necessary part of their extraction process.

Stewart, Chatterji and Smith,[2] however, successfully obtained quantitative adsorption of strychnine by kaolin from solution in trichloroacetic acid. This latter reagent is used as a protein precipitant. Details of the method recommended are as follows:

Grind the original material with an equal volume of 10 per cent trichloroacetic acid solution, allow the mixture to stand for a few minutes and filter through a Büchner funnel. A water-clear filtrate is obtained, almost free from protein and fat. Repeat the grinding and filtration with further portions of the dilute acid. To the combined filtrates add 10 g of kaolin, which has been previously washed successively with ethanol, chloroform and ether. After an hour, filter the kaolin on a Büchner funnel, wash once with water and grind with a little 10 per cent aqueous sodium carbonate solution using enough to make the suspension neutral or slightly alkaline. Then mix the paste so formed with anhydrous sodium sulphate to give a dry powder and extract with chloroform in a Soxhlet apparatus.

The authors obtained a 97 per cent yield from 41 mg of strychnine in

400 g of minced meat by this process and 73 per cent recovery with 5 mg. Using the same method equally good results were obtained with morphine and quinine but atropine showed severe losses, probably by hydrolysis.

Non-basic water-soluble substances will be extracted by the trichloroacetic acid process. Barbitone was shown to be extracted, but it is not adsorbed on kaolin. In admixture with strychnine, after filtration from the kaolin the barbitone was easily adsorbed on animal charcoal. This is eluted by ether (but not by chloroform) after moistening with acetic acid.

It was realised by the authors that effective adsorption of the alkaloid by the kaolin will depend on the quality of the kaolin used and B.D.H. 'levigated powder' brand was specified for use. Confirmation of the efficiency of the particular kaolin to be employed must be obtained before use. Further, particular adsorbents must be expected to vary in effectiveness when the extracts contain high concentrations of electrolytes.

Since strychnine is not affected by either aqueous or ethanolic potash it may often be purified by warming with a few drops of alkali and re-extracting, preferably with ether. Visceral material may be brought into solution by alkali treatment when strychnine is being determined.[3]

Stolman and Stewart[4] extended the application of adsorption methods to the isolation and determination of morphine, codeine and diamorphine from viscera.

For the ethanolic extraction process, macerate 100 g of minced tissue with 200 ml of 95 per cent ethanol and sufficient tartaric acid to give an acid reaction. Mix this mass with another 300 ml of ethanol, filter and wash with ethanol; the filtrate should be clear although coloured. Mix each volume with four volumes of 5 per cent aqueous trichloroacetic acid solution and filter to remove proteins. If aqueous acid extraction is employed, macerate 100 g of minced tissue with 200 ml of 10 per cent trichloroacetic acid solution, filter and wash with more of the acid. Mix with an equal volume of water and to each 100 ml of diluted solution add 25 ml of 95 per cent ethanol. For adsorption, adjust the pH to between 8·0 and 9·0 with dilute sodium hydroxide solution and pass through a 10-cm column of Florisil retained between cotton wool (previously cleaned by refluxing for two hours with a mixture of formic acid 1 volume, ethanol 2 volumes and ethyl acetate 2 volumes) and then wash with 250 ml of water followed by 50 ml of 20 per cent aqueous ethanol.

To avoid large volumes of solvent, elution of the adsorbed alkaloids is carried out in a refluxing apparatus, either that described in the paper or, more simply, by use of the *B.P.* drug extraction apparatus which is similar in principle. Place 25 ml of methanol containing 0·5 g of oxalic acid in the flask and a layer of solid sodium carbonate covered with a cotton-wool pad on the top of the column. Reflux for one hour, the eluting solvent boiling at such a rate as to ensure a constant small layer of fluid above the Florisil. Then evaporate the solvent to a low volume on a water-bath, finally completing the drying, if necessary for colorimetric determination, in a warm air current, since codeine and diamorphine in small quantities can be rapidly destroyed by excessive heat.

Urine filtrates and, to a less degree, tissue extracts still contain pigment which is partially adsorbed under the conditions described, and since the pigments are eluted by methanol, they interfere with the colorimetric determination of the alkaloids. They can, however, be removed by washing the column, prior to elution, with 200 ml of a mixture containing water, ethanol and ethyl acetate in the proportions 10 : 3 : 2 by volume. This treatment removes the pigments from the column without disturbing the alkaloid.

Other methods, using counter-current extraction, ion-exchange resins and other newer techniques, have been published. For general toxicological work, for which this book was not intended, publications in that field, such as Stewart and Stolman[5] and Smith,[6] should be consulted.

1. Daubney, C. G., and Nickolls, L. C., *Analyst*, 1937, **62,** 851; 1938, **63,** 560.
2. Stewart, C. P., Chatterji, S. K., and Smith, S., *B.M.J.*, 1937, 790.
3. Nardu, S. R., and Venkatrao, P., *Analyst*, 1945, **70,** 8.
4. Stolman, A., and Stewart, C. P., *Analyst*, 1949, **74,** 536.
5. Stewart, C. P., and Stolman, A., 'Toxicology', London, Academic Press Inc., 1961.
6. Smith, I., ed., 'Chromatographic and Electrophoretic Techniques', 2nd Edition, London, Heinemann Medical Books, Ltd., 1960.

APPENDIX XIII

Electrometric Titrations

Electrical methods of determining the end-point of titrations are widely used; some of the advantages of the technique are obvious, such as the ability to titrate coloured solutions where the change of a visual indicator would be difficult or impossible to detect and the ability to carry out titrations for which no suitable visual indicator exists. Electrometric end-points may often be employed with greater accuracy than visual ones and with greater sensitivity. It should always be remembered, however, that where a suitable visual method of end-point detection is available, it is usually more rapid and more economical to use. Electrometric methods may be classified into potentiometric, conductometric and amperometric methods.

POTENTIOMETRIC TITRATIONS

If a metal electrode is placed in a solution containing ions of the same metal a potential difference exists between the metal and the solution; there is a simple relation between the potential of the electrode and the corresponding ion exponent of the solution (pM^n, or pH when a hydrogen electrode is used). At the equivalence point of a titration there is a sudden change in the ion exponent and a corresponding abrupt change in the potential of the electrode. It is not practicable to measure the absolute potential between an electrode and a solution but this is not important since it is the change of potential during titration that is significant. This can be determined by making electrolytic contact between the electrode in the unknown solution (referred to as the 'indicator' electrode) and a standard reference electrode; the two electrodes thus serve as half-cells of a Galvanic cell, the e.m.f. of which can be measured simply and with great accuracy. In practice a glass electrode is usually used as indicator electrode in acid-alkali titrations, a silver electrode for titrations in which silver is involved (such as titration of halides) and a platinum electrode in oxidation-reduction titrations. The reference electrode is usually some type of mercury-mercurous ion half-cell, the potential of which is constant throughout the titration, so that changes in e.m.f. are due entirely to changes in the potential of the indicator electrode. For measurement of the e.m.f. any suitable potentiometer may be used, although it is most convenient to use a direct-reading pH-meter having an additional scale graduated in millivolts; it is essential that no current is taken from the electrode system during the voltage measurement otherwise polarisation of the indicator electrode may occur.

For acid-base titrations in aqueous media a glass electrode is used as indicator electrode and a saturated mercury-mercurous chloride half-cell with a potassium chloride bridge as reference electrode. In certain non-aqueous media the same electrode system may be used; for titrations in glacial acetic acid using perchloric acid as titrant care must be taken to prevent leakage of saturated potassium chloride solution into the titration liquid, since the salt would react with the perchloric acid titrant. In the case of titrations with tetrabutylammonium hydroxide and lithium methoxide in pyridine and dimethylformamide respectively more reproducible voltage readings are obtainable if the aqueous salt bridge of the calomel electrode is replaced by a saturated solution of potassium chloride in dry methanol (see p. 794).

For titration of halides the solution is best buffered to about pH 5. The indicator electrode is a piece of silver wire of about 1 mm in diameter and about 3 cm long which has been curled into an open spiral; the reference electrode may be a mercury-mercurous sulphate half-cell with a potassium sulphate bridge. An alternative reference electrode for use in titration of halides, and one which works well in practice and is convenient to use, is the glass electrode; if a glass electrode is used in this way, however, the potentiometer must have a high-impedance, shielded input socket. The following practical details are suitable for halide titrations:

> Before each determination wash the indicator electrode with strong ammonia solution and rinse with water. Transfer the sample to the titration vessel (a beaker of about 250-ml capacity, fitted with a stirrer), and, if a solid, dissolve in a little water; adjust the pH, if necessary, to 5·0 to 6·0 with dilute nitric acid or 20 per cent sodium hydroxide solution. Dilute to 25 ml with water and add 75 ml of an acetate buffer solution prepared by dissolving 13·6 g of sodium acetate trihydrate and 6 ml of glacial acetic acid in water and diluting to 1 litre with water. Insert the glass reference electrode and silver indicator electrode into the solution and titrate with standard silver nitrate solution, stirring continuously. Prepare a graph by plotting e.m.f. against volume of titrant added and read the volume of titrant at the point of maximum slope of the curve. When titrating with weaker solutions of silver nitrate than 0·1N satisfactory results may be obtained by diluting the titration liquid with water to about 200 ml or by adding a colloid such as de-ionised gelatin solution.

In all potentiometric titrations a better method of determining the precise end-point than that given above is to construct a plot of $\Delta E/\Delta V$ against V (where E is the e.m.f. and V the volume of titrant); the point of maximum $\Delta E/\Delta V$ corresponds to the equivalence point of the titration.

APPENDIX XIII

CONDUCTOMETRIC TITRATIONS

In conductometric titrations the electrical conductivity of the solution, in which two platinum electrodes are immersed, is measured by means of a bridge circuit energised by an alternating current having a frequency of about 1,000 to 2,000 cycles per second. Measurements are made after successive additions of titrant and the values recorded are plotted against the volume of titrant added. Usually, two straight lines are obtained which intersect at the equivalence-point. It is frequently possible to apply a conductometric method in cases where other methods fail due, perhaps, to hydrolysis or dissociation of the reaction product; on the other hand large concentrations of foreign electrolytes greatly influence the accuracy and ease of applicability of the method. Perhaps for this reason the conductometric titration does not play any significant part in routine pharmaceutical analysis.

High-frequency methods of titration have been employed in which the electrodes are placed outside the titration vessel and energy at a frequency of several megacycles per second is applied. Measurements on such a system will depend upon the conductance and the dielectric constant of the sample solution, the cell walls and the air spaces between cell walls and electrodes; it is therefore imperative that all factors other than changes in the sample solution during titration are kept constant. Advantages of high-frequency methods over conductometric methods are that possible electrolysis and electrode polarisation are avoided, and that errors due to surface phenomena (such as coating of the electrodes with precipitant) are not possible. A consideration of the possible uses of high-frequency titration methods in pharmaceutical analysis has been made by Allen, Geddes and Stuckey;[1] however, most of the materials to which this method has been applied to date can equally well be assayed by other, simpler, means.

AMPEROMETRIC TITRATIONS

This class of titration is based on the measurement of the diffusion current at a dropping-mercury electrode or at a rotating platinum micro-electrode of the substance being titrated or of the reagent being used. It is known that in polarography the diffusion current obtained from a given ion is proportional to the concentration of that ion at a suitable potential and this fact is used in amperometric titrations.

A suitable potential is applied between a standard half-cell and the micro-electrode and the current flowing through the electrode system during the course of the titration is noted. The current, after the addition of each increment of titrant, is plotted against volume of reagent on each side of the end-point and the latter determined by the intersection of the two straight lines thus produced. The points obtained often give a curve around the end-point, but this is ignored and only the straight portions used.

The apparatus required is simple, comprising the electrodes, a sensitive galvanometer and a variable potential source connected in series. It is usually necessary to remove oxygen from the solutions and this is done by bubbling nitrogen through. This can also be used to stir the solutions between reagent additions; during the measurement there must be no stirring.

Amperometric titrations have a number of advantages over other titrimetric methods; determinations can usually be carried out in very dilute solutions (about 10^{-4}N or even, in certain cases, 10^{-5}N) and they are rapid since only a few measurements of current, before and after the end-point, at a constant applied voltage, need be made. It is often possible to carry out titrations in cases where potentiometric or visual-indicator methods are unsuitable such as in acid-base titrations in which the reaction product is hydrolysed or in precipitation titrations in which the precipitate has a significant solubility. There is, too, no interference from foreign electrolytes.

Some disadvantages are encountered, such as interferences by other elements, supersaturation effects in precipitation reactions or reduction of metal ions by colloidal precipitates, although these can usually be overcome.

DEAD-STOP END-POINT DETECTION

The so-called 'dead-stop' method of end-point detection is a special case and one which is of considerable importance in pharmaceutical work. Two identical platinum electrodes are placed in the solution to be titrated and a current of a few millivolts is applied across them. The end-point of the titration is shown by a sudden change in the current flowing between the two electrodes. In the titration of iodine with a thiosulphate solution both electrodes are depolarised during the titration and hence a current flows through the cell but at the end-point only one of the electrodes remains depolarised and the current ceases to flow. This has given rise to the term 'dead-stop end-point' to describe this type of titration. In practice, however, the converse usually applies; no current passes until the equivalence-point when depolarisation of the electrodes occurs and a current flows, as shown by a sudden permanent deflection on a galvanometer in series. Details of a suitable circuit and procedure are as follows:

Apparatus: A suitable apparatus is as illustrated in the following circuit diagram.

The battery is a 1·5 V dry cell which develops a voltage across the potentiometer P (1,000 ohms) depending on the resistor R_1. Switch S_1 is fitted to save the battery when the equipment is not in use. Two platinum foil electrodes about 0·5 cm square are connected at E and should be about 1·5 cm apart. The galvanometer G is a reflecting spot type, scale length about 15 cm, with a sensitivity such that 1 μA gives a full-scale deflection.

The switch S_2 and resistor R_2 are incorporated so that the galvanometer can be used to measure the approximate voltage applied across the electrodes. If R_2 is 100 Kilohms and R_1 is 10 Kilohms, then about 140 mV is developed across P and with S_2 at position A the galvanometer functions as a voltmeter. A full-scale deflection on the galvanometer is equivalent to 100 mV and intermediate readings are proportional; any voltage up to 100 mV is thus indicated on the galvanometer and P can be adjusted to supply whatever voltage is desired across the

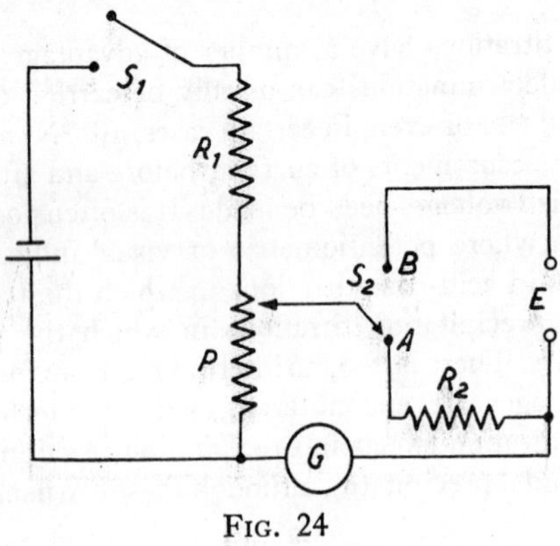

FIG. 24

electrodes. Resetting S_2 to position B then applies this voltage to the electrodes.

It is important that the platinum electrodes are scrupulously clean. This can be achieved by immersing them for about thirty seconds in boiling, concentrated nitric acid containing a small amount of solid ferric chloride.

Method: Transfer the specified volume of the solution to be titrated to a 200-ml beaker fitted with a stirrer. Introduce the electrodes and apply a predetermined polarising voltage,* stirring the solution continuously. The galvanometer will show an immediate small deflection but will then slowly return to zero. Add the specified standard solution slowly from a burette, allowing time for the galvanometer to return to zero after the addition of each increment.

The deflections will become more and more violent as the end-point is approached but there will always be a return to zero until the actual end-point is reached. Depolarisation then occurs causing a flow of current between the electrodes and this is shown by the first permanent deflection on the galvanometer.

Examples of this type of titration are the determination of ascorbic acid

* The optimum polarising voltage is best determined for each type of titration under actual working conditions. It should be sufficiently low to ensure that the galvanometer returns to zero fairly rapidly after the addition of each increment, but high enough to ensure that the end-point deflection is substantial. Usually it will be found that 40 to 100 mV is satisfactory.

with 2,6-dichlorophenolindophenol (see p. 97) and of sulphonamides with sodium nitrite (see p. 608) and the Karl Fischer method for water (see p. 806).

1. ALLEN, J., GEDDES, E. T., and STUCKEY, R. E., *J. Pharm. Pharmacol.*, 1956, **8**, 956.

APPENDIX XIV

Flame Photometry

The coloured radiations produced when the salts of certain elements are introduced into a flame have been used for identification purposes for many years. In flame photometry a solution of a salt is introduced continuously and at a constant rate so that the intensity of the radiation is a constant value which when measured forms the basis of a quantitative procedure. Many instruments have been built for this purpose and the range of work which can be accomplished depends on the design. In the simplest equipment a cool air/coal gas or air/propane flame is used so that few elements are excited and from the simple spectra the required radiations can be isolated by means of filters. The intensity of the transmitted radiation is then measured with a photocell coupled to a galvanometer or amplifier and meter. Such instruments are used for the determination of the alkali metals and in certain cases the alkaline earths. The more versatile instruments employ a monochromator for isolating the required wavelengths and so hotter flames can be used which excite many more elements and therefore produce much more complex spectra. A sensitive detector is required and a photomultiplier coupled to an amplifier satisfies this need.

Two different kinds of source units are used for excitation. In the first the sample is sprayed into a chamber where most of the larger drops fall out of the air-stream and run to waste and the finer particles in the form of a mist pass with the air supply into the burner; here the aerosol is mixed with a fuel gas and the mixture burns at a Meker or Bunsen-type burner top. The gas mixtures normally used with this type of burner are air/coal gas, air/propane, air/hydrogen and air/acetylene, although there seems to be no reason why oxygen could not be used or air/oxygen mixtures with the different fuels. In the second type the spray chamber is eliminated, and the sample is atomised directly into the flame which almost always utilises an oxygen/hydrogen or oxygen/acetylene mixture. This is a much smaller unit and has certain advantages, in that it can be used with solvents other than water and with fairly viscous solutions or fine suspensions. On the other hand it cannot operate with a cool flame, is noisy and the spray itself is very coarse, so that when aqueous solutions are used many of the drops pass right through the flame. Both methods have their own merits and for the greatest versatility it is an advantage if the instrument is capable of using either.

The desired wavelength is isolated by optical or interference filters, or by prism or grating monochromators. The latter give a versatility not obtainable with filters, because in addition to the possibility of setting to any required wavelength from the ultra-violet into the infra-red the band width of the selected radiation is much narrower than with filters and it is therefore possible to isolate lines which lie close together in the spectrum. In addition, the wavelength control can be motorised in order to scan through the spectrum automatically.

The detector and read-out unit depend on whether filters or monochromators are used. With filters a barrier layer photocell and sensitive galvanometer give sufficient sensitivity, whilst with a monochromator photomultipliers are required.

The ideal flame photometer is one which comprises a monochromator with motorised wavelength control, and to which can be attached any type of source unit. The detectors should be capable of responding to emission from 2,000A to 8,000A, and these should feed into an amplifier of wide sensitivity range. The output can be either read on a meter or passed into a recorder. This opinion is not intended to decry the use of simple equipment, but indicates what is required for the estimation of a large number of elements in all kinds of samples.

Whatever method is used to isolate the required lines and bands the light which reaches the detector will include background radiation from the flame itself and from incandescent particles of materials which are present in the sample. When monochromators are used scattered light of wavelengths other than the selected one can break through. These difficulties are all overcome if an examination of the background is made and a recording instrument is most useful for this purpose, particularly when there is a danger that the background radiation characteristics may change from sample to sample or between standard and sample. In addition it is not always possible for the composition of the standard solutions used to calibrate a flame photometer to be similar to that of the samples and this may give rise to considerable problems because the emitted intensity of the lines and bands of elements can be seriously affected by the presence of other materials in the sample and by conditions existing in the flame.

It can be seen then that many factors can affect the readings obtained when a sample is examined and it is essential for anyone undertaking work of this kind to appreciate the difficulties which can exist and to investigate the problems associated with every sample bearing these points in mind. The various interferences are dealt with in detail in books on the subject[1] and may be listed briefly as follows.

1. Spray rate variation due to differences in viscosity, surface tension or temperature of the sample.
2. Optical interference caused by light from elements other than that being determined being accepted through the optical unit.

3. Variation of flame background due to combined effect of all the materials in the sample.
4. Variation of line or band intensity due to chemical combinations occurring within the flame.
5. Variations in the proportion of the element at the excited state at any time due to changes in flame temperature.
6. Ionisation of the element being determined.

Many different procedures are used to provide quantitative results; the simplest one is to compare solutions containing known quantities of the element being determined, with the sample. If there are no interferences the wavelength is set on the monochromator or the correct filter is put into place and with water being sprayed the zero controls are adjusted to bring the instrument reading to zero. The most concentrated standard is then introduced and the sensitivity controls used to give a full-scale reading, the other standards are then sprayed, the readings noted for each and a calibration curve drawn for instrument reading versus concentration. Without altering the instrument settings in any way readings are obtained for the sample solutions and the results obtained by direct reference to the standard curve.

If the samples contain materials which affect the height of the background but not the intensity of the emission from the test element a correction procedure can be used. The best method is to utilise an instrument which gives a recording of intensity against wavelength; a true background reading to one side of the line can then be measured readily or if the background is sloping a base-line method of measuring the line intensity can be employed. This procedure is very useful in that it is not necessary to determine the concentration of the interfering materials in the samples and simple standards can be used to calibrate the instrument.

Buffers are often added to samples and standards in order to eliminate the effect of different concentrations of interfering ions. Perhaps the best known example of this is in the determination of calcium when phosphate is present. Under these conditions the intensities of the calcium lines and bands are reduced, probably due to the formation of compounds which are excited to a less extent than calcium alone. When the molecular ratio of calcium to phosphate is approximately 1 : 1 the depression reaches a limit and the addition of more phosphate has no further effect. It is convenient therefore to add an excess of phosphate to samples and standards alike so that the effect of that ion in the sample is effectively swamped. Other examples of the use of buffers are given in the monograph on calcium (see p. 146).

When a sample of unknown composition is being examined the standard addition technique can often be used providing the calibration curve of the test element is linear. Chow and Thompson[2] have used the method for the determination of strontium in sea water. A number of solutions are produced each containing a similar aliquot of the sample plus steadily increasing additions of the test element. The emissions of the solutions are plotted against added element and the true content of the sample obtained by extrapolation.

Many other techniques can be employed, depending on the nature of the sample and on the instrument being used, for example the test element can be extracted by solvent after complexing and the solvent solution employed directly. Dean[3] has been one of the foremost workers on this method which has been applied to the determination of iron, chromium, lanthanum, aluminium, copper, nickel, manganese, etc. Ion-exchange methods can be used either to extract the test element from interfering materials or to remove interfering materials from solutions of the sample.[4] Internal standard techniques can be employed with recording instruments or with specially designed equipment to avoid problems associated with spray-rate changes and sometimes solution properties.

Providing a careful investigation is made for each type of sample, flame-photometric methods are capable of giving reliable results in a very short time for a large number of elements. It is essential however that the equipment used should be fully capable of the task it is expected to do, particularly with regard to flame temperature and dispersion of the monochromator. It cannot be too greatly emphasised that the simple instruments are in general capable of analysing only relatively simple samples.

Atomic Absorption

The principles of atomic absorption have been known since the early nineteenth century and the technique has been used by astronomers for the approximately quantitative analysis of stellar atmospheres for many years. However, apart from the determination of mercury vapour, it was not used by analytical chemists until 1955 when Walsh[5] realised its potentialities and devised a simple apparatus which could be used for routine analysis. Since that time other equipment has been built and a commercial attachment is available for use with a spectrophotometer.

Walsh showed that when an element is introduced into a flame the temperature of which is between about 2,000° K and 3,000° K only a very small proportion of the atoms at any moment are in the excited state and this proportion varies exponentially with the flame temperature. However, the number of atoms in the ground state remains virtually constant and is independent of temperature. For this reason a measure of the absorption of monochromatic light at the wavelength of the resonance line of the element is a superior analytical technique to the measure of emission spectra.

The apparatus required for such measurements consists of a lamp source emitting the line spectrum of the element being determined, a flame for the vaporisation of the sample, a monochromator or filter to separate the resonance line from all others emitted by the source and photoelectric detecting and measuring equipment. It is necessary that the source should emit lines which are much sharper than the absorption lines in order to obtain a true measure of the maximum absorption and for the alkali metals and mercury a vapour discharge lamp is satisfactory, particularly if operated at currents lower than normal. For other elements hollow cathode discharge tubes are most convenient and are freely available commercially.

The flames used are essentially similar to those employed in flame photometry but as an approximately linear relationship exists between absorption and the number of absorbing atoms it is an advantage to increase the path length of the light from the source through the flame either by using a long burner or by multiple reflections in order to improve sensitivity.

The isolation of the required line can be achieved either with filters or a monochromator. It is necessary only to ensure that the resonance line is separated from others emitted by the source unit, and except for the transition elements which give many lines this is a relatively simple task. A standard spectrophotometer is very conveniently used both for its monochromator and associated measuring circuitry so long as the intensity of the radiation from the source is large compared with that from the flame in the wavelength region accepted through the monochromator. If, however, the flame contributes a significant proportion of the total light falling upon the detector it is necessary to modulate the light source either by supplying the hollow cathode lamp with an alternating current or by inserting a chopper between the source and the flame. If an amplifier tuned to the frequency of the modulated light is used then only the signal due to the radiation from the source is amplified and emission from the flame can be totally ignored.

The principal factor which affects the sensitivity of the method is the fluctuation of the light source. Stabilised power supplies are used but double-beam methods designed to eliminate the effect of these variations have been used and would appear to have sufficient promise to encourage workers to develop them further.

The advantages of this technique over emission flame photometry lie in the fact that the interferences due to physical inter-element effects, background radiation and scattered light are absent. Unfortunately chemical interferences still exist so that the effect of phosphate on the absorption of the calcium line is the same as its effect on the emission.

Twenty elements have been determined by this procedure and David[6] has published a review in which they are listed. The method is probably the best one available for the determination of zinc, magnesium and cadmium amongst the commoner elements and has been applied successfully to the determination of the noble metals.[7] It can be used for the determination of more elements than can emission analysis, is seldom inferior to that technique in sensitivity or precision and is often better. The apparatus required is more complex and it takes some time to change from the determination of one element to another with the commonly used equipment. However, the subject is still in its infancy and the development of comparatively simple inexpensive equipment seems a likely trend in the near future.

1. DEAN, J. A., 'Flame Photometry', New York, London [etc.], McGraw-Hill, 1960.

2. CHOW, T. J., and THOMPSON, T. G., *Anal. Chem.*, 1955, **27,** 18.

3. DEAN, J. A., *Amer. Soc. Testing Materials; Spec. Tech. Publ.*, 1958, **238,** 43.

4. GEHRKE, C. W., AFFSPRUNG, H. E., and WOOD, E. L., *J. Agric. Food Chem.*, 1955, **3,** 48.

5. WALSH, A., *Spectrochim. Acta*, 1955, **7,** 108.

6. DAVID, D. J., (Review) *Analyst*, 1960, **85,** 779.

7. LOCKYER, R., and HAMES, G. E., *Analyst*, 1959, **84,** 385.

APPENDIX XV

Gas Chromatography

Gas chromatography has developed rapidly within the last ten years from a research method to an analytical technique with wide application in the fields of biochemistry, food, essential oils, petroleum chemistry, horticulture and others. The adaptation of adsorption chromatography to mixtures in the form of gases or vapours began in 1943 with the development of gas-solid chromatography. Martin and Synge[1] introduced liquid-liquid chromatography in 1941, and in 1952 Martin and James[2] presented the first application of gas-liquid chromatography. This technique has proved to be more widely applicable than gas-solid chromatography and many commercial instruments are now available utilising a wide variety of columns, ovens and detectors.

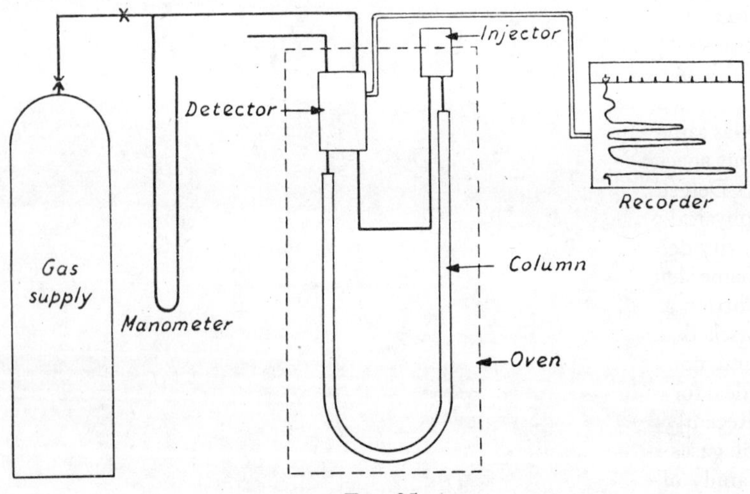

Fig. 25
Apparatus for Gas Chromatography

The simplest equipment consists of a tube, which may be straight, U-shaped or coiled, containing an inert solid acting as a support for the stationary phase. The support usually consists of narrow screen fractions of a diatomaceous earth (Celite, kieselguhr) or ground firebrick (Chromosorb), and the stationary phase is a liquid which has low volatility at the temperature of the experiment. It may be either polar or non-polar depending on the composition of the mixture to be separated. The column is maintained at a suitable temperature and a controlled flow of an inert gas is passed through it. A small sample of the volatile mixture to be separated is introduced to one end of the column by some sort of injection system and the inert gas transports the mixture through the column, where the components are separated as they are retained by the stationary phase to various extents. The eluting gas containing the sample then passes into a sensitive detecting device (Fig. 25).

The resolution of the components of a mixture depends on the length and diameter of the column, the particle size and packing of the support, the type and amount of the stationary phase, the nature and velocity of the carrier gas, the size of the sample and the properties of the components. In analytical applications the sample size is usually small and the introduction of accurate volumes of samples has led to the design of many injection systems. Liquid samples may be introduced into the column by means of a micro-capillary pipette or by hypodermic syringe through a serum cap. An injection system suitable for both these applications has been constructed[3] as an improvement to that described previously by Brealey *et al.*[4] The new system is easier to construct, has no moving parts and will prevent any non-volatile material, present in many pharmaceutical preparations, from reaching the column (Fig. 26). The body of the system (*a*) is mounted in the top of the oven and either of the two heads (*b*) or (*c*) can be used. (*d*) shows a glass micro-pipette suitable for use with head (*c*). Gas samples may be introduced by a gas-tight syringe through a serum cap, but special sampling valves are generally used.[5,6]

Detecting systems are often of a differential type measuring some physical property of the eluted gas. Detectors such as the thermal conductivity detector or Katharometer, the gas-density balance and the hydrogen flame detector give useful results at concentrations of a component in the carrier gas down to approximately 1 in 10^4. They are mainly used with packed columns and sample sizes of about 1 mg. They are robust, reliable and not susceptible to contamination due to overloading, and are thus ideal for routine determination of single components of complex mixtures.[7] Recently-developed detectors utilising changes in the ionisation properties of gases now enable the detection of 6×10^{-14} g/ml. These include a family of detectors utilising argon as carrier gas developed by Lovelock and Lipsky,[8] a hydrogen flame ionisation detector developed by McWilliam and Dewar,[9] and highly selective detectors such as the electron-capture detector which responds with high sensitivity to halogen compounds and has been used for the determination of traces of insecticides.[10,11] The high sensitivity of these detectors necessitated the use of very small samples and this made possible the useful development of capillary columns by Golay[12] and Desty *et al.*[13] These columns, lengths of narrow bore tubes whose walls carry a thin film of stationary phase, have very high resolving power and separations of complex mixtures are completed efficiently and quickly.

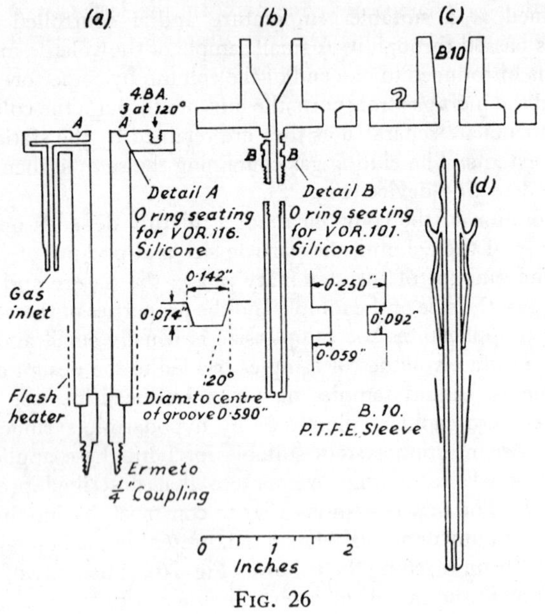

FIG. 26

The length of time before a component appears at the detector and the volume of gas having passed through the column during this time are defined as the retention time and retention volume respectively and, under a standard set of experimental conditions, they are characteristic of the component. In many cases, particularly in routine analysis, the components present in the mixture will be known and can therefore be identified by a comparison of their retention volumes with those found in the analysis of a synthetic mixture. If the components are completely unknown various methods may be used to aid their identification. These methods generally depend on plotting log retention volumes for members of an homologous series against the number of carbon atoms,[14] or retention volumes for members of an homologous series against the retention volumes for the same members using a second stationary phase.[15] In both these methods straight line plots are obtained. Thus if the retention volume of an unknown material is read off a graph previously obtained it may be identified. Fractions can also be collected in cold traps at the end of the column and analysed by other physical or chemical means.

Gas chromatography detectors usually present results as a series of peaks on a recorder chart, and the area of each peak is proportional to the concentration of that component in the sample. The areas of the peaks may be determined by cutting them out of the chart and weighing, by use of a planimeter, by use of an electronic integrating device or by a geometric approximation or triangulation method. In the last case a value proportional to peak area is obtained by multiplying the peak height by the width at half-peak height or by multiplying the peak height by the width at the base given by the inflection tangents. If the peaks obtained are narrow and symmetrical the height alone may be used as a measure of concentration but this method is very sensitive to changes in operating conditions (Fig. 27).

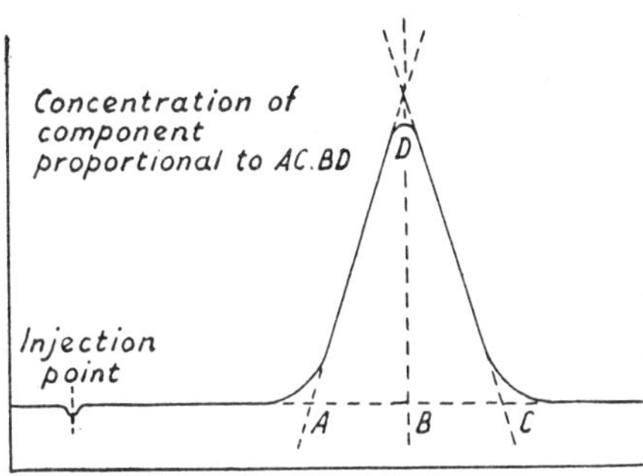

FIG. 27

Quantitative analyses may be carried out by calibrating the detector with pure samples of the components to be detected, by the addition of an internal standard and subsequent measurement of the ratio of internal standard and component peak for samples and synthetic standards, or by summation of all the peak areas and finding the proportion of each area to this total after taking account of the relative response of the detector to the different components.

It would be impossible to list here the wide application of gas chromatography. Applications to pharmaceutical problems are detailed through the text. The literature is still increasing in volume and a full coverage is given in abstract form in Gas Chromatography Abstracts.[16]

1. MARTIN, A. J. P., and SYNGE, R. L. M., *Biochem. J.*, 1941, **35,** 1358.
2. JAMES, A. T., and MARTIN, A. J. P., *Analyst*, 1952, **77,** 915.
3. BAINES, C. B., and BREALEY, L., private communication.
4. BREALEY, L., ELVIDGE, D. A., and PROCTOR, K. A., *Analyst*, 1959, **84,** 221.
5. TIMMS, D. G., KONRATH, H. J., and CHIRNSIDE, R. C., *Analyst*, 1958, **83,** 600.
6. CRAATS, F. VAN DE, *Anal. Chim. Acta*, 1956, **14,** 136.
7. BAINES, C. B., and PROCTOR, K. A., *J. Pharm. Pharmacol.*, 1959, **11,** 230T.
8. LOVELOCK, J. E., and LIPSKY, S. R., *J. Amer. Chem. Soc.*, 1960, **82,** 431.
9. MCWILLIAM, I. G., and DEWAR, R. A., *Nature*, 1958, **181,** 760.
10. LOVELOCK, J. E., Gas Chromatography, edited by R. P. W. Scott. London, Butterworths, 1960, pp. 16–29.
11. 'Gas Chromatography in Medical Research', *Nature*, 1961, **192,** 717.

12. GOLAY, M. J. E., *Anal. Chem.* 1957, **29,** 928; *Nature*, 1957, **180,** 435.
13. DESTY, D. H., GOLDUP, A., and WHYMAN, B. H. F., *J. Inst. Petrol.*, 1959, **45,** 287.
14. JAMES, A. T., and MARTIN, A. J. P., *Biochem. J.*, 1952, **50,** 679.
15. JAMES, A. T., MARTIN, A. J. P., and SMITH, G. H., *Biochem. J.*, 1952, **52,** 238.
16. Gas Chromatography Abstracts, edited by C. E. H. Knapman, London, Butterworths, 1958-1962.

APPENDIX XVI

INFRA-RED SPECTROSCOPY

A light-absorption measurement in the ultra-violet or visible region of the electromagnetic spectrum is the basis of an accepted quantitative analytical technique. It is only in recent years that a similar measurement in the infra-red region has established itself as a complementary tool of equal value to the analyst. Infra-red radiation promotes transitions in a molecule between rotational and vibrational energy levels of the lowest electronic energy state, and the energy that is absorbed from a radiation beam as a result of such a transition and the corresponding frequency or wavelength of an absorption band, is directly associated with the atomic masses, bond forces and spatial geometry of the molecule. The infra-red absorption spectrum thus has a high degree of specificity and no two compounds have identical spectra. Small differences in structure frequently result in significant differences in spectra, and early workers used the technique for material identification and functional group analysis. Improved instrumentation and the development of more efficient source units, monochromators, detectors and measuring systems led to an interest in quantitative organic analysis, and a range of commercial spectrophotometers[1] is now available which satisfies all requirements of industry and university, whether it be rapid qualitative identification, accurate quantitative determination or fundamental high resolution research.

INSTRUMENTATION

The electromagnetic spectrum between 0·78 micron and 300 microns is generally recognised as the infra-red region, and for convenience it is subdivided into three parts as follows:

Region	Wavelength (μ)	Wave-number (cm^{-1})
Near IR	0·78 – 3·0	12,800 – 3,333
Middle IR	3·0 – 30	3,333 – 333
Far IR	30 – 300	333 – 33·3

The unit of wavelength, the micron (μ, $1\mu = 10^{-4}$ cm), and the unit of so-called frequency or wave-number, the reciprocal centimetre (cm^{-1}), are interchangeable [wavelength (μ) = 10^4/wave-number (cm^{-1})], and because it has not been agreed internationally which to adopt as standard nomenclature, analysts must be familiar with both.

Commercial infra-red spectrophotometers cover one or more specific ranges within the above regions, the range defined by the transmission of the prism or the reflection of the grating used in the monochromator. Typical prism materials with their recommended wavelength coverage are glass $0{\cdot}3\mu - 2\mu$, quartz $0{\cdot}3\mu - 2{\cdot}5\mu$, lithium fluoride $0{\cdot}2\mu - 6\mu$, calcium fluoride $0{\cdot}2\mu - 9\mu$, sodium chloride (rocksalt) $2\mu - 15\mu$, potassium bromide $12\mu - 25\mu$ and cæsium bromide $15\mu - 38\mu$. Gratings provide higher resolution than prisms and, with an associated fore-prism or filter system to isolate a particular order, may be manufactured to cover ranges similar to the above.

Two common sources of infra-red radiation are the Nernst filament, an element of rare earth oxides, mainly zirconium oxide, fused together in a rod between 1 mm and 2 mm diameter, and the Globar, a larger diameter rod of silicon-carbide. Both elements are heated electrically, and at temperatures between 1,200° and 2,000° emit radiation with a maximum between $1{\cdot}5\mu$ and $2{\cdot}5\mu$ rather like a black body radiator.

Detection of infra-red radiation is by means of its heating effect, and the thermo-couple, the bolometer and the Golay pneumatic cell are each used by different manufacturers. Photoconductive cells of the lead sulphide type, although having a speed of response superior to the heat-sensitive detectors, are not as yet sufficiently sensitive beyond about 7μ.

All commercial instruments record on a paper chart the percentage transmission or the absorbance against wave-number or wavelength. Double-beam instruments provide a base-line free from atmospheric water vapour and carbon dioxide absorption, and enable compensation to be made for the solvent when recording solution spectra.

QUALITATIVE ANALYSIS

The qualitative interpretation of spectra and structural diagnosis[2] are outside the scope of this book, but since many qualitative techniques can be modified to give quantitative information by, for example, the use of an internal standard, a brief survey is given here of the different methods of sample preparation. Apart from dissolving in a solvent and holding the solution in a fixed thickness cell, four alternative procedures are available for the presentation of solid materials:

(1) Residue—A concentrated solution of the sample in a volatile solvent (ether, chloroform, ethanol, etc.) is fed dropwise on to a rocksalt plate and the solvent allowed to evaporate leaving behind a film of the solid.

(2) Melt—If the sample is of a waxy nature or has a low melting-point a few milligrams may be deposited on a rocksalt plate and heated in an oven. When molten a second rocksalt plate is put over the first and a thin film of the sample in the liquid state is ready for introducing into the sample compartment of the spectrophotometer. Depending upon whether the temperature of the instrument and the heat generated in the sample beam is sufficient to keep the sample in the liquid state, so the spectrum will be of the sample in either the liquid or the solid state.

(3) Mull—About 5 mg of sample is ground in a pestle and mortar with one drop of mulling agent, generally Nujol, a repurified paraffin oil; if the wavelength range in which the CH bands of the Nujol absorb is of interest, perfluorokerosene or hexachlorbutadiene may be used. The paste obtained is squeezed evenly between two rocksalt plates which are then placed in a suitable holder in the sample beam of the spectrophotometer. The spectrum is that of the sample superimposed upon that of the mulling agent.

(4) Disc—About 2 mg of sample is mixed and ground with about 200 mg of pure and dry alkali halide, potassium chloride or potassium bromide, and the mixture loaded into a die. When subjected to vacuum and high pressure a solid and robust glass-like disc is produced in which the sample is uniformly distributed throughout the supporting alkali halide. The disc is mounted in a holder in the spectrophotometer and the spectrum of the sample recorded, the alkali halide contributing nothing to the absorption.

Care must always be taken when interpreting solid state spectra of materials which exist in more than one polymorphic form, because different crystal modifications of the same substance have different infra-red spectra. Also in certain cases there is the possibility of physical or chemical changes induced by grinding with either Nujol or an alkali halide.[3]

Typical materials with their associated absorption bands that may be used as internal standards in either the mull or disc technique are potassium thiocyanate 4·8μ, calcium carbonate 11·4μ and potassium nitrate 12·1μ.

Liquid samples may be presented to an instrument either as capillary films held between two rocksalt plates, in fixed-thickness cells or in a solution in a fixed-thickness cell.

QUANTITATIVE ANALYSIS

The laws governing an infra-red absorption measurement are as follows: Absorbance (A) and transmittance (T) are defined as

$$A = \log_{10} \frac{1}{T} = \log_{10} \frac{I_0}{I}$$

where I_0 is the intensity of radiation incident on the sample and I is the intensity of radiation transmitted by the sample, both measured at the same wavelength and with the same slit width. The radiation beam is understood to be parallel and incident at right angles to plane parallel surfaces of the sample.

For a solution of an absorbing solute results are evaluated by applying the following absorption law, commonly referred to as Beer's Law:

$$A = a\,b\,c$$

where $a =$ absorptivity, a constant characteristic of the solute, solvent and wavelength, $b =$ internal cell length, $c =$ concentration.

The absorbance of a mixture at a particular wavelength is equal to the sum of the absorbances of the individual components. Thus

$$A = a_1\, b\, c_1 + a_2\, b\, c_2 + a_3\, b\, c_3$$

where the subscripts refer to the different components. If for a three component mixture, three suitable wavelengths are chosen such that at each wavelength one component has strong absorption and the other two components weak absorption, and if each wavelength is designated by superscripts 1, 2 and 3, then

$$\text{at } \lambda^1 \; A^1 = a_1^1\, b\, c_1 + a_2^1 b\, c_2 + a_3^1\, b\, c_3$$
$$\lambda^2 \; A^2 = a_1^2\, b\, c_1 + a_2^2\, b\, c_2 + a_3^2\, b\, c_3$$
$$\lambda^3 \; A^3 = a_1^3\, b\, c_1 + a_2^3\, b\, c_2 + a_3^3\, b\, c_3$$

The cell length b is known, the absorbtivity constants a may be obtained from measurements on pure materials, and then a measurement of A^1, A^2 and A^3 on the unknown mixture and a solution of the three equations will give the concentrations of the three components c_1, c_2 and c_3.

The solving of such a set of simultaneous equations may be by the method of successive approximations,[4] or by matrix methods and electronic computors, but whichever method is used, its applicability is dependent upon the extent to which Beer's Law is obeyed.

Hence when developing a method of analysis the factors which affect this relationship should be considered.[5,6] A narrow spectral slit width should be used to bring the radiation as near as possible to monochromatic and the concentration should be as low as possible to reduce intermolecular association. On the other hand a solvent must be chosen which has little or no absorption in the region of measurement and the sample must be sufficiently soluble in that solvent to give a satisfactory spectrum. If the solubility problem proves difficult a longer cell length and more dilute solution may be used, but as this also increases the solvent absorption it may then be necessary to increase the amount of energy reaching the detector by using a wider slit, with a consequent loss of resolution and a larger deviation from Beer's Law. Hence, in the majority of cases, a compromise has to be reached between choice of solvent, cell thickness, concentration and slit width, and this may entail a considerable period of preliminary investigation.

To reduce the possibility of solute-solvent interaction non-polar solvents should be used. This is not always practicable and the more common solvents are carbon disulphide, chloroform, carbon tetrachloride and acetone. Methylene chloride, bromoform, dimethylformamide and pyridine are less commonly used. All organic materials have infra-red absorption and no solvent is completely transparent; it is usual therefore to select one that has a transmission 'window' at the wavelength of measurement. Cell thicknesses between 0·05 mm and 2 mm are generally used.

Instead of relying upon the linearity of Beer's Law and using the associated simultaneous equations, it is often more accurate to compare the absorbances of the sample solution with absorbance measurements made at the same time on a standard solution which contains the different components at approximately the same concentrations as the sample solution.[7] A direct comparison may then be made between absorbance measurements, at the same wavelength, of the sample and standard solutions. This method may be applied to single or multicomponent analyses and it has the advantages that the sample and standard measurements are made under as near identical instrumental conditions as possible. The sample and standard absorbances for each component are then similar and the presence of unwanted impurities in the sample solution are easily detected. These factors enable in general an accuracy of rather better than ± 1 per cent to be attained.

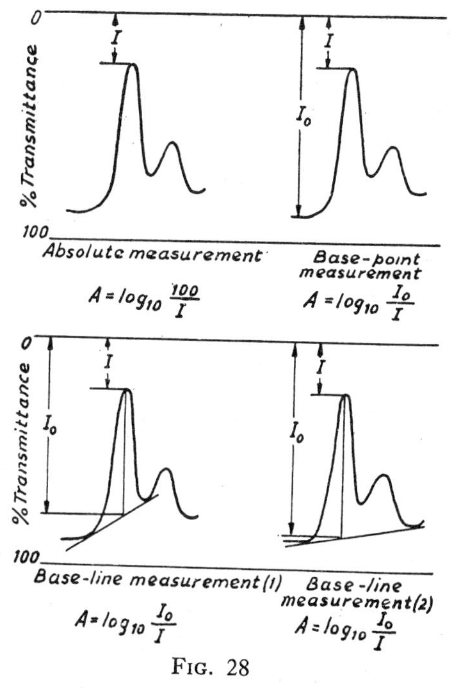

FIG. 28

Instead of measuring the absorbance A of an absorption band as defined above, it is often more convenient to measure its base-line[4] or base-point absorbance. These measurements are designed to minimise or eliminate the effect of interfering materials or of all components except the one of interest at the wavelength concerned, and in selecting the base-point or the points between which the base-line is drawn care must be taken to allow correctly for the unwanted absorption. Four different methods of measuring the absorbance of the same band are shown in Fig. 28.

A difference measurement is a technique that may be used to determine minor constituents. The major component is introduced into the comparison cell (a variable space cell may be useful here) at a concentration equal to its concentration in the sample cell. Its absorption is thereby compensated and the result is a spectrum of the minor constituents. There are several difficulties that must be appreciated when applying this technique. Because of strong absorption in both beams a wider than normal slit width must be used and this will result in poorer resolution and a deviation from Beer's Law. Care must be taken to avoid over- or under-compensation, not only for the major component, but also for the solvent if working in solution. Nevertheless in specific instances it is a most valuable technique.

1. Cross, A. D., An Introduction to Practical Infra-Red Spectroscopy. London, Butterworths Scientific Publications, 1960, p. 18.
2. Bellamy, L. J., The Infra-Red Spectra of Complex Molecules, 2nd. ed. London, Methuen, 1958.
3. Farmer, V. C., *Spectrochim. Acta*, 1957, **8,** 374.
4. Heigl, J. J., Bell, M. F., and White, J. U., *Anal. Chem.*, 1947, **19,** 293.
5. Robinson, D. Z., *Anal. Chem.*, 1951, **23,** 273.
6. Robinson, D. Z., *Anal. Chem.*, 1952, **24,** 619.
7. Ward, W. R., *J. Appl. Chem.*, 1960, **10,** 277.

APPENDIX XVII

Some Hints on the Elimination of Emulsions during Extraction with Immiscible Liquids

The most useful hint on this subject is that 'prevention is better than cure,' and that emulsions should not be allowed to form, *e.g.* chloroform is notorious in forming emulsions, but if it is used mixed with ether, emulsification is less likely. The best way to avoid emulsions is by keeping aqueous layers as small as possible and extracting with liberal quantities of solvent. If emulsions have formed, the following methods have been found useful for destroying them, each depending upon the circumstances.

(*a*) Light emulsions can be broken by shaking a wire in the mixture.

(*b*) Warm the mixture in the steam from a water-bath without agitating the separator.

(*c*) Saponaceous aqueous-ether emulsions can be broken by the addition of ethanolic potassium hydroxide.

(*d*) Bulk the solvent layers containing the emulsion together in another separator. Shake violently, and after separation extract the small residual emulsion layer with a large volume of solvent.

(*e*) The previous method is very successful with the addition of a little ethanol to the bulked emulsions before agitation. When ethanol is used, it must not be added in sufficient quantity seriously to affect the partition between the immiscible layers.

(*f*) For heavy emulsions in water-chloroform mixtures, add the emulsion, a few ml at a time, to a large bulk of chloroform in a second separator, shaking vigorously between each addition.

(*g*) For the majority of aqueous mixtures, likely to give heavy emulsions when extracted by solvent, the emulsions can be avoided by adding an equal bulk of ethanol to the aqueous layer and then twice as much chloroform as ethanol. After vigorous shaking, the chloroform will separate almost at once. The extraction is repeated by the addition of another half volume of ethanol and one of chloroform. After evaporation of the chloroform, the residue must be taken up in aqueous solution and re-extracted with chloroform without ethanol since the above procedure may extract a considerable amount of extraneous matter.

(*h*) If surface-active agents are known to be present, emulsification can be prevented by extraction with light petroleum (b.p. 40° to 60°) from 50 per cent ethanol in the aqueous layer. The surface-active agent remains in the aqueous phase.

APPENDIX XVIII

Sugar Table for the Lane and Eynon Titration Method

ML OF SUGAR SOLUTION REQUIRED	10 ML OF FEHLING'S SOLUTION				25 ML OF FEHLING'S SOLUTION			
	INVERT SUGAR † (NO SUCROSE)	INVERT SUGAR,† SOLUTION CONTAINING IN ADDITION 1 G SUCROSE/100 ML	ANHYDROUS DEXTROSE †	ANHYDROUS LACTOSE †	INVERT SUGAR † (NO SUCROSE)	INVERT SUGAR,† SOLUTION CONTAINING IN ADDITION 1 G SUCROSE/100 ML	ANHYDROUS DEXTROSE †	ANHYDROUS LACTOSE †
15	336	333	327	432	824	817	801	1,093
16	316	312	307	405	772	767	751	1,022
17	298	295	289	381	727	721	707	960
18	282	278	274	359	687	682	668	906
19	267	264	260	340	651	646	633	855
20	254·5	251·0	247·4	323·0	619·0	614·0	601·5	811·8
21	242·9	239·0	235·8	307·6	589·5	584·8	572·9	772·3
22	231·8	228·2	225·5	293·6	563·2	558·2	547·3	735·8
23	222·2	218·7	216·1	280·6	538·7	534·0	523·6	703·0
24	213·3	209·8	207·4	268·8	516·7	512·1	501·9	673·1
25	204·8	201·6	199·3	258·0	496·0	492·0	482·0	645·5
26	197·4	193·8	191·8	248·0	477·3	473·1	463·7	620·1
27	190·4	186·7	184·9	238·5	459·7	455·6	446·8	596·5
28	183·7	180·2	178·5	230·0	443·6	439·6	431·1	574·6
29	177·6	174·1	172·5	222·2	428·3	424·4	416·4	554·1
30	171·7	168·3	167·0	214·7	414·3	410·4	402·7	535·1
31	166·3	163·1	161·8	207·8	401·0	397·4	389·7	517·6
32	161·2	158·1	156·9	201·3	388·7	385·0	377·6	501·0
33	156·6	153·3	152·4	195·3	377·0	373·4	366·3	485·5
34	152·2	148·9	148·0	189·7	366·2	362·6	355·6	470·8
35	147·9	144·7	143·9	184·3	355·8	352·3	345·6	457·0
36	143·9	140·7	140·0	179·2	346·1	342·5	336·3	443·9
37	140·2	137·0	136·4	174·3	336·8	333·5	327·4	431·6
38	136·6	133·5	132·9	169·8	328·1	324·7	318·8	420·0
39	133·3	130·2	129·6	165·4	319·7	316·4	310·7	409·0
40	130·1	127·0	126·5	161·2	311·9	308·6	303·1	398·5
41	127·1	123·9	123·6	157·6	304·4	301·2	295·9	388·6
42	124·2	121·0	120·8	153·8	297·3	294·1	289·0	379·1
43	121·4	118·2	118·1	150·2	290·5	287·3	282·4	370·2
44	118·7	115·6	115·5	147·0	284·1	280·9	276·1	361·7
45	116·1	113·1	113·0	143·7	277·9	274·7	270·1	353·5
46	113·7	110·6	110·6	140·6	272·0	268·7	264·3	345·7
47	111·4	108·2	108·4	137·8	266·3	263·1	258·8	338·2
48	109·2	106·0	106·2	135·0	260·8	257·7	253·5	330·9
49	107·1	104·0	104·1	132·2	255·5	252·5	248·4	324·0
50	105·1	102·0	102·2	129·8	250·6	247·6	243·6	317·5

† mg sugar per 100 ml solution.

APPENDIX XIX

SUCROSE CORRECTIONS IN CHLORAMINE TITRATION OF ALDOSE SUGARS
(Hinton and Macara)

TOTAL CHLORAMINE CONSUMED (ML 0·05N)	AMOUNT (G) OF SUCROSE IN THE SERUM TITRATED						
	0·40	0·44	0·48	0·52	0·56	0·60	0·64
12·0	0·30	0·33	0·36	0·39	0·41	0·44	0·47
14·0	0·25	0·28	0·30	0·33	0·35	0·38	0·40
16·0	0·21	0·24	0·26	0·29	0·31	0·33	0·35
18·0	0·18	0·21	0·23	0·25	0·27	0·28	0·30
20·0	0·16	0·18	0·20	0·21	0·23	0·25	0·26
22·0	0·15	0·17	0·18	0·20	0·21	0·23	0·24

APPENDIX XX

GLYCEROL CONTENT AND SPECIFIC GRAVITY AT 15·5/15·5° OF AQUEOUS SOLUTIONS OF REFINED GLYCERIN*

GLYCEROL PER CENT W/W	SPECIFIC GRAVITY AT 15·5/15·5°	GLYCEROL PER CENT W/W	SPECIFIC GRAVITY AT 15·5/15·5°	GLYCEROL PER CENT W/W	SPECIFIC GRAVITY AT 15·5/15·5°
100	1·26532	66	1·17410	33	1·08355
99	1·26275	65	1·17130	32	1·08085
98	1·26020	64	1·16855	31	1·07815
97	1·25760	63	1·16575	30	1·07545
96	1·25500	62	1·16300	29	1·07285
95	1·25245	61	1·16020	28	1·07025
94	1·24980	60	1·15745	27	1·06760
93	1·24715	59	1·15465	26	1·06500
92	1·24450	58	1·15190	25	1·06240
91	1·24185	57	1·14910	24	1·05980
90	1·23920	56	1·14635	23	1·05715
89	1·23655	55	1·14355	22	1·05455
88	1·23390	54	1·14080	21	1·05195
87	1·23120	53	1·13800	20	1·04935
86	1·22855	52	1·13525	19	1·04680
85	1·22590	51	1·13245	18	1·04430
84	1·22325	50	1·12970	17	1·04180
83	1·22055	49	1·12695	16	1·03925
82	1·21790	48	1·12425	15	1·03675
81	1·21525	47	1·12150	14	1·03420
80	1·21260	46	1·11880	13	1·03170
79	1·20985	45	1·11605	12	1·02920
78	1·20710	44	1·11335	11	1·02665
77	1·20440	43	1·11060	10	1·02415
76	1·20165	42	1·10790	9	1·02175
75	1·19890	41	1·10515	8	1·01930
74	1·19615	40	1·10245	7	1·01690
73	1·19340	39	1·09975	6	1·01450
72	1·19070	38	1·09705	5	1·01205
71	1·18795	37	1·09435	4	1·00965
70	1·18520	36	1·09165	3	1·00725
69	1·18240	35	1·08895	2	1·00485
68	1·17965	34	1·08625	1	1·00240
67	1·17685				

* BOSART, L. W., and SNODDY, A. O., *Ind. Eng. Chem.*, 1927, **19**, 506.

APPENDIX XXI

Atomic Weights, 1961

NAME	SYMBOL	ATOMIC WEIGHT
Aluminium	Al	26·98
Antimony	Sb	121·75
Arsenic	As	74·92
Barium	Ba	137·34
Bismuth	Bi	208·98
Boron	B	10·81
Bromine	Br	79·91
Cadmium	Cd	112·40
Calcium	Ca	40·08
Carbon	C	12·011
Cerium	Ce	140·12
Chlorine	Cl	35·45
Chromium	Cr	52·00
Cobalt	Co	58·93
Copper	Cu	63·54
Fluorine	F	19·00
Gold	Au	196·97
Hydrogen	H	1·008
Iodine	I	126·90
Iron	Fe	55·85
Lead	Pb	207·19
Lithium	Li	6·94
Magnesium	Mg	24·31
Manganese	Mn	54·94
Mercury	Hg	200·59
Molybdenum	Mo	95·94
Nickel	Ni	58·71
Nitrogen	N	14·007
Osmium	Os	190·2
Oxygen	O	15·999
Phosphorus	P	30·97
Platinum	Pt	195·09
Potassium	K	39·10
Selenium	Se	78·96
Silicon	Si	28·09
Silver	Ag	107·87

Atomic Weights, 1961 (*continued*)

NAME	SYMBOL	ATOMIC WEIGHT
Sodium	Na	22·99
Strontium	Sr	87·62
Sulphur	S	32·06
Tin	Sn	118·69
Titanium	Ti	47·90
Tungsten	W	183·85
Uranium	U	238·03
Vanadium	V	50·94
Zinc	Zn	65·37

WEIGHTS AND MEASURES

Imperial (Avoirdupois) Weights

437·5 grains (gr.)	= 1 ounce (oz.)
16 ounces	= 1 pound (lb.)
Hence 7,000 grains	= 1 pound

Imperial Measures of Capacity

60 minims (min.)	= 1 fluid drachm (fl. dr.)
8 fluid drachms	= 1 fluid ounce (fl. oz.)
20 fluid ounces	= 1 pint (pt.)

1 fluid ounce = volume at 62° F of 1 ounce or 437·5 grain
Hence 100 grains is the weight of 109·7 minims of water

Apothecaries' Weights

20 grains (gr.)	= 1 scruple (℈)
3 scruples	= 1 drachm (ʒ)
8 drachms	= 1 ounce (℥)

Apothecaries' Measures of Capacity

60 minims (♏)	= 1 fluid drachm (ʒ)
8 fluid drachms	= 1 fluid ounce (℥)
20 fluid ounces	= 1 pint (O)
8 pints	= 1 gallon (C)

Conversion Factors between some Imperial and Metric Weights and Measures

1 grain	= 0·0648 g
1 ounce (avoir.)	= 28·350 g
1 pound (avoir.)	= 453·59 g
1 minim	= 0·0592 ml
1 fluid drachm	= 3·5515 ml
1 fluid ounce	= 28·4123 ml
1 pint	= 0·5682 litres
1 inch	= 2·5400 cm

1 gramme (g)	= 15·4324 grains
1 kilogram	= 35·274 ounces
1 millilitre (ml)	= 16·89 minims
1 litre	= 35·196 fluid ounces

Grains per fluid ounce × 0·2286 = g per 100 ml

Minims per fluid ounce × 0·208 = ml per 100 ml

WEIGHTS AND MEASURES

Avoirdupois Weight

437.5 grains (gr) = 1 ounce (oz)
16 ounces = 1 pound (lb)
Hence 7,000 grains = 1 pound

Imperial Measure of Capacity

60 minims (min) = 1 fluid drachm (fl. dr.)
8 fluid drachms = 1 fluid ounce (fl. oz.)
20 fluid ounces = 1 pint (pt)
1 fluid ounce = volume of 1 oz. (437.5 gr) [illegible] grains
Hence 480 grains is the weight of [illegible] minims of water

Apothecaries' Weight

20 grains (gr) = 1 scruple (℈)
3 scruples = 1 drachm (ʒ)
8 drachms = 1 ounce (℥)

Apothecaries' Measure of Capacity

60 minims (♏) = 1 fluid drachm (ʒ)
8 fluid drachms = 1 fluid ounce (℥)
20 fluid ounces = 1 pint (O)
8 pints = 1 gallon (C)

Conversion Factors between Imperial and Metric Weights and Measures

1 grain	= 64.8 mg	1 gramme (g)	= 15.432 grains
1 ounce (avoir.)	= 28.350 g	1 kilogram (kg)	= 35.274 ounces
1 pound (avoir.)	= 453.59 g	1 millilitre (ml)	= 16.89 minims
1 minim	= [illegible] ml	1 litre	= 35 fl. [illegible]
1 fluid drachm	= 3.5515 ml		ounces
1 fluid ounce	= 28.4123 ml		
1 pint	= 0.5682 litres	Grains per fluid ounce × 0.228	= g per 100 ml
1 gallon	= 4.5460 litres	Minims per fluid ounce × 0.208	= ml per 100 ml

INDEX

INDEX

INDEX

INDEX

INDEX

MODEL PAPER : 1

1. Space maintainers are usually needed in the **(MAHE:98)**
   a) mandibular primary incisor area
   b) mandibular primary canine teeth area.
   c) mandibular primary second molar area
   d) maxillary primary incisor teeth area
2. The lower lip gets sensory nerve supply through the **(KER:99)**
   a) buccal branch of facial nerve
   b) buccal branch of mandibular nerve
   c) mandibular branch of facial nerve
   d) mental nerve
3. Gout results from a defect in metabolism of **(AIIMS:98)**
   a) Fat b) Pyrine
   c) Pigment d) Glucose
4. In orthodontic treatment, in order to avoid injuries to the tissues, the forces, applied should not exceed the **(MAHE:97)**
   a) arterial blood pressure b) capillary blood pressure
   c) masticatory forces
   d) muscular forces of facial muscles
5. Bacteria whose optimum temperature for growth is between 15° and 20° have been termed **(MAHE:98)**
   a) Autotrophs b) Mesophiles
   c) Chemophiles d) Psychrophiles
6. Measles is transmitted from one person to another via **(PP:117)**
   a) faeces b) insect bites
   c) fomites d) respiratory droplets.
7. The inferior dental artery is a branch of **(CHA:120)**
   a) mandibular artery b) maxillary artery.
   c) pterygomandibular plexus. d) None of the above

Ans. 1. C 2. D 3. B 4. B 5. D 6. D 7. B

8. All of the following muscles are elevators of the mandible except. **(AIIMS:96)**
   a) Digastric b) Masseter
   c) Medial pterygoid d) Temporalis.
9. First evidence of calcification of 3rd molars. **(MP:2(2))**
   a) 1½ years b) 2 years
   c) 4 years d) 8 years.
10. Disturbance during calcification of dentin causes **(ORB:116)**
    a) Cementicles b) Dentine dysplasia
    c) Interglobular dentine. d) None of the above.
11. Ptosis may be caused by a lesion of the
    a) Oculomotor nerve b) Superior oblique nerve.
    c) Trigeminal nerve d) Trochlear nerve.
12. Cystoid bodies and civette bodies are characteristics of **(SHA:810)**
    a) Lichen planus b) Psoriasis.
    c) Pemphigous d) Keratosis follicularis.
13. A high eosinophil count in the peripheral blood is most suggestive of which of the following diseases.
    a) Pulpitis b) Trichinosis
    c) Osteomyelitis d) Pulmonary tuberculosis.
14. All of the following are anatomically related to mandibular nerve except **(CHO:125)**
    a) Inferior alveolar nerve b) Auriculotemporal nerve
    c) Lingual nerve d) Chorda tympani nerve.
15. Cleft palate occurs due to disturbances at ... week of I.U. life. **(KER:98)**
    a) 7-8 b) 8-10
    c) 10-12 d) 12-14.
16. A benign mushroom-like tumor of bone in the metaphyseal area of a young person showing a peripheral cartilage cap is most likely a **(N.B.)**
    a) Osteosarcoma b) Exostosis
    c) Chondroma d) Osteochondroma.
17. Cementum is thickest at **(GLK : 38 (8TH))**
    a) Coronal third. b) Furcation area
    c) Apical third. d) Middle third of root.

Ans. **8. A 9. D 10. C 11. A 12. A 13. B 14. D 15. A 16. D 17. C**

CONTENTS